Pediatrics

Fourth Edition

Pediatrics

Edited by
Mohsen Ziai, M.D.

Professor of Pediatrics, Georgetown University
School of Medicine, Washington, D.C.; Chairman,
Department of Pediatrics, Fairfax Hospital, Falls
Church, Virginia; Lecturer in Pediatrics, Johns
Hopkins University School of Medicine,
Baltimore; Edward H. Townsend, Jr., Chairman
Emeritus, Department of Pediatrics, University of
Rochester Medical Center and Rochester General
Hospital, Rochester, New York

Little, Brown and Company
Boston/Toronto/London

To my wife, Nahid, our children, and our little granddaughter,
a constant reminder of what the love of children is all about.

Contents

viii

Contributing Authors

Silva Arslanian, M.D.
Assistant Professor of Pediatrics, University of Pittsburgh
School of Medicine; Attending Physician, Division of
Endocrinology, Children's Hospital of Pittsburgh, Pittsburgh
Chapter 7

John Baum, M.D.
Professor of Medicine and Pediatrics, The University of
Rochester School of Medicine and Dentistry; Associate
Director, Pediatric Arthritis Clinic, Strong Memorial Hospital,
Rochester, New York
Chapter 18

Paul de Bellefeuille, M.D., F.R.C.P.C.
Former Associate Professor of Pediatrics, University of Ottawa
School of Medicine; Attending Physician, Children's Hospital
of Eastern Ontario, Ottawa, Ontario, Canada
Chapter 10

Robert M. Berger, M.D.
Assistant Clinical Professor of Urology, George Washington
University School of Medicine and Health Sciences,
Washington, D.C.; Active Staff, Pediatrics and Urology,
Fairfax Hospital, Falls Church, Virginia
Chapter 13

Philippe A. Bernard, M.D., Ph.D.
Professor of Otolaryngology, University of Ottawa School
of Medicine; Chief, Division of Otolaryngology, Children's
Hospital of Eastern Ontario, Ottawa, Ontario, Canada
Chapter 10

Susan H. Black, M.D.C.M.
Clinical Assistant Professor, Virginia Commonwealth
University Medical College of Virginia School of Medicine,
Richmond; Clinical Geneticist, Genetics and IVF Institute,
Fairfax, Virginia
Chapter 5

Karina M. Butler, M.B., M.Ch., M.R.C.P.I.
Clinical Assistant Professor of Pediatrics, Georgetown
University School of Medicine, Washington, D.C.; Senior
Staff Fellow, Pediatrics, National Cancer Institute, Bethesda,
Maryland
Chapter 20

J. Julian Chisolm, Jr., M.D.
Associate Professor of Pediatrics, The Johns Hopkins
University School of Medicine; Director, Lead Poisoning
Program, Kennedy Institute, Baltimore, Maryland
Appendix A, Section 1; Appendix B

James E. Clayton, M.D.
Assistant Professor of Pediatrics, Georgetown University
School of Medicine, Washington, D.C.; Director, Infant
Apnea Program, Associate Director, Pediatric Intensive Care
Unit, Fairfax Hospital, Falls Church, Virginia
Chapter 10; Appendix A, Section 5, 8

Solomon J. Cohen, M.D.
Associate Clinical Professor of Pediatrics, Columbia University
College of Physicians and Surgeons, New York; Attending
Pediatrician, Overlook Hospital, Summit, New Jersey
Chapter 15; Appendix A, Sections 2, 10, 12

A. R. Colón, M.D.
Professor of Pediatrics, Georgetown University School of
Medicine, Washington, D.C.
Chapter 8

Thomas E. Cone, Jr., M.D.
Clinical Professor Emeritus of Pediatrics, Harvard Medical
School; Senior Associate in Clinical Genetics and Medicine,
Emeritus, The Children's Hospital Medical Center, Boston
Appendix B

Joann T. Dale, M.D.
Formerly Clinical Assistant Professor of Pediatrics, The
University of Rochester School of Medicine and Dentistry;
Associate Attending Physician in Pediatrics, Rochester General
Hospital, Rochester, New York
Chapter 10

Ihsan Dogramaci, M.D., LL.D., F.R.C.P. (Lond.)
Professor Emeritus of Pediatrics, Hacettepe University School
of Medicine, Ankara, Turkey
Chapter 7

Spyros A. Doxiadis, M.D., F.R.C.P.E.
President, Foundation for Research in Childhood, Athens,
Greece
Appendix A, Sections 3, 9

Allan L. Drash, M.D.
Professor of Pediatrics, University of Pittsburgh School of
Medicine; Director, Division of Pediatric Endocrinology,
Children's Hospital of Pittsburgh, Pittsburgh
Chapter 7

Andrée Durieux-Smith, Ph.D.
Associate Professor of Otolaryngology, University of Ottawa
School of Medicine; Director of Audiology, Children's
Hospital of Eastern Ontario, Ottawa, Ontario, Canada
Chapter 10

Jose Luis Enriquez, M.D.
Assistant Professor of Pediatrics, Division of Pediatric
Nephrology, University of Texas Medical School at Galveston,
Galveston
Chapter 13

Nancy B. Esterly, M.D.
Professor of Pediatrics and Dermatology, Medical College of
Wisconsin; Head, Division of Dermatology, Children's
Hospital of Wisconsin, Milwaukee
Chapter 22; Appendix A, Section 27

Robert D. Fildes, M.D.
Assistant Professor of Pediatrics, Georgetown University
School of Medicine; Director, Pediatric End-Stage Renal
Diseases, Georgetown University Hospital, Washington, D.C.
Chapter 13; Appendix A, Section 19

Laurence Finberg, M.D.
Professor and Chairman of Pediatrics, State University of New
York Health Science Center at Brooklyn College of Medicine,
Brooklyn; Chairman, Department of Pediatrics, Children's
Medical Center of Brooklyn, Brooklyn
Chapter 7

Bishara J. Freij, M.D.
Assistant Professor of Pediatrics, Georgetown University
School of Medicine; Attending Physician, Georgetown
University Hospital, Washington, D.C.
Chapter 20

Bent Friis-Hansen, M.D., Ph.D.
Professor of Pediatrics, University of Copenhagen; Chief,
Department of Neonatology, University Hospital,
Rigshospitalet, Copenhagen, Denmark
Appendix A, Section 17

Ayhan Gocmen, M.D.
Professor of Pediatrics, Hacettepe University School of
Medicine, Ankara, Turkey
Chapter 7

Glenn R. Gourley, M.D.
Associate Professor of Pediatrics, University of Wisconsin
Medical School; Attending Physician, University of Wisconsin
Hospital and Clinics, Madison
Appendix A, Section 14

George G. Graham, M.D.
Professor of Human Nutrition and Pediatrics, Johns Hopkins
University Schools of Public Health and Medicine, Baltimore,
Maryland
Appendix A, Section 4

Richard J. Grand, M.D.
Professor of Pediatrics, Tufts University School of Medicine; Chief, Division of Pediatric Gastroenterology and Nutrition, New England Medical Center Hospital, Boston
Chapter 12

Donald E. Greydanus, M.D.
Director, Pediatric Education and Adolescent Medicine Programs, Kalamazoo Center for Medical Studies, Michigan State University School of Medicine, Kalamazoo
Chapter 24

Niilo Hallman, M.D.
Professor Emeritus of Pediatrics, Faculty of Medicine, University of Helsinki; Chief, Foundation for Pediatric Research, University Central Hospital, Helsinki, Finland
Appendix A, Section 18

Seymour I. Hepner, M.D.
Director, Division of Pediatric Cardiology, Department of Pediatrics, Fairfax Hospital, Falls Church, Virginia
Chapter 11

Ronald S. Illingworth, M.D., D.Sc., F.R.C.P., D.P.H., D.C.H.
Professor Emeritus of Pediatrics, University of Sheffield; Pediatrician, Children's Hospital, Sheffield, England
Chapters 3, 4

Richard A. Insel, M.D.
Associate Professor of Pediatrics, The University of Rochester School of Medicine and Dentistry; Associate Pediatrician, Strong Memorial Hospital, Rochester, New York
Chapter 19

August L. Jung, M.D.
Professor of Pediatrics, University of Utah School of Medicine; Director, Division of Neonatology, University of Utah Medical Center, Salt Lake City
Chapter 9

Alok Kalia, M.B., B.S.
Associate Professor of Pediatrics, Division of Nephrology, University of Texas Medical School at Galveston, Galveston
Chapter 13

Stephen R. Keller, M.D.
Assistant Professor of Pediatrics, Georgetown University School of Medicine, Washington, D.C.; Director, Pediatric Intensive Care Unit, Fairfax Hospital, Falls Church, Virginia
Appendix B

Richard E. Kravath, M.D.
Professor of Clinical Pediatrics, State University of New York Health Science Center at Brooklyn; Director of In-patient Pediatrics, Department of Pediatrics, Kings County Hospital Center, Brooklyn, New York
Chapter 7

Chinh T. Lê, M.D.
Associate Clinical Professor of Pediatrics and Internal Medicine, University of California, Davis, School of Medicine; Staff Pediatrician and Infectious Diseases Consultant, Kaiser Permanente Medical Center, Santa Rosa, California
Chapter 20

Ian Leibowitz, M.D.
Clinical Instructor in Pediatrics, Georgetown University School of Medicine, Washington, D.C.
Chapter 12

Kathleen M. Link, M.D.
Active Member, Department of Pediatrics, Fairfax Hospital, Falls Church, Virginia
Appendix A, Sections 25, 26

Frederick H. Lovejoy, Jr., M.D.
Professor of Pediatrics, Harvard Medical School; Associate Physician-in-Chief, Children's Hospital Medical Center, Boston
Chapter 1

Noni MacDonald, M.D., F.R.C.P.C.
Associate Professor of Pediatrics and Microbiology, University of Ottawa School of Medicine; Head Pediatric Infectious Disease Service, Children's Hospital of Eastern Ontario, Ottawa, Ontario, Canada
Chapter 10

Anne Moddalena, Ph.D.
Director, Molecular Genetics Laboratory, Genetics and IVF Institute, Fairfax, Virginia
Chapter 5

Mohamed K. Mardini, M.D., F.A.C.C.
Assistant Professor of Pediatrics, Division of Pediatric Cardiology, Johns Hopkins University School of Medicine; Consultant Pediatric Cardiologist and Co-director, Pediatric Cardiology Service and Department of Pediatrics, Fairfax Hospital, Falls Church, Virginia
Chapter 11

William T. McLean, Jr., M.D.
Associate Professor of Neurology and Pediatrics, Bowman Gray School of Medicine of Wake Forest University; Head, Section of Pediatric Neurology, North Carolina Baptist Hospital, Winston-Salem
Chapter 14; Appendix A, Section 3

Richard A. Molteni, M.D.
Associate Professor of Pediatrics, University of Utah School of Medicine; Vice Chairman, Pediatrics, Director, Medical Studies, Division of Neonatology, Primary Children's Medical Center, Salt Lake City
Chapter 9

H. David Mosier, Jr., M.D.
Professor of Pediatrics and Pathology, University of California, Irvine, College of Medicine; Irvine
Chapter 6

Fe Del Mundo, M.D., M.A.
Professor Emeritus of Pediatrics, Far Eastern University, Manila; President and Chief Pediatrician Children's Medical Center, Quezon City, Philippines
Appendix A, Section 21

Gerard B. Odell, M.D.
Professor of Pediatrics, University of Wisconsin Medical School; Director, Pediatric Gastroenterology and Nutrition, University of Wisconsin Hospital and Clinics, Madison
Appendix A, Section 14

Thomas E. Oppé, M.B., F.R.C.P.
Professor of Pediatrics, St. Mary's Hospital Medical School; Consultant Pediatrician, St. Mary's Hospital, London, England
Appendix A, Sections 13, 16

Michael E. Pichichero, M.D.
Clinical Professor of Pediatrics, University of Rochester School of Medicine and Dentistry; Attending Pediatrician, Strong Memorial Hospital, Rochester, New York
Chapter 19

F. Stanley Porter, M.D.
Professor of Pediatrics, Eastern Virginia Medical School, Norfolk
Chapter 16

Charles V. Pryles, M.D.
Former Professor of Pediatrics, University of Massachusetts Medical School; Former Attending Physician in Pediatrics, University of Massachusetts Medical Center, Worcester
Chapter 20

V. Balagopal Raju, M.D., D.C.H.
Professor of Pediatrics and Director, Institute of Child Health, Madras Medical College of Madras University, Madras, India
Appendix A, Section 15

Pierre E. Royer, M.D.
Director, International Children's Center, Paris, France
Honorary Consultant Editor

Erkki Savilahti, M.D.
Chief, Research Laboratory, Department of Pediatrics, University of Helsinki; Chief, Department of Gastroenterology and Nutrition, Children's Hospital, University Central Hospital, Helsinki, Finland
Appendix A, Section 18

Henry M. Seidel, M.D.
Professor of Pediatrics, Johns Hopkins University School of Medicine; Pediatrician, Johns Hopkins Hospital, Baltimore, Maryland
Chapters 1, 2, 23

Nasrollah T. Shahidi, M.D.
Professor of Pediatrics, University of Wisconsin Medical School; Head, Division of Pediatric Hematology/Oncology, Children's Hospital of Wisconsin, Madison
Chapter 16

Sunil K. Sood, M.D.
Assistant Professor of Pediatrics, Albert Einstein College of Medicine of Yeshiva University, Bronx, New York; Attending Physician, Division of Infectious Diseases, Scheider Children's Hospital of Long Island Jewish Medical Center, New Hyde Park, New York
Chapter 20

Pierre Soucy, M.D.
Associate Professor of Surgery, University of Ottawa School of Medicine; Head, Division of Pediatric General Surgery, Children's Hospital of Eastern Ontario, Ottawa, Ontario, Canada
Chapter 10

Timur Sumer, M.D.
Associate Professor of Pediatrics, University of Medicine and Dentistry of New Jersey, Piscataway; Attending Physician, Department of Pediatrics, Cooper Hospital/University Medical Center, Camden, New Jersey
Chapter 17

Luther B. Travis, M.D.
Professor of Pediatrics and Director, Divisions of Nephrology and Diabetes, University of Texas Medical School at Galveston, Galveston
Chapter 13

John T. Truman, M.D., M.P.H.
Professor of Clinical Pediatrics, Columbia University College
of Physicians and Surgeons, New York; Chairman,
Department of Pediatrics, Morristown Memorial Hospital,
Morristown, New Jersey
Chapter 16; Appendix A, Section 23

Scott B. Valet, M.D.
Clinical Assistant Professor of Pediatrics, University of
Rochester School of Medicine and Dentistry; Attending
Physician, The Strong Memorial Hospital, Rochester, New
York
Chapter 21

Ali Akbar Velayati, M.D.
Associate Professor of Pediatrics, Tehran University of Health
Sciences; Medical Staff Member, Department of Pediatric
Infectious Diseases, Children's Hospital Medical Center,
Tehran, Iran
Chapter 20; Appendix A, Sections 9, 11, 20, 21, 22, 27

Otto H. Wolff, C.B.E. M.D., F.R.C.P.
Emeritus Nuffield Professor of Child Health, University of
London, Institute of Child Health; Consultant Physician,
Hospital for Sick Children, London, England
Appendix A, Section 24

Mohsen Ziai, M.D.
Professor of Pediatrics, Georgetown University School of
Medicine, Washington, D.C.; Chairman, Department of
Pediatrics, Fairfax Hospital, Falls Church, Virginia; Lecturer in
Pediatrics, Johns Hopkins University School of Medicine,
Baltimore; Edward H. Townsend, Jr., Chairman Emeritus,
Department of Pediatrics, University of Rochester Medical
Center and Rochester General Hospital, Rochester, New York
*Chapters 3, 10, 14, 15, 18, 20; Appendix A, Sections 6, 7, 8, 9,
10, 11, 15, 17, 19, 20, 21, 22, 26, 27*

Preface

The previous editions of *Pediatrics* have been met with overwhelming success. Medical students find the text concise and well-proportioned; residents use it extensively for review, and primary care providers consider it indispensable, particularly because of the inclusion of sections on differential diagnosis and pediatric emergencies.

The task of dealing with the impressive body of new knowledge, yet maintaining the usefulness of the book, has been monumental considering the decision to decrease the size of the text by one-third. Every effort has been made to deal with common and important problems in reasonable detail. Complex issues have been presented from a conceptual point of view, assuming that if they cannot be presented in a few simple words they are not worth the inclusion in a text of this size.

The credit for any success that the present edition might have goes to the distinguished and dedicated contributors. My special thanks are due to the staff of Little, Brown publishers, particularly Mr. Louis C. Bruno, Jr. for his expert assistance. Dr. Paul de Bellefeuille has provided excellent suggestions and honored us by joining as a contributor. The expert secretarial and managerial skills of Mrs. Macel Thompson have been the greatest asset. To her and all those who have made this 4th edition a reality, I am truly indebted.

M. Z.

Notice. The indications and dosages of all drugs in this book have been recommended in the medical literature and conform to the practices of the general medical community. The medications described do not necessarily have specific approval by the Food and Drug Administration for use in the diseases and dosages for which they are recommended. The package insert for each drug should be consulted for use and dosage as approved by the FDA. Because standards for usage change, it is advisable to keep abreast of revised recommendations, particularly those concerning new drugs.

1

The Pediatrician, the Child, and the Family

The Well Child and the Physician

Infancy and childhood have implicit in them the beauty of growth and development and the anticipation of the future — the exquisite blend of nature and nurture, the genetic endowment and the impact of environment.

Pediatrics devotes its attention fully as much to the well child as to the sick child. It strives to preserve well-being or to achieve it when it is lacking, mindful of the present, anticipating the adult to be. The achievement of optimal health is an immediate target of the anticipatory years. The definition of *optimal*, of course, is primarily cultural, and *normal* is an elusive quality varying in the eye of the physician and with the circumstance of the individual patient.

We all, however, use the concept of the normal child, defining the concept in pieces if not in the whole, and we no longer restrict the concept to physical growth and organic development. It encompasses intellectual progress, emotional balance, and social adjustment. The concept underlies a perhaps pretentious goal, that of uniting all these components into a whole, permitting happy progress for the child, seeking the development of a competent, relatively independent being who, for the moment, is quite dependent in a setting of parents, family, and community, each defined by its varying customs and prejudices.

The role of the pediatrician in working toward this goal is shaped and ordered by the consent and cooperation of others. The physician's directives may be implemented only with the support of parents and school, and the pediatrician must be willing to offer support to these others who play a much larger role in the lives of most children. The physician may begin to assist the youth more directly to establish independence and personal identity during the time of middle and late adolescence. It is, however, but assistance, and it gives promise of a successful intervention only to the extent that the physician is able to recognize and to acknowledge constructively the other powerful factors in the patient's life.

Prenatal Period

The physical environment of a child may be said to begin at the moment of conception, but, in fact, it stretches back into infinity. Conception, however, can be reasonably accurately dated, and sometime between this accidental, casual, or planned event and the delivery of the baby, the pediatrician should encourage at least one prenatal visit for expectant primiparous mothers and the fathers. Such a visit gives the chance to explore the hereditary background, to establish rapport, and to inquire into any deviation from normal in the pregnancy. First-time parents are generally excited and apprehensive. The discussion should be open but might include the material needs of the infant — clothing, bedding, bathing, and feeding. Feeding is always of particular significance. Breast feeding is the method of choice the world around, but to make it an inflexible demand would be a mistake. The mother who breast feeds her infant resentfully and because of pressure from family or physician might well have an irritable infant with poor weight gain. The circumstance should be encouraged but not be forced. It is better to have a contented mother who bottle feeds than an unhappy one wrestling with a hungry baby at an inadequate breast. Most women, however, anticipate nursing with joy and require only positive reinforcement from family, friends, and health professionals. The deprived families of the developing areas of the world need special services to assure proper advice concerning nutrition and health education.

The prenatal visit affords the opportunity to assess the temperament and character of the parents. An inquiry into their childhood experiences and feelings is often predictive of their responses to the expected child. This total picture will enable the physician to modify approaches to the problems of an individual child in a particular family setting. The decision concerning nursing, for example, is much facilitated in such an interview. Small brochures or booklets that describe what can be expected of the baby during the first weeks or months of life can complement such interviews prenatally and postnatally, but they cannot substitute for the live interaction of parent and health professional.

Neonatal Period

The initial approach to the newborn infant requires, first, the assessment of the child and the determination of normality and the discovery of abnormality, and, second, the communication of that information to the parents. Then, too, one must offer instruction about the baby and respond to questions. A happy outcome for this interaction requires empathy and a sense of this impressive moment in the life of the family. It requires the conscious effort for good rapport if there is to be an important immediate impact and if satisfactory continuous communication is to be achieved with the family.

The physician must, if problems are discovered, be honest yet sympathetic. It is not necessary to be harshly blunt or determinedly objective all the time. Deception, however, will taint the relationship and undermine confidence. The parents must be given continuing support as they absorb the initial blow, come to understand it, grieve for the loss that the problem with their child imposes, and establish life under the constraints of that problem.

First Year

Contact with the family is ordinarily most frequent during the first year of a child's life. The first-time parent may be somewhat more dependent and insecure; indeed, educational or social advantage does not assure security. Each of us needs direction and the reassurance of competence when the parent's role is assumed.

In particular, one must be ready to protect and support the self-esteem of the woman who becomes unsuccessful at breast feeding. The physician should make the point that the early weeks at the breast are the most important emotionally but that the mother may consider the use of supplementary bottles, early introduction of solid foods, or early weaning with deliberate caution but without guilt or a sense of failure.

Circumstances such as this require access to the pediatrician. Some prefer a set telephone hour for discussion of routine care and minor problems. Indeed, a weekly call by the mother can be helpful during the first month at home, and a home visit at least once during this period has important value for teaching the physician about the family and establishing communication and a base for support. Follow-up visits during the first year have a number of purposes:

1. To examine carefully for undiscovered congenital anomalies or for early signs of developmental abnormality. A checklist, assigning certain tasks to each visit, can help prevent omissions or oversights.
2. To assess growth and development, using measurement of the head size, height, and weight and inquiry into the developmental milestones (see Chaps. 3, 4). Social and cultural pressures are a major source of difficulty, for example, neighborhood competition over the size and weight of contemporary babies. It may be difficult to persuade a mother or grandmother that each child has a constitutional ideal and that one child may quite acceptably weigh as little as 8 kg at 1 year and another as much as 12 kg. Height and weight charts depicting normal upper and lower limits are mandatory in every child's medical record and are valuable educational aids (see Chap. 3). The

estimate of the developmental progress of the infant is vital to the early discovery of problematic states. Each such problem has prepossessing importance, but some are easier to find than others. It is difficult, for example, with "soft" signs to appreciate early that disabling but elusive condition inaptly named minimal brain damage (see Chaps. 3, 4).

3. To counsel concerning the infant's diet. A wide range of variations is possible, but the diet must fulfill the criteria of freedom from pathogens, adequacy in nutritional elements, and sufficiency without excess of vitamins. Poorly tolerated foods must be withdrawn. The potential of food sensitivity must always be considered, and constraint must always be exercised when considering the introduction of any food other than breast milk. Some pediatricians advocate beginning the use of a cup at 5 or 6 months and encourage the child's hand feeding whenever the child seems so inclined. It is a common practice in developing countries to continue breast feeding for 2 years or more since this may be the only source of animal protein for many infants. Socioeconomic factors that delay the introduction of solid foods until late in the first year need to be considered, and cultural factors should be allowed full play within the constraints imposed by the basic needs of the infant. There need certainly be no rush to introduce solid foods, and there is a need to be cautious about excessive parental devotion to particular regimens.

4. To administer immunizing agents that are regionally appropriate. Immunization against diphtheria, whooping cough, tetanus, poliomyelitis, and measles should be included for all normal children in all countries. Booster shots should be planned at proper intervals. In addition, BCG (antituberculosis immunization) and typhoid and yellow fever series are essential in many areas.

5. To provide the parents with an opportunity to ask questions and to discuss problems. A relaxed environment, attentive listening, and a few judicious remarks will provide much useful exchange regarding the parent-child interaction and sociocultural attitudes.

6. To educate regarding the prevention and treatment of accidents and injury. This is in many areas the principal source of morbidity and mortality in children past the age of 2 years.

One can recognize the expression of certain temperaments during the first year. Patterns of reaction and response are being formed that can persist for better or worse throughout life. Frequently these budding characteristics may not be tolerable to parents. Among the most valuable and enduring contributions of the physician are fostering

the parents' understanding of the child's behavior, channeling strengths in positive directions, and ameliorating handicaps to the extent possible so that they do not impede progress toward realistic goals and ambitions. This is not psychotherapy; it is true mental hygiene. Good rapport with the family can be of incalculable assistance at this level of support and primary prevention.

1 to 3 Years of Age

The child from 1 to 3 years is an active, seemingly tireless explorer, striving to examine and to define the world through personal initiative and the use of all of the senses. Accidents and poisonings are common. A discussion with the mother about the potential of aspiration of foreign objects and ingestion of noxious agents is essential; advice regarding prevention of serious falls and street accidents, a must.

Pedal locomotion focuses the attention of parents on the legs and feet of children of this age. Concern about bowlegs, knock knees, and flatfeet is frequently expressed. Most such conditions, perceived as abnormal, are truly phases in development, and many more are of constitutional heritage rather than signs of disease such as rickets. Shoe wedges and other manipulative devices are often unnecessarily prescribed. These interventions cannot substitute for sound education and explanation. Forbearance and rapport make good allies.

Speech is a major developmental feature. The child who is not using phrases at 2 to 2½ years of age becomes suspect for possible difficulties. Hearing problems must be considered early and appropriately investigated in any instance of retarded speech. Always respect and explore a parent's concern about hearing regardless of the age of a child.

The office examination is frequently a wrestling match at this age. The parent's lap rather than table should be relied on so that the child may feel more at ease. Reason, threats, or bribes are not very effective. It is just as well, therefore, for the parent to restrain firmly when necessary and for the doctor to complete the examination swiftly.

Preschool and School Age

The nursery school, day-care center, and kindergarten have, in recent years, given a further dimension to the early care of children, particularly as women have asserted their appropriate societal role in a more determined fashion. The multiple purposes and objectives of early childhood care and educational settings offer advantages to every social level — a safe and secure haven for the children of working mothers; a noonday meal, sometimes government funded, to augment a perhaps limited diet; and an opportunity for children to see and to hear things, to take part in social activities, and thus to learn in a circumstance in which they may not have had previous experience and that the family might not otherwise have been able to provide.

The child's first approach to the school experience is a crucial step. Children are expected to enter school at an empirically established age in many countries. Educators have too often been forced to plan in a manner that establishes the so-called average child as a statistical concept. Curricula are designed to deal with groups and not individuals. Thus, many of the "slow" are laggard not because of an inherent lack of ability but, most often, because of individual physical, emotional, or social handicaps compounded perhaps by societal or institutional limitations or, unhappily, indifference or ignorance. These problems must be recognized. Humiliation and inadequate performance in the first grade of school can effectively establish a hostile, negative attitude, replacing achievement satisfaction with failure and too often resulting in school dropout and behavioral disorganization.

A thorough preschool evaluation, including assessment of visual and auditory acuity, therefore, is essential. Physical and mental handicaps that are to any extent distracting or exhausting should be recognized and properly managed. Children whose defects may warrant special consideration should be grouped for special classes or, if the circumstance suggests, considered for continuation in the mainstream of the childhood experience.

Many children might benefit by an additional year in the preschool setting. We sometimes tend to ignore the fact that future success or failure is far more important than the age of entry into school and that the best for each child must be individually determined. We must resist the tendency of educational institutions to compress the child into preset patterns and predetermined pathways.

The school, after all, controls as many as 30 hours a week of the child's time and constitutes the most compelling demand on his attention outside the family and home. The physician, therefore, should establish a comfortable and cordial relationship with the schools in the vicinity and should, as a child-oriented and an educated member of the community, strive to improve the educational opportunities for children. Talks, meetings, and personal communications with the staffs can be useful in this regard. The provision of appropriate pediatric care also requires full understanding of the method of administration and the significance of psychological tests commonly employed in the school system. In any event, the onset of the school experience, at whatever age in the life of the child, brings into play the need to balance those forces that are often in conflict: the desire for ultimate success and the impulsive reach for immediate gratification. The parent plays a major role here, and the child may often be a pawn. The pediatrician can be the moderating influence, an intermediary, often providing the view that preserves perspective for the child.

A great number of problems can evolve, then, during the preschool and school years. Some of them are discussed here.

BRAIN INJURY. The spectrum extends from evident and severe cerebral palsy, with multiple-system involvement to the extremely subtle conditions of cerebral dysfunction.

MENTAL RETARDATION. Recognition is easy in the severe circumstance. However, quite common borderline handicap may too often escape recognition until problems develop in school. The child then is put at risk for the frustration of efforts, becomes overwhelmed, resents the label of failure, and adopts defensive measures inimical to his or her best interests. The earlier an accurate appraisal, the sooner a more suitable setting can be planned for that child. Still, caution must be taken to assure that borderline manifestations of limited intelligence are truly organic and not psychosocial in origin. There can be difficulty in this instance in an abrupt transition from an illiterate or culturally constrained home to an alien, formal school setting (see also Chap. 4).

EMOTIONAL HANDICAPS. There are emotional problems so overpowering that little energy remains for the tasks of daily living and learning. The attempt to cope, to preserve energy, may result in withdrawal into personal fantasies and "model" behavior. Quite the opposite may occur instead. The expression of school phobia and the adoption of impulsive, disruptive behavior may trap the child in further difficulty if the institutional or parental response is insensitive to the true need and if, as a result, unenlightened discipline is imposed.

In sum, these disabilities are diverse and seemingly infinite in number and complexity and, added to the problems caused by visual defects, hearing disorders, speech defects, cardiac lesions, and epilepsy, among many others, alert attention is required for the earliest possible detection and integration of the management of the problem in a manner least disruptive to the child's and the family's life. The pediatrician as advocate may need to function at the interface of child with family or family and child with school. Appropriate advocacy requires, first, recognition of the fact that this is part of the role of the pediatrician and, after that, a multitude of sensitivities and skills, not the least of which is the ability to balance constantly the life requirements of each of the persons involved. There may be conflicting needs and, in the end, it is the child who is the patient and the child in the context of the family who must be served first. Obviously, in the early years, school is one of the prime imperatives, but, as time passes, the work of adolescence and the struggle for identity and independence — the reach for the future — take center stage.

Adolescence

Adolescence (see also Chap. 22) is one of nature's most fascinating transformations, and it is fair to characterize the period as frequently turbulent and tumultuous. Some children may live it evenly with gradual evolution to maturity; others may endure a tortured, laborious time. There is, however, a Gaussian distribution to the quality of the experience. Certainly the period is a proving ground for the physician, and if there is inherent value in the continuity of the doctor-patient relationship from infancy on, it becomes evident here. A heritage of positive experience with the patient and the family will make possible valuable interaction during the time of adolescence.

The first challenge perhaps is in the wide normal variation in physical growth and development. This is, after all, a time of accelerated growth and of body transformation that heralds the unleashing of sexual interest and desire and the struggle for emancipation. It is imperative to seek acceptance by contemporaries, to set goals, to test values, to explore life's purpose, and to decide on an occupation.

Adolescents may find some of the somatic and parallel emotional transformations overwhelming. Some may face the change earlier than others, and those who must wait need a sensitive, temporizing explanation and reassurance. In any event, when change ensues, the new physical habitus may approach that of the adult, but social acceptance in that status will quite often lag considerably behind.

These are years of physiological and psychological stress and organic vulnerability. Repeated thorough examinations are important since psychic strains may be diversely expressed and somatization is not uncommon. Successful intervention requires intimate knowledge of the individual. Time *must* be taken to achieve this sensitivity; if it is not, the potential for the provision of good medical care is too readily lost.

It is important to respect the adolescent's need for privacy and self-esteem. A first step involves exclusion of the parents from the examining room, a distinct, symbolic change after all the years of working with the child through intermediaries. The youth should be encouraged to take on direct responsibility for health care and for communication with the doctor. The parent can, of course, be invited into the examining room on the patient's expressed desire or as a chaperone when that is necessary. Certainly it is vital to include examination of the genitalia in both males and females. This should, of course, be sensitively done. Too many physicians omit these procedures and, in so doing, lose the opportunity to gain vital information, to reassure, and to give positive messages regarding the body and human sexuality.

Indeed, attention to physical needs should not be lost in the social, behavioral context of adolescence. For example, tuberculin test conversion increases in frequency; urinary tract infections increase in number, particularly in females; and, also in females, anemia associated with the onset of menses and aggravation of abnormal spinal curvatures become more evident. There must, then, be attention to a changing frequency distribution of the kinds of problems encountered. The thyroid gland must be palpated with care. Recurrent headaches may assume the classic pattern of the migraine or tension varieties. Undiagnosed abdominal complaints may develop the periodicity of peptic ulcer or culminate in the bleeding of ulcerative colitis. Above all, anatomical and physiological evidence of gonadal maturation should be observed and recorded. These changes are most likely to cause anxiety. Be it the obvious acne or the concealable masturbation, the mysteries are many and the confusions perplex and preoccupy.

It is essential, therefore, to be ready and willing to discuss all this openly with the adolescent. The wide variations in onset and completion of the physical and emotional processes of this period must be explained with conviction and with honesty.

Age itself is the first clue to the need to give this kind of attention. Physical change also alerts. Breast changes usually precede menstruation by about 2 years. This allows adequate time to engage in anticipatory counseling. Variations in height, from too short to too tall, require reassurance, as do variations in the onset of nocturnal emissions or of menses. Metrorrhagia, menorrhagia, dysmenorrhea, and amenorrhea, both primary and secondary, present a variety of concerns. Primary amenorrhea and short stature arouse suspicion of gonadal dysgenesis. Secondary amenorrhea suggests pregnancy. Unfortunately, there may be reluctance to do a "complete" physical examination — particularly the rectal and pelvic procedures in the female. There are those who advocate a rectal examination for every child. Others fear that this is destructive to the relationship one is attempting to preserve and a violation of the exaggerated modesty quite common at this time. Nevertheless, these examinations are often necessary, and a personally secure, mature, appropriately confident physician can proceed with sensitivity and assurance. It is wise, of course, to explain carefully both the rectal and the vaginal maneuvers, and it is a time when a parent or other chaperone should be present.

Hypertension, in particular, systolic readings of 140 mm of mercury or more, is not infrequently found in the adolescent; this is the result of the mercurial nature of the autonomic system in this age group. There is most often no organic disease, but the persistence of elevated blood pressure demands at least limited investigation. However, probabilistic decision making is justified in the effort to limit invasive studies in this as in other common circumstances that most often have no identifiable organic cause — frequent headaches, abdominal pain, and prolonged fatigue states.

Obesity is also common. The decision to regard it as a problem depends on the degree and on the personal and social attitudes of the patient. Permanent weight reduction is rarely achieved; it requires powerful motivation uncommon at this age level. Chronic ailments of the earlier years, such as rheumatic fever, tuberculosis, diabetes, and asthma, may become exaggerated or complicated during this period, and adjustment to the limitations their treatment imposes may be difficult. The apparent refusal to take greater responsibility for the care of self must be understood and must not try the patience of the physician.

The need for independence and emancipation typifies adolescence. These involve increasing ability to make decisions, to exercise judgment, and to assume responsibility for the results. The youth must have the chance to test this capacity, to explore and try a value system, to stress self-discipline. If not, there will be difficulty in the short run and during adult life. Parents who cannot unfetter a child and who seek vicarious justification in the child's achievements fail to support the adolescent's growth to maturity or to solve the family's problems. The whole process is not facilitated when, in the early days of emancipation, the adolescent tends to look at us and to judge us, to measure our honesty, scale of values, and maturity of judgment, and, being feisty and often a bit dogmatic and unyielding, to emphasize our shortcomings and to exaggerate our defects.

The adolescent needs to cope with the problem of a maturing sexual drive and the establishment of sexual relationships. When? With whom? How? The answers are culturally and experientially based. The physician can play a role if that role is defined by the need to teach and not to preach. Still, the need to develop peer-group adjustment and acceptance is an overriding factor in determining eventual behavior. There is fear of being different and of being rejected. It is a trial to attempt to be identified with one's age group but to preserve, nevertheless, one's individuality. Uniform styles of dress, speech and mannerisms, and music and dance preferences serve to signal group membership. Yet each adolescent will seek some area of competence for special recognition. It might be academic or athletic excellence, heroism, personal charm, material possessions, or rebellious behavior; or it might be the tragic, aberrational call for help implicit in the increased accident and suicide rates in these teen years.

The effort to cope is not infrequently helped by the adoption of a hero. The idealized person is usually not of the immediate family, perhaps being a rather casual acquaintance whose advice the adolescent might be willing to accept. The right person can be an enormous support; the wrong person, a disaster. The search for sharper direction and defined goals is, of course, usually tolerably successful. If the pathway tends to remain vague and the end obscure, the unease is intense and decision making delayed. The pediatrician can play a role, but it cannot be forced; and, of course, a sense of mutual respect with the patient is absolutely necessary.

Events of the past decade have made the pediatrician's role with the adolescent more intense and the establishment of a mutual respect more difficult. Adolescent morbidity today is, in large part, the result of risk-taking behavior. Obviously, exploratory behavior is implicit in the growth and development of the adolescent. Nevertheless, these explorations — these risks — result in injury, suicide, pregnancy, substance abuse, and disease, particularly sexually transmitted disease.

One of the advantages of the care of children is their innocence. We do not often find ourselves blaming children for what happens to them. Now, in many ways, adolescence reflects the loss of innocence, and the pediatrician may discover hidden reserves of resentment that may, if one is not careful, obstruct the establishment of a relationship as a particularly poignant problem confronts the teenage patient and the physician.

Nature of Problems Affecting Wellness

There are other problems that often need the intercession of the pediatrician as the well child grows, develops, and integrates with the family. The issues are not necessarily concerned with a pathophysiological base in physical illness but, rather, in some societal malfunction that has a great impact on the life of the child and that in fact, in its own way, can cause considerable morbidity. We will discuss a few examples, and we will make the point that large numbers of children are affected by many of these examples. It is probable, for example, although the figures are difficult to define with certainty, that almost 2% of children in the United States are adopted and, in the United States at least, 40% of first marriages end in divorce, another source of potential morbidity. There is, on the average, at least one child per divorced family, and since the median duration of marriage prior to divorce is a bit over 7 years, most divorces and the separation implied will affect the young child. In any event, the important point is that children may incur morbidity in a wide variety of ways, and the role of the pediatrician, therefore, is obviously diverse and exciting.

Adoption

The successful adoption of a child requires the coordinated effort of experienced workers in the fields of medicine, law, and social services. Frequently the physician is the first to know of the desire of an expectant mother to place her infant for adoption and also of a childless couple's desire to adopt. The doctor, then, may be at a crucial focal point.

Most adoptions are within families and by close relatives of the child. Other situations include the wide range of so-called black-market adoptions (arranged for illicit personal profit of some third party), "gray" market adoptions (legal, but the adoptive parents assume the costs of the biological mother), variations on both of these themes, and, finally, agency adoptions (arangements consummated under the supervision of certified adoption agencies). "Surrogate motherhood," a circumstance in which a woman agrees to artificial insemination with the sperm of the male in the adopting pair, complicates this picture and is currently being argued in courts and legislatures.

Physicians most often encounter difficulty when an agency is not involved. The guiding principle should be that the first obligation is to the child, and there must be reasonable assurance that the child be accepted into a home in which there is adequate opportunity for a productive life. The physician also has an obligation to the biological parent, or parents, to ascertain that the decision to yield the child is not reached hastily or because of immaturity or insufficient understanding of all aspects of the problem. There is also an obligation to the adoptive parents to assure that all medical information regarding the child, including the genetic, is available. The adoptive parents must be advised as accurately as possible as to the infant's potential for health. If discoverable congenital defects or other problems are present, the adoptive parents must be made fully aware of the consequences and be willing to assume the responsibility. Finally, the physician has an obligation to the community. Every possible effort must be made to ensure that the adoption

will be successful, with little likelihood of legal or social complications in ensuing years. Conflict arises, however, because the physician is most often engaged and paid by the adoptive parents, and too often there can be an implicit assumption that they deserve first consideration.

In any event, if all obligations are to be met, the physician must be thoroughly acquainted with the specific local adoption laws and make certain they are carefully followed. Proper use must be made of the legal and social service facilities of the community. Indeed, many individuals believe that all adoptions must be arranged through approved social agencies. This may not be possible, however, in communities in which the available facilities are not sufficient to meet the demand. Of late, however, the increase in single parents raising their babies and the accessibility of abortion have seriously diminished the number of babies available for adoption. Thus there has been increasing attention to the adoption of handicapped and older children in the foster care setting and to interracial and international adoption. The mandate at all times, however, must be to respect the needs of all the individuals involved, and this will require forbearance and frequent interdisciplinary effort.

Divorce

A major cause of "disability" in our children is divorce, a much more common phenomenon now, certainly in the United States, than in the past. In the United States there was in 1986 almost one divorce for every two marriages. Today, at least 40% of first marriages end in divorce, and, on the average, the incidence of children per divorced family is slightly greater than 1. Seventy-two percent of divorces occur in the first 14 years of marriage, and the median duration of these marriages is 7.1 years. This suggests that most divorces affect young children. In addition, the father becomes the noncustodial parent at least 90% of the time.

The potential for conflict is obvious; but, in the event of behavioral disturbance, there is no single symptom or symptom complex unique to the child of divorce. The response depends on the child's developmental stage, intellectual capacity, personality, and moral capacity. Predominantly, however, divorce means loss, and loss requires grief. This is true for the child and for each of the parents. Their needs in this regard must be met if they are to resolve their anger and their guilt appropriately. It can be a chaotic time, and the pediatrician can, of course, make a positive contribution. The disruption usually peaks about 1 year after the divorce, and when a child is involved, many families will have been to court by that time. The pediatrician should work hard to discourage the child's becoming a pawn in a triangle with the parents. Sensitivity to the varying needs of children at different ages is also required. An egocentric view of the world, which is more particularly the province of the child in the early years, invests the young child of divorce with particular guilt and with the fear of retaliation as payment for his supposed error. And, perhaps a bit surprisingly, the adolescent — older, more competent in the world, less dependent, and less prone to personalized losses — may be hurt and angry but, fortunately, may not feel as guilty as the younger child. The adolescent has a greater facility to detach from the family by engaging in extrafamilial activities and relationships that, if they are harmonious, may help the coping process. Regardless, the pediatrician should be available and prepared to listen and, when necessary, to intervene. In the last analysis, while parents, siblings, and the particular patient must all command the pediatrician's concern, it must in the long run be the child with the problem who has priority; and, unlike the parents, it is the child with the problem who does not have a lawyer for representation in court.

Foster Care

Accurate figures are hard to determine, but there are each day in the United States at least 250,000 to perhaps 400,000 children in foster care, children of all ages, many of them with physical or emotional handicaps. These children are served by social work agencies seriously constrained by inadequate fundings, inadequate staffing, and inadequate experience among the staff. Too many social workers have too many children to supervise. In addition, the law is quite careful in protecting the rights of biological parents. Regardless of the parents' inability to provide or of their indifference, it may not be possible to put children in a circumstance in which they might be adopted; despite an often dire need, legal termination of parental rights is made quite difficult.

The pediatrician must be sensitive to the societal problems and to the need to work constructively toward more effective protection of these large numbers of children. If children were more readily freed for adoption they might have a greater opportunity for a stable and loving home environment than that existing in a foster home or, in many cases, in foster homes that frequently change because they are judged deficient for some reason. The problems here of rejection, of guilt, and of a relative paucity of affection, attention, acceptance, and approval make for greater risk of emotional instability. The pediatrician who cares for the foster child must be alert to the potential for the development of problems and should be prepared to give the

child — and the persons who at the moment are responsible for the child's care — every attention and every opportunity to talk, to ventilate feelings, to anticipate, and, perhaps, to prevent the development of problems.

Henry M. Seidel

Sudden Infant Death Syndrome

One of the most difficult problems facing the pediatrician is the sudden infant death syndrome (SIDS) or crib death. There are perhaps 2 to 4 such deaths per 1000 births worldwide. The syndrome occurs more commonly in males, in the winter and spring months, and in an age range from 3 weeks to 6 months with a peak incidence between 2 and 4 months. The cause or causes are not yet known, and a long list of possibilities has been rejected; it is not hereditary. Vigorous clinical and laboratory study goes on. There has been an insistent effort to identify babies at risk and to "monitor" them closely. Still, there is much to learn.

For the moment, the principal task of the pediatrician is to encourage a fine balance between spontaneity and careful attention in the care of the infant in a world in which media attention to SIDS has been extensive. The concern is real, but it cannot be allowed to undermine the joy of life. The pediatrician must work at this and counsel appropriately, and, when there is tragedy, must be ready and willing to support the grieving and often guilt-ridden parents. The effort of the pediatrician can at this point be complemented by lay groups concerned with the problem.

Henry M. Seidel and Frederick H. Lovejoy

The Sick Child and the Physician

The physician has the responsibility always to attempt to heal, to ease pain, and to prolong useful, comfortable life. This requires an exquisite balance of competence, insight, and compassion. The maturity and motivation of the physician are under constant stress as the formerly well child becomes a sick child.

Acute Illness

Sickness, with its attendant pain and discomfort, is often inexplicable and bewildering to the young (and, too, to those of us who are older). A child usually responds by regressing to the pattern of an earlier age when discomfort was expressed by crying and whining. We must always be sensitive to these infantile manifestations of dependency. There is, after all, a lesser ability with illness at any age to accept with equanimity the anxiety-provoking and sometimes painful manipulations and procedures attendant on it. Thus, the otherwise compliant child may resist examination. Some initial time spent on explanation and reassurance is often helpful. Having known the child prior to illness is invaluable — one of the essences of continuity of care. Deferral of the examination of painful or sensitive areas to the end of the examination may shorten the period of violent resistance.

It has been a time-worn practice to recommend bedrest in an illness, and, indeed, rest, judiciously administered and pleasurably accepted, may well be advantageous. Still, the child playing quietly in a chair or even actively on the floor is using less energy than the bawling, maniacal one struggling to escape from a confining bed. Rigidity in health care and medical management can often be a nuisance, and sometimes it can be harmful; caution must always be taken to define the bounds of an order that, taken literally, may add to the distress of illness.

The school-age child usually accepts a transient illness and may even enjoy it because of the secondary gains of indulgence and rewards. The younger ones, however, often regard it as retribution for misconduct or as punishment for disobedience, particularly when parents use the situation to recall such incidents as their ignored advice about rain and cold weather. The hospitalized child may be distraught with anxiety about operations, mutilation, and death. The adolescent, with some bravado, often denies the illness and resents its recognition. There may be a querulous assertion that there are too many "important" matters to take care of and annoyance at the loss of useful time. Always underlying all of this, be the patient young or old, is uncertainty and partial information, worry about what it all really means, and the gnawing concern that the future is seriously threatened, even in the least threatening pathophysiological circumstance.

Hospital Admission of Sick Children

Most illnesses of childhood are transient and minor, and the decision to hospitalize a child becomes necessary relatively infrequently. Care at home, if it is possible, should always be considered. The separation of the young child from the family and the removal to a strange and threatening environment may often result in disturbed behavior after the return home.

The primary reason for hospitalization should be to provide diagnostic and therapeutic facilities that are not available at home or to provide personal care that, for some reason, may tax the energies of the parents. The physician, through it all, must try to prevent or modify the traumatic experience of hospitalization and must take every practical step to ease the stress of separation from home and to involve the parent in the continuing care of the child. Only those procedures essential to appropriate diagnosis and management should be employed, and the duration of hospitalization should be kept as short as possible. Necessary at any time, these requirements, unheeded, threaten greatest difficulty when the child is between 9 months and 5 years of age. Earlier, any compassionate caretaker may well satisfy the child's undifferentiated needs. Beyond this period, separation anxiety may diminish, but concern over death and mutilation remains. Subsequent disturbed reactions of hospitalized children can be eased by sensitivity to the emotional needs imposed by illness, separation, and the manipulation of the body, by improved understanding and modified procedures in the pediatric wards, and by adoption of in-hospital procedures that allow as much as possible for the resultant constraints. There is much that one can do. The following suggest the central thrust of the effort:

1. At any age, a patient should be hospitalized only when necessary. Full use should be made of outpatient or emergency hospital services. Even the most serious illness can be managed at home if complex equipment is not needed, communication with the family is good, and the parents are competent and willing.
2. The patient and the parents should be prepared for the hospitalization. Every step should be explained clearly and explicitly and, if necessary, repeatedly. Emotional stress may preclude immediate understanding.
3. Hospital areas for children should include:
   a. Cheerful and roomy accommodations
   b. Well-stocked, age-appropriate play areas for ambulatory children
   c. A staff of appropriately educated teachers to facilitate both play and continuing learning for the bedridden and the ambulatory
   d. Flexible grouping arrangements to allow for various situations based on the child's age, ailment, and attitude
   e. Rooming-in arrangements or, at the least, great freedom for parental visits

f. Diet management that respects the theoretical and the practical in preparing food appealing to children

Certainly there must be continuing attention to the instruction and indoctrination of all personnel — doctors, nurses, social workers, play teachers, and other attendants — in the understanding of the anxieties of hospitalized children and in appropriate methods of management.

Bureaucratic procedures should give way at every step if at all possible: Admission practices, in particular, should allow the parent to be with the child as much as possible from the start and when strangers appear. The parent, when it is feasible, should stay in the hospital. In fact, in developing countries, parents are constantly urged to be with the children, for their presence is a major part of health education, fosters increasing confidence in the doctors and nurses, and, of course, adds to the emotional security of the child. This is no less necessary and true in developed countries.

The child with long-term illness of chronic or permanent disability has additional particular needs. Parents and child must grieve for the loss of the eagerly anticipated "healthy" life and must adapt to the long-term consequences of the illness for each of the family members. The continuing participation of the physician in these significant emotional, social, and economic life problems is essential. Unfortunately, most of us have little training in these matters, and the continuing stresses in our own lives make it difficult to become too much immersed in circumstances that may not give immediate positive reward and that often seem to stretch on without resolution. We do not always understand the major contribution of our compassionate attention. We may not always invoke appropriate resources in the community and ask assistance or utilize services of social workers and other helpful professionals. If a social worker is not available, the doctor must be able to complement the efforts of the strong, active, and experienced lay organizations that give attention to handicapping abnormality. Members of these groups have banded together to provide mutual support and concerted effort to improve the care of, knowledge about, and public attention to the needs of these children. The competence gained by personal experience is thus turned to the advantage of others, since most such organizations have abundant participation by parents who have had the same disruptive experience and who, by their courage and example, demonstrate what the best-intentioned doctor may provide most often only peripherally and vicariously. The central point is that the physician must be willing and must participate in the management of *all* aspects of the problem, discovering the necessary resources and invoking and coordinating them so that the full power of a coordinated effort is made available to child and family.

Preoperative and Postoperative Care of the Young

The neonate is plethoric at birth, has a substantially lower water requirement, excretes very little potassium in the urine during the first few days of life, and responds to operative stress with less potassium diuresis than do older infants and children. The surface area relative to the body weight is much greater than in the older person, and there is definite handicap in the infant's inability to turn over or to clear the bronchial tree of mucus or aspirated vomitus by coughing.

Clearly, major operative procedures upon newborn infants require minute-by-minute, intelligent nursing and medical care. Routine pediatric nursing care of neonates in incubators must be supplemented by meticulous attention to the maintenance of a clear airway, and the laryngoscope and appropriate suction apparatus must be readily available for direct aspiration of the posterior pharynx and larynx. A large variety of neonatal problems require the institution of gastric suction as soon as possible after the problem is recognized. A small tube may be passed through the nostrils or a large one through the mouth. Tilting the head of the incubator upward lessens the risk of regurgitation and aspiration. Since respiration is largely diaphragmatic in infants, this position is also helpful in any circumstance with abdominal distention or intestinal obstruction. Some procedures and many conditions with an inherent risk of infection or those associated with an increased risk of pulmonary compromise require the judicious use of "preventive" antimicrobial therapy. All manipulations, as always, should be indicated and careful. The newborn rectum, for example, is a delicate structure that may be readily perforated. The use of rectal tubes, thermometers, and enemas is not free of risk and, whenever ordered, should be implemented or supervised by an experienced person.

FLUID ADMINISTRATION. Administration of fluid during the operative periods is almost entirely by the intravenous route. It is, during major procedures, preferable to use a saphenous vein cutdown just anterior to the internal malleolus. To assure that it is patent and effective during the operation, it is best to perform the cutdown on the operating table just after induction of anesthesia. In older children, the saphenous vein, or the basilic vein in the antecubital fossa, may be large enough so that a large needle can be safely and securely placed percutaneously.

PREMEDICATION. Use of premedication must be judicious and may include atropine (except in a patient with Down syndrome) or scopolamine but not barbiturates or morphine. Older children may be premedicated in their rooms so that the journey to the operating room is made without too sharp awareness. In any event, the order for premedication requires prior consultation with the anesthesiologist or the surgeon or both.

EMOTIONAL CONSIDERATIONS. The approach to the older child is particularly difficult, perhaps, but infants, too, must be managed in a manner designed to avoid fright and pain to the extent possible. Children who have suffered prolonged illness need much attention and sympathy from the nursing staff in spite, at times, of apparent bravado.

The older child must be informed of the operation or possibility of operation before admission to the hospital and should possess some idea of the process. The cardinal rule is directness and honesty. The confidence of a child, once lost, is not easily restored — and the need for cure is increased because the child is not always able to distinguish between deception and oversight.

It is, emotionally speaking, difficult to determine the ideal age for operation on pediatric patients. One can communicate with older children more successfully, yet they are able to formulate more dreadful fears than are younger ones, fears fed by the almost universal feeling that any such event is in some way punishment and retribution for some real or assumed guilt — "the Talionic law." Some may look on hospitalization, including an operation, as a fascinating experience and return to the hospital or to the surgeon with interest and enthusiasm; indeed, the child's reaction to the trauma of hospitalization and operation may be governed as much by the emotional stability of the home and of the parents as by the experience itself. In general, the sooner the operation for an elective and correctable condition is undertaken, the better. Indeed, the sooner the child is freed of a defect or hazard, the less anxiety for all concerned. The sine qua non, however, is the availability of appropriate expertise and facilities. Given this, even infants can tolerate operations of great magnitude surprisingly well, although some special circumstances dictate postponement of some procedures (e.g., open-heart surgery) until the child has grown to a size that will assure the best results with currently available techniques.

ANESTHESIA. Local anesthesia has relatively less place in pediatric than in adult surgery. A properly administered general anesthetic provides a smooth and swift approach and with usually less physical and emotional trauma for the child. All major operations on infants and children should be conducted under intratracheal inhalation anesthesia; the halogenated hydrocarbon anesthetics are currently fashionable and valuable.

There is an absolute need for conserving the body heat of neonates and small infants; the relatively large surface area should be kept in mind. On the other hand, in older children there is greater danger of the development of hyperthermia under the drapes, particularly if a nonrebreathing system is used. In such instances it is valuable to employ a water mattress under the child.

Even with properly administered intratracheal anesthesia, it is not uncommon to find gastric dilatation after operation. A gastric tube with continuous aspiration should, therefore, be in place during general anesthesia in children, or a tube should be inserted at the conclusion of the operation and the stomach evacuated of air.

GASTROSTOMY FEEDING. Gastrostomy feeding has become an important step in the postoperative care of many small infants. The operative procedure is relatively simple, and the results obtained with this approach to alimentation are excellent in selected patients. Certainly the risk of aspiration of vomitus is greatly diminished.

The Physically, Mentally, and Emotionally Handicapped Child

It is admittedly difficult to manage the problems of children with physical, emotional, and mental handicaps. The nature of the handicap is important, of course, but less relevant than the fact that the handicap exists and the dream of the "ideal" child diminished. Therefore, once the parents recognize the problem, their response, which is dependent upon their personal characteristics, becomes a dominant factor. There is often unceasing travel to new clinics or "experts" for refutation or some magic that will obliterate or cure. There may also be rejection of the child, with subsequent guilt and reaction formation leading to overindulgence and overprotection. This may then produce ever-increasing dependency in a demanding child who suffers not only the initial handicap but also the added difficulties of adjustment. In addition, there is always the grieving essential to the ultimate ability to cope, the grieving for the "lost" healthy child.

The patient, too, has similar needs. As the stage of peer recognition and companionship needs is reached, the deformity or disability is soon perceived, and children are blunt in their observations. A child who is shielded, or perhaps hidden, is not likely to surmount this initial reception or any peer harassment that can follow. Ideally, then, the child must from the very beginning recognize the exceptional nature of the circumstance, feel the family's acceptance, appreciate the opportunity to function up to a personal potential, and, at some point, grieve for the loss that the child learns has been imposed by some poorly understood and variously imagined force. Such emotional content is a part of almost every experience. The physician must not make the error of assuming that this may not be so with the retarded.

Nursery schools are desirable testing grounds for early adjustment. Still a matter of some debate is whether it is desirable to place the handicapped child among others with similar disabilities or in an average environment. In the first instance, there is the advantage of feeling part of a group, of some special belonging, and of learning that the "special" problem is not unique. In the second circumstance, adjustment to society from the beginning — the one in which life must be lived — seems more readily accomplished. The latter arrangement, called mainstreaming, offers an additional benefit. It is hoped that the normal companions, growing up with the disabled, may recognize the disadvantage of the handicapped and, through this association, may learn to accept and to assist others who are the innocent victims of an implacable destiny.

Most modern systems of education now provide special classes and teachers as well as facilities and techniques for the physically handicapped and the mentally retarded. There is probably a happy balance to be achieved between this special attention and mainstreaming, and the effort should be made to achieve it.

Those children who become handicapped later in life, for example, by rheumatic heart disease, rheumatoid arthritis, epilepsy, or diabetes, have the additional problem of readjustment. Such diseases tax the courage of the child and of the family; so, too, the strength and ingenuity of the physician who assists in the necessary grieving and in the reconstruction of a way of life that can be productive and satisfying. The adolescent, so sensitive to personal deviation, is especially susceptible to the depressing loneliness that these conditions can impose and may react with rebellion against the therapeutic program. Time spent in anticipatory counseling and discussion with the patient and the family separately may avert a catastrophic reaction.

Fatal Illness

The need to help children and their parents to understand the fatal nature of certain illnesses is an agony that cannot be avoided. Whenever possible, a consultation should be suggested for even those problems that are obvious. Every therapeutic measure, however unlikely, must be considered. The family and the patient should be informed participants in the decision-making process to the extent possible. The physician must be in attendance as often and for as long as possible and should be the person, preferably, who informs

the parents that their vigil is ended and that death has come. All this is to lend support and to emphasize that every appropriate effort had been made.

The older child with a lingering or prolonged but recognizably fatal condition presents a particularly complex series of problems for the physician — problems that involve, as always, the patient, the parents, and any siblings. The parents must be told of the disease and of its nature as soon as this becomes well established. If there is doubt, additional opinions must be sought. Parents respond in different ways, and each of these ways is a legitimate effort to cope with this devastating knowledge. They do their best to conceal the facts from the child, but their altered conduct will be apparent and will cause confusion and anxiety. Some physicians contend that the child should be informed about the nature of the illness. They argue that this knowledge enables living out the final period without the reciprocal strain of concealing anxiety from secretive parents. Others oppose this suggestion, claiming that the child, unlike an adult, has no legal need to make any final disposition of personal effects, and that to encumber an already anxious child with the knowledge of a desperate status is cruel and unnecessary. The deception inherent in this approach, of course, lies in the fact that the child has already learned much from all manner of spoken and unspoken messages and might engage in the game of pretense and anxiously avoid the verbalization of fears. The only consequence is loneliness and fear. The adults may be relieved of some distress, but it is a false relief, and candor is most often preferable. Still, it pays to consider each circumstance and to avoid rigid approaches.

In any event, our personal principles of behavior and our own emotional needs will dictate our attitudes. Is acknowledging the truth honesty or brutality? Is concealing the truth compassion or cruelty? Each physician at this point must be advocate and judge. The goal is to establish and to maintain a channel of communication that provides comfort to all involved.

Henry M. Seidel

References

Allmond, B. W., Buckman, W., and Gofnaught, F. *The Family Is the Patient*. St. Louis: Mosby, 1979.

American Academy of Pediatrics. *Adoption of Children* (3rd ed.). Evanston, IL: American Academy of Pediatrics, 1973.

Brazelton, T. B. *What Every Baby Knows*. Reading, MA: Addison Wesley, 1987.

Friedman, S., and Hoekelman, R. *Behavioral Pediatrics*. New York: McGraw-Hill, 1980.

Illingworth, R. S. *The Normal Child* (9th ed.). Edinburgh: Churchill Livingstone, 1986.

Illingworth, R. S. *The Development of the Infant and Young Child: Normal and Abnormal* (9th ed.). Edinburgh: Churchill Livingstone, 1987.

Kanner, L. *Child Psychiatry* (4th ed.). Springfield, IL: Thomas, 1972.

2

Pediatric History and Physical Examination

The physician usually begins the doctor-patient relationship with the act of history-taking and physical examination and through the performance of these tasks becomes uniquely the physician-artist; by employing all faculties the physician builds the awareness that leads to the educated use of the available scientific, medical, and paramedical tools. This awareness is more firmly rooted if there is consistent effort to go beyond the chief complaint to an understanding of the sources of concern that make the chief complaint a particular problem for a given patient — the "iatrotropic stimuli" that give dimension to the most common problems.

The medical student is given instruction in history-taking and physical diagnosis. What follows are suggested modifications for use with the pediatric patient. There is, after all, a change in pace from the usual adult thrust. The pediatrician is expected to be a counselor and a health-care supervisor as well as a caretaker of the sick, assuring that appropriate preventive measures are meticulously implemented and that anticipatory guidance is given at age-appropriate times. Thus, taking advantage of the benefits implicit in continuity of care, it is useful to have a prenatal interview with a family one is meeting for the first time, a chance to get to know each other in anticipation of the birth of the baby.

History

The child's history is usually obtained from a parent, generally the mother. However, a baby or young child may also provide valuable information if one watches or plays with him or her, as will an older child if given the opportunity to talk. The patient's own account of events is often somewhat less tinged by editorializing and, therefore, possibly more accurate.

If, at the beginning of the interview, considerable anxiety is detected in mother or child, it pays to take the time for a comforting statement, a moment of chatting, a moment to hold and soothe the younger child, or to play with the older child. The simple act of offering a toy, picture, or a wooden tongue blade is often an effective step toward establishing rapport. It may at times be wise to allow the mother or child a chance to talk separately, but it may then be best to arrange for such a visit on a subsequent occasion. In any event, rigid adherence to routine is seldom necessary. Each of the principals must be heard, and there should always be time for review and further questions. Much can be learned of the family constellation and the parent-child relationship by simply observing parent(s) and child during the history-taking and physical examination process — the obvious and more subtle ways in which they signal their habitual patterns of interaction.

The physician must document the history, but it is best first to make brief notes and not to allow copious writing to detract from careful listening and observing. Eyes must often meet; questions should not be read. The participants should be seated comfortably and at an easy distance, and conversation should flow without obvious and restrictive adherence to time requirements and without the intervening barriers of desks or other furniture.

The interview begins with the informant as the principal speaker, but it must also include periods in which the physician allows questions and outlines thoughts and plans. No matter should be left unsettled if a satisfactory explanation can be offered at the moment the question is raised. Of course, it may be necessary to wait for clarification on some issues until more data are obtained. Then, parent and child should receive an explanation regarding the necessary steps so any apprehension may at least be eased. They will, of course, have some doubt and anxiety until the problem is resolved. The physician, therefore, should not take offense at a statement that might seem to question ability or judgment. Most often it stems quite simply from fear and uncertainty.

The physician stands before the patient as an educated adult and before the parents as a well-informed contemporary. In talking with them, the physician can gain most by avoiding pretension and by being mature enough to avoid intimidating with knowledge, attitudes, and use of words and by appreciating the need for mutual respect. There can then be marvelous communication that facilitates problem solving and, beyond, that adds to everyone's pleasure.

There are many pertinent points to cover in any history. The following are some that are particularly relevant to the pediatric patient.

Past History

The life experience of a child begins at least at the moment of conception and not with birth. Many factors, maternal and environmental, can affect the fetus during the period of gestation. It is more realistic to consider the infant's age as the chronological age plus the duration of gestation, although this is not usual clinical practice. The younger the child, the more important the information about the period of intrauterine life. Indeed, the past history stretches back into the cultural traditions and experience of the child's family.

PREGNANCY AND IMMEDIATE POSTNATAL PERIOD. The history of pregnancy should include information about nutrition and medications, prenatal care, serological tests, examinations of blood and urine, weight gain, and bleeding. A vague, perhaps ignored, rash in the first trimester, or suggestions that conception may not have been desired, may be the key to a problem.

The history of labor and delivery should include the duration of labor, drugs, complications, whether the delivery was in the hospital or at home, and whether attended by an obstetrician or a midwife. Whenever necessary, the history should be supplemented by hospital records or by a conversation with the attending personnel.

The history of the immediate postnatal period is frequently revealing when a cardiopulmonary or neurological abnormality is present. Information concerning crying and breathing times, Apgar and Dubowicz scores if available, birth weight, and resuscitation may provide the answer. The mother may be unaware of an unusual event, but a clue may be provided by asking how long was it before she actually saw the baby. In recent years, fathers have participated more in the actual birth event, and they should be queried much more than they were in the past.

NEONATAL PERIOD. Information should be obtained on the type of feedings and vitamins; on the presence of cyanosis, jaundice, pallor, or vomiting; and on bowel and urine habits, crying, and jitteriness. One must begin to think of vitamins and drugs, including "street drugs," as possible etiological factors in the production of disease states; details as to the amounts of all medications administered to the infant and mother are, therefore, helpful. For example, aspirin can cross the placenta, but too often it is not thought of as a drug. The patterns of urination, defecation, and crying in the newborn period may be the first indication of certain difficulties, such as urethral obstruction or congenital megacolon. A dehydrated baby with frequently soaked diapers may have obligatory polyuria.

INFANCY AND CHILDHOOD. Detailed evaluation of growth and development is essential. The student is referred to Chapters 3 and 4 for a brief review of this subject.

When reviewing past illnesses, the physician should ask specifically about diseases endemic to the area. Recent exposure to contagious disease should be recorded; knowledge of its possible incubation may provide the correct diagnosis and spare those who are exposed to the patient the risk of developing the disease.

When there is a history of major operations or minor operations such as circumcision, tonsillectomy, and tooth extractions, one should establish whether excessive bleeding occurred. Injuries and accidents, including the ingestion of toxic substances, fractures, and burns, are common during childhood. Education about their prevention can be provided even as the history is being taken.

Persons with a history of allergic disease such as eczema, hay fever, or asthma have a greater chance of developing a serious, even fatal, drug reaction. Before a drug is prescribed, a history of possible sensitivity should always be elicited and recorded.

There must be a complete record of immunizations already given and a plan for the necessary additional ones to bring the child and, indeed, the whole family up to date.

A history of mouth breathing and persistent nasal discharge is suggestive of adenoid hypertrophy. This condition must be expeditiously treated if one is to prevent complications, including deafness. A child who cannot hear well will not learn to speak well. This may be a clue. In reviewing the digestive system, the physician should pay particular attention to a history of pica and to normal nutritional habits. It is not sufficient to ask whether or not the child eats well. The parent should be asked to describe at least one typical day's diet in detail so that clues to nutritional deficiency might be recognized. In areas in which parasitic infestation is common, it is important to ask if the patient has a history of passing worms.

Family and Social History

Social and environmental factors are of utmost importance to the developing child. The questions should be concerned with family income, number of individuals who are considered part of the family unit, source of water supply, toilet facilities, and exposure to animals and pets. It is essential to know about housing conditions and whether the child has an unshared bedroom or, indeed, an unshared bed. Performance in school and adjustment to playmates are important aspects of the school-age child. The point is simple. The life experience of the child must be understood if the child is to receive appropriate health supervision and attention to illness. That experience involves the family, the physical setting, school, and playmates. All must be queried at age-appropriate times.

The family history must also include the age, sex, and health of other members of the immediate family and if there is consanguinity of parents. Other useful information includes chronological data on pregnancies, deaths, and miscarriages and any history of allergy, cancer, inborn errors of metabolism, convulsions, rheumatic heart disease, tuberculosis, and venereal and neurological diseases.

Physical Examination

Physical examination and the taking of the history are so integrated that the physician need not always do one before the other. The seriously ill child may be examined while pertinent history is being obtained. There is considerable medical artistry in the flexibility and integration of the two procedures. The examiner should consider the value of each step, its sensitivity and specificity, and the likelihood that it will give information of value and, with this, possibly exclude observations of little promise that might disturb the child.

One should at all times observe the interactions of child and parent to discover their attitudes toward each other. The examiner should not hesitate to alter the approach to assure a successful examination. The examining table may very often be the parent's lap. In older children one may begin by looking at the patient's hands or feet — a look toward the periphery first is seen as less threatening. This is comforting to the child and gives a first idea about the state of cleanliness. The examiner may play or sing, sit on the floor, feed the child, do anything reasonable to gain information with almost every act. As trust is earned, the physician begins to touch and to feel and to use the examining equipment. The child may be allowed to play with the instruments and thus be encouraged to gain confidence. Sometimes, however, a child continues to cry or to be unresponsive or uncooperative. The examiner's senses, by constant practice, should be sharpened to probe beyond such obstacles, to be able to hear the heart sounds at a moment when the breath is held, to feel the abdomen in transient seconds of relaxation, and always to be alert for a subjective feeling that a deviation from the normal exists, albeit difficult to articulate or define.

The examiner owes the child the thoughtfulness of warming hands and instruments. Respect should be given to modesty. It is not always necessary to remove all the patient's clothes, although it is often essential in the examination of an acutely ill child. Restraint of the patient is rarely necessary and can usually be provided by a reassuring parent. Procedures that may produce discomfort, such as rectal or pharyngeal examination, or provoke fear and anxiety, such as use of the ophthalmoscope, are generally postponed until the end. The tongue blade is often forbidding. If it must be used, its tendency to cause gagging can be alleviated by moistening it with warm water.

In approaching the physical examination, one must be age oriented and accustomed to normal changes in findings at various age levels. As one feels the liver, listens to the heart, and hears the breath sounds, one must always be aware that these are 3-hour, 3-day, or 3-year-old livers, hearts, and lungs — there is a difference.

The blood pressure should be obtained with an appropriate-sized cuff. Too narrow a cuff tends to give a higher reading. A band one-third to one-half the length of the brachium should do. Absence of or weak femoral pulses suggests the diagnosis of coarctation of the aorta.

It is best to record the patient's height, weight, and head and chest circumference on growth charts (see Chap. 3).

Skin and General Appearance

A gentle pinch over the abdomen will reveal the skin turgor. Yellowness of the skin does not necessarily indicate liver disease. If noted about the nares, palms, or soles, it may be the result of ingestion of carrots and other substances that contain carotene; however, if the sclerae are involved, true jaundice is likely. Intense yellowness of the skin suggests the presence of increased quantities of indirect bilirubin; yellow green, an increase in direct bilirubin. The cyanosis of heart disease will not have the same metallic gray blue quality as that of methemoglobinemia. The distribution and sequence of appearance of erythemas are important diagnostic features of many acute infectious diseases. A small telangiectasis will blanch on pressure; a petechial spot will not. A cover glass pressed gently over a telangiectasis will reveal pulsation.

A description of the general body type is important; departures from the normal may indicate skeletal abnormalities or hormonal imbalance. The state of nutrition and the feel of soft tissues and muscles should be noted.

Breath odor can be the first clue to dental caries, pharyngeal infection, foreign body in the nose, and many metabolic disorders. The first three can give a fetid odor and the last, mousy or sickeningly sweet odors.

There must be particular observation of the respiratory movements. The shape of the thorax and deformities of the sternum are clues to congenital abnormality and respiratory competence. The respiratory excursion and its variations need careful inspection; the laggard movement of the chest induced by an agenetic lung, the deep hyperpnea of a metabolic disturbance, and the retraction of the chest wall at various levels due to respiratory obstruction are among the many observations that can be made. In subcutaneous emphysema the palpation of crepitus may be the only clue to the diagnosis. Flaring of the alae nasi suggests pneumonia. The normal respiratory mechanism is impeded in the child who is using the abdominal muscles for respiration. A lack of abdominal fullness can often be the first clue to a diaphragmatic hernia in the newborn infant. A bulge of the precordium is usually indicative of right ventricular hypertrophy.

Palpation

The child need not be supine. Good examination can be obtained with the child on the mother's lap or in the burping position over her shoulder. Better relaxation can be had if the infant is given a bottle or pacifier during the examination. Deep structures can sometimes be better felt if the infant is doubled over the examiner's hand; this is particularly true in the case of pyloric tumor (see Chap. 11).

The liver and spleen may be normally felt in infancy and even in later childhood. Palpation must be gentle and, at first, superficial. There can then be increasing vigor if the situation demands and the child's relaxation allows. If the child is ticklish, the child's hand should guide the examiner's. The stethoscope can also be used as a palpating instrument (see App. A, Sec. 12).

Percussion

Percussion, because of the relative thinness of the chest wall of the young, must be lighter and the finger a more sensitive instrument than with adults. One must be able, if a child is crying, to detect abnormalities without hearing the sound. The "feel" transmitted to the finger is all that is necessary, and it is preferable to feel rather than to "hear." In any event, only light percussion is necessary. Too vigorous a tap destroys cooperation and may mask minor physical signs. A dull percussion note in a small infant has the same significance as the flat note in the adult, that is, it indicates the presence of fluid. Percussion, however, is not usually a productive exercise and should be incorporated in the examination on a selective basis only.

Auscultation

The stethoscope is a multifaceted instrument. It may, as mentioned, even be used for abdominal palpation. The examiner must become familiar with the variations in sound the stethoscope can offer by the simple act of exerting greater or less pressure with the bell on the body surface. When the child is crying, it is important to listen to the respiratory sounds during the inspiratory phase and to the heart during the pause between respirations. The character and quality of the normal breath sounds and heart sounds vary at different ages. This is important because appreciation of minimal variations from the normal can often provide the first clue to heart failure.

Murmurs must be evaluated in terms of quality, intensity, timing in the cardiac cycle, variation with the respiratory cycle, and response to exercise and to changing position.

One must learn to differentiate the venous hum from an organic or a functional murmur. The venous hum will appear and disappear as the patient's head is turned from side to side.

An astute observer will recognize borborygmi in the chest and none in the abdomen in the instance of a diaphragmatic hernia or the variations that may occur with a tracheo-esophageal fistula or peritonitis. Small clues appreciated by the experienced observer can never be replaced by mechanical diagnostic aids and are invaluable in small or remote clinics or in the patient's home.

Head

Measurement of the head size must be routine. The skull of a newborn infant is subject to many variations in shape as a result of molding, the width of the sutures, and the patency of the fontanels. The fontanel should be lightly palpated to assess the degree of tension. Cephalhematoma, meningocele, and encephalocele are immediately discoverable in the newborn. Craniotabes is often normally present in early life and can be demonstrated posterolaterally on both sides. The skull responds with the "give" of a Ping-Pong ball, but, after a few weeks of age, such a response is abnormal. Macewen's cracked-pot sound is discovered in the presence of increased intracranial pressure by tapping the skull lightly.

The facies may be characteristic in diseases such as Down syndrome, the mucopolysaccharidoses, hypercalcemia, and mandibulofacial dysostosis (Treacher-Collins syndrome) as well as in many of the more recently recognized chromosomal disorders. The symmetry of the face and the smile are neurological clues. Mouth breathing may indicate nasal obstruction. The cheeks in the neonate can be palpated for the fat necrotic lumps produced by forceps.

Ears

The set of the ears should be noted. A low position below the eyes and with a forward sweep may suggest syndromes involving brain defect or congenital kidney abnormality. Is there a brachial cleft cyst? Does the child hear? Hearing can be tested crudely by clapping the hands behind the child and watching for a blink or startle response. The physician should talk to the older child, listen to the quality of the speech, and evaluate the ability to respond to instructions. Many factors may control these skills, but defective hearing must not be missed and, at any age, if it is suspected, must be pursued with more sophisticated diagnostic techniques. If cerumen obstructs visualization of the tympanic membrane, it can be cleaned out with warm water and a syringe or a

Water-Pik. A curet is to be avoided; it may cause bleeding, pain, and alienation and their obvious consequences.

Eyes

Epicanthal folds are frequently present in infancy. These may give the illusion of extraocular muscle imbalance. The fact that the reflection of a distant light source falls in the same spot on both pupils can refute this. Drawing the folds back by pinching them together over the bridge of the nose can also destroy the illusion. These are easy and mandatory tests in every young child if amblyopia ex anopsia is to be avoided.

Skill in ophthalmoscopical examination is possible with children of every age. This examination is best done in the very young when they are drowsy, a bit hungry, and sucking on the bottle. A darkened room is unnecessary. Drugs that dilate the pupils should not be used until observations of the neurological examination have been validated. A crying baby squeezes the eyes shut. If the mother picks up and nestles the baby over her shoulder, the eyes will open, for at least a moment. The examiner must not miss this opportunity to look for the red reflex. It may be distorted in the presence of cataracts and some relatively rare conditions such as retinoblastoma and *Toxocara* infections.

Nose

The child with adenoid hypertrophy usually keeps the mouth open constantly. There may also be characteristic facies and other findings to suggest this condition. The "adenoid salute" is typically seen as the child sweeps the hand upward over the nose in a vain effort to unplug it. The alae nasi will flare on respiration in the compensatory respiratory effort of a child with pneumonia, but not often with other respiratory distress. A foreign body long present in the nose will cause a unilateral discharge with an odor that pervades the room. The most common place to look for the source of a nosebleed is Kiesselbach's triangle. The frontal and maxillary sinuses should be tapped lightly to discover the tenderness of sinusitis. They may be explored further by transillumination and by inspection of the turbinates for swelling. One should not assume that a child may be too young to have fully developed sinuses.

Lips

The examiner should check for weaknesses and the ability to suck. Is there pallor or cyanosis, or are the lips cherry red? Lips should be checked for cleft, herpes, chapping, fissures, rhagades, scars, perleche, and cheilosis.

Mouth

Breath odor, the shape and possible distortions of the palate, and the contour of the jaw are noted. The high-arched palate, often neglected, can alert the examiner to the possibility of mental retardation. The presence or absence of cleft palate must be routinely checked in the newborn infant.

Mucous Membranes

Koplik's spots on the buccal membranes are the time-honored herald of rubeola. Bednar's aphthae, pallor, ulcers, and hemorrhagic phenomena are also important findings. The orifice to the parotid duct is reddened and hypertrophied in the presence of mumps, and a drop of purulent discharge expressed from the duct may solve the problem of unexplained parotid swelling in suppurative parotitis.

Lymph Nodes

Lymph nodes in the cervical, postauricular, occipital, axillary, inguinal, and epitrochlear areas must be felt. It is important to know that childhood represents the period of lymphatic hypertrophy. Glands palpable in an adult that might suggest the presence of a malignant process may in the child suggest only a response to infection and, at the latency age, "normal" hypertrophy.

Muscles

Competence of muscles should be evaluated. The child is simply asked to stand or climb and the manner noted in which these basic movements are accomplished.

Extremities

Toes and fingers are checked for clubbing and cyanosis or pallor. Are the nails disfigured or friable? Are the interphalangeal spaces cracked or eroded? These are ready portals for infection.

Bones and joints are a frequent site of infection or inflammation. In a child with fever, the physician carefully searches for points of local tenderness over bones (osteomyelitis), watches for signs that the child is protecting an inflamed joint by maintaining a fixed position, and manipulates the joints to elicit pain on motion — always gently. There is never a need for brusk handling in the pediatric examination.

Neurological Examination

In the young child, most information is obtained by observing patterns of spontaneous movement and behavior and response to simple stimuli (following a light, startle to a clap of the hands, withdrawal from a gentle pinprick). Certain reflex patterns, like tonic neck reflexes, which are normal in young infants, are signs of abnormality at a later age. The stiff neck, so characteristic of meningeal irritation, is often lacking in the infant with meningitis, but a bulging fontanel may provide the clue. A somewhat older child, fontanel closed, may resist flexion of the neck — pseudomeningismus caused by fear, pleurisy, pneumonia, or adenitis — but will even eagerly bend the head in pursuit of a tongue blade or a finger the examiner has offered for biting. Nerve and muscle function, sensation, reflexes, coordination, and muscle tone should be formally tested, but only after careful observation of the child as a whole.

Rectal Examination

Rectal examination should not be avoided. The physician must use judgment in deciding its need but should never forgo it if abdominal mass or tenderness, bladder distention, or rectal or bowel abnormalities are suspected. It must never be assumed that a newborn infant has a patent anus unless there has been proper passage of meconium.

Genitalia

In the male, the position of the urethral meatus should be noted. An abnormal urinary stream, particularly dribbling, may indicate urethral stricture. Palpation of the testes is important in early detection of an atrophic or undescended testicle. When the child is somewhat older this may best be determined by palpation with the child sitting in the tailor's cross-legged position. Transillumination will reveal the presence of a hydrocele.

In the female, the presence of clitoral hypertrophy, adhesions, or discharge should be noted. There may frequently be hymenal hypertrophy in the newborn and also some vaginal bleeding for a few days as a result of passive hormonal transfer from the mother. Simple labial adhesions are not abnormal, and separation can be easily accomplished. Most important, the pelvic examination of the adolescent is too often eliminated, thus denying to the patient appropriate care and assurance.

The newborn male or female may have lactating breasts; the milk thus secreted is known as witch's milk. Occasionally adolescent boys may temporarily have tender unilateral or bilateral breast development behind the nipple. Great reassurance is required to both sexes — to girls, that unilateral development will eventually be bilateral and symmetrical, and to boys, that breast development will fade away.

The physician should take the opportunity to hold a young baby, to offer a feeding if possible, and to thus increase understanding. It is best not to try to do everything in a single sequence unless the circumstance of the moment mandates it. One can come back to the child at the right moment to supplement the findings.

It is helpful to maintain a front sheet in the child's record containing a condensation of significant information, a historical profile, and a listing of ongoing problems. The value is obvious when various school, camp, and organizational forms must be completed. Essential facts of family and birth history, common diseases and dates, immunizations and tests (i.e., tuberculosis, urine, blood, x ray, vision, hearing), operative procedures, injuries, and miscellaneous items pro-

vide a compact physical profile. Behavioral notes, if added, increase the value of this document. This must also be supplemented with a growth chart on which serial measurements of head circumference in the first year of life and height and weight are plotted.

Henry M. Seidel

References

Judge, R. D., Zuidema, G. D., and Fitzgerald, F. T. *Clinical Diagnosis: A Physiologic Approach* (5th ed.). Boston: Little, Brown, 1989.

Seidel, H. M., Ball, J. W., Dains, J. E., and Benedect, G. W. *Mosby's Guide to Physical Examination*. St. Louis: Mosby, 1987.

Ziai, M. (Ed.). *Bedside Pediatrics: Diagnostic Evaluation of the Child*. Boston: Little, Brown, 1983.

3

Physical Growth
and Development

The term *normal* in relation to growth and development and other measurements, including biochemical data, is incorrectly used. The correct term is *average*. There is a vast difference between the normal and the average. A child may be kilograms (or pounds) below the average in weight, and centimeters (or inches) below the average in height, or weeks later than most children in reaching a milestone of development, and yet may be normal. On the basis of statistical data one may define as normal those biological values that fall within two standard deviations from the mean in either direction. The further a child's development differs from the average, the less likely it is to be normal. It follows that in the study of normal children it is essential to know the average, and the variations from the average that occur without disease — and to try to understand some of the reasons for those variations.

In dealing with biological systems, such as those that determine the rates of growth and development, it is impor-

tant to keep in mind the concept of biological variation. The normal variation can be demonstrated by recording the physical measurements of a large group of apparently normal children who are of exactly the same age. It becomes immediately obvious that there is a wide variation in their heights. If one plots the number of children against their heights on a chart, one obtains a bell-shaped curve (Fig. 3-1). The majority of the children will be found somewhere near the middle of this curve, with its peak representing the mean or fiftieth centile. The farther one gets from the mean in either direction, the fewer children will be found, and the more likely they are to be abnormal. Nevertheless, one can never draw a strict dividing line between normal and abnormal, and it would be wrong to say that because a child's weight or height is in the ninety-fourth centile, the child is necessarily abnormal. (See Fig. 3-4 [growth charts] at the end of this chapter.)

Prenatal Growth

The mean birth weight in the United States is 3405 g (7½ pounds). (For the development of the embryo, see Chap.

Some of the data used in this chapter are derived from *Growth and Development of Children* (7th ed.), by E. H. Watson and G. H. Lowrey. Copyright © 1978 by Year Book Medical Publishers, Chicago.

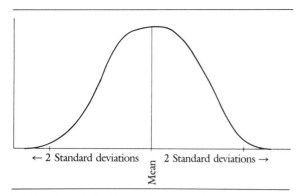

← 2 Standard deviations | 2 Standard deviations →

Mean

Fig. 3-1. Normal distribution of height according to age.

5.) The factors that affect the birth weight are mainly the following:

1. The duration of gestation. The mean birth weight at four periods in the third trimester of gestation is:

WEEK OF GESTATION	MEAN WEIGHT(G)
28	1045 (2 lb 4 oz)
32	1680 (3 lb 8 oz)
36	2478 (5 lb 3 oz)
40	3405 (7 lb 8 oz)

These figures are important because they help to distinguish the preterm from the low-birth-weight baby. The accepted definition of a preterm baby is one who is born before 37 weeks' gestation, and that of a low-birth-weight baby is one who weighs 2500 g (5½ pounds) or less at birth irrespective of the duration of gestation; it is now recognized that the infant who is small in relation to the duration of gestation ("small for dates") is more likely to have mental subnormality or cerebral palsy than the truly preterm baby. Owing to placental insufficiency, there is not usually much weight gain after 40 weeks of gestation.
2. Poverty and malnutrition are associated with both low birth weight and preterm delivery. Malnutrition in the third trimester often results in low birth weight. The mother's weight gain in pregnancy is related to the fetal weight. The mean birth weight of infants in a country is a useful index of that country's nutritional status. In Eastern countries, with poor nutrition, the mean birth weight may be 3000 g (6½ lb) or less.
3. Maternal toxemia and placental insufficiency, commonly associated with low birth weight.
4. Excessive smoking by the mother. The mean birth weight of infants of smokers is less than that of infants of non-smokers.
5. Multiple pregnancy. The mean birth weight of each twin is 2400 g (5 lb 4 oz), of each triplet 1800 g (4 lb), and of each quadruplet 1400 g (3 lb 2 oz).
6. Diabetes (or prediabetes), commonly associated with an unusually large birth weight. Postmature babies are not usually large, because of placental insufficiency.
7. Genetic and chromosome disorders, infections in pregnancy, and unknown factors.

Loss of Weight at Birth

Babies commonly lose 5 to 10% of their body weight in the first 24 to 48 hours. This change in weight is due to loss of water (see Chap. 8). Full-term babies usually regain their birth weight within 10 to 14 days.

PHYSICAL GROWTH AFTER BIRTH. For practical purposes there are two measurements that are essential for assessing body growth — weight and height. The head circumference is important as a guide to assessing mental development. The charts shown on pages 28 to 32 are based on a longitudinal growth study of a number of healthy children.

The adequacy of growth is best shown on the centile chart by serial rather than single measurements. A falling off in the weight gain on the centile chart demands urgent investigation. Disease is unlikely when the weight gain shows a steady increase, retaining its position on the centile chart, though below the average. The most likely explanation of this is a low birth weight or a familial small body build.

It is important to remember that it is easy and common to make mistakes on measuring weight, height, or head circumference. Weighing scales may be faulty, and tape measures of cloth material may stretch and give a wrong measurement.

Changes in Body Proportions

Body growth is not uniform at different ages. The head is considerably larger in relation to other body measurements during infancy. This proportion gradually changes and finally assumes the adult ratio (Fig. 3-2).

The younger the child, the shorter are the extremities in proportion to total height. The measurement is best achieved by comparing sitting height (trunk and head) with total height. The relationship of these two figures is a useful index in the diagnosis of certain conditions that affect growth. In a child with hypothyroidism, for example, body

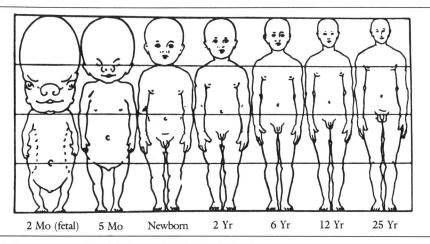

Fig. 3-2. Changes in form and proportion of the human body during fetal and postnatal life.

proportions remain infantile, whereas a hypopituitary dwarf with the same total height is expected to have body proportions corresponding to chronological age.

Figure 3-3 compares the general body growth (general type) with genital, neural, and lymphoid growth at different ages. There are two periods of rapid growth — during infancy and during adolescence. The period of rapid genital growth occurs during adolescence. Neural growth continues fairly rapidly during the first few years of life but then approaches a plateau. Lymphoid growth, shown, for instance, by the size of the tonsils, is rapid during infancy and childhood but quickly drops to adult proportions during adolescence.

The following are the average weight gains in 3-month periods after birth (with prenatal weight gains for comparison):

AGE (MONTHS)	WEIGHT GAIN PER WEEK (g)
Prenatal	
5–8	110 (4 oz)
9	340 (12 oz)
Postnatal	
0–3	200 (7 oz)
4–6	140 (5 oz)
7–9	85 (3 oz)
10–12	70 (2½ oz)

The most rapid weight gain is in the ninth month in utero; thereafter the weight gain is less. The postnatal figures are

Fig. 3-3. Main types of postnatal growth of the various parts and organs of the body. (After R. E. Scammon, The Measurement of the Body in Childhood, *In J. A. Harris,* Measurement of Man. *Minneapolis: University of Minnesota Press, 1930.)*

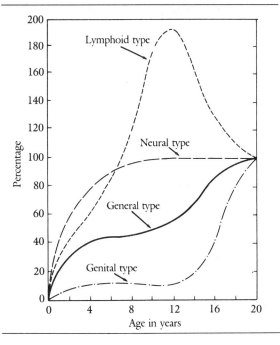

important, for mothers commonly worry about the slowing of the child's weight gain (especially at 6 to 12 months of age) with associated falling off in appetite. It is worthwhile to explain the usual growth curve to these mothers, telling them that if a child had to continue gaining 200 g (7 oz) a week, he would weigh 146 g (322 lb) by the age of 14 years. As a child's weight and height are closely related to the birth weight, it is clearly wrong to state that a child's weight should double or treble by a certain age.

No one can be expected to remember the average weight at each age. The figures listed here are the approximate expected weight of a child at a certain age.

AGE (YEAR)	WEIGHT (LB)
1	20
3	30
5	40
7	50

The average annual increase in height from 2 to 5 years is 7.6 cm (3 in.); from 5 to 10 years, 6.3 cm (2½ in.); at puberty the maximum annual increase is 8.9 to 10.1 cm (3½ to 4 in.).

After about the age of 10, height and weight charts are of little value because of the varying age of puberty. In this age period figures should be related more to the maturity of the child than to chronological age.

Factors Affecting Physical Growth

The following factors affecting physical growth must be remembered:

1. Genetic factors. Whenever a child is smaller than usual in weight and height, it is important to ascertain the weight and height of both parents. Many children are thought to have malnutrition or some disease when in fact they are perfectly well but following an inherited growth pattern.
2. Growth potential. To some extent, the growth potential is shown by the infant's size at birth, particularly in relation to the duration of gestation. The smaller the child at birth (particularly in relation to gestation), the smaller the child is likely to be in later years; the larger at birth, the larger the child is likely to be later.
3. Nutrition. Growth in weight and to a lesser extent in height is reduced by defective food intake, by increased loss of nutrients (vomiting or diarrhea), or by malab-

sorption. Unsatisfactory socioeconomic factors are a major cause of a child's weight being below the average without known disease.
4. Metabolic disorders. Renal acidosis and glycogen storage disease are examples of metabolic disorders that retard growth.
5. Chronic infections. Growth is slowed by chronic infections.
6. Severe chronic disease of the heart (e.g., congenital heart disease), chest (asthma, bronchiectasis), liver (cirrhosis), kidneys (renal insufficiency), or pancreas (diabetes mellitus, cystic fibrosis). These diseases retard growth.
7. Endocrine disorders. Growth is regulated by complex mechanisms, such as growth hormone, somatotropin, and somatomedin. Hypopituitarism is a rare cause of dwarfism. Thyroid deficiency retards the growth in height. Adrenocortical overactivity usually leads to excessive height in early childhood; height is eventually less than average, however, because of premature closure of the epiphyses.
8. Mental deficiency. This is often associated with defective physical growth, which may be extreme.
9. Unknown factors (and rare forms of dwarfism). It is essential to remember that growth is affected by an interrelation of many factors and that there are wide variations in health from the average. It is far more important that a child should be full of energy, free from lassitude, and abounding in joie de vivre than average in weight and height.

The Underweight Child

If the child is well and free from symptoms, the usual factor responsible for small size is a genetic one — the child taking after one parent or both — or low birth weight — especially if the infant was small for dates — or malnutrition. It could be the result of previous illness, now cured. If a child's growth is defective in the first 2 or 3 years as a result of malnutrition or disease, and the cause is corrected, the child is likely to catch up to the average (catch-up growth). Temporary cessation of weight gain, due to an infection for instance, is compensated by an increase of appetite on recovery from the illness, so that the weight recovers its position on the centile charts. If the cause, however, such as malabsorption or a major surgical problem, cannot be corrected until after the age of 2 or 3, the child is likely to remain small in later years. The malnutrition may be due to poverty, but it could also be a form of child abuse. The problem of failure to thrive is one seen by all pediatricians. A convenient classification of the causes is as follows:

Defective intake of food

Defective absorption of fat, carbohydrates, or protein (Hirschsprung's disease)

Increased loss of nutrients (diarrhea, vomiting)

Chronic infection (tuberculosis, malaria, ancylostomiasis)

Organ disease: severe disease of the brain (mental deficiency), heart (congenital heart disease), chest (asthma, bronchiectasis), liver (cirrhosis), kidney (renal insufficiency), pancreas (diabetes, fibrocystic disease)

Metabolic diseases associated with polyuria and constipation (renal tubular acidosis, hypercalcemia, nephrogenic diabetes insipidus)

It follows that investigation is difficult and complex, but when faced with a child with failure to thrive, the first essential is to make sure that it is not due merely to underfeeding or adverse socioeconomic circumstances.

The Overweight Child

The causes of obesity (see also App. A, Sec. 24) are complex and not fully understood, but basically the cause of obesity is intake of more food than is needed. Many children and adults have an enormous appetite but do not become fat; many become or remain fat with a small intake. Underactivity is a risk factor; children who are handicapped by severe hypotonia, the spastic type of cerebral palsy, or meningomyelocele readily become fat with a small calorie intake because they need less food than normally active children. There are many other factors, however, including metabolism by brown fat and hypothalamic and other endocrine factors; frequently there are genetic factors.

Much overeating is related to emotional causes, such as sibling rivalry, and habit. Jealousy and sibling rivalry can cause a child to eat more than he or she really wants, because of the example set by a sibling; and children are encouraged to develop the habit of eating sweets and frequent snacks, following the example set by their parents.

Fat children are almost always tall for their age. Fat boys often appear to have a small penis, but this is mainly because the penis is obscured by fat. Gynecomastia and striae are often found in older fat boys, often before puberty. Puberty tends to be early rather than late. Pituitary dysfunction (e.g., as in Fröhlich's syndrome or adipososkeletogenital dystrophy) is very rare; there is polyuria and altered glucose metabolism.

If a child is small and fat, certain diseases should be considered, i.e., Prader-Willi syndrome, Cushing's syndrome, Turner's syndrome, hypothyroidism, and pituitary disease; the effect of prolonged corticosteroid treatment should also be considered.

Smallness of Stature

Relevant factors are heredity, especially the size of parents and siblings, and social class (the height of children in lower social classes, especially if there is malnutrition, tends to be less than that of children in better social circumstances). A low birth weight, especially if the child were small for dates, is a significant cause of small stature (see also Sec. A-4). The causes of short stature include small for gestational age, chronic infection (e.g., malaria, ancylostomiasis), skeletal abnormality (e.g., achondroplasia, Morquio's disease, vitamin D–resistant rickets), organ disease (heart, chest, liver, kidney, pancreas), endocrine disease (thyroid, pituitary, adrenal), Prader-Willi syndrome, Turner's syndrome, mucopolysaccharidoses, and prolonged corticosteroid treatment. A mother may be comforted by the thought that it is not true that the bigger a baby or child is, the better it is.

Excessive Height

The most common causes of excessive height are genetic. Rare syndromes in which excessive height is present include cerebral gigantism (tallness, odd facies, prognathism, antimongoloid slant of the eyes, mental subnormality), the extra Y chromosome, Marfan's syndrome, homocystinuria, and eosinophilic adenoma of the pituitary. Children with obesity, sexual precocity, or adrenocortical hyperplasia are usually tall for their age, but premature closure of the epiphyses results in early cessation of growth.

Relationship of Height in Childhood to Adult Height

It is of some importance to know the relationship of height at various ages to the expected adult height. This is shown in Table 3-1. When a mother is worried about the unusually low weight and height of her child, it is helpful to calculate the expected adult height. When, as is often the case, this is precisely the same as the height of the (diminutive) mother, worries are likely to disappear. It is important to remove such worries, because they may lead to the forcing of food and so to food refusal and a poor appetite.

Head Circumference

The measurement of the maximum head circumference is a routine part of the examination of any infant. It is important because head size reflects the growth of the brain, and if the brain does not develop normally, as in mental subnormality, the head is likely to be small. If a child develops normally for the first few months and then becomes mentally defective,

Table 3-1. Mean Percentages of Mature Height Reached

| Chronological age (yr) | Mean percentage of mature height reached | |
	Boys	Girls
1	42.2	44.7
3	53.5	57.2
5	61.6	66.2
7	69.1	74.3
9	75.6	81.2
11	81.3	88.7
13	87.3	96.0

Source: Data from N. Bayley, and S. R. Pinneau, Tables for predicting adult height from skeletal age: Revised for use with Greulich-Pyle hand standards. *J. Pediatr.* 40:423, 1952.

*Table 3-2. Correction Factors to Determine Head Circumference**

| Age | Girls | | Boys | |
	in.	cm	in.	cm
Birth	1/3	0.8	1/4	0.6
6 weeks	1/4	0.6	1/4	0.6
6 months	1/8	0.3	1/8	0.3
10 months	1/10	0.3	1/10	0.3

*Amount to be added or subtracted for each pound above or below the average weight.

the head measurements are less likely to be abnormal. The reason is that by the sixth month the brain has reached 50% of adult size; by 1 year, 60%; and by 2 years, 75%.

In all cases, head circumference must be related to the size of the baby, for a small baby is likely to have a smaller head than a large baby, and vice versa. A simple correction for each pound above or below the average weight allows one to determine the expected head size (Table 3-2). The head may be smaller than normal because the baby is small, or smallness of the head may be a familial feature; in other words, it is just a normal variation. The usual cause of microcephaly (which merely means small head) is mental subnormality; a rare cause is craniostenosis. An unusually

large head may be merely a normal variant: it may be because the baby is large, or the largeness of the head may be a familial feature. It can be due to a subdural effusion, hydrocephalus, megalencephaly or hydranencephaly, or a cerebral tumor, or certain rare syndromes. It must be borne in mind that in a preterm baby the head is relatively larger than in a full-term baby. The following are average head circumferences for preterm babies:

WEEK OF GESTATION	HEAD CIRCUMFERENCE (CM)
28	25 (10 in.)
32	29 (11½ in.)
36	32 (12¾ in.)
Full term	33–35.5 (13–14 in.)

It may be useful to relate the head circumference to the birth weight.

BIRTH WEIGHT (g)	HEAD CIRCUMFERENCE (CM)
501–1000	23.3 (9¼ in.)
1001–1500	26.6 (10½ in.)
1501–2000	30.0 (11¾ in.)
2001–2500	32.0 (12½ in.)
2501–3000	33.7 (13¼ in.)
3001–3500	34.7 (13¾ in.)
3501–4000	35.4 (14 in.)
4001 +	36.2 (14¼ in.)

During the first year the head grows approximately 10 cm (4 in.); during the second year, the head grows approximately 2.5 cm (1 in.) in circumference (Table 3-3).

It is important in assessing head circumference to relate it to the size of the mother's and father's heads and to the infant's weight. It is also important to feel the fontanels for undue bulging and the degree of separation of the sutures; serial measurements should be determined to assure normal growth rates. A growth curve that changes in relation to the next centile is more significant than one that remains parallel to the centile. Changes in the physical growth of the infant will be reflected in the head circumference.

When there is malnutrition, the head is relatively large. Normally the circumference of the head is greater than that of the chest until the age of 6 months, but less than that of the chest thereafter.

Table 3-3. Head Circumference
of Children in the United States

Age (mo)	Inches			Centimeters		
	10th Percentile	Mean	90th Percentile	10th Percentile	Mean	90th Percentile
Birth	12.9	13.8	14.7	32.7	35.0	37.3
1	14.0	14.9	15.8	35.3	37.6	39.9
2	14.6	15.5	16.4	37.4	39.7	42.0
3	15.0	15.9	16.8	38.1	40.4	42.7
6	16.3	17.0	17.8	41.3	43.4	45.5
9	16.9	17.8	18.7	42.7	45.0	47.3
12	17.4	18.3	19.2	44.2	46.5	48.8
18	18.1	19.0	19.9	46.1	48.4	50.7
24	18.3	19.2	20.1	46.7	49.0	51.3

Source: Calculated from E. H. Watson and G. H. Lowrey, *Growth and Development of Children* (7th ed.). Copyright © 1978 by Year Book Medical Publishers, Chicago. Used by permission.

The anterior fontanel closes in 90% of boys and 70% of girls by the age of 18 months. It may be closed in rare normal infants by the age of 6 months, however, or open in normal infants at the age of 2 years or even later. These variations are often genetic.

Teeth

Teething cannot be used as a milestone of development. The average age at which the first tooth appears is 6 months, and one tooth commonly appears in each of the next few months (number of teeth = age in months −6). The first permanent teeth, the 6-year molars, are sometimes mistaken for deciduous teeth. This is a serious error, as these teeth represent the foundation of permanent dentition.

About 1 in 1500 children is born with an erupted tooth. In some normal children the first tooth may not appear until the age of 15 months or even later. True anodontia is extremely rare. The age at which teeth appear is commonly related to racial or familial factors.

Normal Changes at Puberty

The average age at which the adolescent spurt growth occurs is 12½ to 15 years in boys and 10½ to 13 years in girls.

The average age of the menarche is 13 years. Growth in height commonly ceases at 18 in boys and at 16 to 17 in girls.

The usual order of changes in girls is as follows: rapid increase in weight and height; breast changes — pigmentation of the areola, enlargement of the nipple, enlargement of the breast tissue; increase in pelvic girth; growth of pubic hair; activity of axillary sweat glands; appearance of axillary hair; menstruation, which commonly starts 2 years after first sign of puberty; and abrupt slowing of increase in height.

The usual order of changes in boys is as follows: rapid increase in weight and height; enlargement of the penis and testicles; appearance of pubic hair followed by axillary hair, hair on the upper lip, and later on the groin, thigh, and between pubis and umbilicus (facial hair commonly appears about 2 years after the appearance of pubic hair); changes in the larynx and, therefore, in the voice; nocturnal emissions of seminal fluid; and abrupt slowing of the increase in height.

In general, children of small build tend to reach puberty later than those of large build. Contrary to popular belief, the onset of puberty is not usually delayed in fat boys; in fat boys and girls it tends to be average or earlier than average in onset. The age of onset of puberty is thought to be strongly influenced by genetic factors, so that when a child reaches puberty earlier than usual, one must inquire about the family history of the age of puberty. To some extent, poor nutrition retards the age of onset of puberty.

Precocious or early puberty in girls is usually benign or "constitutional," although it may be due to disease of the hypothalamus, adrenal glands, or ovaries. In boys, very early puberty is more often due to disease of the hypothalamus, adrenal glands, or testes.

Growth Charts

Growth charts (Figs. 3-4A–H) are normally used to compare an individual with average. Various parameters of physical development are measured and plotted on the charts. (Different charts are used for each sex and age range.) Several growth charts are reproduced here, each showing the distribution pattern of parameters such as height, weight, and head circumference.

Ronald S. Illingworth and Mohsen Ziai

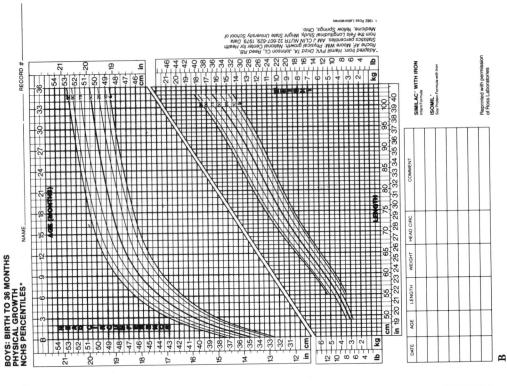

BOYS: BIRTH TO 36 MONTHS PHYSICAL GROWTH NCHS PERCENTILES*

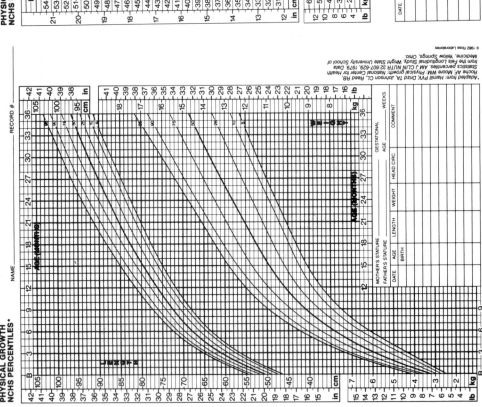

BOYS: BIRTH TO 36 MONTHS PHYSICAL GROWTH NCHS PERCENTILES*

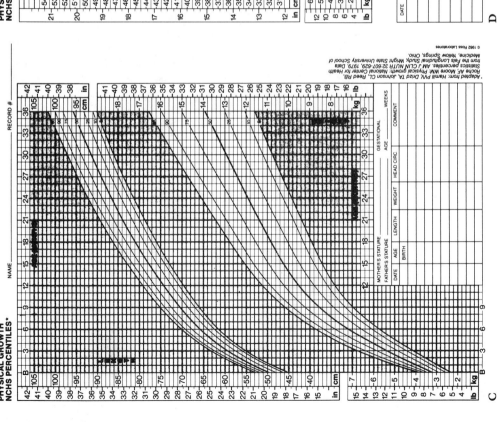

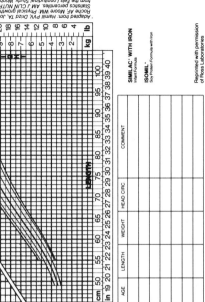

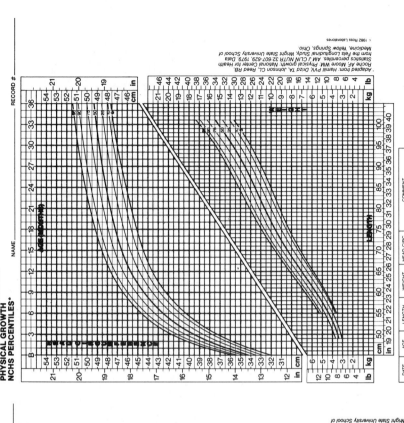

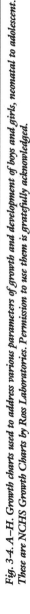

Fig. 3-4. A–H. Growth charts used to address various parameters of growth and development of boys and girls, neonatal to adolescent. These are NCHS Growth Charts by Ross Laboratories. Permission to use them is gratefully acknowledged.

30

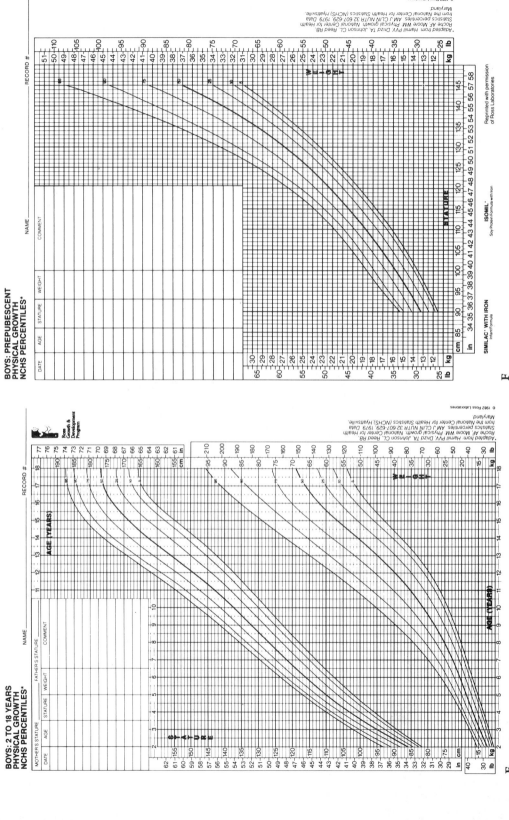

BOYS: PREPUBESCENT
PHYSICAL GROWTH
NCHS PERCENTILES*

BOYS: 2 TO 18 YEARS
PHYSICAL GROWTH
NCHS PERCENTILES*

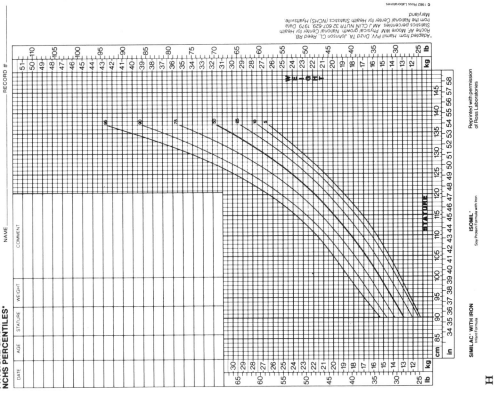

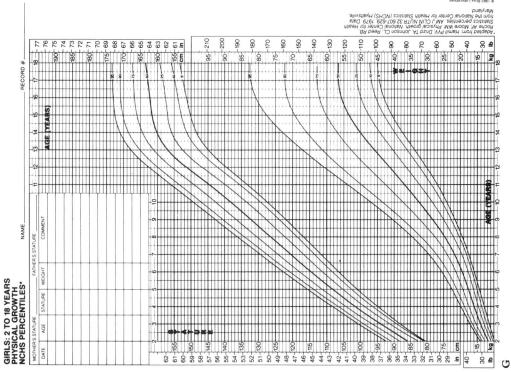

Fig. 3-4. (Continued)

31

References

Falkner, F., and Tanner, J. M. *Human Growth* (2nd ed). New York: Plenum, 1986. (3 Vols.).

Illingworth, R. S. *The Normal Child* (9th ed.) London: Churchill Livingstone, 1987.

Lowrey, G. H. *Growth and Development of Children* (7th ed.). Chicago: Year Book, 1978.

Nellhaus, G. Head circumference from birth to 18 years. *Pediatrics* 41:106, 1968.

Usher, R., and McLean, F. Intrauterine growth of live born Caucasian infants at sea level. *J. Pediatr.* 74:901, 1969.

4

Mental Development

The term *development* is used to describe the spontaneous acquisition of increasingly complex patterns of activity and behavior on the part of the growing child. A child's level of physical or mental development at any age is the end result of complex interaction of prenatal, perinatal, and postnatal factors. Important prenatal factors are genetic (including chromosome defects, hereditary diseases), placental problems (such as maternal toxemia, hypertension, antepartum hemorrhage, intrauterine growth retardation), infections in pregnancy (including rubella and AIDS), and drugs (medicines, drugs of addiction, tobacco or alcohol). Perinatal factors include difficulties in labour or delivery, hypoxia, and trauma. Postnatal factors include socioeconomic problems, the child's health, nutrition, illnesses (especially pyogenic meningitis), personality, the quality of the home, school, friends, neighbourhood, and opportunities.

Evaluation of the child's physical and mental development is an integral part of the work of the pediatrician and others concerned with child welfare. In order to assess development, one must be thoroughly conversant with the average and the normal, normal variations not amounting to disease, and the reasons for those variations.

The following are the main principles of development:

1. Development depends on maturation of the nervous system. No amount of training will enable a child to pass a milestone of development until the nervous system is ready for it; however, lack of opportunity to practice skills can certainly retard the child's development.
2. Development is continuous from conception to maturity, but there may be lulls in development, particularly in speech, when other skills are being learned. The child appears to make no headway at all in one area of development and then suddenly progresses rapidly and makes up lost ground.
3. The direction of development is from the head downward. For instance, the child can do much with the hands before being able to walk.
4. The order of development is the same in all children. For instance, all babies learn to sit before they walk (though some omit the creeping stage), but the rate of development varies from child to child.
5. All children are different. It is never possible to define the exact range of normality; but, the further away a child's

physical or mental development is from the average, the less likely is the child to be "normal." Almost all children vary from the average in some fields of development without being "abnormal."

The principal patterns of development are:

1. Average throughout in all fields (rare)
2. Average, then becoming superior (may be due to slow maturation or may sometimes be explained by the inadequacy of the developmental tests)
3. Advanced in certain fields
4. Advanced in all fields (mental superiority)
5. Average or advanced, then deteriorating
6. Retarded in individual fields
7. Uniformly retarded throughout (mental subnormality)
8. Uniformly retarded, becoming average or superior (delayed maturation, "slow starter"). A mentally subnormal child is retarded in all aspects of development, except occasionally sitting and walking. Advanced motor development does not suggest mental superiority.

The range of intelligence in children is as follows:

IQ	PERCENTAGE
150 or over	0.1
130–149	1.0
120–129	5.0
110–119	14
100–109	30
90–99	30
80–89	14
70–79	5
Below 70	1

Normal Development

The infant's development depends on the maturation of the nervous system. The significance of maturation is clearly shown by the neurological examination of preterm babies at different periods of gestation, compared with that of babies born at term. A baby born prematurely has inevitably missed development in utero; hence, when a baby is born, for example, 3 months early, the infant has missed 3 months' development, and when assessing the baby after birth, full allowance must be made for it. For instance, while a full-term baby usually begins to smile at his mother in response to her overtures by about 6 weeks, the baby born 3 months early would be expected to begin to smile at 6 weeks plus 3

months. Failure to make this allowance for preterm delivery and for development missed in utero inevitably leads to serious errors in developmental assessment.

The newborn baby shows a wide variety of primitive reflexes, such as the asymmetrical tonic neck reflex and the grasp, walking, and Moro responses. There are also many other primitive reflexes that are more of academic interest than of practical use.

At 3 or 4 weeks of age, the infant begins to fix the eyes on the mother as she talks, soon begins to smile, then to vocalize, and later to laugh.

The newborn baby in the sitting position rolls into a ball. The baby soon begins to lift the head up, and to straighten the back, and at 6 months can sit with the hands forward for support, and at 8 months can sit securely. The infant then begins to crawl, to creep, to walk holding on to furniture, and at about 13 months to walk without support. It is not until 3 years of age that the child can stand on one foot.

The newborn baby has a grasp reflex, causing the fingers to close on an object placed in the hand. At about 3 months, he can hold to an object placed in his hand, but cannot pick it up if he drops it. At about 5 months the infant can reach out for an object and get it but cannot pick up a pellet between the tip of the forefinger and the thumb until 10 months. Shortly after this the baby begins throwing one object after another onto the floor. Not until 3 years can the child build a tower of nine to ten 1-inch blocks. From 5 or 6 months, everything the baby gets hold of goes to the mouth; but with maturity in the use of the hands, the mouthing of objects ceases (at 12 or 13 months), a good sign of maturity. In mentally defective children, mouthing continues much longer. At 15 months the child can pick up a cup, drink from it, and put it down without help and eat without assistance. The child can manage buttons at the age of 2 or 3 years and, if given a chance, can dress fully without help (apart from shoelaces) at 3 or 4 years of age. (Children begin to help the mother to dress them at about 10 months, by holding out the arm for a sleeve, and the foot for a shoe.)

The first stage in the acquisition of speech is vocalization, beginning at about 5 or 6 weeks, when the mother talks to the infant. Thereafter the infant goes through a series of well-defined stages (ah-goo, ba, da, and ka, followed by combinations of syllables — baba, dada, mama); by the age of 11 or 12 months the child begins to say words with meaning and by 21 to 24 months combines them into short sentences.

The first stage in the acquisition of sphincter control is at 15 to 18 months of age when children tell their mother that they have wet their pants. Later they tell her that they are going to wet them. By 2 years of age most children are dry by day, and by 3 years of age at night — although some 10% wet the bed occasionally at the age of 5.

Normal Sequence of Development

The following is a brief outline of the average sequence of development in a full-term baby:

Newborn

When prone — pelvis high, knees under abdomen (Fig. 4-1)

When pulled to sitting position, almost complete head lag

4 to 6 weeks

Begins to respond to the mother by smiling; a week or two later begins to vocalize when smiling

When prone — pelvis flat, legs partly extended

At 6 weeks, when held in ventral suspension with the hand under the abdomen, head momentarily in same plane as rest of body (Fig. 4-2)

8 weeks

When prone — lifts chin off bed so that plane of face is at angle of 45 degrees to table

12 weeks

When prone — chest off table; plane of face at angle of 45 to 90 degrees to table

Holds rattle placed in hand

Turns head to sound

16 weeks

When prone — plane of face at angle of 90 degrees to table

Hands join together in play

20 weeks

No head lag when pulled to sitting position

When prone — weight on forearms

Reaches out for objects and gets them

24 weeks

When prone — weight on hands, elbows extended

Bears full weight on legs if given the chance (Fig. 4-3)

28 weeks

Sits on floor with hands forward for support

When supine — lifts head up spontaneously

*Fig. 4-1. Infant in prone position at various ages. (From R. S. Illingworth, **Basic Developmental Screening**. Oxford, Eng.: Blackwell, 1988.)*

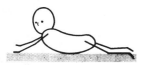

Newborn: prone, pelvis high, knees under abdomen.

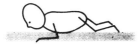

6 weeks: prone, pelvis flat, hips extended.

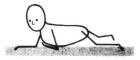

6 weeks: prone, chin intermittently lifted off couch.

3 months: prone, weight on forearms, chest well off couch.

6 months: prone, weight on hands, arms extended.

*Fig. 4-2. Infant in ventral suspension at various ages. (From R. S. Illingworth, **Basic Developmental Screening**. Oxford, Eng.: Blackwell, 1988.)*

Newborn: ventral suspension, head held up a little, elbows flexed, hips partly extended.

6 weeks: ventral suspension, head held up momentarily in same plane as rest of body, hips extended.

10 weeks: ventral suspension, head held up well beyond plane of rest of body.

2 months: abnormal baby in ventral suspension, arms and legs hang down.

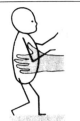

3 months: held standing, sags at knees and hips.

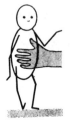

6 months: held standing, bears full weight.

Fig. 4-3. Infant in standing position. (From R. S. Illingworth, **Basic Developmental Screening.** *Oxford, Eng.: Blackwell, 1988.)*

Transfers object from one hand to another
Chews
Begins to imitate — a cough, hand movement
32 weeks
Sits seconds on floor without support
Combines syllables — dada, baba, mama
36 weeks
Stands holding furniture
Pulls self to stand
Sits minutes on floor without rolling over
40 weeks
Crawls on abdomen
Characteristic index finger approach to objects
Picks up pellet between tip of thumb and forefinger
Waves bye-bye, plays pat-a-cake
Holds arm out for coat, foot for shoe
44 weeks
Creeps on hands and knees (Fig. 4-4)
48 weeks
Walks, holding furniture
Gives toys to mother
Says one word with meaning
52 weeks
Walks, one hand held (Fig. 4-5)

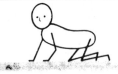

10 months: creep position, on hands and knees.

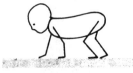

1 year: walking like a bear, on soles of feet and hands.

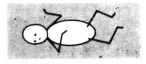

Newborn: supine, flexed position.

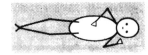

Newborn: spastic, lower limbs extended.

Fig. 4-4. Infant in creeping and supine positions. (From R. S. Illingworth, **Basic Developmental Screening.** *Oxford, Eng.: Blackwell, 1988.)*

Throws one object after another to floor
Says three words with meaning
13 months
Walks without help
Feeds self with spoon
15 to 18 months
Picks up cup, drinks, and puts it down without help
Creeps upstairs
Tells mother of need for potty
Takes shoes and socks off
Points on request to parts of body
Builds tower of two blocks
Has stopped taking toys to mouth
Domestic mimicry — copies mother sweeping, etc.
21 to 24 months
Joins two or three words into sentence
Builds tower of five to six blocks
24 months
Takes some clothes off

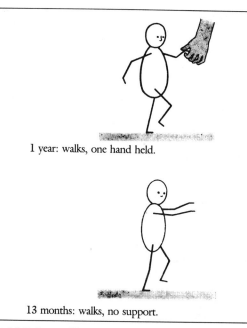

1 year: walks, one hand held.

13 months: walks, no support.

**Fig. 4-5. Infant walking. (From R. S. Illingworth,
Basic Developmental Screening.** *Oxford, Eng.: Blackwell,
1988.)*

Puts on shoes, socks, pants
Dry by day
Builds tower of six or seven blocks
3 years
    Dry by night
    Builds tower of nine blocks
    Knows full name and sex
    Jumps with both feet
    Repeats three numbers (once in three times)
    Stands on one leg for seconds
    Rides tricycle
3 to 4 years
    Dresses self fully

Variations in Development

There may be great variations and extreme ranges in a child's
development. A baby or child should be called retarded only
with caution and (whenever possible) only after consultation with experts.

Assessment of Development

There are many reasons for developmental assessment. Parents want to know whether a baby is developing normally,
especially if a previous child is handicapped, or there had
been a difficult pregnancy or delivery. They are likely to
want an assessment if there is unusual development in any
field, such as lateness in walking, talking, or toilet training,
or if the child has an unusual appearance or behaviour. The
doctor has to assess a baby for suitability for adoption; he
wants to assess obstetrical or neonatal management or the
effect of illness, injury, or drugs. He needs to assess a child's
educational needs, if there is some retardation; and he may
need to look for evidence of deterioration if, for instance,
there is a family history of degenerative disease of the nervous system.

Developmental assessment is a clinical diagnosis, and a
clinical diagnosis should be based on the history, full physical and devlepmental examination, special investigations
where relevant, and interpretation of the results.

The History

The first essential in assessing a child's development is to
obtain a detailed history, encompassing everything that may
have affected the development such as illness, parental neglect, or failure to give the child the opportunity to learn. In
addition, one should inquire about previous development
up to the time of examination to appraise the rate of development (i.e., whether there are indications that the child is a
slow starter and is now catching up or is deteriorating after
previous normal development). One should also note factors that make the child more likely than others to be retarded (e.g., family history of mental deficiency, rubella in
early pregnancy, hyperbilirubinemia or convulsions in the
newborn period, or severe hypoxia at birth). It is essential
that the child's birth weight and the duration of gestation be
known, so that allowance can be made for possible prematurity. If, for instance, the child was born 3 months prematurely, passing of the milestones of development can be
expected to be about 3 months later than in full-term infants.

When relevant to the child's age, the following questions
concerning development must be asked. The average age at
which the various milestones are passed has been placed in
parentheses after the question. When did the child

1. First begin to smile at you when you were talking to him
   or her? (4–6 weeks) It is not sufficient to ask when the
   baby first began to smile, without amplifying the ques-

tion; the mother may refer to any facial movement in sleep or on tickling the face as a smile.

2. Begin to make little noises, such as cooing, as well as smiling, when talked to? (6–8 weeks)
3. Hold on to a rattle for a minute or two when it was placed in the hand? (12 weeks)
4. Begin to turn the head upon hearing a sound? (12 weeks) In the case of suspected hearing defect one should ask about response to squeaky toys, music, being sung to, the telephone, and so on.
5. First able to go for and get a rattle without its being placed in the hand? (20 weeks)
6. Begin to roll completely over from the front to the back? (16–24 weeks) From the back to the front? (up to 28 weeks)
7. Begin to take an object from one hand into the other? (26 weeks)
8. Begin to make chewing movements when given a biscuit or rusk? (26 weeks)
9. Begin to sit on the floor for a few seconds without rolling over? (28 weeks) This is quite different from sitting when some support may be provided, as in a carriage.
10. Begin to imitate you? (28 weeks) In what way? (The baby is likely to imitate a cough, tongue protrusion, or some noise or simple act.)
11. Begin to stand holding on to furniture? (36 weeks)
12. Begin to pull up to the standing position without help (40 weeks), crawl on the abdomen (40 weeks), creep on hands and knees (44 weeks), walk holding on to the furniture (48 weeks), and walk unsupported? (13 months)
13. Begin to wave bye-bye (40 weeks) and play pat-a-cake? (40 weeks)
14. Begin to say a word with meaning — that is, not mere dadada, mumum? (48 weeks)
15. Begin to hand you a block, releasing it into your hand? (48 weeks)
16. Begin throwing one object after another onto the floor? (12 months)
17. Begin to hold out an arm for a coat or a foot out for a shoe? (10–12 months)
18. Learn to pick up a cup, drink from it, and put it down without much spilling? (average, 15 months; some learn by 9 or 10 months)

It is essential to ask each question precisely and accurately to avoid errors. When it is thought that the mother does not know, or is guessing, no answer is recorded. Unless the history is properly taken, it means nothing (see Chap. 2).

The Examination

The examination of the newborn baby includes the Apgar score (reflecting the general condition at birth), the maturity in relation to the duration of gestation, the head circumference in relation to weight and possibly the duration of gestation, the nature of the cry, the anterior fontanelle, the quality, quantity, and symmetry of limb movements, the facial appearance, and alertness. The Brazelton method of neurological assessment of the newborn is commonly used.

After the newborn period the examination must include the head circumference in relation to weight, full physical examination for abnormalities, such as hypotonia or hypertonia, subluxation of the hips, sensory defects (visual and auditory), and any other handicaps that affect development. Omission of such full physical examination is likely to cause serious defects in the assessment.

The method of developmental assessment has been fully reviewed by me elsewhere. A widely used method of scoring is the Denver test. Any developmental tests used, whether the Denver method or otherwise, *must* be used in conjunction with full history-taking and physical examination, for a developmental assessment must cover the child as a whole and not merely the response to certain readily scorable items.

Intelligence tests for older children include visuospatial, memory, speech, and understanding of language.

Special Investigations

Examination of the newborn for phenylketonuria, hypothyroidism, and, often, other metabolic abnormalities is a routine. When an infant is suspected of having brain damage or cerebral palsy, imaging techniques, especially ultrasound, computed tomography (CT scan), and magnetic resonance imaging (MRI) are useful for demonstrating possible prenatal fetal cerebral or vascular abnormalities. As in the case of very low birth weight babies, these techniques give a good indication of the outlook for normal development or residual handicap.

Interpretation

For the assessment, all relevant items in the history, physical and developmental examination, and results of special tests must be considered. Allowance must be made for preterm delivery and any handicaps, physical or environmental (e.g., emotional deprivation). The family history of developmental variations (e.g., lateness in individual fields of development) and evidence, if any, that the rate of development has been changing are important. One must be satisfied that the child's performance in tests was the best of which he was capable.

It is vital to remember that some aspects of development are far more important than others. Gross motor development (e.g., unusually early or late sitting or walking), for instance, is far less important than manipulation (e.g., finger-thumb apposition and the index finger approach to objects from 9 to 12 months of age). The most important of all are unscorable items, such as the child's interest in surroundings, alertness, concentration, responsiveness, and the quality of vocalization.

After considering all these factors, one can calculate the developmental quotient (DQ) — the relation of the child's overall performance or performance in individual fields to his chronological age. This will be considerably modified by various postnatal factors (see p. 37). The intelligence quotient (IQ) is the relation of the mental age to the chronological age.

Retardation in Smiling, Walking, Speech, and Sphincter Control (After Correction for Maturity)

Delay in Onset of Smiling

The usual factors that cause delayed onset of smiling are lack of stimulation by the parents (not talking to the child) or mental subnormality. Rare causes are blindness or infantile autism.

Walking

The common factors responsible for delay in walking are:

Familial pattern. Lateness in walking is often a family characteristic.
Low intelligence. Severely defective children are late in learning to walk; moderately defective ones may sit and walk at the usual age.
Variations in muscle tone. Hypotonia, due to one of many causes, or hypertonia (cerebral palsy).
Lack of opportunity to bear weight on legs, due to neglect at home, illness, or institutional care.
Duchenne muscular dystrophy, blindness. Delay is unlikely to be due to obesity or dislocation of the hip.

Speech

Understanding of speech long precedes the ability to articulate. The child may be thought to be late in speech when his understanding of speech is advanced; he may merely take after one parent in being later than usual in learning to articulate. Delay in speech is not due to tongue-tie, cleft palate, or mere laziness ("Everything is done for him"), and it is not due to jealousy. The common factors responsible for delay in learning to speak are:

Familial pattern. Late speech is frequently a family characteristic.
Low intelligence. Speech is always late in children of low intelligence.
Deafness — for all tones or merely high tones.
Multiple pregnancy. Twins are commonly late in speaking, for unknown reasons, partly, perhaps, because the mother has not as much time to devote to twins as to a singleton. (On the average, the first child of a family learns to speak earlier than do subsequent children.)
Unknown factors. Most children with cerebral palsy are late in speaking, possibly because of low intelligence, hearing defect, or cortical damage. Spasticity or incoordination of the muscles involved in speech may also delay the development of speech.

Sphincter Control

The factors involved in delayed control are:

Familial pattern. Lateness in acquiring control of the bladder is very frequently a familial feature.
Low intelligence. Most, but not all, mentally subnormal children are late in acquiring control of the sphincters.
Psychological factors, e.g., overenthusiastic toilet training, including punishment for accidents. Neglect of the child, in the form of failure to help when the child needs to pass urine, may sometimes be a factor. Emotional stress, especially at the time when sphincter control is normally acquired, is a possible cause, but delayed control is rarely just psychological. Maturation of the relevant part of the nervous system, commonly familial, is far more important, but psychological factors (e.g., due to mismanagement) may be superimposed.
Congenital anomalies of the bladder neck in boys, in which case there is constant dribbling of urine, or an ectopic ureter entering the vagina or a ureterocele in girls, also shown by constant dribbling. Other causes are urinary tract infection, absent sacral segments, and meningomyelocele.

Mental Subnormality

The term *mental subnormality* is commonly defined as a level of intelligence score two standard deviations below the mean for the age: this applies to 3% of the population. Mild mental retardation is usually of socioeconomic origin and commonly corresponds with that of the parents.

Mental subnormality is mainly due to prenatal factors, though the precise cause is commonly unknown. Known causes include scores of genetic conditions, such as mental subnormality in a parent, chromosomal abnormalities (which are mostly associated with a lower than average IQ), degenerative diseases of the nervous system, psychoses, metabolic conditions, and syndromes involving many organs of the body such as the skin (e.g., neurodermatoses). The mental subnormality may be due to cerebral or cerebrovascular malformations, and this child is more likely than others to have other congenital abnormalities (in the eyes, skull, mouth, limbs, heart, or other organs). There may be unusual skin markings on the hands (such as a single palmar crease, but this may occur in normal children) and low-set ears (difficult to define) or other ear malformations, which may also occur in normal children. Mentally subnormal children are on the average smaller than normal ones. Delayed sexual development is common.

There are important prenatal causes of mental subnormality apart from genetic ones. They include placental insufficiency (related to maternal toxemia, hypertension, antepartum hemorrhage, and to intrauterine growth retardation and chronic fetal hypoxia), infections in pregnancy (such as toxoplasmosis, rubella, cytomegalovirus, herpes, AIDS), irradiation of the mother's pelvis, and drugs. Alcohol taken by the mother during pregnancy is the most common preventable cause of mental subnormality.

Perinatal factors, such as hypoxia or cerebral trauma at birth, hyperbilirubinemia, or hypoglycemia in the child, are unusual causes. Postnatal causes include in particular malnutrition, emotional deprivation, pyogenic meningitis, hypoglycemia, hypoxia, lead poisoning and drugs, and severe head injury.

Cerebral palsy, which is usually of prenatal origin, is commonly associated with a lower than average level of intelligence. For instance, the mean IQ score for spastic hemiplegia is around 70. The mean IQ of boys with Duchenne's muscular dystrophy is around 80. The relationship of epilepsy to IQ depends in part on the cause and type of epilepsy, but a prolonged convulsion may cause brain damage. Infantile spasms and, in the older child, Lennox-Gastaut epilepsy are usually associated with mental subnormality.

The diagnosis, as in any developmental assessment, is made on the basis of the history, full physical examination (to include other congenital abnormalities), developmental examination, special investigations if relevant, and the interpretation (see p. 38). Head circumference in relation to weight is of particular importance, for if the brain is not growing normally, the head is likely to be small (unless there is obstruction to the cerebrospinal fluid). It is particularly important to look for sensory defects (visual or auditory), because they are so often associated with mental subnormality and may be confused with it.

As for developmental features, the mentally subnormal child is late in all aspects of development, except occasionally in sitting and walking. The full-term baby at birth, being late in maturation, behaves in many ways like a preterm baby, sleeping a large part of the day and night, failing to demand feedings, often with sucking and swallowing difficulties. Mothers often say that their baby is so good, not a bit of trouble, perfectly content to lie quietly all day without complaint, having little or no interest in the surroundings. The child is then late in beginning to smile at her (average for normal child, 4–6 weeks): the infant is then late in beginning to vocalize as well as smile (normally babies begin to vocalize 7–14 days after beginning to smile in response to the mother). Later the baby is backward in following with the eyes so that the doctor wonders if the infant is blind; and if the optic fundi are examined, the normal pale optic disk may convince the physician that the baby has optic atrophy and confirm the (wrong) diagnosis of blindness. The baby is late in responding and turning to sound (average 3–4 months), and so the doctor may suspect deafness. The baby is late in all aspects of motor development — in holding the head up in ventral suspension, in development in the prone position, and in other aspects of head control. The infant is late in reaching out and getting objects (average 5 months), in beginning to chew (average 6–7 months), and usually in sitting, creeping, and walking. Later there is retardation in speech, sphincter control, and all other fields of development.

A peculiar feature of normal babies between 12 and 20 weeks of age is hand regard: the baby when awake and playing, and with the wrists in front, pronates and supinates them, but retarded children often show this feature much later — 24 weeks of age and older.

Normal babies take all available objects to the mouth from about 3 months of age; this normally stops shortly after 12 to 24 months, but it persists in backward children.

Normal babies deliberately throw one object after another onto the floor from the age of 10 months or so ("casting"), but they cease to do this by 15 to 16 months. Retarded children continue this much longer.

Normal babies usually stop slobbering (drooling) shortly after 15 months of age, but mentally subnormal ones commonly continue longer.

Tooth grinding when awake is a common feature of subnormal children.

The most important developmental features of mentally subnormal children are lack of interest in surroundings, lack of normal responsiveness, and lack of concentration, for instance, in trying to reach a toy. Later this defective concentration leads to boredom and to difficulties for the mother. The child will not play with anything for more than a very short time (though some psychotic children have obsessional play for prolonged periods with a single favorite toy).

After infancy the mentally subnormal child who in the early weeks seemed to be inactive, lying quiet all day, acquires mobility, and then a characteristic feature is constant aimless overactivity.

Errors in the diagnosis of mental subnormality are frequent. Common sources of error are the following:

1. Failure to allow for preterm delivery.
2. Delayed maturation. An occasional baby is backward in many or even all aspects of development in the early weeks, especially after problems of delivery or sometimes after early infantile meningitis or encephalitis, and then catches up to the average. Some, without any history of illness, are just slow starters — backward at first but catching up to the normal later. One occasionally sees delayed visual or auditory maturation; although normal in other aspects of development, the child appears to be blind or deaf at first but later is shown to see and hear normally.
3. Failure to recognize that the child's performance was not the best of which he was capable — perhaps because he was hungry, tired, feeling poorly, or bored.
4. Failure to allow for all handicaps, such as physical and, especially, sensory (visual or auditory).
5. Diagnosis of mental subnormality wrongly based on finding retardation in individual fields of development such as walking, speech, and sphincter control (commonly merely a familial trait), or diagnosis purely on the basis of some developmental tests instead of on the child as a whole. Diagnosis of mental subnormality must never be based on mere clinical impression.
6. Failure to recognize that some aspects of development are far more important than others.
7. Diagnosis based on normal variations, such as later than usual closure of the anterior fontanelle, late teething, and normal variations such as unusual appearance of the ears or single palmar crease on the hands.
8. Cerebral palsy. Since the athetoid child is retarded in most aspects of development, it is extremely easy to make a diagnosis of mental subnormality when, in fact,

intelligence is normal. The spastic child is late in so many aspects of development that it is common to underestimate the child's intelligence. Nevertheless, the majority of spastic children have lower than average intelligence.
9. The effect of drugs used for the treatment of epilepsy, especially barbiturates.
10. The effect of emotional deprivation or child abuse. This can greatly lower a child's level of intelligence. It is likely that the head of such a child would be of normal size; the discerning doctor may notice that the child shows good interest in the surroundings and possibly good responsiveness. The diagnosis, however, can be very difficult.
11. Infantile autism and psychoses. The child's total lack of responsiveness, lack of interest in being picked up, and sometimes persistent unexplained crying may readily lead to a diagnosis of mental subnormality. In fact, the autistic child functions like a mentally subnormal one.

Mental Deterioration

The main causes of mental deterioration are as follows:

Meningitis, encephalitis, cerebral tumor, vascular accidents
Degenerative diseases of the nervous system
Severe hypoglycemia, hypernatremia
Metabolic diseases: hypothyroidism, phenylketonuria, lipoidoses, mucopolysaccharidoses
Lead poisoning
Head injury
Anoxia: anesthetic mishap, near-drowning, carbon monoxide poisoning, epileptic seizures
Emotional deprivation
Poor standard of education, prolonged absence from school
Drugs: drugs used for epilepsy; in the older child, drugs of addiction
Malnutrition

Mental deterioration should be distinguished from the usual slowing down of development in babies with Down syndrome after about 6 months of age.

Mental Superiority

It would be incorrect to assume that the mentally superior child is advanced in all aspects of development, i.e., the opposite of the mentally subnormal child. The child may be advanced in everything but usually is not.

The mentally superior baby is often early in beginning to watch the mother as she speaks, and then early in smiling. From this stage onward the child may show unusual alertness, responsiveness, and interest in surroundings. Commonly, gross motor development is in no way advanced. When able to reach out for objects, the child shows unusual determination and concentration, is not distracted as easily as an average child, and is far less distractible than a mentally subnormal child. There may be early manipulative development — ability to transfer objects from one hand to the other (in an average child, 6 months) and early finger-thumb apposition (on average, 10 months). Vocalization is often advanced — from 6 to 8 weeks or so — and speech is often (but by no means always) early. Even if not advanced in speech, the child is advanced in understanding the meaning of words. Later the child may learn to read early, shows superior imagination in play and questioning, and often shows unusual interest in collecting objects.

Cerebral Palsy

The most common type of cerebral palsy is spasticity; other forms are athetosis, rigidity, ataxia, and a rare hypotonia form.

If the child has the spastic form, the mother may notice stiffness of the limbs, tight clenching of one or both hands, or, later, asymmetry in kicking or creeping. The doctor may detect signs in the newborn period (except in the mildest forms) — relative immobility, undue extension of the lower limbs, or maintained clenching of the hands (or of one hand in the case of spastic hemiplegia). When the child is held up with hands in the axillae, there is undue extension of the lower limbs instead of the normal flexion. There is delayed motor development — as seen in ventral suspension or in the prone position or on pulling the baby up to the sitting position. The muscle tone is increased, so that there is undue resistance to passive movement, reduced range of movement in the joints (especially in abduction of the hip or dorsiflexion of the ankle). When placed sitting forward, the 6-month-old (or older) spastic child repeatedly falls back because of spasm of the erector spinae, the glutei, and the hamstrings; and when pulled into the sitting position the child may rise onto the legs as a result of excessive extensor tone. The knee jerks are exaggerated, and the plantar responses are extensor, there may be ankle clonus. Later the child characteristically walks on the toes. When reaching out for an object, the child characteristically slowly splays the fingers and dorsiflexes the wrist. If there is spastic hemiplegia, there will be shortening of the affected limbs and relative coldness on the affected side. Most children with the spastic form of cerebral palsy have a below average level of intelligence, so that they present the usual signs of mental subnormality (p. 39).

The athetoid child in infancy shows delayed motor development and often excessive muscle tone. The plantar responses are flexor, and the knee jerks are normal. The characteristic athetoid movements may be seen any time after about 6 months of age. When reaching out for an object, the child does not show the splaying that is so characteristic of the spastic child; movements are unsteady and ataxic, and only later do the typical writhing movements of the athetoid appear.

Common errors in the diagnosis of cerebral palsy are the following:

1. Diagnosis on single signs, such as isolated delay in gross motor development, instead of on diagnosis of the child as a whole.
2. Failure to recognize normal variations — unusually brisk tendon jerks or ankle clonus in a young baby.
3. Failure to remember that even abnormally brisk tendon jerks and persistent ankle clonus in the early weeks may disappear. In such cases there would not be other signs of cerebral palsy.
4. Toe walking. The common cause is a mere habit when the child of around 9–15 months is learning to walk. There would not be other signs of cerebral palsy. Toe walking is very common in cerebral palsy of the spastic type, but it also occurs in congenital shortening of the Achilles tendon (in which condition the limited dorsiflexion of the ankle would persist when the knee is flexed; in the spastic form of cerebral palsy it would disappear on flexing the knee). Toe walking may also occur in unilateral dislocation of the hip, Duchenne's muscular dystrophy, dystonia musculorum deformans, and infantile autism.
5. Spinal cord disease. In this case the upper limbs would be normal and mental development would be expected to be normal. True spastic paraplegia (i.e., with no abnormality in the upper limbs) is rare, and a spinal lesion should be considered.
6. Muscle weakness (as in brachial plexus injury) or muscle contracture, as in severe hypotonia.
7. Joint disease, limiting joint movements.
8. Mere clumsiness, sometimes a familial feature.

The Blind Child

The mother may notice a corneal opacity, or roving nystagmus, or failure to follow with the eyes. Although the majority of blind children are of average intelligence, a blind child, especially if the blindness is due to a congenital abnormality or to retrolental fibroplasia, is more likely than others to have a lower than average level of intelligence.

It is likely that the blind child, being unable to see the mother's facial expression and overtures, may be late in smiling. Manipulative development may be late. The child may experience pseudoretardation as a result of over-protection and be late in learning to feed and dress himself, and perhaps in walking because his mother does everything for him instead of letting him learn slowly to do things for himself.

Certain characteristic mannerisms commonly develop in the first year, such as pressing the finger into the eye and symmetrical swaying movements of the body.

Specific Learning Disorders

The term *specific learning disorders* covers a wide spectrum of skills, notably reading, writing, spelling, and arithmetic; speech is often late. Nonspecific learning disorders may be related to many interacting factors as chromosome abnormalities, maternal toxemia, alcohol use, or smoking in pregnancy, low intelligence, hypoxia before or at birth, postmaturity, prematurity, hyperbilirubinemia, malnutrition in early infancy, adverse socioeconomic factors, absence of suitable play material at home, unsatisfactory education, and prolonged absence from school.

The most common learning disorder is *dyslexia,* or impairment of the ability to read. The usual causes of difficulty in learning to read are mental subnormality, poor socioeconomic conditions, and sometimes defective vision and hearing, but there is a "specific" form of dyslexia that is genetic and not associated with subnormal intelligence. In this case, there is a family history — in a parent — of some of the features. It is four times more common in boys than girls. There is very often delay in establishment of laterality, or there is ambidexterity or left-handedness. The child may read from right to left, reverse symbols, omit letters, or insert letters in the wrong place. The child may interpret ";" as "?". The order of letters may be reversed: *was* interpreted as *saw, but* as *tub.* In arithmetic, the child may write or say that $16 + 1 = 71, 14 + 1 = 51$. Mirror writing may occur.

To make the diagnosis, one first excludes mental subnormality, audiovisual defects, emotional and socioeconomic factors, and poor teaching. Next one looks for crossed laterality, difficulties in right-left orientation, and some of the conditions commonly associated with learning difficulties (clumsiness, overactivity, and other features of the attention deficit disorder), and then looks for specific signs in reading and writing (omission or reversal of letters and errors in interpreting the order of letters in a word [*was = saw*]).

Specific learning disorders cause considerable school difficulties, and if the condition is not diagnosed, teachers are apt to think that the child is mentally backward or just naughty and not trying. The result is that children with these learning disorders commonly have behavior problems, such as truancy, aggressiveness, or other signs of insecurity.

Physical defects that may be associated with learning disorders include, in particular, defects of vision and hearing, cerebral palsy, hydrocephalus, phenylketonuria, epilepsy, and Duchenne's muscular dystrophy.

Ronald S. Illingworth

References

Bakwin, H., and Bakwin, R. M. *Behavior Disorders in Children.* Philadelphia: Saunders, 1972.

Boder, E. Developmental Dyslexia: Prevailing Diagnostic Concepts and a New Diagnostic Approach. In H. R. Myklebust (Ed), *Progress in Learning Disorders.* New York: Grune & Stratton, 1971.

Brazelton, T. B. Neonatal Behavioral Assessment Scale. In *Clinics in Developmental Medicine,* No. 50. London: Heinemann, 1964.

Dubowitz, L., and Dubowitz, V. The Neurological Assessment of the Preterm and Full Term Newborn Infant. In *Clinics in Developmental Medicine,* No. 79. London: Heinemann, 1981.

Frankenburg, W. K., Fandal, A. W., Sciarillo, W., and Burgess, D. The newly abbreviated and revised Denver Developmental Screening Test. *J. Pediatr.* 99:995, 1981.

Illingworth, R. S. *Basic Developmental Screening* (4th ed.) Oxford: Blackwell, 1988.

Illingworth, R. S. *Development of the Infant and Young Child* (9th ed). London: Churchill Livingstone, 1987.

Shaywitz, S., Shaywitz, B., and Grossman, H. J. Learning Disorders. *Pediatr. Clin. N. Am.* 31:277 (symposium), 1984.

5

Prenatal Development and Clinical Genetics

Intrauterine Growth and Development

Normal Development

PLACENTA. The fetus derives nourishment through the placenta during intrauterine life. There is normally complete separation of the maternal and fetal circulations in the placenta, although maternal red cells can often be found in the fetal circulation and fetal red cells may be identified in the maternal circulation. Maternal blood coming from the uterus enters the intervillous spaces lined with fetal syncytium, while fetal blood coming from the umbilical cord circulates through the villi, permitting various exchanges to take place across the thin membrane separating the two circulations. The placenta is such a good excretory organ for the fetus that there is no need during intrauterine life for an efficient genitourinary system. A baby may be born alive at term with bilateral renal agenesis (Potter's syndrome) or complete obstruction to urinary outflow.

The fetus excretes urine into the liquor amnii, and oligo-

The author acknowledges the contributions of Thomas E. Cone, Jr., who originally wrote this chapter, many portions of which were left intact.

hydramnios may result from renal agenesis or from congenital obstruction to urinary outflow. At the time of delivery the placenta weighs about 500 g, its diameter ranges between 15 and 20 cm, and its thickness is about 2.0 to 2.5 cm. Figure 5-1 is a schematic cross section of the placenta while it is attached to the uterine wall.

UMBILICAL CORD. The fetal circulation is related to the placenta through the umbilical cord, which is from 1.0 to 2.5 cm in diameter and from 30 to 100 cm long, the average length being about 55 cm. It contains the two umbilical arteries bringing fetal blood to the placenta and a single umbilical vein through which blood returns to the fetus.

A single umbilical artery, found in 0.2 to 1% of all newborns, is frequently associated with major congenital anomalies. There is a positive correlation between single umbilical artery and fetal developmental defects, but it is not a direct one. The frequency of detected anomalies varies greatly in the reports, from 18 to 50%.

STAGES OF FETAL DEVELOPMENT. It may be important for the physician to estimate the age of infants who are born prematurely (Table 5-1). During the first 10 weeks of life, while organogenesis is taking place, the product of concep-

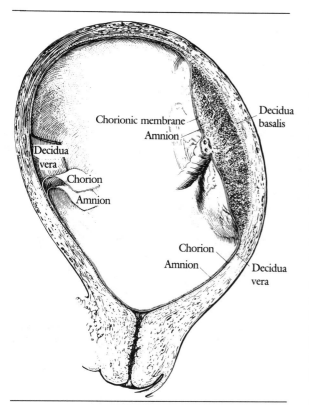

Fig. 5-1. Diagram of pregnant uterus showing normal placenta in situ. (From J. W. Williams, Placenta circumvallata. Am. J. Obstet. Gynecol. 13:1, 1927.)

tion is known as an embryo; during the subsequent months of intrauterine life it is known as a fetus.

Congenital Abnormalities

Congenital abnormalities (malformations, birth defects) are structural defects present at birth and attributable to faulty development. They may be gross or microscopic, on the surface of the body or within it, familial or sporadic, hereditary or nonhereditary, single or multiple. Estimates of their total incidence depend on the inclusion or exclusion of malformed stillborns, the accuracy of diagnosis, the period for which the children are followed, whether minor malformations are included, and whether the estimates refer to hospital births or include births at home as well.

Traditionally, a *major malformation* is defined as a structural abnormality with either surgical or cosmetic significance. The incidence is greater in spontaneous abortions than in liveborn infants. Examples include cleft lip, congenital heart defects, anencephaly, omphalocele, and hypospadias. A *minor anomaly* (or minor dysmorphic feature) is an external physical feature found in less than 4% of the same ethnic population. Examples of such anomalies include epicanthal folds, simian creases, bent fifth fingers, and widely spaced nipples. In contrast, a *deformation* is an abnormal form or position of a body part caused by nondisruptive mechanical (intrinsic or extrinsic) forces. An example is a club foot caused by restricted movement in a twin pregnancy. A *disruption* is a morphologic defect of a body part resulting from a breakdown of or interference with an originally normal developmental process. An example is digital amputation from an amniotic band.

The incidence of children with at least one major malformation present at or soon after birth, stillborns included, is on the order of 15 to 20 per 1000 total births. If the children are followed for a year and minor malformations are included, the incidence rises to about 4%. The proportion of infant deaths due to congenital malformation, in relation to deaths due to all causes, has risen from 7 to 18% during the past 60 years.

Some congenital abnormalities may be so severe that they cause death in utero, resulting in miscarriage or stillbirth, or early neonatal death. On the other hand, certain abnormalities are compatible with long life and may be diagnosed only accidentally in later life. Other congenital abnormalities can be diagnosed early and easily treated. If they remain undetected, they may lead to greater difficulties.

According to the United States National Center for Health, congenital abnormalities are responsible for 4.4 neonatal deaths for every 1000 live births. They are the second most common cause of death in infants and in the 1- to 5-year age group, while deaths from congenital malformations among children ages 5 to 15 years are exceeded in frequency only by those due to accidents and malignant neoplasms. The occasional fetal deaths would raise the total perinatal mortality from this cause.

Factors capable of producing injury to the fetus without killing it may lead to congenital abnormalities. The causes of congenital defects are generally divided into two main groups — genetic and environmental.

GENETIC CAUSES. Genetic factors result from abnormalities of the genes transmitted by the parents or from chromosomal anomalies. There are essentially three agents of genetic predisposition to disease: (1) an abnormal chromosome complement, (2) a single gene (simple Mendelian

Table 5-1. Normal Fetal Development

Age from last menstrual period	Length (cm)	Crown–rump length (cm)	Weight* (g)	Other characteristics
2 weeks	2 or a few cells	—	—	Microscopical: from 2 cells to a vesicular organism
3 weeks		—	—	Embryonal stage—medullary groove and canal, head folds, visceral arches, clefts, cerebral and optic vesicles, limb buds
4 weeks (1 lunar month)	1	—	—	Eye, ear, and nose rudiments are seen; embryo is bent over on its ventral surface
2 lunar months	4	0.23	1.1	Similar to other mammalian fetuses: head enlarges markedly, external genitalia appear in second half of this period
3 lunar months	9	6.1	14.2	Ossification centers and nails appear; fingers and toes can be differentiated; external genitalia show sex characteristics
4 lunar months	16	11.6	108.0	Sex differentiation can be made more easily
5 lunar months	25	16.4	316.0	Skin less transparent: lanugo covers all the body and normal hair has gradually appeared on the head
6 lunar months	30	20.8	630.0	Subcutaneous deposition of fat is noted; head comparatively large; if born, the infant tries to breathe but almost always unsuccessfully
7 lunar months	35	24.7	1045.0	Skin red and covered with vernix caseosa; no pupillary membrane; body very thin; fetus moves extremities; if born, may survive with good care
8 lunar months	40	28.3	1680.0	Skin is red and wrinkled, with old-man appearance
9 lunar months	45	32.1	2478.0	Skin is less wrinkled, with more deposition of fat under the skin
10 lunar months	50	36.2	3405.0	Full-term baby known as normal newborn infant

*The weight will vary in different population groups.

Source: Modified from N. J. Eastman and L. M. Hellman (Eds.), *Williams Obstetrics* (13th ed.). New York: Appleton-Century-Crofts, 1966, p. 193.

diseases), and (3) a marked deviation from the mean for a polygenically (multifactorially) determined predisposition.

Table 5-2 lists the frequency of genetic disorders among patients admitted to a pediatric hospital in Montreal during the period 1969–1970.

ENVIRONMENTAL CAUSES. A single factor may produce different abnormalities, while different factors may produce the same congenital abnormality. The period of organogenesis and differentiation up to 10 to 12 weeks of gestation is when adverse environmental factors are most likely to produce malformations, which will depend upon the nature and intensity of the environmental factor and upon its timing in relation to embryological development.

The incidence of anomalies varies with race, sex, season, and maternal age. There is wide variation in incidence of anencephaly in different parts of the world; it is low among Asians and Africans, intermediate in America, and highest in

Table 5-2. Frequency of Genetic Disorders Among Patients Admitted to a Pediatric Hospital, Montreal, 1969–1970

Condition requiring hospitalization		Percentage of all admissions
Genetic disorders		
Autosomal recessive	2.0	
Autosomal dominant	2.0	
X-linked	2.7	11.0
Chromosomal	0.4	
Multifactorial	3.9	
Congenital malformations		18.4
Unknown		6.9
Nongenetic disorders		63.7

Source: *Genetic Disorders: Prevention, Treatment, and Rehabilitation* (WHO Technical Report Series no. 497). Geneva: World Health Organization, 1972.

western Europe. A recent international study confirms a 40-fold variation in incidence among hospital births in the centers studied. The incidence of anencephaly per 1000 total births (hospital deliveries only) varied from a low of 0.10 in Yugoslavia to a high of 4.48 in Northern Ireland.

The marked variation of birth frequency of mendelian disorders in different populations is puzzling. In the case of small isolates, the "founder effect" may often explain a relatively high frequency of a sublethal dominant disorder or of a recessive disorder, even a recessive disorder that is lethal in childhood. In some instances it has been possible to trace the founder, as in the dominant South African form of porphyria, recessive tyrosinemia (common in a French-Canadian isolate), and Ellis–van Creveld syndrome (common in Old World Amish in the United States). However, there are several instances of high birth frequency for certain recessive disorders that involve large populations and therefore, are not attributable to the founder effect; examples are cystic fibrosis in Europe and in the United States, sickle-cell anemia in West Africa, beta-thalassemia in Italy and the eastern Mediterranean countries, and familial Mediterranean fever in North Africa and the eastern Mediterranean. In the case of sickle-cell anemia, the heterozygote advantage is felt to consist of resistance to infection with *Plasmodium falciparum*. For the other conditions heterozygote advantage must be presumed, but its nature is not known.

There are other conditions with high birth frequency in populations of intermediate size, where the relative parts played by the founder effect (or genetic drift) and heterozygote advantage have not yet been proved. Examples include the high birth frequency of infantile Tay-Sachs disease in Ashkenazi Jews originating in Poland and Lithuania and congenital nephrosis in populations of Finnish extraction. Although accurate comparative data are lacking, it is believed that polydactyly and umbilical hernia are more common in black children, whereas cleft lip and palate, clubfoot, and congenital heart disease occur more frequently in white children. Males have a higher incidence of anomalies than females. The risk of liveborn children with fetal aneuploidy such as Down syndrome (trisomy 21) is higher with advancing maternal age (Table 5-3).

Phenocopy. Some nongenetic disorders may simulate hereditary disease leading to confusion and erroneous prognosis; therefore, drugs taken during pregnancy, intrauterine or perinatal infections, and trauma should always be sought for any pedigree and be kept in mind as possible etiological factors. It is of course important to differentiate these etiologies because (1) the recurrence risk may be very low or (2) the agent responsible for the previous birth defect may be avoided in future pregnancies.

Table 5-3. Risk of Having a Live-Born Child with Chromosomal Abnormalities

Maternal age	Down syndrome	All abnormalities except 47,XXX
20	1/1923	1/526
21	1/1695	1/526
22	1/1538	1/500
23	1/1408	1/500
24	1/1299	1/476
25	1/1205	1/476
26	1/1124	1/478
27	1/1053	1/455
28	1/990	1/435
29	1/935	1/417
30	1/885	1/384
31	1/826	1/384
32	1/725	1/322
33	1/592	1/285
34	1/465	1/243
35	1/365	1/178
36	1/287	1/149
37	1/225	1/123
38	1/177	1/105
39	1/139	1/80
40	1/109	1/63
41	1/85	1/48
42	1/67	1/39
43	1/53	1/31
44	1/41	1/24
45	1/32	1/18
46	1/25	1/15
47	1/20	1/11
48	1/16	1/8
49	1/12	1/7

Because sample size for some intervals is relatively small, 95-percent confidence limits are sometimes relatively large. Nonetheless, these figures are suitable for genetic counseling.
Source: J. L. Simpson, M. S. Golbus, A. O. Martin, and G. S. Sarkin. *Genetics in Obstetrics and Gynecology.* New York: Grune and Stratton, 1982. Data from E. B. Hook. Rates of chromosome abnormalities at different maternal ages. *Obstet. Gynecol.* 58:282, 1981; and E. B. Hook and G. M. Chambers. Estimated rates of Down syndrome in live-births by one year maternal age intervals for mothers aged 20–49 in a New York State study—implications of the risk figures for genetic counseling and cost-benefit analysis of prenatal diagnosis programs. *Birth Defects* 13 (3a):123, 1977.

Although teratologists have been able to produce anomalies in animal fetuses with a wide variety of stimuli applied to the pregnant female at the proper time in gestation, the factors proved to cause congenital malformations in human infants are few in number, and cause cannot be identified in most instances. Although anoxia in the embryo as a result of high altitude or disturbances of the maternal or fetal circulation has been suspected as a cause, its role has not been proved. There is evidence that one of the following types of environmental insult may play an etiological part in certain cases.

Radiation. Babies born to mothers who have been exposed to accidental x irradiation, especially in dosages greater than 50 rads, may exhibit abnormalities of the brain, eyes, or limbs. Diagnostic radiation exposure appears to produce extremely low or negligible risk for malformations in the developing fetus throughout pregnancy. According to the recommendation of American Academy of Pediatrics, however, interruption of pregnancy is *not* justified because of the radiation risk to the embryo/fetus from a diagnostic x-ray examination (American Academy of Pediatrics, 1978). While there is no proof that congenital malformations have been caused by exposure of pregnant women to diagnostic radiography, some authors recommend that to avoid irradiation of the conceptuses of undiagnosed early pregnancies, irradiation should, as far as possible, be performed only during the first half of the menstrual cycle. Pregnant women should be examined roentgenologically only on strong clinical grounds.

Drugs. The administration of certain drugs during pregnancy, particularly in its early stage, is known to be hazardous to the fetus. Drugs recognized as having such effects are thalidomide, alkylating agents, antimetabolites, hydantoins, oral anticoagulants, lithium, alcohol, and Accutane. By contrast, to date *none* of the following have been proved to cause birth defects: Bendectin, aspirin, marijuana, or caffeine.

Fetal Alcohol Syndrome. Over 20 years ago, it was recognized that maternal alcohol ingestion may have multiple effects on the fetus, including a now well-recognized fetal alcohol syndrome. Alcohol is now appreciated as the most common major teratogen to which a fetus is likely to be exposed. Features of fetal alcohol syndrome are variable, but in general consist of pre- and postnatal onset growth deficiency, microcephaly, shortened palpebral fissures, variable mental retardation, irritability in infancy, maxillary hypoplasia, short nose, smooth philtrum and smooth upper lip, and multiple joint anomalies including small distal phalanges. Congenital heart defects are relatively common. In women who may take 4 to 5 ounces of absolute alcohol per day, there is about a 30 to 45% risk of fetal alcohol syndrome in their offspring. It is not specifically known, however, what lower limits are safe in consumption of alcohol; therefore, it is now recommended that alcohol consumption be avoided in pregnancy.

Hormones. Maternal virilizing tumors or fetal adrenal hyperplasia may produce fetal pseudohermaphroditism in females or macrogenitosomia in males. The administration of synthetic progestins to control bleeding or of androgens or estrogens in early pregnancy may also affect development of the genital tract.

Infections. In utero exposure to maternal viral, parasitic, or bacterial infections can be teratogenic. For example, maternal rubella infection, whether or not it is clinically manifest, may lead to infection of the fetus. A syndrome consisting of low birth weight, congenital cataract, deaf-mutism, mental retardation, and congenital heart disease (most frequently patent ductus arteriosus with or without stenosis of the pulmonary valve, pulmonary artery, and its branches) is observed in about 15 to 20% of infants born to mothers infected during the first 10 weeks of pregnancy. Infants infected later in pregnancy may show active disease, with hepatosplenomegaly, thrombocytopenic purpura, and bone lesions. No matter at what stage the fetus becomes infected, virus persists and can be detected in urine or respiratory secretions for months after birth; it may produce infection in contacts. Thus congenital rubella, like congenital toxoplasmosis, syphilis, and cytomegalovirus infection, presents a hazard to the infant even when infection does not produce congenital anomalies.

Genetic Counseling

Genetic counseling is the giving of information by a physician or qualified person on birth defects or hereditary diseases to a patient or the patient's relatives, most likely parents. It involves an exchange of information. Genetic counseling usually involves multiple sessions over a varying period of time. People seeking counseling are frequently prospective parents who have had an affected child, know of relatives suffering from a hereditary condition, or know there are factors in their own background (e.g., advanced maternal age) which increases the risk of a child with birth defects. With all its social, religious, and legal implications, counseling calls for a careful and responsible attitude. It deals with probabilities attending a risk. The final decision rests with those who are seeking the advice. Genetic counseling, like other medical services, should be devoted to the welfare of the individual or the family seeking advice. The person seeking advice should, whenever possible, receive a clear estimate of risk about which the inquiry is made. In genetic counseling answers are sought to the following questions:

1. What is the diagnosis?
2. What is the etiology of the problem?
3. What is the prognosis?
4. Is there a specific treatment available?
5. What are the chances this specific problem will happen again?
6. What can be done to prevent this same problem occurring again in the future?

When counseling families of, for example, a newborn, one should try to have both parents present to be sure that each obtains information firsthand. As in any medical situation, a family history should be obtained. The reaction of individuals to the information as given can vary. Information is also being received in a situation when a family is dealing with mourning an infant or child, whether still living or now deceased, with unexpected problems which can potentially affect family dynamics for many years. Education of patients or parents about themselves or their child's disease is crucial. With rare exceptions patients should be thoroughly familiarized with their disease, because lack of knowledge may be a factor in prognosis. This is not dissimilar to the patient with diabetes mellitus knowing about the variation in his condition. The same understanding should be extended to inherited disorders such as muscular dystrophy, cystic fibrosis, sickle cell anemia, hemophilia, etc.

Part of genetic counseling includes a detailed family history. This history should include parental age, siblings, consanguinity, radiation history, history of drug exposure or viral infection early in pregnancy, and previous pregnancy history. Construction of family pedigrees and Mendelian inheritance will be addressed after Chromosome Abnormalities.

Chromosome Abnormalities

Chromosomes obtain the hereditary material DNA. Their numbers vary with each species; human beings normally have 46 chromosomes. Somatic or body cells are diploid, containing 23 pairs of chromosomes; germ cells or gametes are haploid with only half that number. Somatic cells divide in the usual manner, producing two daughter cells, each with a complement of 46 chromosomes. This is called mitotic division. In contrast, germ cells undergo meiosis or reduction division, producing gametes with 23 chromosomes each. Fertilization, resulting in zygote formation, brings two gametes together, and once again 46 chromosomes are obtained.

The total frequency of all chromosome disorders in newborns is about 0.6%. The sex aneuploidies represent about 0.25%, and the autosomal disorders about 0.36%. About 0.12% of autosomal disorders are autosomal trisomies, about 0.19% are balanced structural rearrangements, and about 0.05% are unbalanced rearrangements. Nearly all unbalanced chromosome aberrations will present with the following triad: multiple external dysmorphic features plus or minus major malformations, pre- and postnatal growth retardation, and mental retardation of varying degrees, often profound. In addition, chromosome analysis should be done if a patient presents with ambiguous genitalia, developmental delay or mental retardation of undefined etiology in the older infant or child, recurrent miscarriages (3 or more), infertility or sterility at reproductive age, continued sexual infantilism, or delayed pubertal development. An inherited but chromosomally defined syndrome called fragile X should also be considered in any male with undefined learning disabilities, autism, and/or mental retardation.

Presently, diagnosis and counseling for a chromosome aberration should be done only when karotype analysis with appropriate resolution, including banding, has been performed. Most G-banded karyotypes have a 300 to 400 band resolution (Fig. 5-2). After growth in culture medium for a few days, cells are processed to free the chromosomes. Trypsin is added which will produce a characteristic banding pattern. Then the chromosomes are stained with Giemsa for analysis under a light microscope. Other staining techniques are available to help define certain areas of some chromosomes if the G-banded chromosome analysis is uncertain. These include different stains with various names: reverse banding, C-banding, NOR staining, etc. Cytogenetic laboratories will generally have these additional techniques available for further study as needed.

Obtaining Tissue for Karyotype Analysis

The procedure for karyotype analysis is simple. Place 1 to 2 ml of whole blood in a sterile sodium heparin tube and notify the appropriate lab as soon as possible. Keep at room temperature. Other tissues such as skin, kidney, pericardium, or liver (in fetal demise or stillborns) can be used as long as they are not infected. Usually in this situation, obtaining several different specimens and placing them in sterile saline or appropriate tissue culture medium until delivery to the lab is necessary. In emergency situations involving an infant with a possible chromosome abnormality, preliminary chromosome results can be obtained as soon as 48 hours after initiation of culture. Using modified techniques this time can be reduced to 24 to 36 hours, at least for a number count with possible identification of excess chromosome material (trisomies, etc.). Bone marrows are still used to provide a 6 to 8 hour preliminary count in some situations.

High Resolution Karyotype Analysis

In the last 15 years, techniques have been developed which allow for higher numbers of bands to appear on chromosomes. This can be achieved by growing lymphocytes in similar culture situations but adding chemicals such as methotrexate or ethidium bromide. This arrests the chromosome earlier in condensation and allows for greater band resolution involving 500 to 600 bands. This method has made possible the identification of microscopic deletions and insertions of some previously undefined genetic syndromes. An example of such a syndrome is Prader-Willi syndrome, generally considered a sporadic genetic disorder which presents with hypotonia in infancy followed by hypogonadism, mental retardation, and onset of obesity in early childhood. In about half of patients presently diagnosed with Prader-Willi syndrome a submicroscopic deletion of the long arm of the 15 chromosome has been seen.

Because these improved techniques allow greater resolution and identification of subtler chromosome abnormalities, repeat chromosome analysis should be considered in

any patient presenting with multiple congenital abnormalities and/or mental retardation of undefined etiology who had karyotype analysis prior to 1975.

Nomenclature for Human Chromosomes

Since the human chromosome complement was originally defined in 1956, numerous international workshops have convened to produce a uniform nomenclature for human cytogenetic studies. The International System for Human Cytogenetic Nomenclature last convened in 1985. Autosomes are numbered from 1 to 22 in order of descending length, position of the centromere, and presence of satellites.

Each chromosome is composed of two chromatids joined together by a central constriction called the centromere. Chromosomes are arranged according to their length, the position of the centromere, and shape and presence of satellites. Identification of the individual chromosome is based on size, position of the centromere, and characteristic banding pattern produced by trypsin. The sex chromosomes are referred to as X (for female) and Y (for male) and are placed at the end of a karyotype as illustrated in Figure 5-2. A simple nomenclature is included here, but for more specific information we refer you to the previously mentioned reference. A description of a karyotype is arranged in the follow-

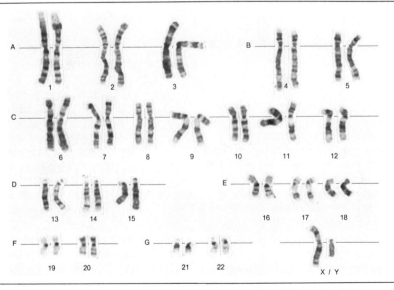

Fig. 5-2. G-banded normal male karyotype (compliments of Dr. Patricia N. Howard-Peebles).

ing order: the first designation is the number of chromosomes seen in the karyotype followed by the sex identification, followed, if applicable, by the type of abnormality seen. The presence of an additional chromosome (trisomy) is indicated by a plus sign (+), followed by the number identifying the extra chromsome; the absence of one chromosome by a minus sign (−). For example, 47,XX,+21 indicates a female with trisomy 21. The long arm of a chromosome is designated by the letter q and the short arm by the letter p; therefore, 46,XX,4p− indicates a male with a deletion of the short arm of one of the 4 chromosomes. A ring chromosome is designated by the letter r. Other chromosome designations include t, translocation; del, deletion; and inv, inversion. If, for example, a translocation were involved, the designation would be t(2;8) with certain identified breakpoints which would then follow t(2;8)(q24;q23). The q would designate the long arm of the involved chromosomes and the numbers the breakpoints in the bands.

Sex Determination

In a normal female karyotype there is a pair of X chromosomes in addition to the 22 pairs of autosomes. The normal male has a single X and a Y chromosome. (A brief mention of some of the sex chromosome aneuploidies will be discussed later.)

Disorders Due to Chromosome Abnormalities

Cytogenetic studies of early spontaneous abortions suggest that one-half of all spontaneously aborted fetuses, once a pregnancy is recognized, have a chromosome abnormality. Many more conceptions with lethal chromosome abnormalities are thought to be lost right after conception and prior to missing the next menstrual period. The normal human complement of chromosomes has only been known in the last 30 years, and now it has become evident that one can have added or missing pieces of chromosomes or an ever-increasing number of described chromosome abnormalities. It is obviously impossible in this chapter to describe cytogenetic disorders extensively. We have restricted choice to some of the most frequent syndromes, which include trisomy 21, trisomy 13, and trisomy 18 and an example of a deletion.

During meiosis, a pair of chromosomes may not part from each other producing nondisjunction. The result is a gamete with 22 or 24 chromosomes; therefore, in fertilization a zygote will have either 45 or 47 chromosomes. Monosomy in general tends to be very lethal. Trisomies,

such as trisomy 21, 18, or 13, are occasionally viable. Nondisjunction sometimes occurs not in meiosis but in early division of the zygote. In this way it is possible not only to have 48 chromosomes, but multiple extra chromosomes. Multiple extra chromosomes are usually confined to the sex chromosomes. It is also possible for pieces of chromosomes to be exchanged between two chromosomes. A person with this rearrangement carries a balanced chromosome translocation. In this situation, there is usually no phenotypic expression in the carrier. There is, however, a higher risk of adverse reproductive outcome from unmatched pairing of these chromosomes resulting in an unbalanced chromosome abnormality in the fetus.

TRISOMY 21 (DOWN SYNDROME). Trisomy 21 (Fig. 5-3) is usually recognizable at birth and is the most common liveborn chromosome abnormality seen. The incidence is around 1 in every 700 to 800 births. About 95% of Down syndrome results from nondisjunction of the 21 chromosomes in either the egg or sperm with the zygote cell then having three 21 chromosomes rather than two after conception. Occasionally post-zygotic nondisjunctional events will occur which will produce mosaicism. The affected individual will often carry at least two cell lines, sometimes more, which may include a normal chromosome cell line in conjunction with an abnormal cell line such as trisomy 21 mosaicism. In the presence of mosaicism, the clinical findings may be somewhat modified, and prognosis for mental development is unpredictable because of the normal cell line. Less than 5% of Down syndrome is secondary to a

Fig. 5-3. A 6-month-old male with Down syndrome.

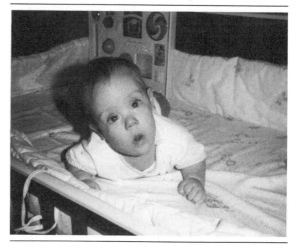

Robertsonian translocation in which a 21 may be attached to chromosomes 13, 14, 15, 21, or 22. The clinical presentation of Down syndrome is similar whether due to translocation or random trisomy. If a parent carries a chromosome translocation for Down syndrome, however, the risk of miscarriage and liveborn children with Down syndrome is significantly increased. For example, for translocation for Down syndrome involving the 14 and 21 chromosomes, the risk for a liveborn with Down syndrome is 10 to 20% for a woman carrying it and for a male carrying it 3 to 5%. This difference in risk between male and female carriers of this translocation is not completely understood.

Down syndrome children have some or all of the following features: external dysmorphic features including mild microcephaly, somewhat box-shaped head, upward slanting palpebral fissures, epicanthal folds (curves on the inside corner of the eye), Brushfield spots in the iris, depressed nasal bridge and protruding tongue, single transverse palmar crease (simian crease), short and bent fifth fingers (clinodactyly), and spacing between the first and second toes. Frequently associated malformations include: congenital heart defects (40–60%), congenital eye problems such as strabismus, and 10 to 20% incidence of gastrointestinal malformations such as duodenal atresia. Less frequently seen are problems such as cataracts, seizures, and atlantoaxial dislocation. All children with Down syndrome exhibit some degree of retarded psychomotor development, but with early intervention, special education, and supportive family environment they very often can lead happy, productive lives. Life expectancy has changed considerably in recent years because of medical intervention which includes heart surgery. Down syndrome children and adults, however, continue to show a higher and earlier mortality than the general population.

TRISOMY 18 (47,XX,+18). Trisomy 18 has an incidence of about 1 in 8000 live births, and there is about 1 : 4 sex ratio (male to female). At least 115 different malformations affecting every organ system have been noted in patients with trisomy 18. The most common abnormalities are growth deficiency (both intrauterine and extrauterine), profound developmental delay, prominent occiput, low-set and usually malformed eyes, micrognathia, flexed fingers (index overlaps 3rd, 5th overlaps 4th), short sternum, limited hip abduction, ventricular septal defect, and rocker-bottom feet. Most also show a single flexion crease on the fifth finger and transverse palmar lines. Affected infants are seriously retarded mentally. They usually die in early infancy. About 30% of patients die in the first 2 months with continued increased mortality in the first year. Few affected children survive childhood or adolescence.

TRISOMY 13 (47,XX,+13). The incidence of trisomy 13 is about 1 in 4000 to 10,000 live births with no sex predilection. The trisomy 13 infants appear more severely malformed than trisomy 18 infants, especially in the face. The phenotype in this syndrome is more variable than in either Down syndrome or the trisomy 18 syndrome.

Affected infants have some abnormalities in common with those of trisomy 18 — low birth weight for gestational age, flexion deformities of fingers, and rocker-bottom feet. Many have congenital heart defects, but characteristic of this group are microcephaly, serious eye defects (e.g., microphthalmia, iris colobomas, and cataracts), cleft palate or lip or both (often bilateral), and often defects of the nose (e.g., single nares). They are usually profoundly retarded mentally and do not usually survive for more than a few months. In a review of 221 patients with trisomy 13, approximately 50% lived to 1 month, 33% to 3 months, and 5% to 3 years of age.

DELETION CHROMOSOME ABNORMALITIES. *Wolf-Hirschhorn Syndrome (46,XX,4p−)*. Patients with this chromosome abnormality usually present with marked prenatal and postnatal growth deficiency, ocular hypertelorism with a broad or beaked nose, microcephaly, cranial asymmetry, cleft lip and palate, simple ears with preauricular tags or pits, skeletal abnormalites, and hypospadias in the male. Many die within the first 2 years of life. Those who have survived beyond early childhood continue to show slow growth and generally profound mental retardation.

As previously stated, patients with many chromosome abnormalities are recognized because the constellation of clinical findings is similar in affected patients and relatively commonly seen. Even in the absence of recognition of a well-known genetic syndrome secondary to a chromosome abnormality, chromosome analysis should be considered in the presentation of any infant with multiple congenital anomalies and/or mental retardation.

SEX CHROMOSOME ABNORMALITIES. Two major clinical syndromes are associated with sex chromosome aberrations in humans: Turner syndrome, which has a 45,X karyotype, and Klinefelter syndrome, which has a 47,XXY karyotype. Both of these chromosome abnormalities may be associated with mosaicism that involves normal karyotype or additional sex chromosome aberrations, for example, missing or additional pieces of whole X chromosomes. In addition, polysomic females are not uncommon.

Triple X females are calculated at an estimated frequency of 1 in 1000. In general females with one extra chromosome do not appear phenotypically different, though a small percentage may be dull normal or moderately retarded. In general, however, the addition of every X chromosome increases the incidence of identified mental retardation.

We will only briefly review Turner syndrome, Klinefelter syndrome, and 47,XYY males.

Turner Syndrome (45,X). About 95% of conceptions of 45,X chromosomes will spontaneously abort. About 50% of the liveborn females with Turner syndrome are the result of complete monosomy X while the other 50% will represent mosaic karyotypes as previously described. The most important mosaicism to rule out in Turner syndrome is the presence of any Y chromosome material: the presence of male gonadal tissue represents an increased risk of testicular tumors. Females with Y chromosome material should be evaluated early in life with potential removal of any identified male gonadal tissue. Newborn infants with Turner syndrome are phenotypically female. They usually present with multiple dysmorphic features which include small size, lymphedema of the hands and feet, low hairline, webbed neck, shield-shaped chest with widely spaced nipples, and cubitus valgus. The most common heart defects are co-arctation of the aorta, valvular aortic stenosis, or bicuspid aortic valve. Sexual infantilism persists through puberty with associated amenorrhea. Generally, Turner syndrome is not associated with mental retardation, but it does have associated learning disabilities.

Treatment for Turner syndrome involves estrogen replacement for sexual infantilism and menstruation. Growth hormone and alternatives are being studied for treatment of short stature. Children with Turner syndrome should be evaluated by pediatric endocrinologists.

Klinefelter Syndrome. When there is nondisjunction involving the X chromosomes, the product of the conception may have 47 chromosomes which include two X chromosomes and one Y. There are often few clinical manifestations until puberty, when somewhat feminizing features, including gynecomastia, cubitus valgus, and female distribution of fat, may be observed. In addition, there may be small testes. Many males with Klinefelter syndrome are only identified after they are married and infertility becomes evident. Most Klinefelter syndrome males have normal intelligence. The incidence in the newborn population is around 1 in 500. Again, if identified prior to puberty, hormone substitution therapy can begin at an appropriate time in order to allow for secondary sexual characteristics to develop.

47,XYY Syndrome. Most studies have shown that the presence of an extra Y chromosome predisposes these males to tall stature, more severe acne in puberty, aggressive behavior, and subnormal adult mentality. Many males with XYY karyotypes, however, are normal. It is presently uncertain to what extent mental defect or the chromosome ab-

normality influences or determines the behavioral traits observed in this syndrome. The frequency is considered to be about 1 in 1000 boys.

Fragile X Syndrome. The fragile X syndrome has been recognized in the last 12 years as a unique disorder because of its atypical X-linked inheritance pattern, and its frequency. It is presently believed to be the most common cause of male mental retardation second to Down syndrome and is the most common familial cause of mental retardation. It is an X-linked inherited disease in which one-third of carrier females manifest similar clinical findings to affected males. Cytogenetically only 40 to 50% of females who are carriers for fragile X actually manifest the fragile site on the X chromosome. The fragile site on the X chromosome is never seen in every cell of an affected person. The percentage of cells that carry this fragile site varies from 1 to 50% and may vary over time. Cytogenetic analysis for fragile X is different from usual chromosome techniques because the blood must be grown in folic acid–deficient or induced folate-deficient media. In general, when analyzing cells for fragile X at least two different media are used to produce the fragile site. On the X chromosome is seen either narrowing or cutting at Xq27.3 band. In doing fragile X screening, around 100 to 150 lymphocytes are screened. Because the culture and screening techniques are different for fragile X syndrome, one must specifically request fragile X screening and not assume it will be done as part of a karyotype analysis. Two to three ml of blood in a sodium heparin tube is sufficient for study.

Clinically, the three classic physical manifestations of fragile X are macroorchidism in the postpubertal male, larger, prominent ears, and a long, narrow face with a protruding chin. About 80% of affected males will have one or more of these features. Behavior problems include poor eye contact, stereotype behavior, and autistic-like mannerisms, hyperactivity, and attention deficit disorders. Affected patients may have mild learning disabilities to severe mental retardation. Speech abnormalities are also an important clinical finding. Fragile X screening should be considered in any male with learning disabilities and/or mental retardation of unknown etiology. In any family history with possible X-linked mental retardation, including affected females, fragile X syndrome should be considered in the differential diagnosis. Because of its X-linked pattern of inheritance, fragile X syndrome represents a significant risk of similarly affected family members. Prenatal diagnosis using both cytogenetic and DNA molecular techniques are now available for fragile X syndrome.

There is no specific cure yet for fragile X syndrome, but treatment using folic acid therapy and appropriate CNS stimulants for behavior problems have been utilized. The associated learning disabilities and behavioral abnormalities are becoming increasingly well-defined. Appropriate behavior modification and educational intervention is now available.

For more detailed information on the presently defined chromosome aberrations, the reference textbooks at the end of this chapter are recommended.

Congenital Malformations

The most important clinical question to be answered with a malformation is whether it is isolated or part of a malformation syndrome. The prognosis and risk of recurrence in future pregnancies can vary greatly according to the answer to this question. The majority of developmental anomalies do not follow a simple pattern of inheritance, and they are secondary to multifactorial or polygenic inheritance. By definition, a multifactorial defect is one due to the additive effect of a genetic predisposition and nongenetic (environmental) factors. Common birth defects include congenital heart anomalies, cleft lip and palate, clubfoot, pyloric stenosis, congenital dislocation of the hip, and hypospadias. Table 5-4 depicts empiric risks for some of the common multifactorial congenital disorders. In general, about 45% of malformations are due to multifactorial inheritance, 31% to a single gene mutation, 15% to chromosomal aberrations, and 9% to infections or teratogens, especially drugs or alcohol intake by the mother.

CONSTRUCTION OF FAMILY PEDIGREE. Even when the exact nature of the disease is in doubt, the family history can provide valuable clues as to its mode of inheritance upon which genetic counseling may be based.

Pedigrees are constructed as follows: circles (O) are used for females; squares (□) for males. Horizontal lines represent matings, and vertical lines their offspring.

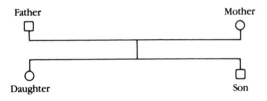

Affected individuals are denoted by solid figures (■, ●). An arrow is used to point to the first case noted (the proband). A large number of symbols are utilized in pedigree construction, usually with a table explaining their meaning. Some examples are: ■, miscarriage; ═, consanguineous; □–□, identical twins; ◇, sex unknown; O O, twins; ■, ▨, or D, dead; S or √, examined; and ◖, carrier of disease.

Suppose a boy is suffering from muscular dystrophy inherited as an X-linked recessive (he is the proband); family history reveals that his maternal grandfather died of the same condition. The rest of the family is examined, and it is discovered that the proband's brother is also affected. The remainder are normal. The pedigree might then look as follows:

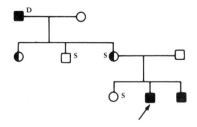

Table 5-4. Empirical Risks for Some Common Disorders (%)

Disorder	Incidence	Sex ratio M:F	Normal parent having second affected child	Affected parent having affected child	Affected parent having second affected child
Anencephaly	0.20	1:3	4–5	—	—
Cleft palate only	0.05	2:3 (Caucasian)	2	7	15
Cleft lip, with or without cleft palate	0.10	3:2 (Caucasian)	4	4	12
Clubfoot	0.10	2:1	3	3	10
Congenital heart disease (all types)	0.8	—	1–4	1–4	—
Pyloric stenosis	0.30	5:1	2	4	13
Male index			2	4	13
Female index			10	17	38
Spina bifida	0.1–0.3	1:1	4	4	—

PARENTAL AGE. The age of parents at the time of a child's birth should also be noted. There is a significant rise in the frequency of fetal aneuploidy with advanced maternal age. An increased incidence of autosomal dominant new mutations such as achondroplasia has been described with advanced paternal age.

ORIGIN AND ETHNIC BACKGROUNDS. Particular attention must be paid to the place of origin and the ethnic background of patients. Certain genetic traits are more common in some areas or races; e.g., familial dysautonomia, Niemann-Pick disease (type A), Gaucher's disease, Bloom's syndrome, and Tay-Sachs disease occur more frequently in Ashkenazi Jews, and sickle-cell anemia occurs most frequently in blacks.

Mendelian Modes of Inheritance

Chromosomes are arranged in homologous pairs, each gene having an opposite number. A mutation can occur at any site (locus) along the chromosome. Competing genes at a locus are called alleles. In certain conditions a single mutation is sufficient to cause a given clinical effect. These disorders are said to be dominant (the effect of the mutant gene dominates over its normal allele). When a double dose of the mutant gene is required to bring about a clinical change, the mode of inheritance is called recessive. The affected person is homozygous for that locus when both genes are of the same kind and, conversely, is heterozygous when the genes are dissimilar. The genes in question may be located on somatic chromosomes (autosomal inheritance) or on the sex chromosomes (X-linked inheritance).

Hereditary diseases, due to mutations at a single locus, tend to follow the Mendelian laws of inheritance. They behave as follows:

AUTOSOMAL DOMINANT INHERITANCE. A pedigree showing typical autosomal dominant inheritance is shown in Figure 5-4. With the autosomal dominant mode of inheritance, a trait may be identified from generation to generation. Each offspring of an affected parent stands a 50% chance of inheriting the trait. The chances are the same for each child independent of birth order or sex. The presence of two or three or only one affected of five children in a family does not negate autosomal dominant inheritance.

Also seen in autosomal dominant inheritance are two important genetic principles: penetrance and expressivity. Penetrance denotes whether someone will have any phenotypic manifestations in carrying a mutant gene. Some autosomal dominantly inherited diseases such as neurofibromatosis have a high degree of penetrance, but some such as dominantly inherited colobomas may have reduced pene-

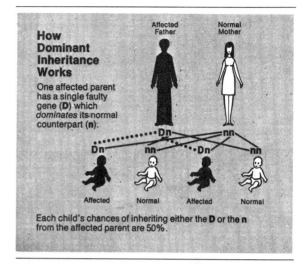

Fig. 5-4. How dominant inheritance works. (From Genetic Counseling. *New York: The National Foundation—March of Dimes.)*

trance; therefore, it is possible for diseases with reduced penetrance to appear to "skip" generations in affected families. The expressivity of a mutant gene means how affected will someone be in having this dominantly inherited condition. It is not uncommon in families in which multiple members are affected with a dominant disease that there be marked variability in expression of the disease within family members.

Genetic diseases can arise de novo; therefore, it is possible and often the most likely explanation in many families that an affected child represents an autosomal dominant new mutation in that family. Their recurrence risk may be extremely low, but the affected child may then go on to have a 50% risk in each pregnancy of similarly affected children. In recent years it has become apparent that germ-line mosaicism exists for some inherited diseases; therefore, when a couple have an affected child with what appears to be autosomal dominant new mutation, the recurrence risk may not be zero.

AUTOSOMAL RECESSIVE INHERITANCE. With autosomal recessive inheritance the clinical effect is apparent in the homozygous state. The affected child inherits one deleterious gene from each parent. Figure 5-5 illustrates the various genotypes in their relative proportions expected from the mating of two heterozygous individuals, N representing the normal gene and r the mutant gene. The chances

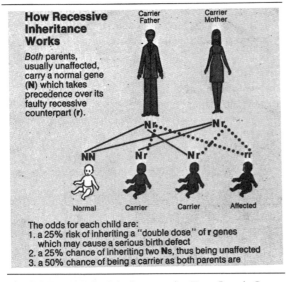

Fig. 5-5. *How recessive inheritance works. (From* Genetic Counseling. *New York: The National Foundation—March of Dimes.)*

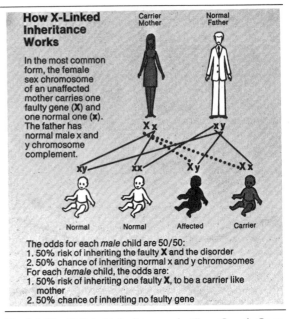

Fig. 5-6. *How X-linked inheritance works. (From* Genetic Counseling. *New York: The National Foundation—March of Dimes.)*

that any offspring will be affected are 1 in 4. Considerable effort is being directed toward heterozygote detection, because it offers a means of identification of high-risk families prior to the birth of an affected child.

X-LINKED INHERITANCE. The cardinal rule in this mode of inheritance (Fig. 5-6) is that the trait cannot be passed by a father to his son. A son, by definition, has inherited the father's Y chromosome and not the X.

X-linked disorders also may be recessive or dominant. Because males have only one X chromosome, a single mutant gene is enough to cause clinical effects. For this reason, X-linked recessive traits are usually confined to the male sex. (See Fragile X Syndrome for atypical X-linked inheritance.)

By drawing a diagram similar to the one used for autosomal recessive inheritance, students can satisfy themselves that each male offspring of a mating between a normal father and a carrier mother has a 50% chance of being affected, and each daughter has a 50% chance of being a carrier.

X-linked dominant traits are uncommon. The same cardinal rule applies. X-linked dominant traits resemble autosomal dominants except that there is no male-to-male transmission. Often in X-linked dominant diseases the trait is lethal in an affected male; therefore, a family with such a disease has affected females, unaffected males, and, perhaps, multiple miscarriages or stillborn males.

CONSANGUINITY. The frequency of recessively inherited diseases among offspring of consanguineous marriages is higher than among children of unrelated couples. People with a common ancestor are more likely to carry identical genes. For example, if an individual who has inherited a deleterious gene from a grandfather were to marry a first cousin, who has a $\frac{1}{8}$ chance of carrying the same gene, the risk of producing a homozygous or affected child is $\frac{1}{8} \times \frac{1}{4} = \frac{1}{32}$. This is a much higher risk than occurs in random mating. However, considering all first-cousin marriages, the actual risk of producing a child with a recessive disorder is not very high, and the majority of children from such marriages are quite healthy. The calculated risk is about 3% greater than the general population risk. Consanguinity is likely to be found in families with children affected by rare recessive disorders. In a more common disorder such as cystic fibrosis, the carrier frequency is about 1 in 20–25 Caucasians; therefore, the majority of affected patients are born to nonconsanguineous couples.

Detection of Carriers

Genetic counseling is becoming less conjectural as we are able to detect the heterozygous or carrier state in more diseases. As more specific etiologies are defined for many inherited diseases, carrier risks become better defined. As will be discussed later, the rapid advancement in molecular genetics which has allowed DNA diagnosis for many diseases will provide in many families accurate information on carrier status and prenatal diagnosis. For example, about 70% of males affected with Duchenne's muscular dystrophy have a deletion in the X chromosome, therefore, allowing much more accurate diagnosis of carrier status. Even in those family members of a living affected patient, in whom a deletion has not been seen, DNA linkage analysis of the X chromosome will allow highly informative carrier or non-carrier status and prenatal diagnosis in pregnancies at risk.

An unaffected sibling of an affected patient with a known autosomal recessively inherited disease has a 2/3 risk of being a carrier of that disease. It is extremely important when identifying an inherited disease in a family history to discuss with a clinical geneticist about the availability of carrier testing for that disease. Rapid advances in diagnostic techniques continue to identify more diseases with enzyme deficiencies, and informative DNA analysis allows carrier detection and prenatal diagnosis.

Inborn Errors of Metabolism

Most metabolic disorders follow a straight Mendelian mode of inheritance: recessive, dominant, or X-linked. Although most inherited genetic diseases are individually rare, they compose a significant fraction of human disease. About 1% of newborns have an inborn error of metabolism. Over 4000 single mutations in human beings have been recorded so far. Most of the inherited metabolic disorders are transmitted as autosomal recessive diseases. Some are X-linked, and a few, for which there is presently a known biochemical abnormality, are inherited as autosomal dominant diseases. In the last 20 years, there has been an exponential increase in our ability to define both enzyme deficiencies and to identify biochemical aberrations; therefore, it is impossible to present all the presently known inherited metabolic diseases in this section. Instead we will focus on clinical presentation and appropriate evaluation in order to rule out or identify the potential of a metabolic disease in a sick neonate, infant, or child.

The diversity of clinical manifestations in inherited metabolic diseases is obvious. There are conditions which hardly interfere with ability or normal lifespan, for example pentosuria and fructosuria, while others, if untreated, may be extremely life-threatening, such as maple syrup urine disease, or cause mental retardation, such as phenylketonuria (PKU). Symptoms may become apparent at birth or appear

at any time thereafter into adulthood. The duration of the symptom-free interval depends on toxicity and rate of accumulation of certain metabolites, although the metabolic error has been present from fetal life. Presently, the inborn errors of metabolism can be classified as errors in amino acids, organic acids, urea cycle defects (nitrogen), carbohydrate, fatty acids, serum proteins, abnormal mineral metabolism, and energy defects. Other classifications include abnormalities within cell organelles such as lysosomal storage diseases, peroxisomal disorders, and mitochondrial diseases.

An inborn error of metabolism may result in failure of formation of certain proteins, accumulation of breakdown products because of a missing enzyme, or a transport defect that does not allow a necessary metabolite into cell organelles for processing. In general, the site of the disturbance is marked by accumulation of a substrate and other metabolites of the substrate and by deficiency of products and their action. Secondary alterations in other enzyme functions may also result from inhibition by increasing levels of substrates.

Many of the inborn errors of metabolism cannot be specifically treated, although one can provide a reduction in substrate load (protein restriction), provide calories in alternate pathways, treat acute symptoms (dialysis), and supplement with cofactors. Some diseases, however, are specifically treatable by restriction of a specific metabolite or addition of supplements. Because some of these diseases are treatable, screening is provided in all of the United States. Most states provide screening for phenylketonuria and hypothyroidism, while many additionally screen for galactosemia, homocystinuria, and maple syrup urine disease. Virginia also screens for biotinidase deficiency, because it, too, is a treatable metabolic disorder.

Metabolic diseases complicate clinical pictures for sick neonates or children, because the symptoms are nonspecific and may mimic sepsis or respiratory disease. It is often advisable, therefore, to evaluate newborns, infants, and children while supportive treatment for acquired diseases is ongoing. Indiscriminate study, however, of all ill newborns or children for metabolic disorders may not be warranted.

Clinical manifestations are not specific to the metabolic disorders. A child with a metabolic disorder may well be susceptible to sepsis, respiratory disease, and intracranial hemorrhage; therefore, one may be treating several problems while awaiting final laboratory evaluations. The general clinical presentation of various groups of inborn errors will be reviewed in order to focus evaluation for the specific disorders. This will be followed by the relevant laboratory investigations for screening and specific diagnosis of these diseases.

Inborn Errors of Amino Acid Metabolism

The clinical presentation of a disorder caused by inborn errors of amino acid metabolism in the neonate usually consists of feeding problems, vomiting, lethargy, and seizures within a few days of life. The feeding problems can include poor suck and vomiting. There may be abnormalities of tone which can vary from examination to examination from hypotonia to hypertonia, and reflexes may be lost.

In the older infant or child one may see a clinical picture of failure to thrive, mental retardation, and seizures. One can also see an intermittent picture of worsening of neurological signs precipitated by infection and fever, which increases endogenous protein catabolism. Some amino acid disorders have associated and distinctive odors, which may be an important diagnostic clue. Examples include the mousy odor of untreated PKU and the peculiar maple syrup or curry odor of maple syrup urine disease (Table 5-5).

Table 5-5. Some Important Treatable Inborn Errors of Metabolism

Disease[a]	Clinical findings	Laboratory findings
Cystinosis	FTT[b], renal failure, Fanconi's syndrome, renal calculi crystals seen on slit lamp exam. Treatment: cysteamine and supportive as per chronic renal disease; renal transplantation	Elevated cystine, arginine, lysine, ornithine, renal tubular acidosis; phosphaturia crystals seen in many body tissues. Lysosomal transport disorder. Carrier testing and prenatal diagnosis available
Nonketotic hyperglycinemia	FTT, MR[c], lethargy, seizures, coma after valine loads, vomiting, acidosis; neurodegenerative presentation is atypical. Treatment: supportive; protein restriction and sodium benzoate tried	Elevated glycine levels in urine, plasma, and cerebrospinal fluid. Ketosis absent. Ammonia elevated in some
Homocystinuria (methioninemia), variable presentation	Newborn screening in many states; Marfan-like, tall stature, ectopic lens, thromboembolus, MR, seizures, dementia, schizophrenia. Treatment: some are pyridoxine responsive; dietary methionine restriction; betaine being tried	Elevated homocystine levels in blood and urine; high or low levels of homocystine methionine in blood; cystathionine beta-synthase, gamma-cystathionase or hepatic methathionine adenosyl-transferase deficiency
Phenylalanine phenylketonuria (PKU)	Newborn screening; incidence is 1/14,000; MR, musty odor, eczema, vomiting, microcephaly. Treatment: restriction of phenylalanine in diet (levels ≤ 5 mg/100 ml); restriction to continue for pregnant PKU females to prevent birth defects of exposed fetuses	Elevated phenylpyruvic acid and phenylacetic acid in urine; plasma phenylalanine >20 mg/ml; deficiency of hepatic phenylalanine hydroxylase (PAH); PAH alleles on chromosome 12q22-24 region with DNA linkage analysis available; carrier testing, prenatal diagnosis available
Hyperphenylalaninemai (non-PKU)	Transient or persistent, less common than PKU, usually benign clinical course. Phenylalanine levels should be reduced in pregnancy to protect fetus	Elevated phenylalanine (Phe) levels in blood. Often no Phe metabolites in urine. DNA allelic mutations on chromosome 12
Hyperphenylalaninemia tetrahydrobiopterin and BH_4 deficient forms	MR, microcephaly, eczema, musty odor; neurologic progression despite phenylalanine restriction. Treatment: BH_4, DOPA, or 5-hydroxytryptophan supplements; for dihydropteridine reductase (DHPR) deficiency, folinic acid or other forms of tetrahydrofolate. Prenatal diagnosis available	Phe metabolites in urine; elevated Phe in blood; variable BH_4 or DHPR deficiencies in various somatic tissues. Allelic mutation on chromosome 4p15. Some unknown

Table 5-5. (Continued)

Disease[a]	Clinical findings	Laboratory findings
Ornithine transcarbamylase (OTC) deficiency, a urea cycle defect	MR, vomiting, lethargy, apnea, seizures, coma; X-linked inheritance, variable course but many males die in infancy. Variable expression in females: many avoid proteins. Treatment: protein restriction, sodium benzoate, and phenylacetate	Hyperammonemia; elevated orotic acid levels; variable deficiency of OTC in liver; carrier studies by protein loading and DNA analysis. DNA deletion and linkage analysis, prenatal diagnosis available
Maple syrup urine disease (MSUD)	Newborn screening in some states. Variable presentation: severe, early onset; mild variant, intermittent. MR, feeding difficulty, CNS deterioration, urine odor of maple syrup when ill. Treatment: restriction of branched-chain AAs as needed	Amino aciduria and amino acidemia; variable elevations of valine, leucine, isoleucine ketonuria; hypoglycemia. In various tissues inherited defects in mitochondrial multienzyme complex, branched-chain alphaketoacid dehydrogenase. Prenatal diagnosis available
Organic Acids		
Propionic acidemia	MR, FTT, vomiting, acidosis; biotin-responsive subtype. Treatment: restriction of protein and, especially, methionine, threonine, valine, and isoleucine	Ketonemia, acidosis, elevated urine tiglyglycine, methylcitrate, beta-hydroxypropionate. Assay of propionyl-CoA carboxylase deficiency (two subunit abnormalities) in leukocytes and fibroblasts. Prenatal diagnosis available
Methylmalonic acidemia	MR, FTT, acidosis, vomiting, lethargy, coma; multiple types. Treatment: some B_{12}-responsive; protein restriction	Ketoacidosis; hyperglycinemia, hypoglycinemia, neutropenia, elevated plasma, and urine methylmalonic acid. Several mutations known: deficiencies of methylmalonyl-CoA mutase and adenosyl cobalamin synthesis abnormalities. Prenatal diagnosis available
Carbohydrate Metabolism		
Galactosemia	Newborn screening; FTT, vomiting, liver disease, cataracts, MR. Treatment: dietary restriction of galactose	Urine reducing substances; generalized aminoaciduria, liver dysfunction, deficiency of galactose-1-phosphate uridyl transferase or generalized diphosphate galactose-4-epimerase. The uridine diphosphate galactose-4-epimerase deficiency limited to red cells and white cells appears to have benign clinical course. Prenatal diagnosis available
Galactokinase deficiency	Picked up on newborn screening; cataracts are main clinical feature	Positive urine reducing substance; galactokinase deficiency

[a] Inheritance is autosomal recessive.
[b] Failure-to-thrive.
[c] Mental retardation.

Inborn Errors of Urea Cycle

Urea cycle disorders will present with clinical findings similar to the inborn errors of amino acid metabolism. In addition, one may see rapid and progressive coma and hyperammonemia. Vomiting in the urea cycle disorders is usually mediated by the central nervous sytem in association with the hyperammonemia. Respiratory distress and apnea seen in urea cycle disorders usually results from the toxic encephalopathy that is the end result of this disease. Organomegaly can also be seen.

Inborn Errors of Organic Acids

These, too, may present with symptoms similar to the inborn errors of amino acid metabolism. In addition, one may see metabolic acidosis with or without ketosis, hypoglycemia, and, therefore, hyperpnea. Respiratory distress and apnea may also be seen. Occasionally cardiac enlargement with failure is also evident.

Inborn Errors of Carbohydrate Metabolism

Clinical presentation is similar to the other inborn errors. In addition, one may see diarrhea or significant hepatotoxicity with jaundice, hepatomegaly, and liver dysfunction. The typical carbohydrate disorder is galactosemia (see Table 5-5).

Laboratory Investigations

Because the clinical presentation of these disorders is not distinct, laboratory evaluation is extremely important. Two general categories of laboratory testing are: (1) those tests that can be done in most hospital clinical settings, and (2) studies that usually should be referred to specialty labs. In a patient suspected of having an inborn error of metabolism, initial studies are:

Complete blood count and differential
Plasma electrolytes and blood pH
Plasma glucose and ammonia
Blood lactate and blood pyruvate
Urine reducing substances and urine ketones

Although abnormal results may not diagnose specifically an inborn error of metabolism, the abnormality usually indicates one category of disease. It is also important to correct an identified abnormality such as hypoglycemia while awaiting more specific diagnostic testing. For example,the organic acidoses can produce bone marrow

dysfunction, which can include pancytopenia requiring treatment. Metabolic acidosis is an important clue to an organic acid disorder, which often needs treatment while awaiting further studies. Ketones in the urine are extremely rare even in the severely ill newborn with hypoglycemia and are an important clue to an organic acid disorder such as maple syrup urine disease, methylmalonic, or propionic acidemia. Ammonia elevations can be seen in defects of the urea cycles or in the organic acidemias. If one sees a combination of elevated ammonia levels with metabolic acidosis, an inborn error of organic acid metabolism is possible, while a normal acid base balance with elevated ammonia suggests a urea cycle problem. Newborns may normally have higher ammonia levels (up to twice the upper limit of normal described for adults).

Elevated blood lactate and pyruvate levels in the presence or absence of metabolic acidosis are present in disorders of the mitochondria such as pyruvate dehydrogenase deficiency.

Testing urine for reducing substance is a fast and simple screening for galactosemia; however, for the urine test to be positive the infant needs to have received a galactose-containing nutrient.

Special Studies

Special studies are often referred to more central labs with greater experience in interpreting results. Special studies include serum or plasma amino acids (2–3 ml of blood), plasma carnitine (2–3 ml of blood), urine amino acids, and urine organic acids (10–20 ml of urine). If one is looking for a specific problem, less urine can be used in diagnosis. If it is difficult to obtain the necessary urine, one can call the refering lab to inquire as to the minimum amount needed so as not to delay diagnosis. Most amino acid studies are done with the amino acid analyzer, which uses ion exchange chromatography or high performance liquid chromatography. Quantitative organic acids are most often studied using automated gas chromatography and mass spectrometry. Urinary screening with spot tests is still used to evaluate quickly some patients. This screening would involve reducing substances for galactosemia, ferric chloride-positive, p-hydroxyphenylpyruvic acid of tyrosinemia, and the dinitrophenylhydrazine-positive ketoacids of maple syrup urine disease.

Carnitine is a micronutrient responsible for the transport of fatty acids into the mitochondria. Carnitine deficiency, whether primary or secondary, is a treatable problem; therefore, measurements of free plasma or acylcarnitine levels in patients with possible organic acidemia are recommended as carnitine supplementation may be indicated.

Once a metabolic disorder is identified by analysis of plasma and urine metabolite levels, enzymatic confirmation for many defects is available. Only certain laboratories may be available to do these studies. Some coordination of efforts may be required to obtain and transport the required tissues for study. It is important, however, to confirm the diagnosis of an inborn error of metabolism in order to provide accurate prenatal diagnosis and to distinguish possible variants of a disorder that may require distinct or different therapies.

If an infant or child is admitted with a rapid fatal disease for which a metabolic problem is even suspected, every attempt to obtain tissue, even at postmortem, should be made. Routine laboratory analyses previously described should be performed. Plasma and urine for amino acid and organic acid analysis should be obtained and frozen. A skin biopsy for fibroblasts should also be requested, and a postmortem exam obtained as soon as possible. Multiple tissues, especially muscle and liver, should be not only processed for microscopy (light and electron histochemistry), but some should be frozen for further study. There are many case reports of deceased patients in which this has been accomplished and diagnoses made after death. These studies have enabled families to obtain appropriate genetic counseling and allowed accurate prenatal diagnosis in future pregnancies.

A few of the treatable inborn errors of metabolism are listed in Table 5-5. The references at the end of this chapter include important and relevant textbooks for further study.

Lysosomal Storage Diseases

Lysosomal storage diseases are generally divided into three categories: the mucopolysaccharidoses, the sphingolipidoses, and the mucolipidoses. Clinical presentation can vary, but in general these diseases are characterized by both physical and mental regression over a variable period of time. Physical findings often include coarsening of facial features, organomegaly, ocular changes like optic atrophy or cherry-red spots, macrocephaly, and often progressive bony abnormalities including shortening of limbs or thickening of joints, actual thickening of skin, and progressive neurologic disease including spasticity. Progression of the disorder may be seen in an affected child who appears clinically normal for some time after birth, but who will then either lose milestones or will fail to progress (i.e., regress). Although low levels or absence of enzyme activity are seen in most of these diseases, progression of the disease can be

highly variable with variable clinical presentation and manifestation in infants, children, or even adults.

Evaluation for the mucopolysaccharidoses can include x rays of hands and lateral spine, where dysostosis multiplex can be found in some of these diseases. Around 20 to 30 ml of urine should be collected for mucopolysaccharide spot test as well as thin layer chromatography. The specific enzyme assays can be performed on leukocytes derived from whole blood (8 to 10 ml) and/or serum (San Filippo type B and I cell disease).

Biochemical testing of white cells or serum may be diagnostic or suggestive of any of these diseases. Confirmation in a second tissue, such as fibroblasts, is recommended. In addition, some patients may present with findings of a storage disease in which the presently known enzymes are not deficient. In this situation, tissue (either skin, rectal biopsy, or sural nerve) may be obtained and studied under the electron microscope for evidence of storage cells, thereby providing a more specific diagnosis. In order to illustrate the variety of clinical presentations and individual enzyme deficiencies in some of the storage diseases, Table 5-6 delineates most of the known spingholipidoses.

In general, these diseases are not curable, but medical treatment offered recently for those diseases without brain involvement has included bone marrow transplantation. Otherwise, treatment is symptomatic.

In both mucopolysaccharidosis and sphingolipidosis, the mode of inheritance is considered autosomal recessive with the exceptions being Hunter disease in the mucopolysaccharide diseases and Fabry disease in sphingolipidosis, both of which are X-linked. There is a recently defined group of storage diseases called the mucolipidoses. These, too, appear to present with a clinical mixture of motor, mental, and physical regression. Enzyme assays have to be correlated with the clinical findings. Specific diagnosis is important not only to identify prognosis but also to provide carrier status and accurate prenatal diagnosis in at-risk pregnancies.

Peroxisomal Disorders

In recent years a new group of genetic diseases has been defined involving disorders of the peroxisome, an essential organelle in the human cell. Rapid advances in this area of human disease have allowed classification of peroxisomal disorders into three groups. Clinical findings in these diseases can range from neonatal presentation with profound hypotonia, multiple congenital anomalies, dwarfism, seizures, and biochemical abnormalities, to slower onset degenerative neurologic disease, ophthalmologic abnormalities such as retinitis pigmentosa, and variable mental

62

Table 5-6. Some Lysosomal Storage Disorders: Sphingolipidoses[a]

Disease	Enzyme deficiency	Clinical findings	Laboratory findings
GM$_1$ gangliosidosis	Acidic beta-galactosidase	Infantile form, type I, MR, coarse facies, corneal opacity, seizures, hypotonicity to decerebrate rigidity, hepatosplenomegaly, macrocephaly, macroglossia, ± cherry-red spot Type II; juvenile ataxia, seizures, strabismus, loss of speech. Motor weakness to decerebrate rigidity, blindness, dysphagia	Vacuolated peripheral leukocytes; foamy histiocytes in bone marrow; DEA in serum, WBC, and fibroblasts
GM$_2$ gangliosidoses Type I: Tay-Sachs disease	Hexosaminidase A	Onset at 3–6 months, cherry-red macula, motor weakness to decerebrate rigidity, blindness, dysphagia	DEA in serum, WBC, and fibroblasts
Type II: Sandhoff's disease	Hexosaminidase A and B	Virtually identical to Tay-Sachs disease	Accumulation of GM$_2$ ganglioside and its asialo derivative in neural tissue and visceral organs. DEA in serum, WBC, and fibroblasts
Type III: Juvenile GM$_2$ gangliosidosis	Hexosaminidase A	Onset at 2–6 years, neurologic deterioration to decerebrate rigidity, ataxia, no cherry-red macula, but blindness from optic atrophy. Adult form also seen	Neuronal lipidosis, DEA WBC, serum, and fibroblasts
Fabry's disease	Alpha-galactosidase A	Corneal opacities, skin lesions (angiokeratomas), X-linked	Myelin-like lamellar cytoplasmic inclusion bodies. DEA in WBC, fibroblasts, and plasma
Gaucher's disease	Beta-glucosidase	Hepatosplenomegaly, delayed development, strabismus, osteoporosis of long bones, anemia, thrombocytopenia. At least 3–4 subtypes with acute/chronic neuropathic and nonneuropathic forms. Bone marrow treatment offered in nonneuropathic	Anemia, thrombocytopenia, DEA in WBC, fibroblasts
Niemann-Pick disease	Syphingomyelinase	Hepatosplenomegaly, MR, growth retardation, anemia, and thrombocytopenia Types A–D depending on progression and neuropathic findings	DEA in WBC and fibroblasts
Krabbe's disease (globoid cell leukodystrophy)	Galactocerebroside beta-galactosidase	Chronic crying, excessive irritability, progressive muscular rigidity, and early death	DEA in leukocytes and cultured fibroblasts
Metachromatic leukodystrophy (MLD)	Arylsulfatase A	Progressive psychomotor and neurologic deterioration, ataxia, blindness, dysphagia, variable onset and progression, infantile, juvenile, and adult types	DEA in WBC and fibroblasts, elevated CSF protein, decreased nerve conduction velocity

MR = mental retardation; DEA = decreased enzyme activity.

retardation or behavioral abnormalities. Peroxisomal disorders can present at any point in life with evidence of neurologic disease that can be rapidly or slowly progressive and evidence of storage problems with hepatomegaly and evidence of adrenal hypofunction.

The first group of disorders involves general peroxisomal dysfunction. This includes Zellweger's syndrome, infantile type of Refsum disease, neonatal adrenoleukodystrophy, and hyperpipecolic acidemia. Chemical abnormalities include elevations of very long chain fatty acids (c26 : c22 ratio) in plasma (or serum). Abnormalities of pipecolic acid and phytanic acid can be seen if initial diagnosis is made, and further specific enzyme studies in white cells or fibroblasts can be pursued.

The second group includes impairment of some but not all peroxisomal functions, which includes rhizomelic chondrodysplasia punctata, a neonatal presentation of disproportionate short stature, cataracts, shortened lifespan, and severe mental retardation. This diagnosis must be made by analysis of plasmalogen in red cells: it is severely decreased in this disease.

The third group includes peroxisomal disorders with impairment of a single peroxisomal function. This includes acatalasemia, X-linked adrenoleukodystrophy, adrenomyeloneuropathy, adult type of Refsum disease, peroxisomal acyl-CoA oxidase deficiency, hyperoxaluria, and others. Here, diagnosis requires analysis of a specific enzyme, such as catalase, or a determination of a specific product such as phytanic acid in adult Refsum disease.

Analysis for these diseases usually involves contacting a specific lab that has expertise with these analyses; therefore, prior to initiating these studies, an evaluation should involve a geneticist or biochemical specialist. In general, one obtains 1 to 5 ml of plasma in an EDTA tube. The sample is centrifuged, separated, and frozen, and then sent to the lab within 24 hours of drawing the blood. A pellet of red cells is obtained from 2 to 10 ml of blood. Five to ten ml of urine from a clean collection issent for N-acetyl-L-aspartic determination. Skin biopsies for fibroblast studies may be obtained. These diseases are amenable to prenatal diagnosis.

Mitochondrial Diseases

In the last few years, abnormalities in mitochondrial function have been found to be responsible for a wide variety of neurologic and neuromuscular conditions. Mitochondria are considered the "power plants" of the cell, generating the high energy phosphate bond in ATP by phosphorylation of ADP. There is a considerable amount of energy required for this reaction which is derived from oxidation of metabolic products of carbohydrates, fatty acids, and proteins. Mitochondrial DNA differs from DNA in the cell nucleus in three important ways: (1) it is transmitted exclusively by mothers, (2) it contains very few noncoding sequences (introns), and (3) it has a slightly different genetic code. Codes for 13 proteins which are part of the mitochondrial respiratory change are known, as well as two ribosomal RNAs and 22 transfer RNAs.

The mitochondrial diseases include both myopathies and encephalopathies, which are clinically and biochemically heterogeneous. Characteristic histologic findings are "ragged red fibers" seen in muscle biopsy specimens. Clinically, they can present from birth to adulthood with findings that include infantile lactic acidosis, progressive external ophthalmoplegia (Kearns-Sayre syndrome), myopathy (with weakness exacerbated by exercise), and Leigh disease (subacute necrotizing encephalomyopathy). These are multisystem disorders that often affect the central nervous system causing seizures, ataxia, dementia, movement disorders, and stroke-like episodes. Retinopathy, deafness, peripheral neuropathy, cardiac conduction defects, and renal dysfunction also occur. This important group of diseases must be considered in the differential diagnosis of any of these clinical presentations.

Initial biochemical evaluation includes blood for pH, lactates, and pyruvates. If abnormalities are considered primary, further biochemical or histologic studies of skin, muscle, and liver are indicated. If initial biochemical findings suggest the likelihood of such a diagnosis, it is important to involve a geneticist or metabolic disease expert in order to optimize evaluation. One of the most important factors of mitochondrial diseases is that mitochondrial DNA is maternally inherited; therefore, for some mitochondrial diseases, there is a 100% risk of affected offspring if the mother is affected. An example is Leber hereditary optic atrophy, which causes acute or subacute blindness in young adults and is much more common in men than women. It is only transmitted maternally and is thus different from X-linked inheritance in that the descendants of affected men are never affected. Point mutations of mitochondrial DNA in affected family members have been delineated in this disease. In those mitochondrial DNA diseases that are not maternally inherited, mutations of the genetic information that resides in nuclear DNA may directly affect formation or structure of mitochondrial proteins or alter mitochondrial gene expression. These diseases, therefore, can appear to be sporadic or in some families inherited.

Fatty Acid Oxidation Abnormalities

Inborn errors involving oxidative metabolism of fatty acids are also a newly recognized area of human disease. These also involve metabolism within mitochondria. Classically, fatty acid oxidation abnormalities present with hypoketotic hypoglycemia. It is important to recognize these diseases, because clinically they may resemble Reye syndrome. There is a high degree of mortality with the first clinical presentation. Family histories can include sudden death in siblings during infancy, and defects of fatty acid metabolism have been implicated as one of the causes of sudden infant death syndrome. Presentation can include acute episodes of vomiting and lethargy, which is produced by fasting from intercurrent illness and may progress to coma. Clinical presentation may vary because usage of fatty acids as a source of energy occurs very late in fasting; therefore, the disease may not present until adulthood, when fasting for 12 to 15 hours may occur. In those with clinical symptoms of myopathy, a history of recurrent aching of muscles, exercise intolerance, myoglobinuria, and cardiomyopathy may be a cause of morbidity. Most laboratories do not have the facilities to diagnose these diseases; therefore, studies should be referred to specialty laboratories. Five to ten ml of urine is assayed for dicarboxylic aciduria and measurement of three glycine conjugates (suberylglycine, hexanylglycine, and phenylpropionic glycine) excreted in excess in the urine. Plasma measurement of carnitine, acetylacetate, and 3-hydroxybutyrate are also available through specialized labs. Treatment of the clinical findings, i.e., treatment of the hypoglycemia or fluid management, is necessary. Dietary management with restricted fat can be instituted if diagnosis is confirmed. Carnitine is a normal intermediate in metabolism required in transport of fatty acids, and its deficiency is a relatively common inherited metabolic disease. Carnitine replacement is a specific treatment for primary carnitine deficiency, but is also a supplement for secondary deficiency.

Carnitine can be measured in plasma, which can be analyzed immediately or frozen (after separating from red cells) awaiting study. Additional special tests are required that can be arranged by the geneticist or an appropriate laboratory. Specific enzyme studies can be performed on white cells or fibroblasts. It is very important to confirm the diagnosis by enzyme biochemical studies. Patients with fatty acid metabolism abnormalities may not demonstrate any biochemical abnormalities of organic acids once the acute episode is over. If this disorder is suspected, however, enzymatic analysis or more specialized biochemical tests should be pursued.

Susan Black

Molecular Genetics

Over 200 genetic disorders are associated with known mapped genes that encode well-defined metabolic enzymes, cellular receptors, or other proteins. For 50 to 100 other genetic disorders of unknown etiology, the responsible gene has been at least tracked to a particular chromosome location where researchers are then able to screen candidate genes. While the ultimate goals of such gene identification studies are the treatment or cure of the disorder, at the present time the primary benefits have been in the area of improved diagnosis.

Diagnosis of disease through gene (DNA) analysis has two features that make it exceptionally powerful. One, because all cell types contain the full complement of genes for that individual, *any tissue can be used*. In practice, peripheral white blood cells are the most convenient DNA source. Second, *the test can be conducted at any time* relative to onset of disease, including prenatally or postmortem, provided that a tissue sample with intact nucleated cells is available. An important corollary of this is that genetic defects can be traced in asymptomatic carriers as well.

In the future, it is hoped that the critical gene can be examined in an individual at risk for a particular disease, and any and all mutations would be detected. At the present, DNA analysis is much more cumbersome and less thorough. Direct detection of mutations is practical for only a few disorders, where the nature of the mutation is predictable. In sickle-cell anemia, all mutant beta globin genes have the same point mutation. While the mutant protein is easy to detect by hemoglobin electrophoresis in a postnatal blood sample, prenatal blood sampling is risky and cannot be performed early in pregnancy. It is a simple matter, however, to detect the corresponding DNA change in a prenatal chorionic villus or amniocyte sample, and many parents have elected to obtain this information. In Duchenne's muscular dystrophy, each new mutation in the X-linked dystrophin gene is unique, but over 70% are large deletions that are readily detectable by DNA analysis. Duchenne's muscular dystrophy thus can be diagnosed from a blood sample in lieu of a full neurological workup and muscle biopsy. Following a positive identification of a DNA deletion in this gene, asymptomatic female relatives can determine whether or not they are carriers, and if so, have the option of prenatal testing. In 1989, a three-base DNA deletion that appears to be responsible for about 70% of cystic fibrosis (CF) mutations was discovered. This now allows for accurate carrier detection and prenatal diagnosis in at-risk family members even if the affected family member is deceased.

For most other genetic disorders that have been mapped to a chromosomal location or to a known gene, DNA-based detection is done by family analysis. Because it is impossible or impractical to detect the mutation itself, the defective gene or the chromosome that carries it must be tracked through the family by comparing DNA patterns of family members who carry the defect to those of members who do not. These DNA patterns are similar to those used for so-called DNA fingerprinting for paternity testing or forensic analysis. The critical difference is that the study must focus on, or in the chromosomal neighborhood of, the gene associated with the disease in question.

For a DNA family analysis, there are certain individuals whose availability and cooperation is essential. For example, if the sister of a child with myotonic dystrophy wishes to know if she is a carrier, a DNA sample is required from the affected child as well as from their parents and other family members. Obviously, such questions may not arise until the affected child, and possibly the parents, are deceased. Similarly, the parents often do not make a decision about future use of prenatal diagnosis until after the death of their affected child. Sadly, many families who perceive an urgent need for a carrier test or prenatal test that is reportedly available for their disorder may find that their particular family is not eligible.

The pediatrician who sees children with hereditary diseases has the opportunity and, increasingly, the obligation, to refer the family to genetic counseling in a timely manner. No commitment to additional testing or notification of relatives need be made; rather, a blood sample from the affected child and other key relatives can be banked for future use if needed. In some cases where death may be precipitous, a preserved DNA sample from the patient may provide a postmortem diagnosis of a specific metabolic defect and allow the parents to be tested for carrier status.

Luckily, DNA is very stable if it is purified before cell autolysis. The ideal sample is 10 to 20 cc of anticoagulated peripheral blood, provided the white count is not depressed. Most molecular genetics laboratories prefer EDTA or ACD as anticoagulants. The white blood cells are stable at room temperature for 48 hours and possibly longer. Once extracted, DNA is stable indefinitely. Alternatively, some laboratories, generally on a research basis, have the capability of establishing cell lines from about 5 ml of heparinized blood or from a skin biopsy. While a carefully prepared, abundant DNA sample increases a family's chances of having a thorough analysis, recovery of material such as formalinized tissue sections and Guthrie cards should not be neglected if no other sample is available.

Anne Maddalena

Gene Therapy

It is now possible in principle to insert genes into human cells. This work is being done in animal models and has application for treatment of human disease. A distinction has to be made between insertion of genes into somatic cells, which would then not be passed on to future generations, and introduction of genes into the germ line cells, in which the new gene would then be inherited by all cells in subsequent generations. This technique involves introducing genes into cells in culture and then transferring the cells into a host. The hematopoietic system cells lend themselves to somatic gene therapy. A focus for consideration would be replacing defective genes for hemoglobin that cause thalassemia or sickle-cell anemia into hematopoietic stem cells and then transferring the genetically engineered cells into the patient. Some diseases that have lent themselves to this type of therapy include the hemoglobinopathies and severe immune deficiency due to adenosine deaminase deficiency. Experimental work also involves an X-linked inborn error of metabolism, hypoxanthine-guaninephosphoribosyl transferase (HGPRT) deficiency, which is responsible for the X-linked inherited Lesch-Nyhan disease. In theory, these treatments could correct clinically recognizable defects, leading to fewer children with abnormalities and, theoretically, to fewer terminations of pregnancy if the disease can be prevented after birth. The technical aspects of gene therapy are presently complex and will require a great deal more work before clinical application.

Prenatal Diagnosis

The last two decades have produced rapid advances in prenatal diagnostic techniques for early and accurate detection of many birth defects and genetic diseases. In many situations, parents now have the option of preventing the birth of an infant with serious disabling abnormalities in hundreds of chromosomal, biochemical, and structural malformation disorders. Fetal therapy has been attempted for a few of these biochemical disorders with limited success; however, ongoing research may identify more successful interventions or specific treatments.

Prenatal diagnosis is available for those diseases in which a specific marker has been identified. Amniocytes, fetal blood, or tissue, such as chorionic villi can be analyzed; therefore, if a disease has a known chromosomal abnormality, enzymatic deficiency or identifiable DNA gene deletion or linkage pattern prenatal diagnosis is possible.

Indications for prenatal diagnosis are multiple. Table 5-7 identifies those patients who should be referred for consideration of prenatal diagnosis.

Prenatal diagnosis is generally divided into two areas: noninvasive or invasive.

Noninvasive Prenatal Diagnosis

Noninvasive prenatal diagnosis presently involves sonography throughout pregnancy and maternal serum alpha-fetoprotein screening in midtrimester.

ULTRASOUND. High frequency, nonelectromagnetic, nonionizing sound waves present an echo-visual picture of inner structures in the pregnant woman. This permits the physician to visualize the fetus, implantation site, uterus, and the fetal structures with little or no discomfort to the patient. This is used in conjunction with invasive prenatal diagnostic procedures at all times. Several different "levels" of sonography are available in pregnancy. Limited scanning (level I) permits identification of fetus, implantation of placenta, multiple gestation, fetal availability, and gestational age of the pregnancy. It is widely available in obstetricians' offices as well as prenatal diagnostic units and radiology departments. This is usually done with a sector scanner

Table 5-7. Indications for Prenatal Diagnosis

Maternal age 35 or greater
Previous child with a chromosome abnormality
Known parental chromosome translocation carrier
Previous child with a known inborn error of metabolism
Previous child or appropriate family member with fragile X syndrome
Parents are known carriers of a metabolic or inherited disease (Tay-Sachs disease, sickle-cell disease)
Sex determination for an X-linked disorder without a known metabolic or DNA diagnosis
Parent, previous child, or a close family member with a neural tube defect
Abnormal maternal serum alpha-fetoprotein screening
Previous child with a diagnosed structural malformation
Abnormal ultrasound findings in pregnancy
Maternal concern
Mosaicism found at chorionic villus sampling (amniocentesis recommended)

transabdominally with real time allowing two-dimensional visualization of the fetus. Vaginal ultrasound is a recent development which permits more detailed evaluation of the uterus and fetus in the first trimester because the ultrasound probe is in close proximity to the uterus and adjacent structures.

Level II ultrasound allows closer scrutiny of fetal structures and can be used to identify structural malformations. Even in experienced hands, however, some of the abnormalities can be missed. This technique has been used in the second and third trimester to diagnose various fetal conditions such as anencephaly, hydrocephaly, renal agenesis, dwarfing syndromes, diaphragmatic hernias, oligohydramnios, polyhydramnios, and others.

Level III ultrasound usually focuses on specific structures such as the fetal heart. Fetal echocardiography has rapidly become an important diagnostic tool in the second or third trimester, especially in families with a risk of congenital heart defects. Both level II and level III ultrasound are usually performed in specialized tertiary centers with a high degree of expertise and equipment with the maximum resolution available. Animal and human studies have failed to demonstrate harmful or untoward effects associated with the use of ultrasound; however, an ultrasound is recommended only as indicated, not as a screening procedure in pregnancies.

MATERNAL SERUM ALPHA-FETOPROTEIN (MSAFP) SCREENING. In recent years, maternal serum for alpha fetoprotein has rapidly become accepted as an important diagnostic tool. Initially developed in the United Kingdom because of the higher risk of neural tube defects, many physicians in the United States include this as part of their prenatal diagnostic care. At present, however, only California has mandated statewide MSAFP screening. Although generally used to rule out neural tube defects, the incidence of which is approximately 1 to 2 per 1000 newborns, alpha-fetoprotein determinations have been a screening tool for other obstetric problems and genetic diseases. In general, the time of screening is at approximately 16 weeks gestation. Any laboratory performing the test has a median number for alpha fetoprotein in a specific gestational week. A multiple of the median greater than or equal to 2.0 is considered elevated. A repeat level should be requested at the same time as an ultrasound examination for fetal viability, gestational age, and number of fetuses. If repeat screening remains elevated, and there is ultrasonographic confirmation of gestational age with single fetus, the risk of a fetal neural tube defect is approximately 1 in 20. At this point, amniocentesis with amniotic fluid alpha-fetoprotein measurement and acetyl-cholinesterase electrophoresis, if indicated, is recommended. High MSAFP can also be indicative of other birth defects such as omphalocele, cystic hygroma, and congenital nephrosis.

Low maternal serum alpha-fetoprotein levels in conjunction with maternal age-related risks for fetal aneuploidy have identified patients at increased risk for Down syndrome. A small proportion of women, therefore, are referred for amniocentesis to rule out Down syndrome, unless ultrasound examination demonstrates a marked discrepancy in gestational age of the fetus between dates from the last menstrual period and ultrasound dates. Two studies have shown that Down syndrome is identified in 1 in 80 to 100 amniocenteses performed for low MSAFP with confirmed gestational dates; trisomy 18 is identified in a smaller percentage.

Invasive Prenatal Diagnosis

By definition, invasive prenatal diagnosis involves obtaining tissue or fluid from the fetus, amniotic fluid, placenta, or chorion. Decisions regarding invasive prenatal diagnosis always include a discussion of the risks and benefits associated with a particular procedure. An important part of prenatal diagnosis, therefore, is genetic counseling, which should examine the identified risk of having an affected fetus as well as the risks of the procedure. Invasive prenatal diagnostic options include chorionic villus sampling in the first trimester, amniocentesis in the second trimester, fetal blood sampling, and fetoscopy usually done in the late second to third trimester. Space limitations permit inclusion of only brief descriptions of these procedures.

CHORIONIC VILLUS SAMPLING (CVS). In the last 10 years, CVS allows earlier prenatal diagnosis and thus continued privacy of a pregnancy until results are available. This procedure is performed at many centers throughout the United States, although it is less commonly available than amniocentesis at this time. Information as to centers performing CVS can be obtained from geneticists or obstetrics departments in hospitals or medical schools.

Chorionic villus sampling is a method of obtaining cells in the first trimester of pregnancy for cytogenetic, biochemical, or DNA analysis. It is a relatively safe and effective technique for early prenatal diagnosis, providing a substantial advantage over amniocentesis in terms of time.

Tissue is usually obtained by two methods. In the first method, a catheter with a flexible metal stylet is inserted transcervically under the guidance of ultrasound after antiseptic cleansing of the vagina. The stylet is removed, and tissue is aspirated by applying suction with a syringe. The second method is similar to amniocentesis: a needle with a removable stylet is inserted through the abdomen under ultrasound guidance. Tissue again is aspirated by applying suction on the syringe while moving the needle in and out several times in the chorionic plate.

Both methods have been used extensively in both the United States and Europe and appear to differ little in associated risk of miscarriage or infection. The risk associated with CVS in the recently published National Institute of Health study appears to be a fraction of a percent higher than amniocentesis. Chorionic villus sampling is most commonly used for the prenatal diagnosis of fetal cytogenetic abnormalities in advanced maternal age.

Confined placental mosaicism appears to occur in around 1% of patients sampled. Thus, around 1% of the women who undergo CVS will have amniocentesis recommended for this reason to confirm the likelihood the fetus is chromosomally normal. Cytogenetic techniques have rapidly improved, so that karyotypes, whether derived from CVS or amniocentesis, appear equally good.

AMNIOCENTESIS. Amniocentesis is usually performed between 15 and 20 weeks gestation, although earlier amniocentesis is being studied. Under ultrasound guidance, a needle is inserted through the maternal abdomen, into the amniotic sac, and approximately 15 to 20 ml of amniotic fluid is obtained for analysis. Amniocentesis has a slightly lower identified risk than CVS. It also can accurately identify chromosome abnormalities and is amenable to molecular genetics studies and assays to detect enzyme abnormalities. In addition, amniocentesis is the most accurate method of ruling out neural tube defects: this is of particular importance in families at specific risk in which either a parent or a previous child has a neural tube defect. Many women are referred for amniocentesis in the second trimester because of abnormal MSAFP screening or ultrasound examination. Amniocentesis has an identified risk of loss of 0.5% or less.

FETAL BLOOD SAMPLING. Fetal blood sampling (periumbilical blood sampling) involves insertion of a needle under ultrasound guidance into the umbilical cord of the fetus, usually at the insertion of the cord into the placenta. It is usually done after 20 weeks gestation because of the rapid growth of the umbilical cord after that time. In experienced hands using advanced ultrasound techniques, the risk of loss is around 1 to 2%. Fetal blood sampling is indicated in situations where rapid karyotype analysis is required: advanced gestation with identified high risk for a chromosome abnormality; some of the X-linked immune diseases or other immune diseases in which analysis of fetal blood components is required; and for accurate diagnosis of some of the in utero infections such as toxoplasmosis. Referral to a physician or center specializing in fetal blood sampling is usually necessary as it is not widely available.

FETOSCOPY. In some select circumstances, it may be indicated to actually insert a fetoscope into the uterus for visualization of the fetus or to obtain specific fetal tissues. Fetoscopy has been used for visualization and biopsy of fetuses with high risk for certain lethal skin conditions, biochemical disorders in which only enzyme analysis of fetal liver is available, or for specific identification of fetal parts not seen on ultrasound examination. In experienced hands, the risk of loss is approximately 5%.

FETAL THERAPY. Because rapid advances in prenatal diagnosis have allowed identification of abnormalities prior to birth, intervention has been attempted with variable success in some metabolic diseases and identified malformations. An example of in utero therapy includes prenatal treatment with steroids for congenital adrenal hyperplasia. In a family at risk, the pregnant mother may be administered dexamethasone very early in pregnancy in order to prevent masculinization of the female fetus. Using a combination of prenatal diagnostic techniques such as CVS or amniocentesis, fetal sex can be determined as well as whether a fetus is affected, and treatment stopped or continued throughout the course of the pregnancy depending upon results. Similar therapy has been used in organic acidemia, such as methylmalonic acidemia, in which vitamin B_{12} may be administered to a mother throughout pregnancy with an identified affected fetus.

In utero surgery has been attempted for identified birth defects such as hydrocephalus, diaphragmatic hernia, and obstructive uropathies. Ongoing research indicates the need for specifically identifying a select isolated abnormality. For example, treatment of obstruction from a posterior urethral valve in an affected male may well be indicated, while shunt placement in a fetus with hydrocephalus associated with a severe brain malformation such as holoprosencephaly is not indicated. Continuing studies of the natural course of these problems in utero are still required before the risks and benefits of these in utero fetal therapies can be accurately assessed. Again, if these problems are identified in utero, however, genetic counseling and specific referral is indicated.

In review, the rapid advances in sonography and other techniques have made prenatal diagnosis available for a wide range of genetic disorders. In any family with identified risks, specific information should be obtained in each pregnancy because of new developments in molecular, cytogenetic, and biochemical techniques. Referral to a genetics center is always indicated in this situation in order to obtain the most recent and up-to-date information on availability of accurate prenatal diagnosis.

Susan Black

References

Antonarakis, S. Diagnosis of genetic disorders at the DNA level. *N. Engl. J. Med.* 320(3):153, 1989.

De Grouchy, J., and Turleau, C. *Clinical Atlas of Human Chromosome Abnormalities.* New York: Wiley, 1984.

Emery, A. E. H., and Rimoin, D. L. (Eds.). *Principles and Practice of Medical Genetics,* Vols. I and II. Edinburgh: Churchill Livingstone, 1983.

Jones, K. L. *Smith's Recognizable Patterns of Human Malformations* (4th ed). Philadelphia: Saunders, 1988.

McKusick, V. A. *Mendelian Inheritance in Man* (8th ed.). Baltimore: Johns Hopkins University Press, 1988.

Nyhan, W. L., and Sakati, N. A., *Diagnostic Recognition of Genetic Disease.* Philadelphia: Lea & Febiger, 1987.

Rhoads, G., Jackson, L., and Schlesselman, S., et al. The safety and efficacy of CVS for early prenatal diagnosis of cytogenetic abnormalities. *N. Engl. J. Med.* 320(10):609, 1989.

Scriver, C. R., Beaudet, A. L., Sly, W. S., et al. (Eds.). *Metabolic Basis of Inherited Disease,* Vols. I and II. New York: McGraw-Hill, 1989.

6

The Endocrine Glands

Adenohypophysis

Hypopituitarism

Pituitary deficiency states in children are rare. They are generally divided into two types, idiopathic and acquired. Idiopathic hypopituitarism is usually manifested clinically by deficiency of growth hormone and gonadotropin deficiency and, less frequently, adrenocorticotropin and thyrotropin deficiency. An infant with this condition tends to be of normal birth weight and size; in most cases growth failure is apparent around the age of 1 to 3 years. The growth failure is typically profound retardation of linear growth with normal body proportions. Skeletal age is delayed. Hypoglycemia may be present. Clinical evidence of hypothyroidism, if present, tends to be slight. Older children tend to retain a juvenile appearance of the facial features. In cases with gonadotropin deficiency, gonadal maturation fails to occur spontaneously, and the patients remain sexually infantile unless given replacement therapy with sex hormones. Monotropic, single hormone, deficiency states have been

described. A patient may, therefore, have only somatotropin deficiency; in this case normal pubertal gonadal maturation would occur.

Hypopituitarism may be acquired as a result of injuries to the skull, intracranial infections, or tumors. Removal of a cyst or tumor in the region of the sella turcica can lead to damage or destruction of the pituitary gland. In contrast to idiopathic hypopituitarism, acquired hypopituitarism tends to include deficiencies of corticotropin and thyrotropin as well as of gonadotropin and somatotropin.

Somatomedin-C (insulin-like growth factor-I [IGF-I]), a polypeptide normally present in human serum, promotes synthesis of proteoglycans and collagen by chondrocytes in vitro. IGF-I is produced in the liver in response to growth hormone stimulation. It is also present in many tissues and may locally carry out paracrine and autocrine functions. It is probable that both growth hormone and IGF-I have direct growth stimulating functions in cartilage. Deficient somatomedin production with normal or elevated circulating growth hormone levels is associated with dwarfism with an autosomal recessive mode of inheritance (Laron dwarfism). Studies indicate that African pygmies may have a defect in production of somatomedin.

DIAGNOSIS. Serum growth hormone is assayed after challenge with a variety of stimuli, including exercise, arginine infusion, insulin hypoglycemia, and glucagon given intravenously or subcutaneously. An adequate response is usually considered to be a peak value of greater than 10 ng/ml. Growth hormone secretory profiles and/or integrated growth hormone level in plasma may be determined by serial sampling of growth hormone levels in blood; however, these have uncertain diagnostic value in the individual patient. Pituitary thyrotropin function is determined by stimulation with thyrotropin releasing factor (TRF) and measurement of resultant circulating thyrotropin levels. Peripheral thyroid function is evaluated by measurement of circulating thyroid hormone levels. Pituitary ACTH function is determined by testing response of plasma concentration of 11-desoxycortisol to oral administration of metyrapone. The absence of gonadotropins in patients with sexual infantilism after the age of normal puberty is presumptive evidence of a gonadotropin defect. Administration of gonadotropin hormone releasing hormone (Gn-RH) permits evaluation of the capability of the pituitary to secrete gonadotropin. Skeletal age is usually retarded in hypopituitarism. The sella turcica may be smaller than average.

TREATMENT. The principal clinical disturbance of idiopathic hypopituitarism in childhood is growth failure due to deficiency of growth hormone. Replacement with pituitary growth hormone has a growth-promoting effect.

Some patients develop hypothyroidism while receiving growth hormone; thus the thyroid hormone level should be monitored during treatment.

Sexual infantilism, hypoadrenalism, and hypothyroidism are treated by appropriate replacement therapy. Patients with hypopituitarism seem to be highly sensitive to ordinary maintenance doses of cortisol (17-hydroxycorticosterone). For this reason, replacement therapy with hydrocortisone or related steroids should be undertaken with smaller doses than are usual in other adrenal insufficiency states. Sex hormone replacement causes appearance of secondary sex features. The patient may have normal sexual relations; males can ejaculate but are not fertile because of the absence of gonadotropins to stimulate gametogenesis. Sex hormone therapy will induce closure of the epiphyses, after which growth hormone replacement fails to cause further increase in height.

Hyperpituitarism

Pituitary gigantism, due to acidophilic tumors, and Cushing syndrome, produced by basophilic tumors of the anterior lobe, are both easily recognizable syndromes of hyperpituitarism. Hyperpituitarism does not cause syndromes related to excessive production of gonadotropins or thyrotropins in children. (See Cushing's Syndrome, p. 78.)

PITUITARY GIGANTISM. Pituitary gigantism results from excessive pituitary growth hormone secretion during childhood prior to epiphyseal closure. In addition to manifesting possible neurological deficiencies and enlargement of the sella turcica due to the presence of a pituitary tumor, patients show excessively rapid growth. Membranous bones, as well as the long bones of the skeleton, are enlarged, but acromegalic changes in the skeleton usually do not occur until after closure of the epiphyses. Evidence of mild hyperthyroidism or hyperadrenalism may be present.

The serum inorganic phosphate concentration is increased in the acromegalic adult, but this finding may not be present in children with pituitary gigantism. Presence of an elevated fasting serum growth hormone level that is not suppressible during a standard oral or intravenous glucose tolerance test is confirmatory of hyperpituitarism. Treatment consists of removal or ablation of the pituitary adenoma.

Neurohypophysis

Diabetes Insipidus

Deficient secretion of antidiuretic hormone leads to excessive water loss in the urine. The resultant polyuria and polydipsia constitute the syndrome known as diabetes insipidus. Primary diabetes insipidus may be a familial disorder without other findings, or it may be produced by hypothalamic lesions or pathological conditions that destroy the neurohypophysis itself.

True diabetes insipidus must be differentiated from compulsive water intake (psychogenic diabetes insipidus) and nephrogenic diabetes insipidus. Individuals with true diabetes insipidus fail to concentrate urine during water deprivation or the infusion of hypertonic saline (Carter-Robbins test), and they respond with increased urinary concentration to an administered antidiuretic hormone.

Nephrogenic diabetes insipidus (see Chap. 12, The Genitourinary System) is an inherited disorder that affects males predominantly. The clinical pattern suggests an X-linked recessive mode of inheritance, but alternate modes of inheritance may occur. Signs of excessive water loss occur soon after birth; large amounts of water must be given if the infant is to survive. Restriction of solute load by dietary management or reduction in body sodium by diet or diuretics (or both) is of some assistance in controlling the excessive drinking. There is no response to vasopressin in this disorder. Diuretics have been used with beneficial effect in limiting water excretion. Diuretics have no long-term effects on the disorder, and the decision to use them is based on the marked inconvenience and social problems generated by the large urinary volume of the untreated children with nephrogenic diabetes insipidus.

Treatment of True Diabetes Insipidus.

Nasal spray containing 1-desamino-D-arginine vasopressin is favored in therapy of diabetic insipidus because of its convenience and relatively prolonged action. The dosage schedule varies with the patient but usually consists of one or two doses daily. Vasopressin, which may be given as the tannate salt in sesame oil by intramuscular injection, controls the polyuria for 18 to 36 hours. When variations of clinical response occur, the cause is usually inadequate suspension of the principal in the oily vehicle or improper injection into subcutaneous fat.

Aqueous preparations of vasopressin for injection have short-term effects and are useful only for diagnostic tests and for early management and determination of the dose requirements.

Thyroid Gland

Developmental Physiology

Uptake of radioactive iodine has been demonstrated in the thyroid gland as early as the fifth month of gestation. The formation of the iodothyronines, thyroxine and triiodothyronine, as well as their increase in proportion to the concentration of iodotyrosine compounds occurs somewhat later. The fetus is probably dependent on an intact thyroid gland for maintenance of normal growth and development in the late stages of fetal life.

At birth the serum thyroxine (T_4) level approximates or is slightly lower than that of the mother. It may rise to 10 to 15 μg/100 ml within a week after birth, and then gradually decline over the next several weeks. The levels may subside to a mean of about 10 μg/100 ml by 4 months and remain at this level. The normal adult range is usually given as 4.5 to 11.5 μg/100 ml. The concentration of thyroid-stimulating hormone (TSH) in cord blood is elevated with respect to maternal concentration. It rises abruptly and peaks around 30 minutes after birth. The TSH concentration drops off rapidly thereafter. At 2 days of age it is slightly above cord blood levels. The 24-hour radioactive iodine uptake during the first week of life has been found in the usual range or elevated by different observers. After the first week of life, the uptake falls in the usual range for children, which is slightly higher than that of adults. Precise limits for uptake values vary in different laboratories, depending on instrumentation and environmental factors such as dietary iodine intake.

The thyroid gland grows during childhood from approximately 2 g at birth to about 35 g in the adult. Variations in size are noted at different stages of development. Physiological enlargement of the thyroid gland occurs at the time of puberty, probably because of the increased metabolic demands at that time; ordinarily the enlargement is relatively greater in females. Requirements for thyroid hormone also increase with growth and development. Thus in cretinism one must periodically adjust the dosages of thyroid hormone to meet new requirements.

Hyperthyroidism

The etiological factor in hyperthyroidism (Graves' disease) is widely accepted to be an autoimmune mechanism. The long-acting thyroid stimulator (LATS), an immunoglobulin, was the first noted of the now several recognized thyroid-stimulating immunoglobulins circulating in patients with hyperthyroidism. Graves' disease is relatively uncommon in childhood and adolescence. The diagnosis is usually not difficult, because the clinical signs are striking. Management presents certain problems unique to pediatrics.

One commonly finds evidence of a predisposition to various thyroid disorders in the families of patients with hyperthyroidism. These range from goiter with hypothyroidism to hyperthyroidism.

CLINICAL FEATURES. Over a period of days or weeks the patient develops irritability and nervousness, hyperactivity, increased appetite, weight loss, and excessive perspiration. Rapid pulse, short attention span, poor school performance, difficulty in sleeping, and occasionally diarrhea may also occur. Prominence of the eyeballs and a stare may be observed; lid lag is occasionally present, and there is often mild weakness of convergence. The thyroid gland is somewhat increased in size during this time, and there may be a slight increase in linear growth, with a corresponding increase of skeletal age, if the condition has existed for several months.

The skin is warm, soft, and moist, with a heightened color. The pulse is full and rapid. Enlargement of the heart and murmurs may lead to confusion with rheumatic myocarditis.

On palpation the thyroid gland is well rounded but is not often markedly enlarged. The lobes are smooth and soft or rubbery in consistency. It is uncommon to hear a distinct bruit in the gland of the hyperthyroid child or adolescent. There is increased cardiovascular activity, however, and one often hears vascular noises transmitted from the thorax and neck vessels. The precordium is occasionally active on visual inspection; percussion and x-ray examination may reveal that the heart borders are enlarged. The heart sounds are intensified, and functional murmurs may be heard. Mild hepatic and splenic enlargement may be noted on abdominal palpation. Exophthalmometry is primarily useful as a reference in the event that exophthalmos appears to increase during the course of the disease.

LABORATORY AIDS IN DIAGNOSIS. The serum thyroxine (T_4) level is elevated in the hyperthyroid patient. Approximately 10% of hyperthyroid subjects, however, have a T_4 level in the normal range. In these the triiodothyronine (T_3) concentration may be increased. The serum T_4 or T_3 value determined by radioimmunoassay is not affected by exogenous intake of iodide or iodine-containing chemicals. The sensitive TSH assay will show suppression of serum TSH in the hyperthyroid individual except those rare cases in which overproduction of TSH is responsible for the disorder.

The rate of uptake of radioactive iodine by the thyroid gland is increased in the hyperthyroid patient. The early uptake of radioactive iodine (e.g., at 2 hours) is usually more distinctly increased than the uptake at 24 hours. A test of suppressibility of the pituitary-thyroid axis with thyroid hormones (T_3 suppression test) is useful for confirming the diagnosis in doubtful cases.

Determination of thyroxine-binding proteins, either directly or by indirect methods such as the competitive in vitro uptake of radioactive-labeled triiodothyronine by resin, is useful in excluding euthyroid elevation of T_4 by an increase in thyroxine-binding protein. Hyperthyroidism must be differentiated from functional behavioral disorders, chronic infections, and other conditions that may result in fever, weight loss, and other signs suggestive of hypermetabolism.

Hyperthyroidism due to a secreting adenoma rarely occurs in childhood. Excessive administration of thyroid hormone to euthyroid children may produce hyperthyroid symptoms. Athyrotic individuals are more sensitive to slight increases of thyroid dosage above physiological requirements than are euthyroid individuals.

TREATMENT. The therapeutic methods in common use are: (1) suppression of thyroid function with chemical agents, (2) surgical removal of the thyroid gland, and (3) irradiation of the gland with radioactive iodine.

Most pediatricians choose modes of therapy other than radioactive iodine because of the concern over possible risk of long-term irradiation effects. Whenever both surgical approach and medical therapy are found to be ineffective or hazardous, radioactive iodine may be indicated.

Antithyroid substances such as propylthiouracil or methimazole (Tapazole) can be used in the early control of the hyperthyroid state. Treatment is carried on continuously with adjustments of the dose as required in order to maintain the patient in a eumetabolic state. In over half the patients, the thyroid gland reduces in size, but many retain their thyroid enlargement; in some cases an actual increase in thyroid size may be observed. Overdosage with these antithyroid drugs, to the extent that the patient becomes hypothyroid, will result in further enlargement of the goiter. The patients must be watched for signs of toxicity, which may consist of malaise, rash, fever, ulcerations of the oral mucosa, splenic enlargement, leukopenia, and diarrhea. The drug should be discontinued if serious toxic signs are present.

After 1 to 2 years of satisfactory response to antithyroid therapy, the drug may be gradually discontinued. Relapses are not uncommon and require further therapy. Approximately 50% of patients relapse and require further treatment.

Preparation for surgery is directed toward reducing the metabolic state to normal and altering the blood supply and consistency of the thyroid gland. Complications of surgery include thyroid storm, hypoparathyroidism due to operative removal of parathyroids, and damage to the recurrent laryngeal nerves. Patients who become hypothyroid because of excessive removal of thyroid tissue can be given substitution therapy with thyroid extract.

The management of hyperthyroidism in the neonate follows the same principles as those given above. The ordinary course of neonatal hyperthyroidism is spontaneous remission, and there is permanent cure after 1 to 3 months of symptoms. Treatment during this period also follows the previously described principles. Respiratory obstruction and cardiac decompensation are the main complications of the disease.

Propranolol has been effective in alleviating hypermetabolism accompanying hyperthyroidism, although the pathophysiological process in the thyroid may continue and the patient continues to have high levels of circulating hormonal iodide. This agent may be of particular use in treatment of thyroid storm or in preparation for surgery of patients in a toxic state.

Neonatal Hyperthyroidism

Hyperthyroidism in the neonatal period accounts for approximately 1% of juvenile Graves' disease. Approximately one infant for every 70 thyrotoxic mothers is affected. The abnormality may present *in utero* with a high fetal heart rate. The tachycardia may persist after birth along with restlessness, warm flushed skin, increased respiratory rate, and increased motor activity. Exophthalmus and thyroid enlargement are usually present. The onset may be delayed for several days after birth and then evolve rapidly. The LATS may be elevated in mothers of affected infants. The affected infants have an increased serum thyroxin level. Bone age may be advanced and cranial sutures show early closure. Initial treatment is carried out with propylthiouracil and iodide. Rapid control of severe symptoms may be accomplished by the addition of propranolol, sedation, and oxygen. Dexamethasone has been employed as adjunctive therapy. Surgical excision of the isthmus of the thyroid gland is necessary if there is trachial obstruction due to thyromegaly. Close observation and long-term follow-up are required.

Hypothyroidism

Hypothyroidism is divided into two varieties, congenital and acquired. Important differences in cause, treatment, and prognosis exist between these types. The clinical signs include a decreased rate of growth, decreased peripheral circulation, poor appetite, constipation, carotenemia, sluggish motor and mental function, dry skin, and coarse scalp hair. Infants show decreased food intake, lethargy, prolonged physiological jaundice, coarse features, hoarse cry, umbilical hernia, a large tongue, and growth failure.

Controlled clinical trials with thyroid hormones may occasionally be helpful in some of the milder clinical states of hypothyroidism and in the presence of conflicting laboratory results. Many misconceptions, however, exist concerning the relationship of thyroid deficiency to obesity, school failures, behavior disorders, and a variety of other problems. In these conditions the indiscriminate use of thyroid hormones should be avoided.

ACQUIRED HYPOTHYROIDISM. Acquired hypothyroidism in children may result from operative removal of the thyroid gland, treatment with antithyroid drugs, or Hashimoto's thyroiditis (lymphocytic thyroiditis). It may also be caused by deficiency of pituitary thyrotropin production (secondary hyperthyroidism).

Clinical manifestations of acquired hypothyroidism depend upon the extent of thyroid deficiency and the age at onset. They include growth disturbances, low body temperature, constipation, decreased physical activity, and signs of myxedema as well as slowing of mental and intellectual processes.

Hashimoto's thyroiditis produces enlargement of the thyroid gland and histological evidence of atrophy of the follicles as well as lymphocytic infiltration. The disease is an autoimmune disorder. There may be a familial predisposition. Circulating thyroid antibodies, elevation of serum gamma globulin levels, and abnormal flocculation tests are common.

CONGENITAL HYPOTHYROIDISM. *Etiology.* In populations with adequate iodine intake the majority of cases of congenital hypothyroidism (cretinism) are due to partial or complete absence of the thyroid gland at birth (athyrotic cretinism). In the remaining cases, the thyroid gland is present but has a defect in the formation or release of thyroid hormone (goitrous cretinism). Endemic cretinism results from deficient dietary intake of iodine by the mother during pregnancy; severe thyroid deficiency and development of goiter in the infant ensue. Radioiodine therapy of thyrotoxicosis in the pregnant woman is likely to destroy the fetal thyroid and produce congenital hypothyroidism. The use of antithyroid drugs or large doses of iodide in the mother during pregnancy may also suppress thyroid function in the fetus and lead to goiter. This does not lead to permanent hypothyroidism after birth; therefore, one does not usually refer to this condition as cretinism.

Clinical Features. Signs of hypothyroidism are usually not present at birth but may make their appearance during the first week of life. With complete athyrosis, lethargy occurs by a few days of age. The food intake is low, and sleep periods are long. There is often a more intense and more prolonged state of physiological jaundice than is usual. Defecation is less frequent. At 2 or 3 weeks of age the infant tends to have characteristic circulatory mottling of the skin, particularly on exposure to room temperature. By 1 month of age, myxedema is often noticeable. The heart sounds may be of poor quality, consistent with cardiac myxedema and decrease of cardiac work. The cry may be of a hoarse quality. By this time, failure of longitudinal growth is apparent. Constipation may be present. By 5 months of age the cretin has assumed the classic features of congenital hypothyroidism with the retention of fetal body proportions and skeletal development. Development of the facial skeleton is retarded, as evidenced by the depressed bridge of the nose. There is poor skeletal muscle tone and a tendency for umbilical hernia. The skin tends to be dry and cool. The tongue may be enlarged because of myxedema. The patient tends to be sluggish, to be slow in motor development, and to have longer than normal sleep periods. In older infants, after the institution of the feeding of solids, carotenemia may develop.

This sequence of signs and symptoms occurs regardless of the cause of the hypothyroid state. Differences in severity will be seen in different degrees of hypothyroidism. The absence of any palpable thyroid tissue overlying the trachea, between the thyroid and cricoid cartilages, should lead one to suspect athyrotic cretinism. The goitrous cretin, even when untreated, may not develop a prominent goiter for some years, but in such cases the thyroid gland is often slightly enlarged and easily palpated, even during the neonatal period.

Differential Diagnosis. Laboratory determinations of the greatest value in the diagnosis of cretinism are serum TSH and T_4 concentrations, thyroidal radioactive iodine uptake, and thyroidal radioisotope scan. By 1 month of age the serum thyroxine level in the athyrotic cretin, and most goitrous cretins, is well below the normal range. The serum TSH concentration is usually well above the normal range in the hypothyroid infant. Allowance should be made for a marked physiological increase of serum TSH during the first few hours after birth. The uptake of radioactive iodine in the neck is less than normal in the athyrotic cretin any time after birth but may be normal or even increased in the goitrous cretin.

Among the important features of cretinism is defective osseous development, including delayed maturation of the skeleton and epiphyseal dysgenesis.

Differentiation of goitrous cretinism from athyrotic cretinism is of importance from the standpoint of genetic counseling. There is no practical value at this time in differentiating the various individual blocks in metabolism, although certain of these are relatively easy to demonstrate.

Consequences of Hypothyroidism in Children. In untreated severe congenital hypothyroidism, neurological damage and mental deficiency tend to occur. Severe stunting of linear growth becomes evident from early infancy, and skeletal maturation is correspondingly delayed, as is manifested clinically by immature facial and skeletal development, with a tendency toward short extremities in comparison with the length of the spine.

Treatment. The aim in therapy is to reinstitute a normal metabolic state as rapidly as can be physiologically tolerated by the patient. In the period before 3 months of age levothyroxine is administered in a dose of 12 to 25 μg daily. Clinical effects resulting from a given dose schedule may not be detected for 1 or 2 weeks. It is necessary to observe the infant frequently for evidence of cardiac decompensation or arrhythmia. With the onset of therapy there is rapid mobilization of myxedema fluid and enlargement of the vascular volume with resultant cardiac failure. As a further complication, the expansion of the vascular volume causes a drop in hemoglobin concentration. When both severe anemia and cardiac failure are present, small transfusions of sedimented red blood cells may aid in management of cardiac failure.

During long-term therapy one aims for normal growth and development. Periodic assessment of skeletal age is of value. Sleeplessness, rapid pulse, excessive perspiration, and irritability suggest that the dose is excessive. The usual signs of underdosage are continued coolness of the skin, constipation, and sluggishness.

The daily requirement of levothyroxine is determined on clinical and laboratory grounds. The levothyroxine dose during the first year may be 5 to 6 μg/kg, after 2 years, 4 μg/kg, and in late childhood and adolescence, between 2 and 3 μg/kg.

Neurological Prognosis After Treatment. In severe congenital hypothyroidism, even with adequate therapy started by the first month of life, some damage to the central nervous system may have occurred. Adequate replacement therapy before 6 months of age significantly reduces the incidence of neurological disorder and mental defect. Replacement therapy after 2 years of age restores the growth rate to normal and produces better performance in most neurological spheres, but basic intelligence is not improved. It is important that the infant be maintained in a euthyroid state. Hyperthyroidism due to overtreatment may promote premature closure of skull sutures.

Carcinoma of the Thyroid Gland

Carcinoma of the thyroid gland is an uncommon disorder of childhood. The cause is usually unknown, but there is a definite relationship between this neoplasm and irradiation to the upper airways, usually for benign conditions such as an enlarged thymus and adenoid hypertrophy. Metastases occur primarily in the lungs, but they also occur in the skeletal system, the mediastinum, and the axillae. Anaplastic thyroid carcinoma is rapidly progressive and usually fatal, but the more differentiated varieties have much better prognoses.

If possible, the entire thyroid gland and local metastatic sites in the neck should be removed surgically. Radioiodine therapy is given in cases of differentiated thyroid carcinoma. Thyroid hormone is then administered to suppress thyrotropic stimulation, as some of these tumors are thyrotropin dependent. Radioiodine treatment is restricted to patients whose local surgical treatment has been unsuccessful and to patients in whom the neoplasm is capable of concentrating quantities of radioiodine. Regardless of the apparent stability of the patient receiving long-term maintenance therapy, it is advisable to reevaluate the therapeutic regimen every 6 to 12 months. Recurrences may be detected by body scintillation scanning. Serial serum thyroglobulin determinations are useful in determining the existence of metastases in the previously treated patient.

Parathyroid Glands

Parathyroid hormone maintains calcium ion concentration in plasma within narrow limits. In addition to mobilizing calcium in bone, it promotes calcium reabsorption and secretion of phosphate by kidney tubules. The parathyroid glands in the newborn infant may show transient hyperplastic changes histologically, a finding that has been interpreted as resulting from the secondary effect of the increased phosphate load in cow's milk.

Calcitonin

Calcitonin is a polypeptide hormone secreted by the C cells in the thyroid gland. It decreases plasma calcium and phosphate. It acutely inhibits bone resorption from the gut and increases renal loss of many electrolytes, including phosphate. It does not influence calcium accretion. Calcitonin concentration in serum is increased in medullary carcinoma of the thyroid. Its role in health is not well defined.

Hypoparathyroidism

IDIOPATHIC HYPOPARATHYROIDISM. The clinical signs of idiopathic hypoparathyroidism appear early in the neonatal period with tetany and convulsions. In older children, chronic diarrhea and skin infections, especially candidiasis, may occur. Other manifestations include scaliness of the skin, sparse, patchy hair, cataracts, and mental retardation. The serum calium level may fall to 4 mg/100 ml and the diffusible calcium level to 3 mg/100 ml; the plasma inorganic phosphate level may rise to 12 mg/100 ml. The teeth show hypoplastic changes with enamel defects, furrows, and grooves. On x-ray examination the bones may appear unusually dense, and calcification may be present in the basal ganglia of the brain.

The diagnosis is confirmed by determining the acute effects of the administration of parathyroid hormone on serum calcium and phosphorus levels. In hypoparathyroidism, parathyroid hormone produces a trend toward normal in the serum chemistry.

Treatment of Tetany and Hypoparathyroidism. Mild tetany may not require treatment. A neonate with a serum calcium below 7.5 mg/100 ml (ionized calcium below 2.8 mg/100 ml) or older child with a serum calcium less than 8 to 8.5 mg/100 ml should be treated to prevent tetany and other symptoms. Severe hypocalcemia should be treated vigorously with intravenous administration of calcium salts; 10% calcium gluconate is given in a dose of 2 ml/kg body weight, the total not to exceed 20 ml. The drug should be administered slowly; if bradycardia occurs the injection is stopped until the heart rate returns to normal and is then continued at a slower rate. Long-term treatment is carried out with vitamin D or 1,25 (OH)$_2$-vitamin D$_3$ until serum calcium values become normal. The dose required for maintenance requires adjustment for the individual patient, depending on the serum calcium and phosphorus values and on the urinary excretion of calcium. Low calcium and decreased intake of phosphorus may be compensated by the use of calcium supplements and dietary regulation. Deficiency of magnesium is often associated with conditions that cause tetany. If the serum magnesium concentration is reduced, magnesium salt supplementation may be given.

ACQUIRED HYPOPARATHYROIDISM. Surgical removal of the parathyroid glands and damage to these glands during thyroid surgery are the most common causes for acquired hypoparathyroidism. Treatment follows the same general rules applying to congenital hypoparathyroidism.

PSEUDOHYPOPARATHYROIDISM. Pseudohypoparathyroidism is a familial disorder in which patients have chemical findings of hypoparathyroidism but have end organ unresponsiveness to parathyroid hormone. The patients often have skeletal anomalies, a round face, short stature with a broad trunk, and short metacarpal and metatarsal bones. The serum calcium levels may return to normal more readily with a high-calcium, low-phosphate diet than is the case in true hypoparathyroidism. Treatment consists in dietary control of calcium and phosphate intake, supplemented with vitamin D therapy as outlined above.

PSEUDOPSEUDOHYPOPARATHYROIDISM. Some patients with anomalies of skeletal and somatic development seen in the syndrome of pseudohypoparathyroidism respond to parathormone. These individuals may have a subclinical form of pseudohypoparathyroidism.

Adrenal Cortex

Hyperfunction of Adrenal Cortex

HYPERALDOSTERONISM. Primary hyperaldosteronism is a rare congenital disorder caused by bilateral adrenocortical hyperplasia. The usual signs are hypertension, edema, and polyuria. Acquired primary hyperaldosteronism may be caused by a benign adenoma of an adrenal gland. Symptoms include polyuria, polydipsia, albuminuria, and paresthesias. Periodic paralysis and occasionally edema may constitute other features of the disorder.

Primary hyperaldosteronism must be differentiated from secondary hyperaldosteronism. The latter may occur in conditions in which there is a reduction in intravascular volume, for example, nephrosis, cirrhosis, congestive heart failure, and malignant hypertension with renal ischemia.

Positive laboratory tests include low serum potassium levels, increased serum sodium levels, hypochloremia, and alkalosis. Proof of hyperaldosteronism is the demonstration of increased plasma or urinary aldosterone or an increased aldosterone secretion rate while a patient receives a normal sodium intake. Low plasma renin activity is a useful confirmatory finding.

Spironolactone treatment may be indicated in hyperaldosteronism due to adrenal hyperplasia. If an adenoma is found the tumor may be removed. Secondary hyperaldosteronism is treated by managing the primary condition.

CONGENITAL ADRENAL HYPERPLASIA. Congenital adrenal hyperplasia (adrenogenital syndrome) is manifested by bilateral hypertrophy of the adrenal glands, structural abnormalities of the external genitalia of the female (for exception, see Desmolase Defect, 3-Beta-Hydroxysteroid Dehydrogenase Defect), early virilization, and accelerated somatic growth. In some cases a salt-losing tendency or systemic arterial hypertension may also be present. The disorder is inherited as an autosomal recessive condition; not uncommonly, more than one member of a sibship may be affected.

The disorder results from a defect in the synthesis of hydrocortisone by the adrenal glands. The salt-losing tendency is the result of a more severe defect that may be present in some cases.

Adrenal hyperplasia results from increased secretion of pituitary ACTH in response to deficient blood levels of hydrocortisone. Depending on the particular enzymatic block, various precursors of hydrocortisone are produced in excess and account for the majority of the striking clinical symptoms of this disorder.

Enzymatic blocks that give rise to congenital adrenal hyperplasia have been identified at several steps of cortisol synthesis:

Desmolase Defect. Desmolase defect (lipoid adrenal hyperplasia) blocks the conversion of cholesterol to Δ^5-pregnenolone. Most affected individuals have died in infancy. Profound salt loss is associated with the condition. In males, masculinization of the genitalia tends to be incomplete.

21-Hydroxylation Defect. Deficiency in 21-hydroxylase is the most common type of congenital adrenal hyperplasia. Approximately one-third of the patients have deficient aldosterone production and a salt-losing syndrome. Excessive excretion of 17-ketosteroids, pregnanetriol, and other precursors of cortisol may be demonstrable. Virilization begins in fetal life. In the female fetus there is formation of a urogenital sinus and enlargement of the genital tubercle to form a penile structure; thus the infant may erroneously be considered a male. The majority of males with this condition show no apparent defect at birth, although there may be increased pigmentation of the skin of the sexual organs.

In the untreated condition, sexual hair appears at about the age of 2 to 3 years. Throughout infancy and childhood the rate of skeletal growth and maturation is increased because of the stimulation by androgens produced by the adrenal glands. Complete skeletal fusion may occur by the age of 8 years, and although these patients may be increased in height for their age, their ultimate stature in adulthood may be quite stunted. Excessive sex steroids are produced and tend to inhibit gonadotropin production by the pituitary. Thus, untreated boys have small testes in spite of a large penis. (A deceptive clinical picture exists in the rare male in whom hypertrophied adrenal rest tissue in the scrotum gives the appearance of enlarged testes.)

The salt-losing syndrome may appear as early as the second or third week of life with rapid urinary salt loss and polyuria, dehydration, collapse, and death. The infants during the phase of active salt loss are frequently irritable and have episodes of cyanosis along with the dehydration. Collapse without salt loss may occur during periods of stress such as severe illness or surgery. These episodes can terminate fatally unless the patient is given vigorous supportive treatment with glucocorticoids such as hydrocortisone or its analogues.

3-Beta-Hydroxysteroid Dehydrogenase Defect. A less common form of congenital adrenal hyperplasia, this defect is associated in males with incomplete penile development, resulting in hypospadias with shortening of the anal-genital distance, and in females with varying degrees of virilization, which is usually less severe than in the 21-hydroxylation and

11-hydroxylation defects. During infancy there may be profound adrenal cortical insufficiency with sodium loss.

11-Hydroxylation Defect. Characterized by lack of hydroxylation at the 11-carbon position of the steroid molecule, this syndrome is a hypertensive form of congenital adrenal hyperplasia. The defect leads to an increase in 11-desoxycorticosterone, a potent salt-retaining steroid. In the untreated patient, masculinization and hypertension develop, but salt loss does not occur.

17-Hydroxylase Defect. This defect results in increased desoxycorticosterone secretion. Affected females have normal genitalia at birth but remain sexually infantile. Affected males have incomplete masculinization of genitalia. Hypertension, hypokalemic alkalosis, and low levels of urinary 17-ketosteroids are associated findings.

Diagnosis of Congenital Adrenal Hyperplasia. Congenital adrenal hyperplasia should be considered in any infant with ambiguous genitalia (see App. A, Sec. 25).

Genetic sex should be determined by chromosomal analysis. A genetic female with ambiguous genitalia may have congenital virilizing adrenal hyperplasia, virilization on the basis of hormones administered to the mother during the pregnancy, or true hermaphroditism. The levels of plasma 17-hydroxyprogesterone or urinary 17-ketosteroids and pregnanetriol should be determined. These are invariably elevated in the untreated state of virilizing adrenal hyperplasia in the C-21 and C-11 defects. Urinary 17-ketosteroids and 5-pregnanetriol and plasma 17-OH-pregnenolone are elevated in the 3-beta-hydroxysteroid dehydrogenase defect. The 17-ketosteroids tend to be excreted at higher levels for a few days after birth than later in the first month; therefore, determinations after the first week of age produce a sharper differentiation. Radiological demonstration of the extent of the urogenital sinus by filling the cavity with radiopaque dye assists in establishing the nature of the defect of the genital duct system. The decrease in the excretion of 17-ketosteroids and pregnanetriol in response to exogenous administration of dexamethasone serves to confirm the diagnosis of adrenal hyperplasia and firmly differentiates this disorder from a virilizing adrenal tumor.

Newborn males with the adrenogenital syndrome do not show obvious clinical signs unless they have a salt-losing crisis or a poor response to acute stress. Later the effects of masculinization, in the form of increased skeletal growth and maturation as well as the appearance of pubic hair and continued enlargement of the phallus, call attention to the syndrome. Newborn male siblings of affected patients should be investigated, and 17-ketosteroid and pregnanetriol excretion measured to establish the diagnosis as early in life as possible.

A deficiency of desmolase or of 3-beta-hydroxysteroid dehydrogenase may be suspected in infants with male genitalia and hypospadias. Recognition of adrenal insufficiency in early infancy requires alertness on the part of the physician to this possibility and readiness to institute prompt adrenal replacement should signs of adrenal insufficiency or of salt loss occur.

Treatment of Congenital Adrenal Hyperplasia. The aims of treatment are:

1. Replacement of the usual metabolic needs for cortisol (hydrocortisone, compound F) by administration of optimal doses of hydrocortisone or glucocorticoid analogues.
2. Replacement of salt loss, if this occurs, by increasing the salt intake or by administration of mineralocorticoids or by both.
3. Achievement of normal physical growth and development.

The replacement of cortisol deficiency consists in administering hydrocortisone or a glucocorticoid analogue in sufficient doses to meet the patient's metabolic needs and to suppress pituitary corticotropin. This may be given in the form of oral medication, intramuscular injections of short-acting preparations, or injections of long-acting preparations. The dosage in children depends on evaluation of plasma and urinary steroids and on linear growth and skeletal development; the required amount of orally administered hydrocortisone is usually in the range of 20 to 30 mg/m^2/day. The average long-range replacement oral dosage of hydrocortisone is 25 mg/m^2/day given in two or three doses. More potent analogues, such as prednisone, may be given in doses corresponding to the different glucocorticoid effect relative to hydrocortisone.

The acute phase of the salt-losing syndrome is treated by replacement of salt and water. Long-term maintenance consists of adding to the therapy a potent mineralocorticoid such as 9-alpha-fluorohydrocortisone. Desoxycorticosterone acetate may be given parenterally for short-term management, or desoxycorticosterone trimethylacetate in oil may be given for long-term management. In addition to serum sodium and potassium concentration, plasma renin activity (PRA) is useful in monitoring adequacy of mineralocorticoid therapy. The PRA may be elevated in instances of inadequate replacement therapy with normal serum electrolyte concentrations.

The salt-losing tendency decreases somewhat with age, but episodes of salt loss may occur during childhood with febrile illnesses. Although adolescent and adult patients with a history of the salt-losing form of the adrenogenital syndrome may not necessarily require mineralocorticoid therapy, its continuous administration seems warranted in those patients having continued increased salt appetite.

During acute febrile illnesses, surgery, or other forms of stress, the maintenance replacement therapy should be increased.

Regular x-ray measurement of linear growth and skeletal development should be carried out throughout the growing years. This provides further control over the adequacy of the maintenance therapy. At the time the skeletal development attains pubertal maturation, gonadal activation occurs, regardless of the chronological age. Plastic repair of abnormal external genitalia should be undertaken before the child reaches 4 years of age.

Experience has shown that with proper maintenance therapy, normal growth and development may be expected, and normal maturation of gonads and reproduction may be attained.

Late-Onset Virilizing Adrenal Hyperplasia. Delayed-onset virilizing adrenal hyperplasia (non-classical congenital hyperplasia), is a variant of classical congenital virilizing adrenal hyperplasia. It is characterized by development of virilization in late childhood but does not present with evidence of fetal virilization. Premature adrenarche or early development of sexual hair may be the first evidence of the disorder. Other clinical signs consist of acne, hirsutism, amenorrhea or menstrual irregularity, anovulation, and reduced fertility. ACTH stimulation produces an elevation of serum 17-OH-progesterone concentration into a range which is appropriate for classical congenital adrenal hyperplasia. The gene for classical as well as late-onset 21-hydroxylase deficiency is linked to HLA. Transmission is by an autosomal recessive trait. Treatment consists of glucocorticoid suppression of adrenal androgens before virilization progresses and ovaries become polycystic.

CUSHING'S SYNDROME. Cushing's syndrome is a complex clinical syndrome attributable to increased production of cortisol. The condition is rare in childhood. When it occurs, the underlying cause is usually an adrenal cortical carcinoma, although hyperplasia and benign adenoma are also seen. The clinical signs of Cushing's syndrome may also be produced by administration of hydrocortisone or other glucocorticoids in amounts in excess of physiological requirements.

Clinical Signs and Symptoms. Certain typical changes are observed in the patients. There is broadening of the face with temporal fat padding, giving the characteristic moon facies. Skin changes are evident in acne, seborrhea, increased growth of hair, especially pubic hair, and the appearance of dark-colored striae due to weakening of collagenous connective tissue in the skin. Truncal obesity and the "buffalo hump" are characteristic; the latter is due to increased fat padding between the scapulae. Vascular changes consist of hypertension, increased capillary fragility, and easy bruising. Abnormalities of bone metabolism with demineralization of the skeleton lead to pathological fractures. A tendency toward poor wound healing and growth retardation is common. Interference with other pituitary target relationships occurs; this is particularly notable in the adolescent or adult female, who manifests disturbance of the menstrual cycle. In infants and children one may not find the marked difference in obesity between the trunk and extremities that is often noted in adults.

Differential Diagnosis. The most useful laboratory tests in confirming the diagnosis of Cushing's syndrome consist in measuring plasma levels and urinary excretion levels of 17-hydroxycorticosteroids (both are increased) and the responses of these levels to stimulation with corticotropin. In Cushing's syndrome due to adrenal hyperplasia there is usually a greater than normal response to corticotropin infusion. In carcinoma the response is subnormal, indicating the autonomy of the carcinoma from pituitary control. Adenomas are less predictable in type of response. Suppression tests with administration of dexamethasone are of value in differentiating the adrenal lesion. There may also be excessive loss of body potassium, negative nitrogen balance, retention of sodium, and a tendency for a diabetic glucose tolerance curve. Localization of tumors is accomplished by a variety of ultrasound and roentgen imaging procedures. Arteriography and venography with sampling of adrenal veins for differential determinations of steroid levels between the effluents of the two adrenals are helpful procedures.

The disease may result from hypersecretion of ACTH by the pituitary gland. In some instances the condition is associated with a basophilic adenoma of the pituitary gland that may enlarge and erode the sella turcica, but in pituitary-induced Cushing's syndrome the gland is often not frankly adenomatous. Cytological changes may be seen in the pituitary gland in the majority of such cases; whether these represent primary alterations or are secondarily induced by increased levels of adrenal hormones is not always clear.

Treatment. Bilateral adrenalectomy is the treatment of choice, unless a pituitary adenoma is demonstrable. With the availability of the transsphenoidal surgical approach, removal of a pituitary microadenoma may be the first choice of treatment. Expert preoperative and postoperative care and optimal replacement therapy are essential for successful management. Children treated with bilateral adrenalectomy for Cushing's syndrome with adrenal hyperplasia may post-operatively develop Nelson's syndrome (expanding sella turcica and hyperpigmentation).

ANDROGENIC AND ESTROGENIC TUMORS. *Feminizing adrenal tumors* in children are rare. They may be either benign or malignant. They produce increased plasma estradiol concentration and increased urinary 17-ketosteroid excretion. Treatment consists of surgical removal of the adenoma.

Masculinizing adrenal tumors may occur throughout childhood and may be either benign or malignant. Usually the first clinical signs are the precocious appearance of pubic hair and an increased rate of linear growth. The effects on growth and appearance of other signs mimic those of congenital virilizing adrenal hyperplasia. Masculinizing tumors are invariably acquired after birth and, therefore, are not associated in the female with anomalous genitalia. Plasma concentrations of adrenal androgens and urinary 17-ketosteroid levels are elevated. This condition is differentiated from adrenal hyperplasia by the suppression test with dexamethasone. The plasma concentrations of adrenal androgens and urinary 17-ketosteroids are not suppressed in virilizing tumors, in contrast to virilizing adrenal hyperplasia.

Hypofunction of Adrenal Cortex

CONGENITAL HYPOADRENALISM. Congenital adrenal insufficiency occasionally occurs in newborn infants. The signs of adrenal insufficiency may appear rapidly, and the disorder progresses in a few hours through cyanosis, collapse, and death. If congenital adrenal hypoplasia is suspected, adrenal cortical steroids should be administered promptly.

ADDISON'S DISEASE. Acquired adrenal insufficiency, or Addison's disease, may occur throughout childhood as a result of destruction of the adrenals by autoimmunization, by infection (e.g., tuberculosis or moniliasis), or by unknown mechanisms. The onset in children is usually gradual; the earliest clinical signs are growth failure, weakness, and easy fatigability. Pigmentation of the skin, particularly of creases, develops slowly. There may be hypoglycemic attacks, weight loss, dehydration, and other evidence of salt loss. Some children may complain of abdominal pain. Measurements of the secretion rate of cortisol and its derivatives, their plasma levels and urinary excretion, and the adrenal reserve capacity upon corticotropin stimulation are the specific values that demonstrate adrenal cortical insufficiency.

Treatment. The treatment of adrenal cortical insufficiency consists in replacement therapy with a glucocorticoid such as hydrocortisone or one of its analogues. A mineralocorti-

coid such as 9-alpha-fluorohydrocortisone is administered in doses of 0.05 to 0.1 mg daily by mouth in event of aldosterone deficiency with inadequate sodium retention. The parents of children with Addison's disease should be supplied with an injectable form of glucocorticoid with instructions for administering supplements parenterally in the event of severe illness or trauma to the patient when medical attention is not immediately available. Replacement dosages of hydrocortisone acetate or cortisone acetate by mouth should be 25 mg/m^2/day given in two or three doses.

The prognosis of well-managed adrenal cortical insufficiency is good. Normal gonadal function will occur in the adolescent and adult.

SECONDARY HYPOADRENALISM. Secondary adrenal insufficiency is not associated with hyperpigmentation of the skin. Stimulation with corticotropin may produce elevations of plasma or urinary excretion of 17-hydroxycorticosteroids; however, the response often is sluggish on the first few days of such stimulation. The test for pituitary reserve with the administration of metyrapone will confirm the decreased blood levels of cortisol. Replacement therapy in secondary hypoadrenalism is carried out as in primary hypoadrenalism. In panhypopituitarism, replacement with adrenal hormones should always be given in conjunction with thyroid hormone replacement, although the dose required is less than in primary adrenal insufficiency.

HYPOALDOSTERONISM. Hypoaldosteronism may rarely occur as an isolated defect, although its manifestations — hypotension, shock, hyponatremia, hyperkalemia, and cardiac arrhythmias — may simulate Addison's disease. The diagnosis is confirmed by failure to observe an increase in urinary aldosterone excretion during a low salt intake or, alternatively, after injection of angiotensin intramuscularly. Treatment is by administration of mineralocorticoids and addition of salt in the diet. A familial type of aldosterone deficiency, manifested by growth retardation with defective conversion of 18-hydroxycorticosterone to aldosterone, has been described.

Adrenal Medulla

Pheochromocytoma

This is a functional tumor of chromaffin tissue, most often originating in the adrenal medulla. Pheochromocytoma is uncommon in children, but it should be considered in cases of hypertension that do not have a renal or other basis. The majority of children with pheochromocytoma have sustained hypertension, although paroxysmal attacks may occur with the symptoms of sweating, visual complaints, constipation, and Raynaud's phenomenon. Pheochromocytoma may become malignant.

DIAGNOSIS. Determination of catecholamines in the blood or urine provides a specific means of confirming the diagnosis. A single voided urine sample collected during a period of hypertension is preferred over a 24-hour collection. Vanillyl-mandelic acid (VMA) is a breakdown product of epinephrine and norepinephrine. The quantitation of VMA in urine is of value in supporting the diagnosis of pheochromocytoma, especially in occasional patients with normal catecholamine values. Increased catecholamine and VMA secretion may occur with neuroblastoma and other tumors of neural crest origin. False-positive VMA results may occur with ingestion of foods containing vanilla. Pharmacological tests such as alpha-receptor blockade with phentolamine (Regitine) or phenoxybenzamine (Dibenzyline) are useful in supporting the diagnosis but are usually not required.

Testes

Cryptorchidism

PATHOGENESIS. Cryptorchidism is the failure of one or both testes to descend into the scrotal sac. The testes may remain in the abdomen or at various points in the inguinal canal. Abdominal testes are frequently associated with maldevelopment of the genital ducts. It is not uncommon in bilateral abdominal cryptorchidism to have associated anomalies of the external genitalia, such as hypospadias or urogenital sinus. A remnant of vaginal pouch communicating with the posterior urethra may be present. When the testes are located in the canals, it is less likely that internal duct anomalies exist. In cryptorchidism there is an increased frequency of indirect inguinal hernia.

DIAGNOSIS. The diagnosis of cryptorchidism is made after determining that the testis cannot be brought into the scrotum by pressure or by relaxation of the cremaster muscle. If the testes are in the scrotum at birth, true cryptorchidism does not exist, even though the testes may be located in the inguinal canal at the time of examination. In the majority of such cases one may simply push the testes into the scrotum or, by warming the patient, allow the testes to settle into the scrotum spontaneously.

One cannot be certain without further study that the gonads located in the abdominal cavity are actually testes. Radiologic imaging techniques are useful in defining the internal anatomy. Serum testosterone determination before and after a course of human chorionic gonadotropin injections is useful to determine whether functional testicular tissue is present. The karyotype should be determined to exclude chromosomal abnormalities and to resolve the chromosomal sex of the patient. In evaluation of the phenotypic male with nonpalpable gonads one should also differentiate cryptorchidism from congenital adrenal hyperplasia, pseudohermaphroditism, and true hermaphroditism.

TREATMENT. Definitive treatment should be carried out prior to the age of 4 to 5 years. Initially, one may administer a short course of human chorionic gonadotropin, 1000 to 4000 I.U. three times weekly for 3 weeks. If the testes descend, one can predict that orchiopexy will not be required. In some cases the testes remain in the scrotum after this course of chorionic gonadotropin. Repeated trials of chorionic gonadotropin are usually futile and may lead only to damage to the seminiferous tubules. Orchiopexy should be carried out if stimulation by gonadotropin fails to correct the cryptorchidism. There is no assurance that the patient will be left with normally functioning testes even if surgery is carried out in early childhood.

TREATMENT OF HYPOGONADISM. Replacement therapy for testicular dysfunction is not required until the prepubertal period. Patients with anorchism should receive prosthetic testicular implants during childhood. As puberty approaches, replacement therapy with an oral or parenteral androgen preparation should be begun in order to assure the normal sequence of sex development.

When puberty is markedly delayed in patients with testes, an assessment of pituitary function is indicated. Replacement therapy must be considered in any marked delay of adolescence to prevent eunuchoid body proportions and to assure proper psychosocial development.

Ovary

Delayed Puberty

The mean age of menarche in North American girls is approximately 12.5 years. If secondary sexual characteristics have not appeared in girls by 15 years of age, the delay should be evaluated. Possible etiological factors include central nervous system abnormalities, hypopituitarism, primary ovarian abnormalities, and chronic systemic diseases. Rigorous physical training in girls with a lean body mass will tend to suppress the hypothalamic-pituitary-gonadal axis and cause a delay in menarche or oligomenorrhea in postmenarchic adolescents.

Secondary Amenorrhea

Secondary amenorrhea may result from central nervous system, pituitary, or ovarian abnormalities as well as from chronic systemic illnesses. The possibility of pregnancy must not be overlooked.

Diagnosis

The evaluation of ovarian dysfunction will depend on the presenting symptoms; however, a careful history and physical examination are required in all cases. This should include examination of the external genitalia and introitus and pelvic imaging for an estimate of uterine size and presence of adnexal organs or masses. In delayed puberty, a bone age determination can be useful in deciding whether the level of skeletal maturity is appropriate for the menarche. Ovarian estrogen production is assessed by the determination of plasma or urinary estrogens and estrogenization of the vaginal mucosa and cervical mucus. Plasma LH and FSH levels and their response to gonadotropin hormone stimulation will indicate the state of pituitary gonadotropin function. A karyotype is a useful adjunct in diagnosing Turner's syndrome, associated forms of mosaicism, and other anomalies of the X chromosome. Replacement therapy with estrogen should be undertaken only after a careful clinical assessment. Long-term replacement should be undertaken with minimal effective doses of estrogen given cyclically to permit menstrual bleeding. The combination of estrogen with a progestin in the premenstrual phase may be necessary to maintain a normal pattern of menstrual bleeding.

Sexual Precocity, Abnormal Sexual Development, Obesity, Failure to Thrive, and Dwarfism

The above topics are discussed in Appendix A, Differential Diagnosis, in Sections 25, 24, and 4, respectively.

H. David Mosier, Jr.

References

Collu, R., Ducharme, J. R., and Harvey, J. G. (Eds.). *Pediatric Endocrinology* (2nd ed.). Comprehensive Endocrinology Series. New York: Raven, 1989.

Hung, W., August, G. P., and Glasgow, A. M. (Eds.). *Pediatric Endocrinology: An Advanced Testbook* (2nd ed.). New Hyde Park, NY: Medical Examination Publishing Co., 1983.

Kaplan, S. A. (Ed.). *Clinical Pediatric and Adolescent Endocrinology* (2nd ed.). Philadelphia: Saunders, 1990.

Lifshitz, F. (Ed.). *Pediatric Endocrinology: A Clinical Guide*. New York: Dekker, 1985.

Styne, D. M., and Brook, C. G. D. (Eds.). *Current Concepts in Pediatric Endocrinology*. New York: Elsevier, 1987.

Wilkins, L. (Ed.). *The Diagnosis and Treatment of Endocrine Disorders in Childhood and Adolescence* (3rd ed.). Springfield, IL: Thomas, 1965.

7

Disorders of Metabolism

Energy Metabolism

Normal Physiology

The ultimate source of energy for human biological processes is the dietary nutrient intake. Despite feeding intermittently, humans expend energy continuously; hence they must store nutrients for consumption between meals, during prolonged fasting and exercise. The major endogenous energy depositories are the triglycerides in adipose tissue, protein in muscle, and glycogen in muscle and liver. During postprandial phases and short-term fasts, most tissues meet their energy requirements by using glucose derived from liver glycogen or free fatty acids (FFAs) from triglycerides, while the central nervous system depends almost exclusively on glucose metabolism. Most of the disorders of energy metabolism result in excessive falls (hypoglycemia) or elevation (diabetes mellitus) in blood glucose concentration. In normal humans the maintenance of normal energy homeostasis is achieved by a complex synchronized interaction between neural and hormonal factors in the context of environmental factors.

Digestive Process

The average diet in the Western world consists of approximately 50% carbohydrate, 35% fat, and 15% protein. After food ingestion about 90% of foodstuffs is absorbed in the course of passage through the small intestine, which is the main digestive and absorptive organ. Within the gut and intestinal brush border, the complex carbohydrates are hydrolyzed to monosaccharides, glucose, fructose, and galactose, which are actively transported to the portal circulation and delivered directly to the liver. Proteins and fats are cleaved enzymatically within the gut and transported as amino acids to the portal circulation, and as mono- and diglycerides in the form of chylomicrons into the general circulation through the thoracic duct.

Storage Forms of Energy

The energy derived from dietary nutrient intake is stored in the body in various forms. Carbohydrates are stored in the form of glycogen, which is found in the liver at concentrations of up to 5% in the postprandial period and in muscle tissue where glycogen content rarely exceeds 1%. While hepatic glycogen is readily degraded to glucose (glycogenolysis) and released in the general circulation to sustain blood glucose concentration, the glycogen present in muscle can not be released as free glucose; rather it is released as lactate. The total energy available as preformed glycogen in the healthy 70-kg man is between 1000 and 2000 calories, an amount inadequate to meet total energy needs for a single day.

The body's capacity to store energy in the form of fat is essentially unlimited, leading to one of the major diseases of the Western world, obesity. Fat is an ideal storage form of energy. It contains 9 cal/g, is stored with minimal associated water or protein, and is readily convertible to FFA when needed for energy.

There is no storage form of protein in the human organism. Protein is the major constituent of muscle and organs and is also the source of all tissue enzymes. Gluconeogenesis involves the degradation of structural protein to provide new sources of glucose. In periods of prolonged caloric deprivation, 30 to 50% of the structural proteins may be degraded for energy requirements prior to death of the organism.

The energy control system of the body must be able to rapidly adapt to remarkably varying conditions. For the average adult, adaptive requirements are not great but must include the efficient handling of nutrients and energy intermediates under basal conditions, during periods of digestion of food with greater variability in composition, and in periods of short-term fasting such as that associated with overnight sleep. The system, however, is readily adaptable to more extreme demands, including extremes of exercise, prolonged starvation and stress, the special requirements of febrile illness and surgery, and the unique requirements associated with birth and the adaptation to intermittent feeding after the abrupt termination of the continuous nutrient supply from the mother to the fetus via the placenta. With all of these alterations and demands, nutrient concentrations such as glucose, amino acids, and lipids as well as energy intermediates are kept within narrow and safe concentrations. This results from the remarkably efficient mechanism of energy storage, retrieval, and interconversion.

The following brief discussion of biochemistry of energy metabolism is separated into presentation of the salient points of metabolism of carbohydrates, proteins, and fats. One must always keep in mind, however, that there is a dynamic flux and a tight interrelationship in the metabolism of these various energy intermediates.

Biochemistry of Carbohydrate Metabolism

The metabolism of carbohydrate (Fig. 7-1) in the mammals can be subdivided as follows:

1. Glycolysis. The oxidation of glucose or glycogen to pyruvate and lactate by the Embden-Meyerhof pathway. This process occurs in virtually all tissues.
2. Glycogenolysis. The breakdown of glycogen to glucose in the liver, and to pyruvate and lactate in the muscle.
3. Glycogenesis. The synthesis of glycogen from glucose.
4. The oxidation of pyruvate to acetyl CoA prior to the entrance of the products of glycolysis into the citric acid (TCA) cycle, which is the final common pathway for the oxidation of carbohydrate, fat, and protein. The metabolism of pyruvate through the TCA cycle is an oxidative reaction, yielding high energy in the form of ATP and water and CO_2 as the respiratory end products. In the presence of inadequate oxygen to efficiently turn the TCA cycle (as occurs in extreme exercise exertion), pyruvate is reduced to lactic acid.
5. Gluconeogenesis. The formation of glucose or glycogen from noncarbohydrate sources. The principal substrates for gluconeogenesis are glucogenic amino acids, lactate, and glycerol.
6. The hexose monophosphate shunt (pentose phosphate pathway) is an alternative pathway to the Embden-Meyerhof pathway for the oxidation of glucose. Although quantitatively less important than glycolysis, one of its end products, nicotinamide adenine dinucleotide phosphate (NADPH), reduced form, is the essential hydrogen donor in lipid synthesis.

The monosaccharides derived from dietary carbohydrates include glucose, galactose, and fructose. Only glucose is used as a direct energy source. Galactose is readily converted into the glucose pool and stored as glycogen, and fructose is either directly metabolized for energy needs down the Embden-Meyerhof pathway or converted upstream into the glucose pool. The initial enzymatic alteration of each of these monosaccharides is phosphorylation, either by a nonspecific hexokinase or, in the case of glucose, a specific glucokinase. The central energy intermediate in carbohydrate metabolism is glucose 6-phosphate.

In summary, carbohydrate nutrient sources are converted in the liver into glucose, which is then stored in the form of glycogen, released to the general circulation to maintain blood glucose concentration within normal limits, utilized as a direct energy source by metabolism through the TCA cycle, or converted into lipids for energy storage when intake is in excess of immediate needs.

84

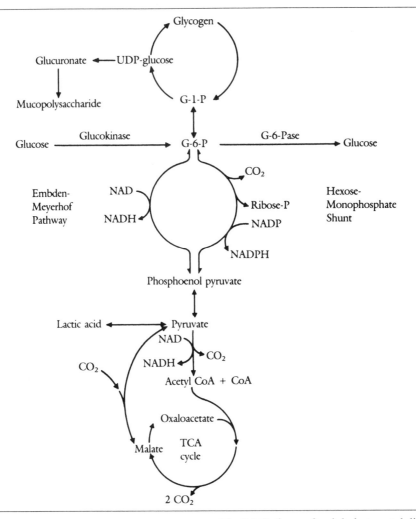

Fig. 7-1. Pathways of carbohydrate metabolism. NADP = nicotinamide adenine dinucleotide phosphate; NADPH = nicotinamide adenine dinucleotide phosphate, reduced form; NAD =
nicotinamide adenine dinucleotide; NADH = nicotinamide
adenine dinucleotide, reduced form; UDP-glucose = uridine
diphosphate glucose; TCA cycle = tricarboxylic acid cycle. (Modified from W. W. Moore, Endocrine Functions of the Pancreas. In
E. E. Selkurt [Ed.], Physiology [3d ed.]. Boston: Little, Brown,
1971.)

Biochemistry of Fat Metabolism

Lipids are important dietary constituents not only because
of their high energy value but also because of the fat-soluble
vitamins and the essential fatty acids contained in the fat of
natural foods. Dietary fats are predominantly triglycerides
with very small amounts of cholesterol and phospholipids.
Lipids circulate bound to specific lipoprotein carriers,
including very-low-density lipoprotein (VLDL), low-
density lipoprotein (LDL), and high-density lipoprotein
(HDL).

The relative proportions of triglyceride, cholesterol, and
phospholipids vary with the specific carrier protein, with
triglyceride primarily carried on VLDL and cholesterol on

LDL and HDL. The FFAs are loosely bound to serum
albumin. Dietarily derived triglycerides, circulating in the
postprandial period as chylomicrons, are "cleared" from the
circulation by enzymatic degradation to long-chain FFAs
and glycerol, which are then taken up by the liver, adipose

tissue, and muscle for either direct energy purposes or storage. De novo synthesis goes on actively in both liver and adipose tissue. The essential building blocks for lipid synthesis include the three-carbon backbone derived from alpha-glycerophosphate; an intermediary of glucose metabolism, acetyl CoA; the two-carbon fragment necessary for elongation of the fatty acid chain, which may be derived from glucose metabolism, amino acids, or fat; and the hydrogen derived from the hexose monophosphate shunt. Lipogenesis is an active process, highly sensitive to hormone concentration. It occurs in the postprandial period under the direction of insulin.

The lipids of metabolic significance to mammals include triglycerides, phospholipids, and steroids, together with products of their metabolism such as long-chain FFAs, glycerol, and ketone bodies. An overview of their metabolic interrelationships and their relationship to carbohydrate metabolism is shown in Figure 7-2.

Lipolysis is the degradative side of lipid metabolism, resulting from beta oxidation and leading to the release of FFAs and glycerol from both adipose tissue and liver. The FFAs provide the alternate fuel to glucose and can be readily and completely metabolized by most of the tissues of the body. The glycerol moiety can be reincorporated into the

Embden-Meyerhof pathway as a gluconeogenic source. Lipolysis is also highly sensitive to endocrine alterations resulting from insulin deficiency or excess of one of several of the counterinsulin hormones, including growth hormone, adrenocorticotropic hormone (ACTH), epinephrine, and glucagon. Cortisol may play a permissive role in lipolysis.

As in the metabolism of glucose, fatty acids must first be converted in a reaction with ATP to an active intermediate before they will react with the enzymes responsible for their further metabolism. This is the only step in the complete degradation of a fatty acid that requires energy from ATP. In the presence of ATP and coenzyme A, the enzyme acyl-CoA synthetase catalyzes the conversion of a fatty acid (or FFA) to an "active fatty acid" or acyl CoA, accompanied by the expenditure of one high-energy phosphate bond. Acyl-CoA synthetases are found both inside and outside the mitochondria. Several acyl-CoA synthetases have been described, each specific for fatty acids of different chain length.

Carnitine (β-hydroxy-γ-trimethylammonium butyrate), stimulates the oxidation of long-chain fatty acids by mitochondria. It is widely distributed, being particularly abundant in muscle. Activation of long-chain fatty acids to acyl CoA occurs in microsomes and on the outer membranes of mitochondria. Long-chain acyl CoA does not penetrate mi-

Fig. 7-2. Relationship of certain phases of lipid and protein metabolism with carbohydrate metabolism. EMP = Embden-Meyerhof pathway; HMP = hexose monophosphate shunt. (From W. W. Moore, Endocrine Functions of the Pancreas. In E. E. Selkurt [Ed.], Physiology *[3d ed.]. Boston: Little, Brown, 1971.)*

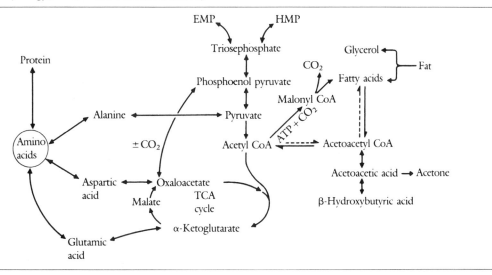

tochondria and become oxidized unless carnitine is present. An enzyme, carnitine palmitoyl transferase I, is associated with the outer side of the inner mitochondrial membrane and allows long-chain acyl groups (as acylcarnitine) to penetrate the mitochondria and gain access to the β-oxidation system of enzymes. A deficiency of carnitine impairs fatty acid oxidation, and triacyglycerol accumulates. Carnitine is synthesized from lysine in liver and kidney. Activation of lower fatty acids may occur within the mitochondria, independently of carnitine.

Several enzymes, known collectively as fatty acid oxidase, are found in the mitochondrial matrix adjacent to the respiratory chain, which is found in the inner membrane. These catalyze the oxidation of acyl CoA to acetyl CoA, the system being coupled with the phosphorylation of ADP to ATP. As acetyl CoA can be oxidized to CO_2 and water via the citric acid cycle (which is also found within the mitochondria) the complete oxidation of fatty acids is achieved. Fatty acids with an odd number of carbon atoms are oxidized by the pathway of β-oxidation until a 3-carbon (propionyl CoA) residue remains. This compound is converted to succinyl CoA, a constituent of the citric acid cycle. Thus, the complete oxidation of long-chain fatty acids is through the TCA cycle, yielding high energy in the form of ATP, CO_2, and water. The incomplete oxidation of long-chain fatty acids may occur under a variety of circumstances, most typically prolonged starvation and insulin deficiency. When acetyl CoA derived from beta oxidation of long-chain fatty acids cannot be fully metabolized through the TCA cycle, then it is short-circuited to acetoacetyl CoA and then on to ketone bodies, including acetoacetic acid, beta-hydroxybutyric acid, and acetone. Insulin deficiency and glucagon excess are highly significant factors in the production of ketone bodies (see Fig. 7-2) and, potentially, ketoacidosis.

In summary, dietary fat is an important source of energy. Circulating and stored fat may be derived from dietary fat and produced from other carbon sources such as carbohydrates and protein. Lipid synthesis and storage occur when calorie intake is excessive. Lipolysis yields FFAs, which are essential alternate fuel sources during intervals when glucose metabolism is reduced. Pathological alterations in complete lipid oxidation result in ketone body formation with the danger of ketoacidosis.

Biochemistry of Protein Metabolism

Protein synthesis is a complex process, utilizing dietarily derived amino acids for the development of specialized enzymes, for the repair of degraded structural protein, and for

cell replication and growth. Amino acid transport into the cell is stimulated by insulin and intracellular protein synthesis, and cell replication and growth are jointly stimulated by growth hormone and insulin. Proteolysis, or protein degradation, is an active process that occurs during periods of starvation. Proteolysis leads to the increase in concentration of amino acids within the cell and the release of amino acids into the general circulation. The degradation and release of amino acids are highly specialized biochemical processes. The old concepts of glucogenic and ketogenic amino acids have been largely replaced with the awareness that essentially all amino acids, with the possible exception of leucine, can be directed into the glucose metabolic pathway by appropriate deamination and transamination. The release of amino acids from muscle tissue during periods of stress and starvation does not reflect the muscle amino acid content. The major amino acids released for potential use in gluconeogenesis are alanine and glutamine. Alanine is the major amino acid taken up by the liver for the formation of glucose, while glutamine is preferentially used by the gastrointestinal tract and kidney. The glucose-alanine cycle is an important biochemical pathway that is the primary mechanism for transferring both carbon atoms and amino terminal groups from muscle to liver. The branched-chain amino acids (leucine, isoleucine, and valine) also receive specialized handling. These amino acids are used for endogenous energy sources within the muscle following prolonged exercise and stress and are released in increased concentrations in the circulation during situations of insulin deficiency and starvation.

As indicated in Figure 7-2, amino acids readily enter the energy pathway by metabolism through the TCA cycle or by conversion to pyruvate and then upstream to glucose. The direction and rate of amino acid metabolism are controlled by the endocrine system.

Hormonal Regulation of Energy Metabolism

Figure 7-3 summarizes some of the major effects of those hormonal agents that are primarily involved in control of intermediary metabolism and energy regulation. Insulin is the primary regulator of energy homeostasis. Insulin is an anabolic hormone that promotes the uptake and storage of energy substrates and the synthesis of protein. Although glucose enters the liver along a concentration gradient, the initial intracellular biochemical reaction, phosphorylation by glucokinase, is promoted by insulin as is the primary glycogen synthetic step, the activation of glycogen synthase. Conversely, the degradation of preformed glycogen is inhibited by insulin action as are the major enzymatic steps in

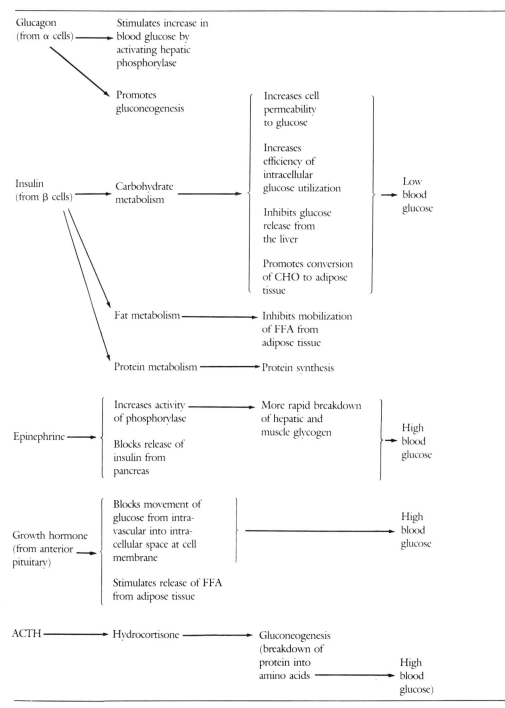

Fig. 7-3. Effects of hormones on intermediary metabolism.

gluconeogenesis, thus effectively reducing hepatic glucose output. In peripheral tissue, specifically muscle, adipose tissue, and organs excluding the brain and liver, insulin has a direct cell membrane effect, promoting increased entry of glucose into the cell. Considerable controversy exists about the possible postreceptor effects of insulin, but increasing evidence points toward intracellular anabolic action of insulin in peripheral tissue.

Insulin affects lipid metabolism in a number of essential ways. Lipoprotein lipase, the tissue-fixed enzyme system responsible for "clearing" dietary fat, is activated by insulin, leading to triglyceride degradation and the uptake of FFA by tissues. Further, calorically excessive carbohydrate is very efficiently converted into triglyceride under the direction of insulin in both liver and adipose tissue. The overall effect of insulin action on lipid metabolism is to promote synthesis and storage of extra calories in the form of triglyceride and to decrease circulating lipid levels.

In terms of protein metabolism, insulin acts synergistically with growth hormone to promote amino acid uptake with the overall effect being anabolic in nature.

While insulin has been called the hormone of feasting, glucagon has been considered the hormone of fasting because its release is suppressed during carbohydrate intake and stimulated during periods of stress, starvation, and exercise. Glucagon stimulates the cascade of enzymatic events that lead to hepatic glycogenolysis and the increase in release of glucose from the liver. Glucagon is the most efficient biological agent in terms of stimulation of the enzyme systems responsible for reversal of the Embden-Meyerhof pathway and the promotion of gluconeogenesis. The latter results in increased hepatic uptake of gluconeogenic substrates including amino acids, principally alanine, but also including lactate, pyruvate, and glycerol. Glucagon stimulates lipolysis and the release of FFA and, more importantly, directs the "set" of hepatic enzymes involved in lipid oxidation away from the TCA cycle and toward ketone body production. The net effect of glucagon release is catabolic in nature, resulting in degradation of preformed glycogen, the conversion of amino acids into glucose (both leading to an increase in the concentration of blood glucose), the degradation of triglycerides, and the promotion of ketosis. The gastrointestinal hormones, subjects of intense current research, are intimately involved in the enteroinsular axis and the release of insulin and glucagon.

Growth hormone affects energy metabolism in several ways, as is clinically demonstrable by the increased frequency of hypoglycemia in the hypopituitary child and the frequent occurrence of carbohydrate intolerance in the acromegalic adult. The actions of growth hormone, like that of insulin, are mediated through direct hormone attachment to specific receptors located on cell membranes of essentially all tissues of the body. The release of growth hormone results in impairment of glucose uptake at the cellular level. Whether this is direct or indirect inhibition of insulin action is unclear. Growth hormone stimulates some systems responsible for lipolysis, leading to the release of FFA from adipose tissues, effectively opposing the action of insulin in terms of amino acid metabolism, and stimulating both amino acid transport into the cell and the synthesis of protein. ACTH has an effect on energy metabolism, primarily through the stimulation of synthesis and release of adrenocortical hormones, principally cortisone; however, ACTH is known to have an extra-adrenal effect similar to that of growth hormone in stimulating the enzyme systems responsible for lipolysis. The primary effect of cortisol on energy homeostasis appears to be permissive in nature, increasing the counterinsulin action of growth hormone, epinephrine, and glucagon. Cortisol, however, has a separate, independent action on proteolysis, or the degradation of preformed protein to amino acids. In conjunction with glucagon, it stimulates those enzyme systems important in gluconeogenesis, leading to increased blood glucose concentration.

The catecholamines epinephrine and norepinephrine are synthesized and released from the adrenal medulla and from chromaffin tissue throughout the sympathetic nervous chain. Although both of these biochemical agents similarly affect energy metabolism, epinephrine is clearly the more potent of the two. The catecholamines are the only naturally occurring inhibitors of insulin release. Further, epinephrine is a highly potent stimulator of the enzyme systems involved in glycogenolysis in both liver and muscle, the end result being release of glucose from the liver and lactate from muscle tissue. The release of epinephrine also rapidly stimulates the breakdown of preformed triglyceride and the release of FFA into the general circulation. The overall effect of catecholamine release is to prepare the organism for emergency action and is catabolic in nature.

Integration of Energy Homeostasis

The objectives of the regulation of energy metabolism are to provide a continuous and adequate supply of energy to the organism at all times while maintaining energy substrate concentrations within a narrow physiological range. These objectives must be met under several highly different environmental circumstances, characterized by food ingestion, basal postprandial state, short- and long-term starvation, exercise, and stress.

HOMEOSTASIS IN THE FED STATE. After the ingestion of a mixed meal, several gastrointestinal hormones are released that, in conjunction with the increased nutrient concentrations (most importantly glucose and amino acids), reach the islet cells of the pancreas, resulting in the release of insulin and, in most cases, the inhibition of glucagon release. Intracellular glucose is the primary substrate that evokes the release of insulin. Several amino acids, notably arginine, lysine, and leucine, act synergistically with glucose to stimulate insulin secretion. A number of gastrointestinal hormones that influence gut motility, digestion, and absorption of nutrients also enhance the secretion of islet cell hormones, including insulin, glucagon, somatostatin (SRIF), and pancreatic polypeptide. The term "incretin" denotes one or more gastrointestinal hormones that augment glucose-mediated insulin release (enteroinsular axis). The best characterized of these is gastric inhibitory polypeptide (GIP), which is secreted by the gut cells during absorption of nutrients and by HCl. In addition, increased cholinergic activity occurring during alimentation may enhance the secretion of insulin by direct vagal innervation of B cells. Consequently, following the ingestion of a mixed meal, an array of factors contribute to augment the release of insulin, which has a predominant anabolic action on fuel utilization and storage. In normal persons, elevated insulin levels are usually demonstrable in the peripheral blood within 20 minutes after carbohydrate ingestion. The effects of increased insulin, in conjunction with a decline in glucagon, in the immediate postprandial period and continuing for 2 to 3 hours after food ingestion, include the following:

1. Promotion of glucose uptake in liver and muscle with glycogen production, catalyzed by a cascade of enzyme reactions, including glycogen synthase, which is regulated by insulin.
2. Glucose metabolism through the Embden-Meyerhof pathway and the TCA cycle for energy generation. Glucose is first phosphorylated to glucose 6-phosphate by the action of glucokinase (hexokinase), a reaction controlled by insulin.
3. Decreased hepatic glucose output by inhibition of glycogenolysis and gluconeogenesis.

In the fed state, therefore, the liver, in the presence of insulin, constitutes an important reservoir for glucose storage.

Sugar, which is not sequestered in the liver, eventually is distributed within the extracellular space, accounting for the increasing plasma glucose levels. Hyperglycemia stimulates additional release of insulin, thereby promoting the translocation of extracellular glucose, primarily into muscle and fat. In these tissues, insulin also enhances glucose oxidation, glycogen synthesis, amino acid transport, protein synthesis, and potassium and phosphate influx. In addition, insulin inhibits the release of amino acids from muscle; in adipose cells, it also restrains lipolysis and enhances lipogenesis. These anabolic effects on fat are readily demonstrated by a decrease in circulating FFAs derived from triglyceride, coinciding with the ascending plasma sugar concentration. Concurrent with the decline in plasma glucose, there is a gradual resumption of hepatic glucose production. This reflects a fall in ambient insulin levels, a decrease in insulin receptors, and increased release of hormones that counter-regulate the action of insulin on both glucose output from the liver and uptake by peripheral tissue, preventing a continued drop in plasma sugar during the postabsorptive phase.

HOMEOSTASIS DURING FASTING. In the postabsorptive phase, which gradually evolves within 4 to 6 hours after eating, and in short-term fasting, such as in overnight sleep, hepatic glycogen is the primary source for maintaining glucose concentrations, with gluconeogenesis contributing 25%. With prolonged fasting, depletion of glycogen necessitates the switching over to gluconeogenesis for almost all glucose produced. The body attempts to conserve protein for mechanical catalytic processes within the cell; consequently, FFA and ketones from the liver are the major fuels used by most tissues. Most of the generated glucose is diverted to the brain and oxidized internally to CO_2 and water. The remainder goes to skeletal muscle, the cellular elements of the blood, peripheral nerves, and renal medullae, where it is utilized through glycolytic pathways. When food deprivation is extended, muscle becomes almost entirely dependent upon FFAs and ketoacids for its energy needs.

Under physiologic conditions, glycogenolysis in the liver is stimulated by glucagon and probably catecholamines, which activate phosphorylase. In the immediate postabsorptive period, 75 to 80% of net glucose balance is furnished by glycogen, but usually within 24 to 48 hours glycogen reserves are dissipated with only around 10 g preserved for emergency use. The glucose pool, therefore, must be replenished by de novo synthesis of glucose from precursors derived from other fuels. During brief fasting, 90% of total gluconeogenesis occurs in the liver, with the kidney assuming importance as a source of glucose during protracted starvation. Of the gluconeogenic precursors in humans, glycerol is only a minor contributor. Resynthesis of glucose from pyruvate and lactate represents a major route of disposal of lactate originating from glycolytic processes in blood cells and nervous tissue.

Within the period extending from the postabsorptive phase through brief fasting, it is clear that the gradual decline of insulin and the rise in glucagon are the major determinants favoring augmented hepatic glycogenolysis and gluconeogenesis. In addition, the lowered insulin concentration leads to diminished glucose uptake in muscle and adipose tissue with concomitant increased lipolysis and proteolysis thereby providing a flow of glucogenic precursors.

With prolonged periods of fasting, glucose output gradually falls with a concurrent decline in protein catabolism. In order to sustain the metabolic requirements of brain and other tissues and to conserve body protein, fat is burned as an energy source. Lipolysis is augmented as a function of the reduced availability of insulin and coincident increased release of counter-regulatory hormones. From the immediate postabsorptive period into early and late starvation, FFA influx into plasma is doubled. The FFAs are taken up by the liver and oxidized via acetyl CoA to ketoacids, are metabolized to CO_2 and water, or are re-esterified to form triglycerides. Ketoacids are minor metabolic fuels during the early postprandial stage; however, in later phases of fasting, ketogenesis is doubled and ketoacids assume major importance as energy sources. These adaptative processes, whereby fat substitutes for glucose in muscle, are also applicable to the central nervous system (CNS). In the past, the brain was considered to have a chronic obligate requirement for glucose; now, during protracted fasting and in the early neonatal period, ketoacids are recognized as the principal fuels utilized by brain. Hence, during starvation, the adaptation of virtually all tissues to fat as energy sources, concurrent with restriction in gluconeogenesis, may be explained teleologically as a compensatory mechanism to minimize protein breakdown for survival.

In contrast to the adult, the newborn infant and young child are particularly vulnerable to disturbances in glucose homeostasis as a result of the dramatic metabolic changes occurring during transition from intrauterine to extrauterine life. At birth the transfer of maternal fuel to the fetus is acutely interrupted and endogenous glucose production is activated via glycogenolysis and gluconeogenesis to provide energy requirements for the newborn. The general principles of fuel utilization observed in the adult apply to the infant; however, the glucose turnover in the immediate newborn period is of the order of 5 to 10 mg/kg/min, about two- to fourfold the rate in adults. It is thought that the high glucose needs are due to the relative increase in the ratio of brain to total body mass. Because most of the gluconeogenic precursors originate from protein stores that are smaller in the newborn infant and young child, and in

the face of increased glucose needs compared to adults, sustained glucose production may be compromised, accounting for the susceptibility of neonates to develop fasting hypoglycemia.

Hypoglycemia

Hypoglycemia occurs when the rate of peripheral utilization of glucose exceeds the supply. This condition may arise under one of three basic situations: (1) increased peripheral uptake and utilization of glucose, (2) deficiency or impairment in gluconeogenesis, and (3) defects in glycogen breakdown and release from the liver. One or more of these situations may pertain in a great variety of very dissimilar pathological conditions.

Disorders Associated with Hypoglycemia

I. Transient neonatal
  A. Decreased production
    1. Small for dates
    2. Prematurity
  B. Increased utilization
    1. Hyperinsulinism
      a. Infant of diabetic mother
      b. Erythroblastosis
      c. "Infant giant" (Beckwith syndrome)
      d. Rapid discontinuation of IV glucose
      e. ? Beta-cell hyperplasia
  C. Decreased production and increased utilization
    1. Birth asphyxia
    2. hypothermia
II. Neonatal and infancy
  A. Decreased production or release of hepatic glucose
    1. Enzyme deficiency
      a. Glycogen storage diseases
      b. Galactosemia
      c. Fructose 1,6-diphosphatase deficiency
      d. Phosphoenolpyruvate carboxykinase deficiency
      e. Pyruvate dehydrogenase deficiency
      f. Pyruvate carboxylase deficiency
      g. Hereditary fructose intolerance
    2. Hormone deficiency
      a. Growth horme (GH) deficiency or hypopituitarism
      b. Glucocorticoid deficiency (ACTH deficiency, congenital adrenal hyperplasia, primary adrenal insufficiency)
      c. Hypothyroidism
      e. Glucagon deficiency
      f. "Adrenal medullary unresponsiveness"

3. Decreased alternate fuel production
   a. Defects in fatty acid oxidation
     (1). Primary carnitine deficiency
     (2). Fatty acid acyl-CoA dehydrogenase deficiency
   b. Defects in amino acid metabolism
     (1). Maple syrup urine disease
     (2). Propionic acidemia
     (3). Methylmalonic acidemia
     (4). Tyrosinosis
B. Increased utilization
  1. Hyperinsulinism
   a. Nesidioblastosis
   b. Islet cell hyperplasia or adenoma
   c. Beckwith-Wiedemann syndrome
   e. Leucine sensitivity
   f. Insulin reaction in diabetes mellitus
   g. Child abuse with insulin
III. Childhood
  A. Decreased production
   1. Enzyme deficiencies listed under II.A.1.
   2. Reye's syndrome
   3. Toxins: Alcohol, Jamaican vomiting sickness
   4. Hormone deficiencies listed under II.A.2.
   5. Defects in fatty acid oxidation II.A.3.a.
   6. Idiopathic-ketotic hypoglycemia
  B. Increased utilization
   1. Hyperinsulinism
    a. Islet cell adenoma
    b. Insulin administration
    c. Oral hypoglycemics
  C. Miscellaneous
   1. Reactive hypoglycemia
   2. Starvation
   3. Salicylate intoxication

Hypoglycemia is diagnosed when the blood glucose is found to be clearly below the normal range for the particular laboratory. A fasting true blood glucose value below 45 mg/100 ml for the older child and 30 mg/100 ml for the normal newborn or premature infant should be considered pathological. Repeat determinations are important for confirmation and to rule out the possibility of laboratory error. Depression of blood sugar is accompanied by certain symptoms which in the neonate include tremors, apnea, hypotonia, irritability, pallor, tachypnea, coma, and convulsions. In the infant and older child hypoglycemic symptoms include pallor, sweating, hunger, nausea, abdominal discomfort, mental confusion or irritability, headaches, visual disturbance, convulsion, and coma. It is important to realize

that these symptoms may or may not be present in the child with hypoglycemia or may occur in a transient manner. In the newborn infant, biochemical hypoglycemia may not be associated with any demonstrable symptoms, or at times it may be associated only with apnea. The older child frequently presents with a convulsive disorder; however, he may come to medical attention initially with a behavior problem or with complaints of a newly acquired ravenous appetite, extreme lethargy, somnolence, or transitory neurological abnormalities.

The importance of early recognition of and therapy for the child with hypoglycemia cannot be overemphasized. Glucose is the primary source of energy to the brain, and in the absence of glucose, there may be rapid and irreversible CNS damage, particularly in infants who have hypoglycemia prior to 6 months of age.

NEONATAL HYPOGLYCEMIA. In the great majority of cases, hypoglycemia is limited to the immediate neonatal period. Cases that fall into this category include infants of diabetic mothers, premature infants, and infants with the syndrome of symptomatic neonatal hypoglycemia.

The association between maternal diabetes and neonatal hypoglycemia has long been recognized. Because the hypoglycemia is often asymptomatic, it was considered by some to be of no particular significance. Recently, however, there has been increasing evidence that asymptomatic neonatal hypoglycemia may be injurious to the central nervous system and should be treated. These infants have hypoglycemia on the basis of hyperinsulinism.

The premature infant frequently has blood glucose values less than 20 mg/100 ml but may remain without symptoms. Hypoglycemia in such an infant results from deficiency of hepatic glycogen stores and immaturity of the enzyme systems involved in gluconeogenesis.

The syndrome of symptomatic neonatal hypoglycemia more commonly occurs in males, in the smaller of twins, and in the offspring of mothers whose pregnancy was complicated by toxemia. These infants weigh much less than expected for their gestational age. For the first 7 to 10 days of life they may have very severe symptomatic hypoglycemia, which requires active therapeutic intervention. The mechanism of hypoglycemia in these infants is not clear, but they appear to be suffering from intrauterine malnutrition.

HYPOGLYCEMIA ASSOCIATED WITH INBORN ERRORS OF METABOLISM. A number of metabolic defects are associated with hypoglycemia. In many cases, hypoglycemia occurs in early infancy with a tendency to persistence or recurrence. The metabolic defects include glycogen storage diseases, galactosemia, hereditary fructose intolerance, maple syrup urine disease, and abnormalities of fatty acid oxidation.

Inborn Errors of Carbohydrate Metabolism. The glycogen storage diseases are classic examples of genetically determined specific enzyme deficiencies that result in major alterations in energy homeostasis. Type I glycogen storage disease, or Von Gierke's disease, results from a deficiency of the enzyme glucose 6-phosphatase, which leads to almost complete impairment of release of glucose from the liver and, consequently, severe hypoglycemia. The typical clinical features include physical retardation, hepatic enlargement, and frequently intellectual impairment. Classic symptoms of hypoglycemia are surprisingly infrequent despite the extraordinarily low blood glucose concentrations. Biochemically, children with this condition frequently have blood glucose values less than 20 mg/100 ml associated with lactic acidosis, hyperlipidemia, and hyperuricemia. Clinically and biochemically, some patients have been described with normal glucose 6-phosphatase concentrations present in liver biopsy specimens. This condition, now referred to as Ib, has been identified as a deficiency of glucose 6-phosphatase translocase, the enzyme responsible for moving the enzyme glucose 6-phosphatase from the intracellular cytoplasm to the microsomes where it is activated. Glycogen storage diseases types III and VI are clinically similar to type I but generally are milder. Both are a result of impairments in hepatic glycogen degradation secondary to enzyme deficiency. Type III glycogen storage disease results from a deficiency in the debranching enzyme system so that the hepatic glycogen molecule can be only partially degraded during periods of fasting or stress. Type VI glycogen storage disease results from an enzymatic deficiency in the phosphorylase activating system. Several possible enzyme deficiencies can theoretically be involved, leading to identical clinical and biochemical alterations. Finally, glycogen synthase deficiency, an extremely rare metabolic disorder, is associated with inability to synthesize or store glycogen and is consequently associated with severe hypoglycemia on fasting.

Galactosemia and fructose pathway defects are similar metabolic conditions, both of which result from an enzyme deficiency leading to the accumulation of an abnormal sugar. Galactosemia may be associated with symptomatic hypoglycemia; however, it is usually a minor manifestation and appears to be dependent on significant liver dysfunction.

Hereditary fructose intolerance is associated with a deficiency of fructose-1-phosphate-aldolase, and symptoms depend on intake of fructose. No symptoms occur in the absence of fructose ingestion (e.g., breast feeding). Symptoms include poor feeding, vomiting, and failure to thrive in almost all affected infants. Other problems may include lethargy, irritability, bleeding tendencies, abdominal distention, and diarrhea. These children protect themselves by developing a marked aversion to sweets. The hypoglycemia response to an intravenous fructose challenge is diagnostic in the presence of a significant history. Oral fructose should be avoided as resulting symptoms may be extremely severe. Most of the symptoms are reversed with the institution of a fructose-free diet. If unrecognized, the liver damage may be fatal.

Fructose 1,6-diphosphatase deficiency is associated with episodes of hypoglycemia and acidosis during times of stress such as infections or prolonged starvation. When not having an acute episode, the children may be slightly acidotic and have hepatomegaly, hypotonia, and obesity. These children do not develop fasting hypoglycemia. At the time of hypoglycemia, serum alanine levels are high. Again, oral fructose should be avoided in children with this syndrome not only as part of the diet but also for diagnostic tests. A specific leukocyte assay for the enzyme may be diagnostic.

Inborn Errors of Amino Acid Metabolism. In maple syrup urine disease there is inability to metabolize the branched-chain amino acids completely. This causes an accumulation of these compounds and their associated keto acids. Hypoglycemia may result from accumulation of leucine, an amino acid that stimulates insulin release.

Inborn Errors of Fatty Acid Oxidation. These represent a newly recognized area of human disease. Despite their recent discovery, these disorders in the aggregate appear to be relatively common. The classic presentation of systemic abnormalities of fatty acid oxidation includes hypoketotic hypoglycemia. Acute episodes of vomiting and lethargy may occur, after fasting induced by intercurrent illness, and may progress to coma. These manifestations have led to the misdiagnosis of Reye's syndrome in many patients. Mortality may approach 60% during the first episode. Defects in the metabolism of fatty acids have been implicated as a cause of the sudden infant death syndrome. In other occasions, especially when the defect is confined to muscle, patients present with myopathy, recurrent aching of muscles, exercise intolerance, and myoglobinuria. Cardiomyopathy may be a major cause of morbidity.

The normal endogenous metabolism of fats begins with lipolysis, which releases free fatty acids and increases their concentrations in plasma where they are bound to albumin and transported to other tissues, particularly the liver and muscle. Fatty acids are then converted to their acyl-CoA derivatives and transported inside the mitochondria for β-oxidation. Long-chain fatty acids require carnitine to enter the mitochondria, whereby short- and medium-chain fatty acids cross the mitochondrial membrane without esterification with carnitine. Three mitochondrial enzymes catalyze the initial step in β-oxidation of fatty acids; short-chain acyl-CoA dehydrogenase, medium-chain acyl-CoA dehydrogenase, and long-chain acyl-CoA dehydrogenase. Deficiencies of each of these enzymes have been described and each may produce the syndrome of hypoketotic hypoglycemia. Additionally, primary or secondary carnitine deficiency can lead to similar clinical manifestations. In these patients with inborn errors of fatty acid oxidation, hypoglycemia is induced by an abnormally long (12–15 hours) overnight fast. The hypoglycemia presumably reflects an inability to reduce glucose consumption by substituting fatty acid oxidation as a source of energy in the later stages of fasting when glycogen stores are depleted. Additional laboratory findings include mild metabolic acidosis, elevation of aminotransferases, prolonged prothrombin time, and hyperammonemia. Diagnosis of fatty acid oxidation defects is made by the detection of elevated levels of urinary acylglycines (abnormal byproducts of fatty acid oxidation) during acute episodes and remissions. The definitive diagnosis is made by enzyme assay in patient's cells.

HYPOGLYCEMIA ASSOCIATED WITH ABNORMALITIES OF HORMONAL HOMEOSTASIS. Hypoglycemia may be a significant clinical feature of a number of endocrine deficiency diseases. Hypoglycemia, either symptomatic or detected on provocative testing, occurs in well over half of the children with hypopituitary dwarfism. The mechanism for hypoglycemia may be due to growth hormone deficiency alone or to a combination of growth hormone, ACTH, and cortisol deficiency in the younger hypopituitary child. As the child increases in age, there is generally an increase in adiposity, and both are associated with declining frequency of symptomatic and asymptomatic hypoglycemia. Addison's disease, an uncommon endocrine disorder of childhood, is characterized by fasting hypoglycemia. Rarely, hypoglycemia occurs in congenital adrenal hyperplasia when the metabolic block of cortisol production is essentially complete. Zetterstrøm's syndrome, a condition associated with hypoglycemia in the younger child, is thought to be secondary to impairment in the synthesis and release of catecholamines from the adrenal medulla or peripheral chromaffin tissue or both. The frequency and importance of glucagon deficiency as a factor in recurrent hypoglycemia remain unclear.

ORGANIC HYPERINSULINISM. Spontaneous overproduction of insulin by the beta cells of the pancreas may occur under one of several circumstances. Histologically discrete insulin-producing tumors may take the form of islet cell adenomas or carcinomas. Islet cell adenomas of the pancreas are uncommon causes for hypoglycemia in childhood. Adenomas have been identified throughout the body and

head of the pancreas in hypoglycemic children ranging in age from the neonatal period to late adolescence. Proper diagnosis in such patients is imperative because surgical removal of the tumor or tumors is the only therapeutic technique that yields a complete cure.

Islet cell hyperplasia is a pathological condition resulting from increase in size and number of the beta cells without disturbance in islet or parenchymal architecture and is associated with increased insulin production. This condition is regularly seen in infants of diabetic mothers as well as infants with erythroblastosis fetalis. In both circumstances, histological changes as well as the overproduction of insulin are transitory and spontaneously reversible. Similar histological changes of a more persistent nature have been described in patients with leucine-sensitive hypoglycemia.

Nesidioblastosis is a histological diagnosis applied to those cases in which there is islet cell hyperplasia with disruption of the islet architecture and proliferation of hyperplastic beta cells in parenchymal and ductal tissue without identifiable discrete tumors. Some pathologists contend that nesidioblastosis does not occur as a pathological entity because the apparent histological changes may be seen as normal developmental histology of the fetal and neonatal pancreas.

Hyperinsulinism is the most common cause of persistent hypoglycemia in infants under the age of 1 year. All the infants with documented nesidioblastosis develop severe intractable hyperinsulinemic hypoglycemia which requires laparotomy and partial or total pancreatectomy. The majority present with symptoms of hypoglycemia, including convulsions, during the first 3 days of life; many of them having a striking physical resemblance to an infant of a diabetic mother. Hyperinsulinism occurring outside the first 6 months is more likely to be due to a localized form of the disease.

Hypoglycemia has been reported in more than 200 adults with large solid tumors of the abdomen or chest. It is an uncommon but definite cause of hypoglycemia in infants and children, being reported in association with fibromas, fibrosarcomas, neuroblastomas, and Wilms' tumors. The exact mechanism for hypoglycemia in most of these patients is not clear. In most cases the primary tumor diagnosis is well established prior to the appearance of hypoglycemia.

IDIOPATHIC HYPOGLYCEMIA OF INFANCY AND CHILDHOOD. Hypoglycemia is of decreasing frequency as the infant and child increase in age. In the great majority of infants with neonatal hypoglycemia there is spontaneous cure by 10 to 14 days of age. Persistent or recurrent hypoglycemia in the infant or toddler is uncommon and requires evaluation. The great majority of cases fit into the category of ketotic hypoglycemia, a condition of recurrent episodic hypoglycemia seen most commonly in children between 1 and 3 years of age and usually associated with intercurrent illness or alteration in dietary intake. These children are frequently small for age, underweight for height, and have a history of prematurity or low birth weight for gestational age. Modest intellectual impairment is not uncommon. The precise definition of the mechanism for hypoglycemia in these children is frequently difficult. Urinary ketones are usually present at diagnosis and characteristically increase with fasting, which leads to an excessively rapid fall in blood glucose concentration. These children have accelerated depletion of hepatic glycogen stores and decreased efficiency of gluconeogenesis. The latter may occur because of (1) impairment in peripheral protein stores; (2) decreased rate of proteolysis as is seen in those patients reported to have hypoalaninemia; (3) partial defects in the enzymes involved in gluconeogenesis; or (4) partial hormone deficiency, e.g., cortisol, glucagon, or growth hormone. Hypoglycemic symptoms gradually decrease and are rare beyond age 6 years.

A specific subset of infants and children with idiopathic hypoglycemia are those who may be classified as leucine sensitive. Although the frequency of this condition is unclear, leucine sensitivity may be present in 10% of those infants and children with recurrent or persistent hypoglycemia. In some cases, it is definitely genetic, with two or more siblings in the same family affected. Amino acid–stimulated insulin release occurs in the postprandial period. Leucine is present in high concentration in cow's milk and eggs. Its ingestion is specifically associated with excessive insulin release and postprandial hypoglycemia in these patients. Several patients have had a pancreatectomy, and islet cell hyperplasia usually has been observed.

MISCELLANEOUS CAUSES. Hypoglycemia may occur in association with severe hepatic disease such as chronic cirrhosis, extensive hepatitis, or acute yellow atrophy. Extreme malnutrition may have marked unresponsive hypoglycemia as a terminal manifestation. Alcohol, salicylates, sulfonylurea compounds, and insulin have all been implicated in the production of acute hypoglycemia. Hypoglycemia has been occasionally reported as a complication of lymphocytic leukemia, as a side effect of a phenylalanine-deficient diet in children treated for phenylketonuria, and in association with intestinal disaccharidase deficiency.

Differential Diagnosis

The appropriate therapy for hypoglycemia is dependent on the specific identification of the pathological physiology.

The majority of cases of neonatal hypoglycemia, such as those seen in infants of diabetic mothers and in premature infants, are transitory in nature and clear spontaneously within the first 10 days of life. Intensive diagnostic evaluation is, therefore, rarely indicated in the neonate. Studies are difficult to make and frequently even more difficult to interpret. The primary concern should be the control of hypoglycemia.

Appropriate studies should be made to rule out metabolic defects, endocrine deficiency states, and organic hyperinsulinism. Metabolic causes for hypoglycemia are usually readily diagnosed. Galactosemia presents a characteristic picture in the neonatal period, that is, jaundice, cataracts, severe seizures, and hypoglycemia. The infants have increased blood galactose and galactosuria. Specific diagnosis is made by red blood cell enzyme studies defining a deficiency of the enzyme galactose 1-phosphate uridyl transferase. Hereditary fructose intolerance is a condition somewhat more difficult to diagnose. The symptoms, including vomiting and diarrhea, vascular collapse, and hypoglycemia, are associated with the ingestion of foods containing a high content of fructose, such as fruits and table sugar. Patients have elevation of the blood fructose level and fructosuria in association with a precipitous decrease in blood glucose following the oral fructose tolerance test. Maple syrup urine disease commonly results in severe neurological morbidity and mortality in the immediate neonatal period. The characteristic odor of the urine should lead to suspicion of the diagnosis. Specific diagnosis is made by examining the urine for ketoacids with the use of chromatography. Von Gierke's disease is characterized by hepatomegaly, growth retardation, mild ketosis, and hypoglycemia. Hypoglycemia is rare in the other forms of glycogen storage disease. Only a minimal rise in blood glucose level following epinephrine or glucagon tolerance tests is expected in glycogen storage diseases. A definitive diagnosis, however, depends on demonstrating specific glycogen enzyme deficiency in the liver biopsy specimen.

Hypoglycemia in the child with growth retardation suggests hypopituitary dwarfism. Appropriate studies to rule out endocrine causes of hypoglycemia include determination of serum growth hormone levels, assessment of the pituitary-adrenal axis by blood and urinary steroid studies, determination of insulin sensitivity, and measurement of bone maturation. Evaluation of the adrenal medulla and sympathetic nervous system response can be carried out by studying urinary catecholamine excretion before and after insulin-induced hypoglycemia. A diagnosis of glucagon deficiency depends on measurement of serum glucagon levels or demonstration of the absence of alpha cells in the pancreatic biopsy specimen.

Life-threatening episodes of coma and hypoglycemia induced by fasting are a common presenting feature in most of the fatty acid oxidation disorders. The hypoglycemia in these disorders is most easily explained by the inability of affected patients to use fatty acids as a fuel substitute for glucose. Severe disturbances of muscle function are a feature in several of the disorders; hypertrophic cardiomyopathy and chronic skeletal muscle weakness occur in both the mild and severe forms. Because the presence of an underlying defect in fatty acid oxidation is unlikely to be appreciated with routine laboratory tests, the genetic defects in fatty acid oxidation are easily and often misdiagnosed as other diseases, such as Reye's syndrome and sudden infant death syndrome. The possibility of a defect in fatty acid oxidation should be considered in all patients with coma and hypoglycemia associated with fasting and in patients with skeletal muscle weakness or cardiomyopathy. The demonstration of inappropriately low urinary ketones (i.e., anything less than large) at a time of illness is a simple clue to the diagnosis. The most powerful tool in the diagnosis of the defects in fatty acid oxidation is an examination of the urinary organic acid profile by gas chromatography or gas chromatography–mass spectroscopy. Specific enzyme deficiencies for most of the disorders can be demonstrated in peripheral blood leukocytes or cultured skin fibroblasts. Clinical studies of fasting adaptation can be useful in demonstrating an impairment of fatty acid oxidation but should be done only with great caution because fasting may provoke a life-threatening illness in these patients.

By careful clinical evaluation, the recognized causes for hypoglycemia can usually be differentiated. The cause of the hypoglycemia cannot be determined by measurement of blood glucose alone. Blood glucose concentration can only be evaluated fully in relation to the concentration of other metabolic fuels and hormones. The diagnostic workup begins with a critical blood sample drawn at the time of hypoglycemia before glucose is given to correct the low blood glucose level. This critical blood sample should be analyzed for blood glucose, ketone bodies, free fatty acids, lactate, alanine, uric acid, insulin, growth hormone, cortisol, and glucagon. If all of these substances cannot be measured initially, then the minimum must be blood glucose and plasma insulin with urinary ketone bodies. The blood sample drawn at the time of hypoglycemia is of crucial importance for a speedy diagnosis. Further information can be obtained by studying endocrine and metabolic interrelations during a typical 24-hour period, and following specific tolerance tests (glucose tolerance test, intravenous insulin tolerance test, glucagon tolerance test, etc.). The reader is referred to larger texts for details of these tests and the interpretation of results.

Treatment

Management of hypoglycemia includes the consideration of both acute and long-term problems. Acute hypoglycemic reactions require prompt measures to increase the blood glucose. This is most efficiently accomplished by intravenous injection of 50% dextrose at a dosage of 0.5 to 1.0 ml/kg of body weight. If the patient is still conscious and relatively cooperative, a trial with an oral glucose solution may be useful; however, if the patient is semicomatose or combative, it is unwise to attempt to administer oral fluids because of the danger of aspiration. Crystalline glucagon may be given intravenously or subcutaneously at a dosage of 50 μg/kg (maximum dose, 1 mg); aqueous epinephrine 1 : 1000 at a dosage of 0.05 ml/kg (maximum dose, 0.5 ml) may also be given subcutaneously. These measures promptly increase blood sugar in patients who have adequate glycogen stores and no inherent defect in glycogen mobilization. Once the blood glucose level is normalized, intravenous glucose should be continued at an infusion rate calculated to provide approximately 150% of the hepatic glucose production rate. The rate is 5 to 10 mg/kg/min for neonates and 3 to 5 mg/kg/min for older infants and children. It is important to ensure that the plasma glucose concentration remain above 50 mg/dl to prevent the sequelae of hypoglycemia, mental retardation, and neurologic damage.

The principal goal of long-term management of hypoglycemia is prevention. Dietary therapy is frequently the cornerstone to management. Neonates with transient hypoglycemia require only supportive intravenous glucose until gluconeogenic enzymes mature, glycogen stores are maintained with oral feedings, and transient hyperinsulinism, if present, resolves. A galactose-free diet is the specific therapy for galactosemia, while avoidance of fructose is essential in patients with hereditary fructose intolerance and fructose 1,6-diphosphatase deficiency. Infants with the more severe forms of glycogen storage disease, such as glucose 6-phosphatase deficiency, require a high carbohydrate diet with frequent daytime feedings and constant nighttime nasogastric glucose feedings at a rate of 8 to 9 mg/kg/min. The milder gluconeogenic enzyme deficiencies, and the disorders of glycogenolysis, fatty acid oxidation, and ketogenesis may only require avoidance of prolonged fasting and nighttime enteral feedings in infancy. Cornstarch or tapioca starch oral feedings have resulted in longer euglycemia in some of those disorders.

Specific therapy is indicated in endocrine deficiency states. Growth hormone and cortisone are administered in hypopituitary dwarfism. Cortisone in physiological replacement doses is the specific therapy in Addison's disease, virilizing adrenal hyperplasia, and congenital unresponsiveness to ACTH. Glucagon is used in the control of hypoglycemia associated with glucagon deficiency.

With hyperinsulinism, medical therapy may be tried initially with frequent feedings and diazoxide, which inhibits glucose-stimulated insulin secretion. If a medical trial is unsuccessful in maintaining plasma glucose above 50 mg/dl, or in the older child, in whom an adenoma is more likely, surgical exploration should be undertaken. If an adenoma is found, removal may be curative. In the absence of an adenoma, a 90 to 95% pancreatectomy should be performed. In a few cases even this is not curative, and reoperation with a total pancreatectomy is necessary. In these latter cases, long-acting somatostatin analogue offers a treatment option.

Idiopathic ketotic hypoglycemia is managed with frequent high-carbohydrate and high-protein feedings. This condition usually resolves spontaneously by 6 to 10 years of age.

Prognosis

Severe or recurrent hypoglycemia may produce seizures and coma and lead to irreversible CNS damage. Death has been reported rarely as a complication of hypoglycemia. There are no adequate long-term, carefully controlled, follow-up studies that accurately predict outcome in terms of neurological development and CNS function in children who have experienced hypoglycemic episodes. The prognosis apparently depends greatly, however, on the age of onset of hypoglycemia, the severity and frequency of hypoglycemic episodes, the underlying diagnosis, and the adequacy of management. Several studies have confirmed that recurrent hypoglycemia in more than 50% of children under 6 months of age is associated with significant and irreversible brain damage; while in hypoglycemia that initially occurs after 6 months of age, the frequency of CNS damage appears to be, in general, diminishing.

Disorders Associated with Hyperglycemia

Hyperglycemia occurs when there is an imbalance between the hypoglycemic effects of insulin and hyperglycemic ef-

fects of other hormonal agents (see Fig. 7-1). Hyperglycemia is regularly associated with increased release of growth hormone, which causes gigantism in the child or acromegaly in the adult. Cushing syndrome, whether resulting from endogenous ACTH overproduction, adrenal hyperplasia, tumor, or steroid therapy, is also associated with decreased carbohydrate tolerance and occasionally mild diabetes mellitus. Pheochromocytoma, with increased epinephrine production, is accompanied by mild to moderate carbohydrate intolerance. Excessive production of glucagon results in hyperglycemia. Although these endocrine conditions may cause a picture indistinguishable from diabetes mellitus, they represent a very small percentage of the total cases of that disease.

Diabetes Mellitus

Diabetes mellitus is a chronic systemic disorder of energy metabolism, frequently genetic in origin, secondary to an absolute or relative deficiency in insulin, and characterized by carbohydrate intolerance as well as alterations in lipid and protein metabolism. Diabetes mellitus, formerly felt to be a single homogeneous disease, is now known to be several basically different diseases, the most common of which are insulin-dependent diabetes mellitus (IDDM), formerly referred to as juvenile or juvenile-onset diabetes mellitus, and noninsulin-dependent diabetes mellitus (NIDDM), formerly referred to as maturity-onset or obesity-related diabetes. More than 80% of the known diabetics in the United States have this form of diabetes, while less than 15% have complete insulin deficiency.

IDDM is the characteristic form of diabetes seen in the child and adolescent, occurring in greater than 95% of such patients. The disorder results from destruction of the beta cells of the pancreas, eventually leading to essentially complete loss of the ability to synthesize and release insulin. The underlying pathophysiology appears to result from a genetic defect in immunological integrity so that environmentally induced inflammatory changes lead to autoimmune destruction of the beta cells. Insulin deficiency leads to major alterations in all phases of energy homeostasis. Peripheral glucose uptake is impaired, and hepatic glucose production is increased, leading initially to postprandial hyperglycemia but eventually to persistent and marked hyperglycemia. Elevation in glucose concentration in excess of the renal threshold results in urinary glucose losses that may be substantial, producing the classic symptoms of diabetes mellitus, that is, polyuria, polydipsia, and polyphagia. As the insulin-mediated "brakes" on lipid mobilization are lost, hyperlipidemia and ketonemia intervene. Diabetic ketoacidosis becomes a potentially highly dangerous metabolic complication. Impairment in protein metabolism secondary to chronic insulin deficiency leads to declining growth and maturation.

The current view regarding the pathophysiology of IDDM is that multiple factors which may be operative in different proportions lead to the expression of diabetes in any one individual. Those factors include genetic predisposition, environmental chemical and infectious agents, autoimmune events, nutrition, physical activity, and psychologic stress. In favor of genetics playing an important role is the observation that predisposition to IDDM is linked to the HLA-D locus on the short arm of chromosome 6. Both HLA-DR3 and -DR4 alleles increase the risk for IDDM, while -DR2 may have a possible protective effect. Among environmental factors, infectious agents and more specifically viruses are the most likely candidates. Viruses that are reported to be associated with IDDM include Coxsackie B, mumps, congenital rubella, infectious mononucleosis, varicella, cytomegalovirus, and infectious hepatitis. In support of an autoimmune destruction of the pancreas is (1) evidence of insulitis with lymphocytic infiltration; (2) the presence of autoantibodies against islet-cell antigens, including anticytoplasmic antibodies (ICA), islet-cell surface antibodies (ICSA), and insulin autoantibodies (IAA); and (3) T-lymphocyte abnormalities.

Clinical Manifestations

In the great majority of children and adolescents found to have diabetes mellitus, clinical symptoms have existed for fewer than 4 weeks and in some instances do not exceed 2 or 3 days. In addition to polyuria, polydipsia, and polyphagia, weight loss, fatigue, and visual disturbances are common. Approximately 40% of our patients with newly diagnosed diabetes have diabetic ketoacidosis requiring initial intensive therapy.

Following initial stabilization and initiation of therapy with insulin and diet, a decline in insulin requirement associated with improvement in metabolic status occurs spontaneously in approximately two-thirds of all patients; this is referred to as the "honeymoon phase" or the period of remission. During this period there is transient partial recovery of pancreatic B-cell function as detected by increased C-peptide levels, and there is improved insulin sensitivity. The nadir of insulin requirement is characteristically seen 3 to 4 months after diagnosis and is followed either by a gradual or abrupt increase in insulin needs so that by 12 to 18 months after diagnosis, the patients are, for all practical purposes, totally insulin deficient, at which point most require insulin at a daily rate of approximately 1 U/kg of body weight.

Diagnosis

The diagnosis of diabetes in the child or adolescent is rarely difficult. The presence of glucosuria, ketonuria, and hyperglycemia in a child with some combination of the clinical symptoms described above should lead to a prompt diagnosis of diabetes and initiation of therapy. In the older child, overt diabetes mellitus is rarely misdiagnosed. Diagnosis in the infant or toddler, however, may be inordinately delayed because of the rarity of diabetes in that age group, the lack of clinically characteristic symptoms, and the infrequency with which urinalysis is done routinely by the pediatrician or family physician. The possibility of diabetes mellitus in the infant and younger child must be kept in mind if excessive morbidity and mortality are to be prevented. Specific studies to diagnose diabetes mellitus are rarely indicated in the symptomatic child. Hyperglycemia may be seen occasionally in the otherwise normal child during a period of intercurrent infection. Fasting or 2-hour postprandial glucose determinations, or both, may be appropriate in patients after they have returned to a state of good health. Fasting blood glucose in excess of 140 mg/100 ml and 2-hour postprandial values in excess of 200 mg/100 ml are almost invariably associated with a diagnosis of diabetes mellitus. Under such circumstances, testing should be repeated, or a standard oral glucose tolerance test should be done under controlled circumstances, or both should be done. The recommended glucose dose is 1.75 g/kg of body weight up to a maximum of 100 g. The child should be clinically well and active for a period of several days, if not weeks, prior to testing and should have a high-carbohydrate diet for a minimum of 3 days before the glucose tolerance test. Fasting blood glucose concentration in excess of 120 mg/100 ml and peak values in excess of 180 mg/100 ml are indicative of carbohydrate intolerance, while fasting values exceeding 140 mg/100 ml and peak values of 200 mg/100 ml are diagnostic of diabetes mellitus.

Management of Diabetic Ketoacidosis

Approximately 40% of patients with newly diagnosed diabetes present with a severe metabolic disturbance associated with metabolic acidosis, ketonemia, and ketonuria. Diabetic ketoacidosis is an acute medical emergency requiring prompt and vigorous therapy. The metabolic disturbances in such patients include the following:

1. Hyperglycemia
2. Dehydration
3. Electrolyte depletion
4. Acidosis
5. Hyperlipidemia

Correction of these alterations requires specific therapy directed toward each of the pathological entities. The most critical initial aspect of therapy is fluid and electrolyte replacement. Potassium replacement is of special importance. Insulin therapy in association with adequate rehydration leads to normalization of energy homeostasis with correction of hyperglycemia and hyperlipidemia as well as elimination of ketonemia. Specific therapy for acidosis may be accomplished with sodium bicarbonate administration but is not always necessary.

The use of continuous intravenous insulin infusion in the initial stages of treatment of diabetic ketoacidosis has been accepted by essentially all diabetologists. We recommend that an initial dose of 0.1 U/kg/hour of crystalline insulin be given preferably by an infusion pump. Blood glucose concentration should be monitored at least hourly, and the rate of glucose fall kept between 50 and 100 mg/100 ml/hour. If the rate of fall is in excess of this then glucose should be added to the intravenous infusion. On the other hand, if the rate of glucose fall is distinctly less than 50 mg/100 ml/hour, an increased rate of insulin infusion should be considered. As the concentration of blood glucose approaches 300 mg/100 ml, the rate of fall should be decreased by the addition of glucose to the infusion medium with the intent of maintaining blood glucose concentration around 150 mg/100 ml during the first 24 hours or so of therapy.

Most children with clinically significant diabetic ketoacidosis have a water deficit of 100 to 120 ml/kg and deficits of 8 to 10 mEq of sodium, 5 to 7 mEq of potassium, and 6 to 8 mEq of chloride per kilogram of body weight. These overall deficits must be corrected, and adequate replacement for continuing losses and basal requirements must be provided. It is recommended that the estimated deficits be replaced during the initial 8 hours of therapy while the calculated continuing losses and 24-hour maintenance requirement be provided during the remaining 16 hours of the initial day of therapy.

Therapy is begun with administration of isotonic saline at a rate of 20 ml/kg/hour to promptly increase intravascular volume and treat or prevent shock. Following this, the solution should be changed to 0.5N saline with sodium bicarbonate added if needed for the treatment of acidosis, or to sodium chloride with a sodium concentration of 100 to 120 mEq/L to provide a modest amount of "free water" for hydration purposes.

The dose of sodium bicarbonate may be calculated, based on the knowledge that the eventual sodium bicarbonate distribution space is 60% of the body weight in kilograms. Bicarbonate should be administered intravenously continuously over the initial 6 to 8 hours of therapy as sodium bicarbonate added to the hydrating solution. Potassium must be provided as soon as adequacy of renal function is established. It is added to the intravenous hydrating solution at a concentration of 20 to 40 mEq/L and can be administered as potassium chloride, potassium phosphate, or a mixture of the two. Glucose may be provided in the intravenous fluids from the initiation of therapy, but most investigators recommend withholding glucose until the blood glucose concentration approaches 200 mg/100 ml, at which time 5% glucose is added.

Continuous intravenous insulin therapy can be reasonably continued as long as intravenous fluid therapy is necessary, in most cases as long as 16 hours or so. When the patient, however, is ready for increasing amounts of oral nutrients as well as to begin mobilization, intravenous fluid and insulin therapy should be discontinued. Subcutaneous administration of insulin should be initiated at least 1 hour prior to termination of intravenous insulin therapy to ensure continuous coverage. Crystalline insulin in a dose of 0.1 to 0.2 U/kg should be administered subcutaneously not less often than every 4 hours with alteration in dosage depending upon clinical and biochemical response. As acidosis and ketosis clear, insulin sensitivity increases as does the danger of hypoglycemia. Careful monitoring of blood glucose, pH, and electrolytes is necessary over the first several days of management. While ketonemia and ketonuria may continue for 2 to 3 days, acidosis should be corrected by the end of the first day of therapy. Persistence of acidosis for a longer period necessitates careful reevaluation of the patient's status; the persistence probably results from one or more of the following:

1. Intercurrent infection
2. Inadequate fluid replacement
3. Inadequate insulin therapy
4. Inadequate nutrient replacement (glucose)

Prompt attention to these factors usually results in clearing of acidosis in a few hours.

Principles of Ambulatory Management

The principles of therapy include:

1. Insulin adminstration in quantity and timing to achieve near-metabolic normality
2. A diet designed to minimize both hyperglycemia and hypoglycemia, provide adequate nutrients for growth and development, and prevent hyperlipidemia
3. Exercise integrated with insulin adminstration and diet to promote a high level of physical fitness while minimizing excessive variations in blood glucose concentration
4. Emotional support to minimize the psychiatric disabilities commonly associated with the chronic stress of diabetes mellitus and its management

The therapeutic objectives include prevention of the classic symptoms of diabetes mellitus, avoidance of diabetic ketoacidosis, avoidance of hypoglycemia, prevention of both acute and chronic complications of diabetes mellitus, and insurance of the patient's physical and emotional well-being.

INSULIN THERAPY. Insulin administration on a daily basis is mandatory in the management of the individual with insulin-dependent diabetes mellitus. A variety of insulin preparations, varying in time of onset and duration of action, are available. Major improvements have been achieved in the purity of commercially available insulin preparations, so the problems of insulin contamination with other pancreatic hormones and nonhormonal protein materials leading to the development of insulin antibodies have been greatly minimized. Probably of greater clinical importance is the development of techniques for the production of human insulin, utilizing recombinant DNA methodology or chemical substitution of highly purified pork insulin to produce an insulin compound identical to that produced by the human pancreas.

There is increasing emphasis upon an acceptance of multiple-dose insulin therapy in the patient with IDDM. In our clinic, approximately 15% of our patients are currently treated with a single injection of NPH insulin or a combination of NPH and regular insulins given daily before breakfast. Around 83% receive split-dose insulin, using a combination of NPH and regular before breakfast and NPH or NPH plus regular before the evening meal or bedtime. Most of the patients receiving split-dose therapy are adolescents, but we find that this approach is also of special value in younger children. Insulin dosage requirements vary with age, weight, duration of diabetes, level of

sexual maturation, exercise, level of physical fitness, general health status, state of nutrition, emotional state, and level of insulin antibodies as well as other factors. Adequacy of insulin dosage should be assessed at least weekly by the patient and family, with review by the physician every 3 to 4 months or more often if major changes are occurring. Insulin therapy should be increased if the degree of glucosuria or glycemia is persistently excessive. An overall increase by 10% of the insulin dose is usually safe, with adjustments between the intermediate and short-acting insulins, depending upon the timing of glucose excess. Symptomatic or asymptomatic hypoglycemia, if persistent or if not understood by virtue of missed meals, excessive exercise, and the like, should result in a prompt 10% decrease in insulin dose.

DIETARY MANAGEMENT. The importance of diet in the management of the child and adolescent has been inadequately appreciated by many pediatricians and family physicians. Reasonable control of energy homeostasis in the child with IDDM cannot be achieved without significant attention to certain principles of diet. We recommend the following:

The diet must be entirely adequate to meet all nutritional needs of the active, growing child. An approximation of the caloric need utilizes the simple formula of 1000 calories as base requirement with the addition of 100 calories for each year of age up to adolescence. Caloric requirements of the adolescent may vary greatly, depending upon activity level. The diet should include between 1.5 and 2.0 g/kg of protein or between 15 and 20% of total calories derived from high-quality protein. It has been traditional in the past to limit carbohydrates in the diet of the diabetic patient. Increasingly there is evidence that absolute limitation in carbohydrates is both unnecessary and possibly detrimental in the patient with diabetes mellitus; however, limitation of "free sugars" remains an accepted principle of management. We recommend that carbohydrates make up 50 to 55% of total calories, with at least 75% of carbohydrate calories being derived from complex starches and the remainder from lactose, sucrose, and fructose. Of the remaining noncarbohydrate calories, 30 to 35% should be derived from dietary fat. This is a reduction in total fat content compared with the average American diet with particular focus on reducing saturated fat (S) and proportionately increasing polyunsaturated fat (P) so that a P/S ratio in excess of 1.0 is obtained. Cholesterol should be limited to less than 250 mg/day. The most recent revision of the dietary recommendation of the American Diabetes Association with the diet exchange list is a valuable source of information for constructing the diet of the child with diabetes mellitus.

Particular attention should be paid to the distribution of total calories throughout the waking hours of the day, which includes three meals and three snacks for the younger child and three meals and two snacks — midafternoon and bedtime — for the older child and adolescent. Because of the tendency toward marked postprandial hyperglycemia following breakfast, total calories for breakfast should be decreased below the total for lunch and dinner. Although calorie estimates are used to develop the initial dietary recommendations and to make periodic alterations, we suggest that the child's appetite be the primary indicator of quantity of food ingested at each meal and our specific recommendations be followed in regard to the composition of the meals. This appears to be a satisfactory arrangement as long as the child's weight gain is not excessive. Caloric excess, however, particularly excess carbohydrate ingestion, appears to be a major factor in inadequacy of control resulting in hyperglycemia and excessive glucosuria. When such is clearly the case, a more restricted dietary program is necessary.

EXERCISE. Increasingly there is evidence that the metabolic control regularly achieved in the diabetic individual who remains physically fit is closer to normal than in those diabetic individuals who do not follow an active daily program of physical fitness. We encourage our diabetic patients to exercise vigorously on a daily basis. We encourage participation in both competitive and noncompetitive athletic programs but realize that some children, by their emotional makeup, are not so inclined. Those children should be encouraged to work out their own physical fitness program at home. Hypoglycemia must be prevented by the proper adjustment of insulin dose and the intake of extra calories prior to and during exercise if needed.

GENERAL MEDICAL MANAGEMENT. The diabetic child requires closer medical supervision, especially for the management of intercurrent infections, than does the normal child. Tonsillitis and other infections such as those involving the skin, can rapidly induce a state of diabetic ketoacidosis and dehydration. Most febrile illnesses result in a transient increase in insulin requirement. The patient's parents must be advised to contact the physician freely when in doubt regarding the child's general health. Early diagnosis and management of a minor illness may avoid serious complications and hospitalization.

Assessment of Metabolic Control

The many controversies surrounding the relationship between metabolic control and chronic vascular complications of diabetes mellitus have resulted in large part because of the inadequacies of accurate techniques for the assessment of metabolic control over time. This has been, in large measure, corrected by the development of several techniques for the measurement of glycosylated hemoglobin, an accurate index of glycemic control over a period of 2 to 4 months. Glycosylated hemoglobin is hemoglobin to which glucose has been coupled nonenzymatically. The reaction occurs in the blood stream after hemoglobin is synthesized in bone marrow. Because the reaction is proportional to the prevailing blood glucose concentration, and continues irreversibly throughout the 120-day life span of the red blood cell, the level of glycosylated hemoglobin is a reflection of the integrated blood glucose concentration over the preceding 2 to 3 months. It is recommended that the glycosylated hemoglobin level be determined for each diabetic child every 3 to 4 months. In addition, daily self-monitoring of blood glucose before three major meals and bedtime is recommended using glucose oxidase strips in conjunction with a reflectance meter. Appropriate insulin adjustment is based on blood glucose level. Additionally the patient is instructed to check urine ketones once daily in the morning and throughout periods of illness. A carefully maintained record charting blood glucose levels is desirable but rarely accurately maintained by children. These records are notoriously unreliable for several reasons including self-delusion, reliance on patient's memory, or attempts to please the physician. Lipids and thyroid function should be analyzed annually. The eyes should be carefully examined on each clinic visit, and retinal examination by an ophthalmologist is indicated annually for the adolescent. Stereocolor photography and fluorescein angiography should probably be accomplished during the adolescent years to document the presence or absence of early microvascular disease. Screening for urinary protein should be part of each clinic visit, and quantitative 24-hour urinary protein excretion should be evaluated if protein is present on spot screening. Persistent proteinuria, even at low levels, should result in detailed evaluation of renal function, including creatinine clearance and possibly renal biopsy.

Factors in the Success of Long-Term Management

Diabetes mellitus is a serious chronic disease with significant morbidity and mortality. The etiology of the chronic complications of diabetes remains unclear, but there is increasing evidence of a relationship between chronic metabolic alterations and the frequency and severity of vascular complications. Consequently there is increasing pressure on the physician to improve the level of metabolic control achieved in patients while avoiding the clear dangers of hypoglycemia and the psychological hazards of excessively restrictive therapeutic regimens. Few physicians have the time or expertise to provide total care for the child with diabetes mellitus and his or her family.

The diabetes therapeutic team is becoming an integral part of patient management in most centers. The team is comprised of a physician well versed in the most up-to-date and accepted modes of therapy and assessment; a diabetes nurse-educator who takes responsibility for primary contact with the patient and family and their education in all aspects of diabetes management; a nutritionist-dietitian who meets with the family initially and annually and is available if necessary for follow-up consultations to insure that the dietary aspects of management are adequate; a psychiatric social worker who can assess the family strengths and weaknesses and also provide guidance to community and institutional resources that may be of value to the family. Additional members of the therapeutic team who should be available for consultation as necessary include a psychologist or psychiatrist experienced with the particular problems of the child with diabetes, an ophthalmologist who would work closely with the physician in routine assessment of patients, and an obstetrician-gynecologist to provide guidance and direction for the teenage diabetic girl as questions regarding contraception, marriage, and pregnancy become of increasing importance.

The achievement of good metabolic control is difficult in the child with diabetes and is of increasing difficulty and complexity in the diabetic teenager whose natural tendency is toward noncompliance and a decreasingly disciplined lifestyle. The emotional hazards of diabetes, particularly during the adolescent years, are great. It is important that the entire therapeutic team have patience and understanding and provide continued support for the diabetic child and family even when therapeutic goals are regularly not achieved. Late adolescence not infrequently is associated with increasing maturity and understanding and an increasing sense of responsibility for future health. Remarkable improvement in metabolic control may be seen in this period, a gratifying experience for all.

The future holds increasing promise for the patient with diabetes mellitus. The new molecular biology approach with advancements in immunology offer the promise for unmasking the primary cause of IDDM and point the direction for attempts at preventing its appearance in genetically predisposed individuals. Transplantation of pancreas (whole, segmental, isolated islets) has been performed with limited success; however, with improving surgical methods and safer techniques for immunosuppression, transplantation may become a clinically feasible therapeutic method.

As we all anxiously await the clinical improvements from scientific advancements, it is imperative that our diabetic patients continue to achieve and maintain optimal metabolic control.

Silva Arslanian and Allan L. Drash

Disorders of Porphyrin Metabolism: The Porphyrias

Porphyria is caused by disturbances of porphyrin synthesis. As every cell in the body has its own porphyrin metabolism, these disturbances usually cause symptoms involving different organs or systems.

Porphyria may be divided into three main groups, depending on the nature of the primary metabolic disturbance: erythropoietic, hepatic, and nonhereditary toxic porphyrin. Several distinct clinical entities fall within each of the three main forms. Each of the porphrias has characteristic patterns and elevated concentrations of porphyrins or porphyrin precursors, excreted or in tissue, as a result of enzyme defects, most of which have been identified.

The congenital erythropoietic and the Turkish type of the hepatic form are of special interest to students of pediatrics because of their relatively greater frequency in infancy and childhood.

Erythropoietic Porphyria

CONGENITAL ERYTHROPOIETIC PORPHYRIA. The congenital erythropoietic form of the disease is one of the rarest inborn errors of metabolism; it is inherited through a autosomal recessive gene. It is caused by a deficiency of uroporphyrinogen III cosynthetase. The disease manifests itself early in life, often at birth.

This type of porphyria is due to the synthesis of an abnormal type of porphyrin (isomers of type I) in certain series of erythrocytes. The patient seems to have two strains of erythrocytes, one synthesizing the normal isomer (type III and the other the unusual isomer (type I). This unusual synthesis is manifest only in erthrocytes and can be seen by fluorescent microscopy. Bone marrow and peripheral blood examinations clearly show the presence of fluorescent type I uroporphyrinogen (uroporphyrin)-loaded erythrocytic cells (fluorocytes) as well as completely normal ones. The abnormal cells seem to produce type I isomer; hence they contain an excessive amount of uroporphyrin I and coproporphyrin I. As synthesis of type I isomers cannot yield hemin, the metabolic pathway ends at the coproporphyrinogen I step. This compound, as well as uroporphy-rinogen, is easily oxidized, and uroporphyrin I and copro-porphyrin I are produced (Fig. 7-4).

Symptoms. The accumulation in the blood stream of uro-porphyrin I and coproporphyrin I, which are fluorescent, leads to symptoms of the erythropoietic system and the skin. In fact, uroporphyrinemia of all types is the main cause for light sensitivity and secondary skin symptoms. These include erythematous spots, which become vesicular or bullous eruptions (called hydroa aestivale), on exposed parts of the body. The vesicles tend to heal slowly, leaving pigmented scars and deformity, particularly of the fingertips, ears, nose and eyelids, and may even lead to severe mutilation. Hypertrichosis and pigmentation of the skin are common. Both deciduous and permanent teeth may show red or brownish discoloration on ultraviolet fluorescence (erythrodontia). The most constant and the earliest sign is the dark red "Burgundy wine" color of the urine. A hemolytic type of anemia with splenomegaly and requiring transfusions is usually present and is the first sign of the disease in some cases.

Treatment. The patient is condemned to live with the disease, and the aim of treatment is to ameliorate the symptoms. Avoidance of sunlight has been the only sure way to prevent or retard photosensitivity. Some porphyrin binding drugs, such as activated charcoal and choles-tyramine, are effective for lowering the porphyrin levels, thus ameliorating the symptoms. Removal of the spleen not only prevents the anemia but reduces the photosensitivity by stabilizing the fluorocytes with a slower release of porphyrins into the plasma.

Erythropoietic Protoporphyria

Erythropoietic protoporphyria is caused by a deficiency of ferrochetase (heme synthetase), and biochemical determinations reveal increased levels of plasma, erythrocyte, and stool protoporphyrin but normal urinary levels of porphyrins. Inheritance is autosomal dominant. Both sexes are equally affected.

The first cutaneous lesions tend to appear at the age of 3 or 4, after sun exposure. The characteristic symptom is a burning sensation or pruritus, followed by edema within the 5 to 30 minutes after sun exposure (solar urticaria). Cutaneous lesions consist of erythematous, erythemato-purpuric, or vesicular elements. Prolonged exposure produces thickening of skin. Hyperpigmentation and hypertrichosis are unusual. The patient may present with severe chronic hepatic dysfunction resulting in fatal cirrhosis. Cholelithiasis caused by protoporphyrin deposition is a frequent complication in this type of porphyria.

Avoidance of sunlight and long-term treatment with β-carotene help to ameliorate the symptoms.

Fig. 7-4. Abbreviated scheme for heme synthesis. (→ indicates formation of porphyrins of normal isomeric series.)

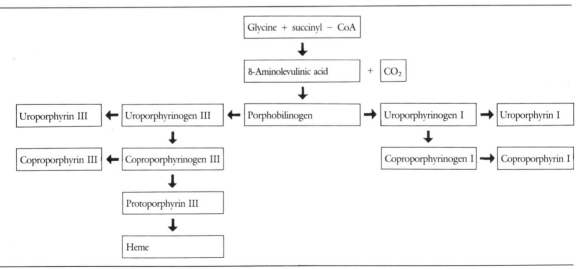

Hepatoerythropoietic Porphyria

Hepatoerythropoietic porphyria is the most recently recognized type of porphyria. Clinical features appear in early infancy, before the age of 2, as dark urine or porphyrinuria; subsequent exposure to sunlight is associated with edema, burning, pruritus, and vesiculation. With continued exposure to sunlight, these lesions lead to scarring, sclerodactyly, hyperpigmentation, and hypertrichosis. Marked mutilations appear. Although this disease is clinically similar to congenital erythropoietic porphyria, biochemically it is different. The enzyme deficient in hepatoerythropoietic porphyria is uroporphyrinogen decarboxylase.

Hepatic Porphyrias

Symptoms of most types of the hepatic form of porphyrias (Swedish, South African, cutaneous, multiform) are rarely seen before puberty. One exception is the Turkish type.

TURKISH PORPHYRIA. In this type of hepatic porphyria 90% of the patients are under the age of 16, and hence it is also called the juvenile form of hepatic porphyria. The adjective *Turkish* is used because the first epidemic occurred in southeastern Turkey as a result of ingestion of wheat seed treated with the fungicide hexachlorobenzene. Although hexachlorobenzene is definitely a porphyria-inducing agent, a hereditary factor may possibly predispose individuals to the disease.

Clinical Features. This type of porphyria is characterized by cutaneous photosensitivity, with blistering, scarring, and mutilation of exposed parts of the body, hyperpigmentation, hypertrichosis, interphalangeal arthritis, hepatomegaly, red or dark brown urine, increased amounts of urinary and fecal porphyrin, and absence of early pyrrole precursor (delta-aminolevulinic acid, porphobilinogen) in the urine.

In most cases at least 6 months elapse after the ingestion of hexachlorobenzene before the onset of the disease. The skin symptoms resemble those of porphyria erythropoietica and can be explained by the uroporphyrinemia. Patients do not manifest the neurological signs of the adult hepatic forms of the disease. There is some hepatomegaly in the early stages of the disease. Apart from the cutaneous symptoms and their complications, the disease is not debilitating.

Rheumatoid arthritic changes of the joints, which are peculiar to the Turkish form of the disease, are detected in about one-third of all the patients in the early stages of porphyria. The joint changes become more prominent as the disease progresses into the chronic stage and are manifest even long after the porphyrinuria subsides. Joint involvement is symmetrical, with surprisingly little pain or tenderness.

The clinical course of Turkish porphyria is that of a chronic disease. After cessation of exposure to hexachlorobenzene, dermatological, orthopedic, and neurological abnormalities have persisted. In a follow-up study in southeastern Turkey 20 to 30 years after the epidemic, most of the patients continued to have severe residual scarring, pinched facies, fragile skin, hyperpigmentation, and hypertrichosis. Some patients affected before puberty had small hands and painless arthritis. Neurological symptoms included weakness, paresthesia, myotonia, and cogwheeling. These findings indicated that long after cessation of exposure to the agent, in this case hexachlorobenzene, porphyrin metabolism continues to be disturbed.

Diagnosis. There is increased uroporphyrin and coproporphyrin excretion in urine and feces. Photodermia is strongly suggestive of the disease, and diagnosis is confirmed with detection of porphyrins in the urine. X-ray examination may reveal rheumatoid arthritic changes.

Treatment. No specific treatment is available except protection of the patient from sunlight and the elimination of any exposure to hexachlorobenzene.

ACUTE INTERMITTENT PORPHYRIA. Acute intermittent porphyria is also called acute porphyria or "Swedish type." This type of porphyria without rash but with marked CNS and abdominal manifestations, is occasionally seen in later childhood. Red urine and dental staining may be seen in the patient and in relatives. The porphyrins present in the urine in great excess are porphobilinogen and delta-aminolevulinic acid. Avoidance of precipitating agents such as barbiturates, sulfonamides, and estrogens is essential. Therapy with chlorpromazine (Thorazine) may be effective.

PORPHYRIA VARIEGATA. Porphyria variegata is also known as mixed porphyria, South African porphyria, or protocoproporphyria. It is a dominant inherited disease. The clinical diagnosis depends on the family history of porphyria, neurological and visceral symptoms similar to acute intermittent porphyria, and cutaneous features of chronic photosensitivity similar to porphyria cutanea tarda.

PORPHYRIA CUTANEA TARDA. Porphyria cutanea tarda is the most frequently encountered type of porphyria. Most cases are observed in males between 40 and 60 years. There is usually a history of above-average alcohol consumption in patients. The clinical features of disease are cutaneous fragility, actinic and traumatic blisters, premature aging of the skin, scleroderma-like lesions, hyperpigmentation, and hypertrichosis. There is usually evidence of liver damage with fatty changes, hemosiderosis, fibrosis, and cirrhosis. Acute intermittent attacks are not observed.

Porphyria cutanea tarda is treated with phleobotomy alone or in combination with chloroquine.

Nonhereditary Toxic Porphyria

Lead poisoning is a well-known example of nonhereditary toxic porphyria. In this instance, deranged porphyrin metabolism is of secondary importance to the basic pathology produced by lead. The disease can be encountered in all age groups with no sex preponderance.

Ihsan Dogramaci and Ayhan Gocmen

Disorders of Fluid and Electrolyte Metabolism

Normal Composition of Body Water

Water accounts for approximately 70% of the lean body mass. Adipose tissue contains relatively little water so that the percentage of water in the body is less in obese children. In rough terms, the plasma is about 6% of the weight and the interstitial fluid about 19%; together they form the extracellular fluid (ECF), or approximately 25% of the body weight. The remaining 45% is intracellular water. For practical purposes it may be assumed that changes in weight over any 24-hour period are all due to loss or gain of water. Such changes should not be cumulative over several days, however. Serious errors can be introduced by neglecting other tissue changes.

The inorganic chemical anatomy of the newborn infant differs from that of older infants primarily because of an "expanded" ECF compartment. Between 30 and 35% of the weight is extracellular water, bringing the total water content to 70 to 75% of the body weight. The relative content of extracellular sodium and chloride is, therefore, greater in the newborn infant.

The "excess" water of the neonate largely disappears by about 10 days of age. This rapidly changing composition, which represents the extrauterine adjustment, should be taken into account in planning fluid therapy for the newborn infant.

Hydrogen Ion Metabolism and Acid-Base Balance

ACIDOSIS AND ALKALOSIS. The hydrogen ion (H^+) concentration, as expressed in pH units (the log of the reciprocal of H+ concentration), must be kept within the narrow range of 7.30 to 7.45; outside these limits, cellular functions are impaired. pH values below 7.30 signify acidemia, and those above 7.45 alkalemia. Using modern terminology, one may say that a substance is acid if it is a proton ($H+$) donor (carbonic acid, lactic acid, ammonium ion NH_4, etc.) and base if it is a proton acceptor (HCO_3^-, NH_3, $HPO_4^=$, etc.). Such ions as Na^+, Cl^-, and K^+ are neither acids nor bases.

Deviations from normal pH are stringently guarded by the buffers and other mechanisms in the lungs and kidneys.

Measurement Systems — Blood Gases

Over the past two decades the measurement of acid-base status has improved technically so that clinicians may now have readily available at the bedside what previously was available only to research laboratories. The principal instrument is the glass electrode, which measures pH by determining the electrical potential difference after hydrogen ions — but not others — diffuse across the glass membrane. This is best done on arterial (or "arteriolized") capillary blood so that the equilibrium with alveolar CO_2 is represented.

An adaptation of the glass electrode allows direct measurement of PCO_2, the partial pressure (tension) of CO_2 in millimeters of Hg. For practical purposes the CO_2 pressure may be converted into the concentration of dissolved H_2CO_3 through use of a solubility constant. In vivo, the enzyme carbonic anhydrase (CA) accelerates the reaction:

$$H_2O + CO_2 \underset{CA}{\rightleftharpoons} H_2CO_3$$

The PCO_2 is a direct measure of the respiratory component of acid-base balance.

The second number that can be derived is the base excess (or deficit). This is the number of hydrogen ions necessary to add or subtract to a liter of blood to bring the pH to 7.4 when the PCO_2 is at the normal value of 40 mm. This determination is not a true physiological quantity, but it is useful, nonetheless. The system is too complex, with several buffers and several body spaces, to allow for such a simple calculation. On the other hand, empirical data have shown that for short-term (up to 30 min) correction of H^+ ion disturbance, if a volume of distribution of bicarbonate equal to $0.3 \times$ body weight is used, the correction is close. For calculation of the total correction needed over hours, one must use a larger distribution space of $0.6 \times$ body weight. In practice, over hours, other adjustments occur, making precision in calculation not possible. This approach, however, is useful in gauging the approximate degree of metabolic disturbance just as the PCO_2 denotes the respiratory disturbance. The base excess (or deficit) then approximates the quantitative *metabolic* correction needed, which is clinically useful as a guide to the amount of bicarbonate deficit.

An oxygen-sensitive electrode is also used to measure PO_2. This gives valuable information about pulmonary and circulatory function that assists in assessment of the causal relationships in a disturbance of H^+ ion metabolism.

Buffers. Buffers are made up of weak acids and their salts. When approximately equal quantities of these acids and their salts are present, there is maximum resistance to changes in pH. The Henderson-Hasselbalch equation defines the relationship for pH:

$$pH = pK + \log \frac{base}{acid}$$

pK is the negative logarithm of the dissociation constant, K, which characterizes this buffer system.

$$K = \frac{H^+ A^-}{HA}$$

There are four buffer systems that are of physiological importance: (1) the bicarbonate–carbonic system, (2) phosphoric acid, (3) the serum proteins, and (4) hemoglobin.

Bicarbonate–Carbonic Acid System. This is the most important buffer system in the body. Production of H^+ occurs in complete metabolism of carbohydrate and fat to CO_2 and H_2O. Here H^+ is accompanied by a base because $CO_2 + H_2O \rightleftharpoons H_2CO_3 \rightleftharpoons H^+; +HCO_3^-$. H+ production also occurs in incomplete metabolism when organic acids are formed; as they may be completely ionized at physiological pH, they increase the free H^+. The intestinal tract also represents a production site for H^+ through bacterial fermentation of sugars. The main advantage of the carbonic acid–bicarbonate system is the ease of its operation as a fine adjuster by pulmonary control of PCO_2, which determines the concentration of carbonic acid in the system.

The lung, through the excretion CO_2, is an important organ for H^+ removal, because carbonic acid (H_2CO_3) is a proton donor. The kidney, on the other hand, can remove H^+ without HCO_3^- (urine with acid pH) and thus compensate for acid production unaccompanied by HCO_3^- production (chiefly organic acid, phosphate, and sulfate).

In various respiratory or metabolic conditions causing acidosis or alkalosis the following relationships exist between the bicarbonate and carbonic acid (PCO_2) values:

1. Rise of bicarbonate in relation to PCO_2 results in a rise of pH (metabolic alkalosis).
2. Fall of bicarbonate in relation to PCO_2 results in a fall of pH (metabolic acidosis).
3. Rise of PCO_2 in relation to bicarbonate results in a fall of pH (respiratory acidosis).
4. Fall of PCO_2 in relation to bicarbonate results in a rise of pH (respiratory alkalosis).

Phosphoric Acid. The relationship of $HPO_4^=$ to $H_2PO_4^-$ constitutes a dissociation constant and is of importance as a buffering system.

Serum Proteins. Proteins are amphoteric substances and carry negative as well as positive charges. They, therefore, act as buffers by taking up ions of positive or negative charge and forming neutral salts at those points.

Hemoglobin. There are two ways in which hemoglobin is useful as a buffer. As a protein it has the properties mentioned above; additionally, the relationship of oxidized to reduced hemoglobin is that of a weak acid to its salt.

Kidneys. The carbonic acid–bicarbonate system is operative in the kidneys as well as in the lungs. Ammonia formation, which is an important function of the kidneys, serves as a way of removing H^+ and conserving sodium. The end products of normal or abnormal metabolism are also excreted by the kidneys, as for example, in the excretion of ketone bodies in diabetic acidosis. The excretion of phosphates may be carried out as $H_2PO_4^-$ or $HPO_4^=$. A more acid urine can be excreted when the kidney adds one hydrogen ion to $HPO_4^=$ and forms $H_2PO_4^-$. This is also a mechanism for conservation of sodium and potassium ions.

Physiological Derangements During Acidosis and Alkalosis. Normal physiological and enzymatic functions of the body take place optimally when the pH is normal. Moderate derangements cause disordered function; great variations are incompatible with life. The maintenance of a normal level for ionized calcium is one example; with alkalosis, the amount of ionized calcium decreases slightly, but the major cause of alkalotic tetany is the low hydrogen ion concentration. Another example is the permeability of cell membranes, which is affected by pH changes leading to the movement of potassium from the cell to the extracellular fluid (ECF).

Causes of Acidosis and Alkalosis. In infancy the most common cause of acidosis is diarrheal dehydration. In addition to the loss of electrolytes through the gastrointestinal tract, they are certain other factors that are contributory. The most important of these is decreased circulatory volume, which impairs renal function. The lack of nutrients normally derived through the intestinal tract necessitates the utilization of fats as the main source of energy, causing the accumulation of organic acids, the ketone bodies. As the acidosis progresses and tissue cells die, acidosis is augmented.

The sequence of events in diabetic acidosis is similar except that the losses of extracellular and intracellular electrolytes and water take place through the kidneys rather than the intestines, on account of osmotic diuresis resulting from the excretion of unutilized glucose.

The main cause of metabolic alkalosis is severe, prolonged vomiting, if the vomitus consists mainly of gastric juice. Pyloric stenosis is a good example of this situation. A high intake of sodium bicarbonate or other alkalinizing salt may also increase extracellular bicarbonate concentrations, particularly if renal function is poor.

Respiratory acidosis results from impairment of respiratory function and retention of carbon dioxide due to any cause, such as pulmonary disease, cardiac failure, or respiratory obstruction. Respiratory alkalosis results from hyperventilation. This may occur in encephalitis and in early salicylate intoxication, as a consequence of hyperpyrexia, or it may be of psychogenic origin.

In states of dehydration a metabolic acidosis usually occurs for the following reasons:

1. Cellular breakdown leads to organic acid and mineral acid release.
2. Starvation leads to fat breakdown with organic acid (ketone) production.
3. In diarrhea, some excess of HCO_3^- without H^+ is lost in the stool (sodium and potassium in excess of chloride).
4. Perhaps most important, renal impairment prevents excretion of the acid load.

When dehydration occurs in a patient with reasonably well-functioning kidneys and lungs, it is seldom necessary to correct the hydrogen ion excess by means other than restoring the circulation; the kidneys and lungs may then resume their function.

The basic principles that guide the management of fluid balance are based on three dimensions.

1. One must assess the deficit of water and electrolyte from losses already incurred; this dimension consists of quantitative differences from the physiological state, and hence it is measured in relation to weight.
2. One needs knowledge of the ordinary requirements of water and electrolytes per unit of time in order to replace usual losses as they occur; these are a summation of insensible evaporation, urine production, and stool

losses. All such loss is proportional to the energy expanded to produce heat; hence, the second dimension relates to calories expended and not to weight.
3. The third factor is made up of abnormal losses as in vomiting, diarrhea, or drainage from a tube in the gastrointestinal tract (or, rarely, abnormal gains) during the period of management. These are variable but can be measured.

Corrections of Disordered Composition. Loss of extracellular fluid is the common disturbance requiring treatment. Sodium and chloride may be lost from the gastrointestinal tract in diarrheal disease, in vomiting from any cause, in intestinal obstruction, or in fistulas. The loss may occur in the urine, as in diabetic acidosis and adrenal insufficiency. Whatever the mechanism, the end result is reduction of intestitial fluid volume and of plasma volume. If these losses are great enough, circulatory insufficiency, with reduction of renal blood flow, and oliguria develop. In addition to reduction of ECF volume, distortions of the extracellular ions occur, because the losses of sodium, chloride, and water may be disproportionate to those normally found in body fluids. If renal function is simultaneously impaired, the usual compensation mechanism — that is, by selective retention or excretion of specific ions — will also be defective. Thus there may be a relative deficit of sodium with respect to the anions (chloride, phosphate, sulfate, and organic acids). This is associated with hydrogen ion excess and a metabolic acidosis with reduction of serum bicarbonate. With high-intestinal or pyloric obstruction, there may be a relative chloride (and hydrogen ion) deficit, causing a metabolic alkalosis and elevation of serum bicarbonate. The losses of sodium and water may be disproportionate, so that the sodium concentration in plasma may be reduced or increased. Treatment is basically directed toward replacement of the sodium, chloride, and water loss from the body; improvement of the circulation; and restoration of renal function. The final correction of body fluids to normal is accomplished by the kidneys, if sufficient water and electrolytes are supplied. When permanent or temporary derangement of renal function is present, the restoration of composition calls for added care and precision during therapy. Serial measurements of body weight can be used as an index of water balance and are, therefore, valuable guides to fluid therapy.

Loss of sodium and chloride are usually associated with intracellular losses of potassium and phosphate. Internal shifts of ions also occur, with replacement of potassium by sodium in the cells. If potassium deficit is marked, final restoration of the normal extracellular electrolyte pattern is delayed until this ion is restored in the cells. Abnormal losses of chloride through the urine occur in hypokalemia. Potassium deficiency, therefore, is accompanied by persistent hypochloremia and elevated serum bicarbonate, as is particularly apparent when the acidosis and water deficit are corrected. Other manifestations of potassium deficiency are muscle weakness, abdominal distention (even to the point of paralytic ileus), and disturbances in cardiac function associated with abnormalities of the electrocardiogram. The serum potassium concentration may be low, but prior to restoration of renal function, the serum potassium concentration can be high even in the face of a marked intracellular deficit.

NORMAL WATER AND ELECTROLYTE REQUIREMENTS. Water requirement is based on losses engendered by metabolism (primarily heat production). The amount of water loss is approximately 1 ml/calorie metabolized (100 ml/100 calories metabolized). Water formed by metabolism, the water of oxidation, is approximately 12 ml/100 calories.

Because heat loss is a function of body surface area, this dimension is sometimes used to calculate requirements. In the presence of high fever or excessive muscular activity, the use of body surface area for such calculations may lead to significant error. We, therefore, prefer the fundamental basis of reference, i.e., caloric expenditure.

Calories expended (actually kilocalories) can be expressed for convenience in terms of weight at a given age. (Even though the relationship is not fundamental, the convenience is obvious.) Darrow has recommended a basal figure of 45 to 50 calories/kg of body weight per 24 hours for newborn infants. After a week or so, the number of basal calories expended per kilogram goes up to the range of 60 to 80 calories/24 hours. Fever increases total metabolism about 13%/degree centigrade. Activity in the newborn infant,

particularly one who is sick, may be taken as negligible; in the older infant a reasonable allowance is an excess of 50% over the basal metabolism. One cannot be expected to achieve precision in these estimates, nor is it clinically necessary. The purpose of the calculations is to avoid large errors. Table 7-1 gives a résumé of water requirements in several dimensions.

Under fasting conditions, the only solute load comes from tissue breakdown; therefore, no additional allowance is needed. The requirements for sodium, chloride, and potassium are about 2 mEq/100 calories metabolized. These needs are easily met by a parenteral solution containing 42 mEq of sodium, 28 mEq of chloride, and 14 mEq of bicarbonate per liter. These can be supplied as a solution of lactate and saline plus 5% glucose in water, to which the appropriate quantities of potassium may be added as chloride or acetate salts. Such a solution is useful for the maintenance of fluid in almost all situations. It is similar to the solutions devised by Darrow and others for this purpose.

It should be appreciated that the fasting requirements for water in the newborn infant is smaller because the body composition is undergoing a transition to a lower water volume, and the metabolism is comparatively low. Electrolyte requirements are similarly small.

Prolonged Maintenance Therapy. The electrolyte needs of the fasting child maintained with parental fluids can usually be met by the provision of about 2 or 3 mEq each of sodium, chloride, and potassium per 100 calories metabolized. A solution containing 20 mEq each of sodium and potassium per liter would provide this requirement. Such solutions are available commercially or can be prepared from Ringer's lactate solution (Hartmann) or lactate-saline (1 part M/6 sodium lactate and 2 parts 0.85% saline) by dilution of the

Table 7-1. Basal Water Requirements in Relation to Age, Weight, and Body-Surface Area

Age	Weight (lb)	Weight (kg)	Body-surface area (m²)	cal/kg	Basal metabolism (cal/24 hr)	Minimal basal water requirement (ml/24 hr)	(ml/m²)	(ml/kg)
1 wk	7.5	3.3	0.20	60	200	200	1000	60
2 mo	11.0	5.0	0.25	54	270	270	1080	54
6 mo	17.5	8.0	0.35	50	400	400	1140	50
12 mo	22.0	10.0	0.45	50	500	500	1110	50
3 yr	33.0	15.0	0.60	47	700	700	1170	47
5 yr	44.0	20.0	0.80	45	900	900	1120	45
8 yr	66.0	30.0	1.05	37	1100	1100	1050	37
13 yr	132.0	60.0	1.70	27	1600	1600	840	27

solution with 7 volumes of 5 or 10% glucose in water and addition of 1.5 g of potassium chloride per liter. Alternatively, individual solutions may be made by adding sodium chloride and potassium acetate to 5% glucose in water. When given in appropriate quantities, these solutions provide the water and electrolyte needs during periods of fasting and also supply sufficient glucose to prevent glycogen depletion and ketosis.

In some situations, prolonged parenteral fluid therapy may be needed for up to several weeks. To provide more calories and to prevent extreme breakdown of cell protein, the simple solutions of electrolytes and glucose just described must be supplemented. Whole blood, plasma, and albumin can be used as sources of protein. Extra calories can also be given in the form of fat emulsions for intravenous use. This has become safer in recent years. Amino acid mixtures can also be given. Twenty to thirty milliliters of 5% amino acid solution per kilogram will provide the equivalent of 1.0 to 1.5 g/kg/ day of protein.

Such amino acid solutions are excellent culture media for bacteria; therefore, meticulous aseptic technique must be observed to prevent bacterial contamination. The solutions should be given from closed bottles and never mixed with other solutions.

Total parenteral nutrition with concentrated nutrients has become routine. Precautions against contamination and local vessel injury must be observed. For most patients the use of more dilute infusions through peripheral veins suffices. Total parenteral nutrition at present should be utilized in the previously well-nourished patient only when more than 2 weeks of enteral starvation is mandatory.

By means of all these additional sources of nutrients, children with peritonitis, intestinal obstruction, and other problems can be maintained with parenteral fluids for many weeks. Table 7-2 lists and describes the solutions that are commonly used for parenteral fluid administration.

When shock is present, parenteral fluids must be administered intravenously because the defective circulation does not allow their absorption from the gut. In children who are not severely dehydrated or who have received sufficient fluids to overcome severe circulatory deficits, the fluid administration can be carried out by subcutaneous clysis. One should never administer, however, solutions that are hypertonic or that contain no electrolytes.

Clinical Evaluation

Application of the foregoing principles to practical problems is readily achieved through a systematic approach. The next few paragraphs contain suggestions for diagnostic observation and initiation of therapeutic procedures. The status of the patient must be evaluated from four points of view before fluid therapy is begun: (1) fluid volume deficit,

Table 7-2. Solutions for Parenteral Fluid and Electrolyte Administration

Solution	Composition	Na (mEq/L)	Cl (mEq/L)	K (mEq/L)
Group A: Solutions for replacement of extracellular ions, sodium, and chloride	0.85% NaCl	145	145	—
	Ringer's lactate (Hartmann)	131	107	4
	Lactate-saline (1 part M/6 Na lactate and 2 parts 0.85% NaCl)	152	97	—
	1,2,6 solution (1 part M/6 Na lactate, 2 parts 0.85% NaCl, and 6 parts 5% glucose in water)	50	32	—
Group B: Potassium-containing solutions	Darrow's	122	104	35
	Potassium-lactate-saline-glucose (1 part M/6 Na lactate, 2 parts 0.85% NaCl, 18 parts 10% glucose in water, and 1.5 g KCl/100 ml mixture)	22	35	20
	Sodium and potassium chloride (1 part 0.85% saline and 1 part 0.3% KCl in glucose solution)	73	93	20
	0.3% KCl in 10% glucose	—	40	40

(2) osmolality of body fluids, (3) ECF ionic relationships, and (4) cellular ion and skeletal ion disturbances.

FLUID VOLUME DEFICIT. First and by far the most important point is the volume of water to be given in therapy. The therapeutic volume for 24 hours equals the estimated deficit, plus the estimated usual losses over the next 24 hours, plus any addition for continued abnormal losses. The deficit is estimated clinically from the decrease in weight. The difference between two weights within 24 hours may be safely assumed to be water so long as this deficit is not estimated cumulatively over several days. When weights are not available, the deficit is estimated by clinical criteria as follows:

1. In loss of water volume equal to 5% of body weight, the earliest objective signs of dehydration are dryness of skin and mucous membranes, oliguria, and slight depression of fontanel.
2. Loss of water volume equal to 10% of body weight means moderately severe dehydration. Circulatory disturbances, manifested by mottled skin, cool extremities, tachycardia, and severe oliguria, are detectable. Depression of fontanel and eyeballs, loss of elasticity and turgor of abdominal skin, and facial pallor are additional signs. In practice, the 10% may be calculated from the dehydrated weight at the time of initial examination.
3. Loss of 15% of body weight as water within 24 hours produces a seriously ill to moribund patient.

Deficit replacement is then estimated on the basis of the above clinical findings. The problems involved in estimating the maintenance requirements have already been reviewed; the appropriate figure for 24 hours (based on estimated caloric expenditure) is added to the deficit. Again in practice, calculation may be based on the dehydrated weight, an "error" that roughly compensates for another "error" in the opposite direction, the water of oxidation, not usually calculated. Abnormal losses continuing after the initiation of therapy are periodically measured and added.

OSMOLALITY OF BODY FLUIDS. Next in importance come the estimation and correction or maintenance of physiological osmolality of body fluids. Disturbances in osmolality result from disproportionate losses of water and electrolytes. Circulatory disturbances occur early in the illness when electrolyte losses are either in proportion to or greater than water loss. When electrolyte losses are disproportionately smaller than water losses (hypernatremic dehydration), neurological disturbances are likely to appear. Small infants, because of their large surface area and immature renal function, are especially prone to hypernatremic dehydration when water intake is curtailed. The predisposition is somewhat offset in the neonate by the lower metabolism and the unique composition already discussed.

If the dehydration is judged to be isotonic (about 65% of problems in temperate regions) or hypotonic (about 10% of problems), the deficit fraction of the therapy should contain physiological amounts of sodium. If hypernatremia is diagnosed (about 25% of infants), the deficit fraction should be very dilute in electrolyte (sodium 40 to 50 mEq/L). The requirement portion is water without electrolyte in either case because maintenance electrolyte is negligible during fasting. Thus the combined (deficit + requirement) portions may, when mixed, have a sodium concentration varying from 15 to 75 mEq/L.

EXTRACELLULAR FLUID IONIC RELATIONSHIPS. The third point of evaluation is an estimate of the chemical "anatomy" of the ECF in the disease state. Traditionally this has been called acid-base balance. In the neonate with renal and pulmonary limitation, this parameter is more significant than in older infants but still clearly less important than changes in volume and osmolality.

Neonates and especially premature infants have a lower carbon dioxide content of the plasma by 3 to 5 mEq/L than do older infants, children, and adults. This physiological "acidosis" may be looked upon as another fragility of homeostasis because the infants' buffering system has, therefore, slightly less capacity to handle increased acid metabolites or decreased carbon dioxide excretion through the lung.

Aggravation of this physiological liability is not readily diagnosed by clinical means. Because small infants do not ordinarily excrete significant amounts of ketone bodies in the urine, acetonuria is not a helpful clue, nor is hyperpnea a reliable concomitant of acidosis at this age.

It is unnecessary to treat even an infant's moderate degree of acidosis with precision. If kidney and lung functions are reasonably good, even by neonatal standards, correction of the volume and osmolar disturbances will take place; the ratio of sodium to chloride and to bicarbonate will be accordingly self-corrected. On the other hand, there is every reason to avoid aggravating the disturbance; therefore, we recommend that, in all but the special situations discussed later, parenteral fluids contain a physiological excess of sodium to chloride ions in a ratio of 3 : 2. The remaining anion may be bicarbonate or lactate or acetate, which will metabolize to bicarbonate.

If there is serious renal impairment or concomitant respiratory acidosis, additional sodium bicarbonate is advisable. Approximately 0.7 mEq/kg (0.06 g) of $NaHCO_3$ will raise the bicarbonate concentration by 1 mEq/L.

CELLULAR ION AND SKELETAL ION DISTURBANCES. The fourth and final clinical appraisal should be in terms of the ions of intracellular fluid (potassium, magnesium, and phosphate) and of those in equilibrium with the skeleton (calcium and phosphate). It has already been stressed that homeostatic mechanism for control of these ions may be immature.

If pronounced muscle weakness and abdominal distention are present, potassium deficit must be considered; however, potassium can be given parenterally with safety if the following precautions are kept in mind. Potassium should ordinarily not be given until extracellular water and electrolyte are partially replaced and some renal function is restored as indicated by moderate urine output or decrease in blood urea nitrogen. The concentration of potassium in the infusion fluid should not be greater than 40 mEq/L; it can usually be given at concentrations of 20 mEq/L. The solutions containing potassium should be administered slowly so that the potassium requirement for the day is given over a period of at least 6 to 8 hours; preferably it should be distributed over the entire 24 hours. Excessively rapid administration of potassium-containing solutions, particularly in the oliguric patient, can produce cardiac arrest and death.

If muscular hyperirritability is present the possibility of hypocalcemia or hypomagnesemia should be considered. These conditions occur more often in neonates and young infants.

Therapeutic Procedure

EXPANSION OF PLASMA VOLUME. It is important to initiate therapy in a way that will best protect physiological homeostasis. Some individuals are severely ill at the outset of therapy and have marked constriction of the plasma volume. The emergency phase is concerned with immediate restoration of the vascular (plasma) volume to maintain the oxygen-carrying capacity of the blood and renal function and to ensure nutrition. When shock or impending shock is present, the first step is rapid intravenous infusion of plasma (20 ml/kg, given in a 30-min period), which will expand the vascular space and, by its protein content, maintain it. This fluid and its electrolyte content may be considered as replacement for a portion of the "deficit" fraction.

The second step is to maintain the vascular expansion and to provide water for rapid urine formation and calories for starving cells. For this purpose, 10% glucose in water is well suited. The glucose molecule is slower to diffuse than crystalloid ions and, therefore, remains in the intravascular space for longer periods. This is a helpful measure even at the temporary sacrifice of interstitial fluid. Rapid infusion of 10% glucose solution (20 ml/kg given in a 30-min period) supports plasma volume for a period of 1 or 2 hours; this support of blood volume, blood pressure, and urine output constitutes the most important immediate course of action. By the time the glucose, followed by water, diffuses out of the vascular system, the other replacement measures are well under way, and no further compromise of circulation should occur. In making the calculations for total fluid management, the volume given here may be conveniently thought of as coming from the "requirement" fraction because no electrolyte is included.

REPLETION OF EXTRACELLULAR FLUID. The two steps described in the preceding section should be completed quickly, in about 30 minutes each, roughly 20 ml/kg of body weight being given in each step. The first (plasma) may be omitted if shock is not present. Taken together these two infusions also fill the ECF to some extent beyond the intravascular portion. Some authorities substitute a solution resembling ECF for these two steps, i.e., a solution containing 120 to 140 mEq/Liter of sodium. In this case, the infusion should be on the order of 40 to 50 ml/kg given rapidly (1 to 2 hr). In either system speed is essential because vascular volume is being restored.

The third step is the more gradual infusion of the remaining fluid over the next 18 to 24 hours. In general, the deficit volume is infused within 6 to 8 hours and the remainder over the next 18 hours. The residual "deficit" and "requirement" fractions (after subtraction of the solution already given) may, for convenience, be mixed together in the same bottle.

Diarrheal Disease

The requisite skill for management of this condition is great, and special emphasis is warranted. Increased loss of water and electrolytes through frequent or large watery stools, with or without accompanying vomiting, places great stress on the young infant. Regardless of cause, success in therapy depends more upon management of the resultant physiological disturbances than upon removal of the cause. The precipitating cause for admission to the hospital is usually marked anorexia or vomiting. When either of these occurs, home treatment should never be attempted.

The approach to and initiation of therapy has been covered in the preceding pages. The infant usually has moderate to severe metabolic acidosis. The intention ordinarily is (1) to restore vascular volume so that oxygen and metabolite transport is resumed immediately to provide substrate (glucose) for starving cells and (2) to expand the extracellular space generally. In most cases one gives a volume of fluid equal to one-half the day's estimate in the first 6 to 8 hours, the remainder being given more gradually. Oral intake may be withheld during this time; a brief period of starvation is usually helpful in reducing stool water losses. Even very sick infants can sometimes resume oral intake after a brief period of parenteral dehydration (6 to 12 hours), and there are a number of advantages in giving the fluid orally at this point. In particular, the administration of potassium is made much safer; indeed parenteral administration of potassium may be avoided altogether. Oral electrolyte solutions, as suggested in Table 7-3, are traditionally used at this stage of therapy. These solutions are now being reevaluated and improved upon (see p. 113). Milk feedings or other high-calorie intake is best delayed for at least 24 hours lest the stool losses become enormous, although it is generally safe to continue breast feeding.

For those infants who do not have circulatory deficits and who will take oral fluid, an oral rehydration solution (ORS) may be used to repair the deficit, 100 ml/kg or the estimated deficit being given over 6 hours. Two such solutions are listed in Table 7-3. The WHO solution has had wide distribution under various trade names. After administration of the solution, one may continue oral therapy with a maintenance solution such as III in Table 7-3 (ion mixture 49-20) or by offering alternate feedings of ORS and plain water (some have recommended two ORS feedings to one of plain water). Although the maintenance solution is theoretically preferable, the alternate system may be more practical outside of large cities. The rate should be slowed after initial hydration just as in the parenteral regimens, with the remainder of the first day's volume being given evenly over the 16 to 18 hours after the rehydration.

The maintenance solution (ion mixture 49-20) is also ideal to give to infants at the onset of illness before they become dehydrated. It is well tolerated at a rate of 150 ml/kg/day and can be given for a day or so until resumption of feeding is desirable, after which gradual replacement with milk may be safely initiated.

During the period of early parenteral therapy the neonate should not be given oral fluids. At this period of life it is particularly important not to risk exacerbating stool water losses, which may rapidly become unmanageable. Oral feedings to premature infants and neonates with diarrhea pose considerable risk during the first 24 hours of treatment. On subsequent days oral feedings are resumed, as in older infants, beginning with a water solution of electrolyte and followed by gradual introduction of milk or modified milk feedings.

During the course of infectious diarrhea the intestinal mucosa may be so badly damaged that the brush border enzyme, lactase, becomes deficient for periods of a few days up to several months. In some racial groups there is an ontogenic disappearance of this enzyme beginning about the second year of life. Consequently the early refeeding

Table 7-3. Oral Electrolyte-Carbohydrate Mixtures

Solution	Composition	Amount of ingredient (g)	Na (mEq/L)	K (mEq/L)	Cl (mEq/L)	HCO$_3$ (mEq/L)	H$_2$PO$_4$ citrate (mEq/L)	Glucose (mM/L)
I. Oral rehydration solution (ORS-WHO)	Sodium chloride	3.5						
	Sodium bicarbonate	2.5						
	Potassium chloride	1.5						
	Glucose	20						
	Water to 1 L		90	15	75	30	—	111
II. Alternate oral rehydration solution (ion mixture 75-15)	Sodium chloride	2.63						
	Potassium chloride	1.12						
	Sodium citrate	2.58						
	Glucose	20						
	Water to 1 L		75	15	60	30	—	111
III. Maintenance or preventive oral solution (ion mixture 49-20)	Sodium chloride	0.61						
	Sodium biphosphate	1.42						
	Sodium citrate	2.49						
	Potassium chloride	1.54						
	Glucose	30						
	Water to 1 L		49	20	30	29	10	167

following a severe bout of diarrhea should not (optimally) contain lactose as the carbohydrate. Glucose and fructose are preferable, at least until an adequate state of nutrition has been achieved.

THERAPY IN SEVERE DIARRHEAL DEHYDRATION. *Emergency Treatment.* The basic program is shown in Table 7-4. If peripheral circulation improves rapidly after infusion of 10% glucose in water and the infant seems more alert, the plasma or blood may be omitted and the 1,2,3 (lactate-saline-glucose) solution or Ringer's lactate solution with equal volume of 5% glucose in water given. When whole blood is administered, the glucose solution is flushed out of the infusion set with saline or lactate-saline before the blood is added. This program is useful in the large group of infants in whom water deficit and sodium depletion are roughly in the proportions in which they are present in ECF, and it provides enough sodium and chloride to replace most of the extracellular deficit. When the laboratory data cannot be obtained rapidly, and the clinical appraisal does not suggest unusual sodium depletion or disproportionate water deficit, this program of therapy is the one of choice.

No specific treatment for the metabolic acidosis is used in this regimen. If the ECF volume is expanded by a solution such as the lactate-saline or 1,2,3 solution that contains sodium in excess of chloride, and the total water intake is adequate so that diuresis occurs, the acidosis will gradually be corrected. In some clinics a priming dose of sodium lactate or bicarbonate is given, followed by a solution of half 0.85% saline and half glucose in water. Although large amounts of sodium bicarbonate or sodium lactate solution given initially increases the serum carbon dioxide content more rapidly than the treatment just outlined, there is no evidence that any advantage is gained, whereas excessive

alkali administration can be harmful. Instead of the 1,2,3 solution, a prepared solution such as Ringer's lactate diluted with 5% glucose in water can be used as previously outlined. The amount of potassium in this solution is small and can be given in the early phase of treatment, although by itself it is not adequate for potassium replacement in patients with potassium deficiency.

If the infant has an extreme degree of sodium depletion as indicated by clinical evidence of marked loss of interstitial fluid and circulatory collapse, and if serum analyses show reduction of concentration of sodium (or carbon dioxide plus chloride), lactate-saline solution is used instead of the 1,2,3 solution in the same volume. This can be given by continuous intravenous drip at a rate of 0.5 to 1.0 ml/minute.

Maintenance Treatment. A few hours after the patient's admission the emergency treatment is completed, and the infant should be considerably improved as evidenced by good peripheral circulation, more normal tissue turgor, increased reactivity and alertness, and frequent voiding of urine. The stools may still be watery and frequent, but the infant is often thirsty and can now take fluids orally in adequate amounts without vomiting. In most instances, at this stage the maintenance water, electrolyte, and carbohydrate requirements can be given by mouth in the form of an electrolyte-carbohydrate solution such as the ones listed in Table 7-3. These solutions contain potassium as well as sodium and chloride. There is ordinarily no urgency about the administration of potassium, and it can wait until this phase of treatment. The maintenance solution is given in amounts of about 150 ml/kg/day, divided into equal portions given every 3 or 4 hours. Thus the patient is provided about 3 mEq/kg/day of potassium, which is sufficient to prevent progressive potassium deficiency even though a considerable fraction of the intake is lost in the diarrheal stools. The sodium intake is also high enough so that sodium deficits ordinarily do not occur despite sodium loss in the voluminous stools.

As mentioned before, early resumption of milk feedings may exacerbate the diarrhea and so cause negative water and sodium balances unless supplemental fluids are given parenterally. The administration of oral electrolyte solution, however, does not appear to exacerbate or prolong the diarrhea, and most patients can be kept in good balance with such a regimen. Solutions containing phosphate or phosphate, magnesium, and calcium have also been tried, because losses of these ions occur in the watery stools, but no evidence has been obtained that addition of these ions increases the efficiency of treatment.

During the first 24 hours of treatment the total water

Table 7-4. Emergency Treatment of Diarrheal Dehydration in Infant

Solution	Route of administration	Amount (ml/kg)
10% glucose in water	Intravenous	20
Plasma or whole blood	Intravenous	20
Lactate-saline-glucose* (1,2,3 solution), or equal parts of Ringer's lactate solution and 5% glucose in water	Intravenous	80

* Oral rehydration solution (Table 7-3) may be substituted in many instances.

intake is about 200 ml/kg, of which about 40 to 120 ml is given parenterally and about 80 to 160 ml orally. Larger amounts of sodium salts can be given but are usually not necessary, and in some infants administration of large amounts can be harmful.

The maintenance oral solution can be continued for several days. Usually small amounts of milk feedings are started by the third day of treatment and increased gradually as tolerated until maintenance calories are provided. As milk feedings are increased, the oral electrolyte solution is decreased and then discontinued. The total fluid requirements are then met by milk and water intake. During this period whole-blood transfusions may be required in severely malnourished or anemic infants to hasten recovery.

Daily weighing of the infant on this regimen helps in evaluation of the water balance. The initial treatment should cause an increase of 8 to 10% of the admission weight of the severely dehydrated infant. Progressive early weight gain of more than 10 to 15% of the initial weight indicates excessive water retention due to overloading with sodium. Sharp weight loss indicates body water depletion and inadequate sodium intake. In addition to the weight of the patient, the excretion of copious amounts of urine is an index of adequate water intake. Finally, analyses should show a return of blood urea nitrogen and serum carbon dioxide, chloride, and sodium contents to normal.

The diarrheal disease, particularly in the well-nourished infant, may be treated in the early stages by withholding of milk feedings and substitution of an electrolyte-carbohydrate mixture. Parenteral fluid therapy is usually not necessary. The use of colloidal water-binding agents such as pectins, cellulose derivatives, and kaolin has been advocated in the treatment of this stage of diarrhea. These substances are sometimes combined with sulfonamide derivatives of the poorly absorbable type. Some of the preparations also contain sodium and potassium salts, so that they provide a source of these ions. We have not used these agents in acute diarrhea, because in the milder diarrheas the oral electrolyte-carbohydrate mixture alone has given satisfactory results. In severe diarrheal diseases the emphasis must be on proper parenteral replacement of water and electrolyte losses.

Modification of the Above Recommendations. The following points are reasons for altering the regimens described in the preceding section:

1. Breast-fed babies rarely need to stop breast feeding because of diarrhea.
2. For less severely ill patients, step 1 (plasma or whole blood) or even step 2 (10% glucose) may be omitted, but the deficit must be replaced rapidly. Oral rehydration using ORS (Table 7-3) followed by administration of oral maintenance solution frequently is sufficient for treatment of infants who do not have circulatory disturbances.
3. If hypernatremia is suspected, the sodium content of the repair solution should be reduced (see following section, Hypernatremic Dehydration in Diarrheal Disease).
4. If oliguria persists, potassium should be withheld from therapy until urine output approaches normal amounts.
5. If weight gain is inadequate or too much, the volume for the next 24 hours should be reassessed.
6. If vomiting prevents oral intake, parenteral administration is continued, potassium being added with great caution.
7. Treatment of malnourished infants with diarrhea requires special precautions.
8. Instead of milk, nonlactose-containing protein hydrolysates sometimes seem better tolerated.

HYPERNATREMIC DEHYDRATION IN DIARRHEAL DISEASE. A significant group of infants with diarrheal disease, fever, and vomiting show the picture of hypernatremic (hypertonic) dehydration. This is particularly the case in dry, hot climates. In hypernatremia (a sodium concentration of 150 mEq/L or more) a physiological defect ensues because of the relative exclusion of sodium and chloride ions from the great mass of body cells. Because water moves to achieve osmolal equilibrium quickly, there is an obligatory intracellular dehydration — that is, the proportion of intracellular fluid goes down and the proportion of extracellular fluid rises, even though there may be a large absolute loss of water from the body, a state designated as hypernatremic dehydration. The clinical signs differ from those of classic dehydration in part because the ECF (and plasma) volume is relatively well preserved until the process is quite severe. The severity of the disturbance depends upon the degree of hypernatremia and also upon the rate of water loss. Marked hypernatremia may not be particularly symptomatic if the water loss is gradual; conversely, a moderate elevation of sodium concentration may cause striking symptoms if the rate of development is rapid.

Clinical Signs. The first clinical sign is either abrupt cessation of oral intake or high solute intake as the predisposing factor. The infants may show neurological manifestations such as muscle spasticity, twitchings, and stupor. Intracranial bleeding, although it is not the usual reason for the neurological signs, may occur in hypernatremia. It is caused by rupture of venules and capillaries secondary to a drop in cerebrospinal fluid pressure. This bleeding may lead to subdural effusion in some cases. As noted earlier, because these infants are less likely to show the classic manifestations of dehydration, the degree of water loss is often underestimated until the patients become quite sick.

Treatment. Treatment requires replacement of water with less sodium than is needed in the treatment of classic dehydration (a deficit fraction having 40 to 50 mEq of sodium per liter). Solutions containing (upon adding deficit to requirement portions) about 20 mEq of sodium per liter are given, and the amount of water replacement is about the same as that for the other types of dehydration of comparable degree. This consists of a deficit fraction of 100 ml/kg for the clinical entity of disturbed consciousness, dry mucous membranes, and "velvety" or "doughy" abdominal skin, plus a maintenance fraction for 48 hours. The fluid should be portioned out evenly over 48 hours, in contrast to the procedure in classic dehydration, in which the first portion is given rapidly. This scheme prevents sudden changes in cerebrospinal fluid pressure that may otherwise occur with such hypotonic infusions. Convulsions are not uncommon during hypernatremic dehydration; they may be precipitated by treatment when rapid solute dilution is produced by an injudicious rate of fluid administration.

These infants may have a greater degree of potassium deficit than infants with isonatremic dehydration; potassium should be added to the solution as soon as urine output or adequate renal function has been confirmed. The potassium concentration should be 40 mEq/L. Hypocalcemia may also be a complication when potassium deficits are marked, so that 10 to 20 ml of 10% calcium gluconate solution should be added to the total intravenous fluid given during the 24-hour period. Serum analyses, when available, confirm or eliminate this need. Maintenance fluids may have to be given intravenously for several days because of the complicating neurological symptoms that may contraindicate oral feedings.

SURGICAL CONDITIONS. *Dehydration Due to Intestinal Obstruction Other than Pyloric Stenosis.* Initial fluid replacement is essentially the same as that for dehydration due to diarrhea. The more difficult problem is maintenance therapy, because affected infants and children may need prolonged parenteral fluid therapy postoperatively while intestinal secretions continue to be removed by suction. The water, sodium, and chloride in the aspirated fluid must be replaced. In addition, potassium deficiencies can become severe because of continued loss of potassium in the gastrointestinal fluid plus the excessive losses of potassium in urine following the trauma of surgery. After the initial deficits have been replaced and circulation and renal function are improved, the total daily fluid requirement is given as described previously. The volume of fluid obtained by gastric

suction is measured and is replaced by an equal volume of a solution supplying about 75 mEq of sodium and 20 mEq of potassium per liter. The total fluid given daily is, therefore, the calculated maintenance requirement plus the replacement of aspirated gastric contents. If intestinal fluids are lost through an ileostomy or a fistula, the volume discharged should be measured and replaced by an equal volume of lactate-saline or lactate-Ringer's solution to which is added potassium chloride to a total concentration of 20 mEq/L. It should be noted that the concentration of sodium is higher in fluids lost by ileostomy than by gastric suction.

Dehydration Due to Pyloric Stenosis. Dehydration resulting from losses of gastric secretions due to pyloric obstruction differs from the previously discussed state in that hydrogen ion is lost and the chloride deficit is in excess of sodium deficit so that the deficiency of ECF volume is associated with hypochloremia and metabolic alkalosis. Replacement therapy requires larger amounts of chloride than that for other forms of ECF deficit. If the dehydration is severe, the estimated water deficit is about 100 ml/kg. If this volume plus the maintenance requirement of 80 to 100 ml/kg is replaced by a solution supplying 75 mEq of sodium and 75 mEq of chloride per liter, a total of 15 mEq each per kilogram of sodium and of chloride is given in the first 24 hours. This is an excessive amount of sodium, but the sodium surplus is lost with HCO_3^- through the excretion of alkaline urine, while the needed chloride is retained. A solution of equal parts of 0.85% saline and of glucose in water is, therefore, the one of choice. This is given in a volume corresponding to deficit plus maintenance requirement. A more precise solution of ammonium chloride and sodium chloride may be used, but, although theoretically advantageous, it does not prove to be necessary clinically. Whole-blood transfusions, 20 ml/kg, are given preoperatively to infants who have been severely malnourished and dehydrated. Oral feedings can usually be given by 12 to 24 hours postoperatively, and potassium requirements can, therefore, be supplied by oral electrolyte solutions or in milk feedings. Deficiencies of potassium may be unusually great, however, in infants in whom the course has been prolonged and who have shown marked metabolic alkalosis. An indication of such severe potassium deficiency is persistent hypochloremia despite treatment with large amounts of sodium chloride. Under these circumstances potassium is given by the parenteral route preoperatively after therapy with saline and glucose in water has improved the circulation and urine output. A solution of 0.3% potassium chloride in glucose can be added to the parenteral fluids; 75 ml of this solution per kilogram supplies 3 mEq of potassium per kilogram, which can be given over a period of 6 to 8 hours. At least partial correction of the potassium deficit and metabolic alkalosis in such cases should be attempted before operation; however, in the majority of infants in whom the diagnosis of pyloric stenosis is made without undue delay, parenteral administration of potassium is not necessary.

Dehydration in Megacolon. Infants with congenital megacolon present a special problem because they lose water to a transcellular space, the colon, which loss may lead to ECF depletion without change in weight. In this regard, the physiological defect (and the problem in clinical estimate) is much like that encountered in the burned patient. Accurate estimation of the deficit is even more difficult. Considerable skill is needed because the dehydration must be estimated by clinical criteria alone.

Dehydration in Burns. See Appendix B.

Dehydration Due to Diabetic Acidosis. See Management of Diabetic Ketoacidosis on page 97.

SEPSIS. One might expect that the increased metabolism caused by fever, in addition to the hyperventilation, would lead to solute concentration during sepsis. In fact, the increased cell breakdown and probably other poorly understood factors, possibly including ADH (antidiuretic hormone) secretion, often lead to a hyponatremic state. While fluids are needed, there is danger in giving them to excess. The mild hyponatremia does not require immediate correction and is self-limited to the acute phase of the illness if management is conservative.

Neonatal Problems

RESPIRATORY DISTRESS SYNDROME. This condition, mixed in etiology, sometimes poses problems in fluid therapy because of increased ventilatory losses of water combined with reduced intake. The most important point is the prevention of dehydration by administration of adequate parenteral fluids containing glucose to provide needed water and calories. Because the increased losses do not contain electrolytes, no added electrolyte is indicated, and all of the increase is given as glucose in water. In this way at least one type of complication is avoided.

Unless the situation is observed late, there should be little or no deficit to consider. The usual losses are increased by the hyperventilation and by the increased muscular activity of labored breathing. In moderately severe respiratory distress with considerable retractions the calculated usual losses can be safely doubled to determine the volume to be administered by continuous intravenous infusion. Measured weight changes are the best guide to volume of continued therapy.

When there is significant pulmonary insufficiency, respiratory acidosis resulting from inadequate excretion of carbon dioxide complicates the hypoxic and hypoperfusion metabolic acidosis. The increase in catabolism from muscular activity may add "acid" metabolites, further aggravating the precarious condition of the homeostatic buffering reserve. There is no way completely to reverse this situation satisfactorily by fluid or electrolyte administration because of the respiratory component.

The accompanying hypoxia gives rise to organic acid production, thus producing complicating metabolic acidosis. This portion of the disturbance can be corrected by alkali (HCO_3^-) therapy; there is a slight hazard of overloading with accompanying cation (Na^+). Therapy directed toward raising plasma pH by administration of sodium bicarbonate ($NaHCO_3$) may be warranted as an emergency measure. In prolonged cardiac arrest 2 mEq/kg of a solution of $NaHCO_3$ with a concentration of 0.5 mEq/ml may be given once by slow intravenous push.

The infants with respiratory distress who have become dehydrated have often shown hyperkalemia. It is doubtful that this represents anything special for these babies; in any event, untoward effects can be avoided by adequate hydration during the period of respiratory difficulty. If already present, this disturbance is also ameliorated by the administration of $NaHCO_3$ as described above.

Finally, when dehydration from hyperventilation occurs, hypernatremia often results. Under these circumstances additional sodium may be aggravating; therefore laboratory studies should be made before vigorous measures are instituted.

INFANT OF A DIABETIC MOTHER. Some infants of diabetic mothers appear normal; others are clearly abnormal. The body composition of those in the abnormal group differs significantly from that of the normal infant. Knowledge is far from complete concerning the differences, but a few significant ones are documented. There is an increase in body fat and a proportionate decrease in water. Thus these large puffy-looking babies are deficient in ECF and perhaps may be hypovolemic; total water needs should include a deficit fraction of about 2 or 3% of weight as fluids containing a physiological concentration of sodium. Losses of water are not unusually great in these infants, except when respiratory distress produces hyperventilation. There are frequently special problems arising from disturbances of homeostatic mechanisms for glucose and calcium. Both hypoglycemia and hypocalcemia may occur and should be corrected promptly.

These infants are all potentially sick; they need meticulous observation and immediate supportive therapy. No specific measures are known. One series of infants has been reported in whom the mortality was significantly reduced by the simple routine use of 5% glucose in 0.45% saline solution (66 ml/kg/day) through a gastric tube. The implication is that careful hydration to offset the low ECF volume and the high rate of water loss is of great importance.

ADRENAL INSUFFICIENCY. The majority of pediatric patients with adrenal insufficiency are those with the salt-losing form of congenital adrenal hyperplasia. Initially there is usually a picture of vomiting, electrolyte disturbances, and shock during the neonatal period.

In addition to the hyponatremia, hypochloremia, and hyperkalemia, another important feature of adrenal insufficiency is the greater loss of intracellular fluid than is apparent by changes in body weight. Losses of sodium and water are primarily extracellular and are produced by the diversion of those substances into the urine and intracellular compartment.

The use of potassium is contraindicated during the initial phases of therapy. Intravenous fluids should consist of isotonic saline in 10% glucose solution. Patients weighing up to 7.5 kg can receive about 120 ml of this fluid per kilogram, those weighing between 8 and 16 kg can receive 100 ml/kg, and those weighing more than 20 kg can receive 75 ml/kg during the first 24 hours. About 20% of the total volume can be given during the first 2 hours. Simultaneous administration of adrenocortical hormones helps to bring the adrenal insufficiency to a halt. After the first 24 hours, half-isotonic saline in 5% glucose may be substituted.

WATER INTOXICATION. Water intoxication is a condition that is produced by improper fluid administration, i.e., insufficient content of electrolytes included in the fluid given to the patient.

Patients who have a serum sodium concentration of less than 125 mEq/L often show clinical manifestations of hyponatremia, including impairment of cardiac and renal function and seizures; the last result from cerebral edema.

Specific treatment is often not necessary unless significant symptoms persist and consists of correcting the sodium and chloride deficiency. This can be accomplished by intravenous administration of a 3% saline solution at the rate of 1 ml/min up to a maximum of 13 ml/kg until the seizures stop.

Laurence Finberg and Richard E. Kravath

References

Brown, K. H., et al. Infant-feeding practices and their relationship with diarrheal and other diseases in Huascar (Lima), Peru. *Pediatrics* 83:31, 1989.

Chameides, L. *Textbook of Pediatric Advanced Life Support*. Elk Grove Village, IL: American Academy of Pediatrics, 1988. Chaps. 5 and 7.

Drash, A. L. Diabetes Mellitus in the Child and Adolescent. In J. A. Galloway, J. H. Potvin, and C. R. Shuman, *Diabetes Mellitus* (9th ed.). Indianapolis: Lilly Research Lab, 1988.

Finberg, L., Kravath, R. E., and Fleischman, A. R. *Water and Electrolytes in Pediatrics*. Philadelphia: Saunders, 1982. Chaps. 10–12, 15–17, 20, and 21.

Finberg, L. Oral electrolyte/glucose solutions: 1984. *J. Pediatr.* 105:939, 1984.

Haymond, M. W. Hypoglycemia in infants and children. *Endocrin. Metabol. Clin. N. Am.* 18:211, 1989.

Martin, D. W., Mayes, P. A., Rodwell, V. W., and Glanner, D. K. *Harper's Review of Biochemistry* (20th ed.). Los Altos, CA: Lange, 1985.

Stanley, C. A. New genetic defects in mitochondrial fatty acid oxidation and carnitine deficiency. *Adv. Pediatr.* 34:59, 1987.

Trucco, M., and Dorman, J. S. Immunogenetics of insulin-dependent diabetes mellitus in human. *CRC Immunological Reviews*. In press, 1989.

8

Nutrition

It is the task of children to grow, and inherent in this process is proper nutrition. The definition of nutrition, seemingly simple on the surface, is fluid and dynamic, changing with every year as our biochemical and physiologic understanding of growth and development changes. With that caveat, what follows is a current understanding of what nutrients children need to sustain healthy growth and reach physical maturity. One must bear in mind that the needs are colored by the child's body size, physical activity, and state of health.

Energy and Nutritional Requirements

Caloric needs vary depending on the body size and rate of growth, but generally one and one-half of the basic metabolic needs are required in order to account for the multiple energy variables and waste. Preterm infants have a caloric requirement of approximately 75 kcal/kg/day, which can be broken down as 33 to 40 kcal for growth allowance, 12 kcal for fecal loss, 10 kcal for cold stress (thermogenesis), and 15 kcal for intermittent activity. The higher metabolic rate of a newborn gradually diminishes as the months roll by. The term baby needs 100 to 120 kcal/kg/day in the first 10 months of life, but thereafter the need decreases from 80 to 100 kcal for months 10 through 12. Into childhood and early adolescence there is a relative stability of caloric needs, but with adolescence and increased activity, caloric needs increase, particularly in boys. Growth consumes approximately 5 kcal for every gram of weight that is gained. This number fluctuates with the degree of physical activity. Preadolescent males spend approximately 31% of their calories on physical activity compared to 25% for girls in the same age group. The child who because of social, deprivational, organic, or malnutritive reasons has failure to thrive, requires 150 to 200 kcal/kg for catch-up growth. These calories should be provided as carbohydrate and fat, efficient energy moieties, which are completely oxidized to carbon dioxide and water. Protein utilized for energy is made unavailable for growth, and when it is habitually used for energy, the result is cachexia and marasmus. The caloric guidelines in Table 8-1 should be tempered according to the variables already expressed, so that the child who has failure to thrive needs excess calories as does the child who is physically active or in a catabolic state.

Table 8-1. Estimated Daily Energy Needs

Age	Kcal/kg
Preterm baby	75
Term baby	100–120
1–3 years	100
4–6 years	90
(For catch-up growth)	100–200
7–10 years	80
Boys 11–14	60
15–18	50
Girls 11–14	55
15–18	40
Pregnant adolescents	+300/day
Lactating adolescents	+500/day

Proteins

The child grows by both cellular hypertrophy and cellular hyperplasia. Each cell is a microscopic building block of protein, contributing to the average protein increment of 3.5 g/day in the newborn. As growth continues, protein requirements (Table 8-2) gradually decrease, so that an adolescent male may require 0.8 g/kg, while a 1-year-old requires 2.0 g/kg. These are not absolutes, and it should be noted that the breast-fed baby grows very well on just 1.8 g/kg/day of protein. Some researchers feel that infants can attain good growth and development on 1.1 g/kg/day.

Protein contributes about 4 kcal/g or about half of what fat yields; however, amino acids essential for adults are found in protein. These include isoleucine, leucine, lysine, methionine, phenylalanine, tryptophan, valine, histidine,

Table 8-2. Estimated Daily Protein
Requirements for the Healthy Child

Age	G/kg/day
Preterm 26–28 weeks	3.1
29–31 weeks	2.7
Infant to 5 months	1.8–2.2
5 months to 1 year	1.0–2.0
1 to 3 years	0.8–1.6
3 to 6 years	0.8–1.5
6 to 10 years	1.1
10 to 14 years	0.9
14 to 18 years	0.8
18 to adult	0.5

and, in part, cysteine and tyrosine. The preterm infant requires special consideration. Protein intake greater than 4 g/kg/day may produce lethargy, acidosis, azotemia, and hyperammonemia. Additionally, the premature infant is unable to metabolize effectively phenylalanine, tyrosine, homogentisic acid, and methionine to cysteine. In these babies the feeding of cow protein (whey-casein [18 : 82 ratio] formulas) can increase plasma phenylalanine and tyrosine; human milk (whey-casein ratio 60 : 40) is safer. Overall in all age groups, 15% of the diet should consist of protein. Children fed lacto, lactoovovegetarian, and semivegetarian diets grow well with normal development. Those infants and children fed purely vegan diet should be assured good dietary guidance. Infants raised on macrobiotic diet demonstrate growth failure and no catch-up growth. This form of dietary habituation is dangerous.

Lipids

Fat contributes 40 to 50% of energy consumed by the infant, generally at about 9 kcal/g. In common with proteins, essential moieties are contributed by lipids. These are the fatty acids; polyunsaturated linoleic, linolenic, and arachidonic acids. These fatty acids are essential components of cell membranes, are prostaglandin precursors, and should provide 3 to 4% of the actual caloric intake. The preterm infant bears special considerations: 40 to 50% of calories should come as fat, but greater than 60% may produce ketosis. Linoleic acid should be given at 300 mg/100 kcal. Because bile salt synthesis is low, unsaturated fatty acids are best, and because pancreatic lipase base is low, medium-chain triglycerides are best. Lingual, gastric, and breast milk lipase base, however, all facilitate fat absorption. Table 8-3 lists recommended fat needs as percent of calories and grams per kilogram.

Carbohydrates

Forty to fifty percent of calories consumed are from carbohydrates, providing about 4 kcal/g. The main carbohydrates consumed in childhood are lactose, sucrose, and starch. For

Table 8-3. Recommended Fat Needs

Age	G/kg	% of calories
Preterm	3.0–5.0	40–50
Infant	2.5–5.0	30–50
Child/adolescent	1.4–1.8	30–50

the preterm infant lactose is generally the major source. The preterm infant has some physiologic limitations. By 28 weeks most disacchardidases are active, but pancreatic amylase is low. Salivary amylase, however, is present and breast milk is high in amylase supplying up to 450 I.U./kg/day of the enzyme. In addition, brush border glucoamylase is present. All three of these amylases, therefore, help to compensate for the low pancreatic amylase present in the preterm infant.

The dietary fibers are generally categorized under carbohydrates and include cellulose, pectin, gums, mucilages, algal polysaccharides, and lignin. These moieties are present in all plant cell walls. With the exception of lignan and cellulose, most fibers are somewhat degraded by gut flora to short-chain fatty acids such as acetic, propionic, and butyric acids.

Some fibers (gums, pectins) are soluble and can lower serum cholesterol levels. Others (cellulose, algal polysaccharides) promote intestinal transit time and defecation. While these features seem desirable it should be remembered that some fibers bind cations, while other fibers can bind iron, calcium, magnesium, and zinc inhibiting their absorption. Furthermore, fibers may promote satiety and diminish caloric intake. In the older child, therefore, fiber intake should not exceed 10 g/1000 kcal calories consumed, and the soluble to insoluble ratio of fiber should be one to three, approximating what is normally found in nature.

Water and Electrolytes

The newborn is 75% water at birth, but by 1 year of age this percentage is decreased to 60%. Water is in constant flux both through insensible (skin and respiratory tract) and sensible loss (renal, fecal). The newborn may have insensible losses of 150 to 200 ml/day and the 1-year-old 500 ml/day. By late adolescence this number is up to 800 to 1000 ml/day. Insensible losses increase with temperature and decrease with humidity. Taking into account both insensible and sensible water loss, metabolic water, and activity, the average child consumes 0.7 ml of water/kcal/day.

Metabolic water is generated endogenously through the oxidation of nutrients. One gram of protein yields 4.1 ml of water, 1 g of carbohydrate yields 5.5 ml, and 1 g of fat yields 1.07 ml. Table 8-4 is a list of water and electrolyte requirements in children under normal circumstances.

Vitamins and Minerals

The fat-soluble vitamins are retinol (vitamin A), ergocalciferol and cholecalciferol (D_2 and D_3), tocopherols (E),

Table 8-4. Maintenance Water and Electrolyte Requirements

Age	Water (ml/kg/day)	NA (mEq/kg)	K (mEq/kg)	Cl (mEq/kg)
Preterm	54–94	3.5	2.5	3.1
Term	125	3.0	2.5	2.5
6 Months	130			
1 Year	120			
5 Years	100	2.5	2.0	2.0
10 Years	85			
Adolescent	50	1.5	1.5	1.5

and phylloquinone and menaquinone (K_1 and K_3). All these vitamins are soluble in lipid and organic solvents, and deficiency occurs with decreased fat intake or malabsorption of fat. As opposed to water-soluble vitamins, these can be toxic.

The water-soluble vitamins are thiamin, riboflavin, niacin, pyroxidine, folacin, cyanobalamin, ascorbic acid, pantothenic acid, biotin, choline, inositol, carnitine, and bioflavanoids. These vitamins tend to be ubiquitous in natural foods and deficiency occurs predominantly from malnutrition. Choline, inositol, carnitine, and bioflavanoids are not true vitamins but rather enzymatic cofactors.

The elements of established nutritional importance are the major elements C, O, Ca, Cl, N, Na, P, Mg, H, K, S, and the minor or trace elements Fe, Cu, Se, Ni, Si, I, Co, Mn, Va, F, Zn, Mo, Cr, Sb, and Ar.

Table 8-5 summarizes the roles and requirements of essential vitamins and minerals.

Maternal Milk

The components of human breast milk (BM) are proteins, carbohydrates, lipids, vitamins, hormones, ions, water, and cells. It is secreted in three phases: colostrum, transitional, and mature milk. Lactose is the major osmol and citrate the major buffer. Enzymes found in BM include xanthine oxidase, aldolase, and alkaline phosphatase found in lipid globules. Lipase, amylase, catalase, and peroxidase are present via mammary capillaries. Lysozymes and lactoferrin are secreted by macrophages, and immunoproteins come from cellular elements.

Colostrum has 67 kcal/100 ml compared to mature milk with 75 kcal/100 ml. It is yellowish in color due to betacarotene. It is high in protein, low in fat, and rich in IgA (1740 mg/100 ml). Colostrum facilitates *Lactobacillus bifidus* colonization.

Table 8-5. Summary of Salient Vitamin and Mineral Factors

Name	Role	Deficiency	Excess	Sources	Age (years)	RDA Amount
Vitamins						
Vitamin A* (retinol)	Component of retinal pigments; needed for growth	Nyctalopia, xerophthalmia, photophobia, defective bones and teeth	Hepatomegaly, splenomegaly, ↑ ICP, bone pain	Liver, fish, oil, milk, eggs	1–5 7–10 11–18	400 µg 700 µg 1000 µg
Vitamins B, B_1 (thiamin)	Coenzyme of pyruvic acid oxidation	Beriberi	—	Liver, meat, milk, grains	1–5 7–10 11–18	0.5–0.7mg 1.2 mg 1.4 mg
B_2 (riboflavin)	Flavoprotein coenzyme participating in hydrogen transfer	Photophobia, corneal vascularization	—	Milk, liver, eggs, fish, vegetable greens	1–5 7–10 11–18	0.6–1.0 mg 1.2 mg 1.6 mg
Niacin	Coenzyme of dehydrogenase	Pellagra, dementia	Flushing, pruritis	Meat, fish, grains, vegetable greens	1–5 7–10 11–18	8–11 mg 16 mg 18 mg
Folacin	Purine, pyrimidine, nucleoprotein, and methyl group synthesis	Megaloblastic anemia	—	Liver, vegetable greens	1–5 7–10 11–18	100 µg 300 µg 400 µg
B_6 (pyridoxine)	Coenzyme for decarboxylation, transamination, transsulfuration, and fatty acid metabolism	CNS symptoms, anemia	Neuropathy	Meat, liver, grains	1–5 7–10 11–18	0.6–1.2mg 1.6 mg 2.0 mg
B_{12} (cobalamin)	Purine and methyl group metabolism; RBC maturation	Pernicious anemia	—	Meat, fish, eggs, milk	1–5 7–10 11–18	2 µg 3 µg 3 µg
Biotin	Coenzyme of acetyl-CoA carboxylase	Dermatitis, anorexia, myalgia	—	Yeast, liver, egg yolk	Unknown, for deficiency use 10 mg/day	
Vitamin C (ascorbic acid)	Metabolism of folacin, iron, tyrosine, and collagen	Scurvy, poor wound healing	Oxaluria	Citrus fruits, tomatos, berries	1–5 7–10 11–18	40 mg 45 mg 50 mg
Vitamin D*	Regulates metabolism of Ca, P, and alkaline phosphatase	Rickets	Toxic syndrome	Fortified milk, fish oils, sunlight	All ages	10 µg
Vitamin E*	Decreases oxidation of carotene, vitamin A, and linoleic acid	Hemolysis, neurologic syndrome	—	Grain oils, vegetable greens	1–5 7–10 11–18	5 mg 10 mg 10 mg

Nutrient	Function	Deficiency symptoms	Excess	Sources	Requirements
Vitamin K*	Prothrombin formation; Factor II, VII, IX, X, osteocalcin, and vitamin K dependent	Hemorrhagic symptoms	—	Leafy green vegetables	Infants 5 µg/day; Other ages unknown
Pantothenic acid	Component of acetyl CoA	Hypotension, muscle weakness	—	Meats, fish, vegetables	5–10 mg/day?
Minerals					
Calcium	Bone and teeth formation; cellular transport integrity	Osteomalacia, porosis, tetany, FTT	Stones	Milk, leafy vegetables, bivalves	1–5 500 mg; 7–10 800 mg; 11–18 1200 mg
Chloride	Critical electrolyte, acid-base, and HCl balance	Alkalosis	—	Salt, milk, meats	(See Table 8-3)
Chromium	Insulin cofactor	Impaired glucose metabolism, hyperlipidemia	—	Yeast, water	Uncertain 0.02–0.20 mg
Cobalt	B_{12} component	?	—	Water	?
Copper	Cuproenzyme factor to cytochrome oxidase and ferroxidase	Anemia, osteoporosis, neutropenia	Cardiomyopathy, Cirrhosis	Liver, oysters, meat, fish	1–5 1–2 mg; 7–10 1–3 mg; 11–18 2–3 mg
Fluorine	Cariostatic	Caries	Fluorosis	Water, seafood	1 ppm in water
Iodine	Component of T_3 and T_4	Goiter	—	Iodized salt, seafood	1–5 60 µg; 7–10 120 µg; 11–18 150 µg
Iron	Component of hemoglobin, myoglobin, cytochrome C, and catalase	Anemia	Hemosiderosis	Liver, meats, egg yolk	1–5 15 mg; 7–10 10 mg; 11–18 18 mg
Magnesium	Intracellular cation	Tetany	—	Cereals, legumes	1–5 100 mg; 7–10 200 mg; 11–18 350 mg
Manganese	Metalloenzyme of oxidative phosphorylation	Dermatitis, decreased cholesterol	—	Organ meats	1–5 1–3 mg; 7–10 1–5 mg; 11–18 2–5 mg
Molybdenum	Metalloenzyme to xanthine oxidase and sulfite oxidase	Headache, lethargy	—	Legumes, grains	0.1–0.5 µg?
Nickle	(Present as trace element, function and requirements unknown)				
Phosphorus	Bone and teeth formation, acid-base balance	Rickets, hypotonia	—	Milk, egg yolk	1–5 500 mg; 7–10 700 mg; 11–18 1200 mg
Potassium	Critical electrolyte and intracellular ion	Weakness, ileus, irritable, tachycardia	Heart block	Ubiquitous	(See Table 8-3)

Table 8-5. (Continued)

Name	Role	Deficiency	Excess	Sources	RDA Age (years)	RDA Amount
Selenium	Glutathione peroxidase cofactor	Muscle pain, pancreas degeneration	—	Seafood, organ meats, vegetables	1–5 7–10 11–18	10 μg 20 μg 60 μg
Sodium	Critical electrolyte, osmotic regulator, acid-base balance	Nausea, diarrhea, muscle cramps, dehydration	Edema	Salt	(See Table 8-3)	
Sulfur	Part of all cellular proteins	—	—	Meats, vegetables		
Vanadium	(Present as trace element, function and requirements unknown)					
Zinc	Metalloenzyme for alkaline phosphatase, carbonic anhydrase, DNA and RNA, polymerase	FTT, anemia, hepatomegaly, splenomegaly, dermatitis	Nausea vomiting, low Cu	Meats, grains, nuts, seafood	1–5 7–10 11–18	7 mg 10 mg 15 mg

* A fat-soluble vitamin.

FTT = failure to thrive; ICP = intracranial pressure.

Adopted and amended from L. A. Barnes, Nutrition and Nutritional Disorders. In *Nelson Textbook of Pediatrics*. Philadelphia-Saunders, 1987.

The main proteins of BM are casein, serum albumin, alpha-lactalbumin, beta-lactoglobulin, and immunoglobulins. Taurine, which is needed for bile conjugation and neuroregulation, is present at 34 μmol/100 ml. The initial high levels of IgA found in colostrum decrease in mature milk to 100 mg/100 ml. IgG is present in mature milk at 4 mg/100 ml. Breast milk is high in cysteine and low in methionine (the converse of cow milk). The protein composition ranges of BM are nitrogen, 180 to 250 mg/100 ml; total amino acids, 0.9 to 1.3 g/100 ml; nonnitrogenous protein, 0.3 g/100 ml; and whey, 0.2 g/100 ml.

Lipids in BM provide the major fraction of calories (30–55%). Lipid concentration varies from 3.5 to 4.5 g/100 ml. Fifty-six percent of the fatty acids are C18 (oleic, linoleic, and linolenic) and C16 (palmitic). Linoleic acid yields arachindonic acid (C20) and docosahexaenoic acid (C22), both needed for myelin formation. Cholesterol concentration is 240 mg/100 g of lipid or a range of 9.0 to 41.0 mg/100 ml. Breast milk carnitine concentration is 70 to 90 nmol/ml.

The carbohydrates in BM are variable. Lactose concentration is about 6.8 g/100 ml, glucose 14 mg/100 ml, and galactose 12 mg/100 ml. Fucose is present which together with colostrum helps to establish *L. bifidus* in the gut. Other oligosaccharides are present in a concentration 10 times greater than in cow milk.

Breast milk is rich in hormones including gonadotropin releasing hormone, thyroid releasing factor, thyroid stimulating hormone, thyroxine, prolactin, estrogen, progesterone, corticosteroids, erythropoietin, cAMP, and cGMP. Prostaglandins, both PGE and PGF, are found in a concentration 100 times that of plasma or at about 700 pg/ml. The role is uncertain. Epidermal growth factor is present at 50 to 90 ngm/ml.

With this overview of childhood nutrition, we can now briefly touch on undernutrition, a problem of unimaginable magnitude throughout much of the world.

Malnutrition

Kwashiorkor is protein malnutrition. Typically the child shows edema, anasarca, growth failure, misery, apathy, skin and hair changes, proximal wasting, and hepatomegaly. Pallor, stomatitis, and pellagra are common, particularly in mixed kwashiorkor-marasmus malnutrition. Hypothermia may be noted in severe states. Laboratory studies reveal anemia, hyponatremia, hypoalbuminemia, low blood sugar, and abnormal levels of aminotransferases, alkaline phosphatase, and bilirubin. Liver biopsy shows steatosis. The protein- and energy-starved child has diminished barriers against infections, with decreases in antibody production, leukocytic phagocytosis, and cell-mediated immunity. Among children with vitamin-A deficiency, mortality rates are 4 to 12 times higher than among nondeficient children, and supplementation of vitamin A can reduce mortality in these children by 30%.

Treatment must be individualized and based on facilities available. Hospitalization is preferable, if possible. Debilitated children may require nasogastric feedings by drop method and, in some cases, initial parenteral nutrition. Those children who are able to take oral feedings profit from the following formula: full-cream dried milk, 27 g/L; arachis oil, 20 g/L; and sugar, 100 g/L, given at a dosage rate of 136 ml/kg/day in hourly feedings. Supplemental vitamins and minerals are provided. In place of this protocol, a chemically defined diet can be used.

Outside the hospital, a simple but effective formula is dried skim milk, 20 level teaspoons; sugar, 4 level teaspoons; and oil, 6 level teaspoons in 20 oz of boiled water. This is given as tolerated by the child. Recovery may take a year.

Marasmus is protein-calorie malnutrition. Physically, these children are extremely cachectic with thin muscles, marked reduction of subcutaneous fat, and severe growth failure. No hair changes or edema are evident and the liver is small and atrophic. Treatment is similar to that used in kwashiorkor, and recovery is much slower. Osmotic diarrhea is a common problem requiring slow feedings. Secondary infections such are tuberculosis and parasitosis are common.

A. R. Colón

References

Barness, L. A. Nutrition and Nutritional Disorders. In *Nelson Textbook of Pediatrics*. Philadelphia: Saunders, 1987.

Beaton, G. H., and Chery, A. Protein requirements of infants. *Am. J. Clin. Nutr.* 48:1403, 1988.

Gleason, W. A., and Kerr, G. R. Questions about quinones in infant nutrition *J. Pediatr. Gastroent. Nutr.* 8:285, 1989.

Howard, R. B., and Winter, H. S. *Nutrition and Feeding of Infants and Toddlers*. Boston: Little, Brown, 1984.

Jacobs, C., and Dwyer, J. T. Vegetarian children. *Am. J. Clin. Nutr.* 48:811, 1988.

Paige, D. M. *Maunal of Clinical Nutrition*. Pleasantville, NJ: Nutrition Publications, 1985.

Pediatric Nutrition Handbook. Elkgrove, IL: American Academy of Pediatrics, 1985.

Pipes, P. L. *Nutrition in Infants and Childhood.* St. Louis: Mosby, 1989.

Sokol, R. J. The coming age of vitamin E. *Hepatol.* 9:649, 1989.

Somer, A., et al. Impact of vitamin A supplement on childhood mortality. *Lancet* I:1169, 1984.

Suskind, R. M. *Textbook of Pediatric Nutrition.* New York: Raven, 1981.

Van Staveren, W. A., and Dagnelie, P. C. Food consumption, growth, and development of Dutch children fed on alternative diets. *Am. J. Clin. Nutr.* 48:819, 1988.

Walker, W. A., and Watkins, J. B. *Nutrition in Pediatrics.* Boston: Little, Brown, 1984.

9

The Newborn Infant

This chapter concerns the newborn period, the first month of life, a period of inordinately high mortality and morbidity and physiologic activities peculiar to adaptation to extra-uterine life.

A newborn infant is a passive object of a number of different pathogenic factors. The infant may be structurally or physiologically imperfect because of chromosomal or genetic defects. During gestation the fetus has been subjected to all the ills that beset the mother: infections, hormone imbalances, drugs, ethanol, or radiation and diseases such as diabetes, preeeclampsia, hypertension, or other maternal problems that may lead to placental nutritional and oxygen deprivation. The newborn may undergo the considerable hazards of labor and delivery: prolonged, precipitate, or dysfunctional labor; early rupture of the membranes; cord entanglements; fetal distress; premature separation of the placenta; fetal monitoring complications; chorioamnionitis; anesthetic exposure; and difficult forceps delivery or cesarean section. Incompatibility between fetal and ma-

ternal blood cells may cause serious disease. The infant may have been born prematurely, and the handicaps of immature organs and enzyme systems make survival over these first days and weeks a risky matter.

Considerable expertise in the total care of children during the first year of life has produced a fall in infant mortality in the United States from almost 100 per 1000 live births in 1915 to the present rate of approximately 10 per 1000 live births. During this same time, neonatal mortality rates (death before 28 days) has decreased from 36 to 6 to 7 per 1000 live births. The perinatal mortality rate (PMR), which represents both fetal and early neonatal deaths, has fallen dramatically from 60 per 1000 in 1935 to its present rate of 11 per 1000. In most newborn weight categories, perinatal mortality is equally distributed between both components. The continued cooperation of all health care providers invested in maternal and infant well-being is necessary to continue this downward trend in perinatal mortality in the United States.

Evaluation of the Newborn Infant

Family History

Prenatal care provides an invaluable opportunity to meet with the expectant family. The family may evaluate the personality, practice routines, and style of the individual pediatrician. Likewise, the practitioner is provided with an invaluable tool with which to judge the expectations, interactions, and preparation of the family for the birth of the child. Much of the data given below may be provided by the parents on a standard form at their leisure; however, the opportunity for direct contact and observation of parental interactions is important.

1. Parent expectations
   a. Planned or unexpected pregnancy?
   b. Replacement child: new marriage, neonatal or infant death, retarded child?
   c. Home, hospital, or "birthing room" delivery; natural, Leboyer, repeat cesarean?
   d. Rooming-in or early discharge from the hospital?
   e. Sibling visitation in the hospital?
   f. Breast feeding?
   g. Early maternal return to work and defined caretaker or babysitter?
   h. Infant feeding peculiarities, "natural" foods, vegetarians, megavitamins?
   i. Sudden infant death syndrome concerns?
   j. Sibling rivalry questions?
2. Past pregnancy history
   a. Number of miscarriages, abortions, live births, premature births, neonatal deaths, and living children
   b. Vaginal or operative deliveries
   c. Gestational age and birth weight of previous children: small or large for gestational age
   d. Postpartum complications: bleeding, infections, depression
   e. Drug therapy for infertility
3. Siblings' nursery course
   a. Days in the nursery
   b. Medical problems recognized in the nursery
   c. Jaundice, its cause and therapy
4. Siblings' infancy history
   a. Anomalies
   b. Developmental milestones
   c. Retardation; special education; hearing, vision, or coordination problems
   d. Specialists or visits to specialty clinics
   e. Weight and height at 1 year, failure to thrive
   f. Special diet
   g. Present medications or medical problems
   h. Attitudes toward present pregnancy
5. Family history
   a. Genetic backgrounds of parents
   b. Mental retardation, institutional care, seizures
   c. Anemia, splenectomy, bleeding
   d. Hyperlipidemia
   e. Hypertension
   f. Medical conditions common to other family members
6. Present pregnancy history
   a. Parental ages
   b. Medications and over-the-counter drugs utilized
   c. Alcohol, drug, and smoking history
   d. Hypertension, chronic or pregnancy associated
   e. Urinary tract infection
   f. Viral syndrome
   g. Weight gain (polyhydramnios or oligohydramnios)
   h. Serology, Rh type, antibody screen, and PPD
   i. Vaginal bleeding
   j. Thrombocytopenia, past or present
   k. Diabetes; renal, thyroid, or connective tissue disease
   l. Perceptions of fetal movement
   m. Amniocentesis
   n. Ultrasound screening
   o. Nonstress or stress tests
   p. Biophysical profile
   q. Expected date of confinement

This information when not obtained prenatally must be reviewed with the mother or both parents as soon as possible after the delivery of the child.

Intrapartum Appraisal

A careful appraisal of the intrapartum period often provides significant insight into problems recognized in the newborn infant. Mortality and morbidity in the newborn, when prematurity and congenital anomalies are excluded, are often a corollary of acute or chronic hypoxemia. By modern obstetric standards an atraumatic delivery is synonymous with a "normoxemic" delivery. Recognition of this association has led to an explosion of prepartum and intrapartum tests of fetal well-being. Early identification of a hypoxic uterine environment was primarily responsible for the rapidly escalating cesarean section rate noted in most obstetrical services. A recognition that vaginal delivery is possible for most women who have had a previous section is causing a gradual fall in this rate nationally. Some of the more commonly employed tests with which to judge the adequacy of fetal oxygenation are discussed below.

TESTS OF FETAL WELL-BEING. *Prelabor.*

1. *Estriol.* The concentration of estriol, as measured in either urine or plasma, is of value in determining the function of the entire maternal-placental-fetal unit. Precursors (cholesterol or acetate) are manufactured in the placenta, metabolized in the fetal liver and adrenal, and excreted transplacentally into the maternal circulation and eventually excreted into the urine. Estriol normally rises with increasing gestational age. Persistently subnormal values or values that fall over successive days are prognostically worrisome for growth retardation or placental insufficiency.

2. *Fetal movements.* Quickening, or the perception of fetal movement, usually occurs at about the eighteenth to twentieth week of gestation. Although the number of movements is regulated by a variety of factors (for example, time of day, meals, glucose level, smoking), diminished fetal activity over days or weeks is indicative of fetal hypoxemia or impending fetal death.

3. *Ultrasound.* Used to monitor high-risk pregnancies defined prenatally, ultrasound can provide information on fetal growth patterns and identify intrauterine growth retardation indicative of placental dysfunction. Fetal ultrasonography may also identify the presence of congenital anomalies, twinning, hydrops, abnormal volumes of amniotic fluid, fetal cardiac disease, disorders of placental vascular resistance, and blood flow (seen with fetal hypoxia) and other anatomical abnormalities of the placenta such as placenta previa or abruptio placentae.

4. *Nonstress test.* Normal fetal movements, either spontaneous or induced, are frequently followed by a reflex sympathetic increase in fetal heart rate. Monitored externally by tocodynamometry, the test is noninvasive. A positive test (increase in heart rate with movement) is reassuring evidence of fetal health.

5. *Stress test or oxytocin challenge test (OCT).* Artificial uterine contractions are produced by infusion of oxytocin (Pitocin) while the fetal heart rate is monitored externally. A pattern of consistent "late" decelerations (a decrease in the fetal pulse rate near the end of a contraction that persists well after the contraction is completed) indicates a fetus with a poor oxygen reserve. When such a result is obtained, monitoring of spontaneous labor should be extremely diligent, and delivery by cesarean section might be indicated.

6. *Amniocentesis.* Transabdominal needle aspiration of the amniotic fluid is used to determine fetal maturity (e.g., amniotic fluid creatinine), organ maturity (e.g., for the lungs, the lecithin-sphingomyelin [L/S] ratio), genetic and chromosomal abnormalities, amnionitis (bacteria and white blood cells), and degree of Rh sensitization (bilirubin). The presence of meconium in aspirated amniotic fluid may indicate fetal hypoxemia.

7. *Biophysical profile.* The fetal equivalent of the Apgar score. Each of five determinants of fetal well-being are appraised by ultrasound: fetal tone, fetal movements, fetal breathing activity, heart rate acceleration, and amniotic fluid volume. Each characteristic is rated zero to two with a total of ten representing a perfect score.

8. Percutaneous umbilical blood (PUB) sampling. Under ultrasound guidance a needle is passed transabdominally into the amniotic sac and advanced into the umbilical vein. Direct sampling of fetal hematocrit, platelet count, and blood gases may identify the extent of fetal disease or provide a route for direct fetal therapy (e.g., packed red cell transfusion for erythroblastosis).

Intrapartum

1. *Meconium.* Although meconium passage occurs in 6 to 18% of all deliveries, passage of very thick meconium early in labor is frequently indicative of true fetal compromise.

2. *Fetal heart rate monitoring.* Hypoxemia during labor may be indicated by fetal tachycardia, persistent bradycardia, and deep variable or late decelerations with uterine contractions.

3. Measurement of pH by fetal *scalp blood sampling.* The hydrogen ion concentration of blood from the fetal scalp, as determined by sampling after rupture of the membranes and descent of the fetal head into the pelvis, correlates well with Apgar scores at birth. If fetal heart rate patterns are difficult to obtain, inconsistent, or difficult to accurately interpret, this test may determine whether labor should be allowed to proceed.

Etiologies of Fetal Distress

Placental Abnormalities

ABNORMALITIES OF PLACENTAL GROWTH. An unusually small placenta is commonly associated with states of fetal growth retardation. Impaired oxygenation, accentuated by the stresses of labor, accompanies the associated nutritional deficiency and increases the hypoxic risk to the fetus. A small dysfunctional placenta with multiple areas of infarction is also observed during states of maternal hypertension (essential hypertension, preeclampsia, and secondary to renal and collagen vascular disease). An exceptionally large placenta is seen with maternal diabetes, Rh incompatibility, and congenital infections (syphilis, toxoplasmosis, and cytomegalic inclusion disease). Classified as "hydropic," these placentas are functionally impaired, their excessive volume representing edema, not trophoblastic mass.

ABNORMALITIES OF PLACENTAL ATTACHMENT. The two most common conditions affecting fetal well-being are placenta previa and abruptio placentae. The initial symptom of both is usually vaginal bleeding. In placenta previa the placenta lies partially or completely over the cervical os. With progression of labor and continued cervical dilatation, detachment of the placenta and vaginal bleeding occurs. Abruption of the placenta indicates premature separation from the uterine wall. Usually painful, it may be associated with an enlarging or tender uterus. In both conditions bleeding may represent fetal as well as maternal blood loss. Fetal hypoxemia, therefore, may result from maternal or fetal hypovolemia as well as from impaired oxygen exchange due to physical separation from the maternal circulation.

ABNORMALITIES OF PLACENTAL SHAPE. An accessory lobe of the placenta (succenturiate lobe) possesses fetal blood vessels (vasa previa) that transverse the fetal membranes. Rupture of these vessels by the presenting fetal part during labor can result in rapid fetal exsanguination or hypovolemic shock at birth.

Abnormalities of Uteroplacental Perfusion

ANESTHETIC COMPLICATIONS. Maternal hypotension may follow administration of high doses of analgesics or sedatives and is a common complication of caudal and epidural blocks. Decreased uterine artery blood flow and diminished oxygen delivery to the fetus may follow rapidly.

MATERNAL BLOOD LOSS. Seen in abruptio placentae, placenta previa, and uterine rupture, decreased circulating maternal blood volume and uterine artery flow impede oxygen transfer to the fetus.

TETANIC UTERINE CONTRACTIONS. Diminished uterine blood flow usually follows excessive doses of Pitocin during induction or augmentation of labor.

MATERNAL HYPERTENSION. Any form of maternal vascular disease, including toxemia, diabetes, and renal and collagen vascular disease, may also involve the uterine and placental microvasculature and thus impair fetal oxygen exchange.

VENA CAVAL OBSTRUCTION. When the mother is in the supine position the weight of the gravid uterus may compress the inferior vena cava or aorta impairing and, thereby, influencing placental blood flow and oxygen delivery to the fetus.

Abnormalities of the Umbilical Cord

PROLAPSE OF THE CORD. More common in states of polyhydramnios, complete prolapse may occur through the cervical os or occult prolapse may occur between the fetal head and shoulder. If intervention is not expeditious, fetal death may result rapidly from anoxia.

TRUE KNOTS. True knots, unless associated with an unusually short umbilical cord, are uncommonly a cause of fetal hypoxia.

SHORT CORD. An abnormally short cord may cause early separation of the placenta and be symptomatically indistinguishable from placental abruption.

FUNISITIS. An ascending infection of the fetal membranes (chorioamnionitis) and amniotic fluid (amnionitis) that involves the cord as well (funisitis) may impair fetal oxygenation through direct action on the umbilical vessels.

Abnormal Presentations

BREECH. More common with decreasing maturity and with serious congenital anomalies, this presentation may increase an already high risk to the preterm infant. Failure to complete full dilatation of the cervix by the largest presenting part (the fetal head) may lead to entrapment of the head at the cervical os. Vigorous manual delivery may lead to osseous, peripheral nerve, cerebral, or visceral damage.

TRANSVERSE LIE. Failure of external version necessitates operative delivery.

HYPEREXTENSION OF THE HEAD. Failure to recognize this complication may lead to a greatly prolonged second stage of labor with traumatic and/or anoxic harm to the fetus.

Fetal Abnormalities

FETAL MACROSOMIA. Macrosomia of the fetus is usually a complication of maternal diabetes leading to dysfunction in the second stage of labor. A traumatic delivery by forceps or vacuum extraction may further compromise fetal oxygenation during the intrapartum period.

VERY LOW BIRTH WEIGHT. Fetal hypoxemia, during what might otherwise be considered a nonstressful labor, is more common in the infant weighing less than 1500 g.

CONGENITAL ANOMALIES. Hydrocephalus, ascites, hygroma, meningomyelocele, omphalocele, gastroschisis, encephalocele, sacral teratoma, and other fetal masses may delay delivery and compromise the already stressed infant.

The Normal Newborn

Growth Patterns

ESTIMATION OF GESTATIONAL AGE. The scoring system devised by the Dubowitzes and Goldberg (1970) (Fig. 9-1), combining both physical and neurological parameters, enjoys widespread use because of its ease of administration and overall reliability. Because age and maturity do not necessarily progress concomitantly, estimates include a standard deviation of almost 2 weeks. Because neonatal transition, adaptation, behavior, and pathology may vary directly with gestational age and organ maturity, an approximation of postconceptual age is essential as a guide to the correct interpretation of postnatal normalcy.

INTRAUTERINE GROWTH PATTERNS. In addition to gestational age, intrauterine growth patterns are highly predictive of a variety of neonatal adaptive disturbances. Within a particular gestational age the anthropometric measurements of weight, height, and head circumference define the particular fetal growth pattern. Normal intrauterine growth patterns with tenth and ninetieth percentile limits are extrapolated from the data of Lubchenco and associates (1972) (Fig. 9-2) and described below:

1. *Appropriate for gestational age (AGA)*. Birth weight and weight-length ratio fall within 2 standard deviations (SD) of the mean for the gestational age in question.
2. *Small for gestational age (SGA)*. The birth weight and weight-length ratio fall 2 SD or more below the mean.
3. *Large for gestational age (LGA)*. The birth weight and weight-length ratio fall 2 SD or more above the mean.

With this classification system the infant must first be described as term (38–42 weeks), preterm (less than 38 weeks), or postterm (more than 42 weeks). Within each of these classifications, and based upon the week of gestation and birth weight, the infant will then be classified as AGA, SGA, or LGA.

SGA Infant. This growth disturbance may be one that was operative early in gestation, inducing symmetrical reduction of weight, length, and head circumference. This pattern is often seen in chromosomal aberrations (trisomies), early acquisition of congenital viral diseases, radiation exposure, or early drug (including alcohol) exposures. In the majority of cases growth retardation occurs later in gestation, is milder in degree, and leads to selective retardation of birth weight alone. In utero, ultrasound examinations detect sluggish growth of the biparietal diameter of the fetal head, shortened femurs, or discrepancy in the trunk-head ratio. In addition to later occurring viral infections, maternal toxemia, hypertension, twinning, drug and alcohol addiction, and primary placental abnormalities (e.g., chorioangioma, infarctions) may be responsible. These neonates are particularly susceptible to cold stress and hypoglycemia from deficient fat stores (dermal insulation and brown fat) and deficient liver glycogen. Polycythemia, presumably related to chronic in utero hypoxia, is also observed. Because of borderline availability of nutrients and oxygen, the stress of labor is particularly hazardous to these infants, making fetal distress and its postnatal sequelae particularly common.

LGA Infant. The most common condition predictably leading to excessive infant birth weight is maternal diabetes. Macrosomia is particularly common in infants of mothers with class A, B, and C diabetes. With longstanding diabetes, and especially with associated maternal vascular or renal disease, the incidence of growth-retarded (SGA) fetuses increases while macrosomia becomes less prominent. Fetal overgrowth is presumably related to maternal hyperglycemia leading to a state of chronic fetal insulin excess. Insulin is just one of many fetal "growth hormones."

Other conditions associated with macrosomia and hyperinsulinemia include Rh sensitization, other forms of fetal hydrops, and the Beckwith syndrome. Neonates with transposition of the great vessels tend to fall into the LGA category, though the reason for this association is unknown. The majority of LGA infants are otherwise normal. A relationship to maternal prepregnancy weight has been observed; neonatal hypoglycemia and polycythemia are slightly more common in these infants. The major risks for LGA infants arise from prolonged and dysfunctional labor with birth trauma and resulting neurological, orthopedic, and asphyxial complications.

Postterm Infant. After 42 completed weeks of gestation the placenta appears to undergo progressive degeneration. The postmature infant begins to take on some of the characteristics of growth retardation. At birth these infants demonstrate cracked peeling skin, meconium staining of nails, skin, and cord, and some discrepancy of the weight-length ratio. As in other forms of growth retardation, the incidence of intrapartum hypoxia, meconium staining (and aspiration), and birth asphyxia is high.

Resuscitation at Birth

Preparation. Prepartum identification of the high-risk mother will not include identification of all infants requiring resuscitative measures at birth. At least one-third of all high-risk deliveries will not be identified until labor is in progress;

ESTIMATION OF GESTATIONAL AGE BY MATURITY RATING

Side 1

Symbols: X - 1st Exam   O - 2nd Exam

NEUROMUSCULAR MATURITY

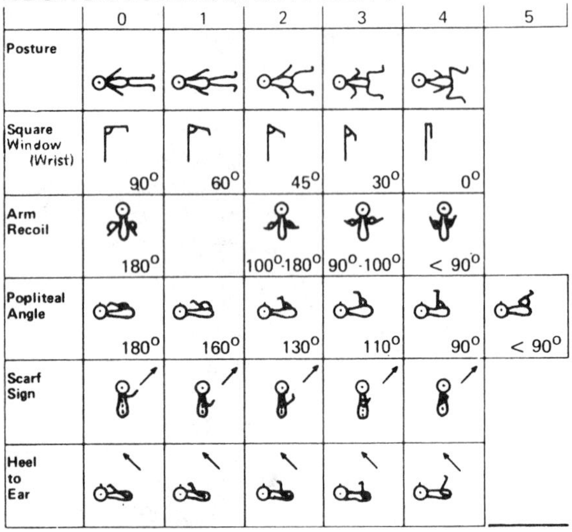

	0	1	2	3	4	5
Posture						
Square Window (Wrist)	90°	60°	45°	30°	0°	
Arm Recoil	180°		100°-180°	90°-100°	< 90°	
Popliteal Angle	180°	160°	130°	110°	90°	< 90°
Scarf Sign						
Heel to Ear						

Gestation by Dates _____ wks

Birth Date _____ Hour _____ am / pm

APGAR _____ 1 min _____ 5 min

MATURITY RATING

Score	Wks
5	26
10	28
15	30
20	32
25	34
30	36
35	38
40	40
45	42
50	44

PHYSICAL MATURITY

	0	1	2	3	4	5
SKIN	gelatinous red, transparent	smooth pink, visible veins	superficial peeling &/or rash, few veins	cracking pale area, rare veins	parchment, deep cracking, no vessels	leathery, cracked, wrinkled
LANUGO	none	abundant	thinning	bald areas	mostly bald	
PLANTAR CREASES	no crease	faint red marks	anterior transverse crease only	creases ant. 2/3	creases cover entire sole	
BREAST	barely percept.	flat areola, no bud	stippled areola, 1–2 mm bud	raised areola, 3–4 mm bud	full areola, 5–10 mm bud	
EAR	pinna flat, stays folded	sl. curved pinna, soft with slow recoil	well-curv. pinna, soft but ready recoil	formed & firm with instant recoil	thick cartilage, ear stiff	
GENITALS Male	scrotum empty, no rugae		testes descending, few rugae	testes down, good rugae	testes pendulous, deep rugae	
GENITALS Female	prominent clitoris & labia minora		majora & minora equally prominent	majora large, minora small	clitoris & minora completely covered	

SCORING SECTION

	1st Exam=X	2nd Exam=O
Estimating Gest Age by Maturity Rating	_____ Weeks	_____ Weeks
Time of Exam	Date _____ am Hour _____ pm	Date _____ am Hour _____ pm
Age at Exam	_____ Hours	_____ Hours
Signature of Examiner	_____ M.D.	_____ M.D.

Fig. 9-1. Newborn maturity rating and classification. (From M. H. Klaus. The Care of the High-Risk Infant [2nd ed.]. Philadelphia: Saunders, 1979.)

Name _____

Birth date _____

Hospital number _____

Date _____

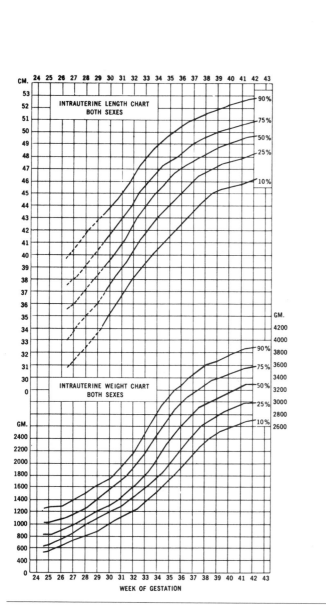

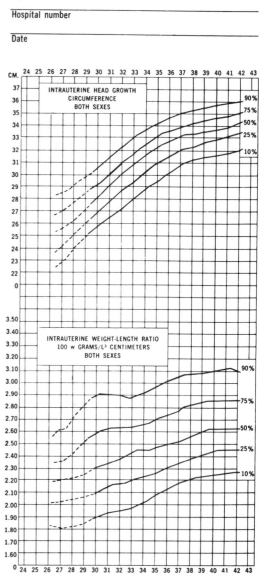

Fig. 9-2. Colorado intrauterine growth charts. (From L. O. Lubchenco, et al., Colorado Intrauterine Growth Charts. Pediatrics 37:403, 1966. Copyright © 1966 by The American Academy of Pediatrics.)

a smaller proportion of neonates will not be recognized as hypoxic until birth is completed, even when fetal monitoring is employed.

When certain fetal conditions are recognized prenatally (by ultrasound) or early in labor (fetal monitoring) that will necessitate intensive care of the neonate (birth weight less than 1500 g, a significant congenital anomaly, hydrops fetalis, or a surgical condition requiring immediate intervention), all attempts should be made to transfer the pregnant woman with the fetus in utero to a perinatal referral center. When this is not possible, predelivery contact with a tertiary nursery and its neonatal transport team will often expedite transfer of the infant postnatally.

An individual (preferably two) proficient in resuscitation should be present in the delivery room when certain complications are recognized. These include:

Prematurity
Intrapartum fetal distress
Cesarean section
Meconium staining
Severe growth retardation
Maternal diabetes
Rh incompatibility with hydrops
Fetal anomalies
Multiple births
Profuse vaginal bleeding
Abnormal presentations

If unable to be present the pediatrician must be certain that a qualified in-house individual (obstetrician, anesthesiologist, anesthetist, respiratory therapist, or neonatal nurse) is present in the delivery room. Each delivery room must be completely equipped. The minimum requirements for adequate resuscitation are:

A radiant heat source
Resuscitation bag capable of delivering 100% oxygen
A variety of soft pliable face masks suitable for full-term and preterm neonates
A laryngoscope with Miller 0 and 1 blades
Endotracheal tubes (2.5, 3.0, 3.5 F)
Adjustable wall suction
Suction catheters to fit endotracheal tubes
Umbilical catheters (3.5, 5.0, and 8.0 F) and tray
Volume expanders (Ringer's lactate, Plasmanate, albumin, normal saline)
Nasogastric tubes (5.0 and 8.0 F)

Drugs, including glucose (diluted to 10%), calcium, epinephrine (1 : 10,000) sodium bicarbonate, and naloxone hydrochloride (Narcan)
Tape, tincture benzoin, butterflies (25 gauge), needles, syringes, stopcocks)

APPROACH TO RESUSCITATION. When fetal distress is recognized prior to delivery, resuscitative measures can begin before birth. The mother is placed on her left side to remove the weight of the gravid uterus from the vena cava, thereby improving uterine blood flow. She is also asked to breathe 100% oxygen by face mask. A small increase in fetal oxygen tension (PaO_2) will occur unless complete cord strangulation is present. Additionally, expansion of maternal blood volume, transfusion of lost red blood cells, and other measures to support maternal blood pressure and uterine perfusion pressure may be indicated. Most importantly, any contributing factors such as oxytocin (Pitocin) infusions should be discontinued.

In the presence of meconium staining, the obstetrician should thoroughly suction both the oropharynx and the nasopharynx of all meconium with a suction catheter before completing delivery of the infant. This simple maneuver essentially eliminates meconium aspiration syndrome in the postnatal period.

Unless there has been significant maternal bleeding, clamping of the cord should not be delayed and the cord should not be stripped.

When the infant is placed on the warmer, suctioning of the mouth, pharynx, and anterior nares should be rapidly performed with a bulb syringe or suction catheter. The catheter should not be passed completely through the nares to the nasopharynx or deeply into the hypopharynx or stomach. Such catheter stimulation may easily provoke vagal bradycardia and complicate resuscitative efforts.

The Apgar score (Table 9-1) at 1 minute adequately dictates the resuscitative approach. A neonate with a score of 7 to 10 will be compromised by any major intervention. Drying, clearing the oropharynx and nasopharynx of secretions, and holding oxygen near the face to counteract cyanosis should suffice.

Conversely, a score of 0 to 3 dictates immediate and maximal resuscitative efforts. Thorough drying, suctioning, and rapid appraisal for anomalies should precede any intervention. Bag-and-mask ventilation with 100% oxygen should then rapidly be commenced. In the absence of airway obstruction (meconium or mucus) and with a tight seal of the face mask, this method of ventilation should be successful. Successful bag-and-mask ventilation is apparent when

Table 9-1. Apgar Scoring

Score	Heart rate	Respiratory effort	Muscle tone	Reflex irritability (catheter in nostril)	Color
0	Absent	Absent	Limp	No response	Blue or pale
1	Less than 100	Slow, irregular	Some flexion	Grimace	Body pink, extremities blue
2	Over 100	Good	Good motion	Cough or sneeze	Completely pink

the hypopharynx bulges forward, the chest moves, and breath sounds are auscultated by an assistant. The first few breaths may require high pressures—in the range of 35 to 40 mm Hg or greater. Pressures of 20 to 25 mm Hg and rates of 25 to 30 breaths/min will then usually suffice. The minimum pressure sufficient to inflate the lungs is the only real guideline. Bags with manometers attached help to maintain an appropriate inspiratory pressure and thereby decrease the risk of pneumothorax.

If the heart rate does not quickly rise above 100 beats/min orotracheal intubation with a 3.0 or 3.5 endotracheal tube should be completed. Suctioning of this tube should follow to ensure a patent airway. A breathing rate of 40 breaths/min with an inspiratory hold of 1 second should be utilized. Absence of an immediate increase in heart rate necessitates cardiac massage as the next priority. A rate of 100 to 120 compressions/min should be used with one-half the cycle time in full compression. A two-finger technique over the midsternum is preferred. Care should be exercised to avoid direct compression over the lower sternum and xiphoid which might lacerate the liver.

If improvement is not rapid and progressive an access line is essential for volume and drug therapy. A 5 F catheter passed into the umbilical vein just far enough to obtain blood return is sufficient. A volume expander such as Plasmanate or Ringer's lactate in a dose of 20 ml/kg should be given initially and repeated if necessary. Calcium gluconate, epinephrine, or sodium bicarbonate may occasionally be required in the delivery room. Other vasoactive pressors require more sophisticated monitoring that is available only in an intensive care area, to which the infant should be transported.

Infants with an Apgar score of 4 to 7 can usually be resuscitated with bag-and-mask ventilation with 100% oxygen. In association with adequate ventilation, continued poor color or perfusion usually implies a volume-deficient state and necessitates the interventions described in the previous paragraph.

Some of the numerous reasons for resuscitative failure are listed below:

1. *Infant never improves*
   a. Resuscitation bag broken, oxygen source disconnected, or less than 100% oxygen delivered
   b. Airway obstruction that requires direct airway suction
   c. Poor seal or inappropriate sized face mask
   d. Compression of tongue and occlusion of posterior hypopharynx by the hand
   e. Esophageal intubation
   f. Insufficient initial inflation pressure
   g. Significant blood loss or volume depletion
   h. Prolonged severe intrapartum asphyxia
2. *Infant improves then deteriorates*
   a. Equipment failure (bag or oxygen)
   b. Endotracheal tube misplaced in esophagus or right main-stem bronchus
   c. Resuscitation-induced pneumothorax
   d. Plugging of the endotracheal tube with secretions
   e. Cold stress
   f. Narcotic depression
3. *Infant initially well then deteriorates*
   a. Anesthetic or analgesic effect
   b. Choanal atresia
   c. Diaphragmatic hernia
   d. Spontaneous pneumothorax

Fetal Transition

PHYSIOLOGICAL ADAPTATIONS. The fetal cardiopulmonary conversion from a passive placental circulation to an air-breathing independent organism requires a highly sophisticated intertwining of complex physiological events.

During fetal life the placenta, which receives 40% of fetal cardiac output, acts as a low-resistance circuit providing the total oxygen and nutrient requirements of the fetus. Umbilical venous (oxygenated) blood is distributed primarily across the foramen ovale to the left side, providing blood of maximal oxygen saturation for critical fetal organs such as the heart and brain. Right ventricular blood, with the exception of 4 to 6% of total fetal cardiac output, bypasses the fetal lung and shunts directly across the ductus arteriosus to the descending aorta. This pattern of blood flow is maintained by vasoconstriction of the fetal pulmonary vessels due to the relatively low oxygen tension of the fetal blood. The peculiarities of placental diffusion characteristics combined with these normal fetal shunts preclude the attainment of a high fetal PaO_2 and thereby prevent prenatal increases in pulmonary artery blood flow and major redistribution of cardiac output.

Maintenance of adequate cardiac output, oxygenation, and perfusion after birth requires three simultaneous events: (1) ventilation and alveolar expansion increasing arterial PaO_2, (2) increased PaO_2 and lung expansion dilate the pulmonary vessels and increase pulmonary blood flow, and (3) peripheral vascular resistance must then increase to compensate for the loss of the low-resistance placental circuit. Following these initial events, subsequent transitional events lead to closure of the foramen ovale and ductus arteriosus within hours or days.

PHYSICAL FINDINGS RELATED TO TRANSITION. In the preterm infant, an initial period of reactivity may be shortened and the following period of deep sleep or diminished reactivity prolonged. Failure to appreciate variations in this pattern may lead to overaggressive treatment (e.g., oxygen, intubation, intravenous therapy, multiple cultures) stressing the neonate. On the other hand, application of standard management routines to an infant with abnormal transition leads to delay in diagnosis and therapy or to iatrogenic complications such as vomiting, aspiration, cold stress, hypoglycemia, or untreated sepsis.

Examination of the Newborn

The routine initial examination of the newborn is best performed after completion of this period of stabilization and transition. The infant should be examined in a warm environment completely undressed.

Behavior and General Activity

The physical findings must be interpreted initially in light of the neonate's stage of transition and later in terms of the state of alertness. After the initial transition period has passed the infant should normally progress through periods of deep sleep, rapid eye movement (REM) sleep, drowsiness, quiet alertness, active awakeness, and fussiness. The examiner must be aware of the infant's particular sleep-wake stage to correctly interpret physical findings. Lethargy during deep sleep and irritability during prefeeding fussy periods are considered normal behavior when transiently related to these events. Twitching limb movements during REM sleep are normal and not indicative of seizure activity. Tachycardia, tachypnea, perioral cyanosis, and increased muscle tonus are also normal during the prefeeding fussy period as is hypotonia in the postfeeding drowsy period.

The initial examination is best performed with the infant in the quiet-alert period, that is, awake, alert, looking about, fixing on objects, and demonstrating slow, controlled limb movements. Physical neurological, and behavioral examinations are most productive when performed at this time.

Posture

The infant's normal resting posture should be observed, note being taken of generalized dystonia (CNS damage, congenital muscle disease), lower limb dystonia (prematurity, lower spinal cord disease), or postural changes in a single limb (peripheral nerve damage, fracture).

Color

Though acrocyanosis (cyanosis of the hands and feet) may be normal during cold stress for the first day or two of life, central cyanosis during rest is always abnormal. Jaundice and the ruddy appearance of polycythemia should be looked for. Following a difficult vaginal delivery, especially during a face or mentum presentation, petechiae may be observed about the face, neck, and upper chest. Petechiae, bruising, or ecchymosis in other areas is suggestive of bacterial or viral infection, congenital thrombocytopenia, maternal medication (warfarin sodium [Coumadin], aspirin, thiazides) or heritable forms of clotting disorders. Cracking, peeling or meconium staining of the skin and thin subcutaneous fat are suggestive of postmaturity and fetal growth retardation. Multiple skin agiomas, although normal in the glabellar or suboccipital region, in other areas may be indicative of more occult generalized hemangiomatosis involving multiple organ systems. Single or multiple pustular lesions may be the first clue to herpes simplex infection or staphylococcal pustulosis.

Head

If delivery has been spontaneous and easy or a cesarean section performed the skull may be symmetrical and regular with little evidence of molding. The anterior fontanel should be widely open, the posterior one smaller but patent. The suture lines should be palpable. If delivery of the head has been somewhat difficult, however, it is not truly abnormal to find:

1. Overriding of cranial bones at the sutures
2. Caput succedaneum, molding of the skull with lengthening in the anterior-posterior direction and subcutaneous edema in one or both occipital regions
3. Cephalohematoma, a collection of blood beneath the periosteum of the cranial bone, sharply delineated by the suture outlining this bone

Craniotabes (Ping-Pong-ball skull) is seen with bone thinning from congenital hydrocephalus. An especially wide anterior fontanel occurs with certain trisomies, congenital hypothyroidism, and osteogenesis imperfecta congenita. Depressed skull fractures require immediate recognition and surgical intervention. Asymmetrical shape of the skull may be indicative of craniosynostosis (fusion of a cranial suture). Occipitofrontal diameters greater than the ninetieth percentile for age or markedly divergent from other anthropometric measurements require evaluation by transillumination and ultrasonography.

Eyes

Excessively wide-spaced eyes, slanting (mongoloid or antimongoloid), or small globes are common in many chromosomal abnormalities. Similar associations exist for corneal opacities, colobomas, or cataracts. Examination of the vascular pattern of the immature lens may provide valuable information relating to gestational age. Retinal and choroidal changes are observed frequently in congenital viral infections.

Ears

Low position, rotational abnormalities, and abnormal configurations of the pinnae are seen in many neonatal syndromes, particularly abnormalities of the renal system. Patency of the external canals must be confirmed at this time.

Nose

Dislocation of the nasal cartilage occurs in face, mentum, and occiput-posterior deliveries. Patency must be confirmed by holding strands of cotton from a cotton applicator in front of the nares to detect air movement or by *careful* passage of a small catheter.

Mouth

Facial nerve palsies should be looked for during crying. An excessively large tongue (macroglossia) occurs with cretinism, Beckwith's syndrome, glycogen storage diseases, and mucopolysaccharidoses. The hard and soft palate should be palpated for defects and the gag and sucking reflex evaluated.

Neck

Webbing of the neck (pterygium colli) in Turner's syndrome and short neck in Klippel-Feil syndrome are diagnosed by inspection. Prenatally acquired positional deformities of the neck resulting from shortening of the sternocleidomastoid muscle (torticollis) are frequently encountered. Branchial (lateral) and thyroglossal (midline) cysts are recognized occasionally. A congenital goiter may be present with thyroid enlargement.

Chest

Pectus carinatum (pigeon chest) and pectus excavatum (concave chest) is evident at birth and, if severe, may lead to later restrictive lung problems. A shield-type chest and wide-spaced nipples are characteristic of Turner's syndrome. The degree of expansion of the chest should be next evaluated. In the immediate postnatal period, failure to assume a barrel-chest appearance is observed in situations of underexpansion or atelectasis such as central nervous system disease, drug depression, generalized muscle disease, or diseases with diminished lung compliance such as hyaline membrane disease. Exaggeration of this phenomenon is seen in conditions involving air trapping or ball-valve obstruction (meconium or blood aspiration). Unilateral hyperexpansion may be noted contralaterally with complete lung collapse and pneumothorax, or ipsilaterally with lobar emphysema, diaphragmatic hernia, or cystic adenomatoid malformation.

Respirations should be counted for a full minute to determine the rate. Resting levels above 60 breaths/min are abnormal. Tachypnea alone may be indicative of neurologic, metabolic, cardiac, or pulmonary disease in addition bacterial sepsis. The breathing pattern should be regular without long rest periods or apnea. Deep rapid respirations are indicative of states of metabolic acidemia. Shallow rapid respirations are noted with pulmonary congestion. Retractions, or the utilization of accessory muscles of respiration, are graded by severity—intercostal, subcostal, or suprasternal—and are typical of primary lung disease and increased work of breathing.

Audible grunting, expiration against a partially closed glottis, is heard in states of diminished functional residual capacity (FRC) or atelectasis.

Flaring of the alae nasi frequently accompanies retractions and grunting. Auscultation of the newborn chest is usually successful only during deep inspiration. The inspiration occurring after a cry provides an excellent listening period. During the first stage of transition, pulmonary rales are normal findings as lung fluid is reabsorbed. Pulmonary rales at other times, when distinguished from transmitted upper airway sounds, are always abnormal, and usually indicative of neonatal pneumonia. Absence of breath sounds (atelectasis, pneumothorax) and prolonged expiration or wheezes (ball-valve obstruction) may also be noted during lung auscultation.

Heart

Because of transitional changes in the neonatal circulation, examination of the heart, especially auscultation, is challenging. The infant should first be observed for cyanosis (visible to the eye when saturation is 75–85% or less) or the ruddiness of polycythemia. The precordium should be observed for the presence of heaves or thrusts at the apex or at the right parasternal line. Palpation should detect obvious thrills and confirm the location of the cardiac pulse on the left side. A resting heart rate of less than 160 beats/min and the absence of significant arrhythmias should be confirmed. Absence of cardiac murmurs at birth unfortunately is no guarantee against underlying heart disease. Likewise a number of vibratory murmurs, especially in the pulmonary artery and ductal areas, are normal variants during the transition period. Infants with asphyxia or pulmonary disease may have prolonged elevation of pulmonary artery pressure and accentuation or persistence of these transitional murmurs. Accentuation of the second cardiac sound usually accompanies such states of persistent pulmonary artery hypertension. Fluctuation in pulmonary artery pressure and flow dynamics leads to rapid auscultatory changes complicating the cardiac examination. In addition, the femoral and brachial pulses should be carefully palpated simultaneously to detect major obstructive lesions of the left side of the heart or aorta. Palpated differences should be confirmed with blood pressure measurements of the upper and lower extremities and the left and right arms.

Abdomen

The abdomen of the normal neonate becomes distended with air swallowed during crying but never tensely so. Abdominal distention *at birth* is abnormal. Maternal polyhydramnios and aspiration of 25 ml or more of fluid from the infant's stomach at birth are pathognomonic of upper intestinal obstruction. A scaphoid abdomen in an actively crying infant is an early sign of congenital diaphragmatic hernia. Spitting and emesis with the first few feedings can be considered normal, but true vomiting that persists beyond this period especially if bilious is always abnormal and requires immediate investigation. Extensive mucus production in the mouth after the first period of transition is suspicious of tracheoesophageal fistula. With crying at birth, active bowel sounds should be present within the first 30 minutes of life, becoming less prominent during second transition and deep sleep. The abdomen should be observed for generalized fullness (ascites), flank fullness (hydronephrosis, polycystic disease), or midline fullness (hydrometrocolpos) and should be lightly palpated to detect tenderness or rebound. Hepatic or splenic enlargement may be indicative of hemolytic disease, congenital viral infection with hepatitis, or metabolic or storage disease. The normal liver may be palpated 1 to 2 cm below the right costal margin except in states of hyperexpansion when it is felt even lower in the abdomen. The spleen should not normally be palpable. The kidneys should be carefully examined and the width, thickness, contour, and consistency of the lower poles noted. Other abdominal masses should be excluded and a normal position and patency of the anus confirmed.

Genitalia

Ambiguity, clitoromegaly, cryptorchidism, and hypospadias may be important clues to more serious endocrine abnormalities. A small amount of vaginal bleeding and discharge is normal and linked to maternal pregnancy-related hormones transferred to the infant.

Spine

Dimples, cysts, hemangiomas, and nevi in the midline may be indicative of occult spinal cord disease, as are clubfoot deformity and abnormal lower limb reflexes.

Joints

The hips should be carefully examined for instability or dislocation during abduction (Ortolani's sign). Flexure contraction of other joints (oligohydramnios from prolonged rupture of the membranes or renal agenesis) may be related to in utero positional effects, primary hypotonic muscle disease, or a genetically transmitted disease.

Extremities

Lack of spontaneous movement of an extremity may indicate dislocation, fracture, or peripheral nerve or cord damage. Abnormalities are most commonly seen when fetal macrosomia, breech presentation, or difficult forceps extraction complicate the delivery process.

Neurological Examination

The neurological examination can be extremely misleading when performed in an infant of less than 24 hours postnatal age, especially if it is not repeated. Likewise the child's state of arousal is important in interpreting observed deficiencies. The quiet-alert period represents the optimal behavioral state for accurate interpretation of results.

Initially the child should be closely observed for diminished or asymmetrical limb movement. The basic components of a neurological examination of a newborn should include notation of the following:

1. Behavioral state, responsiveness, fixation and following, ease of arousal, and ability to be consoled
2. Tremulousness, jittery movements, or clonus, either spontaneous or stimulated
3. Diminished movement of a limb
4. Facial asymmetry, indicating cranial nerve dysfunction
5. Postural deficits in the supine or prone position
6. Alerting response to noise and light

Muscle tone and strength should be evaluated next. This evaluation must include truncal tone in horizontal and vertical suspension, neck flexors during pull-to-sit position, and limb recoil and response to traction. A series of basic primitive reflexes also require evaluation. These include:

1. *Sucking reflex.* If a finger is inserted between the lips of the mature neonate, the infant will engage it and suck vigorously.
2. *Rooting reflex.* If one strokes the cheek or chin of a normal full-term newborn, the infant will open his mouth and turn his head toward the finger in a searching movement.
3. *Righting movements.* When held with his back to the examiner's chest, the infant will straighten his spine and hold his head upright for a short period.

4. *Moro reflex.* If suddenly jolted or allowed to fall the infant will grimace, extend his arms convulsively outward, and then bring them inward rigidly in an embrace motion, while his legs react somewhat similarly.
5. *Stepping and placing response.* When the infant is held in vertical suspension and his feet are touched to a firm surface, he will flex his legs. If the child is then placed on a flat surface, he will extend his legs and produce stepping movements.

Care of the Full-Term Newborn

The last 15 years have produced profound changes in the manner in which infants are cared for in nursery settings. Emphasis has been placed on the importance of maternal-infant bonding in the immediate postpartum period, and older isolation nurseries have been converted into family-oriented care centers. In the obstetrical unit this philosophy has led to use of homelike labor, delivery, recovery (LDR) rooms, birthing rooms and natural, Lamaze, and Leboyer delivery methods and even to home births. Family-centered delivery suites within the hospital are far safer alternatives to home delivery and should be preferentially encouraged. Fathers now routinely "coach" deliveries and are present during most births including cesarean sections. Mothers hold their infants and breast-feed in the delivery room. Rooming-in facilities and sibling visitation are now commonplace.

An observational period may be as efficiently managed in a birthing room or recovery area as in the newborn nursery if experienced staff are utilized. When normal transition of the neonate and postpartum recovery of the mother are assured, both may easily move to rooming-in facilities with no interruption in bonding. Both eye prophylaxis (silver nitrate, erythromycin, or tetracycline) and administration of vitamin K (AquaMEPHYTON) may be safely delayed until the initial bonding and recovery process has been completed. Other routine procedures that should be completed during the initial hours after birth include bathing, cord care, blood typing and Coombs' testing of all infants of mothers with Rh negative or O blood type, and notation of urine and meconium passage. In infants with a prolonged period of starvation (greater than 4 hours) and in SGA, infants of diabetic mothers, and asphyxiated infants, blood glucose determinations (Dextrostix) should be obtained routinely and frequently. In this same group, early feeding should be encouraged. In any infant born to a mother with Rh-negative blood or a mother with vaginal bleeding the hematocrit should be checked soon after birth and repeated at 4 to 6 hours of age. Likewise in an infant with birth asphyxia or respiratory distress or an infant who is SGA, LGA, or plethoric, a hematocrit should be determined shortly after delivery.

Feeding the Full-Term Infant

BREAST FEEDING. In many parts of the world it is assumed that the mother will breast-feed her infant; in others the decision of whether or not she will nurse is left up to her. The obstetrician and pediatrician must be responsible to convince the new mother that breast feeding is a preferable alternative to artificial feedings.

Human milk is superior to cow's milk in several respects. Its protein content is lower; therefore, it places less metabolic load upon the kidney. Yet its quality is so high that the baby's protein and growth requirements are easily met. The total solute load is lower, again sparing the kidney excess work. While its total calcium and phosphorus contents are low, absorbtion is high and its calcium-phosphorus ratio is high, a fact that precludes neonatal tetany. It contains most known needed vitamins and perhaps even some unknown ones that might be of benefit. It provides opsonins, antibodies, and immune protection to the otherwise vulnerable newborn. It is sterile, thereby minimizing intestinal infections. It is inexpensive. Nursing periodically brings baby and mother into repeated intimate physical contact. Thus mother, too, derives much satisfaction.

ARTIFICIAL FEEDING. It is ironic that formula feeding, once largely limited to upper socioeconomic groups, has now been largely abandoned by the economically deprived population groups while the incidence continues to climb in middle and upper social strata. Although there are compelling reasons for breast feeding, complete nutritional requirements including iron and vitamins can be met by these commercial formulas. Although an explosion of new formulas specifically designed for the premature infant or the child with feeding disorders has occurred, the typical formula is 20 cal/ounce (67 kcal/100 ml), representing 290 mOsm/L. It is composed of lactose as the primary carbohydrate at approximately 7 g/100 ml, representing 40 to 45% of the total caloric value. The protein (1.5 g/100 ml) is prepared from nonfat cow's milk and represents 9 to 10% of the caloric value of the formula. The remainder of the caloric value (45 to 50%) is composed of vegetable fat (corn, coconut, soy) with a fat concentration of 3.5 g/100 ml of formula. At a caloric requirement of 120 cal/kg/day, maintenance needs and growth in a 3-kg neonate will require a minimum of 12 to 15 ounces/day. This quantity is usually exceeded after the first day or two of life, especially during periods of rapid growth and increased activity. Indeed, over-

feeding produces an array of annoying yet common symptoms, including spitting, vomiting, diarrhea, and diaper rash, in addition to speculative late sequelae, including obesity, hypertension, and atherosclerosis. There is no real evidence that early introduction of solid foods (before 3–4 months of age) is nutritionally beneficial. A demand feeding schedule dependent on the individual neonate's needs is usually adopted, with a total intake over 24 hours being the best judge of total nutritional adequacy.

Planning for Discharge

In most nurseries an observational period of 3 to 4 days is common, although shorter stays (at times less than 24 hours) are becoming less unusual. To be judged ready for discharge the neonate must meet certain conditions:

1. Show no signs of cardiorespiratory distress
2. Demonstrate a functional gastrointestinal tract with normal stooling patterns
3. Maintain adequate temperature when bundled in an open bassinet
4. Demonstrate ability to suck effectively to ensure normal weight gain at home
5. Show no signs of bacterial sepsis
6. Have no evidence of hyperbilirubinemia (greater than 12 mg/100 ml in a full-term infant on day 3). (In some instances, in the absence of hemolytic disease, arrangements can be made for discharge of an infant with borderline levels and for return to the nursery the next day for a repeat bilirubin determination. In some areas of the country home phototherapy for uncomplicated hyperbilirubinemia is also available.)
7. Have demonstrated adequate bonding with the mother

The discharge examination is best performed at the mother's bedside. This enables the physician to answer maternal questions about routine child care and to formulate a plan for follow-up of the infant. Concepts of child safety (for example, car seats) should be introduced at this time.

The Abnormal or Sick Newborn and Common Causes of Neonatal Mortality

Although significant reductions in neonatal and perinatal mortality have been realized in the last few decades and the absolute number of neonatal deaths has declined, the causes of these deaths remain essentially unchanged: (1) prematurity and its sequelae, (2) congenital anomalies, (3) asphyxia and related complications, and (4) sepsis. Each of these topics will be addressed in some detail in the following section.

Prematurity

Declining neonatal mortality rates, fertility rates, and birth rates have not been matched with a similar decline in the incidence of prematurity. The rate of low birth weight varies dramatically from one geographical area to another, being strongly dependent upon the socioeconomic status of the population served. In most areas of this country prematurity rates of 5 to 15% fill 50 to 60% of neonatal intensive care beds and account for 75% of total perinatal mortality. Survival of this group of neonates has presented pediatricians with a series of previously uncommon or unrecognized diseases often iatrogenic in origin. A small percentage of these infants also suffer either temporary or permanent physical or developmental handicaps requiring close medical and emotional follow-up after discharge. Based on presently available data, it is encouraging that as the rate of surviving infants continues to increase and overall mortality continues to decline across all birth weight categories, the incidence of significant developmental, motor, or intellectual handicap does not appear to be rising.

Improved outcomes in the LBW infant, though in part due to the high technology so visible in the intensive care unit, can largely be attributed to recently acquired knowledge of basic physiological biochemical and developmental principles and their application to premature care.

LABOR AND DELIVERY. The lowest mortality-morbidity in the LBW group of infants is realized when principles of labor management and operative intervention are applied equally to the full-term and preterm infant. Survival is no longer the only issue—ensuring the quality of survival demands a unified approach to prenatal and labor management.

"PREVIABLE" INFANTS. Mortality changes dramatically in 100-g increments in infants below 1000 g birth weight. Previability adjudged categorically by inexact methods are often misleading. Decisions related to the management of labor and delivery in this group of infants demand a close working relationship among the family, the perinatal obstetrician, and the pediatrician or neonatologist. Except in the very smallest neonates (<600 g or 24 weeks) morbidity can not be judged visually but rather by the infant's response to resuscitation.

TEMPERATURE MAINTENANCE. The effort to maintain core temperature within a normal range imposes significant stress upon the LBW infant. Reasons for this poor adaptation to cold stress *include*, large surface area to weight ratio,

diminished insulating subcutaneous fat, absent deep energy-efficient brown fat, and absence of shivering. In addition, the frequent requirement for resuscitation and stabilization in the delivery room with inadequate drying and high evaporative heat losses adds to this cold stress. Vascular control of peripheral blood flow is inadequate either as a result of prematurity alone or as a response to hypoxia.

The effects of cold stress include apnea, hypoglycemia, acidosis, hypoxia, increased metabolic rate, and increased mortality.

The aim of therapy is to maintain normal body temperature in a "neutral thermal environment," defined as one in which the metabolic rate of the infant is minimal. It varies with birth weight, gestational age, and postnatal age. The VLBW infant is limited in ability to raise metabolic rate and increase heat production; high skin temperatures (often close to the core temperature in the very small infant) are required to prevent a dramatic decrease in rectal temperature.

The physical properties of heat loss are countered during care of the premature infant by various nursing techniques: (1) *Radiant* losses are prevented by provision of radiant heat to the skin surface by an infant warmer or through utilization of double-wall isolettes or heat shields. In the latter instance the inner isolette wall (or heat shield) is maintained at the same temperature as the ambient air, thereby preventing radiant losses from the infant's skin to a cooler surface. (2) *Convective losses* are difficult to eliminate with open radiant warmers. In the isolette, warm air is convected over the surface of the neonate at the same temperature as the skin. (3) *Conductive losses* are eliminated if the surface upon which the infant rests is at the same temperature as that of the incubator. Placing the neonate on a water mattress heated to skin temperature assures minimal losses by this mechanism. (4) *Evaporative losses* are minimized by utilizing warmed air or oxygen of high humidity within the isolette or head box or through the endotracheal tube.

Most heating devices utilize a Servocontrol mechanism to maintain abdominal skin temperature; the heating element is activated when the skin temperature falls below a preselected value and then shuts off automatically when this temperature is reached. With a Servocontrol mechanism the infant's temperature remains stable while thermal instability is reflected by wide fluctuations in the isolette temperature. Likewise difficulties with the probe or its attachment to the skin may be mistaken for problems with the neonate leading to unnecessary interventions.

FLUID AND ELECTROLYTE REQUIREMENTS. The content of total body water varies inversely with gestational age; therefore, the most immature infant tends to demonstrate the largest weight loss, expressed as a percent of body weight. In the VLBW infant normal loss can approach 15 to 20%; however, the rate at which body weight (that is, water) is lost is of critical importance. Additionally, failure to allow for a normal decrease in body weight leads to tissue edema, not simply confined to the skin but involving other organ systems that may already be compromised by accompanying disease states. The thin skin of the LBW infant, in whom a well-developed cornified layer of skin is absent, accounts for these large transepidermal water losses.

In the LBW infant renal immaturity is evident by the inability to concentrate urine in the face of volume depletion or excrete a high free-water load when so challenged. Balanced hydration becomes a tedious process in these small infants. "Sure" judges of dehydration such as urine volume, specific gravity, cool, mottled extremities, mucous membranes, blood pressure, and tachycardia are unreliable indices in LBW infants, while changes in body weight, when diligently followed, are indispensable guides to hydration. Likewise serum sodium and chloride concentrations rise rapidly with water depletion and fall profoundly with overhydration. Rapid and significant changes in serum osmolality related to changes in serum sodium (including sodium added in the form of bicarbonate) and glucose present a distinct hazard to the central nervous system. A universally applicable formula for water and electrolyte therapy cannot be prescribed for these infants. Water requirements may range from 60 to 250 ml/kg/day dependent strongly upon the attention paid to controlling insensible water losses (isolette, heat shield, heat, and humidity). Although 10% glucose is the usual infusion, at high flow rates hyperglycemia, glycosuria, and osmotic diuresis may necessitate conversion to a 5% infusion.

The LBW infant also faces potential hazards from hyperkalemia. Blood drawing, intracranial bleeding, bleeding diatheses, or septic shock may lead to the need for frequent blood transfusions and concurrent high potassium loads. In addition, tender skin easily bruised during vaginal delivery adds to the risk of hyperkalemia as extravasated blood is reabsorbed into the sera. Perinatal hypoxia and temporary renal failure may further interfere with the excretion of this cation. Although the LBW infant is tolerant of higher levels of extracellular potassium than the older child or adult, life-threatening bradyarrhythmias may occur.

Calcium homeostasis is also impaired in these infants, and symptomatic hypocalcemia (seizures, apnea) or ECG abnormalities (prolonged corrected QT interval) are common and usually require early replacement therapy.

FEEDING AND NUTRITION. Nutritional philosophies and feeding techniques in the small infant vary widely with little objective evidence available to strongly recommend one approach over another. Whether it is appropriate to continue intrauterine rates of growth postnatally by the use of artificial formulas or breast milk in conjunction with total parenteral nutrition is still debated. Normal third-trimester storage of a substantial number of nutrients, vitamins, and minerals is substantially compromised with preterm delivery. Postnatal provision of these substances often proves a challenge. The infant is frequently too sick for early feedings, the gastric volume is small, and there is risk from ischemic bowel complications. Inability of the LBW infant to regulate intake has led to alternate feeding regimens, including total parenteral nutrition, intermittent gavage tube feeding, constant infusion gastric feeding, and transpyloric duodenal or jejunal feeding. With each method the intention is to provide appropriate calories to meet basal needs while attaining a daily weight gain of 10 to 20 g. For the majority of small premature infants this will be met when 110 to 125 cal/kg/day are provided. In the sick LBW infant the fluid (water) load entailed may be excessive. More highly concentrated formulas (24 cal/ounce or 81 kcal/100 ml), addition of glucose polymers or medium-chain triglycerides (to improve the poor absorption of long-chain fats in the immature neonate) are all utilized to circumvent this problem and ensure adequate growth rates.

The premature neonate is also robbed of the third-trimester storage of iron, folate, most vitamins, calcium, and a variety of trace minerals that must be provided in the selected formula.

The status of breast feeding in the premature infant continues to be debated. After a premature delivery breast milk is different in composition from that after a full-term pregnancy. Although breast milk is used regularly in many nurseries, the caloric value, electrolyte concentration, and calcium-phosphorus content may occasionally be inadequate: however, the benefits provided to the infant in the form of enhancement of maternal-infant bonding and gastrointestinal protection (lysozymes, antibodies, lymphocytes, secretory IgA) may outweigh other risks.

Three other metabolic abnormalities are seen with some regularity in the VLBW infant during periods of rapid growth. Increased velocity of growth combined with an immature renal sodium reabsorptive mechanism may increase sodium maintenance requirements to 5 to 6 mEq/kg/day; if this level is not provided in the formula, hyponatremia and sluggish growth may result. Impaired excretion of metabolic acid and hydrogen ion in the renal tubule, combined with increased hydrogen ion release as calcium is laid down in new bone formation, can add to metabolic acidemia and poor growth. Fractional reabsorption of sodium and bicarbonate are impaired accentuating potential hyponatremia and acidemia in the smallest preterm babies. Increased oral bicarbonate provided in feedings usually corrects this defect. Late-onset rickets due to vitamin D and calcium deficiency in formula-fed infants and phosphate deficiency in breast-fed infants can be prevented with vitamin D, calcium, and/or phosphate replacement.

The formulation and the route of administration of feedings for the VLBW infant varies from nursery to nursery; however, equally important and universally accepted are criteria for beginning and advancing those feedings. The LBW infant should be fed only after adequate gastrointestinal function has been demonstrated, with intravenous nutrition sufficing in the interim. Excellent bowel sounds, normal and consistent meconium passage, and a soft nontender abdomen must be demonstrated. The feedings, when started, must be of small volume and increased slowly and cautiously as tolerated. The infant should be closely observed for signs of gastric residuals, vomiting, abdominal distention, and melena.

SEPSIS. The LBW infant possesses limited immunologic and white cell defenses against bacterial invasion. The infant suffers from deficient chemotaxis, phagocytosis, opsonization, and antibody and secretory IgA production. Premature and prolonged rupture of the membranes, which frequently precedes premature births, often follows or leads to chorioamnionitis and significant bacterial colonization of the infant at the time of birth. Horizontal infection from maternal bacteremia and placental localization with subsequent spread to the fetal vessels characterizes some forms of neonatal infection. Aspiration of infected fluid into the lungs and bacteremia related to easily excoriated skin, resuscitative procedures, or blood vessel catheterization are the usual routes of infection. The prodromal signs of sepsis, easily recognized in the more mature infant, are often masked by other disease states or completely absent in the LBW infant. Septic disease frequently appears initially as catastrophic deterioration with hypotension, apnea, myocardial failure, renal failure, and major clotting abnormalities. When septic disease is unrecognized before cardiovascular collapse has intervened, mortality is exceedingly high. Late nursery-acquired infections are equally dangerous to these neonates because frequently a highly resistant organism, prevalent in intensive care units due to heavy antibiotic usage, is the causative agent.

JAUNDICE. The etiology of hyperbilirubinemia is similar, though accentuated, in the LBW infant. Liver immaturity, skin bruising, delayed feedings, frequent transfusions, and hypoxia tend to accentuate "physiological" jaundice. In the preterm infant, especially when stressed by asphyxia or sepsis, an immature and ineffective blood-brain barrier is demonstrated. In these LBW infants pathological yellow staining of the basal ganglia (kernicterus) has occurred with significantly lower levels of bilirubin than are usually assumed necessary for this occurrence in term infants. Bilirubin levels at which phototherapy is initiated must be adjusted in proportion to degree of immaturity. A significant increase in insensible water loss (10–20%) can be expected during phototherapy and must be considered when the infant's fluid requirements are determined.

ANEMIA. The normal physiological anemia of the neonate due to prolonged bone marrow suppression is accentuated in the preterm infant. In addition to blood drawing, deficiencies of vitamin E (alpha-tocopherol) and occasionally of folate intensify the decrease in the hematocrit value if not prophylactically treated.

APNEA. The pathogenesis of apnea is multifactorial. Apnea appearing in the immediate postnatal period may be due to pulmonary insufficiency (major atelectasis, decreased lung compliance, poor chest wall stability), primary parenchymal lung disease, maternal drug or anesthetic effect, hypoxic central nervous system disease, cold stress, or early-onset sepsis. The preterm neonate's respiratory center is relatively insensitive to hypoxia and hypercarbia. This immature central ventilatory control makes identification (heart rate and respiratory monitoring) and treatment (tactile stimulation, mechanical ventilation, or drug therapy) of critical importance in the LBW infant.

Other conditions in which apnea may appear within the first few days of life include hyperthermia, hypoglycemia, sepsis, hypocalcemia, anemia, postnatally acquired infections, seizures, intraventricular hemorrhage, necrotizing enterocolitis, gastroesophageal reflux, and chronic lung disease.

SPECIFIC DISEASES RELATED TO PREMATURITY. *Respiratory Distress Syndrome (RDS)*. RDS is not the inevitable end result of premature birth. Although RDS is rarely observed in the neonate beyond 35 weeks' gestation, its highest incidence is expected in the neonate of 28 to 32 weeks. The clinical symptoms of tachypnea, audible grunting, chest-wall retractions, nasal flaring, and cyanosis in room air are coupled with the radiological appearance of lung hypoexpansion (microatelectasis) and a characteristic ground-glass appearance to the lungs with air bronchograms. Anatomically, immaturity of the lung with deficient branching of alveolar ducts into saccules or alveoli, combined with incomplete capillary invagination leading to deficient alveolar-capillary continuity, impairs oxygen exchange. Biochemically, deficiency of lung phospholipids (surfactant) leads to "stiff" and poorly compliant lungs. Large inflation pressures are required to expand the lungs of affected infants, and lung collapse occurs at higher airway closing pressures. Small-airway collapse leads to major ventilation-perfusion abnormalities and a requirement for high inspired oxygen (FIO_2). Continued hypoxemia compromises tissue oxygen delivery, and metabolic acidemia supervenes. Significantly increased breathing work leads to respiratory muscle fatigue, a decrease in minute ventilation (the product of respiratory rate and tidal volume), hypercarbia, and/or apnea.

In recent years major efforts have been expended to diminish the incidence and severity of this disease. An accurate appraisal of the risk of the disease can be made prenatally by employing amniocentesis to measure the ratio of lung phospholipids in the amniotic fluid (the lecithin-sphingomyelin, or L/S ratio) as well as the quantification of other phospholipids (phosphatidylglycerol and phosphatidylinositol) indicative of lung maturity. The universal availability of this test has led to a diminished incidence of iatrogenic RDS due to inappropriately timed elective induction or repeat cesarean section.

Clinical application of drug therapy for labor inhibition when premature labor commences, prenatal induction of lung maturity by maternal injection of corticosteroids, and early recognition and prevention of fetal distress have all led to diminishing the incidence and severity of this disease.

Clinical Management. Treatment of RDS begins in the delivery room with rapid and effective resuscitation. The primary aims of therapy are maintenance of normoxemia (PaO_2 of 50–90 mm Hg), systemic perfusion, and normocarbia ($PaCO_2$ of 40–45 mm Hg) until lung maturation occurs by the third or fourth postnatal day. Application of continuous positive airway pressure (CPAP) by face mask, nasal prongs, or endotracheal tube may suffice in neonates with mild to moderate disease. CPAP increases functional residual capacity (FRC) and stabilizes the nonrigid (compliant) chest wall, thereby decreasing the work of breathing, the incidence of atelectasis, and subsequent ventilation-perfusion abnormalities. Increasing FIO_2 requirements despite increasing $PaCO_2$ or apnea requires the addition of mechanical ventilation. When present-day ventilatory techniques are utilized in conjunction with strict supportive management (temperature, fluids, electrolytes, blood volume, nutrition), the majority of infants with RDS will be expected to survive their initial disease.

Most recently the use of replacement surfactant offers great promise as a form of therapy.

Retinopathy of Prematurity (ROP). The vasospastic response of the retinal vessels with subsequent capillary proliferation and neovascularization during exposure to a high PaO_2 is unique to the preterm infant. The disease can be mild and transient, or it can result in total blindness. Strict attempts to normalize the PaO_2 are employed in the LBW infant to minimize this complication. Intermittent PaO_2 sampling through an umbilical or radial artery catheter and transcutaneous pulseoximetry are the most commonly utilized monitoring techniques. Despite these techniques, ROP is still seen in the premature infant of less than 1500 g. We now recognize that other stimuli such as hypotension, hypocarbia, and hypercarbia may play a strong contributory role.

Cerebral Intraventricular Hemorrhage. With the advent of computed axial tomography (CAT scan) and portable ultrasound units for diagnosis, the incidence of this disease appears to approach 30 to 40% in infants weighing less than 1500 g at birth.

The bleeding originates in the subependymal layer of the germinal matrix near the lateral surface of the third ventricle. This area is sensitive to hypoxemic and major vascular (venous and arterial) pressure changes. Rupture of this capillary network may remain confined to the subependymal area, or it may rupture medially into the ventricular cavity or laterally into the surrounding white matter. The ventricles may dilate with blood, and either communicating or noncommunicating hydrocephalus may result.

The clinical presentation may be catastrophic, with sudden profound shock, hypoxemia, seizures, flaccid paralysis, and rapid death. The majority of bleeding is silent, though the event may be suspected by sudden changes in clinical condition, unexplained major decreases in the hematocrit value, or transient abnormalities in neurological function. Most bleeding appears to occur in the first postnatal day and usually before 72 hours of life. Outcomes in terms of mortality and morbidity appear closely tied to the severity of the bleeding. A number of contributing factors have been proposed—hypoxia, clotting abnormalities, hyperosmolality, hypertension, hypercarbia, high ventilatory pressures, and pneumothorax, to name a few. Therapy at the present time is directed toward the early recognition and management of subsequent hydrocephalus.

Necrotizing Enterocolitis. Necrotizing enterocolitis is a transmural ischemic bowel disease that affects primarily LBW infants on the second to twentieth day of life. Early symptoms include abdominal distention, gastric residuals, bilious vomiting, Hematest-positive stools, and apnea. As the disease progresses, symptoms of septic cardiovascular shock predominate—temperature instability, hypotension, skin mottling, and metabolic acidemia. Radiological examination of the abdomen shows distention and thickening of bowel loops, ileus, linear streaks or bubbles of air within the bowel wall (pneumatosis intestinalis), air within the portal venous system, or free air within the abdomen. A single etiological factor has not been described. An ischemic insult, combined with pathogenic bacterial colonization and enteral feedings, is present in most affected infants. The incidence appears lower in breast-fed infants and higher in those given hypertonic feedings. Rapid introduction of large-volume feedings in infants with diminished intestinal contractility may also be a contributing factor. Infants with cyanotic congenital heart disease who have been administered hypertonic dye during catheterization studies are also at risk.

Initially therapy is symptomatic and supportive. Feedings are stopped, intravenous fluid therapy is begun, nasogastric suction started, vascular volume maintained, and the child is investigated for the possibility of bacterial infection. If peritonitis or perforation is observed, surgical intervention is indicated. The usual location for the lesion is at the terminal ileum, ileocecal valve, and proximal right colon; however, the disease may occur anywhere from stomach to anus and can include large portions of the bowel. Residual bowel function depends upon the length of intestine resected. Not uncommonly late strictures are recognized during the healing phase.

Patent Ductus Arteriosus (PDA). The ductus arteriosus fails to close functionally in the first 48 hours of life in 50% of infants weighing less than 1500 g. In many of these neonates the defect produces few clinical symptoms and eventually closes within the neonatal period. In the VLBW group and in some larger infants with significant respiratory disease, however, frank congestive heart failure with further deterioration in pulmonary function may occur. Tachycardia, full bounding peripheral pulses, and a hyperdynamic precordium are all noted while a pansystolic or continuous to-and-fro (machinery-type) murmur is auscultated. With frank congestive heart failure, hepatomegaly, pulmonary rales, fluid retention, and deteriorating arterial blood gases are observed. Fluid restriction and administration of diuretics are first-line therapy. When this form of medical management is insufficient or attempts to establish a caloric intake sufficient for growth lead to further congestive heart failure, pharmacological or surgical therapy is indicated. The ductal tissue is sensitive to prostaglandins, which tend to maintain ductal patency. Use of a prostaglandin synthetase inhibitor such as indomethacin has proved effective in inducing closure in many infants. In other neonates surgical ligation is required to correct the defect and allow normal growth to resume.

Bronchopulmonary Dysplasia (BPD). The premature infant appears to be at particular risk for developing BPD, and the incidence of this disease is closely tied to decreasing gestational age. Related to pulmonary oxygen toxicity and barotrauma, BPD is seen usually in the preterm infant requiring a protracted period of high inspired oxygen concentration (not PaO_2) and mechanical ventilation. During the improvement phase of the original pulmonary diseae an increased and persistent requirement for oxygen is demonstrated concomitant with a radiological pattern of diffusely hazy lung fields that progress to some degree of cystic change and, finally, fibrosis and emphysematous blebs. BPD occurs in 8 to 30% of mechanically ventilated LBW infants exposed to FiO_2s greater than 40%. With continued lung growth and maturation the disease may be self-limiting. Treatment consists of prevention of hypoxemia, careful management of fluid states, provision of sufficient caloric intake for growth, and the use of diuretics and systemic or aerosolized bronchodilators when indicated.

Asphyxia and Birth Trauma

ASPHYXIA NEONATORUM. Prenatal recognition of the possibility of fetal hypoxia, intrapartum monitoring, and resuscitative management of hypoxic infants at birth has already been discussed.

In affected neonates, postnatal transition is significantly impaired. The asphyxiated infant may not enter the hyperactive first stage of transition and may experience a prolonged second, or deep-sleep, stage. A series of abnormal behavioral patterns coexists in these neonates. Excessive sleepiness or lethargy and hyperirritability may be observed with rapid fluctuation from one phase to the other. The infant's ability to fix and attend to stimuli (visual or auditory) is impaired. Normal quiet-alert periods are unusual, and instead, a distant stare is observed during wakeful periods. The infant feeds poorly; there are absence of or slow nippling and disinterest in feeding; sucking and swallowing incoordination and vomiting are frequent. Dusky spells, hypoventilation, and apnea are alarming symptoms and may be indicative of seizures. Extreme jitteriness, hyperirritability, and a high-pitched cry are more prominent symptoms than lethargy in some infants.

On neurological examination, abnormal primitive reflexes and muscle tone are usually identified. Initially, hypotonia or increased extensor tone predominates. The rapidity of conversion to normal or slightly increased flexor tone can be a useful criterion in predicting outcome. Certainly prolonged periods of seizure activity early in the neonatal period are a poor prognostic sign. Because no single finding correlates well with long-term intellectual developmental or motor handicaps, however, extreme caution must be exercised in assigning exact prognostic significance to any of these findings. The major organ systems requiring close scrutiny after identification of a hypoxic insult are discussed below.

BRAIN. Although intraventricular hemorrhage is usually limited to the LBW infant, hypoxic-ischemic encephalopathy in the term infant may lead to intracerebral white matter bleeding, subarachnoid bleeding, and local or generalized neuronal death or "dropout." The first may lead to porencephaly, or a cystic communication with the ventricular system, while the last may result in major degrees of leukomalacia and cerebral atrophy. Focal deficits may occur, with auditory and visual areas being particularly vulnerable. Periods of prolonged anoxia lead to recalcitrant seizure disorders and, later, true hypsarrhythmia; motor deficits including spastic diplegia, quadriplegia, or hemiparesis; and severe retardation of mental and motor development. Early deficits that appear and disappear quickly postnatally may be more related to the degree of cerebral edema than to underlying permanent ischemic damage. In addition, varying degrees of cerebral edema in these infants may lead to major fluid and electrolyte disturbances, usually related to inappropriate secretion of antidiuretic hormone or renal dysfunction or both.

HEART. A period of diminished myocardial contractility may follow a hypoxic event. If prolonged, necrosis of the papillary muscles of the tricuspid valve with tricuspid insufficiency and heart failure may result. Cardiac output and oxygen delivery to other organs is then compromised, complicating the infant's recovery phase. Posterior-wall myocardial infarction, nodal arrhythmias, and heart block have all been described in the postnatal period following severe hypoxic insults.

KIDNEYS. Varying degrees of renal failure are frequent and often the cause of death of the most severely affected infants. Frank hypotension and shock at birth often lead to anuria from birth and pathologically represent acute cortical necrosis. Milder or more rapidly reversible impairments of renal oxygen delivery appear as acute tubular necrosis. An initial period of oliguria may be accompanied by fluid retention, hyponatremia, hyperkalemia, increase in blood urea nitrogen and creatinine, and subsequently hypertension. The urine demonstrates poor concentrating ability and impaired reabsorption of sugar, amino acids, bicarbonate, calcium, phosphorus, sodium, and potassium. These abnormalities may persist in varying degrees for a number of postnatal months.

LUNGS. As in adults, significant hypoxia may lead to "shock lung," with temporary impairment of surfactant production, a leaky capillary bed, interstitial edema, impaired oxygen diffusion, and pulmonary hemorrhage.

GASTROINTESTINAL TRACT. A common sequela of asphyxia in the LBW infant is necrotizing enterocolitis (NEC), which was discussed previously. Though NEC is uncommon in the term infant, malabsorption, diarrhea, and hypomotility with distention may complicate enteral feedings in this hypoxic group.

Liver. Asphyxial liver disease may, in its mildest forms, by recognized only by impaired bilirubin uptake, conjugation, or excretion by the damaged hepatocyte. More extensive liver cell necrosis may induce bleeding diatheses due to clotting factor deficiencies. Hyperammonemia may result from impaired hepatic detoxification of ingested or infused protein.

ADRENALS. Adrenal hemorrhage, though an infrequent event, may be seen in this oxygen-deprived group of neonates and may precipitate acute adrenal insufficiency.

HEMATOPOIETIC SYSTEM. Anemia, or polycythemia, consumptive coagulopathy, and thrombocytopenia may be recognized in these infants.

TREATMENT. The mainstay of treatment is prevention. If circulating blood volume and myocardial function are normal, fluid restriction and careful monitoring of electrolytes, body weight, urine output, and central nervous system function are essential to minimize the effects of rapidly developing cerebral edema. Hypoxia, hypercarbia, and apnea must be prevented, and this often requires a temporary period of mechanical ventilation. Anticonvulsants are indicated for extreme central nervous system irritability or frank seizures. In the face of myocardial dysfunction, digitalis or inotropic agents may be employed. Renal function may be impaired, and replacement fluid and electrolytes must be carefully selected and frequently adjusted. Feedings should be withheld until normal intestinal tract function has been demonstrated. Accentuation of physiological hyperbilirubinemia may necessitate earlier therapeutic intervention. The neonate should be observed for any signs of abnormal bleeding that may require replacement of clotting factors. The most severely affected infants demonstrate a baffling array of physiological and metabolic abnormalities; only strict attention to small details will ensure a successful outcome.

Birth Trauma

HEMORRHAGE. Subdural hemorrhage in the full-term infant is almost exclusively due to trauma. In the primiparous mother, cephalopelvic disproportion, fetal macrocephaly, prolonged or precipitous delivery, breech presentation, and difficult forceps or vacuum extractions all predispose to this lesion. Bleeding may occur from rupture of the tentorium, the falx, and the superficial bridging cerebral veins. The first two lesions can be catastrophic and rapidly fatal. The last may be asymptomatic, may occur initially with seizures on the second or third day of life, or may result in chronic subdural effusion recognized only after the neonatal period.

In primary subarachnoid hemorrhage a wide clinical spectrum may also exist. The majority of infants but certainly not all of these are preterm. Minor degrees of hemorrhage are usually clinically silent. Some infants, clinically well on examination, may have sudden seizures on the second day of life or recurrent apnea if preterm. The massive, rapidly fatal form of subarachnoid hemorrhage is rare. More unusual forms of visceral hemorrhage such as adrenal, pulmonary, and hepatic appear to be related to a combination of asphyxia and trauma.

TRAUMA TO THE HEAD. The major causes of trauma were noted previously. Molding, cephalohematoma, and caput succedaneum have been described. Linear fractures of the skull sometimes underlie cephalohematomas; these fractures are of little importance. Depressed skull fractures, which may follow forceps extraction, may correct themselves within 24 hours; significant depression of bone fragments, however, demands early neurosurgical intervention.

TRAUMA TO THE PERIPHERAL NERVES. *Erb-Duchenne Palsy.* Erb-Duchenne palsy (upper-arm type of brachial palsy) is the most common peripheral nerve injury. This lesion follows forceps extraction, manual extraction of breech presentation, or shoulder dystocia. It is due to stretching or avulsion of the anterior roots of the fifth and sixth cervical nerves. Diagnosis is obvious at birth. The affected arm is held close to the chest, is not flexed at the elbow, and is internally rotated with the forearm pronated. Abduction and external rotation at the shoulder are impossible; the elbow cannot be flexed or the forearm supinated. The strength of the hand and wrist is impaired. Treatment consists of placing the paralyzed muscles in a position of rest. The arm should be secured in a position of abduction, external rotation, and supination.

Klumpke's Palsy. Klumpke's palsy (lower-arm type of brachiopalsy) is much more serious, and many of the infants do not recover full use of the paralyzed part. In this form of palsy the damage has been to the anterior roots of the eighth cervical and first thoracic nerves. Paralysis is limited to the wrist and hand. Grasp is abolished, the hand falls limp at a position of flexion, and no wrist movements can be performed. Treatment consists of supporting the hand and wrist by binding them firmly and placing a flat splint under the palm and forearm.

Facial Palsy. Paralyses of one side of the face are not uncommon after spontaneous or forceps deliveries. Most commonly this lesion is caused by pressure of the sacral promontory on the posterior portion of the cheek (peripheral VIIIth nerve) as the head moves through the birth canal. The affected side of the face appears smooth, and the corner of the mouth on that side droops. The nasolabial fold is obliterated. The eye cannot be closed firmly, and the forehead on that side does not wrinkle. Crying brings out these signs more sharply.

Phrenic Nerve Palsy. Stretching of the third, fourth, and fifth cervical roots of the cord from lateral hyperextension of the neck results in diaphragmatic paralysis, usually in conjunction with other brachial plexus injuries. The lesion almost always is unilateral, and on chest radiograph a high-riding diaphragm is seen. Fluoroscopy reveals paralysis and paradoxical movement during inspiration. Clinical symptoms include tachypnea, retractions, and cyanosis, necessitating at times mechanical ventilation in the most severe cases. Spontaneous recovery is usual over weeks to months, though surgical intervention with plication or electrical pacing of the affected diaphragm is occasionally required.

Vocal Cord Paralysis. Though uncommon in the neonate, injury to the recurrent laryngeal branch of the vagus nerve due to excessive neck traction from forceps or during breech delivery is occasionally seen. Hoarseness and stridor are the prominent symptoms. Bilateral paralysis is usually of central origin and related to cerebral hypoxia, or hydrecephalus hemorrhage.

TRAUMA TO THE VISCERA. *Rupture of the Liver.* Hepatic rupture is not as rare as it was once thought to be. The cause is possibly trauma superimposed on asphyxia (for example, macrosomia, prolonged labor, or difficult delivery), although it may occur in small premature infants as well. The infants usually seem well at birth and for the next 1 or 2 days. Then abdominal distention and pallor develop, and shock rapidly supervenes. If the hemorrhage is only subcapsular, a mass may be palpable contiguous to the liver. If the capsule is also ruptured, free fluid may be demonstrated within the peritoneal cavity by physical and x-ray examinations. If there is doubt, a needle tap of the abdomen or careful ultrasound examination may be done to verify the diagnosis.

Rupture of the Spleen. In conditions of splenomegaly there is an increased incidence of rupture from rough handling at the time of delivery. In neonates with erythroblastosis fetalis, other forms of congenital hemolytic anemia, or congenital viral disease this hazard exists. The clinical findings are identical to those of hepatic rupture.

Rupture of a Hollow Viscus. Gastric perforation is especially prominent along the greater curvature and may occur spontaneously when there is weakness of the muscle wall, or it may be present in conditions of gastric overdistention. The latter may occur after prolonged bag-and-mask ventilation without adequate decompression of the stomach. Additionally, perforation of the stomach may occur after passage of a stiff gavage catheter used to lavage the stomach or feed the infant.

Rupture of a hollow viscus may or may not be preceded by hematemesis and melena. If it follows intestinal obstruction there is usually a precedent period of vomiting. The actual rupture is marked by sudden vomiting, abdominal distention, and the rapid appearance of shock. X-ray examination shows free air within the abdomen, usually between the diaphragm and the dome of the liver.

Such a complication requires immediate laparotomy and repair of the torn tissue.

TRAUMA TO THE BONES. Fracture of the clavicle is the most common bone injury at birth. It usually follows vigorous manipulation, shoulder dystocia, or in a fetus with breech presentations delivered by manual extraction. It may be completely asymptomatic and recognized only after 1 to 2 weeks by the formation of callus, or it may cause a constant cry and refusal to move the involved arm. It can be appreciated by point tenderness, hypomobility, and a grating or crepitant sound when the shoulder is moved. This condition requires virtually no treatment, but if pain is present the shoulder should be immobilized.

Congenital Malformations

Chromosomal Aberrations

It would appear that approximately one of four conceptions will end in abortion, the majority during the first trimester. In this group of abortuses approximately two-thirds are karyotypically abnormal. About half represent various trisomies, with triploidies and XO carrier types equally compris-

ing the remainder. Errors of blastogenesis, cleavage, and nondisjunction also account for early pregnancy losses. These usually occur before pregnancy is recognized by the mother.

In those karyotypically abnormal infants who complete gestation, the diversity of described chromosomal aberrations has broadened expansively because of technical advances in cell-culturing and chromosomal-banding techniques. A complete discussion of gross chromosomal aberrations is included in Chapter 5.

Dysmorphic Conditions

Any number of dysmorphic conditions may be recognized at or shortly after birth. Some of these are described in Chapter 5.

Infections of the Fetus

Early Onset Bacterial Infections

Septic mortality and morbidity are increased in the neonate because of impaired chemotaxis, phagocytosis, opsonization, and antibody production. Early clinical symptomatology is subtle, difficult to recognize, and easily confused with that of other disease states.

The majority of neonatal infections occur by vertical transmission, either prenatal or intrapartum, from the mother to the infant. Colonization may occur through the amniotic fluid in the presence of ruptured membranes or during passage through the birth canal. The quantity of colonizing organisms as well as the type and pathogenicity of the bacterial species are crucial in determining the neonate's risk of infection. Bacterial infections may reach the fetus by invasion of the fetal membranes, umbilical cord, and blood stream or by aspiration of infected amniotic fluid during fetal breathing or gasping during in utero hypoxia. The incidence of early bacterial sepsis ranges from 0.5 to 2%. Prenatal risk factors include prolonged rupture of membranes (>12 hr), prematurity, chorioamnionitis, prolonged difficult labor, and fetal instrumentation.

The Infant at Risk

Certain historical and clinical symptoms help to identify the infant in whom infection is suspected or who is actively sick in the early phase of disease. These symptoms include:

1. Significant depression at birth (low Apgar score) with obligatory resuscitation

2. Malodorous skin
3. Failure to pass normally through the early postnatal transition phase
4. Significant lethargy, jitteriness, or hyperirritability
5. Temperature instability
6. Feeding disinterest, sluggishness, or vomiting
7. Tachypnea, cyanosis, periodic breathing, or apnea
8. Abdominal distention or ileus
9. Skin mottling, cool extremities, or poor capillary filling
10. Hypotonia or absence of primitive reflexes

As the infective process progresses, more definitive signs of bacterial sepsis intervene, including hypothermia, hypotension, seizures, increasing hypoxemia, metabolic acidemia, and, finally, shock.

In the early stages, laboratory tests may provide some confirmation of bacteremia. Significant colonization is recognized by the presence of large numbers of polymorphonuclear cells and bacteria in Gram's stains of the gastric aspirate, external ear, the trachea, or in frozen sections of the fetal membranes or umbilical cord. Neutropenia (<2000) and thrombocytopenia are extremely suggestive of early bacteremia. The microsedimentation rate, the presence of C-reactive protein, and counter immunoelectrophoresis, which identify bacterial antigens, may also prove helpful in early identification. If after assessment the risk of infection appears high, cultures of the blood, urine, and cerebrospinal fluid must be obtained in addition to a diagnostic chest radiograph.

In most areas of the country the incidence of group B streptococcal infection appears to have surpassed that due to gram-negative enteric bacilli (*Escherichia coli, Klebsiella, Proteus,* and *Enterobactero*). *Staphylococcus aureus* and *Listeria monocytogenes* remain common pathogens in some geographical areas. Although anaerobic organisms have been recovered in up to 25% of neonatal blood cultures, bacteremia is usually transient and septic complications rare.

In most situations, initial antibiotic management usually combines a penicillin (aqueous penicillin G, ampicillin sodium) with an aminoglycoside such as gentamicin. Most recently interest in the use of white cell transfusion and intravenous immunoglobulin therapy as adjuncts to antibiotic therapy is increasing in the neonate with overwhelming infection. When no evidence of septic localization has occurred and initial cultures show no growth, therapy is often discontinued after 72 hours of parenteral administration. Positive "central" cultures (blood, urine) or observation of the presence of pneumonia on the chest roentgenogram require 10 to 14 days of parenteral therapy. Infection of the

central nervous system (meningitis, ventriculitis) demands prolonged therapy of at least 21 days.

The mortality in early-onset infections may reach 30 to 50%, with morbidity common, especially in neonates with meningitis.

Specific Bacterial Infections

INTRAUTERINE PNEUMONIA. In most cases this condition leads to the birth of an asphyxiated infant, who, after resuscitation, demonstrates tachypnea, retractions, and cyanosis. At times the syndrome develops more slowly over the first 8 hours. Pulmonary rales are usually present and do not disappear as transition progresses. The chest roentgenogram shows characteristic alterations; linear, at times fluffy, areas of opacification are concentrated around the hili, often obscuring the sharp cardiac silhouette. These radiodense regions spread fanwise in diminishing concentration toward the lung periphery. At times, significant patchy infiltrates are seen diffusely through both lung fields.

MENINGITIS. Bacterial meningitis in the neonate usually follows bacteremia, most commonly due to group B streptococci or gram-negative bacilli. Clinical presentation is often indistinguishable from sepsis alone. Seizures and a full fontanel may point to the presence of meningitis. When the suspicion of infection arises, a lumbar puncture must be promptly performed.

Neonatal meningitis is still fatal in a large proportion of cases. The best results are obtained when appropriate antibiotic treatment is begun very early in the course of the disease.

ACUTE PYELONEPHRITIS. This is another relatively common complication of sepsis neonatorum. The diagnosis is suspected on the basis of the same criteria applied to other neonatal infections and is verified by the presence of pyuria or bacteruria (more than 100,000 colonies) or both.

Appropriate antibiotic treatment usually effects cure. In the neonatal form of pyelonephritis, males are affected as often as females, and pyelograms demonstrate congenital obstructive malformations of the genitourinary tract in a minority of patients.

GROUP B STREPTOCOCCAL DISEASE. The incidence of septicemia due to group B streptococcus (GBS) has been rising in recent years. In most areas of the country the reported rate of sepsis varies from 1 to 3/1000 live births. The rate of sepsis due to GBS is 6 to 10 times higher in LBW infants; mortality is proportionally higher as well.

Colonization rates vary widely by area of the country, the culture media employed, the number and location of culture sites, and the stage of gestation. At the time of parturition, apparent recovery rates of 5 to 25% have been reported. At least one-half of infants born by vaginal delivery to mothers in whom colonization has occurred will themselves demonstrate colonization. In a further group of neonates, acquisition occurs during the first postnatal days from colonization in nursery personnel. The colonization-sepsis rate is approximately 200 : 1; it is higher, however, in LBW infants. It appears that the organism's serotype, the quantity of colonization, and the presence of protective maternal antibodies may all determine the risk of sepsis and/or death.

Attempts to identify and treat maternal carriers prior to delivery has been hampered by two major problems: (1) the carrier state is difficult to eradicate from mucous membranes, and (2) infection may recur through venereal transmission. Maternal therapy during labor to diminish the bacterial load to the neonate and intramuscular treatment with aqueous penicillin of the neonate in the delivery room are both practiced in some areas. At the present time, prevention of mortality depends upon early identification of the bacteremic infant. Soon after birth septic shock may be present and death may occur; clinical and radiological similarity to HMD makes differentiation at times impossible. The presence of leukopenia, neutropenia with or without immature forms (bands), or thrombocytopenia appears to be the most selective discriminator of infection. The rapidity of onset, the high mortality, and the lack of a single predictive test for neonatal infection have led many pediatricians to routinely treat sick infants (especially those with respiratory symptoms) for this potential complication. Although GBS is the most common organism recovered in this early-onset rapidly fatal form of bacterial sepsis, this same pattern may be seen in infections due to *Listeria monocytogenes, Hemophilus influenzae, Streptococcus pneumoniae,* and *Neisseria meningitidis.*

POSTNATALLY ACQUIRED BACTERIAL INFECTIONS. The majority of staphylococcal infections are contracted postnatally either from ward personnel who have respiratory or skin lesions due to this organism or from family contamination. Pathogenic staphylococci are almost always hemolytic and coagulase positive and fall into one of a comparatively small number of antibody and phage types.

Common types of staphylococcal infection include impetigo or staphylococcal pustulosis and its variants—conjunctivitis, umbilical infection, mastitis, pneumonitis, and osteomyelitis. This disease is usually caused by a staphylococcus acquired during the neonatal period. It usually begins 2 to 10 days after birth with the appearance of scattered vesicles in the diaper area. These may spread to any part of the body. At first they are loosely filled with clear fluid; later they become turbid, the skin excoriates, and round, red, moist areas are left; they do not crust.

Treatment begins with strict isolation from other infants. Cleansing of the skin with soap or a diluted solution of hexachlorophene is usually indicated. Until bacteremia is excluded, parenteral therapy with an antistaphylococcal antibiotic such as methicillin or nafcillin is indicated.

The neonatal variant of scalded skin syndrome (Ritter's disease) due to erythrogenic toxin producing phage types may be seen. In this form of the disease vesiculation and bulla formation may proceed to rapid exfoliation of the dermis; virtually all of the skin may be lost. Loss of fluids and serum proteins and secondary bacterial invasion complicate this variant of staphylococcal disease.

CONJUNCTIVITIS. Conjunctivitis in the newborn may be caused by many bacteria and some viruses (herpes). Staphylococci, *Hemophilus, Streptococcus pneumonia, Enterococci,* and *Pseudomonas* are the usual etiological agents. There is nothing to distinguish this form from the others. Local treatment with a broad spectrum antibiotic ointment usually suffices.

The incidence of gonococcal ophthalmia has been rising in the nation as a whole. A higher incidence of asymptomatic gonococcal carriers and inadequate eye prophylaxis may be the underlying reasons for this rise. Systemic and local antibiotic therapy are indicated when this disease is identified. *Chlamydia* conjuctivitis is discussed later in this chapter.

UMBILICAL INFECTIONS. Umbilical infections become manifest as a discharge, at first serosanguineous and later purulent, from the base of the cord or from the navel, with or without redness of the surrounding skin. Systemic antibiotic therapy should be started and continued until all signs of local cellulitis diminish.

OSTEOMYELITIS. Both the staphylococcus and group B streptococcus are principally responsible for osteomyelitis in the neonatal period. Portal of entry may be the skin, umbilicus, or respiratory tract. Some cases are caused by injury to the bone in the course of attempted femoral vein or artery puncture. Infection begins at the end of long bones and often ruptures into the neighboring joint to cause purulent arthritis.

Unlike osteomyelitis in the young child, the neonatal disease usually involves multiple small bones. When the disease is progressive there may be swelling about the joint or brawny edema encompassing the entire extremity; the limb may be motionless, with pain occurring on passive movement.

Suggestive findings may not be present on a plain radiograph of the limb until 10 to 14 days after infection has begun. In this situation a radionuclide bone scan may be helpful in early identification of osteomyelitis.

Systemic antibiotic therapy must be begun immediately and continued for a minimum of 2 to 3 weeks. In addition, if there are signs of joint involvement, aspiration and decompression of the joint space are indicated to prevent later deformity.

DIARRHEA OF BACTERIAL ORIGIN. Bacterial diarrhea is not especially common in the newborn period; however, infection with *Shigella, Salmonella, Campylobacter* and enterotoxigenic *Escherichia coli* may occur. Cases may be sporadic, but frightening epidemics have been reported in nurseries. An adult carrier is usually the source of infection.

Shigella infections in this age group are likely to be comparatively mild. *Salmonella* infections, however, are somewhat more serious. They have a greater tendency to cause epidemics and are harder to eradicate. They are more prone to invade the bloodstream, and they have a strong affinity for the meninges. Treatment must be with the antibiotic that has proved to be effectively bactericidal against the specific organism in vitro.

Fluid and electrolyte therapy are of paramount importance in the newborn infant, because dehydration and acidemia quickly follow vomiting and diarrhea in this age group.

Spirochetal Infections of the Fetus

SYPHILIS. The manifestations of syphilis may be present at birth or may appear within the first 2 weeks. Snuffles or nasal obstruction occurs, plus a discharge that is at first serous, later serosanguineous. Rashes made up of round or oval copper-colored macules are confined to, or most profuse, about the mouth, nose, genitalia, or buttocks. Lesions about the mouth tend to become radiating linear ulcerations called rhagades. Jaundice may appear, and the liver and spleen may enlarge. General lymph node enlargement is common. Central nervous system invasion (meningoencephalitis) takes place in one-third of cases and may or may not give rise to the expected signs. Bones become involved in a widespread process in which epiphyseal destruction, periosteal thickening, and erosions of the shaft may be seen on x-ray films. A not uncommon presentation in the first month of life is pseudoparalysis of the limb due to a painful periosteal reaction.

This stage may subside with or without treatment; it is sometimes bypassed, only to be followed after a few years by a group of signs characteristic of late congenital syphilis. Routine maternal screening at delivery makes such unrecognized fetal infection rare today.

Protozoal Infection of the Fetus

TOXOPLASMA GONDII. This is the only protozoan responsible for significant morbidity and mortality in the newborn infant by virtue of hematogenous transplacental passage from mother to fetus. In the mother the infection is usually asymptomatic.

The newborn has signs and symptoms very similar to those of cytomegalic inclusion disease. Jaundice, hepatosplenomegaly, and thrombocytopenia are common to both. Pneumonitis is less frequent and meningoencephalitis and chorioretinitis are considerably more frequent in toxoplasmosis than in cytomegalic inclusion disease. Myocarditis is not rare in toxoplasmosis.

Many fetal infections have run their course by the time of birth, leaving the infants with late effects, the most striking of which are microcephaly, with disseminated areas of intracranial calcification visible throughout the brain on x-ray examination, and blindness resulting from severe chorioretinitis.

Diagnosis is verified by a positive Sabin dye test, finding antibodies to *Toxoplasma* in the mother and infant; a positive complement fixation test; or by an IgM-specific immunofluorescent antibody test. The organism can be visualized on properly stained biopsy or autopsy specimens. It cannot, however, be grown in vitro.

Fungal Infection of the Fetus

POSTNATAL OR PERINATAL CANDIDIASIS OR MONILIASIS. *Candida* (formerly *Monilia albicans*) is by far the most common fungal pathogen of the newborn infant. Its usual manifestation is thrush, which becomes manifest a few days or weeks after birth. Thrush consists of round or oval elevated plaques on the buccal, gingival, and lingual mucous membranes that may become confluent.

The disease may rarely spread down into the esophagus. If it does, swallowing becomes difficult, and aspiration follows, resulting in pneumonia. More often, however, the swallowed fungus leads to monilial enteritis, causing diarrhea. Monilial dermatitis is characterized first by maceration of the skin about the anus, the raw red areas becoming covered with a pseudomembrane. Satellite maculopapules appear about the periphery and later excoriate to leave red erythematous patches surrounded by a white collar. In some infants, lesions may spread to involve the entire surface of the body; rarely, monilial septicemia supervenes, usually in the immunosuppressed infant or the VLBW infant with a central venous catheter receiving total parenteral hyperalimentation.

A few cases have been reported in which the infant was covered with lesions of cutaneous moniliasis at birth. This must represent ascending amniotic infection with the vaginal organism.

Diagnosis is verified by identifying the fungus in appropriate specimens. Finding the mycelial form in the stools or urine is more significant than finding the yeast form.

Treatment may be local, with 2% nystatin (Mycostatin) ointment, or oral, using Mycostatin oral suspension. Systemic therapy involves the use of either amphotericin B or 5-flucytosine.

Chlamydial Infection

Chlamydia trachomatis is the most common sexually transmitted disease manifest in the neonate, the spectrum of disease has expanded in recent years. Chlamydial conjunctivitis appears from the fourth to tenth day of life and is usually acquired during passage of the infant through an infected cervix. Mild conjunctivitis and chemosis may be the only symptoms, and are usually self-limiting over a period of 6 to 8 weeks. Only rarely does progression to scarring of the cornea occur. The diagnosis is made by detecting typical inclusion bodies or positive monoclonal antibody slide test on conjunctival scrapings. The conjunctivitis usually responds to local application of erythromycin or tetracyline.

Chlamydia has now been demonstrated by direct culturing techniques and serum immunofluorescence titers to be responsible for late neonatal pneumonia, usually occurring during the fourth to eighth week of life. Systemic symptoms are minimal, but a constant harsh dry cough, chest hyperinflation, eosinophilia, and hypergammaglobulinemia are seen. Patchy pulmonary infiltrates are present in addition to hyperexpansion noted on chest x-ray film. As with chlamydial conjunctivitis, pneumonia is due to infection acquired during the intrapartum period.

Viral Infections of the Fetus

Virtually all of the agents that attack the fetus in the first trimester of gestation are viruses. The effect may be either lethal (embryonic death and spontaneous abortion) or teratogenic (damage of the developing organs or organ systems), leading to the birth of congenitally malformed infants. Rubella is a prime example of the latter group.

RUBELLA (GERMAN MEASLES). The mother who contracts rubella develops viremia. Virus then infects the placenta. Either the embryo is killed (spontaneous abortion) or the embryo survives with perhaps one or more patterns of congenital infection. Infection in the first 4 weeks may damage the fetus, leading to the birth of a malformed infant in as many as 40% of cases. The risks decrease with advancing gestation, to 20% in the second 4 weeks, and 10% in the third 4 weeks. Some damage may possibly result from infections transmitted even later than this.

The triad that is commonly associated with congenital rubella includes cataracts, congenital heart defects, and deafness. During the 1964–65 rubella epidemic in the United States, it was learned that many other defects may also result. Congenital glaucoma, microcephaly, thrombocytopenic purpura, neonatal hepatitis, immunodeficiency states, and disseminated osteitis are but a few of these.

Diagnosis is based on the finding of several of these characteristic defects in addition to a history of maternal febrile illness with a rash early in pregnancy. A positive history may not always be obtainable. Diagnosis can now be verified by growth of rubella virus from the nasopharyngeal washings, urine, or tissue samples or by demonstration in the infant's serum of neutralizing rubella antibody, the titer of which remains high for many months, indicating that it has been actively, not passively, acquired.

CYTOMEGALIC INCLUSION DISEASE. Cytomegalovirus is one of the more common viruses and causes dramatic forms of disease in the newborn infant; it seldom produces clinical effects in the mother.

In the acute disseminated form, the infant is sick at birth or shortly thereafter. Among the important manifestations are microcephaly, anemia, jaundice, petechiae, and hepatosplenomegaly. The disease is often rapidly progressive, resulting in death within a few days. In addition to hepatosplenomegaly, there may be signs of pneumonitis and of meningoencephalitis. X-ray films may show bronchopneumonic alterations and changes in the skull, including periventricular calcification. Chorioretinitis may be seen early or may develop after a few months.

There are less typical varieties. The liver may be large at birth; over the course of months, deepening jaundice and progressive enlargement of the liver and spleen may be seen. Meningoencephalitis and chorioretinitis may or may not follow. These less fulminant types may subside spontaneously but may lead to late hearing defects or mild degrees of developmental delay.

The majority of infections in neonates, however, are asymptomatic. In the premature nursery, breast milk, blood transfusions, and long-term debilitated infants excreting virus present additional infective risks. Even in the asymptomatic child, later defects have been described, in particular, auditory problems and school behavioral difficulties.

Diagnosis can be verified by growing the virus from

urine, nasopharynx, or stool. In addition, an IgM-specific immunofluorescence test can be utilized. Demonstration of inclusion cells in the urine can be extremely misleading.

OTHER VIRAL INFECTIONS AFFECTING THE FETUS BY HEMATOGENOUS SPREAD. When the mother develops measles, German measles, varicella, mumps, poliomyelitis, echovirus, herpes, or coxsackie viral disease, they may cause spontaneous abortion or may appear in the newborn infant within the first 10 days of life. The time of onset of disease in the infant depends upon the timing of infection in the mother; that is, the first signs of the disease in the infant appear after approximately the usual incubation period for that particular infection. Many neonatal virus diseases are mild, but the great portion are severe in susceptible neonates. There is little that can be done in the way of treatment or prevention. In some, pooled immune globulin may modify the clinical course in the neonate.

Perinatal Viral Infection: Herpes Simplex

Herpes simplex is the only important example in this group. If the mother has herpes progenitalis, produced by *Herpesvirus hominus* type II, the fetus may acquire infection by contact during delivery. Local (mucous membrane, eye, skin), isolated central nervous system, disseminated herpes simplex may follow. Herpes simplex begins to be manifest from the second to the tenth day of life. In half of the infected group, onset may be marked by scattered vesicular or pustular lesions. Conjunctivitis, fever, hypothermia, bleeding (DIC), pneumonia, and shock may all be noted, in addition to poor feeding and lethargy. The liver becomes enlarged, and jaundice develops. Meningeal signs may be observed before death, which may occur very rapidly.

Cultures from vesicles, pustules, mouth and conjunctiva reveal the virus. Virus can also be cultured in some cases from urine and cerebrospinal fluid. Lesions are frequently disseminated throughout the liver, brain, lungs, and elsewhere. At the present time, treatment regimens with antiviral drugs including Vidarabine and Acyclovir appear to reduce both mortality and morbidity if started early in the disease.

When herpes lesions are recognized or cultured from the maternal labia or cervix prior to delivery, cesarean section is protective to the fetus if the membranes have been ruptured for less than 4 hours. Fetuses at highest risk are those whose mothers experience a primary herpetic infection at the time of birth. The risk to the fetus whose mother experiences a recurrent flare-up at delivery is considerably lower than what had previously been assumed.

Neonatal Jaundice

Elevated levels of bilirubin remain a common, annoying, and usually benign problem in the neonate. Abnormal timing of elevations, peak level, or type (conjugated) of bilirubin, however, can be an important early warning sign of life-threatening disease.

Jaundice is clinically recognized at levels of 5 to 6 mg/100 ml, and further elevation of levels usually leads to progressive skin staining in a head-to-toe fashion. The neonate is at particular disadvantage in handling this pigment for a number of reasons: Total red blood cell mass is great at birth, and the life span of the red blood cell is shortened to 70 to 90 days. Because each gram of hemoglobin accounts for 34 mg of bilirubin, a large potential load of pigment may be presented to the immature organism.

A further source of nonhemoglobin-heme protein located in the cytochromes adds to this bilirubin influx. At birth, reabsorption of bilirubin in meconium, relative bowel ileus, and diminished bacterial gut flora all increase the enterohepatic bilirubin load. To offset this gastrointestinal recirculation, early feedings, activated charcoal, and agar gel have all be utilized.

After dissociation from albumin, to which it is tightly bound, bilirubin must diffuse through the liver cell membrane and bind to an intracellular transport protein (Y protein) known as ligand. Depressed levels of Y protein in the neonate further accentuate problems in bilirubin handling. Glucuronyl transferase catalyzes the transfer of glucuronic acid from uridine diphosphoglucuronic acid (UDPGA) to unconjugated bilirubin to form a more polar water soluble complex. This enzyme is deficient in the newly born and premature infant, adding to unconjugated hyperbilirubinemia. Lastly, in the neonate, ability to excrete the conjugated compound from the liver cell into the bile duct is limited.

Together these defects comprise what has been termed physiological jaundice of the newborn. Bilirubin levels up to 6 mg/100 ml on the third day of life are considered physiological in the term infant. In the premature infant these defects in bilirubin handling are exaggerated, and higher peak values (10–12 mg/100 ml) with a later peak are more typical.

Particularly worrisome alterations in bilirubin level necessitating early and complete evaluation include the following: (1) jaundice in an infant less than 24 hours of age; (2) increases greater than 5 mg/day; (3) total bilirubin greater than 12 mg/100 ml in the full-term infant and 14 mg/100 ml in the larger, healthy preterm infant; (4) a direct-reacting fraction greater than 1.5 mg/100 ml;

152

(5) jaundice lasting more than 10 days in the term infant or more than 14 days in the preterm infant.

In the evaluation of neonatal jaundice, certain general categories of disease need to be considered and thoroughly investigated. Some of these are discussed below.

Hemolytic Diseases

BLOOD GROUP INCOMPATIBILITIES. *Rh Incompatibility; Erythroblastosis Fetalis.* Any of a number of Rh factors may be responsible for blood group incompatibility between fetus and mother, but D is the one responsible for the overwhelming majority of cases.

The disturbance occurs with the conception of an Rh-positive fetus in an Rh-negative mother. If the father is homozygous D, all the offspring will be Rh positive; if he is heterozygous, one-half will be. The D antigen is attached to the fetal red cells, some of which cross the placenta and enter the mother's circulation. In some mothers, as little as 0.5 ml of fetal blood cells may provoke the maternal reticuloendothelial system to form anti-D antibodies (7 S and 19 S). The "incomplete" 7 S antibody can recross the placenta into the fetal circulation and sensitize the D-positive red blood cells of the fetus, thereby inducing hemolysis.

First pregnancies are immune to the development of erythroblastosis, because fetal red cells rarely cross the placenta in sufficient amounts to provoke an antibody response during gestation unless the mother has been previously sensitized. To limit this possibility Rh-negative mothers are now immunized with anti-Rh globulin (RhoGAM) at 24 to 26 weeks gestation. Also, if anti-Rh globulin had not been given after previous abortions, miscarriages, or incompatible blood transfusions, sensitization may occur during the initial pregnancy. With labor and delivery, large quantities of fetal erythrocytes may be transfused into the maternal circulation. These erythrocytes may provoke antibody formation during the succeeding weeks in the mother and are responsible for her initial Rh sensitization. Succeeding pregnancies may not result in hemolytic disease (1) if too little fetal blood crosses the placenta or (2) if ABO incompatibility was also present during the first pregnancy between mother and fetus, because the circulating anti-A or anti-B antibodies of the mother may have destroyed the transfused fetal red cells before they stimulated production of anti-D antibody. For these reasons, many Rh-incompatible fetuses do not develop the disease. Allelic forms of D have varying capacity to induce antibody response, and the host has variable capacity to respond to the antigenic stimulus. Thus, as a result of these variables, if the disease develops, it may be mild, severe, or lethal.

In the mild form, the baby is normal at birth. Visible jaundice appears within 24 hours, Coombs' test is positive, indicating Rh sensitization, and serum bilirubin concentrations do not exceed 20 mg/100 ml. Jaundice subsides within a week. Hemoglobin concentration remains within normal values. No treatment is indicated except that the infant often requires a small blood transfusion at 3 to 4 weeks of age. Phototherapy may be utilized early, when the rate of increase of bilirubin is still unknown, to prevent an increase toward a level requiring exchange transfusion.

In the severe form the infant becomes jaundiced within a few hours after birth and intensely so by the end of the first day. The liver and spleen are enlarged. Anemia may be marked. The bilirubin level in the umbilical cord blood exceeds 5 mg/100 ml and rises rapidly, at a rate of more than 1 mg/hour. If this form is untreated, serum bilirubin concentrations may reach 30 to 50 mg/100 ml. The hemoglobin in the umbilical cord blood is less than 14 g/100 ml and frequently falls to much lower levels. Reticulocytes are numerous, and many nucleated red blood cells may be present in the peripheral blood (hence the name erythroblastosis). In the more severe form, early exchange transfusion may be indicated to remove sensitized red cells and free antibody, thereby preventing further hemolysis and sudden rise in bilirubin levels. One exchange transfusion may not suffice if sufficient sensitization has occurred prior to delivery. After the first exchange is completed, however, the child may receive phototherapy in an attempt to limit the risk of further exchanges. Continued hemolysis, however, may require simple transfusion therapy at a later date if phototherapy is chosen.

In hydrops fetalis (massive edema of the newborn), the most severe form of hemolytic disease, intense blood destruction occurs in utero. The bilirubin level in the amniotic fluid is closely monitored by amniocentesis from about the twentieth week of gestation onward. If a significant rise is detected (a small rise in the amniotic fluid bilirubin level occurs normally as gestation proceeds), either intrauterine transfusion (into the fetal peritoneum or directly into the umbilical vein under ultrasound guidance) or preterm delivery must be contemplated. The risk of such a procedure must be weighed against the expected survival rate at the fetus's particular gestational age. If the condition is uncorrected, the infant is born with massive head-to-foot edema (including ascites and bilateral hydrothorax), profound anemia, respiratory distress, and high output heart failure. At delivery, intubation and ventilation are mandatory, and if hydrothorax exists it must be evacuated by thoracentesis. Massive abdominal ascites impeding lung expansion may also require drainage in the delivery room. The anemia and depressed oxygen-carrying capacity must be corrected immediately after birth by a partial exchange transfusion using compatible O-negative packed red blood cells through the umbilical vein. After these stabilizing procedures and return of the infant to a nursery setting, an initial exchange transfusion can be performed.

The development of and widespread use of anti-D antibodies (RhoGAM) in Rh-negative mothers during gestation in an Rh-negative mother or after delivery of an Rh-positive fetus or miscarriage has led to a marked diminution in the incidence of this disease. Failure to produce passive immunity after proper use of this therapy is uncommon.

ABO Incompatibility. If the mother and her baby are of different ABO blood groups or incompatibility to the Kell, Duffy, or Lewis system exists, hemolytic disease may occur in the baby. This occurrence is most likely when the mother is type O and her baby type B. This condition differs from Rh-induced disease in the following respects: (1) the disease rarely results in intrauterine death or anemia at birth; (2) the first born is as liable to be affected as later children; (3) the hemolytic processes are usually less severe; (4) the direct Coombs' test may be negative or only weakly positive; (5) many of the infant's red blood cells are spherocytic in shape.

If sensitization of the infant is confirmed after birth, exchange transfusion is rarely indicated. In most situations, phototherapy alone is sufficient treatment; however, hemolysis may continue after the child is discharged home, and close follow-up of the hemoglobin level is necessary over the first 6 weeks of life.

KERNICTERUS. This pathological entity refers to yellow staining of the nuclear areas of the brain, predominantly the basal ganglia, subthalamic nuclei, and inferior olives. Glial replacement and neuronal atrophy are dominant findings in pathologic brain sections.

Clinical findings, in addition to deep jaundice, begin with a sluggish, incomplete Moro response. When the infant is startled, the neck often become hyperextended. Sucking becomes poor and feeding slow. With further progression, genereralized hypotonia and regurgitation are noted. The eyes are fixed in a downward gaze because of paresis of the extraocular muscles (setting-sun sign). The cry is weak; later it is high pitched; oculogyric crises may be observed intermittently. Within a few days, rigidity replaces the hypotonia, producing opisthotonos. The arms are pronated and fixed at the elbows, the fists tightly clinched. In severely affected infants, hyperpyrexia and convulsions are commonly noted. In the terminal stages pulmonary and gastric hemorrhages occur.

Should the infant survive, extrapyramidal signs appear

between the ages of 6 and 12 weeks. Severely affected children have rigidity, while in the milder forms of the disease hypotonia, ataxia, and choreoathetosis are observed. High-tone nerve deafness, dental malocclusion, and deficient formation of tooth enamel are noted in a large percentage of those infants who survive. Some degree of mental deficiency will be almost universally found in infants who manifest detectable signs during the neonatal period.

Other Causes of Jaundice

See Chapter 15, The Blood and Appendix A, section 14, Jaundice.

Common Metabolic Abnormalities of the Neonate

HYPOGLYCEMIA. When infants of diabetic mothers are excluded, symptomatic hypoglycemia (see also Chap. 7) is estimated to occur in 2 to 3 per 1000 live full-term infants and in 5 to 10% of preterm infants.

At birth the neonate loses the intravenous placenta supply of glucose and gluconeogenic precursors, leading to depletion of liver glycogen in 6 to 8 postnatal hours. Lipase is then activated leading to the release of glycerol, fatty acids, and ketone bodies. High basal metabolic rates and oxygen consumption, high brain-weight-to-body-weight ratios (the brain being a major source of glucose utilization), and high insensible water loss (and caloric losses) increase the neonate's need for a readily available glucose supply. Glucose requirements (utilization rates) vary from 5 to 8 mg/kg/min in the immediate postnatal period. These needs must be met by glycogen breakdown, gluconeogenesis (including production of gluconeogenic precursors such as alanine), or oral or intravenous glucose replacement.

Classically, hypoglycemia is defined as a blood sugar content less than 30 mg/100 ml (serum or plasma value; whole blood is 15% lower) in the first 48 hours and less than 40 to 50 mg/100 ml thereafter. In the preterm neonate the respective values are 20 mg and 30 mg/100 ml.

A variety of symptoms have been ascribed to low glucose concentration—for example, lethargy, poor feeding, cyanosis, jitteriness, seizures, cyanosis and tachypnea. In the majority of infants, however, this complication is asymptomatic. Although there is significant disagreement concerning the future neurological status of hypoglycemic infants, there is no evidence to suggest that hypoglycemia is beneficial. The first step toward prevention is identification of the high-risk infant. Although the list is long, prematurity, growth retardation, infants born to diabetic mothers, Rh sensitization, sepsis, and perinatal asphyxia represent particularly high risks.

In the premature and growth retarded infant, deficient substrate stores are responsible. In erythroblastotic and diabetic infants, endogenous oversecretion of insulin is the primary defect. Infection, extensive muscular exercise (seizures, narcotic withdrawal), elevated basal metabolic rate (hyperthyroidism), and glycosuria are representative of excessive tissue utilization or excretion. States of reduced gluconeogenesis include growth retardation, adrenal insufficiency, hypopituitarism, fructose intolerance, and ketotic hypoglycemia. Disorders of glucose release include the glycogenoses and galactosemia. These and other inborn errors of metabolism associated with hypoglycemia will be discussed later.

Once the high-risk infant is identified, blood sugar (Dextrostix readings with corroborating blood sugar determinations for low values) should be monitored regularly *before* feedings. In infants who are neurologically normal, early feeding should be encouraged. If blood sugar levels remain borderline or low, an intravenous infusion should be started (100 ml/kg of D10W in a full-term infant of 3 kg is equivalent to 7 mg/kg/min of glucose) and continued until the infant's condition is stable, Dextrostix readings are elevated, and a reasonable feeding pattern is established. If hypoglycemia persists for longer than 72 hours, abnormalities of the islet cells (nesidioblastosis or adenoma) or carbohydrate intolerance must be seriously considered.

Hypocalcemia

Calcium accumulation by the fetus occurs against an uphill gradient even in the presence of deficient maternal calcium intake. Increased maternal calcium absorption and parathyroid levels lead to maternal skeletal utilization and enable the fetus to maintain calcium levels above maternal values. These high fetal levels of ionized calcium lower fetal parathyroid activity and favor fetal bone deposition. Elevated fetal calcitonin and estrogen levels also aid in bone mineralization.

Calcium levels may be depressed as a result of a number of factors. Calcium intake may be low, especially in the LBW infant. The neonates high fecal fat loss may bind calcium and increase intestinal losses. In breast-fed infants fat losses are decreased and calcium absorption is equivalently higher than in formula-fed infants. In sick LBW infants, infants of diabetic mothers, and infants with birth asphyxia, a low calcium intake compounds other hypocalcemic stresses. Inadequate intake of vitamin D, inadequate conversion in the liver (immaturity or liver disease) to 25-hydroxyvitamin D or in the kidney to 1,25-dihydroxyvitamin D may lead to early rickets, especially in the VLBW infant. The response of

the parathyroid gland to low calcium levels is sluggish at birth, especially in LBW and diabetic infants. Formulas with a high phosphate content or cow's milk can produce hyperphosphatemia and hypocalcemia in the first week of life.

Other causes of neonatal hypocalcemia include intestinal malabsorption, hypomagnesemia, metabolic alkalosis, increased blood citrate (transfusion with CPD blood), severe renal disease, absence of the parathyroid glands (usually associated with DiGeorge's syndrome), and high free-fatty-acid concentrations (intralipid). In the last situation, only ionized levels of calcium may be depressed.

In most cases, hypocalcemia is asymptomatic, though irritability, jitteriness, apnea, bradycardia, or frank seizures are occasionally noted. Serum ionized calcium levels or electrocardiographic prolongation of the corrected QT interval confirm the diagnosis. Oral or intravenous calcium therapy combined with a low-phosphate formula corrects this condition. When hypocalcemia leads to neonatal seizures a slow intravenous infusion of 10% calcium gluconate is required and is corrective.

Inborn Errors of Metabolism

Identification of infants with inborn metabolic errors is accomplished from a familial history of previously affected children or physical findings at birth suggestive of recognized syndromes or as part of the total evaluation of the status of a "sick" neonate. With many syndromes when there is a history of previously affected children, prenatal diagnosis is now possible. Amniocentesis is completed at the fourteenth to sixteenth week of gestation, and the level of metabolic byproducts is determined either directly in the amniotic fluid or after growth of fibroblasts in tissue culture. A number of these diseases are amenable to dietary manipulations and occasionally to vitamin or drug therapy. In suspicious cases, careful formula introduction with close observation of the infant's metabolic status allows earlier intervention at a stage when reversibility is possible.

A number of inherited syndromes possess a striking similarity of clinical symptoms—disinterest in feeding, vomiting, lethargy progressing to coma, seizures, metabolic acidemia, hepatitis, and jaundice. These symptoms are most easily confused with those of neonatal sepsis. Unlike bacterial infections, however, symptoms are usually related to the introduction of adequate feeding regimens and thereby delayed until the second or third day of life. In many areas of the United States, legislation requires neonatal screening for a number of conditions in addition to phenylketonuria; thus, neonates are being identified for therapeutic intervention long before complications such as mental retardation intervene. Some of the more common areas of altered metabolism are discussed in Chapter 5.

DISORDERS OF PROTEIN METABOLISM. See Chapter 5, Prenatal Development and Clinical Genetics.

Major Neonatal Diseases

In the section that follows diseases will be categorized by the major organ system or body area affected. Though certainly not intended to be all-encompassing the major diseases occurring in the early neonatal period will be briefly discussed.

Central Nervous System

NEONATAL SEIZURES. Unlike seizures in the older child, typical tonic-clonic movements are rare manifestations of neuronal irritability in the neonatal patient. Subtle seizure equivalents include eye blinking, lip smacking, sucking movements, apnea, and eye deviations (vertical or horizontal). Movement disorders include rhythmic slow twisting limb movements, which are repetitive and said to resemble swimming or bicycling activities. Unlike the high-frequency low-amplitude jittery movements common in many neonates, these movements are of high amplitude and low frequency, are not stimulus sensitive and cannot be interrupted by an examiner by actively moving the limb.

Common metabolic causes of seizures should be carefully searched for—hypoglycemia, hypocalcemia, hyponatremia, and hypomagnesemia. Infection including meningitis is an important consideration, as early recognition and treatment are essential for intact survival. Subarachnoid and subdural bleeding require consideration (intraventricular bleeding in the LBW) when a traumatic birth is recognized. Although extreme irritability and jitteriness are more common than frank seizures in the infant undergoing withdrawal from maternal narcotics or other psychotropic agents, frank seizures occur, and a careful history of maternal drug use is necessary.

By far the most common inducer (80% of cases or more) of neonatal seizure activity is prolonged perinatal hypoxia. When this is the cause the onset of seizure activity is rarely before 4 hours of age or prolonged after 12 hours. The signs of cerebral edema (lethargy progressing to coma, full fontanel, disconjugate gaze, and ocular palsies) usually precede or are concurrent with seizure activity.

Recognition and appropriate treatment of metabolic or infective causes is of paramount importance. Provision of adequate oxygenation and circulating blood volume represents important supportive therapy. If feeding difficulties, vomiting, or metabolic acidemia is also present urine and

blood sampling is appropriate to eliminate an inborn error of metabolism. Polycythemia and hyperviscosity should also be included in the differential diagnosis.

Once the seizure is identified, close monitoring of fluid intake, urine output, and serum electrolytes is essential. The cessation of seizures in situations other than of metabolic cause is best attempted with a loading dose of phenobarbital (20 mg/kg). A similar dose of diphenylhydantoin (Dilantin) can be given if seizures persist. Diazepam (Valium) may be effective in recalcitrant seizures, though respiratory and circulatory collapse and bilirubin displacement from protein are recognized side effects.

CONGENITAL HYDROCEPHALUS. See Chapter 13, The Nervous System.

Upper Airway and Oral Cavity

CHOANAL ATRESIA. Obstruction to air passage from the nares to the posterior nasopharynx may be either unilateral or bilateral and due to a bony plate or a thin membrane. Bilateral obstruction may be present at birth with cyanosis at rest, which clears with crying. Unilateral obstruction is commonly recognized as a constant nasal discharge present since birth. Feeding problems, including duskiness, choking, and gagging, are common. Diagnosis is suspected by the absence of air movement through the nares and failure to pass a catheter through to the nasopharynx. Radiographic confirmation is obtained after dye instillation into the nares. The membranous defects are easily ruptured, but bony defects require surgical removal and prolonged implantation of plastic stents until growth and adequate scarring have occurred.

CLEFT LIP AND PALATE. Cleft lip and palate represent developmental defects of the first branchial arch and in some cases may be recessively inherited. Defects may be unilateral, bilateral, or midline. Teratogenic exposure, dietary deficiencies, and chromosomal aberrations have all been implicated in pathogenesis. Other midline facial defects may be present. Cleft palate may be represented by simple bifid uvula, submucous cleft of the soft palate, or extensive cleavage of the entire hard palate, which may extend through the alveolar ridge and nares. Feeding difficulties, recurrent bouts of otitis media, and audiological and phonetic problems may ensue. Timing of surgical correction depends upon the extent of the defect and the child's ability to thrive at home.

LARYNGEAL OBSTRUCTION. Significant stridor and dyspnea from birth frequently indicate a developmental defect of the airway, including laryngeal and aryepiglottic cysts, webs, hemangioma, lymphangioma, papilloma, and vocal cord paralysis. The majority of these lesions are visible during direct laryngoscopy performed when respiratory difficulties are first noted.

TRACHEAL OBSTRUCTION. With the exception of inspissated mucus and meconium, intratracheal obstruction (hemangioma, lymphangioma, web, stenosis) is rare. A deficiency of supporting cartilage (tracheomalacia) is a more common cause of stridor in the neonate. Although the condition frequently is asymptomatic when the infant is at rest, hoarseness, dyspnea, stridor, and retractions are typical with agitation and crying. Extratracheal causes include bronchogenic and enteric cysts and duplications, mediastinal masses, and aberrant major blood vessels.

Respiratory System

ASPIRATION SYNDROMES. Until very recently meconium aspiration had remained one of the more common admission diagnoses in neonatal intensive care units and represents an important causative agent in asphyxial deaths. Mortality rates of 25 to 30% are still common in neonates with meconium aspiration. When proper obstetrical suctioning before delivery is combined with rapid airway suctioning during postnatal resuscitation, mortality and morbidity from this disease are minimal. The pulmonary complications result from airway obstruction, ball-valve obstruction with distal hyperinflation, or atelectasis, chemical pneumonitis, and major ventilation-perfusion defects leading to hypoxemia and hypercarbia. Because intrapartum asphyxia has existed in the majority of these neonates, these mechanical disadvantages may be complicated by surfactant deficiency, leaky pulmonary capillaries (shock lung), pulmonary edema, and severe persistent pulmonary hypertension. The initial chest roentgenogram demonstrates marked hyperexpansion with fluffy or patchy infiltrates throughout both lung fields.

Mechanical ventilation is necessary though hazardous: The risk of pneumothorax is high. Steroids do not appear helpful and may increase mortality. Because meconium readily supports bacterial growth, antibiotic coverage is usually provided. In addition to pulmonary complications, hypoxemic damage to other organ systems must be carefully searched for and appropriately managed.

Aspiration of clear amniotic fluid due to fetal gasping movements delays postnatal conversion from a fluid-blood interface to an air-blood interface at the alveolar level. Typical respiratory distress and mild hypoxemia are seen from birth. The chest roentgenogram demonstrates a diffuse alveolar infiltrate resembling pulmonary edema, though usually without cardiomegaly. Treatment is symptomatic, with provision of oxygen to diminish cyanosis and occasionally application of continuous distending airway pressure. A secondary surfactant loss may occur with a delayed clinical picture compatible with hyaline membrane disease.

TRANSIENT TACHYPNEA. A delay in the normal reabsorption of amniotic fluid through lymphatic channels produces symptoms of mild to moderate respiratory distress, usually in term or near-term infants. Tachypnea is more prominent than grunting and retractions. Cyanosis is usually mild. Symptoms may persist for 24 to 72 hours, and treatment is symptomatic. The chest roentgenogram is diagnostic, with increased interstitial markings and prominence of the major and minor fissures due to fluid accumulation. A small percentage of these infants demonstrate pneumothorax, and close observation for this complication is indicated.

LOBAR EMPHYSEMA. Partial obstruction of a main-stem or subsegmental branch of the airway leads to overdistention of the distal air spaces behind the obstruction. A ball-valve obstruction may impede expiration and eventually produce compression and collapse of adjacent normal lobes and alveoli with mediastinal shift toward the unaffected side. This condition may arise from a developmental defect in branching of the conducting airway system, inflammatory edema and scarring due to infection, local trauma, oxygen toxicity, cardiac chamber enlargement (particularly the left atrium), aberrant mediastinal vessels, or intrapulmonary lesions.

Respiratory distress is usually present. In addition, hyperinflation or poor mobility of the affected side of the chest may be observed. Auscultatory findings include diminution of breath sounds over the emphysematous lobe and a shift of heart sounds away from their usual location. The chest radiograph shows localized overexpansion with atelectasis of normal parenchyma and mediastinal shift. If conservative management (bronchopulmonary segmental drainage) fails to dislodge the entrapped material or respiratory distress progresses, surgical resection of the involved lobe will be required.

PNEUMOTHORAX. In older radiographic screening studies, pneumothorax was demonstrated in 1% of all neonates; it was symptomatic in half of this group. Unequal distribution of inspired air during the initial large intrathoracic pressure changes typical of the first breaths was felt to overdistend and rupture distal alveoli. With alveolar rupture, air dissects along the peribronchial tissues toward the hilum, rupturing through the mediastinum and proceeding from there to the pleura, producing the typical appearance of free air in the intrathoracic space compressing the normal lung. Excessive pressures during resuscitation, air-block syndromes (meconium aspiration), congenital lung cysts,

CPAP, and mechanical ventilation with high mean airway pressures (Paw) are the most common antecedents of pneumothorax. Overinflation of one side of the thorax, diminished chest-wall movement on the affected side, diminished breath sounds, and mediastinal shift are clinical clues. Fiberoptic transillumination of the chest and anteroposterior and cross-table lateral radiographs are confirmatory. Treatment includes nitrogen washout with 100% oxygen (contraindicated in the preterm infant because of the risk of ROP), needle thoracentesis, or placement of a pleural drainage tube.

INTRAPULMONARY LESIONS. Bronchogenic cysts are clear fluid-filled masses that usually fail to communicate with the tracheobronchial tree. They are usually located close to the carina and may produce respiratory distress by airway compression. In the posterior mediastinum, cysts representing detached duplicated segments of gut are occasionally encountered. They are filled with fluid typical of their original intestinal location. Esophageal indentation and narrowing may produce swallowing difficulties or vomiting, while tracheal impingement leads to dyspnea and stridor. Intrapulmonary fluid and/or air-filled cystic adenomatoid malformations may involve one or more lobes, compress normal lung parenchyma, and displace the mediastinum to the contralateral side.

Accessory and sequestered lobes may be difficult to distinguish from pneumonia and atelectasis. Aortography demonstrates anomalous blood supply to these lobes from the aorta rather than the pulmonary circulation.

Heart: Congenital Heart Disease

The signs and symptoms indicative of heart disease in the neonate have been previously reviewed. Some form of cardiac defect, many of which are self-limiting, is present in approximately 1% of live births. Patent ductus arteriosus and ventricular septal defect are the lesions most commonly encountered. In the neonatal period, however, these lesions are usually asymptomatic except in the preterm infant or when present in association with other cardiac defects. When either is detected as an isolated lesion, spontaneous closure of the defect is common.

Clinical symptoms in the neonatal period may be due either to outflow obstruction or to large right-to-left shunts. Increased pulmonary blood flow and consequent congestive failure may be delayed until after the neonatal period because of "physiological banding" from normally elevated pulmonary artery pressures. As pulmonary resistance decreases postnatally, left-to-right shunting increases and symptoms of congestive failure supervene.

Diagnosis depends upon the combined input from physical examination, electrocardiography, roentgenography of the chest, and echocardiography. When the diagnosis remains in doubt or surgical correction is anticipated, early cardiac catheterization is recommended to thoroughly describe the abnormal cardiac anatomy and blood flow patterns to allow the cardiac surgeon to choose the most appropriate palliative or definitive repair.

Symptoms of congestive heart failure in the newborn are predominantly related to difficulties associated with feeding and breathing. The infant with congestive heart failure is alternately lethargic and irritable, feeds poorly and slowly, often with cyanosis, is diaphoretic, and has significant tachypnea and tachycardia. Physical examination may reveal a hyperdynamic precordium, an S_3 or S_4 gallop rhythm, lung congestion and rales, and hepatomegaly. Although edema about the face and eyes is not infrequently noted, dependent edema in the lower limbs is unusual. A chest x-ray examination confirms cardiomegaly with increased vascular markings throughout both lung fields. Specific forms of congenital heart disease are discussed in Chapter 10, The Heart and Great Vessels.

PERSISTENCE OF THE TRANSITIONAL CIRCULATION. In this syndrome, high pulmonary artery pressure, typical of in utero existence, persists postnatally, thereby maintaining fetal blood flow patterns through the ductus arteriosus and foramen ovale. The infant is usually born near term, but frequently is postmature or growth retarded and often demonstrates evidence of some degree of in utero hypoxia. The medial muscle mass of the fifth and sixth generation pulmonary arteries is increased, and the internal diameter of the vessels narrowed, thereby limiting pulmonary flow. Cyanosis begins at or shortly after birth with tachypnea and mild hypercarbia but little metabolic acidemia. Hypoxemia becomes progressively severe with little response to breathing of 100% oxygen or mechanical ventilation.

Chest x-ray examination demonstrates little or no cardiomegaly and diminished pulmonary vascularity. An ECG confirms right ventricular hypertrophy. The murmur of patent ductus arteriosus (PDA), ventricular septal defect (VSD), or tricuspid insufficiency may be present, but true congestive failure is uncommon. The echocardiogram demonstrates normal cardiac anatomy, but right ventricular systolic time intervals are typical of increased afterload due to high pulmonary artery pressure. A venous injection of saline that has been shaken to produce microbubbles can be seen flowing from right to left across the foramen. A much higher level of PaO_2 in the right radial artery than umbilical artery confirms shunting at the ductal level. Resolution gradually occurs in 5 to 7 days as involution of the medial muscular hypertrophy occurs. Mechanical ventilation, induction of respiratory and metabolic acidosis, intravascular volume expansion, and pulmonary vasodilators are the mainstays of therapy. Recently the application of extracorporeal membrane oxygenation (ECMO) to neonates has offered further options to the critically ill neonate suffering from this self-limiting process.

Gastrointestinal Tract

ESOPHAGEAL ATRESIA WITH TRACHEOESOPHAGEAL FISTULA. Occurring once in 4000 live births, this anomaly represents an interruption in the normal division of the foregut into the dorsal esophagus and ventral trachea during the third week of embryonic development. The various combinations of defects are presented in Figure 9-3. A blind atretic proximal esophageal pouch and a fistulous connection from the distal esophagus to the trachea represent 85% of cases. In 10% of cases either isolated esophageal atresia or an H-type fistula exists. In 15% of infants with this defect the VACTERL syndrome is present (vertebral, anal, cardiac, tracheoesophageal, renal, and limb anomalies). Prematurity complicates the course and repair in 30% of the infants, and associated cardiac anomalies usually include either VSD or ASD.

Frequently a maternal history of polyhydramnios is elicited. Abundant mucous secretion at the mouth, respiratory distress with aspiration pneumonia, and vomiting during feedings are frequent clinical clues to diagnosis. Inability to pass a catheter to the stomach is diagnostic and confirmed by x-ray examination. Often the blind pouch can be visualized on the plain radiograph. When a blind pouch is demonstrated, the presence of gas within the intestinal tract confirms the presence of a fistula.

Surgical correction includes primary anastomosis if the blind ends are apposable, with ligation of the fistula and gastrostomy. If the blind ends are widely separated, mercury-filled or magnetic bougies may aid in their approximation. If apposition by these techniques is unsuccessful, colonic interposition between the two segments can be utilized.

DIAPHRAGMATIC HERNIA. Usually a posterolateral defect (Bochdalek) on the left side, this occurs once in 5000 live births and represents failure of fusion of the diaphragmatic membrane during the tenth week of gestation. The fusion coincides with the return of the intestines into the abdominal cavity from the umbilical pouch. If significant bowel herniation into the chest occurs, pulmonary paren-

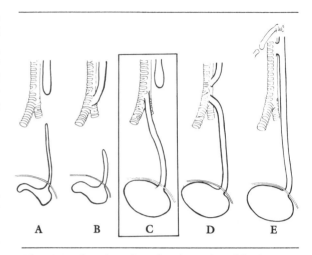

Fig. 9-3. Esophageal atresia and tracheoesophageal fistula.
A. Esophageal atresia without fistula. Respiratory difficulty is relatively less because there is no gastric regurgitation into the trachea and no gastric distention with air.
B. The proximal end of the esophagus terminates in a tracheal fistula, and the distal end is blind superiorly. Continuous aspiration of saliva into the trachea makes this one of the forms for which treatment is most urgently required.
C. The most common form (85–95% of cases), in which the proximal end of the esophagus terminates blind high in the thorax and the distal end communicates with the trachea or either main bronchus. The diagnosis is made by the bubbling of spittle at the mouth, strangulation on attempted feeding, repeated respiratory difficulty, and distention of the stomach with gas blown through the distal fistula.
D. Double fistula.
E. The H fistula, more often high than low. Both are always difficult to diagnose in the absence of atresia.

chymal hypoplasia as well as hypoplasia of the pulmonary artery on the affected side may follow. Likewise, compression of the mediastinum to the contralateral side may produce changes in growth in the normal lung. Although in 5% of cases this lesion may be present without early herniation of abdominal contents into the thorax, most infants have respiratory distress and increasing cyanosis shortly after birth. Significant crying with air swallowing or bag-and-mask ventilation produces gaseous distention of the entrapped bowel and further compromise ventilation. The presence and degree of pulmonary hypoplasia (both parenchymal and arterial) often determine the severity of the course and mortality risk.

Diminished chest-wall movement, absence of breath sounds or bowel sounds on the ipsilateral side, scaphoid abdomen, and mediastinal shift are signs frequently detectable clinically. Kinking of the mediastinum leads to impairment of venous return to the right side of the heart and consequently compromises systemic cardiac output. The chest roentgenogram confirms the presence of bowel loops in the thorax and demonstrates shift of the heart toward the contralateral side. Immediate surgical intervention and repair of the diaphragmatic defect are standard treatment practices. In some neonates with severe pulmonary hypertension, a period of ECMO support before or after surgical correction is suggested. Careful monitoring of oxygen tension, with attention toward preventing major mediastinal shifts, are critical aspects of postoperative management.

INTESTINAL OBSTRUCTION. High intestinal obstruction is often present in the neonate with a history of maternal polyhydramnios, a large gastric residual at the time of stomach lavage (more than 30 ml), distention of the epigastrium, and vomiting (frequently bile stained). Early onset of symptoms is typical. Associated malrotation is frequently present, and on barium enema examination the cecum may be displaced out of the right lower quadrant. On x-ray examination the bowel loops are distended, widely separated (bowel-wall edema), fixed in location, and, if obstruction is complete, devoid of air in the colon and rectum. In utero vascular accidents leading to bowel-wall ischemia and subsequent scarring are the usual pathogenic mechanisms.

Duodenal stenosis may be due to congenital webs, annular pancreas, or malrotation with Ladd's bands. This form of stenosis often occurs concomitantly with Down syndrome. In this lesion an abdominal x-ray examination demonstrates a double-bubble pattern.

Ileal atresia is more common than jejunal obstruction. In utero vascular accidents, volvulus, and intussusception may lead to these small-bowel obstructions. Absence of, delayed, or infrequent stool passage in the first day of life is typical. The cecum is usually displaced on barium enema. Significant abdominal distention is often followed by bile-stained vomiting, though the clinical presentation may be delayed for 24 hours or more after birth when the atresia is low.

Midgut volvulus results from an abnormal twist of malrotated unfixed midgut and may lead to vascular compromise of the entire small intestine and a portion of the ascending colon. The sudden appearance of vomiting, usually bilious, with each feeding on the third or fourth (up to thirtieth) day of life is associated with sudden abdominal distention. Immediate recognition and surgical intervention are necessary to maintain bowel viability.

MECONIUM ILEUS. Obstruction of the terminal ileum with thick viscid meconium is a presenting symptom in 10% of neonates with cystic fibrosis. The typical symptoms of intestinal obstruction are combined with failure to pass stool and an abnormal palpable mass in the abdomen. The bowel loops on the roentgenogram have a soap-bubble appearance representing air mixed with meconium. A Gastrografin enema may be successful in separating the thick meconium from the bowel wall, thereby facilitating passage. If this is unsuccessful, operative removal of the meconium through an ileostomy may be required. Meconium ileus may lead to in utero perforation with sterile meconium peritonitis and a meconium cyst present at birth. Calcifications are usually seen on the plain radiograph. Again this lesion carries a strong association with cystic fibrosis.

HIRSCHSPRUNG'S DISEASE. Arrest in migration of the ganglion cells during the fifth to twelfth week of embryonic development impairs neuromuscular conduction in the sigmoid colon (85% of cases), in the entire colon, or entire intestine (total aganglionosis). Failure to pass stool or establish a normal defecation pattern may be present from birth. Barium enema study demonstrates a narrow "transitional" zone with distention of the normal colon proximal to the obstruction. Barium retention 24 hours after the radiographic procedures is typical. Rectal manometry may demonstrate dysfunction of the internal rectal sphincter, and rectal biopsy with cholinesterase staining demonstrates absence of ganglion cells and enzyme activity. A colostomy proximal to the aganglionic section is done at the initial surgery; complete correction of the defect is planned after the infant's body has grown considerably.

IMPERFORATE ANUS. This defect is usually related to maldevelopment of the urorectal septum that results in incomplete separation of the cloaca into the urogenital and anorectal portions. The defect may be less complex, however, with failure of the anal membrane to perforate at the seventh to eighth week of gestation. Simple rectal atresia or stenosis represents a low defect without associated anomalies, but high atresia (above the puborectalis sling) usually contains a fistulous connection to the bladder, vagina, urethra, or perineum. Failure to pass meconium, an external perineal deformity, meconium passage through the urethra or vagina, and discovery of a blind pouch on rectal examination confirm the diagnosis. A strong association with urinary tract malformations also exists. Low defects may be primarily repaired, while high defects usually require resection of the fistulous tract and colostomy.

Spine and Spinal Cord

MENINGOCELE, MYELOMENINGOCELE. Spina bifida refers to failure of the spinal column to complete normal closure because of a defect in the somatic development of the vertebrae. It is usually associated with a saclike protrusion of the skin and meninges (meningocele) or portion of the spinal cord (myelomeningocele). Occult spina bifida or meningocele is usually asymptomatic at birth, though associated anomalies are commonly present when myelomeningocele exists. Congenital or rapidly developing hydrocephalus, clubfoot deformity, lower-limb palsies, dislocation of hips, and bowel and bladder dysfunction frequently coexist when the spinal cord is present in the protruding sac. The defect is most common in the lumbar region, followed by lumbosacral, sacral, thoracolumbar, thoracic, and cervical defects.

The long-term prognosis for physical and intellectual health is dismal in high spinal lesions, especially when combined with congenital hydrocephalus and significant lower-motor neuron disease. Orthopedic and renal disabilities are chronic medical concerns in these children. Control of existing or developing hydrocephalus and prevention of bacterial contamination of the sac and subsequent meningitis are major concerns early in the neonatal period. Closure of the skin defect is accomplished at the earliest possible date. Increasing ventricular dilatation is an indication for early placement of a ventriculoperitoneal shunt when treatment is deemed genetically and ethically indicated.

Genitourinary System

See Chapter 12, The Genitourinary System.

Hematopoietic System

See Chapter 15, The Blood, and Appendix A, section 22, Pallor and Anemia.

POLYCYTHEMIA. An increased number of circulating red cells may be due to delayed clamping or stripping of the umbilical cord after birth. In this situation, hematocrit is normal, total blood volume is increased, and the major risk to the neonate is an increased bilirubin load potentiating physiological jaundice. In other neonates, circulating blood volume is normal, though the red cell mass and hematocrit are increased. In this case, hyperviscosity with impairment of the microcirculation may result. This condition is common in growth-retarded fetuses (SGA), infants of diabetic mothers, and fetuses exposed to chronic hypoxia in utero. Increased red cell mass and diminished plasma volume combined with decreased deformability of the fetal red blood cells can lead to sluggish flow and diminished oxygen delivery to various fetal organs.

In the absence of viscosity measurements, diagnosis is suspected when central hematocrit values greater than 65% are obtained. Viscosity begins to increase linearly near this value. Symptoms include lethargy, jitteriness, irritability, poor feeding, tachypnea, tachycardia, cyanosis, cardiomegaly, gastrointestinal dysfunction, clotting abnormalities, and hypoglycemia. Symptomatic elevation of the hematocrit above this level is best treated with partial exchange transfusion through the umbilical vein with fresh frozen plasma to lower the hematocrit toward 50%.

IDIOPATHIC THROMBOCYTOPENIC PURPURA. Although thrombocytopenia is not uncommon in the sick neonate during bacterial and viral sepsis, bowel ischemia, or any disease process leading to disseminated intravascular coagulation, its presence in the full-term healthy neonate is most unusual.

Scattered petechiae are not uncommon over the head, face, and neck of infants born by abnormal presentation (face, brow, or mentum). Extension of petechiae to other areas of the body or frank ecchymotic lesions are suggestive of clotting abnormalities or platelet dysfunction. Maternal drug use, especially of the thiazides, has been implicated in neonatal thrombocytopenia. The phenomenon may also be observed with erythroblastosis fetalis, ABO incompatibility, repetitive exchange transfusions, congenital leukemia with Down syndrome, and the Wiskott-Aldrich syndrome.

In most instances in which infection is unlikely to explain a low platelet count, either isoimmune or autoimmune thrombocytopenia is responsible. Isoimmune thrombocytopenia should be suspected in any otherwise healthy thrombocytopenic infant whose mother has a normal platelet count and no history of drug therapy. In this situation, the antibody present in the infant's serum attacks both the infant's and father's platelets, and successive pregnancies may result in thrombocytopenic infants. In the autoimmune situation the mother's platelet count is low or has been low in the past because of the presence of an antiplatelet antibody in her sera. Frequently the mother has a history of either chronic corticosteroid usage or splenectomy. Even when the maternal platelet count is near normal, transplacental passage of maternal antibody may produce thrombocytopenia in the infant. Added risks to the extremely thrombocytopenic infant include central nervous system and other organ bleeding during labor or in the first few postnatal days. When severe fetal thrombocytopenia is recognized before delivery (scalp blood sample, umbilical vein blood sampling under ultrasound guidance), cesarean section should be strongly considered. Therapy after birth includes carefully typed platelet transfusions or steroid administration in the infant. When thrombocytopenia is produced by abnormal maternal platelet antibodies the disease is self-limiting.

Endocrine Glands

See Chapter 6, The Endocrine Glands.

Richard A. Molteni and August L. Jung

References

Avery, G. B. (Ed.). *Neonatology: Pathophysiology and Management of the Newborn* (3rd ed.). Philadelphia: Lippincott, 1987.

Avery, M. E., and First, L. R. *Diseases of the Newborn. Pediatric Medicine,* Baltimore: Williams & Wilkins, 1989.

Dubowitz, L. M. S., Dubowitz, V., and Goldberg, C. Clinical assessment of gestational age in the newborn infant. *J. Pediatr.* 77:1, 1970.

Klaus, M. H., and Fanarof, A. A. *Care of the High Risk Neonate* (3rd ed.). Philadelphia: Saunders, 1986.

Lubchenco, L. O., Searls, D. T., and Brazic, J. B. Neonatal mortality rate: Relationship to birthweight and gestational age. *J. Pediatr.* 81:814, 1972.

10

The Neck, Ears, and Respiratory System

The Neck

Cysts, Sinuses, and Solid Lesions

MAINLY MIDLINE LESIONS. *Ranula.* This cystic swelling arises in the floor of the mouth from an obstruction of sublingual salivary ducts. It may protrude intraorally or in the submental triangle. It is thin-walled and translucent and is treated by drainage into the mouth by a wide incision (marsupialization).

Thyroglossal Duct Cyst. The thyroid gland develops from a midline diverticulum at the base of the embryonic tongue, which is represented in the adult by the foramen cecum. As the neck elongates and straightens, the gland assumes a position in the lower neck, and normally all continuity is lost with the foramen cecum. Occasionally a tract is left behind that runs downwards from the foramen cecum through the tongue musculature, hooks around the front of the hyoid bone, to which it is very intimately adherent, and ends blindly a short distance below.

This tract is tubular and lined by a respiratory-type, mucus-secreting epithelium. As mucus is produced, it gives rise to progressive dilatation of the blind distal end, resulting eventually in a midline, subcutaneous "pseudocyst," a couple of centimeters in diameter, filled with turbid, mucoid secretions and lined by a fibrous tissue wall often poorly defined from surrounding normal tissue. The cyst is usually located just below the hyoid and often closely attached to it.

Because it takes a while for the mucus to accumulate and the cyst to form, thyroglossal duct cysts are usually not seen in the neonatal period but tend to appear around 2 to 3 years of age.

Because of their communication with the mouth, they may become infected and present as a midline prehyoid abscess. *Hemophilus influenzae* is the organism most commonly recovered. Drainage (spontaneous or surgical) of the abscess may result in a chronic fistula to the skin; the fistula itself is not congenital.

Simple removal of the cyst is inadequate, because a new blind-ending tract is left which forms a new cyst. The whole tract must be removed up to the foramen cecum including the midportion of the hyoid bone.

Midline Ectopic Thyroid. Sometimes an individual's thyroid gland consists only of a small midline nodule of tissue which may lie anywhere along the course of the thyroglossal tract. This small amount of thyroid tissue may be adequate for a while but eventually, because of the increased demands imposed by growth, puberty, pregnancy, etc., enlarges under TSH stimulation to form a palpable mass in the back of the tongue or the cervical midline. It is important to recognize that such patients are borderline hypothyroid and require permanent thyroid hormone replacement, which results in disappearance of the mass and obviates surgery.

If the diagnosis is suspected clinically, radionuclide scan confirms the diagnosis and shows absence of a normally situated thyroid gland. Thyroid function tests usually show some degree of hypothyroidism. If the diagnosis is made at the time of surgical exploration, the gland is left in place and thyroid replacement therapy is instituted.

Epidermoid Cyst. Epidermoids are thought to be a result of entrapment of epidermis under the skin during development of the embryo. Their walls are formed of stratified squamous epithelium with all the normal skin appendages. The cyst may be entirely closed off, in which case it presents as a very discrete, mobile, firm, round subcutaneous mass which may appear vaguely yellow through the skin because of its sebaceous contents. It may also communicate with the skin through a tiny, often inconspicuous opening (dermoid sinus), which may allow bacteria to enter and lead to abscess formation.

Sites of predilection for *closed* epidermoid cysts are (1) the anterior cervical midline, often just above the sternal notch, (2) the submental area, (3) a prehyoid position where they may mimic a thyroglossal duct cyst, (4) the supraciliary area, especially its lateral end (lateral angular dermoid), and (5) the scalp away from the midline. Treatment is by simple excision.

Sites of predilection for *open* epidermoid cysts (dermoid sinuses) are (1) the preauricular area (congenital preauricular sinus), (2) the left presternoclavicular area, and (3) the midline of the body from the nose up along the cranium and down along the spine to the sacrum. In this instance there may also be an internal sinus passing towards the meninges, which may be the cause of repeated episodes of meningitis. The sinus must be totally removed for cure.

LATERAL LESIONS. *Lymphangioma*. In the neck, lymphangiomas are often referred to as cystic hygroma colli. The most common site is the posterior triangle in relation to the accessory nerve, but in newborns they may occur as a huge mass often causing acute embarrassment to breathing and swallowing. They may appear, often suddenly, later on, as a result of small, spontaneous hemorrhages and consequent rapid accumulation of fluid within presumably preformed but collapsed cysts. This is a common occurrence, which may also be responsible for sudden life-threatening enlarge-

ment of previously documented lesions in confined areas such as the neck or mediastinum.

In any location lymphangioma appears as a relatively soft, mobile, polylobulated subcutaneous mass of variable size, often with a slightly bluish tinge as seen through the skin. The lesion is multicystic and does not respect tissue planes. In particular it is often intimately related to major nerves (facial, accessory, brachial plexus, phrenic), which course through it and render complete excision difficult and hazardous.

Because of their relationships with the lymphatic system, lymphangiomas occasionally become infected, although not as often as one would fear. Their appearance may follow a respiratory tract infection. Their ultrasound appearance is usually diagnostic. They can be distinguished from deep hemangiomas, which they may resemble closely, by a "cold" appearance on the blood pool phase of a technetium radionuclide scan.

Unlike hemangiomas, lymphangiomas seldom resolve spontaneously. Complete or partial excision is necessary, sometimes associated with such procedures as tracheostomy or gastrostomy.

STERNOMASTOID TUMOR. This is an idiopathic fibromatosis of the sternomastoid muscle, almost always unilateral, presenting in the newborn period as a very firm, rather large, ovoid swelling within the muscle and associated with a variable degree of contracture of the muscle and cervical fascia. Because of the origin of the muscle in the sternoclavicular area and its insertion on the mastoid, this contracture results in lateral flexion of the neck towards the affected side and rotation of the chin to the opposite side, the so-called sternomastoid torticollis.

The sternomastoid tumor is often associated with variable degrees of plagiocephaly (cranial asymmetry along a diagonal axis, with flattening of the occiput on the side opposite to the lesion and flattening of the frons on the same side) and facial hemihypoplasia on the same side.

The mass is composed mainly of young fibroblasts. Regardless of treatment, it disappears after a few months as the fibroblasts mature and contract. This results in a fixed contracture requiring surgical release (sternomastoid myotomy). Because the diagnosis is now usually made quite early, however, treatment is directed towards keeping the muscle stretched to its full length until the tumor has completely resolved, by stretching exercises under the direction of the surgeon and physiotherapist for 6 months or more, and discouraging, by various maneuvers, the child's natural tendency to keep the head in the same position. For example, use may be made of the fact that a baby lying in bed tends to turn its head towards the door. The plagiocephaly and facial hemihypoplasia usually then remodel almost completely after a few years.

BRANCHIAL LESIONS. Branchial cysts, fistulae, and sinuses are thought to be aberrant derivatives of the first and second branchial cleft.

A *second branchial cleft fistula* presents as a tiny, inconspicuous opening draining crystal-clear, mucoid material in small amounts intermittently and situated along the anterior border of the sternomastoid usually at the level of its middle third. It is usually unilateral. Deep to this opening is a tract that may simply end blindly at a variable distance up in the neck but in its full expression ascends as a fairly substantial tube lined by a respiratory-type epithelium upwards towards the bifurcation of the carotid artery. At this point it hooks inwards, passes within the bifurcation, and ends in the tonsillar fossa. Despite its apparently formidable anatomical relationships, it is easy to excise completely.

First branchial cleft cysts are lined with keratinizing squamous epithelium and may be mistaken for epidermoids or sebaceous cysts by the uninitiated, leading to incomplete removal and recurrence, or sometimes disastrous results because of their intimate relationship with the facial nerve. They are flask-shaped and take two different configurations. In some, the bulbous end presents as a cystic swelling behind the ear lobe, with the other extremity coursing parallel to and underneath the external ear canal to end blindly in the area of the tympanum. In others, the dilated end presents lower down towards the angle of the jaw; the narrow segment courses upwards and enters the inferior wall of the external ear canal at right angles to it, as a sinus. As in thyroglossal duct cyst, an external fistula to the skin does not develop unless the lesion has formed an abscess that has drained to the outside.

LYMPHOEPITHELIAL CYSTS. Usually referred to as branchial cysts, these are probably not branchial at all. They are now thought to arise from inclusions of parotid epithelium within the nodes of the upper deep jugular lymph node chain. Clinically they present at the time of adolescence and beyond as a large mass deep to the upper third of the sternomastoid, often appearing following an upper respiratory infection. They have no communication with the skin or the pharynx and are quite distinct from the occasional fusiform dilatation that one may see along the course of a branchial fistula. They are unilocular with a thick wall of fibrous tissue, very abundant lymphoid material, and an ulcerated, rudimentary epithelial lining. The contents are liquid and characteristically contain cholesterol crystals.

Pierre Soucy

The Ears

Congenital Conditions

Any deformity of the head and neck, including the branchial cleft lesions just described, even simple preauricular tags, should be reason to suspect sensorineural deafness. Some inherited disorders and certain intrauterine infections (cytomegalovirus, mumps) interfere with the development of the labyrinth. Microtia with or without middle ear malformation is associated with conductive hearing loss. Bilateral outward projection of the pinnae (lop ears) is best treated by plastic surgery before school entry, so as to spare the child much embarrassment.

Trauma to the Ears

A thin object inserted into the canal, a blow on the ear, or a loud explosion can rupture the eardrum. It can also be torn with a skull fracture; cerebrospinal fluid or perilymph may drain from the ear. A ruptured tympanic membrane is allowed to heal spontaneously; antibiotics are given prophylactically against the organisms usually involved in otitis media (see Acute Otitis Media) until healing is complete, and the ear canal is protected with a sterile dressing. Ear drops are prohibited, because of the risk of ototoxicity. If audiometry demonstrates a sensorineural hearing loss, either profound or fluctuant, the middle ear must be explored in order to discover and obliterate a perilymphatic fistula which carries the risk of life-threatening meningioencephalitis should acute otitis media supervene. If no spontaneous healing of the ruptured eardrum takes place, tympanoplasty may be required; persistence of a conductive hearing loss may indicate repair of a dislocated ossicular chain (ossiculoplasty).

Foreign Bodies and Cerumen

An insect trapped in the canal can easily be killed by inserting a few drops of alcohol. Small objects placed in the canal by the child may be well tolerated, may impair hearing, or may produce a purulent secretion. If syringing fails to remove the object, it can be extracted by various microinstruments; general anesthesia may be necessary.

Cerumen is, of course, a normal secretion that contributes to the cleanliness of the ear canal by trapping dust. It often accumulates and occasionally becomes dry and hard (inspissation). Sometimes there is an actual impaction. The condition, quite often, does not bother the child in the least; or he may not hear as well on that side or complain of a sensation of fullness, tickling, or noise when chewing. The cerumen may interfere with drainage of water after bathing or swimming, and this is a contributory factor in the development of otitis externa. If the plug is troublesome or its removal is necessary to permit inspection of the eardrum, it is first softened by warm water with or without 10% sodium bicarbonate; the child is advised to let the shower water go alternately in and out of the canal. Detergent preparations advertised for that purpose should be avoided, because they often produce a troublesome contact dermatitis; hydrogen peroxide turns cerumen into a glue which is difficult to remove and prevents proper examination. If the impaction persists, syringing with warm water is quite often effective. The jet is not directed into the axis of the canal, but against one of its walls, in such a way as to produce a gyrating motion and to avoid pressure upon the drum. A word of caution: syringing must *not* be undertaken unless one is certain that the eardrum is not perforated and that the child does not have ventilation tubes. A mass of hard cerumen which is well localized and stands clear of the drum can be taken out by a small blunt curette under otoscopic control, but this should not be attempted in the preschool child in whom it may cause bleeding from the canal. Cerumen that is close to the outside can often be removed by a cotton applicator; but the tuft of cotton must be very small, otherwise it will only push the cerumen further in.

Infection of the External Ear

Otitis externa is dermatitis of the canal. It may be due to a wide variety, and often a mix, of gram-negative and gram-positive bacteria and fungi, especially *Candida*. Among local causes one may mention middle ear disease with drainage of pus through a perforation of the drum or a ventilation tube, as well as the presence of impacted cerumen which may cause retention of water. Infection from the latter cause is likely to follow swimming in a river or in water of doubtful cleanliness. A point must be made: though this is the original meaning of the expression "swimmer's ear," swimming even in clean water (e.g., in a pool) is often followed by the development of acute myringitis if the child carries ventilation tubes. The child who has not learned to close the nasal passage when under water may let water come through the eustachian tube into the middle ear cavity, bringing with it bacteria from the pharynx. Furthermore, hypotonic water is probably irritating for the mucosa of the middle ear, which

must be just as sensitive to chlorine as the conjunctiva of the eye!

Returning to otitis externa, examination shows redness and tenderness of the canal with swelling. Pain may be present and enhanced by mobilization of the pinna. The lumen is narrowed by exudate and by edema of the skin. In *treatment,* gentamicin drops or an antibiotic wick may be inserted; systemic therapy with cloxacillin may be required for *Staphylococcus aureus* infection. The presence of fungi or any opportunistic organisms should lead one to suspect immunologic incompetence, e.g., from diabetes mellitus or immunosuppressive drugs.

Prevention of otitis externa in the predisposed child may be effected by the instillation of an acidic antiseptic solution (e.g., benzethonium chloride) after swimming.

A furuncle of the skin of the canal may be seen as part of otitis externa or in an otherwise healthy canal. It should not be incised, even when "ripe," as this would cut across blood and lymphatic vessels and favor the spread of infection. Warm saline compresses, with the soaked absorbent cotton pulled out into a point that will fit into the canal, are applied for 15 minutes every 2 or 3 hours. An antistaphylococcal penicillin is prescribed for 10 days.

Infection of the Middle Ear

EPIDEMIOLOGY AND PATHOGENESIS. The various forms of otitis media are among the most frequent complaints with which a child comes to the doctor. It is seen in the infant of a few weeks of age; the incidence then rises to reach a peak around 1 year of age, but it remains high throughout childhood. Otitis media most often accompanies or follows a viral infection of the nasal passages. Measles and scarlet fever frequently, and less often varicella, are complicated by otitis media. The great susceptibility of the young child to middle ear infections is usually explained by the short, wide, and straight eustachian tube, but this ought also to make drainage from the middle ear easier! More to the point is the notion that the eustachian tube is lined by a loose submucosa, rich in lymphoid tissue, which in response to infection swells readily, leading to obliteration of the lumen. Bacteria are then aspirated into the middle ear cleft by the negative pressure thus created. Infection also induces a cessation of the metachronic beating of eustachian tube cilia and impairs local immunity in the middle ear space. Another factor in infancy may be related to immaturity of deglutition. It is known that in the normal infant, while swallowing, there is a reflux of milk toward the nasopharynx and perhaps the eustachian tube; this is one reason why infants should nurse (at the breast or the bottle) in a sitting, not supine, position. The relationship of diseased adenoids and tonsils to otitis media is controversial; simple hypertrophy of these structures is *not* a cause of frequent or protracted middle ear infection. In the newborn, middle ear infection may be hematogenous, as part of sepsis; other manifestations of sepsis, for example meningitis, may be present. Rupture of the eardrum and the trauma of adenoidectomy may lead to infection.

Significant risk factors for frequent attacks of otitis media and for otitis media with effusion are prematurity, Down syndrome, and craniofacial anomalies, particularly cleft palate. Incidence is high in native Americans; the reasons for this are probably environmental rather than structural.

The most common causal organism at all ages after the neonatal period is *Streptococcus pneumoniae*, followed by *Hemophilus influenzae*; the proportion of cases due to the latter is higher in the preschool child. Group A beta-hemolytic streptococci, *S. aureus*, and *Branhamella catarrhalis* are also encountered, and some reports suggest that *Mycoplasma* and certain viruses may be the pathogens.

Rupture of the eardrum may lead to the direct implantation into the tympanic cavity of gram-negative organisms from the ear canal. Such organisms are also found in mixed growth with the original inciting bacteria when, in the course of an acute otitis media, the eardrum has been incised or has ruptured spontaneously. Such superinfection occurs in a few hours.

ACUTE OTITIS MEDIA. Clinical manifestations vary with age and with the patient. The small-for-dates newborn and the premature are prone to otitis media, especially if intubated. They may have diarrhea and failure to thrive or more subtle signs of illness. The occurrence of meningitis must be kept in mind.

After the neonatal period, pain is the main symptom. In the infant pain may not be obvious. The baby may be irritable, crying, and feverish. The cry is often shrill. One pattern occasionally seen is that the baby cries suddenly while being laid down, presumably because of the effect of hydrostatic pressure. The infant may begin to cry at the first swallow when fed, which suggests that pressure changes transmitted to the middle ear through the eustachian tubes are painful. Many an infant prefers to lie on one side; another may jerk the head sideways while crying. From the age of about 6 months the child may tap, scratch, or tug at the ears. The child usually has had a nose cold for 2 or 3 days, or the otitic condition may appear in a hitherto healthy one. Fever and decrease of appetite are quite variable. With marked temperature elevation, convulsions may occur; in such cases coincident meningitis must be ruled out. Vomiting is seen. Diarrhea if present is probably due to the initial viral infection but may be enhanced by antibiotics, especially ampicillin or amoxicillin.

Past infancy, the only systemic symptom is usually fever. Pain is felt deeply in the ear; the pain may be intensified by coughing or by lying on the affected side. The child may be aware of decreased hearing, but that is not usually the case; crackling or bubbling sounds may be heard, especially when chewing. Pain immediately behind the ear does not necessarily mean mastoiditis, but this should be kept in mind (see Infection of the Mastoid). Pain in front of the ear may result from strain on the temporomandibular joint due to the habit of grinding the teeth, to malocclusion, or to gum chewing. Involvement of that joint in juvenile rheumatoid arthritis is not unusual.

Physical Signs. The essential diagnostic step is otoscopy. Easy to perform in the school-age child, it is problematic in the infant who is irritable and whose canal is narrow. The child of 1 to 5 years may resist too, because he or she fears the instrument and does not see what is being done. It is a good idea for the doctor first to simulate an otoscopic examination of the parent. The child is examined sitting sideways on the lap of the parent, who is asked to hold the child's arm in one hand and, with the other, to hold the head against her or his own upper chest. This gives the examiner two free hands. In any case the examination is often uncomfortable, due to the sensitive, thin skin of the canal. The speculum does not have to be inserted far into the canal. If it is poised at the meatus, the canal being made straight by taking the pinna between two fingers as close as possible to the meatus and pulling it gently towards the examiner's eye, the eardrum comes into view unless there is intervening cerumen or exudate.

In an infant, the eardrum is difficult to visualize, being almost horizontal; a common mistake is to confuse its usually well vascularized upper part (pars flaccida) for an inflamed membrane. In a child with a cold and sore ears, one is often surprised to find no sign of inflammation, and even to see that the membrane is retracted; both the otalgia and the retraction can be ascribed to decreased eustachian permeability. Signs of inflammation, in order of appearance, are hyperemia (sometimes with dilated vessels converging from the edge to the center, or forming a grid); loss of sheen of the membrane which looks uneven, thickened and opaque; bulging, first of the pars flaccida, which then overhangs the remainder of the drum; and later inflammation of the entire drum with disappearance of the handle of the malleus, marked redness, and convexity of the drum, which is much closer to the outside than normally. Parallel with these are changes in the light reflex, from the normal pencil-like shape to a rounded one in the center of the drum, through a crescent or ring near the outside rim, to its complete disappearance. Simple hyperemia without progression to the other changes is often seen in colds. This "congestive myringitis" should not be called otitis media, but needs to be watched. A serous or hemorrhagic bulla on the membrane is sometimes the initial sign of otitis media.

The pneumatic otoscope, used with the largest possible speculum, allows observation of the mobility of the eardrum as pressure or suction is exerted by means of a bulb. The normal membrane demonstrates a crisp, fluttering movement in response to pressure change; this may also be seen when the child coughs. Decreased movement suggests thickening or retraction of the drum, scarring, or effusion of fluid into the middle ear.

When the drum cannot be seen adequately, the physician must exercise judgment in deciding to diagnose otitis media and treat it. Marked, continuous pain with fever is often sufficient. Pressure on the tragus applied against the meatus may evoke or worsen pain. A small retroauricular lymph node may be present.

Otorrhea, or suppuration from the ear, results from spontaneous perforation or from incision of the eardrum. Sometimes it appears suddenly in a young child who has shown no definite symptoms of otitis. In other cases, there has been much pain, which quickly subsides when the perforation occurs. The discharge is often bloody at first. The bacteria it may contain have been listed previously. It may be difficult to tell whether the pus comes from the middle or the external ear. Discharge from a furuncle of the canal is scanty; but a dermatitis of the external ear is sometimes associated with much discharge. In such a case the edema of the skin and tenderness on mobilization of the pinna are of help in diagnosis. Indeed, a marked difficulty in clearing the canal sufficiently to permit otoscopy is suggestive of external otitis, as is the absence of constitutional symptoms. In favor of middle-ear origin of the pus are (1) pulsatile pus — the light dancing on the surface of the fluid is evidence for the dilatation of middle-ear arterioles, which are close branches of the internal and external carotid arteries, and (2) apparently not hitherto described in print, air bubbling through the pus, indicating the continuity from the nasopharynx through the eustachian tube and the middle-ear cavity to the outside.

The perforation itself is usually not visible, because of the intervening pus, until the inflammation has subsided greatly under treatment. By that time it has quite often closed.

Treatment. In acute otitis media an antibacterial is always necessary, its choice taking into account the local and temporal prevalence of beta-lactamase-secreting organisms. Equally recommended at this time are amoxicillin, trimethoprim-sulfamethoxazole (Bactrim, Septra), and erythromycin-ethylsuccinate-acetylsulfixazole (Pediazole). The latter should not be given before the age of 2 months. Relief of pain is usually effected by the use of acetaminophen; if necessary, codeine may be given orally. Antihistamines and decongestants are not effective. If perforation appears imminent or the pain is intractable, myringotomy may be considered. A culture can then be done. In any case the antibacterial treatment should be continued for at least 10 days, and follow-up within 2 weeks is imperative to ascertain that the condition is cured or on the way to a cure.

Complications. Acute complications such as mastoiditis (see Infection of the Mastoid), lateral sinus thrombosis, septicemia, meningitis (particularly pneumococcal), brain abscess, labyrinthitis, and facial paralysis, have become quite rare since the dawn of the antibiotic era. Conversely, atrophic otitis with ossicular chain rupture is more common.

Chronic otitis media results from the inadequate treatment of acute otitis media. Poor living conditions and especially nutritional factors may be suspected, especially in native American children. There may be tuberculous or mycotic infection. The tympanic membrane is always perforated. The presence of a polyp in the external canal necessitates a biopsy, because of the possibility of Langherhans cell histiocytosis. Chronic mastoiditis must be suspected and investigated. In long-standing cases, an epidermal cyst (cholesteatoma) of the tympanic cavity may form; it is difficult to treat.

SEROUS OTITIS MEDIA. Sometimes called secretory otitis media or glue ear, serous otitis media is an effusion of serous or seromucous exudate in the middle ear. It can cause hearing impairment. The tympanic membrane is dull, opaque, and an air-fluid level may be seen. Tympanometry measures compliance and middle-ear pressure by means of an electroacoustical impedance bridge. This simple and rapid method can diagnose middle-ear effusions painlessly and with ease.

Treatment. Antihistamines and decongestants have been shown to be of no value. Controlled trials have documented that long-term chemoprophylaxis should be undertaken first. If failure is evident after 6 months, insertion of ventilation (tympanostomy) tubes should be considered.

Infection of the Mastoid

Acute mastoiditis usually follows acute otitis media. The pain is constant, the fever is oscillating, and toxicity is frequent. Otoscopy demonstrates a bulging eardrum and the retroauricular sulcus is filled with a red and painful swelling.

A wide myringotomy under topical anesthesia (cocaine 4%) is made, and systemic antibiotic therapy (e.g., cefuroxime 200 mg/kg/day along with clindamycin 40 mg/kg/day)

168

is instituted. In the absence of a clinical response within 24 hours, cortical mastoidectomy with drainage avoids the development of life-threatening complications (meningitis, peridural or brain abscesses, thrombophlebitis of the sigmoid sinus).

Philippe A. Bernard and Paul de Bellefeuille

Hearing Loss

Deafness may be congenital or acquired. Congenital deafness, though rarer, occurs in 1 per 1000 live births. Unless there is reason to suspect deafness at birth, the diagnosis can unfortunately be delayed for several years until failure to develop normal speech becomes apparent.

DEFINITION. Because hearing loss is seldom a total defect, deafness normally refers to a partial hearing loss. The intensity of sound is measured in decibels (db). Mild hearing loss refers to audiometric thresholds of 20–40 db hearing level (ANSI, 1969). A hearing loss of 70 to 85 db is severe. Hearing losses greater than 90 db are profound. Very few deaf children are totally deaf.

Two general types of hearing loss are recognized.

1. Conductive hearing loss. There is interference with the transmission of sound from the external ear through the middle ear to the oval window, so that the energy reaching the inner ear is reduced. The perception of sound is better by bone conduction than by air conduction.
2. Sensorineural hearing loss. There is impairment of the inner ear, the eighth cranial nerve, or the pathways beyond. This may be further divided into sensory loss in which the abnormality is in the hair cells of the organ of Corti, and neural loss in which the defect lies in the nerve pathways. In sensorineural loss, sound conduction is the same for air conduction as for bone conduction.

CAUSES OF HEARING LOSS/DEAFNESS. Nearly half the cases of congenital deafness are due to an insult to the fetus in utero or to the infant during the immediate postnatal period. One-fifth are genetic, and the remainder are due to as yet unknown causes. A list of many of the known etiologies follows.

Congenital infections
 Rubella
 Herpes simplex
 Cytomegalovirus
 Toxoplasmosis
 Varicella

Teratogens, toxic substances
Prematurity
Asphyxia at birth
Hyperbilirubinemia
Congenital malformations of the auditory apparatus
Inherited deafness
Associated with recognizable syndromes
Birth trauma

Deafness is a frequent finding in infants born with congenital infections, particularly the rubella syndrome. Certain drugs ingested by the pregnant woman may cause in sensorineural deafness in the baby. These include streptomycin, thalidomide, chloroquine, and quinine. A number of patterns of malformation involving facial abnormalities are associated with deafness such as trisomy 13, the 18q syndrome, and the Treacher Collins syndrome. In the Treacher Collins syndrome there is an abnormality of the canals, tympanic membrane, incus, and malleus, and a conductive hearing loss.

Meningitis is the leading cause of permanent acquired deafness in children. In many cases this is the result of extension of the infection into the labyrinth. The ototoxicity of the aminoglycoside antibiotics is responsible for some of the deafness. A number of viral illnesses may also produce deafness. Mumps is the most common of these; when it produces deafness, this is usually unilateral.

The more common causes of acquired deafness follow.

I. Sensorineural
 A. Inflammatory
  1. Meningitis (bacterial)
  2. Encephalitis
  3. Viral infection
   a. Mumps
   b. Rubeola
   c. Rubella
   d. Herpes zoster
   e. Influenza
   f. Adenovirus
   g. Chickenpox
   h. Poliomyelitis
  4. Congenital syphilis
 B. Traumatic
  1. Overstimulation by loud noises
  2. Direct disruptive force
  3. Postoperative
  4. Spontaneous rupture of inner ear membranes
 C. Neurological disorders
  1. Multiple sclerosis
  2. Leukodystrophies

D. Systemic disorders

E. Drugs: aminoglycosides, aspirin

II. Conductive

  A. Infection

    1. Middle-ear infection and its sequelae

    2. External otitis

    3. Viral myringitis

    4. Furunculosis of canal

  B. Foreign body obstruction

  C. Trauma

  D. Tumor

Congenital syphilis is included here because deafness does not occur until late childhood or adulthood.

Temporary acquired hearing loss is most frequently associated with middle-ear infections and is of the conductive type. Repeated bouts of otitis may lead to permanent damage to the structures of the middle ear (fixation of the ossicles, scarred immobile tympanic membrane) and permanent hearing loss. Significant risk factors for otitis media with effusion are listed in Acute Otitis Media.

Trauma is another important cause of acquired hearing loss. A loud explosion may disrupt the ossicles. Continued exposure to loud noise may lead to progressive deafness due to a gradual loss of parts of the organ of Corti and its neural connections. Head trauma or a direct blow on the ear may damage the auditory apparatus, and spontaneous rupture of the membranes of the inner ear has been reported after vigorous activity.

INCIDENCE. Audiometric screening is the usual method utilized to determine hearing loss. The incidence of permanent hearing loss in high-risk infants is approximately 2%. In school-age children the frequency of hearing loss is about 3%. Approximately 1 in 1000 school-age children has severe to profound deafness.

CLINICAL MANIFESTATIONS. Acquired hearing loss is more readily apparent than the congenital form. Failure to respond to otherwise adequate auditory stimuli, behavior problems, and poor school performance are common. Simple attempted solutions such as playing the radio or television at loud volumes may suggest hearing loss.

It is difficult to diagnose hearing loss in infants. Because hearing and speech are intimately related, many of the symptoms of hearing deficiency are associated with speech and its pattern of development in the child.

The deaf infant does not respond to sounds but may babble. The child may experience frustration and show behavior problems if the hearing loss is not recognized. Failure to develop normal speech sounds in early childhood should prompt consideration of hearing loss as the explanation.

The profoundly deaf preschool child appears alert but does not speak. The partially deaf child behaves in different ways, depending on the hearing deficit. With high-tone deafness, the child does not hear certain consonants, and the absence of these from the speech make it appear garbled and unintelligible. The child with conductive hearing loss often speaks very softly (because his or her voice is so loud) and be shy and withdrawn. One should never wait for a delay in speech and language development before referring a child for hearing evaluation.

DIAGNOSIS. Early diagnosis of hearing loss is critical to successful habilitation. Brainstem electric response audiometry (BERA) is the most accurate method to assess auditory function in infants; even newborns can be tested. The pediatrician and family physician have a very important role to play in the early identification of hearing loss. Infants who present risk factors should be screened with BERA. This leads to the recognition of some 65% of hearing-impaired children. The 35% of them who have no risk factors can be identified by the primary-care physician. During well-baby visits, questions should be asked about auditory development. At 3 months old, does the infant awaken or quiet to the sound of the mother's voice, and does he or she react to it without seeing her? At 11 to 15 months, does the child turn to face familiar sounds, and does he or she point to objects when asked to? Does the 18-month-old toddler enjoy certain sounds and imitate them, does he or she point to parts of the body, and can he or she obey commands? If the parents are concerned about the child's hearing, take them seriously: they are indeed the best diagnosticians!

Andrée Durieux-Smith and Joann T. Dale

Upper Respiratory Tract

Growth and Development

In the newborn, the upper orifice of the larynx is more directly related to the nose than to the mouth (Fig. 10-1). Because the mouth is completely filled by the tongue (and by the nipple while sucking), the baby is an obligatory nose-breather and tolerates nasal obstruction very poorly. It interferes with sleep and feeding; in order to breathe the mouth must be opened, which the child does only when awake.

Grateful thanks for valuable suggestions and help in the preparation of this section to Dr. William Feldman, Dr. Peter McDonald, and Dr. Jeffrey Simons.

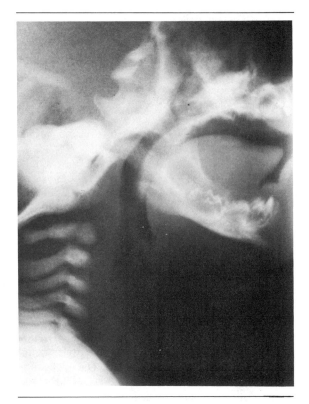

Fig. 10-1. Lateral radiograph of the neck of a healthy, 4-week-old girl. The tracheal airway is in a straight line with the nasal passage; the mouth is filled by the tongue. (Courtesy of Dr. Peter McDonald.)

Knowledge of the development of the craniofacial air cavities and of pharyngeal lymphoid tissue may help in understanding disorders affecting these (Table 10-1).

Nasal Passage and Paranasal Sinus Disorders

NASAL DISCHARGE. Clear (serous) nasal discharge is usually a viral condition (common cold). Wind, dust, and crying (nasal drainage of tears) may also produce transient sniffling. As a cold progresses, the coryza becomes thicker (seromucous, often mucopurulent, see below).

A serous or seromucous discharge that is prolonged and without signs of infection (fever) suggests *allergy*, particularly if it is seasonal and accompanied by spasmodic sneezing, tearing, and itchy nose and eyes. The child often shows a purplish-grey discoloration of the lower eyelids (so-called allergic shiners) and tends to rub his hand upward against

his nose (the "allergic salute"). The nasal mucosa is pale and edematous; the secretions may contain eosinophils.

Bloody nasal discharge results from local trauma (nose-picking, forcible nose blowing) or inflammation (see below). The hemorrhagic coryza ("snuffles") of the newborn with congenital syphilis is now very rare.

Unilateral discharge, usually purulent and fetid, strongly suggests a foreign body (pencil eraser, toothpaste tube cap, etc.), which is easily removed with or without the gentle use of a bivalve nasal speculum.

Bilateral *mucopurulent* secretion denotes bacterial infection with or without sinusitis, as described below. The secretion contains pus cells and bacteria.

NASAL OBSTRUCTION. All of the conditions just mentioned bring about a measure of interference with air flow by virtue of swollen mucosa and retained secretions.

As explained above, nasal obstruction is poorly tolerated by the newborn; its cause may be infection, congenital hypothyroidism, or a malformation. *Choanal atresia* is manifested from the time of birth especially if it is bilateral: the baby makes vigorous inspiratory efforts. When attempting to feed, and when asleep, the baby may be cyanosed. The diagnosis is suspected when a fine catheter cannot be passed up the nose into the pharynx.

Structural causes comprise *septal deviation,* though a marked degree of this is often surprisingly well tolerated; it should then be left alone. *Adenoid hyperplasia* and *chronic infection* will be discussed later. *Polyps* occur in nasal allergy and in cystic fibrosis. *Allergy* to inhalants or, sometimes, to food, e.g. cow's milk, can produce troublesome obstruction, often with coughing or even wheezing.

EPISTAXIS. Many children have repeated nosebleeds, often apparently spontaneous, which are commonly ascribed to vascular fragility in Kiesselbach's area of the septum. Viral or bacterial rhinitis may play a part. The finger-in-nose habit is to blame more often than the parents realize! Not very often, nosebleed, especially if frequently recurrent or severe, reveals a blood dyscrasia or bleeding disorder. The most common of the latter, and usually not otherwise manifested, is von Willebrand factor abnormality; it is best screened by the bleeding time and does not usually require particular treatment.

The bleeding almost always comes from the lower part of the septum. It can be stopped by placing in the nostril, up a centimeter or two, a cotton pledget soaked with hydrogen peroxide solution and pressing laterally on the wing of the nostril. This pressure is maintained for 5 to 10 minutes. The pledget is removed after 15 minutes; with it comes a clot, and the bleeding has stopped.

Cauterization of dilated vessels in Kiesselbach's area is

Table 10-1. The Mean Ages at Which Aeration of Craniofacial Cavities Becomes Radiologically and Clinically Significant, and the Relative Size of Pharyngeal Lymphoid Tissue.

Structure	Birth	1 year	3–4 yrs	6–7 yrs	10 yrs	13 yrs
Sinuses (aeration)	Maxillary antrum Ethmoid cells		Sphenoid	Frontal	Maxillary & zygomatic air cells	—
Mastoids (aeration)	Antrum	—	Mastoid process air cells	—	—	—
Adenoids (relative size)	±	++	+++	++	+	+
Tonsils (relative size)	−	+	++	+++	++	++

(Adapted from B. F. Jaffe. Development of the Respiratory Tract. In T. R. Johnson, et al. [Eds.]. *Children are Different. Developmental Physiology* [2nd ed.]. Columbus: Ross Laboratories, 1978; and F. N. Silverman. *Caffey's Pediatric X-Ray Diagnosis: An Integrated Approach* [8th ed.], Vol. II. Chicago: Year Book, 1984.)

seldom necessary and is not always effective. When not done well, it carries the danger of mucosal ulceration and atrophy and even of septal perforation.

Viral Upper Respiratory Infections

THE COMMON COLD. This expression, though avoided by some as nonscientific, conveys well what it means, and is more precise than upper respiratory infection (URI), which comprises almost all that will be described in the remainder of this section!

Though a serous or seromucous coryza may be due to irritation or allergy, the common cold is caused mostly by a large number of viruses, notably rhinoviruses, with a high rate of communicability. Coryza is a constant feature of measles, preceding the eruption by 3 or 4 days, during which there is much fever, and is common also at the onset of varicella and rubella. This discussion will focus on the colds of the infant and young child.

Sneezing in the newborn is normal and almost never means infection. In the infant, colds become frequent at 3 or 4 months of age. One of the earliest symptoms is difficulty in nursing at the breast or bottle, as obstruction of the nose makes it necessary for him to breathe through the mouth. Irritability, crying, and restlessness are the result. Within 3 or 4 days the secretions may become thick and tenacious, due to irritation of mucous glands (catarrhal inflammation), making the obstruction more troublesome. Fever in the uncomplicated cold rarely exceeds 38.5°C. There is a decreased desire for fluids or solids and sleeplessness or frequent awakening. Coughing in short spells and sometimes vomiting of food or mucus may occur, due to pooling of secretions in the hypopharynx. A degree of conjunctivitis is often present with redness and tearing. Mild hyperemia is seen in the oropharynx and on the eardrums. This, in the absence of tympanic edema, bulging, reduced mobility, and obscured landmarks, must not be mistaken for otitis media

(see pages 166–167); but it is a good reason to watch the ears for its possible development. In all of the mucosal areas mentioned, secondary bacterial invasion may produce conditions that are described in this chapter.

There is, of course, no specific *treatment* for a cold. Positioning of the infant (on the sides or the stomach) may be quite helpful in easing drainage of secretions. A rolled blanket placed against the back may facilitate lying on the side. Sometimes a round-ended dropper may be used to remove secretions, but it should never be introduced into the nostrils. In high latitudes, where the air in a heated house may be quite dry, use of a humidifier or boiling some water often helps. An ultrasonic cold-vapor apparatus must be cleaned often and used only with distilled water. The ideal temperature of the room is 20°C, and the ideal humidity is from 40 to 60%. Feeding may have to be fractionated; sufficient intake of fluids is especially important. Smoking in the room, even in the home, is best avoided. Medication (dosage carefully adapted to body size, see Appendix C) should be limited to acetaminophen for fever higher than 38°C and possibly one of the decongestant mixtures. Though there is no evidence that the latter's routine use is beneficial, the impression is that they sometimes give relief when congestion is quite marked. One that is well tolerated combines an antihistaminic with two sympathomimetics. Other preparations, notably pseudoephedrine, may cause agitation and are best avoided; vasoconstrictor nose drops too, for the same reason, and because of the rebound effect and the local irritation they produce. Normal saline drops are harmless and may be helpful. Prophylactic antibiotics are never needed in the otherwise healthy child; but, of course, one must be on the alert for secondary bacterial infection.

A common cold may well last more than the proverbial "1 week or 7 days." If it does the parents may need reassurance, as often their patience is severely exercised. Beyond 2 weeks, especially if cough is a feature, and before that time, in the presence of persistent fever, increasing cough or dyspnea, pain in the ears, and purulent nasal or ocular secretions, a medical visit is indicated.

RECURRENT, PROLONGED, AND CHRONIC COLDS: EPIDEMIOLOGY. During the first 3 years of life, the normal child living in a temperate climate has 3 to 8 colds per year. This fact may be invoked in reassuring parents who fear that their child is having too many. At the same time, if colds are really frequent or tend to linger, the physician thinks of the factors that may come into play. One is *day care* in homes or facilities where there are many preschoolers. That such children are prone to frequent infections (respiratory and intestinal mainly) is undisputed, although not a valid argument against day care when it is necessary or advantageous to the parents. Another possible factor is *allergy,* alluded to above and fully discussed in Chap. 21. While the role of inhalants in asthma is often considered, their not infrequent responsibility or that of foods (e.g., cow's milk or soybean allergies) in protracted upper respiratory symptoms must not be discounted. The diagnosis of such allergy in infancy and early childhood does not rest on skin testing, but on history, dietary change, and effect of reintroducing a food that has been withheld. *Ambient factors* need to be examined: house air (too dry, too warm); clothing (too little or too much; often a bundled-up youngster in wintertime is overdressed); and dust and smoke, especially "passive smoking." The efforts of the doctor in persuading a parent to give up smoking in the child's (and the parent's) interest may be very rewarding.

Suppurative Infections in the Nasal and Paranasal Areas

These are characterized by thick mucoid or mucopurulent secretions, cough of variable severity and frequency, and obstruction leading to mouth breathing. This may result from mucosal swelling, lymphoid hyperplasia, and viscid secretions. It may seem to complicate a viral cold or supervene on its own. Involvement of the middle ears is common.

Sinusitis accompanies any catarrhal inflammation of the nasal passages. The cavities that are involved depend on the patient's age (see Table 10-1). Suppuration within a sinus is suggested by fever, headache, pain, and tenderness over the cavity involved. Antral pain may be referred to the cheekbone or upper teeth. Ethmoid infection produces pain between the eyes, and in young children can cause puffiness of the eyelids, which may be mistaken for blepharitis or conjunctivitis. Osteomyelitis of facial bones, meningitis, and cavernous sinus thrombosis are serious complications; fortunately they are now infrequent. Radiography and transillumination are not always reliable in the young child: they may suggest opacification when the child is in good health.

Bacterial infection of the nasopharynx must be suspected when there is fever and the secretions are purulent, often with crusting of the nostril rims. Impetiginization of the upper lip suggests the presence of hemolytic streptococci. There may be a drop of yellowish or greenish pus in the inner canthus, if not frank purulent conjunctivitis with marked hyperemia of the mucosa and edema of the eyelids. When this occurs, *H. influenzae* is often isolated from the eye and nasopharynx; there may well be an otitis media. Also frequently found in prolonged nasopharyngitis are *B. catarrhalis* and *S. pneumoniae.*

Nasal swabs are painful and often yield a skin-type flora, including staphylococci that are not necessarily the cause of infection. Much to be preferred is nasopharyngeal intubation (Auger suction), which is easily and almost painlessly done with a premature-size feeding tube inserted to a depth of some 5 to 7 cm (according to age) and fitted to a syringe. Although the presence of bacteria, even in heavy growth, does not exactly satisfy Koch's postulates, it suggests that bacterial infection is quite possibly causal. That suitable antibiotic therapy is often beneficial in such circumstances adds weight to this view. Attention needs to be paid to the epidemiological factors mentioned above, all of which may play a part in a "chronic cold."

Infections of the Oropharynx

ACUTE PHARYNGITIS. Sore throats in children may be due to viruses (Chap. 20) as well as to bacteria, the most important of which are the betahemolytic streptococci of group A. The pathogenesis, epidemiology, and treatment of infections with these streptococci are fully discussed in Chap. 20. These organisms are frequently found in nasopharyngitis in infants, as described earlier; they are a common cause of oropharyngitis with tonsillitis from the age of 4 years onwards. Pharyngitis is also one of the signs of Kawasaki disease (Chap. 18).

Clinical Features. Pharyngitis is usually manifested by fever (mild to marked), irritability, coughing, disinclination to feed and to drink sometimes to the point of dysphagia, and even drooling: in the last instance acute epiglottitis may be suspected (see Acute Epiglottitis). A child old enough (about 2 years old) to do so may say that his throat is sore. Vomiting and abdominal pain (diffuse or periumbilical) are common.

In viral pharyngitis, the entire oropharynx is red and swollen to a variable degree. Rhinitis is often present as well. The disease lasts from 1 to 5 days. Papules and vesicles of 1 to 2 mm diameter may appear on the soft palate and anterior faucial pillars and soon form shallow greyish or yellowish ulcers surrounded by a rim of erythema: this, originally described by Marfan as pustular pharyngitis, was later rediscovered by Zahorski who called it herpangina, an unfortunate name, because it is not due to herpes simplex (whose vesicles appear in the anterior parts of the mouth) but to some coxsackie A viruses (see Chap. 20). When in addition the child has a maculopapular rash on the palms and soles, one speaks of hand-foot-and-mouth disease.

Clinicians differ on whether streptococcal sore throat can be distinguished clinically, with some confidence, from the viral. In favor of the streptococcal form are sudden onset (often with such constitutional symptoms as abdominal pain and initial vomiting); sustained fever; subjective symptoms of sore throat and painful swallowing; bright red swelling of the faucial pillars, tonsils, uvula, and free edge of the soft palate; a fine macular rash on the soft palate; the "strawberry tongue" (with a whitish coat through which enlarged red papillae are showing); and a typical smell of the breath. A scarlatinal rash on the skin is pathognomonic. But lymph node enlargement in the anterior triangle of the neck can just as likely be due to adenoviral or Epstein-Barr virus infection. Whitish or yellowish exudate on the tonsils, usually in discrete patches centered by cryptic openings, is quite suggestive of streptococcal infection, although it is also consistent (and the more so if it is extensive or confluent) with infectious mononucleosis. Pharyngeal diphtheria, though now exceptional in many areas, must be considered (see Chap. 20). It is common to mistake for exudate the punctate white plugs, consisting of desquamated epithelium, which normally occupy the cryptic openings; these may become prominent by contrast whenever there is hyperemia of the tonsillar mucosa.

Management. The child's malaise and irritability can be very trying for the parents, and they must be reassured. Acetaminophen is a valuable antipyretic and analgesic. It is preferred to aspirin whose synergistic effect with certain viruses may cause Reye's syndrome. Sucking crushed ice or frozen fruit juice on a stick helps to numb the pain and to maintain hydration. Sufficient fluid intake is often effective in keeping the temperature down. Warm sponge baths followed by brisk rubbing are relaxing and help in the dissipation of body heat.

When practical, especially in the presence of exudate and in a child over the age of 3, a culture or a latex agglutination test for streptococcal antigen from a throat swab is advised, and a blood antibody test for infectious mononucleosis is often useful in diagnosis. In the many areas where rheumatic fever has become rare, the main reasons for penicillin therapy in streptococcal infections are to relieve the child's symptoms and perhaps to check the spread of infection in

home and school. For that purpose, one of the salts of penicillin V, given orally for 10 days, is preferred. It is not certain that such therapy lessens the likelihood of the child remaining a carrier of beta-hemolytic streptococci of group A. This carrier state is common; indeed, the finding of these bacteria on culture does not always mean that a child's sore throat is due to them, and many an instance of reputed persistent or recurrent streptococcal throat infection may merely represent a carrier state.

PERITONSILLAR ABSCESS. Peritonsillar abscess (tonsillar abscess, quinsy) is a localized collection of pus within the deep parts of a tonsillar crypt, which passes to peritonsillar areas by extension. It is seen less frequently since the advent of antibiotics. The condition is frequently unilateral, is well circumscribed, and tends to recur.

Fever and constitutional symptoms are present. There is a sore throat. Pain on swallowing and enlarged cervical lymph nodes are evident.

The tonsil is enlarged and inflamed, and the tonsillar pillar is displaced to one side beyond the midline by edema and an accumulation of pus. By the time the infection is localized, the abscess may be seen pointing to the palate at the upper pole of the tonsil.

Antibiotics if given early will abort the condition. Gargles help relieve the pain. Once the abscess is formed, surgical drainage is required.

RETROPHARYNGEAL ABSCESS. A retropharyngeal abscess is a suppurative lesion of one or more of the lymph nodes that lie behind the pharynx. It is secondary to infection in this area and occurs most frequently in children during the first 2 years of life. Onset usually follows an infection of the upper respiratory tract and is heralded by a sudden rise in temperature. Symptoms depend to a large degree on the position of the suppurating node. If it is high, the nose is blocked; if low, respirations are impaired. There may be difficulty in swallowing, and respirations are often noisy and bubbling in character. The child cannot rest because of difficulty in breathing and when exhausted allows his head to fall back. Each time this happens the abscess is pushed forward by the curvature of the cervical spine, the airway is blocked, and the child becomes terrified from momentary suffocation. Torticollis and cervical adenitis may also be present.

Inspection of the throat reveals distinct bulging of the posterior wall of the pharynx, perhaps more marked on one side than the other. The fluctuation can be detected by palpation. Danger from a viscerovagal reflex and cardiac arrest is ever present. Rupture of the abscess may lead to aspiration. Digital examination should be conducted with extreme caution. A lateral roentgenogram of the neck demonstrates the forward bulge in the posterior pharyngeal wall (Fig. 10-2).

Treatment. Antibiotic therapy should be instituted promptly. If the abscess is fluctuant, surgical drainage should be performed with the patient under anesthesia and in the Trendelenburg position to prevent aspiration of the abscess contents.

Hypertrophy of Adenoids and Tonsils

Much that has been printed and taught in the past concerning these organs and the need for their removal was based on ignorance of the fact that the tremendous growth they show in childhood is a physiological process. The present tendency is to respect immunologic role of the tissues and to spare the child the pain and possible complications attendant upon the operation.

THE ADENOIDS. Adenoids show clinically significant hyperplasia earlier than do the tonsils (see Table 10-1). This, combined with the effects of infection, may produce mouth breathing, irritability, and difficulty in feeding. In most cases the symptoms tends to decrease under treatment and with time. Surgical removal of the adenoids is of advantage only if, after an adequate period of care and observation, there is a significant degree of functional impairment. This is manifested mainly by agitation at night with snoring and frequent awakening, somnolence in the daytime, and lack of appetite. A tape recorder placed beside the child's bed is a good way to document the interference with sleep. In a few cases, the obstruction to the airway leads to hypoventilation, sleep apnea, hypoxia, and even to right heart failure.

The classical "adenoid facies" with open mouth and prominent upper lip often has nothing to do with nasopharyngeal obstruction: it may be related to maxillodental malocclusion or to abnormal position or mobility of the tongue. Mouth breathing seems to be a habit in some children who have no nasal obstruction. Frequent nasal infection would be an indication for adequate treatment of each episode, and for correction of the contributory factors outlined above, not for adenoidectomy. Nor is there any evidence, contrary to what is often stated, that the operation is beneficial in chronic or recurrent middle ear infections.

THE TONSILS. Usually invisible at birth, tonsils normally show much growth in childhood, reaching a maximum around 5 to 7 years of age (Fig. 10-3). Their size alone is of no concern; many a pair of round, juicy-looking tonsils that touch each other in midline is perfectly well tolerated. As is true of adenoids, they too tend to swell like sponges in the presence of infection and, often, allergy. Their removal

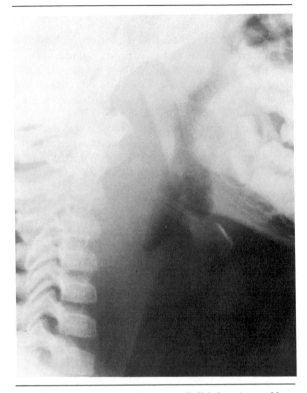

Fig. 10-2. Retropharyngeal abscess or cellulitis in a 4-year-old girl: widening of space between cervical vertebrae and pharyngeal lumen. (Courtesy of Dr. Peter McDonald.)

should not be considered before the age of 4 years, some say 5 to 7, and before a few months' treatment or observation. Many a time, the child who has been referred for tonsillectomy does not need it by the time he is seen by the specialist. Infection as such is not an indication; there is no evidence supporting often-stated criteria such as 3 throat infections in 1 year. Tonsillectomy does *not* prevent subsequent throat infections, though the infections do present differently in the absence of tonsils. Nor does it lessen the number of days lost in school because of sore throats, especially if one takes into account the postoperative sore throat.

Tonsillectomy is indicated (1) if significant obstruction interfering with feeding and sleep is present and persistent despite adequate observation and treatment (e.g., a long course of a suitable antibacterial if infection is a factor), (2) after a peritonsillar abscess that has recurred in spite of adequate antibiotic treatment, and (3) in marked hyper-

child lives, ultimately result in deformities of the chest. The infant has difficulty sucking and taking foods because of dyspnea. Direct visualization of the larynx by a laryngoscopy and roentgenography is required to make the diagnosis in most instances.

Laryngeal web must be dilated at birth or the infant may not survive. Stenosis of the larynx may require tracheostomy. Pressure on the larynx and trachea by such *extrinsic masses* as teratoma and cystic hygroma necessitates their surgical removal. *Vascular ring,* caused by a complete or incomplete double aortic arch, may also constrict the trachea and cause stridor. Hypoplasia of the mandible with or without cleft palate (*Pierre Robin syndrome*) and the resulting respiratory difficulty associated with the poorly functioning musculature of the tongue and pharynx may also produce stridor. A *subglottic hemangioma* is congenital, but like cutaneous capillary hemangiomata, which may be present, grows during the first months. It may produce dyspnea in the same age range with similar manifestations as viral laryngitis, and it may respond likewise to steroids. In case of doubt, laryngoscopy is advised. Pressure of the thymus on the larynx and trachea is no longer considered a problem. In the past, many infants were treated by radiation for "enlarged thymus," but there has been an increase in thyroid carcinoma in this group of children secondary to the irradiation, and this procedure is no longer performed.

Birth injury resulting in dislocation of the cricoid cartilages of the larynx may require manipulative replacement and tracheostomy. Unilateral or bilateral birth trauma due to instrumentation may cause paralysis of the recurrent laryngeal and/or phrenic nerve.

Congenital laryngeal stridor (laryngomalacia) may appear at or shortly after birth, persist for months, and then disappear. It is more common than the congenital malformations noted above. The infant appears to suffer no great inconvenience. The stridor diminishes in intensity when the infant is quiet or asleep. No specific treatment is required, but mothers need reassurance. The cause is floppiness of the epiglottis and the supraglottic aperture.

Papillomas may grow on the vocal cords and cause dyspnea and hoarseness. This distressing condition may require frequent surgical removal of the tumors from the vocal cords and prolonged tracheostomy. At puberty the lesions regress.

FOREIGN BODIES. Frequently lodged in larynx and trachea, foreign bodies produce hoarseness, stridor, tracheal tug, and dyspnea. If the child cannot breathe, speak, or cough there is an emergency. An infant should be placed face down at an angle of 60 degrees, and four blows given with the heel of the hand high in the interscapular area. If

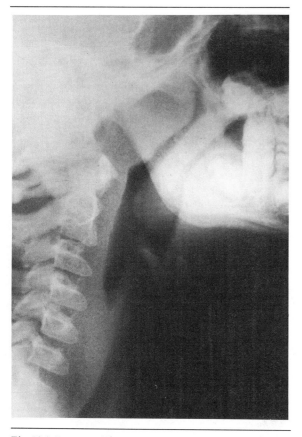

Fig. 10-3. Large tonsils and adenoid in a 6-year-old boy. (Courtesy of Dr. Peter McDonald.)

trophy of only one tonsil, if required for biopsy purposes. Some clinicians are not convinced indication 1 ever exists.

The child who is to have nose or throat surgery should be prepared psychologically for it. A preliminary visit to the operating suite and familiarization with the anesthetic gear are of much help.

Larynx

CONGENITAL MALFORMATIONS. Congenital malformations (see Chap. 9) of the larynx and the organs adjacent to it are promptly manifest in the newborn period by stridor and dyspnea. The laryngeal "crow," or hoarseness, is so characteristic as hardly to need description. The cyanosis, dyspnea, and severe supraclavicular, intercostal, and subcostal retractions that accompany these conditions, if the

the obstruction persists, the infant is placed supine on a table and four rapid thrusts are given to the sternum. (After 1 year of age, the Heimlich maneuver is done.) If the obstruction persists, one may try to draw the tongue away from the fauces and thus reveal the foreign body. A foreign body in the trachea will be shown by radiography in most instances; endoscopy is necessary to remove it.

ANGIOEDEMA OF THE GLOTTIS. Glottal angioedema is an immediate allergic response to a food, injection, bee sting, etc. Prompt treatment with epinephrine subcutaneously followed by an antihistamine intramuscularly is necessary. Preventive treatment by desensitization to the insect responsible should be considered.

SPASM OF THE LARYNX. So-called spasmodic croup, of unknown cause, may be distinct from acute viral laryngitis, described later, which it resembles except for the absence of fever and signs of inflammation. It appears suddenly in a child of 1 to 3 years, mostly in the evening or at night, and recedes in the daytime. It may reappear the following evening or two. Principles of treatment are the same as for subglottic laryngitis (see Inflammation of the Larynx).

Spasm of the glottis, or *laryngismus stridulosus,* was common in former years in children of 6 to 18 months of age as a manifestation of rachitic tetany. It would supervene mostly about the vernal equinox, when skin synthesis of vitamin D under the sun's rays would precipitate hypocalcemia and deposition of mineral in osteoid tissue. Convulsions could also occur. Immediate treatment was calcium gluconate intravenously.

INFLAMMATION OF THE LARYNX. *Acute Subglottic Laryngitis.* "Viral croup" or acute laryngotracheobronchitis is most often due to para-influenza viruses. It usually has a gradual onset in an infant or young child who has had a cold for a few days. The voice and cough become hoarse, and the inspiration may be stridulous. With significant restriction to air flow, there are tachypnea, nasal flaring, and retractions that are suprasternal at first. As the condition worsens retractions are also intercostal and infracostal. In severe cases the child is quite dyspneic and agitated. Auscultation may detect decreases in air movement. A radiograph of the neck in the anteroposterior position may show narrowing of the subglottic airway (the "steeple sign," Fig. 10-4).

It is important to rule out other causes of upper airway obstruction, such as retropharyngeal abscess, foreign body, angioedema of the glottis, subglottic hemangioma, infectious mononucleosis, acute epiglottitis, and bacterial tracheitis.

Initial treatment consists of placing the child in a moist, cool environment, close to a reassured parent. Oxygen is given in the presence of dyspnea or agitation. Most children respond well to this therapy. Marked obstruction should be treated in an intensive-care environment. Especially important are such signs of hypoxia as increasing agitation, altered level of consciousness, and cyanosis that persists in 40% oxygen. One may resort to the administration of racemic epinephrine 2.25% solution by nebulization in a dose of 0.5 ml in 3.5 ml of normal saline; if this is effective it may be repeated in 30 to 60 minutes. One must be on guard for a rebound effect. Dexamethasone may be given intravenously or intramuscularly, but its value has not been conclusively proved. Rarely, if insufficient relief has not been obtained, endotracheal intubation is necessary.

Acute Epiglottitis. In reality supraglottic laryngitis, epiglottitis is due most often to *H. influenzae* type B. It supervenes mostly in children from 2 to 7 years of age. Inflammatory swelling causes the epiglottis to protrude backward and downard over the glottic opening. Onset is usually sudden and symptoms progress rapidly. The child is feverish and appears ill. Inspiratory stridor may be low-pitched, gurgling, or hissing in quality. The child drools and does not attempt to swallow. He or she tends to sit up, leaning on the arms, with mouth open and lower jaw in a forward position. The child should not be made to lie down but rather to sit on a parent's lap. Inspection of the throat of a cooperative child often reveals the typical cherry-like mass of the inflamed epiglottis, but *no* attempt should be made to depress the tongue in order to see it. A lateral radiograph of the neck shows the swollen epiglottis (Fig. 10-5), but it should not be obtained at the expense of delaying treatment.

No time should be wasted in performing endotracheal intubation under general anesthesia. The nasotracheal route is preferred. Cultures of the secretions and the blood are obtained and antibiotic therapy started intravenously. At this time, the recommended choice is ampicillin and chloramphenicol. In some areas, because of the pattern of the organism's resistance to antibiotics, cefuroxime is perferred. Extubation is usually done in 1 or 2 days. The possible presence of concomitant meningitis or arthritis due to invasive *H. influenzae* should be kept in mind.

INFLAMMATION OF THE TRACHEA. *Bacterial Tracheitis.* An uncommon condition due mostly to *S. aureus, H. influenzae,* and *S. pneumoniae,* it clinically resembles a severe laryngitis. The child is quite ill. Direct laryngoscoy reveals inflammation with thick sticky secretions and membrane formation. Antibiotics are required. If nasotracheal intubation is done, one must guard against obstruction of the tube by membranes. For this purpose frequent instillation of saline solution is advised.

Paul de Bellefeuille, Joann T. Dale, and Mohsen Ziai

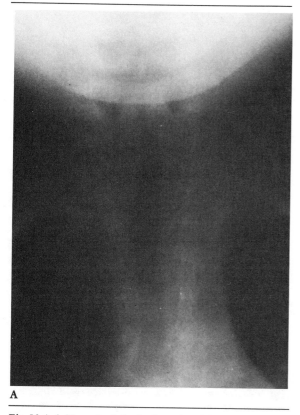

A

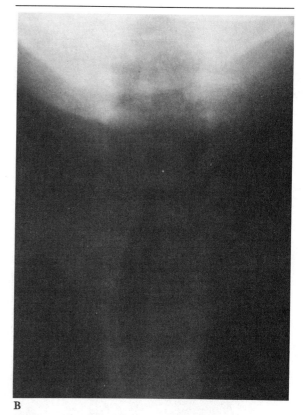

B

Fig. 10-4. A. Normal subglottic airway in a 16-month-old boy.
B. Subglottic edema in a 21-month-old boy: the "steeple sign."
(Courtesy of Dr. Peter McDonald.)

Lower Respiratory Tract

Bronchial Infections

BRONCHITIS. Bronchitis, usually accompanied by some degree of tracheitis, is often preceded by an upper respiratory tract infection. The primary cause in most cases is viral. The respiratory syncytial virus (RSV), adenovirus, influenza or parainfluenza viruses, and coxsackie virus groups A and B have all been associated with bronchitis. In addition, bronchitis occurs with measles, myocplasma infections, and pertussis. Secondary bacterial infection is not uncommon. The condition usually affects children in the first 4 years of life.

Clinical Manifestations. The onset is abrupt, with rhinorrhea and a temperature about 38.5°C that lasts for 2 or 3 days. There is a harsh cough that is worse at night, in a warm stuffy room, aggravated by cigarette smoke, and that becomes productive in 2 or 3 days; it may be paroxysmal or followed by vomiting. In the presence of a past or family history of respiratory allergy, wheezing may occur. Physical examination reveals audible and at times palpable rhonchi, with some moist rales and wheezing.

Course and Prognosis. The cough resolves spontaneously in 1 or 2 weeks. Secondary infections such as otitis media may complicate the condition.

Laboratory Investigations. Chest roentgenograms are normal or show increased lung markings. The leukocyte count is usually normal. Leukocytosis suggests secondary infection. Bacterial nasopharyngeal culture yields nonspecific organisms and are not helpful. Nasopharyngeal viral cultures or rapid viral diagnostic tests may identify the offending viral agent.

Treatment. No specific treatment is indicated unless secondary infection is present, in which case an appropriate antibacterial drug may be given if necessary. An adequate fluid intake should be provided, and fine mist may help secretions. Antihistamines, decongestants, and antitussives

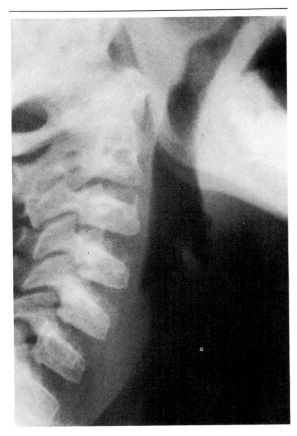

A

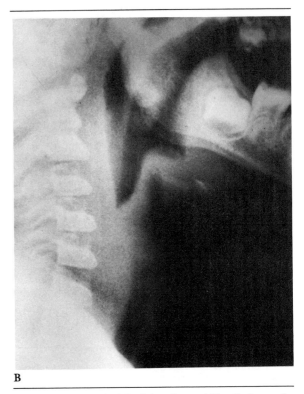

B

Fig. 10-5. A. Normal epiglottis in a 6-year-old boy. B. Acute epiglottitis in a 2-year-old boy. (Courtesy of Dr. Peter McDonald.)

have no proven efficacy in bronchitis and may retard recovery. Sedatives are not usually indicated because of the danger of excessive suppression of the cough, with retention of mucus in the lungs. Analgesic therapy with acetaminophen may be helpful.

BRONCHIOLITIS. Bronchiolitis mainly affects infants under 2 years and most often 2 to 12 months of age. It is characterized by inflammatory changes in the lower respiratory tract, predominantly involving the bronchioles. The bronchiolar lumen is narrowed by mucosal thickening, mucous plugs, cellular debris, and in some cases spasm, leading to small areas of atelectasis and emphysema and resulting in hypoventilation. This important disease is responsible for hospitalization of large numbers of seriously ill infants, chiefly in winter and spring.

Pathophysiology. In the already narrow bronchioles of infants, even a small diminution in the radius secondary to inflammation greatly decreases the surface area. Hypoventilation causes a decline in alveolar oxygen tension (PO_2),

which falls at a much steeper rate than does blood oxygen saturation. In severe cases, oxygen saturation may diminish sufficiently to result in clinical cyanosis. The arterial carbon dioxide tension (PCO_2) tends to rise, leading to respiratory acidosis, although in milder cases this trend is controlled by increased ventilation of normally functioning alveoli. With clinical recovery, arterial PO_2 is usually normal within 2 weeks, but in a few cases hypoxemia has persisted for 4 to 8 weeks after the height of the illness.

Etiology. The respiratory syncytial virus, considered by many to be the single most important viral agent in the respiratory tract during infancy and childhood, is the cause in the majority of instances. Other agents associated with bronchiolitis are parainfluenza viruses, adenoviruses, influenza viruses, and *Mycoplasma pneumoniae.* In about a third of the cases bronchiolitis is later followed by bronchial asthma, and in some of these patients there is a family history of respiratory allergy.

Clinical Manifestations. The onset is initiated by an infection of the upper respiratory tract, followed by a cough and a few days later by the sudden onset of tachypnea, expiratory wheezing, and a variable degree of intercostal and sternal retraction. The infant may be pale or cyanotic. Fever is usually low grade and lasts only about 3 days. Respirations are rapid (40–80/min) and shallow, with an expiratory wheeze and grunt, and tachycardia is present. The lungs may be hyperresonant to percussion. In the early stages rales may be absent, but scattered fine rales, and later, as the cough loosens, moist rales are heard. Breath sounds may be reduced in intensity. Overinflation of the lungs may cause the liver and at times the spleen to be displaced downward, raising the possibility of congestive cardiac failure, particularly when significant tachycardia is present. Mild conjunctivitis is present in about one-third of cases, otitis media in 5 to 10%, and pharyngitis of varied severity in about 50%.

Chest roentgenograms show signs of generalized obstructive emphysema with depressed diaphragms, increased radiolucency of the lung fields; increased lung markings; and in some cases areas of collapse or consolidation. The heart usually appears small.

Course and Prognosis. Most symptoms subside in 3 to 5 days, though cough may persist for a week or more. The mortality is about 1% or less, varying in different series and epidemics.

Laboratory Investigations. Nasopharyngeal cultures for bacterial pathogens yield organisms no more frequently in these patients than in controls. The viral agent, usually RSV, can be grown from nasopharyngeal secretions or identified by rapid viral diagnostic tests. The leukocyte count is normal or mildly elevated with a left shift. This latter finding does not necessarily mean secondary bacterial infection.

Diagnosis and Treatment. In the differential diagnosis, allergic bronchitis should be considered in the presence of a past or family history of allergy or when attacks are recurrent. Left-sided heart failure due to congenital heart disease, especially as a result of patent ductus, ventricular septal defect, or, rarely, endocardial fibroelastosis, may cause wheezing and fine rales. The chest x-ray film shows cardiac enlargement; electrocardiographic changes are present; and in the case of ventricular septal defect and patent ductus, a murmur is present. Cystic fibrosis should be considered when recovery is delayed or the child has diarrhea or malnutrition. The sweat chloride test can confirm this diagnosis.

A small infant is often better managed in an incubator than in a tent. The baby should be kept with the head and shoulders partially raised. Hydration should be well maintained if necessary by careful administration of intraveneous fluids. This helps to prevent thickening of secretions. If the baby is not too ill to take feedings by mouth, frequent small feedings are better tolerated than larger feedings; the latter further embarrass respiration and cause regurgitation and aspiration. Nasal secretions may be removed with a rubber suction bulb.

Most important in the management is the continuous and uninterrupted administration of oxygen, even in the absence of cyanosis. In most cases, concentrations in the incubator of 40% are adequate to control hypoxemia. The PaO_2 should be maintained at 70 to 90 mm Hg. Blood gases or cutaneous oxygen saturation determinations should be done as clinically indicated.

Specific anti-RSV therapy in the form of ribavirin is recommended for infants with severe disease (decreasing PaO_2, increasing PCO_2) and for those predisposed to serious disease (congenital heart disease with pulmonary hypertension, chronic lung disease such as bronchopulmonary dysplasia). Ribavirin is given by small particle aerosol in a tent or headbox for 12 to 18 hours/day for 3 to 7 days. The efficacy of this treatment is not fully established but it does appear to increase PaO_2.

If respiratory failure occurs, rising $PaCO_2$ is greater than or equal to 65 mm Hg with falling arterial pH, despite oxygen and ribavirin therapy, then the infant should be intubated and ventilated. Ribavirin therapy may be continued but with extreme caution, because it may clog the ventilator values or tubes and cause obstruction. In infants with marked tachycardia, tachypnea, and hepatomegaly, congenital heart disease with heart failure complicating the infection must be ruled out. An electrocardiogram, echocardiogram, and chest roentgenograms are often helpful. If heart failure is present, digoxin and judicious use of diuretics and fluid restriction may be necessary.

Antibacterial drugs are unnecessary because this is a viral disease, and secondary bacterial infections are unusual. Adrenergic bronchodilators including salbutamol and steroid agents such as dexamethasone have been tried but without objective effect when compared to placebo. Some authorities, however, recommend a trial of salbutamol aerosol and/or intravenous aminophylline in severe cases. Sedatives and cough suppressants should be avoided because they may aggravate hypoventilation. Restlessness is more likely an indication of increasing hypoxemia and impending respiratory failure. Appropriate isolation procedures especially good handwashing must be utilized with all hospitalized bronchiolitis infants to minimize nosocomial spread of the virus.

BRONCHIECTASIS. Bronchiectasis is abnormal dilatation of the bronchi and may be cylindrical, fusiform, or saccular, and localized or widespread. It was previously thought that collapse of a segment or lobe of the lung was an essential precursor of bronchiectasis, but there is now evidence that the disease may result from damage to the bronchial wall without atelectasis.

Bronchiectasis in childhood may be associated with a predisposing congenital problem such as cystic fibrosis, ciliary dyskinesis syndrome, immunodeficiency, or congenital lung cysts. Secondary local infection leads to damage to the bronchial wall with resultant bronchiectasis. Some children without underlying congenital abnormalities also develop bronchiectasis, but this is now relatively unusual. It may occur following foreign body aspiration or more rarely, measles, pertussis, or pneumonia. In patients with underlying conditions, bronchiectasis may be generalized or localized. In patients without underlying abnormalities it is usually localized and, therfore, more amenable to surgery.

CLINICAL MANIFESTATIONS. Persistent rhinorrhea, recurrent or persistent moist cough, recurrent fever, anorexia, pallor, failure to gain weight, and clubbing of the fingers are typical. Wheezing or rattling in the chest is sometimes present. Older children may produce purulent sputum. Exacerbations, with bronchitis or pneumonia, tend to occur during winter months. If there is a predisposing condition such as cystic fibrosis, relentless progression of symptoms is usually seen. Physical examination reveals rales over the affected areas. With atelectasis there may be impaired breath sounds and dullness to percussion. Complications consist of recurrent attacks of pneumonia and occasionally empyema, more rarely brain abscess, or purulent meningitis. Hemoptysis is rare in children.

Course and Prognosis. The prognosis for life depends upon whether an underlying predisposing condition is present. If not, prognosis is generally good, but symptoms persist to a variable extent. Most symptomatic patients are undersized and underweight. The prognosis is more favorable in cylindrical bronchiectasis than in saccular bronchiectasis.

Diagnosis and Treatment. The diagnosis can often be made by computerized axial tomography of the lungs. Occasionally, bronchography is necessary. When the diagnosis of bronchiectasis is considered in any child, one must rule out predisposing conditions such as cystic fibrosis or immunodeficiency. A high index of suspicion should be maintained when respiratory symptoms tend to persist after adequate treatment of infants with bronchiolitis, interstitial pneumonia, measles, or pertussis. In the case of foreign body, the obstructing object should be removed without delay by bronchoscopy. The history of inhalation may be difficult to obtain but is usually one of sudden choking when the child had something in the mouth, followed by a cough or wheeze. The acute episode tends to be forgotten.

Antibiotics, according to sensitivity studies of organisms cultured from sputum or tracheal secretions, may be given intermittently for exacerbations or may be given for prolonged periods. The former is preferred on account of the potential development of drug-resistant organisms or side effects from the drugs. In addition to specific treatment, it is important to direct attention to restoration of a good nutritional state. Postural drainage, with percurssion over the affected area, should be carried out daily. This is more likely to be successful, because of superior cooperation, in the older child. Mucolytic agents such as *N*-acetylcysteine are not helpful but bronchodilators such as aerosolized salbutamol may facilitate postural drainage during acute exacerbations in some patients.

Surgical treatment is most effective when applied to removal of functionless lobes in patients with localized severe bronchiectasis. When extensive surgical removal is carried out, hypoventilation and persistent dyspnea may follow. Spread of bronchiectasis after it is established is uncommon.

Pneumonia

Acute respiratory infections are one of the most common problems in pediatrics. Although a normal child may have six to eight respiratory illnesses a year, these are usually self-limited upper-tract infections with minimal morbidity. In contrast, pneumonias account for less than 10% of acute respiratory illnesses but can cause significant morbidity and mortality, especially in infants.

Pneumonia is inflammation of the lung parenchyma. This does not occur often because of the efficient host defense mechanisms of the lower respiratory tract. These include the epiglottic reflex, which prevents aspiration of infectious or noxious materials; the mucus-secreting cells, mucosal antibody, ciliated epithelium, and cough reflex, which serve to trap and propel or expel aspirated material from the lower tract; the phagocytic cells — macrophages and polymorphonuclear leukocytes — and opsonins; and the lymphatics, which try to destroy and eliminate microorganisms and foreign matter from the terminal bronchioles and alveoli.

Viruses are the most common agents that upset these host defense mechanisms and lead to inflammation and pneumonia; however, many other infectious agents can cause childhood pneumonia, including bacteria, mycoplasmas, rickettsiae, chlamydiae, fungi, and protozoa. Lung infiltrates, inflammation, or both can also be seen with foreign body aspiration, congestive heart failure, hypersensitivity reactions, hydrocarbon inhalation, and tumor metastases.

The diagnosis of pneumonia may be made when there are clinical signs of lower respiratory tract disease (cough, tachypnea, dyspnea, cyanosis, decreased breath sounds, rales, or wheezes) associated with radiographic evidence of lung infiltrates. Although the clinical syndromes of bacterial and viral pneumonia overlap, a classification of "typical" and "atypical" pneumonia is often helpful in practice (see Table 10-1). The atypical pneumonia syndrome is seen with mycoplasma infection as well as with other agents.

The organisms commonly causing pneumonia vary with the age of the patient, the season of the year, the environment, and individual host factors. In the neonate, the organisms found in the maternal genital tract, especially group B streptococcus and *Escherichia coli,* are the most common pathogens. Although *Chlamydia trachomatis* may also be acquired during delivery, the infected infants are usually asymptomatic until 3 to 16 weeks of age. In older infants and preschool children, viruses, such as RSV, parainfluenza virus, adenovirus, and enterovirus, predominate. *M. pneumoniae* assumes the dominant role in school-age children and adolescents. A recently recognized chlamydial agent called Taiwan acute respiratory (TWAR) agent can cause both endemic and epidemic pneumonia in children. In all of the age groups except neonates, primary and secondary bacterial pneumonias are uncommon and account for less than 10% of cases. Beyond the neonatal period, the major bacterial pathogens include *S. pneumoniae, H. influenzae* type B, *S. aureus,* and group A streptococcus. Bacteria such as *Legionella,* in contrast to adults, rarely cause pneumonia in children.

There is marked seasonal variation in the viral causes of childhood pneumonia. Influenza virus and RSV predominate in the winter-spring, parainfluenza virus in the fall and spring, enteroviruses in the summer-fall, and cytomegalovirus (CMV) and adenovirus are common in all seasons. In certain geographical locations, fungi may play a dominant role, for example, *Coccidioides immitis* in the southwestern United States. Similarly, environmental factors may suggest a particular pathogen, for example, psitticosis is associated with handling of infected birds or their feathers or inhalation of dust contaminated with their feces. Recurrent pneumonias, slowly resolving pneumonias, or pneumonia caused by an unusual agent or an organism unusual for the age of the patient should suggest that the child's host defense mechanisms may have been altered, and conditions such as cystic fibrosis, immunodeficiency disorders, and malignant disease should be considered.

VIRAL PNEUMONIAS. The development of viral culture techniques has led to increased awareness of the major role of viruses in infant and childhood pneumonias. This is in contrast to adult pneumonia in which viruses do not appear to be common pathogens. In infants the major cause of pneumonia is RSV. Other agents such as parainfluenza virus, adenovirus, and influenza virus play a significant role, while enterovirus, rhinovirus, CMV, and herpes simplex virus are less common pathogens. Pneumonia may also be associated with systemic viral infections such as measles or chickenpox.

Pathogenesis. The offending virus usually reaches the lower respiratory tract by direct spread from the infected upper tract, by inhalation of infected particles, or occasionally by hematogenous spread (viremia). Viral pneumonias are usually interstitial during the acute stage, and there is involvement of the airways as well as of the parenchyma. The infiltrate is generally mononuclear in type, and with some viruses there may also be necrosis of tracheal and bronchial epithelium.

Clinical Features. There is a wide range of clinical patterns with viral pneumonia, varying with the agent as well as with the age, sex, and any underlying illnesses of the infant or child. Most viral pneumonias are preceded by several days of upper respiratory tract symptoms such as rhinorrhea, cough, and low-grade fever. Frequently other members of the family are also ill. In the early stages, the cough is likely to be unproductive or productive of only a small amount of whitish sputum. Although cough and fever are prominent symptoms, they are usually not as pronounced as in cases of bacterial pneumonia. Dyspnea, which is ordinarily delayed in onset for several days, is mild to moderate. In younger children and infants with associated bronchiolitis or with plugging of the bronchioles with necrotic debris, dyspnea may be prominent.

Physical examination is often unremarkable or reveals only meager chest findings such as occasional rales and wheezing; however, with severe pneumonia, such as RSV causes in very young infants, the patient may be cyanotic and in severe respiratory distress. Clinical findings alone do not help differentiate between viral and mycoplasma pneumonia. In infants, bacterial and viral pneumonias may also have identical clinical patterns, but viral pneumonia is far more common.

Diagnosis. The chest roentgenogram in viral pneumonia is usually characterized by a diffuse infiltrate, often very prominent in the perihilar areas. Hyperinflation may occur if bronchiolitis is associated with the pneumonia. Transient lobar infiltrates and effusions may also be seen in some cases.

The offending virus can usually be cultured from the nasopharynx or throat. The RSV is rarely, if ever, present in the respiratory secretions of healthy children, and parainfluenza and adenovirus are only occasionally found in healthy, asymptomatic children. Isolation of rhinovirus, enterovirus, CMV, or herpes simplex virus from the upper respiratory tree (e.g., nasopharynx, throat) does not necessarily imply that the agent is the cause of the pneumonia. Definitive diagnosis requires isolation of the virus from the lung by biopsy or aspiration. Both of these procedures carry some risk and should be done only in an appropriate clinical situation by experienced personnel. Indirect retrospective evidence of the viral etiology can be shown by demonstrating a specific fourfold rise in antibody titers.

Rapid viral diagnostic techniques, including direct or indirect immunofluorescent slide tests and enzyme immunoassays, have been developed for several of the respiratory viruses, for example, RSV and influenza virus. These tests are very helpful and are available in many laboratories.

The peripheral white count and differential count may reveal mild leukopenia or mild leukocytosis, or they may be normal. In severe cases, there may be marked leukocytosis with a left shift. This does not necessarily imply a secondary bacterial suprainfection. The arterial blood gases provide an indication of the severity of the hypoxia.

Treatment. Most cases of viral pneumonia require only simple general supportive care, which can be given at home. Infants with significant hypoxia or respiratory distress may need hospitalization for supplemental oxygen therapy, intravenous fluids, and occasionally assisted ventilation. Antibacterial agents are indicated if a secondary bacterial infection is suspected. When an infant is admitted to the hospital, appropriate isolation procedures, especially good hand washing, must be encouraged to prevent nosocomial virus spread.

Specific antiviral agents are available including rimantadine and amantadine for symptomatic management of influenza A respiratory tract infections. Because widespread use of these agents may result in an increase in incidence of resistant virus, their use should be restricted to patients with severe influenza A infection. Ribavirin can be used to treat patients with RSV pneumonia, particularly those with severe disease. Research is ongoing to evaluate this and other new antiviral agents.

Immunoprophylaxis against many of the agents of viral pneumonia is currently under active investigation in several centers. Influenza vaccines are available, although the protection offered is only against the particular strains included in the preparation and must be repeated yearly. Amantadine can also be used for prophylaxis against influenza A.

Respiratory Syncytial Virus. RSV is now recognized as the major cause of serious lower-tract disease in infants and young children. Most cases of pneumonia or bronchiolitis occur in infants less than 6 months of age with a peak incidence at 2 to 3 months. Infection can occur in the neonatal period. Premature infants, infants with certain types of congenital heart disease, and immunocompromised children and infants with cystic fibrosis may be at risk for more severe and even fatal disease with RSV infection. The virus is usually acquired in the community during yearly winter-spring epidemics; however, nosocomial infection is a major problem in pediatric infant wards. Because primary infection does not confer lifelong immunity, repeat infections are common. The severity of the infection seems to moderate with age. At present ribavirin therapy is recommended for those with severe disease. Its efficacy is not completely established. Efforts are ongoing to develop a safe and effective RSV vaccine.

Parainfluenza Virus. In the absence of an influenza epidemic, parainfluenza virus is the second most common cause of serious lower respiratory tract disease in infants and young children. Infants with parainfluenza pneumonia are usually slightly older than those with RSV pneumonia and usually have milder disease. Type 3 parainfluenza virus is the most frequent offender, although type 1 is also associated with lower respiratory tract infection. Type 3 is endemic, while type 1 tends to occur in epidemics in the late fall or early spring. Immunocompromised older children may manifest severe or even fatal infections with parainfluenza virus.

Influenza Virus. Although attack rates with influenza virus are higher in infants and young children than in adults, the illness is usually milder, with few lower respiratory complications. Influenza, however, can cause bronchiolitis and pneumonia in young children. In contrast to RSV and parainfluenza virus, influenza virus infection tends to cause more systemic manifestations, especially myalgias. Fever, cough, vomiting, diarrhea, and conjunctivitis may be prominent features in the very young. Epidemics with strains of A virus tend to occur every year or two, while those of B virus occur less frequently. Although most infections are community acquired, nosocomial infection is also an important route. Amantadine or rimantadine is recommended for patients with severe disease.

The childhood population at risk for severe or fatal lower respiratory tract infection with influenza virus is not well defined. Data, primarily extracted from studies of adults, suggest that children with the following disease categories should receive annual influenza immunization: (1) cardiovascular disease (congenital, hypertensive, or rheumatic heart disease), (2) chronic bronchopulmonary disease such as cystic fibrosis, (3) chronic metabolic disease, (4) chronic glomerulonephritis or nephrosis, (5) chronic neurological disorders, and (6) malignant disease or immunodeficiency disorders. Alternatively, amantadine chemoprophylaxis may be given during an influenza A epidemic to these high-risk infants.

Adenovirus. Adenoviruses are common respiratory pathogens and may cause sporadic or epidemic pneumonia in children. Pneumonia is usually seen only in children under 4 years of age; severe disease, only in the very young. Of the more than 30 types of adenovirus, types 1, 3, and 7 are most commonly associated with childhood pneumonia. Disease may be especially severe if there is a coinfection with RSV. Most outbreaks occur in the summer, but peaks are also seen in the winter and spring. Characteristic associated clinical findings include exudative pharyngitis, conjunctivitis, and posterior cervical lymphadenopathy. There may also be abdominal pain, vomiting, and diarrhea.

Cytomegalovirus. See Chapter 20.

Herpes Simplex Virus. See Chapter 20.

Rhinovirus. See Chapter 20.

Enterovirus. See Chapter 20.

PNEUMOCOCCAL PNEUMONIA. *Streptococcus pneumoniae* is still responsible for the great majority of bacterial pneumonias in children, but because of the availability of potent antibacterial agents this type of pneumonia is not the serious problem it was in the preantibiotic era. Indeed, most cases of pneumococcal pneumonia can now be treated at home.

Although pneumococcal pneumonia occurs throughout the year, there is a peak prevalence in the late winter and early spring that coincides with the winter respiratory virus season. In childhood the disease usually occurs as a sporadic illness with highest attack rates during the first 4 years of life. Although there are more than 80 types of *S. pneumoniae,* only about a dozen commonly cause disease in children, particularly types 1, 3, 6, 7, 14, 18, 19, and 23. In general, the pathogenicity of the pneumococcus is slight, and the organism may be recovered from the upper respiratory tract of up to 70% of healthy people. Asymptomatic carriers of pathogenic types play an important role in transmission and spread of the disease. Upon a person's recovery from pneumococcal infection, the development of type-specific antibody protects from reinfection with that type and also decreases the likelihood of carriage of that specific serotype of organism.

Pathogenesis. Initially there is an infection of the upper respiratory tract, often due to a virus, that is associated with increased respiratory secretions containing large numbers of pneumococci. These secretions are probably aspirated into the peripheral lung area from the upper airway or nasopharynx. Initially there is a reactive edema that supports the multiplication and spread of the organisms along the airway and through the pores of Kohn until a natural barrier, such as the interlobar fissure, is reached. In older children the infection usually remains localized to one lobe or segment of a lobe. In infants the infection may be more widely disseminated and follow a bronchial distribution. The involved lobe undergoes early consolidation — red hepatization with polymorphonuclear leukocytes, fibrin, red cells, edema fluid, and pneumococci packing the alveoli. In untreated cases, this is followed by gray hepatization in which the central areas show a fibrinous reaction with phagocytosis of the organisms. During resolution, increasing numbers of macrophages digest and remove the fibrin, dead polymorphonuclear leukocytes, and organisms. In untreated cases the crisis occurs at about the seventh day, but complete resolution takes another 2 to 3 weeks. The alveolar walls escape with surprisingly little damage. Resolution of antibiotic-treated cases is usually complete and rapid.

Bacteremia occurs in only 30 to 50% of the cases, and metastatic infection is uncommon. Small sterile effusions are common, but empyema is only occasionally a late complication.

Clinical Manifestations. In lobar pneumonia, the pattern usually seen in children and adolescents, the onset is usually preceded by an upper respiratory tract infection. This may be associated with conjunctivitis, which is frequently unilateral, or with otitis media, or both. The first symptoms of the systemic infection may be heralded by abrupt onset of headache and a shaking chill followed by a high fever. Occasionally, as the temperature rises, delirium, convulsions, or meningismus occur. The fever is accompanied by rapid respirations, anxiety, periods of restlessness, malaise, and anorexia. Cough is not conspicuous before the second day and is initially harsh and either unproductive or productive of a little whitish sputum. Rusty sputum and chills are less common in children than adults. There is often pleuritic pain from which the child tries to obtain relief by lying on the affected side. Vomiting may occur early and be followed by abdominal distention due to mild ileus. Abdominal pain is a frequent complaint if the lower lobes are involved.

Examination in a typical case shows a flushed child with shallow rapid respirations, occasional grunting, and with relatively less tachycardia than expected from the respiratory rate. Mild cyanosis may occur later. Dullness to percussion and crepitant rales are often absent on the first day, but they become increasingly obvious with time. Breath sounds are slightly diminished in the early stages, and later bronchophony and whispering pectoriloquy may be heard. During the stage of resolution, rales become moist and the cough becomes more productive and disturbing to the patient. Two common findings in adults, herpes labialis and a pleural rub, are uncommon in children.

In infants, disseminated pneumonia is the more common pattern. The onset of the infection is more gradual and is manifested by refusal to eat, vomiting or diarrhea or both, and fever or hypothermia. The temperature pattern is remittent rather than continuous. There is sometimes little to suggest a pulmonary infection; however, close observation often reveals rapid, grunting respirations with intercostal retractions and nasal flaring. The physical findings may otherwise not be helpful. Percussion is usually not informative because there are scattered areas of involvement. In this age group, dullness to percussion usually indicates pleural effusion and not localized pneumonia. On auscultation there may be areas of decreased breath sounds and rales, but these are not always present and may be variable.

Laboratory Findings. The leukocyte count is characteristically 15,000 to 40,000/mm^3, with a preponderance of mature polymorphonuclear leukocytes and band cells. Counts below 5000/mm^3 are often associated with a grave prognosis. The hemoglobin level is usually normal or slightly low. Urine examination may indicate proteineuria and ketonuria with occasional red and white cells and casts.

Although nasopharyngeal cultures frequently yield a predominant growth of pneumococci, this finding cannot be considered proof of a causative relationship, because normal healthy children frequently carry this organism. Definitive diagnosis rests with the culture of the organism from the blood, pleural fluid, sputum, tracheal aspirate, or lung aspirate. Unfortunately, this is often difficult. Blood cultures are positive in only about 30% of the cases. Many children are unable to produce sputum and provide saliva instead. Tracheal and lung aspiration and thoracentesis carry added risks for the patient.

Latex particle agglutination positive for pneumococcal antigen with serum or concentrated urine is a significant finding. This test, however, is not positive in all cases of pneumococcal infection, and it is not universally available.

Roentgenographic Findings. The roentgenographic changes in pneumococcal pneumonia do not always correspond to the clinical observations. The chest roentgenogram in a typical case shows consolidation of a lobe or even a whole lung. In some cases there is also evidence of partial atelectasis in the affected lobe. As a result of early medical treatment, the fully developed picture of lobar pneumonia is infrequently observed, and consolidation may involve only a portion of a lobe. During the stage of resolution, clearing of the area of consolidation may be patchy and may even suggest the presence of cavities. In the dissemi-

nated type of infection seen in infants, the initial appearance is usually that of scattered areas of clouding. If these coalesce, the picture of homogeneous consolidation may be seen. Pleural reaction with demonstration of fluid on the roentgenogram is not uncommon.

A follow-up roentgenogram may be helpful when recovery does not proceed as expected. If complete resolution is not present, an underlying problem such as immunodeficiency disorder, cystic fibrosis, or foreign body aspiration must be considered.

Differential Diagnosis. The picture of lobar pneumonia may also be caused by *H. influenzae.* In those cases in which areas of consolidation coalesce, streptococcus group A should be considered. Other conditions that may be confused with pneumococcal pneumonia include bronchiolitis, foreign body aspiration, congestive heart failure, pulmonary abscess, sequestered lobe, and bronchiectasis.

Treatment. The drug of choice is penicillin, because most pneumococci are exquisitely sensitive to it. Pneumococci resistant to penicillin have been reported in the Far East, Africa, and Australia but are exceedingly rare. Other antimicrobial agents are indicated only if there is a definite contraindication to penicillin. Strains of pneumococci resistant to erythromycin and tetracycline are not uncommon, so these drugs should not be used unless the sensitivity of the organism has been specifically tested.

Penicillin should be given intravenously or intramuscularly initially if the patient is vomiting or unable to take the medicine orally. Treatment should be continued for 5 to 7 days after the temperature is normal. Most older children can be treated at home. Pneumonia in very young infants, however, is best treated in the hospital because fluids and antibiotics may have to be given intravenously.

Polyvalent pneumococcal vaccines have proved efficacious in certain adult populations at risk for severe pneumococcal infections. The vaccines have also been suggested for use in specific at-risk children, e.g., those with sickle-cell disease, and in postsplenectomy patients. One must be aware, however, that vaccine failures do occur because not all types of pneumococci are included in the vaccine.

Course and Prognosis. Before antimicrobial agents were available the mortality for lobar pneumonia was approximately 5% and for disseminated pneumonia 50%. With the use of penicillin and good supportive care, the mortality is less than 1%. The natural course of pneumococcal lobar pneumonia with resolution by crisis or, less commonly, by lysis is now rarely seen.

Complications. Pleurisy is essentially a part of the disease, but occasionally it may progress to significant pleural effusion or empyema. Pericarditis is rare. Hematogenous spread is unusual but may result in meningitis and rarely in arthritis or peritonitis.

STAPHYLOCOCCAL PNEUMONIA. Pneumonia due to *S. aureus* is a serious and rapidly progressive infection, which even with early diagnosis and treatment may still cause significant and prolonged morbidity. Staphylococcal pneumonia occurs less frequently than pneumococcal or viral pneumonia. Over 75% of cases occur in infants less than 1 year of age, and more than 30% of these infants are less than 3 months of age. Boys are more commonly infected than girls. Although staphylococcal pneumonia is unusual in children over 2 years of age, older infants and children with other respiratory diseases, such as cystic fibrosis, whooping cough, influenza, and measles, or those with immunodeficiency disorders or diabetes mellitus, are at an increased risk to develop it.

The organism is commonly found on normal skin and mucous membranes. Nearly 90% of normal healthy infants become nasal carriers in the neonatal period. The carrier rate declines to about 20% over the first 2 years and subsequently climbs to adult levels of 40 to 50% by 4 to 5 years of age.

The peak incidence of staphylococcal pneumonia is in winter and early spring. As with other bacterial pneumonias it parallels the winter respiratory virus season and is often preceded by an upper-tract viral infection. Viral respiratory tract infections may play an important role in dissemination of the organisms and in the conversion of colonization to disease.

Pathogenesis. Staphylococci produce a number of toxins and enzymes, including coagulase, hemolysins, leukocidin, staphylokinase, hyaluronidase, and penicillinase. These products are important factors in the rapid destructive spread of the organism in the lung. Virulence correlates well with coagulase production. Organisms without the ability to produce coagulase only rarely produce serious disease.

The staphylococci most commonly reach the lower respiratory tract by inhalation. In about 20% of cases they reach it by hematogenous spread from another site. Aspirated organisms invade the walls of the secondary bronchi and cause peribronchial abscesses. These may coalesce to form areas of severe hemorrhagic consolidation. Frequently the peribronchial abscesses in turn erode through the bronchial walls, allowing air to enter the abscesses. A check-valve mechanism is initiated that results in formation of pneumatoceles. Subpleural abscesses may rupture into the pleural cavity, causing empyema or pyopneumothorax when a bronchopleural fistula is present. Both the pneumatoceles and pneumothorax are frequently only unilateral.

Thus with staphylococcal pneumonia the common features are bronchial ulceration, parenchymal necrosis, and cyst and abscess formation. Invasion of blood vessels with septicemia may occur.

Clinical Manifestations. Most commonly the patient is a young infant with a personal or family history of staphylococcal infection or colonization. The onset of pneumonia is usually insidious as mild upper respiratory signs progress, after a few days, to serious lower-tract disease. In the infant, anorexia, irritability, or lethargy may be the earliest symptom. Diarrhea and vomiting may also herald the onset of pneumonia. Tachypnea, grunting, and gray color or cyanosis rapidly follow.

The patient's temperature is usually elevated, but neonates may be afebrile. The infant has a toxic appearance and is prostrate early in the disease. Examination of the chest often reveals less conspicuous findings than are seen on the roentgenogram, especially later in the course of the disease when pneumatoceles are present. Pulmonary findings include the presence of rales, impaired breath sounds, bronchial breathing, and dullness to percussion. Pneumatoceles with pneumothorax should be suspected when there is a sudden onset or severe exacerbation of dyspnea. Abdominal pain or distention may be present. Rapid progression of signs and symptoms is characteristic.

Laboratory Findings. In older infants and children a leukocyte count of 20,000/mm^3 or more with a prominent polymorphonuclear reaction is common. In young infants the white blood count may stay within the normal range. Leukocyte counts of less than 5000/mm^3 are associated with a grave prognosis. Moderate anemia is present in many patients, but it is not usually severe enough to require blood transfusion.

In the early stages, blood cultures may be positive; however, in later stages, in the absence of associated extrapulmonary infections or other complications, blood cultures are often sterile. When blood cultures obtained late in the illness are positive, this may suggest that the lung involvement is secondary and that a primary-focus infection exists elsewhere. Material for diagnostic cultures may be obtained from a pleural tap or by tracheal aspiration. The finding of staphylococci in the nasopharynx is of no diagnostic value. Examination of pleural fluid usually reveals an exudate with protein content greater than 2.5 g/100 ml, pH less than 7.2, specific gravity greater than 1.018, and lactate dehydrogenase level above 550 units.

Roentgenographic Findings. Early in the illness in most patients the picture is one of nonspecific bronchopneumonia. The infiltrate soon becomes patchy and localized or dense and homogenous and may involve an entire lobe or lung. In about 65% of cases only the right lung is involved.

Bilateral involvement is seen in only about 20% of patients. Pneumatoceles appear as thin-walled, rounded translucent areas, typically varying in size over a period of days or weeks. Pyopneumothorax occurs in about 25% of cases. Accumulation of pleural fluid is common.

Roentgenographically the condition frequently progresses over a matter of hours from bronchopneumonia to effusion with pneumatoceles with or without pyopneumothorax. Thus, frequent follow-up films are helpful in suspected staphylococcal pneumonia. Roentgenographic improvement lags behind clinical improvement. Asymptomatic pneumatoceles may persist for weeks or months.

Differential Diagnosis. The diagnosis of early staphylococcal pneumonia is often difficult in infants. An abrupt onset and rapid progression of symptoms of pneumonia are highly suggestive. Rapidly changing roentgenographic findings and the presence of pneumatoceles and pleural effusions are helpful diagnostically; however, other types of bacterial pneumonia must be considered. Tuberculous pneumonia may cause abscess and cavity formation. *H. influenzae* pneumonia may be accompanied by empyema. Pneumatoceles may be seen with *Klebsiella, E. coli,* and pneumococcal pneumonia. Foreign body aspiration may result in a similar roentgenogram, but the infant or child is usually afebrile and well when symptoms abruptly begin.

Treatment. Staphylococcal pneumonia can only rarely be managed on an outpatient basis. Hospitalization is indicated because of the severity and rapid progression of the disease. Appropriate therapy includes parenteral administration of antibiotics, drainage of large collections of pus that are compromising respiratory efforts, and supportive care of fluid, calorie, electrolyte, and oxygen requirements. Occasionally, assisted ventilation may be needed. This may be associated with a higher incidence of pneumothorax. If severe anemia is present, transfusion of packed red cells may be beneficial.

A semisynthetic, penicillinase-resistant penicillin is indicated pending determination of the specific sensitivities of the organism (e.g., nafcillin or methicillin, 100 mg/kg/24 hr). If subsequent culture results show that the organism is sensitive to penicillin, then penicillin G (100,000 units/kg/24 hr) may be used. Initially the antibiotic should be given intravenously because oral absorption may be variable. If patients are allergic to penicillins, a cephalosporin or vancomycin may be considered.

If a significant amount of pus is present in the pleural cavity, it should be drained without delay by chest-tube placement. Frequently the fluid is loculated, making drainage difficult. In general, tubes should not remain in place more than 5 to 7 days. Pneumatoceles, when causing serious respiratory embarrassment by pressure, may require intercostal decompression, but this is rarely indicated.

Course and Prognosis. Because the course of the disease may change within a few hours, constant surveillance is necessary. The course of the pneumatocele is usually benign, with spontaneous resolution over a period of a few weeks to 3 months. Rupture of a pneumatocele or emphysematous bleb into the pleural cavity may cause tension pneumothorax, which requires urgent treatment. In most patients some degree of emphysema develops, and about one-third acquire pneumatoceles.

The prognosis is poor in infants under 3 months of age, in debilitated children, and in children with disseminated disease. Leukopenia is often associated with a fatal outcome. Mortality still ranges from 10 to 30%.

In children with staphylococcal pneumonia who have no significant underlying disease, prognosis for complete recovery is excellent, although the hospitalizaton may be prolonged. At long-term follow-up, pulmonary function is normal, and there is no increased susceptibility to pulmonary infections.

Complications. Empyema, pneumatoceles, and pyopneumothorax are part of the disease. Metastatic foci, including osteomyelitis, abscesses, and pericarditis, are unusual except in neonates and young infants. In adolescents, however, staphylococcal pneumonia may not be primary but only part of a generalized staphylococcal disease with involvement of other organ systems.

STREPTOCOCCAL PNEUMONIA. Group A streptococcal pneumonia is uncommon. It usually occurs secondary to another illness such as influenza, measles, pertussis, or an upper respiratory tract infection. It may occur as a primary infection but only rarely complicates streptococcal pharyngitis. Most children with group A streptococcal pneumonia are between 3 and 5 years of age. Group B streptococci are a common cause of neonatal pneumonia and respiratory distress (see Chap 9).

Involvement of the lower tract may result in tracheitis, bronchitis, or interstitial pneumonia. Interstitial bronchopneumonia may be hemorrhagic and may spread by the lymphatics to the mediastinum and hilar lymph nodes. Retrograde lymphatic spread to the pleural surfaces is common. The pleural effusion produced may be large and serous, serosanguineous, or thinly purulent.

Clinical Manifestations. The clinical picture is similar to that of pneumococcal pneumonia of the disseminated type. Cough, high temperature, tachypnea, and prostration are typical. Occasionally the illness is more insidious with a low-grade fever and mild toxicity similar to the clinical syndrome with *H. influenzae* pneumonia.

Because streptococcal pneumonia often follows another illness, the symptoms and signs of the initial illness may merge with those of the pneumonia; however, progression of the cough, persistent or increased fever, or the onset of pleuritic pain is suggestive. When streptococcal pneumonia occurs as a primary infection, the clinical picture is similar to lobar pneumococcal pneumonia with abrupt onset of fever, chills, cough, and pleuritic pain.

Laboratory Investigations. Polymorphonuclear leukocytosis is characteristically present. Although an increase in antistreptolysin titer is suggestive of the etiology, this may not occur for 1 to 2 weeks. Blood cultures are positive in 10 to 15% of cases. The definitive diagnosis rests with isolation of the organism from blood, pleural fluid, or lung aspirate. Nasopharyngeal cultures are often positive, but this finding does not constitute proof of the diagnosis.

Roentgenographic Findings. The chest roentgenogram reveals diffuse interstitial bronchopneumonia and often a large pleural effusion. The hilar lymph nodes are commonly enlarged. Pneumatoceles may be present. The findings, however, may be indistinguishable from those seen with viral or myocplasmal pneumonia.

Differential Diagnosis. Because streptococcal pneumonia is an interstitial process, the primary differential diagnosis is with viral and *M. pneumoniae* infections, which have a similar roentgenographic picture and may have a similar clinical presentation. The leukocyte count may be normal in viral or *Mycoplasma* pneumonia. Diagnosis of the specific virus is dependent upon the ability of the laboratory to culture viruses. Even if a virus is isolated, one must remember that streptococcal pneumonmia may complicate viral infections. When this occurs, the illness may appear to be biphasic, and this may suggest the diagnosis. Patients with *Mycoplasma* pneumonia usually do not appear as ill as those with streptococcal pneumonia, and a fourfold rise in mycoplasma titer confirms the diagnosis.

Treatment. Parenteral administration of penicillin G (100,000 units/kg/24 hr) in the appropriate therapy. Usually a 2- to 3-week course is given. Oral penicillin may be used when tolerated. Although this is a serious disease without treatment, the response to penicillin is usually rapid, and recovery is complete. If empyema is present, therapeutic thoracentesis may be indicated.

Course and Prognosis. Bacterial complications are common in untreated patients but are rare after appropriate antibiotic therapy is started. Empyema is the most common complication and occurs in 20 to 30% of children. Other complications include osteomyelitis, septic arthritis, and very occasionally acute glomerulonephritis.

Prior to the antibiotic era, mortality was 30 to 40%. With appropriate therapy, fatal cases are now rare. Final clearing of the roentgenographic changes may be slow, but the roentgenogram is usually normal after 3 months.

HEMOPHILUS INFLUENZAE TYPE B PNEUMONIA. *H. influenzae* type b pneumonia is uncommon, although infants and young children may be affected following an upper respiratory tract infection, laryngotracheobronchitis, epiglottitis, or pertussis. It may also occur after hematogenous spread from another focus. Most cases occur in children under 5 and often less than 2 years old. This infection most commonly occurs in the winter and spring.

Pneumonia due to *H. influenzae* may be either lobar or bronchopneumonic. Involved areas show a hemorrhagic exudate with a polymorphonuclear leukocyte or lymphocytic inflammatory reaction. Destruction of the bronchial and bronchiolar epithelium is prominent and may evolve into bronchiectasis. Empyema may occur.

Clinical Manifestations. The onset may be gradual or abrupt. Prostration is often more marked than would be expected from the extent of the infection. Cough is almost always present but may not be productive. Fever, tachypnea, and decreased breath sounds over the affected lobe are the most common signs. There may be localized areas of dullness to percussion and rales and tubular breath sounds. Otitis media is a very common associated finding. Occasionally involvement of another organ system overshadows the pneumonia, e.g., meningitis, pericarditis, and epiglottitis.

Laboratory Findings. The leukocyte count is characteristically 20,000 to 40,000/mm^3 with polymorphonuclear leukocyte predominance. A positive blood culture is the most consistent method of confirmation and is noted in about 75% of cases. If empyema is present, this fluid may be cultured. Serum, urine, and pleural fluid may be positive by countercurrent immunoelectrophoresis for *H. influenzae* type b antigen. Positive nasopharyngeal cultures are not diagnostic.

Roentgenographic Findings. The typical picture is usually one of lobar pneumonia and less commonly interstitial bronchopneumonia. Pleural fluid is frequently present.

Differential Diagnosis. The possibility of *H. influenzae* should be considered when lobar or interstitial pneumonia in an infant or young child with polymorphonuclear leukocytosis has not responded to penicillin therapy. A positive blood culture confirms the diagnosis.

Treatment. Therapy involves both general supportive

measures and specific antimicrobial agents. Because ampicillin-resistant organisms are common, chloramphenicol (75 mg/kg/24 hr) or cefotaxime (150 mg/kg/24 hr) is the initial drug of choice until the sensitivities are known. Therapy should be continued for 5 to 7 days after the fever has subsided. If empyema is present, prolonged therapy may be necessary.

Course and Prognosis. Complications are frequent, especially in infants, and include bacteremia, meningitis, osteomyelitis, pericarditis, and septic arthritis, as well as others. With early appropriate therapy, complete resolution is the rule. If there is delay in treatment there may be extensive airway damage, which may progress to bronchiectasis.

BACTERIAL PNEUMONIAS CAUSED BY OTHER GRAM-NEGATIVE ORGANISMS. After the neonatal period a small percentage of childhood and infant pneumonias are due to opportunistic gram-negative organisms such as *Klebsiella, E. coli,* or *Pseudomonas aeruginosa.* These pneumonias are rarely seen in healthy children but may occur in children with altered host resistance, e.g., cystic fibrosis or malignant disease, those on a prolonged regimen of broad-spectrum antibiotics, and those using mechanical ventilators or humidification equipment for lung disorders. Occasionally these organisms will cause epidemics in nurseries.

Klebsiella Pneumonia. The characteristic features of *Klebsiella* pneumonia are marked alveolar destruction with abscess formation, and copious, thick purulent secretions. Pneumonia due to *Klebsiella* organisms may be difficult to distinguish from other bacterial pneumonias. Diarrhea and vomiting may be prominent symptoms in nursery epidemics. The respiratory symptoms usually start abruptly, and the course is fulminant. Roentgenograms characteristically show a lobar infiltrate with bulging fissures. Complications frequently occur and include empyema, bacteremia, and residual pulmonary damage.

Isolation of the organism from blood, pleural fluid, or tracheal secretions is diagnostic. Because *Klebsiella* may be carried in the upper respiratory tract of healthy children, nasopharyngeal cultures are not helpful.

Treatment includes supportive care, drainage of empyema and abscesses, and appropriate antimicrobial therapy. Aminoglycosides are the agents of choice, although many organisms are also sensitive to the newer cephalosporins, e.g., cefotaxime. Primary *Klebsiella* pneumonia is a very serious illness and may be fulminating and fatal despite appropriate therapy. Residual pleural and pulmonary damage is not uncommon. The prognosis for secondary pneumonia depends upon the underlying disease. The mortality in sporadic cases is about 50% and in epidemics much less.

Escherichia coli Pneumonia. E. coli pneumonia is rare after the neonatal period but may be seen in children after bowel or kidney surgery. The organism is blood borne from an infectious focus elsewhere such as pyelonephritis. Children with impaired resistance are also at risk.

The characteristic pathological features include bilateral interstitial bronchopneumonia with a mixed cellular infiltrate, and edema, fluid, and fibrin in the alveoli. The children are very ill with gram-negative endotoxic shock. Empyema is common, and pneumatoceles and abscesses may occur.

The organism can usually be isolated from the blood and frequently shows multiple antibiotic resistance. Aminoglycosides are the antibiotics of choice for initial therapy. Despite aggressive supportive care and appropriate antimicrobial therapy, the mortality in *E. coli* pneumonia is high, up to 60%.

Tularemia and Q fever as causes of pneumonia are discussed in Chapter 20.

Pseudomonas aeruginosa Pneumonia. P. aeruginosa causes severe, necrotizing bronchopneumonia that frequently is fatal; it is rarely a primary pathogen, but as a secondary invader it is not uncommon. It is primarily seen in children with chronic debilitating diseases such as cystic fibrosis or cancer. An aminoglycoside combined with ticarcillin is appropriate antimicrobial treatment.

Legionnaires' disease caused by *Legionella* sp. is an uncommon cause of necrotizing pneumonia in children. Those with hematologic malignancies have rarely been afflicted.

MYCOPLASMA PNEUMONIAE PNEUMONIA. *M. pneumoniae* (Eaton agent pneumonia, primary atypical pneumonia) accounts for about 20 to 25% of cases of clinically apparent pneumonia in school-age children and adolescents, but it is only an occasional cause in infants and preschool children.

M. pneumoniae is an organism, 3 to 150 μm in size, that can grow in a cell-free agar medium and that has the three-layered unit membrane characteristic of animal cells. Because *M. pneumoniae* infection is rarely fatal, the pathological changes in the lung have not been well described; however, peribronchial and perivascular lymphoid infiltrates, acute bronchitis, and bronchiolitis are frequent findings in the respiratory mucosa.

Clinical Manifestations. Clinically apparent pneumonia is most commonly seen in school-age children and adolescents. Other family members are often affected too. The incubation period is 1 to 3 weeks, with an average of 12 to 14 days. The onset is abrupt, with headache, chills, and a hacking, paroxysmal cough that may be delayed in onset and becomes productive of whitish mucoid sputum. Generally, few physical signs are present. The temperature may rise as high as 40°C, although tachypnea is not prominent, and bradycardia relative to the degree of temperature elevation is characteristic. Rales, if present, are generally unilateral and are exaggerated by deep inspiration.

Laboratory Findings. The leukocyte count is normal or only slightly elevated. Hypoxemia has been reported in some patients. The organism may be cultured from the nasopharynx with special culture media. This, however, may take 4 to 6 days, and the technique is not available in many laboratories. Although the presence of a cold agglutinin titer equal to or greater than 64 is suggestive of *M. pneumoniae,* in children this test is not always reliable. False negatives and false positives occur. The diagnosis is usually made retrospectively from a fourfold rise in mycoplasma antibody titer in paired sera.

Roentgenographic Findings. The roentgenographic findings are similar to those in viral pneumonia, including a peribronchial infiltrate and patchy areas of clouding, particularly in the lower lobes. Small effusions can be shown in at least 20% of patients with use of lateral decubitus chest roentgenograms. The roentgenographic findings are frequently disproportionately greater than those on physical examination.

Differential Diagnosis. A prolonged course may be the only feature distinguishing *Mycoplasma* pneumonia from viral pneumonia. The diagnosis must be confirmed in the laboratory. Patients with bacterial pneumonia appear sicker and have more marked pulmonary physical signs, tachycardia, a lobar distribution of involvement on the roentgenogram, and leukocytosis.

Treatment. Erythromycin therapy decreases the duration of respiratory symptoms. The response may be delayed for 3 to 4 days, and the drug must not be discontinued too soon. Even with specific therapy, cough and chest signs may persist for a month or more.

Course and Prognosis. The course is variable in duration, but signs, symptoms, and roentgenographic findings may last 3 or 4 weeks with spontaneous resolution. Occasional complications include CNS involvement such as encephalitis, ascending paralysis (Guillain-Barré syndrome), transverse myelitis, cerebellar ataxia, and others. Some cases have been fatal. About 30% of patients with CNS involvement are left with permanent or persistent neurological deficit. The exact role of *M. pneumoniae* in these disorders is not understood. Mycoplasmal pneumonia may also be associated with hematological abnormalities (e.g., hemolytic anemia, paroxysmal cold hemoglobinemia); mucocutaneous lesions (e.g., erythema multiforme, Stevens-Johnson syndrome); musculoskeletal symptoms (e.g., arthralgias and myalgias); gastrointestinal symptoms (e.g.,

anorexia, nausea, vomiting, and diarrhea); and cardiac abnormalities (e.g., pericarditis).

FUNGAL PNEUMONIA. See Chapter 20.

PNEUMOCYSTIS CARINII PNEUMONIA. See Chapter 20.

CHLAMYDIA PNEUMONIA. *Chlamydia trachomatis* can cause a distinctive pneumonia syndrome in young infants. The organism is acquired at birth from the maternal genital tract, but the onset of symptoms is usually delayed until 3 to 6 weeks of age, and it may be as late as 16 weeks.

Clinical Features. The infant may be noted on a routine well-baby check to be gaining weight poorly. There is minimal toxicity and usually no fever. More than 50% have a history of conjunctivitis, and more than 75% have associated serous otitis media. Cough may not be a prominent feature early, but it is distinctive and staccatolike, occurring in a series but without an inspiratory whoop.

Laboratory Findings. The total leukocyte count is usually normal, but half of the patients have an absolute eosinophil count greater than 300/mm^3. Arterial blood gas analysis frequently shows decreased PaO$_2$ with normal PaCO$_2$. Serum immunoglobulin analysis reveals that the IgM is nearly always equal to or greater than 100 mg/100 ml, the IgG is usually also elevated ($\geq$500 mg/100 ml), and IgA is often greater than 30 mg/100 ml. Demonstration of inclusion bodies in Giemsa-stained epithelial cells from scrapings of the infected conjunctiva adds weight to the diagnosis. Because concurrent viral infection may be found in about 30% of the infants, virus isolation from the nasopharynx does not rule out the diagnosis. Definitive diagnosis rests with the isolation of *C. trachomatis* from the nasopharynx by culture techniques or *Chlamydia* antigen detection tests. These procedures are not available in many routine laboratories. Serological diagnosis with demonstration of a fourfold rise in antibody titer to *C. trachomatis* is also specific, but frequently the infant is not seen until well into the course of the illness. In these patients a serum antibody titer to *C. trachomatis* equal to or greater than 1 : 32 is highly suggestive of the diagnosis.

Roentgenographic Findings. The characteristic pattern is of diffuse interstitial pneumonia involving all lobes. There is usually hyperinflation of the chest.

Treatment. Both the respiratory disease and the conjunctivitis require systemic therapy. The preferred agent is erythromycin or sulfisoxazole for 2 weeks. Clinical improvement is usually noted in 5 to 6 days with decreased cough and resumption of weight gain. It may be several weeks before the chest roentgenogram returns to normal.

TWAR PNEUMONIA. Taiwan acute respiratory (TWAR) agent is a recently recognized organism similar but distinct from *Chlamydia psittaci.* Clinically TWAR has been associated with epidemic and endemic pneumonia in older children and adults. The pneumonia is usually mild with cough and fever as presenting complaints. Rales are usually present, and a peribronchial infiltrate with patchy areas of clouding are noted on chest roentgenogram. The infection may be biphasic with severe pharyngitis and laryngitis preceding the pneumonia by a week or two. TWAR pneumonia may also run a relapsing course with persistent cough. Confirmation of the diagnosis is difficult because chlamydia serology for *C. psittaci* and TWAR overlap and the immunofluorescence tests, while better, are still not specific enough. Erythromycin appears to be the drug of choice in children.

Special Considerations

NEONATAL PNEUMONIA. In neonates the presence of a pulmonary infiltrate and respiratory distress does not always imply an infectious etiology. Respiratory distress syndrome, meconium aspiration, congenital heart disease, transient tachypnea of the newborn, and tracheoesophageal fistula are among the more common and important considerations.

Pneumonia due to infection may be acquired transplacentally, perinatally (onset of illness in the first few days of life), or postnatally (onset of symptoms after several days of life).

Transplacentally acquired pneumonia is usually part of a generalized intrauterine infection due to CMV, rubella, *Taxoplasma gondii*, or *Treponema pallidum*. Clues to the diagnosis lie in the maternal history and the neonatal physical examination. Frequently the infant has other stigmata of such an infection.

Perinatal pneumonia is usually acquired after aspiration of infected amniotic fluid or birth canal secretions. The primary organisms involved are group B streptococcus, *E. coli* and other gram-negative organisms, and herpes simplex virus. Group B streptococcal pneumonia is especially important because it may mimic the respiratory distress syndrome and, if untreated, may be fatal.

Postnatally acquired pneumonia is usually due to *S. aureus*, *P. aeruginosa*, *Klebsiella*, or *Serratia* or other gram-negative organisms; however, respiratory viruses, especially RSV, can cause significant disease. CMV has also been implicated in late-onset respiratory illness in neonates who usually have a history of multiple blood transfusions.

PNEUMONIA IN IMMUNOCOMPROMISED CHILDREN. Children who are immunocompromised as a result of cancer, irradiation, or cytotoxic or immunosuppressive drugs pose a complex diagnostic problem. All of the common pathogens must be considered along with other "peculiar" microorganisms.

Important pathogens to consider include *Pneumocystis carinii*, *Mycoplasma*, and gram-negative organisms such as *Pseudmonas*, *Klebsiella*, *Enterobacter*, *E. coli*, *Proteus*, and *Bacteroides*. Fungi such as *Candida*, *Coccidioides*, *Aspergillus*, and *Histoplasma* are also important. Viral pneumonia, especially if due to CMV, herpes simplex virus, varicella virus, or RSV, may be particularly severe in these children.

To compound the problem, the signs and symptoms may be significantly altered because of the underlying condition. Mixed infections can occur. Lung biopsy or lung aspiration, although associated with some significant risks, is often indicated in these children.

PNEUMONIA IN CHILDREN WITH AIDS. Pneumonia in infants and children with AIDS may be due to the wide variety of agents seen in immunocompromised children with further additions such as atypical mycobacteria. Furthermore, lymphoid interstitial pneumonitis is a common problem and it can mimic infection due to organisms like *Pneumocystis*. Aspirates obtained at bronchoscopy or lung biopsy may help delineate infectious from noninfectious causes.

PNEUMONIA IN SICKLE-CELL DISEASE AND IN PATIENTS WITH SPLENECTOMY. Children with hemoglobinopathies such as sickle-cell disease (hemoglobin SS), hemoglobin SC disease, or thalassemia as well as patients with splenectomy may have fulminant and frequently fatal infections with encapsulated organisms such as pneumococcus, *H. influenzae* type b, *E. coli*, and meningococcus. In these patients there appears to be a marked, and probably critical, decrease in the functional mass of the reticuloendothelial system, as well as a defect in opsonizing activity for encapsulated organisms with poor complement activation resulting in delayed clearance of the bacteria from the blood stream. Although patients with fulminant septicemia rarely live long enough to develop evidence of pneumonia, children with sickle-cell disease are prone to all forms of infection with these organisms, including pneumonia.

If pneumonia or septicemia is suspected in such a child, prompt and aggressive therapy is indicated pending laboratory results. Treatment delay may be fatal for the child.

RECURRENT PNEUMONIA. Although pneumonia is a relatively common occurrence in childhood, recurrent or severe and prolonged pneumonia despite appropriate therapy is distinctly unusual. If either of these situations occurs an abnormality in the host defense mechanism must be considered. These would include congenital metabolic disorders such as cystic fibrosis; congenital structural abnormalities, e.g., tracheoesophageal fistula, the immotile cilia syndrome; mechanical or anatomical obstruction such as foreign body aspiration; reactive conditions such as asthma; or immunodeficiency disorders such as cancer or immunological defects. Each child must be carefully assessed to rule out a significant underlying disorder.

GIANT-CELL PNEUMONIA. This uncommon subacute or chronic pneumonia has been observed in patients with measles, and Enders has isolated the measles virus from lung tissue of patients with giant-cell pneumonia. The condition has been described in patients with leukemia in partial remission who were receiving aminopterin. The lesion is a diffuse bronchiolitis and interstitial pneumonia characterized histologically by the presence of multinucleated giant cells containing intranuclear or cytoplasmic inclusion bodies. The diagnosis can be made by the finding of giant cells in the sputum. There is no specific treatment.

Noni E. MacDonald

Löffler's Syndrome

Löffler's syndrome is a clinical entity characterized by fleeting migratory pulmonary infiltrates associated with a marked eosinophilia. The radiographic findings of clouding, fine mottling, and increased bronchovascular markings are thought to be caused by local inflammatory response of the eosinophil. The syndrome is usually associated with parasitic infection with *Toxocara canis, Ascaris lumbricoides,* hookworm, tropical eosinophilia (occult filiariasis); it may be associated with aspergillosis. This syndrome may also be associated with various collagen vascular diseases.

Symptoms are nonspecific. The most remarkable finding is a marked eosinophilia exceeding 3000 total eosinophil count. IgE levels may be quite high as well.

Treatment is etiology specific.

Pulmonary Metastases

Because some neoplasms have as their first physical manifestations metastases to the lungs, it is important to know which tumors tend to develop pulmonary metastases and where the primary tumor is likely to be located. Although pulmonary metastases are commonly treated palliatively, in a few cases small solitary metastases have been treated by wedge resection or lobectomy. Such a procedure is usually preceded and followed by chemotherapy, irradiation, or both.

Atelectasis

Atelectasis is a condition in which a segment, lobe, or whole lung fails to expand at birth or collapses after having expanded completely. It may follow obstruction of one or more bronchi or bronchioles; it may also result from direct compression of the lung from without. Weakness of the chest muscles or diaphragm on the affected side may be a contributory factor.

Volume loss of the atelectatic segment occurs when an airway is completely obstructed and the trapped gas is absorbed into the capillaries. Atelectatic areas contain variable amounts of serous fluid, which tends to restrict collapse. The amount of fluid is greater in the acute stage or in the presence of inflammation. The blood flow through an airless segment is likely to be reduced because of increased resistance, but if the atelectatic area is large, unoxygenated blood, passing through airless lung tissue into the pulmonary veins, may cause cyanosis.

Bronchial obstruction may be due to direct blockage in the lumen, changes in the bronchial wall, or extrinsic compression. In the lumen, inspissated mucus, especially in the presence of mucosal edema, foreign bodies, or blood, may cause atelectasis. Aspirated foreign bodies may be chemically inert or, in the case of vegetable matter, especially nuts, may cause intense inflammatory change in the bronchus and a febrile reaction. Causative factors in the wall of the bronchus are mucosal edema, endobronchial tuberculous tissue, and tumors. Extrinsic bronchial compression by lymph nodes or tumors also may lead to atelectasis. Massive pericardial effusion, a very large heart, enlarged left atrium, or dilated pulmonary outflow tract may cause compression of bronchi, resulting in atelectasis. More commonly the left lower lobe or right upper lobe is affected. An anomalous left pulmonary artery may compress the right main bronchus, causing atelectasis on the right side. Atelectasis is common in the newborn because of the relative small airway diameters.

CLINICAL MANIFESTATIONS. The symptoms depend on the extent of pulmonary atelectasis and the time taken for its formation. Symptoms are more pronounced with an acute onset or when a significant degree of atelectasis has occurred. This may result in dyspnea, tachypnea, cyanosis, and, in severe cases, shock and collapse; sudden death may even result from massive bilateral atelectasis. If the area of collapse is extensive, the ipsilateral hemithorax may appear smaller, and there may be diminished chest wall movement. Dullness, diminished breath sounds, and mediastinal shift to the affected side may also be noted. In the presence of secondary infection crackles may be heard. Because the bronchus is obstructed, bronchial breathing is uncommon.

DIAGNOSIS. The diagnosis is suggested by the findings of reduced breath sounds, dullness on percussion, and a shift of the mediastinum, best indicated by a shift of the maximal cardiac impulse toward the affected side.

An x-ray examination of the chest is essential for confirmation of the diagnosis. The atelectatic lobe or segment is opacified and, except in the case of the middle lobe (which shrinks from both borders toward the center of the lobe), collapses toward the midline. Subsegmental atelectasis may appear as linear streaks. The process of collapse is usually gradual. The hemithorax becomes smaller, its ribs are approximated, and its diaphragm is elevated. In all cases the apex of the wedge is at the hilus of the lung.

TREATMENT. Therapy is directed toward removal of the underlying cause. If it is thought to be a foreign body, bronchoscopy is indicated without delay. If the cause is thought to be mucus obstruction, which is commonly the case with respiratory infections, postoperatively, and with cystic fibrosis, postural drainage and chest percussion in conjunction with aerolized bronchodilators must be performed at least 3 to 4 times daily. Adequate hydration and an atmosphere of fine mist help to keep the mucus liquefied, thus assisting drainage. If the atelectasis persists after 1 or 2 weeks of postural drainage, bronchoscopy may be indicated; however, this procedure must be carried out sooner when the atelectasis is extensive. In the presence of possible infection, antimicrobial therapy for atelectasis is important, as atelectatic pneumonia may lead to bronchiectasis.

Pulmonary Emphysema

Pulmonary emphysema or "air trapping" may be obstructive or interstitial. The obstructive type consists of overdistention of the alveoli, resulting in stretching of connective tissue. When extensive, it causes a reduction in the capillary flow, damage to elastic fibers, and alveolar rupture. Interstitial emphysema is the presence of air in the interstitial tissue of the lung as a result of alveolar or airway rupture.

OBSTRUCTIVE EMPHYSEMA. Obstructive emphysema may affect a segment, a lobe, or all of one or both lungs. It may be patchy. It results from relative expiratory air flow obstruction in an airway caused by intralumenal contents (i.e., mucus, foreign body, or tumor), airway wall abnormalities (mucosal edema, stenosis), or extrinsic compression by nodes, vessels, or tumors. In children the process is commonly acute and reversible, but if the cause persists, chronic lung damage may occur. Because airways are tethered open during inspiration, gas passes distal to the obstruction, but on expiration positive pressure exerted on the airway and its natural recoil reduce the diameter of and, hence, emptying of the given distal lung unit, thus creating trapped air.

Obstructive emphysema causes reduction in effective ventilation. If the condition is sufficiently severe, hypoxemia occurs first, followed by hypercarbia and subsequent development of respiratory acidosis, especially if an acute process is superimposed on a chronic condition. If, however, pulmonary ventilation suddenly decreases, as with an acute lower respiratory tract infection, there may be a decrease in pH.

The acute condition is seen characteristically in children with bronchiolitis, asthma, interstitial pneumonia in the infant, or foreign body inhalation (localized obstructive emphysema) and the chronic condition with cystic fibrosis, asthma, or endobronchial tuberculosis (localized). Lobar emphysema is relatively common in newborn infants (see Chap. 9).

Clinical Manifestations. The cardinal symptom of emphysema is dyspnea. If the condition is sufficiently severe, the chest may appear barrel-shaped. The percussion note is hyperresonant. Chest roentgenograms show horizontal ribs, depressed diaphragms, and translucent lung fields. In the infant there may be bowing of the sternum and increased translucency behind the sternum and the heart. Complications are pneumothorax, interstitial emphysema, subcutaneous emphysema, and cor pulmonale.

Treatment. Treatment is primarily directed toward the cause. Oxygen should be administered with caution in severe cases in which the arterial PCO_2 is significantly elevated; it may cause respiratory depression by removal of the hypoxic stimulus to respiration, resulting in further hypercapnia, coma, and even death, although this is rare in children.

CONGENITAL LOBAR EMPHYSEMA. Congenital lobar emphysema is an obstructive emphysema affecting a selected lobe or lobar segment. The symptom complex may be caused by deficient bronchial cartilage, allowing bronchial collapse during expiration, or by mucus obstruction. Less common causes are bronchial compression by an anomalous pulmonary artery or by a bronchogenic cyst.

Clinical features are the early onset of dyspnea, cyanosis, and localized wheezing. Roentgenograms of the chest show hyperinflation of the affected lobe, which may herniate across the midline, and on the affected side the diaphragm may be flattened and the lower lobe collapsed. In the neonate this may present as an emergency like a tension pneumothorax or may be found incidentally.

Treatment. Treatment may be expectant in the mild cases, but more frequently the condition is recognized as an emergency, and aggressive intervention is necessary. Bronchoscopy with lavage may relieve bronchial plugging. Acute decompression and lobectomy are indicated if there is sudden cardiac compromise pathophysiologically similar to a tension pneumothorax.

INTERSTITIAL EMPHYSEMA. Pulmonary interstitial emphysema is most common in the sick neonate with respiratory distress syndrome receiving ventilatory support with high inspiratory pressures. Leakage of air from distended alveoli or ruptured conducting airways into the pulmonary connective tissue results in interstitial emphysema. The air may also track along perivascular sheaths to the hilus, where it may leave the sheath and enter the mediastinum. The resulting mediastinal emphysema may cause dyspnea and precordial pain especially noted in the older child. Auscultation reveals a crunching sound over the mediastinal area similar to the sound of walking on snow. Air may spread from the mediastinum along fascial planes, causing subcutaneous emphysema in the neck. Pneumothorax may be another complication. Pneumomediastinum is a relatively frequent complication of status asthmaticus.

Treatment of mediastinal emphysema is usually conservative. The air is absorbed in a few days. Rarely is it necessary to aspirate the mediastinum.

Lung Cysts

A lung cyst is a rounded space in the lung, typically thin-walled (unless acutely or chronically infected), and containing air or fluid. Because lung cysts are rarely found in neonates, the great majority are probably acquired and infective in origin. The congenital origin of lung cysts is difficult to prove, but it may be suspected when they are found in neonates in whom anomalous fissures, sequestered lobes, or other congenital anomalies are present. Lung cysts are seldom found in association with cysts in other organs. The presence of columnar epithelium is not necessarily proof of congenital origin. Pneumatoceles are most commonly found with staphylococcal pneumonia and occasionally follow pneumococcal, streptococcal, or coliform infection. In areas where echinococcus disease is prevalent, hydatid cysts occur.

COURSE. The course of pneumatoceles is one of regression, given appropriate antibiotic therapy. Lung cysts, on the other hand, rarely resolve spontaneously and ulti-mately require surgical excision, especially once they have become infected.

SYMPTOMS AND PRESENTING FEATURES. Patients may initially have symptoms of pneumonia (i.e., cough, fever, and wheezing), or they may have hemoptysis, or the cyst (or cysts) may be discovered on a routine x-ray examination. Pneumothorax may be an initial feature.

DIAGNOSIS. The roentgenographic picture of a single large cyst is that of a rounded or oval translucent area, usually bounded by a thin wall. Sometimes resembling pneumothorax, a large lung cyst is separated from the lateral thoracic wall by at least a thin rim of lung tissue, though an oblique view or even bronchography may be necessary to demonstrate this. Whether or not lung markings are seen depends on the presence of lung tissue in front of or behind the translucent area. Lung markings are uncommonly seen on a posteroanterior view of pneumothorax, in which the margin of collapsed lung is usually visualized easily. An area of emphysema is bounded by the borders of a lobe and may herniate across the midline.

Computerized axial tomography of the chest has largely replaced bronchography as a confirmatory test. Though either eosinophilia or a positive Casoni test may be lacking, a positive Casoni test confirms the diagnosis of a hydatid (echinococcal) cyst.

TREATMENT. An infected cyst should be treated with appropriate antibacterial agents. A large, space-filling cyst, not regressing in size and causing significant symptoms, should be surgically removed. Cysts communicating with bronchi are liable to infection and should be excised. Surgical treatment of pneumatoceles, rarely necessary, takes the form of decompression of large cysts causing symptoms.

Congenital Anomalies of the Lung

Congenital anomalies of the lung are infrequently seen, but they may pose serious diagnostic problems to the clinician.

PULMONARY SEQUESTRATION. Pulmonary sequestration, an uncommon congenital abnormality, is an isolated, poorly differentiated, solid or cystic body of lung tissue with anomalous blood supply. There are two main types, intralobar sequestration and extrapulmonic accessory lobes. Both types are more commonly found in the lower lobes, on the left more frequently than on the right. They are both usually supplied by systemic arteries from the aorta and occasionally transdiaphragmatically from the celiac plexus. Venous drainage is into the pulmonary veins.

A clinical feature of pulmonary sequestration is recurrent or persistent infection. Diagnosis is confirmed by angiography, subtraction angiography, and bronchography.

PRIMARY AGENESIS OR APLASIA. Primary agenesis or aplasia represents functional absence of the lung. A single, normal, functional lung is consistent with absence of symptoms.

Pulmonary hypoplasia may be primary, or it may be secondary to a diaphragmatic hernia on the same side. The scimitar syndrome (anomalous right pulmonary venous return to the inferior vena cava), anomalous arterial supply to the lungs from the aorta, or abnormal bronchial communications may be associated with pulmonary hypoplasia. The hypoplastic lung may grow spontaneously to a normal size and is often characterized by absence of symptoms.

ABNORMAL FISSURE FORMATION OR LOBULATION. Abnormal fissures are not uncommon. Examples are the azygos lobe, left middle lobe, and absence of or incomplete fissures. Multilobular lungs are often associated with severe congenital cardiac abnormalities. Isomerism (or mirror image) of the lungs may be associated with visceral situs inversus or with splenic or cardiac abnormalities. Skeletal, cardiovascular, or urinary tract anomalies may also be associated with congenital malformations of the lung.

Diseases of the Pleura

Diseases of the pleura are seldom primary. They commonly arise by extension from the lung.

PLEURISY. Dry pleurisy is a pleural reaction to an irritant that is usually bacterial, the pneumococcus being the major cause. Pleurisy often follows thoracotomy. It is found with rheumatic pneumonitis, which is rare, and with a pulmonary embolism (rare in children) when infarction is adjacent to the pleura.

Clinical Manifestations. The most prominent symptom of acute bacterial pleurisy is a sharp pain over the affected side of the thorax, which is due to involvement of the parietal pleura and is exaggerated by deep inspiration. The pain may be referred to the hypochondrium or to the shoulder tip when the central portion of the diaphragmatic pleura is involved. Grunting respirations may result from pleural irritation. Auscultation and occasionally palpation reveal a pleural friction rub, usually heard best in the midaxillary or posterior basal area. The presence of crackles indicates involvement of the underlying lung. With the formation of a significant amount of pleural fluid, both the pain and the pleural rub disappear.

Diagnosis. The presence of a pleural rub substantiates the diagnosis of pleurisy. The characteristic pain may also be caused by epidemic pleurodynia, a feature of Coxsackie virus group B infection. This disease occurs in epidemics in the summer or fall and is characterized by unilateral or bilateral

chest pain simulating pleurisy but usually without a pleural rub. A history of trauma with point tenderness, and at times crepitus, helps to differentiate a fractured rib from pleurisy; rib fracture may be confirmed by roentgenographic examination. Subphrenic abscess should be considered in the differential diagnosis. Although rare in children, it most often follows suppurative appendicitis or septicemia. The diaphragm may be high and its movement diminished on the affected side.

Treatment. The treatment of pleurisy is directed to the primary cause. Splinting of the chest is seldom indicated.

PLEURAL EFFUSION. A clear pleural effusion may be a transudate, with a specific gravity of 1.015 or less and low protein content, without significant pleocytosis. It is most commonly seen in congestive cardiac failure, the effusion usually being on the right side, in the nephrotic syndrome or acute glomerulonephritis, or in association with effusion into other serous cavities (e.g., acute pancreatitis).

Alternatively, the fluid may be an exudate, with a specific gravity greater than 1.015 and high protein content. Polymorphonuclear leukocytes or lymphocytes may be present in excess, but when the fluid is frankly purulent it is referred to as empyema. Common causes of exudative pleural effusion in children are primary tuberculosis, pneumococcal pneumonia, and streptococcal pneumonia.

Hemothorax may follow trauma, either surgical or accidental, and is seen occasionally in malignant diseases of the lung and pleura. Chylothorax, a rare condition, results from trauma to the thoracic duct or from its obstruction to it by neoplasms or enlarged lymph nodes.

Clinical Manifestations. Pleural effusion is usually asymptomatic, but if large, it may cause tachypnea or dyspnea. Movement of the chest is reduced on the affected side. If the effusion is of long duration, the chest may be flat on the side of the effusion. The percussion note is flat or stony dull, breath sounds are reduced, and egophony may be detected at the upper border of the effusion. A large effusion displaces the heart and mediastinum to the opposite side.

Roentgenograms of the chest reveal diffuse clouding, the upper border of which is concave but not discretely bounded. The costophrenic angle is obscured, and a pleural line may extend up the lateral chest wall. If the effusion is large, the heart and mediastinum are seen to be displaced to the opposite side, and one entire lung field may be clouded.

Diagnosis and Treatment. Indications for thoracentesis are diagnostic or therapeutic. Diagnostic thoracentesis is important for the diagnosis of empyema, in which direct examination and culture for organisms are necessary. In addition, cell counts, pH, protein content, amylase, and lactic dehydrogenase are determined. The pH of the effusion when acidic (< 7.20) may be an indication for chest-tube closed drainage. Therapeutic thoracentesis is performed for relief of dyspnea due to a large pleural effusion. Complications of thoracentesis are pneumothorax, air embolism, hemoptysis, and pulmonary edema when large quantities of fluid are withdrawn rapidly. When thoracentesis is carefully performed, complications are rare.

Pneumothorax

The occurrence of pneumothorax is not common in children. Most frequently it is seen in the neonatal period, with staphylococcal pneumonia or during attacks of asthma. In neonates it is likely to occur after difficult delivery, vigorous resuscitation, or cesarean section. It may complicate tracheostomy, penetrating chest injury, fractured rib, or blunt chest trauma.

The mechanism is usually alveolar rupture followed by air tracking along pulmonary vascular sheaths to the visceral pleura, which ruptures, allowing air to enter the pleural space. Alternatively, pneumothorax may be due to rupture of subpleural blebs or trauma to the visceral pleura.

CLINICAL MANIFESTATIONS. In a neonate who may have had preceding respiratory symptoms, the onset is marked by sudden occurrence or exacerbation of dyspnea, with cyanosis and shock. Physical signs include decreased or absent breath sounds, a shift of apex of the heart, and a shift of the trachea. Tension pneumothorax is life threatening and may present as shock.

The older child usually complains of localized sharp pain followed by dyspnea in addition to the symptoms mentioned for the neonate. Important signs are unilateral hyperresonance to percussion, reduced breath sounds on the same side of the chest, and displacement of the maximum cardiac impulse to the opposite side. Spontaneous pneumothorax is more common in tall slender adolescents and especially with those intraconnective tissue disorders such as Marfan's syndrome.

DIAGNOSIS AND TREATMENT. Suspicion of pneumothorax is sufficient indication to take an x-ray film of the chest immediately. Better delineation of the collapsed lung is obtained with the expiratory film. A translucent area is seen around the sharply outlined periphery of the lung, which collapses toward the hilus.

If the pneumothorax is small (less than 20% of the hemithorax) and is causing no serious symptoms, it may be left alone, the air usually being absorbed rapidly. Increasing the fraction of inspired oxygen may hasten the resolution.

Relief of pressure may be called for, generally when progressive dyspnea is present and the pneumothorax is greater than 20% of the hemithorax. When there is considerable disturbance of lung function, however, as in staphylococcal pneumonia, it may be necessary to relieve pressure from the pneumothorax.

In an emergency, often as a lifesaving measure, a needle may be inserted into an intercostal space, usually at the second lateral to the midclavicular line. After air emerges under pressure, a syringe is attached and all the air aspirated. This procedure should be followed by an x-ray examination of the chest to assess the degree of lung expansion.

When pneumothorax recurs or fails to resolve spontaneously, an intercostal tube should be inserted and left in situ. For this purpose a chest tube can be inserted in the sixth intercostal space in the midaxillary line or third intercostal space just lateral to the midclavicular line. Underwater drainage through a plastic tube is then established and continued until bubbles have ceased for 12 to 24 hours and the lung has reexpanded. Recurrent spontaneous pneumothorax is an indication for pleurodesis.

Mediastinal Masses

Although certain generalizations can be made about the probable nature of a given mass in the chest of a child, the diagnosis cannot be made with certainty. A substantial proportion of tumors within the chest in children are malignant but may be curable; even those that are histologically benign may be life threatening because of increase in size and pressure on vital structures or because infection may develop in them. The discovery of a tumor within the chest of a child is, therefore, an indication for operation. Some large cysts may be asymptomatic; others may cause difficulty because of compression of the trachea, displacement of the mediastinum, irritation of a bronchus, or compression of the esophagus. Computerized axial tomography, after a barium swallow, is usually the extent of diagnostic study required, although occasionally bronchography is helpful. If there is a reasonable possibility that the lesion involves the heart or great vessels, angiocardiography is advsiable. A few cases, with tracheal compression and respiratory obstruction, demand emergent operative intervention.

In the anterior mediastinum the principal tumors are the teratomas, both the solid variety known as teratomas and the cystic tumors commonly called dermoids. The solid tumors are more likely to become malignant; the cystic ones more often become infected. Either variety may reach very great size.

In the superior mediastinum, malignant lymphomas occur, and operation may be required to establish the diagnosis. In the posterior mediastinum, dense, sharply rounded tumors are probably neurogenic in origin. The presence of the masses suggests ganglioneuromas, which are usually benign; the smaller ones are generally either neuroblastomas, which are malignant, or neurofibromas, which are potentially malignant. For all these, including the benign lesions, a curative operation must be undertaken because they may grow so huge as to threaten life.

An interesting lesion in the posterio mediastinum is the enteric cyst of foregut origin, sometimes called a duplication of the esophagus. It is usually lined with gastric mucosa and is situated close to the esophagus. It tends to be associated with vertebral anomalies in the same area and frequently with intestinal "duplications." It does not communicate with the esophagus but may pass down through the diaphragm and communicate with the duodenum or jejunum.

Other cysts, such as bronchogenic cysts and pericardial cysts, are much less likely to be found in children than in adults.

James E. Clayton and Mohsen Ziai

References

American Academy of Pediatrics Committee on Accident and Poison Prevention. First aid for the choking child. *Pediatrics* 81:740, 1988.

Bernard, P., Stenstrom, R., Feldman, W., and Smith, A. Sulfonamide prophylaxis vs. ventilation tubes in hearing loss due to recurrent otitis media with effusion: Preliminary results of a randomized controlled trial. *Am. J. Dis. Child.* 141:389, 1987.

Bhui, P. S. Respiratory emergencies in infants and young children. *Can. Fam. Phys.* 34:2203, 1988.

Bluestone, C. D., and Stool, S. E. (Eds). *Pediatric Otolaryngology,* Vol I and II. Philadelphia: Saunders, 1983. Chapters 14–21.

Bodor, F. F. Conjunctivitis-otitis syndrome. *Pediatrics* 69:695, 1982.

Brouillette, R. T., Fernbach, S. K., and Hunt, C. E. Obstructive sleep apnea in infants and children. *J. Pediatr.* 100:31, 1982.

Durieux-Smith, A., Picton, T. W., et al. Brainstem electric response audiometry in infants of a neonatal intensive care unit. *Audiology* 26:284, 1987.

Feigin, R. D., and Cherry, J. D. (Eds.) *Textbook of Pediatric Infectious Disease* (2nd ed.), Vols. I and II. Philadelphia: Saunders, 1987.

Feldman, W., Momy, J., and Dulberg, C. Trimethoprim-sulfamethoxazole v. amoxicillin in the treatment of acute otitis media. *Can. Med. Assoc. J.* 139:961, 1988.

Feldman, W., Rosser, W., and McGrath, P. *Primary Medical Care of Children and Adolescents.* New York: Oxford University Press 1987. Pp. 9–22.

Gerber, J. Latex agglutination to identify streptococcal antigen. *J. Pediatr.* 107:85, 1985.

Heaf, D. P., et al. Nasopharyngeal airways in Pierre Robin syndrome. *J. Pediatr.* 100:698, 1982.

Hutton, N., Wilson, M. H., et al. Effectiveness of prescribing an antihistamine-decongestatnt for young children with a common cold (abstract). *Am. J. Dis. Child.* 141:38, 1987.

Jaffe, B. F. (Ed.). *Hearing Loss in Children.* Baltimore: University Park Press, 1977.

Jaffe, B. F. Development of the Respiratory Tract. In T. R. Johnson, et al. (Eds.). *Children Are Different. Developmental Physiology* (2nd ed.). Columbus: Ross Laboratories, 1978.

Joint Committee on Infant Hearing. Position statement. *Pediatrics* 70:496, 1982.

Kasian, J. F., Bringham, W. T., et al. Bacterial tracheitis in children. *Can. Med. Assoc. J.* 140:46, 1989.

Katsanis, E., Luke, K. H., et al. Prevalence and significance of mild bleeding disorder in children with recurrent epistaxis. *J. Pediatr.* 113:73, 1988.

Kendig, E. L., and Chernick, V. (Eds.). *Disorders of the Respiratory Tract in Children* (4th ed.). Philadelphia: Saunders, 1983.

Kveton, J. F., and Pillbury, H. C. Conservative treatment of infantile subglottic hemangioma with corticosteroids. *Arch. Otolaryngol.* 108:117, 1982.

Laraya-Cuasay, L. R., and Hughes, W. T. (Eds.). *Interstitial Lung Diseases in Children.* Boca Raton, FL: CRC Press, 1988.

Lim, D. J. Recent advances in otitis media. *Ann. Otol. Rhinol. Laryngol.* [*Suppl.*] 139:98, 1989.

Northern, J. L., and Downs, M. P. *Hearing Loss in Children* (2nd ed.). Baltimore: Williams & Wilkins, 1978.

Nussbaum, E., and Galant, S. P. (Eds.). *Pediatric Respiratory Disorders: Clinical Approaches.* Orlando, FL: Grune and Stratton, 1984.

Paradise, J. C., Bluestone, C. D., et al. Efficacy of tonsillectomy for recurrent throat infection in severely affected children. *N. Engl. J. Med.* 310: 674, 1984.

Schwartz, R. H. Prevention of otitis media: A multitude of yellow brick roads. *Pediatr. Infect. Dis.* 1:3, 1982.

Schwartz, R. H. Pneumatic ototoscopy: Getting the most out of the ear exam. *J. Respir. Dis.* 4:82, 1983.

Schwartz, R. H., Rodriguez, W. J., and Grundfast, K. M. Duration of middle ear effusion after acute otitis media. *Pediatr. Infect. Dis.* 3:204, 1984.

Silverman, F. N. *Caffey's Pediatric X-Ray Diagnosis: An Integrated Approach* (8th ed.), Vol. II. Chicago: Year Book, 1984.

Soucy, P., and Penning, J. The clinical relevance of certain observations on the histology of the thyroglossal tract. *J. Pediatr. Surg.* 19:506, 1984.

Stiehm, E. *Immunologic Disorders in Infants and Children* (3rd ed). Philadelphia: Saunders, 1989.

Telander, R. L., and Deane, S. A. Thyroglossal and branchial cleft cysts and sinuses. *Surg. Clin. North Am.* 57:779, 1977.

Visudhiphan, P., et al. Torticollis as the presenting sign in cervical spine infection and tumor. *Clin. Pediatr.* 21:71, 1982.

11

The Heart and
Great Vessels

Pediatric cardiology deals principally with congenital heart disease. This occurs in 7 to 8/1000 liveborn children. In the majority of cases, the cause is that of multifactorial inheritance. In a minority of cases, there is a specific genetic (e.g., Down syndrome) or environmental (e.g., rubella) cause. Rhythm disorders and acquired cardiac disease make up the rest of the problems that one usually sees. Acute rheumatic fever is in a resurgence in this country today. Congenital heart disease, rhythm disturbances, and some acquired disorders are discussed in this chapter.

Evaluation of Heart Disease

More than ever, accurate anatomical and physiological diagnosis of congenital cardiac malformations can be made in a broad age range. Prenatally, the ultrasound diagnosis (fetal echocardiography) of congenital heart disease has enabled physicians to better plan for postnatal therapy. After repair of complex congenital heart defects, physicians are better able to follow the functional status of patients as they approach adulthood. To a greater extent, this has been possible because of improved ultrasound techniques that help resolve questions concerning the structural and functional status of the patient.

Most of the more severe congenital heart defects clinically manifest themselves in the neonatal or early infancy periods. These are usually recognized by the presence of a murmur, cyanosis, or congestive heart failure.

Although innocent heart murmurs occur universally in children, they infrequently manifest themselves in early infancy. Murmurs associated with significant defects may be affected by perinatal changes in the physiology of the cardiovascular system, mainly due to a gradual decrease in high neonatal pulmonary vascular resistance. Thus, the absence of a murmur does not rule out the presence of severe congenital heart disease, especially when other clues such as cyanosis or congestive heart failure are present.

Cyanosis in the neonatal period, if not caused by respiratory disease, persistent pulmonary hypertension of the newborn, a central nervous system insult, or sepsis, almost assures the diagnosis of congenital heart disease. The remainder of the physical examination is often not helpful in defining the exact structural problem. The electrocardiogram (ECG) can help determine the presence or absence of ventricular hypertrophy. The chest x ray may help by determining the shape and size of the heart and great vessels and whether pulmonary blood flow is diminished or increased. Color-flow, Doppler, two-dimensional echocardiography is the best diagnostic tool to determine precisely the structural and physiological problem. Despite that, there is still role for cardiac catheterization with angiography. Specific anatomic and physiologic details may be needed by the cardiovascular surgeon before palliative or reparative surgery is attempted. In addition therapeutic procedures may be performed during the catheterization (e.g., Rashkind balloon septostomy or balloon valvuloplasty) in order to palliate or fully treat the problem.

Congestive heart failure in children most commonly occurs in infancy. The clinical presentation is one of cardiomegaly, tachycardia, a ventricular diastolic gallop, tachypnea, and hepatomegaly. Cardiac failure may be the first clinical manifestation of a left-to-right shunt, obstructive lesion, or myocardial problem. Management is initially medical, with possible therapeutic catheterization and/or surgery to follow.

On an outpatient basis, the most common cause for referral to a pediatric cardiologist that leads to the diagnosis of a congenital heart problem is the presence of a murmur. This makes it necessary for the primary-care physician to recognize the different types of innocent murmurs. The presence of respiratory and cardiovascular symptoms or growth failure may aid in the diagnosis of a congenital heart problem.

Laboratory Aids to Diagnosis

The ECG is a useful tool in the diagnosis of congenital heart disease. The presence of ventricular hypertrophy may be evidence of a significant pressure or volume overload of one or both ventricles. Enlargement of the atria is less commonly seen. Occasionally, the frontal plane ventricular axis (e.g., left axis deviation in a newborn with tricuspid atresia) or the presence of an arrhythmia (e.g., paroxysmal supraventricular tachycardia with an atrial septal defect) may aid in the diagnosis.

The plain chest x ray is used to confirm the presence of cardiomegaly and evaluate the pulmonary vascularity. Specific cardiac chamber enlargement may be noted. Other features such as a right aortic arch (in tetralogy of Fallot) or extracardiac anomalies (e.g., vertebral anomalies) may be good diagnostic clues.

Echocardiography has changed the nature of the diagnostic work-up for a potential congenital cardiac malformation. It has provided a safe, readily repeatable, specific tool to evaluate the structure and physiology of the heart. The evolution of M-mode, two-dimensional, Doppler, and, finally, color-flow echocardiography has refined the technique over a relatively brief period of time. Screening of patients for subtle defects can be accomplished painlessly with a great degree of safety. In some instances, echocardiography has supplanted cardiac catheterization as the ultimate diagnostic tool used to prepare a patient for reparative surgery. It has virtually eliminated the need for routine postoperative catheterizations to evaluate surgical outcome.

Cardiac catheterization with angiography is still the ultimate diagnostic tool used in preparing patients with complex congenital or acquired heart problems for surgery. Newer catheters and contrast materials have lowered the morbidity and mortality. They may not decrease further in the future because it is now the most critically ill patients who often need to undergo this procedure. The addition of therapeutic modalities that replace or supplement surgical procedures has enabled the pediatric cardiologist to become the therapist as well as the diagnostician. The Rashkind balloon atrial septostomy was the first technique at the start this tradition. Now blade atrial septostomy, balloon valvuloplasty and angioplasty, and closure of left-to-right shunts are all within the realm of therapeutic possibilities.

Disturbances of Rate and Rhythm

In the pediatric age group the disturbances of rate and rhythm produced during cardiac surgery are more numerous than naturally occurring arrhythmias. While all forms of arrhythmia occur spontaneously in infants and children, only the more common problems are discussed here.

For a patient with an irregularity of rate or rhythm, electrocardiography is initially required for an accurate diagnosis. Twenty-four-hour Holter monitoring may be essential to detect an unsustained arrhythmia.

The clinician can estimate the immediate danger of an arrhythmia by clinically judging the adequacy of the cardiac output. Poorly palpable pulses, reduced blood pressure, signs of congestive heart failure, peripheral vasoconstriction, shock, and syncope indicate gross impairment of cardiac function. In contrast, a bizarre ECG is at times encountered in association with apparently normal circulation.

Sinus Tachycardia

Sinus tachycardia is a rapid heart rate with an otherwise normal conduction mechanism. It is the expected response to fever, exercise, excitement, and anemia.

An extremely ill child at times has a sinus tachycardia of sufficient rate to suggest a paroxysmal supraventricular tachycardia. If the underlying cause is obscure, the presence of a heart rate over 200 beats/min may seem to account for all signs and symptoms. Variation in the heart rate is strong evidence against this conclusion. An ECG generally helps to provide the solution to this diagnostic problem.

In the majority of infants sinus tachycardia is a transient phenomenon caused by anemia, hypoxemia, anxiety, and possibly hyperthyroidism. Except in the latter, it usually resolves spontaneously.

Paroxysmal Supraventricular Tachycardia

Paroxysmal supraventricular tachycardia is characterized by the sudden onset of a very rapid heart rate (> 200 beats/min in infants) that may persist for minutes to hours. In general the heart rate does not vary. Following a normal heart rate there is a sudden occurrence of a fixed rapid rate generally with a narrow QRS complex on the ECG. A P wave may or may not be visualized. The conversion of this tachyarrhythmia to a normal rhythm is as abrupt as the onset. Neonates and young infants are more often symptomatic and may develop congestive heart failure earlier than older children. Symptoms may include feeding difficulties, tachypnea, pallor, and irritability. Older children may complain of palpitations and lightheadedness. This arrhythmia may be triggered by an intercurrent infection, fever, sympathomimetic drugs, and caffeine. If the tachycardia is associated with a wide QRS complex, it could be confused with ventricular tachycardia. This may be the result of supraventricular tachycardia associated with a preexcitation syndrome (Wolff-Parkinson-White syndrome). Other predisposing factors may include congenital heart disease (Ebstein's anomaly, congenitally corrected transposition of the great vessels, and atrial septal defect) and a postoperative state.

Treatment of this tachycardia involves utilization of the diving reflex (a bag of ice on the face) in infants and carotid massage in older children. Severely symptomatic infants may require synchronized direct-current (DC) cardioversion. Digoxin remains the most common pharmacologic agent because of its ease of administration. In the presence of Wolff-Parkinson-White syndrome a beta blocker is the agent of choice, because digoxin may shorten the refractory period of the bypass tract and lead to a malignant ventricular arrhythmia. Calcium channel blockers (Verapamil) have been used in the acute situation in older infants and children.

Ectopic Beats

The discovery of a basically regular heart rhythm interspersed with premature atrial or ventricular contractions is a common finding. This condition may be present for years. In the absence of an underlying structural heart problem the situation is generally a benign one. Occasionally the child may complain of palpitations. Pharmacologic agents are rarely necessary to control these premature beats. Removing caffeine from the diet is often helpful in treatment. Premature supraventricular contractions are generally not treated unless they are associated with short bursts of supraventricular tachycardia in infants and long symptomatic runs of supraventricular tachycardia in older children. Unifocal premature ventricular contractions are usually benign and in most cases disappear with exercise.

Atrial Flutter

Spontaneously occurring atrial flutter is very rare in the pediatric age group. It is usually associated with congenital structural cardiac defects or a postoperative state. Appropriate efforts should be made to convert the patient to sinus rhythm.

Atrial Fibrillation

Atrial fibrillation generally results from chronic atrial enlargement secondary to mitral or tricuspid valve disease. The aim of treatment is to bring the ventricular rate to a reasonable level and then to convert the patient to sinus rhythm by either digoxin alone or by adding quinidine to the treatment. Occasionally synchronized electrical cardioversion may be required. Special attention to and treatment of the cause of the arrhythmia is required to prevent a recurrence. Untreated, this condition may lead to congestive heart failure and possibly death.

Congenital Complete Heart Block

This condition is recognized by a fixed, slow heart rate usually less than 70 to 80 beats/min. With greater frequency this is being noted prenatally and documented by fetal echocardiography. The rate increases little with exercise or excitement. Clinically there are associated systolic murmurs secondary to the greater stroke volume needed to maintain normal cardiac output. The ECG is typically diagnostic. There is a 40 to 60% possibility of a structural congenital heart lesion that warrants further evaluation with ultrasound.

There is a well recognized association between congenital complete heart block and maternal connective tissue disease. Most children with uncomplicated complete heart block are asymptomatic. An exceedingly low heart rate, syncope, or presyncope may be the first indication that an electronic pacemaker should be implanted.

Congenital Heart Disease

Patent Ductus Arteriosus (PDA)

In the fetus, the ductus arteriosus is a normal vascular connection between the main pulmonary artery and descending aorta (Fig. 11-1). Persistent patency of the ductus arteriosus after birth is abnormal.

PHYSIOLOGY. In the fetus the ductus arteriosus carries the majority of right ventricular output into the descending aorta. At birth, the resistance to blood flow in the lungs is dramatically decreased. As a result, the flow of blood through the ductus is reversed. In a normal newborn, the left-to-right shunt may be identified during the first day of life. Increased blood levels of oxygen prompt functional and subsequent anatomic closure of the ductus. In some infants, the ductus remains patent and left-to-right shunting persists. With a further drop in pulmonary vascular resistance during the next several weeks, the amount of left-to-right shunting through the patent ductus gradually increases. The classic continuous murmur may only then become clinically evident. Maternal rubella during the first trimester of pregnancy is an established cause of a patent ductus arteriosus (PDA).

Among premature infants delayed closure of the ductus arteriosus is a common finding. This is generally thought to be associated with the hypoxemia associated with respiratory distress syndrome and incomplete smooth muscle formation of the wall of the ductus arteriosus. The typical presentation in the premature infant is that of a nonspecific systolic murmur that develops when the respiratory distress syndrome is improving. Fluid restriction and treatment with intravenous indomethacin (a prostaglandin synthetase inhibitor) effects closure in approximately 70% of the cases. In the other 30% surgical ligation may be necessary.

CLINICAL MANIFESTATIONS. Most patients with a small to moderate PDA are asymptomatic. With a large left-to-right shunt, congestive heart failure and multiple respiratory infections may be present. Typically, a murmur is discovered on a routine examination.

On physical examination, the pulse pressure is wide and the peripheral pulses readily palpable. A continuous murmur, heard maximally at the second left intercostal space, reaches its peak intensity at the second heart sound and tapers off into diastole. With significant pulmonary hypertension, only a systolic murmur may be present with a loud pulmonary component to the second heart sound.

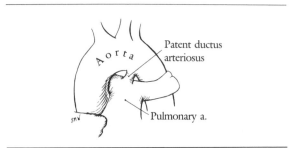

Fig. 11-1. Patent ductus arteriosus.

ELECTROCARDIOGRAPHIC AND X-RAY FINDINGS. In a moderate to large PDA, left ventricular hypertrophy is present secondary to the volume overload of the left ventricle. Pulmonary hypertension may cause a varying degree of right ventricular hypertrophy. Radiographically there may be cardiomegaly and increased pulmonary vascularity with at least a moderate shunt. The echocardiogram is usually diagnostic.

DIFFERENTIAL DIAGNOSIS. In the absence of typical clinical findings, other less common diagnoses should be considered. These include aorticopulmonary window, arteriovenous fistula, aneurysm of the sinus of Valsalva, and even a loud, innocent jugular venous hum. Doppler, two-dimensional echocardiography is typically diagnostic. Occasionally, cardiac catheterization may need to be performed, specifically in the presence of significant pulmonary hypertension or coexisting congential heart disease.

TREATMENT. Symptomatic infants with large left-to-right shunts should have surgical division of the patent ductus when the diagnosis is made. If the shunt is small, one should wait until 9 months or 1 year of age because spontaneous closure may still occur. Even small PDAs should be surgically closed to avoid the chance of infective endarteritis. Children with long-standing left-to-right shunts and severe pulmonary hypertension secondary to increased pulmonary vascular resistance may not benefit from surgical therapy.

Truncus Arteriosus

Persistent truncus arteriosus is characterized by the presence of a single great artery and single semilunar valve. The artery rising from the base of the heart gives rise to the pulmonary, systemic, and coronary arteries. This results from failure of separation of the embryonic truncus arteriosus into a pulmonary artery and aorta. The pulmonary arteries may arise as a single remnant of the main pulmonary artery (Type I), as adjacent posterior vessels (Type II), or as laterally placed vessels on the truncus (Type III) (Fig. 11-2). For clinical purposes the forms of truncus arteriosus with unrestricted communication with the lungs are best considered together. An associated ventricular septal defect is universal.

PHYSIOLOGY. The entire output of both ventricles is ejected into the common truncus. Ventricular pressures are identical and complete mixing of the systemic and pulmonary venous blood occurs in the truncus. The resistance to pulmonary blood flow is usually less than that in the systemic circulation resulting in a left-to-right shunt.

CLINICAL MANIFESTATIONS. The majority of patients develop congestive heart failure and cyanosis in early infancy. Pulmonary vascular disease may occur within several months. Typically the precordium is overactive. A single loud second heart sound is audible. A harsh systolic murmur is present and diastolic murmur as well if there is truncal valve incompetence.

ELECTROCARDIOGRAPHIC AND X-RAY FINDINGS. The ECG typically shows right axis deviation and right ventricular or biventricular hypertrophy. Mild to moderate cardiac enlargement and increased pulmonary vascularity are noted on the chest x ray. In 25% of cases the aorta arches over the right mainstem bronchus.

DIFFERENTIAL DIAGNOSIS. In children with mild arterial oxygen desaturation and congestive heart failure, ventricular septal defect with pulmonary hypertension, aortic-pulmonary window, and transposition of the great vessels with a ventricular septal defect should be considered. Doppler, two-dimensional echocardiography typically demonstrates the anatomy. Further preoperative evaluation should involve diagnostic cardiac catheterization.

TREATMENT. Primary surgical repair of the various types of truncus should be accomplished within the first few months of life after the congestive heart failure is controlled.

Ventricular Septal Defect

Ventricular septal defect (VSD) provides a direct communication between the right and left ventricles. This defect may occupy any portion of the intraventricular septum. Many of these defects close spontaneously.

PHYSIOLOGY. Early in life a left-to-right shunt is the physiologic hallmark of a ventricular septal defect, if the defect is not surgically closed or does not spontaneously close. When high pulmonary vascular resistance is present, the shunt may reverse and produce arterial desaturation. Various associated cardiac defects may modify the basic physiologic pattern.

CLINICAL MANIFESTATIONS. With a small VSD there may be no symptoms. A murmur may not be present during

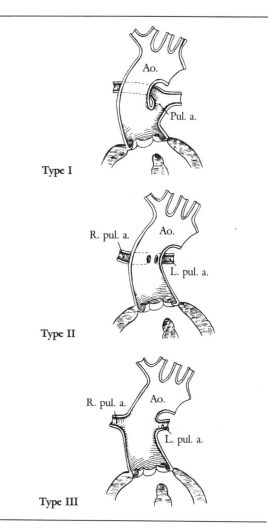

Fig. 11-2. Truncus arteriosus. (Ao. = aorta; Pul. a. = pulmonary artery.) (Courtesy Karl W. Schmidt, M.D.)

the first days of life, appearing only in the first 6 weeks. This is due to transient pulmonary hypertension of the neonate which subsides early in infancy. In the presence of a moderate or large shunt, the precordium may be overactive. A systolic thrill may be palpable at the lower left sternal border. The first heart sound (S_1) is masked by the murmur. The second heart sound (S_2) is usually normally split and of normal intensity. A third heart sound (S_3) and mid-diastolic flow rumble may be audible at the apex in the presence of a large left-to-right shunt. The systolic murmur is holosystolic, loud, and harsh, being heard best at the lower left sternal border.

ELECTROCARDIOGRAPHIC AND X-RAY FINDINGS. The ECG may be normal with a small ventricular septal defect, or it may demonstrate left ventricular hypertrophy in the presence of a moderate to large defect. With a moderate to large shunt there may be mild cardiomegaly with increased pulmonary vascularity.

DIFFERENTIAL DIAGNOSIS. The typical harsh holosystolic murmur makes the diagnosis almost certain. Consideration should be given to associated lesions such as valvular pulmonic stenosis, or PDA. Occasionally a patient with tetralogy of Fallot may be acyanotic and appear to have an uncomplicated VSD. Subaortic stenosis may also present with a murmur at the lower left sternal border. Associated defects need to be ruled out.

CARDIAC CATHETERIZATION. Cardiac catheterization should be performed prior to surgery in order to detail the location of the defect, exclude possible associated lesions, and determine the presence or absence of pulmonary vascular disease.

TREATMENT. Many of these defects close spontaneously, usually within the first 2 years of life. Congestive heart failure should be treated with digoxin and diuretics. Growth failure in the presence of medically treated congestive heart failure is an indication for reparative surgery. In the older child the presence of a pulmonary-to-systemic flow ratio of 2 : 1 or greater is also an indication for reparative surgery. In most medical centers, primary repair of the VSD is the procedure of choice even in young infants.

PROGNOSIS. Patients with a small unoperated defect should have a normal life span and remain asymptomatic. Successful surgical repair of a larger defect should result in the same length and quality of life. Varying degrees of pulmonary hypertension may develop in patients with large left-to-right shunts. This may lead to pulmonary vascular obstruction due to high pulmonary vascular resistance. Irreversible PVD typically does not occur before 6 to 12 months of age except in children with Down syndrome, probably due to chronic hypoxemia caused by alveolar hypoventilation. With maximal pulmonary vascular obstruction none of the typical clinical findings of the ventricular defect is present. A spectrum of clinical observations is encountered in the classic extreme state. With a greater elevation of pulmonary vascular resistance the systolic murmur becomes less intense, shorter in duration, and less localized. The pulmonary component of the S_2 is usually loud and palpable. A diastolic murmur of pulmonary insufficiency may be present. Cyanosis may be hard to detect until late stages of the disease.

The degree of reversibility of pulmonary hypertension depends on the degree of pulmonary vascular resistance.

This may be determined by cardiac catheterization prior to reparative surgery. Children with increased pulmonary vascular resistance are at higher risk in surgical repair with both increased morbidity and mortality.

Ventricular Septal Defect and Pulmonary Stenosis

Mild pulmonary stenosis, both valvular and infundibular, is commonly seen in association with VSD. These patients are typically acyanotic unless the degree of right ventricular outflow tract obstruction becomes severe. In that case the clinical picture may be similar to that of tetralogy of Fallot. Mild obstruction may protect the pulmonary arteries from increased flow and, therefore, decrease the chance of congestive heart failure and pulmonary vascular disease.

VENTRICULAR SEPTAL DEFECT AND AORTIC INSUFFICIENCY. An uncommon, but important complication of VSD is the appearance of associated aortic insufficiency. This is especially true when the VSD is supracristal in location. The defect may not be large and is typically located immediately adjacent to an aortic valve cusp. Surgical therapy is generally indicated.

Atrioventricular Canal Defects

Embryologically, the anterior leaflet of the mitral and septal leaflet of the tricuspid valves and the contiguous portions of the atrial and ventricular septa are formed from four endocardial cushions. Abnormal maturation of these growth centers results in a group of lesions known as atrioventricular (AV) canal defects. The defect may involve primarily the atrial septum (ostium primum defect) or the ventricular septum or both (common AV canal). The anterior leaflet of the mitral valve is almost always cleft, and with a common AV canal there may be a common AV valve.

PHYSIOLOGY. If there is a ventricular component the children typically present with a picture of a large left-to-right shunt with AV valve insufficiency. This leads to congestive heart failure and failure to thrive. Pulmonary vascular disease is often seen relatively early in life in children with Down syndrome.

CLINICAL MANIFESTATIONS. Children with left-to-right shunts predominantly at the atrial level may be entirely asymptomatic. With a significant shunt at the ventricular level, there may be congestive heart failure and recurrent respiratory infections in early infancy. One should look for clinical evidence of Down syndrome. The precordium is typically overactive with a murmur similar to that of a VSD with or without pulmonary hypertension. The pulmonary component to the second sound may be increased in amplitude due to pulmonary hypertension. Mid-diastolic rumbles across the atrioventricular valve(s) are frequently present.

ELECTROCARDIOGRAPHIC AND X-RAY FINDINGS. In the majority of cases the ECG shows a superior frontal plane QRS axis. A significant right ventricular conduction delay and evidence of left ventricular hypertrophy may be present. On the chest x ray the heart may be enlarged with increased pulmonary vascularity.

ECHOCARDIOGRAPHY. Doppler, two-dimensional echocardiography is helpful in confirming the diagnosis and differentiating the various types of defects. The anatomy of the septal defect and nature of the AV valves is often well defined.

CARDIAC CATHETERIZATION. The anatomic diagnosis is typically confirmed at the time of the cardiac catheterization. The presence of pulmonary hypertension should be determined prior to surgical repair.

SURGICAL TREATMENT. Surgical therapy is aimed at eliminating the left-to-right shunt and repairing the AV valve. The physiological results are usually excellent. Complete anatomical repair with no residual mitral regurgitation is somewhat less common. Surgery should be performed before pulmonary vascular disease develops. This generally requires an operation during the first 6 months of life.

Patent Foramen Ovale

The foramen ovale is probe patent in about 50% of infants under 1 year of age and in approximately 20% of adults (Fig. 11-3A): the higher left atrial pressure holds a flap of tissue over the orifice. Occasionally when right atrial pressure becomes elevated, a right-to-left shunt across the foramen ovale may ensue yielding clinical cyanosis. With an increase of pressure and volume of the left atrium, the foramen ovale may actually stretch enough to allow some degree of left-to-right shunting.

Atrial Septal Defect (Ostium Secundum Variety)

An ostium secundum atrial septal defect (ASD) is one in the mid to upper portion of the interatrial septum (Fig. 11-3B).

PHYSIOLOGY. In early infancy, due to the relative non-compliance of the right ventricle, a significant amount of left-to-right shunting across the ASD does not occur. Pulmonary hypertension is extremely uncommon during childhood. The S_2 is typically widely split throughout the respiratory cycle, occasionally being totally fixed. A systolic ejection murmur due to an increased volume of flow through a normal pulmonary valve annulus is heard at the second left intercostal space. With a moderate-to-large de-

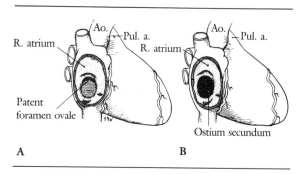

Fig. 11-3. A. Patent foramen ovale. B. Ostium secundum. (Ao. = aorta; Pul. a. = pulmonary artery.)

fect, a mid-diastolic flow rumble across the tricuspid valve may be present at the lower left sternal border.

ELECTROCARDIOGRAPHIC AND X-RAY FINDINGS. The ECG typically shows mild right axis deviation with a right ventricular conduction delay. The chest x ray shows increased pulmonary vascularity. The ascending aorta may be smaller than usual. Doppler, two-dimensional echocardiography may secure the diagnosis. The location of the ASD and associated lesions may be defined.

DIFFERENTIAL DIAGNOSIS. Valvular pulmonic stenosis is the most commonly encountered differential abnormality.

CARDIAC CATHETERIZATION. Cardiac catheterization may be optional in preparing a patient for reparative surgery. Associated abnormalities, such as partial anomalous pulmonary connection, may be well defined.

SURGICAL TREATMENT. To avoid potential complications that may be encountered in adulthood, surgery may be performed as early as infancy with low morbidity and mortality.

PROGNOSIS. Unrepaired, most patients remain asymptomatic until at least middle age. Surgery helps to prevent the possibility of pulmonary vascular disease late in life.

Isolated Pulmonary Stenosis

Pulmonary stenosis without an associated defect is typically valvular. Occasionally, infundibular hypertrophy leading to dynamic obstruction can develop as a secondary phenomenon associated with a severe valvular pulmonary stenosis (Fig. 11-4).

CLINICAL MANIFESTATIONS. Most patients with less than severe pulmonary stenosis remain asymptomatic. With moderate to severe stenosis, easy fatigability, and limited exercise tolerance may develop. Signs of cyanosis and a low cardiac output develop late in the course of the disease.

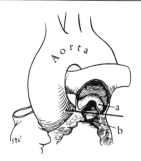

Fig. 11-4. Pulmonary valvular (a) *and infundibular* (b) *stenosis.*

ELECTROCARDIOGRAPHIC AND X-RAY FINDINGS. The ECG reveals right axis deviation and right ventricular hypertrophy in proportion to the degree of right ventricular outflow tract obstruction. On the chest x ray the overall heart size is typically normal. The right ventricle may fill in the retrosternal area on the lateral film. There may be poststenotic dilatation of the main pulmonary artery.

Doppler, two-dimensional echocardiography helps to determine noninvasively the degree of right ventricular outflow tract obstruction. Doppler measurements accurately grade the degree of stenosis.

CARDIAC CATHETERIZATION. Cardiac catheterization is both diagnostic and therapeutic. Percutaneous transluminal balloon valvuloplasty is the treatment of choice for moderate to severe valvular pulmonic stenosis. This may be achieved in all age groups with low morbidity and mortality.

SURGICAL TREATMENT. Surgical valvotomy is reserved for neonates with critical pulmonic stenosis in whom balloon valvuloplasty is not possible or has been unsuccessful. As with balloon valvuloplasty, secondary infundibular hypertrophy spontaneously resolves following surgical therapy.

Aortic Stenosis

Obstruction to outflow from the left ventricle may occur below the valve, at the level of the valve, and above the valve (Fig. 11-5). Valvular stenosis is the most common congenital abnormality. Physiologically, the main problem is that of left ventricular systolic hypertension.

CLINICAL MANIFESTATIONS. Most patients are well developed, athletically active, and asymptomatic. With severe obstruction episodes of syncope, presyncope, or chest pain may be present. With valvular stenosis the murmur is typi-

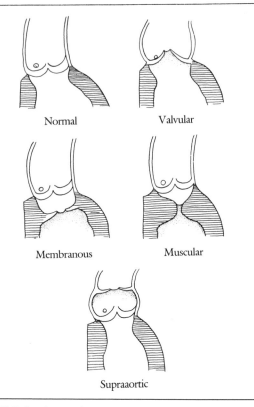

Fig. 11-5. Aortic stenosis.

cally diamond shaped, peaking in mid systole, and heard best at the second right intercostal space. It may be preceded by an early systolic ejection sound (click) if the valvular stenosis is mild or moderate. An early diastolic murmur caused by aortic insufficiency may be present along the left sternal border. Subvalvular and supravalvular stenosis may present with a murmur below or above the level of the aortic valve. Supravalvular aortic stenosis is most commonly seen in children with William's syndrome (elfin facies, mild mental retardation, and possible idopathic hypercalcemia).

ELECTROCARDIOGRAPHIC AND X-RAY FINDINGS. The ECG is usually normal or suggestive of left ventricular hypertrophy. Changes of the ST-T wave consistent with myocardial hypertrophy and ischemia may be present in severe forms of obstruction. On the chest x ray the heart is not commonly enlarged unless there is severe obstruction. There may be poststenotic dilatation of the aorta.

Doppler, two-dimensional echocardiography helps to determine the level of left ventricular outflow tract obstruction and noninvasively measure the actual gradient.

CARDIAC CATHETERIZATION. Cardiac catheterization is most commonly performed as a part of a preoperative evaluation. Percutaneous transluminal balloon valvuloplasty is being performed in some medical centers to relieve severe valvular stenosis.

CLINICAL COURSE. Aortic stenosis may become progressively more severe over a period of years. Calcification of a stenotic aortic valve may occur as early as in adolescence. Sudden death may occur during intensive exercise among children with moderate-to-severe left ventricular outflow tract obstruction. Accordingly, a patient should be counseled as to the type and intensity of exercise in which he or she may participate.

SURGICAL TREATMENT. Surgery is required if there is severe obstruction that is not amenable to balloon valvuloplasty. There is usually some residual left ventricular outflow tract obstruction and mild aortic regurgitation present postoperatively. Reoperation for restenosis may be necessary as may be valve replacement in later life.

Coarctation of the Aorta

Coarctation of the aorta is an obstructive lesion of the distal aortic arch at the site of entry of the ductus arteriosus (Fig. 11-6). This may occur just prior to or just after insertion of the ductus into the descending aorta. Variable collateral circulation usually develops around the obstruction. Physiologically there is a loss of systolic blood pressure below the obstruction. The systolic hypertension proximal to the obstruction may cause problems with left ventricular function.

CLINICAL MANIFESTATIONS. With severe obstruction infants may manifest congestive heart failure. Older children are generally asymptomatic and weak or absent femoral pulses usually lead to the diagnosis. Blood pressure measurements generally reveal a difference between the upper and lower extremities. A systolic murmur may be heard between the scapulae posteriorly.

ELECTROCARDIOGRAPHIC AND X-RAY FINDINGS. The ECG may be normal or demonstrate right ventricular hypertrophy in neonates and left ventricular hypertrophy in older infants and children, especially if there is significant systolic hypertension proximal to the narrowing. On the chest x ray the heart size is often normal. An indented area in the descending aorta may be identified. In older children rib notching may indicate intercostal collaterals.

SURGICAL TREATMENT. Surgical repair of a coarctation is often accomplished during the first few years of life. This may be necessary in infancy if severe congestive heart failure is present. Various methods of surgical relief are available. Reoperation for restenosis is uncommon even if the initial

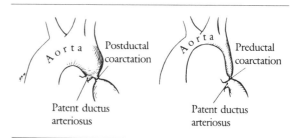

Fig. 11-6. Postductal and preductal coarctation of the aorta.

operation occurred early in infancy. In general, the earlier the surgery, the less likely there will be persistent systemic hypertension in later life.

Congenital Mitral Valve Malformation

Congenital deformity of the mitral valve as either stenosis or insufficiency is rarely encountered in childhood. Diagnostic criteria are far more difficult and less typical than in rheumatic mitral lesions. The murmur typically is present before 2 years of age. Surgical repair is occasionally required.

Hypertrophic Cardiomyopathy

Hypertrophic cardiomyopathy is often familial, being transmitted as an autosomal dominant lesion. It may present in infancy or childhood and appears to be progressive in nature. The majority of patients have little or no left ventricular outflow tract obstruction under basal conditions.

CLINICAL MANIFESTATIONS. The cardinal physical signs of hypertrophic cardiomyopathy are (1) a rapidly rising, double contour pulse with a double or triple left ventricular apical impulse, (2) mild to moderate cardiomegaly, (3) a systolic murmur heard best at the lower left sternal border, and (4) electrocardiographic evidence of left ventricular hypertrophy with deep Q waves in the left precordial leads. Evidence of Wolff-Parkinson-White syndrome may be present. Unfortunately, sudden death may be the first manifestation of this problem.

Echocardiography is typically diagnostic demonstrating asymmetric septal hypertrophy at least 1.3 times the thickness of the left ventricular posterior free wall. There may be systolic anterior motion of the anterior leaflet of the mitral valve secondary to ventricular outflow tract obstruction. Doppler interrogation may reveal evidence of left ventricular outflow tract obstruction.

The prognosis in this condition is variable and guarded.

Sudden death may occur during intensive exercise due to left ventricular outflow tract obstruction or a malignant arrhythmia. Patients should be carefully counseled concerning intensive exercise. Pharmacologic therapy with beta-blockers or calcium antagonists is usually the initial form of therapy. Surgical therapy to relieve severe obstruction is usually left for patients for whom medical management fails.

Infants born to diabetic mothers may manifest a transient form of this disease, which disappears later in infancy.

Cyanotic Congenital Heart Disease

Cyanosis due to a congenital heart defect is caused by inadequate pulmonary blood flow and/or inadequate admixture of the pulmonary and systemic circulations. The former is exemplified by lesions that reduce flow to the pulmonary artery, e.g., tetralogy of Fallot and tricuspid or pulmonary atresia. The best example of the latter is dextro-transposition of the great arteries. Often, these two categories may be differentiated by evaluation of the pulmonary blood flow on the chest x ray.

Tetralogy of Fallot

Tetralogy is the most common of the cyanotic heart lesions. The tetrad consists of severe infundibular pulmonic stenosis, a large VSD, dextroposition of the aorta, and right ventricular hypertrophy (Fig. 11-7) — the first two being more important. The right ventricular hypertrophy is a result of the ventricular outflow obstruction, and the degree of dextroposition of the aorta is very variable.

In tetralogy, the reduction in pulmonary blood flow is caused by the subvalvular right ventricular outflow tract obstruction. This may be accentuated by valvular or supravalvular pulmonic stenosis and even pulmonary valve atresia. The resistance to flow across the VSD is less and, therefore, a right-to-left shunt develops. At times of hypoxic spells, the degree of right ventricular outflow tract obstruction may increase, reducing pulmonary blood flow even further. Patients find that squatting helps to relieve this condition.

Only patients with the most severe forms of right ventricular outflow tract obstruction present with intense cyanosis in the neonatal period. Most children manifest it when they become more active during the second half of the first year of life. Some never manifest cyanosis (pink tetralogy). Auscultation reveals a single S_2 and a loud, harsh, long systolic ejection murmur at the mid-left sternal border. During a tetralogy spell, this murmur may diminish in intensity or even disappear.

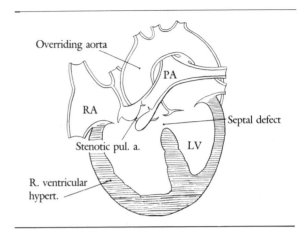

Fig. 11-7 Tetralogy of Fallot. (**LV** = *left ventricle;* **PA** = *pulmonary artery;* **RA** = *right atrium.*)

Laboratory aids help to differentiate tetralogy from an uncomplicated VSD with which it may be confused. The ECG shows right axis deviation and right ventricular hypertrophy. The chest x ray demonstrates a normal-sized, boot-shaped heart with diminished pulmonary vascularity and a concave main pulmonary artery segment. There is a right aortic arch in one-quarter of the cases. Echocardiography confirms the large aorta overriding the subaortic VSD and the presence of right ventricular outflow tract obstruction.

Treatment is surgical. In early infancy, a palliative procedure such as a modified Blalock-Taussig anastomosis may be necessary. In the older child, a primary complete repair is desirable. This consists of relieving the right ventricular outflow tract obstruction at all levels and closing the large VSD. When pulmonary atresia is present, an extracardiac conduit may be necessary to provide adequate right ventricular outflow.

Pulmonary Atresia with an Intact Ventricular Septum

This is a lesion where there is no antegrade flow into the pulmonary artery. The little pulmonary blood flow that is present is supplied by a smaller than usual ductus arteriosus. In the majority of cases the right ventricle is significantly hypoplastic. Due to the precarious nature of the pulmonary blood flow, the patient usually presents in the early neonatal period.

Laboratory tests are extremely helpful in making the diagnosis. The ECG often shows a normal or a leftward QRS axis and less right and more left ventricular precordial forces than normal for a newborn. The chest x ray shows diminished pulmonary blood flow. The degree of hypoxia is often severe and metabolic acidosis may be present. The Doppler, two-dimensional echocardiogram usually confirms the lack of antegrade pulmonary flow and confirms the presence of a thickened, hypoplastic right ventricle. Prostaglandin E_1 (PGE_1) should be started intravenously (IV) to maintain the ductus patent. Cardiac catheterization is useful to determine if the right ventricle is large enough to attempt a primary repair in the neonatal period. If not, the pulmonary arteries should be evaluated to determine the type of palliative shunt that should be attempted.

Tricuspid Atresia

In this abnormality, pulmonary blood flow is diminished due to lack of adequate flow into the right ventricle and subsequently the pulmonary artery (Fig. 11-8A). If the ventricular septum is intact, the ductus arteriosus is the only route for pulmonary blood flow; therefore, the patients typically present as cyanotic newborns.

The ECG in tricuspid atresia typically demonstrates significant left axis deviation, left ventricular hypertrophy, and a lack of dominant right ventricular forces. On the chest x ray, the heart size may be variable, but usually the pulmonary blood flow is diminished. Paradoxically, if the great arteries are transposed (Fig. 11-8B), the pulmonary flow may appear increased. The Doppler, two-dimensional echocardiogram confirms the lack of flow from the right atrium to the right ventricle. Cardiac catheterization is usually necessary to detail the anatomy and document that the pulmonary arteries are of adequate size to accept a palliative shunt. A palliative shunt is necessary to provide for adequate pulmonary blood flow. In case of TGV, pulmonary artery banding may be necessary. At a later date, a Fontan operation (right atrial to pulmonary artery anastomosis) may provide a near "normal" physiologic repair.

Transposition of Great Vessels

This structural abnormality is the best example of the situation in which there is inadequate admixture of the systemic and pulmonary circulations. The aorta emanates from the right ventricle and pulmonary artery from the left (Fig. 11-9). Because the pulmonary and systemic circulations run parallel to each other, there must be a communication between them to sustain life; therefore, adequate interatrial communication is essential. If the ventricular septum is intact, the ductus arteriosus may provide for this in the early neonatal period. In some cases once the ductus closes, the patient may become intensely cyanotic. Transposition of the

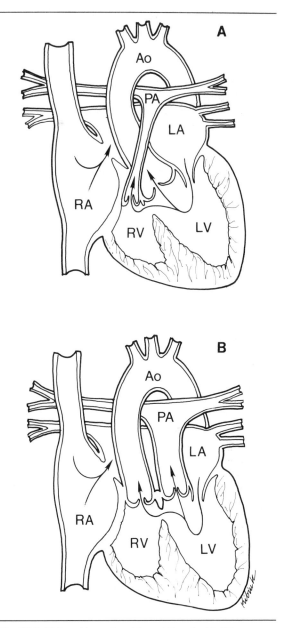

Fig. 11-8. Tricuspid atresia without (A) and with (B) transposition. (Ao. = aorta; LA = left atrium; LV = left ventricle; RV = right ventricle; PA = pulmonary artery; RA = right atrium.)

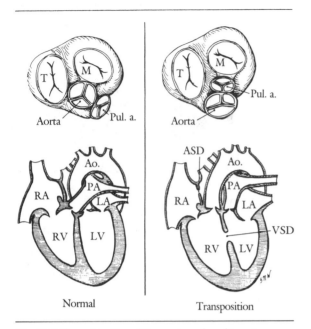

*Fig. 11-9. Normal position of the great vessels and transposition of the great vessels. (*Ao. = *aorta;* ASD = *atrial septal defect;* LA = *left atrium;* LV = *left ventricle;* M = *mitral valve;* PA [Pul. a.] = *pulmonary artery;* RA = *right atrium;* RV = *right ventricle;* T = *tricuspid valve;* VSD = *ventricular septal defect.)*

great vessels is the most common cyanotic congenital heart lesion that presents in the neonatal period. Tachypnea may be present so that the clinical picture may be confused with some form of respiratory distress. The ECG shows dominance of right atrial and right ventricular forces that still may be within normal limits for the neonatal period. The chest x ray may show a narrow base to the heart due to the aorta and pulmonary artery being "in line" with each other. The pulmonary vascularity is increased. Doppler, two-dimensional echocardiography confirms the transposed great vessels and usually helps in diagnosing coexisting defects. Once diagnosis is made, IV PGE$_1$ infusion is recommended to maintain patency of the ductus and increase blood admixture. Cardiac catheterization is both diagnostic and therapeutic. Once again, coexisting defects may be identified (e.g., VSD, pulmonic stenosis). A Rashkind balloon atrial septostomy should be performed to increase admixture at the atrial level. This helps palliate the situation until definitive surgery can be performed.

Surgery for simple transposition of the great vessels is in a period of transition. Many medical centers have progressed

to the arterial switch operation designed by Jatene. It affords a more physiologic repair than the intraatrial baffle of Mustard or Senning that leaves the right ventricle as the systemic ventricle. Long-term follow-up indicates that this is more physiologic and desirable. By transposing the great vessels (and coronary arteries) to their normal position, it is hoped that the late morbidity and mortality with this lesion will improve. Complex transposition with a ventricular septal defect and pulmonic stenosis may necessitate an extra cardiac conduit (Rastelli operation) to bypass the left ventricular outflow tract obstruction.

Total Anomalous Pulmonary Venous Connection

In this malformation, all the pulmonary veins drain into the systemic venous circulation. This usually occurs above or below the diaphragm or as a mixed type. Most commonly when the drainage is above the diaphragm, it is to the superior vena cava, the right atrium, a left innominate vein, the azygous system, or the coronary sinus. Drainage below the diaphragm is to the portal vein, ductus venosus, inferior vena cava, or hepatic vein. In this case, there is often obstruction at some point of flow in the common pulmonary venous channel.

Physiologically, the clinical presentation depends on whether pulmonary venous obstruction is present. When the anomalous drainage is of the infradiaphragmatic type, that is a virtual certainty. Pulmonary hypertension results. When no obstruction is present, the cardiac physiology is that of increased pulmonary flow leading to congestive heart failure.

If a patient presents in the neonatal period with this anomaly, then it is likely that pulmonary venous obstruction is present. The clinical picture is dominated by cyanosis and pulmonary edema. If unobstructed, an infant may elude detection for several weeks or months of life. He or she may manifest only mild cyanosis growth failure due to chronic congestive heart failure. A systolic murmur of pulmonary overcirculation is usually present along with a diastolic rumble generated in the right heart due to increased flow through a normal tricuspid valve. The ECG in the neonatal period or later typically shows a rightward axis with right ventricular hypertrophy and right atrial enlargement. In the neonatal period, the chest x ray shows pulmonary venous obstruction greater than that seen in virtually any other lesion. In the older child, cardiomegaly and increased pulmonary arterial flow dominate. A "snowman" appearance may be seen in the patient with supradiaphragmatic drainage of the pulmonary veins feeding the left innominate vein. Doppler, two-dimensional echocardiography in the neonatal period may be hard to interpret to confirm the diagnosis. The features one looks for are a lack of pulmonary venous return to the left atrium, a small left atrium and left ventricle, and a confluence of pulmonary veins behind the left atrium. In the older child, the ultrasound findings may be easier to interpret. The cardiac catheterization is diagnostic. A Rashkind balloon atrial septostomy may be necessary to allow for better flow of blood to the left heart and the systemic arterial circulation.

Surgical therapy involves a reanastamosis of the pulmonary venous channel to the left atrium. The risk is considerably higher in the neonatal period when pulmonary hypertension complicates recovery. In the neonate or older child, a small left heart has trouble accommodating a higher preload, and severe congestive heart failure may be present postoperatively. Ultimately, the surgical outcome is successful in the overwhelming majority of patients.

Other Forms of Heart Disease

Infective Endocarditis

Infective endocarditis is an uncommon illness in the pediatric population. Rarely does it occur de novo on a structurally normal heart. Usually there is an underlying congenital or acquired heart defect. Lesions with large pressure gradients and a great degree of resulting turbulence place the patient at greater risk for such an infection. Many different organisms have been implicated in endocarditis. Acute endocarditis, most commonly in the postoperative period, is frequently due to a *Staphylococcus aureus* infection. Subacute endocarditis, most commonly after dental work, is usually caused by *Streptococcus viridans*.

The recommendation of prophylactic antibiotics for dental work and certain other invasive procedures is a routine part of the long-term supervision of patients with congenital and acquired cardiac defects. The antibiotic is the physician's best armament against the development of infective endocarditis.

Endocarditis that is more acute, typically after cardiac surgery, is a short-term, more distinct illness. The fever is high and the patient "sicker" than in the subacute form. In the subacute form, the patient usually presents with an indolent illness, involving a long-term, low-grade fever, lethargy, and anorexia. A history of previous dental work or other surgery can usually be elicited. The murmur of the underlying heart defect is usually noted. The remainder of the positive physical findings are related to embolic phenomena. Roth spots, peripheral petechiae, splenomegaly, and splinter hemorrhages should be looked for.

Endocarditis is primarily a clinical diagnosis. It should be suspected in the presence of a prolonged fever in the setting of an underlying structural heart defect. The laboratory is used primarily to confirm a strong clinical impression. The organism should be sought by a series of successive blood cultures, at least six in 24 hours. A complete blood count indicates an acute infection and possibly anemia. The urine should be screened for microscopic hematuria. Nonspecific indicators of acute inflammation are usually elevated. An echocardiogram should be obtained with emphasis on evaluating the site(s) of the underlying heart defect. Vegetations may be demonstrated in this manner.

The treatment of infective endocarditis is aimed at the specific organism present. A protracted course of antibiotics, 4 to 6 weeks, is needed to render the heart sterile. Fortunately, today, one is often able to accomplish a large part of the treatment on an outpatient basis. Complications of septic emboli need to be directed to the organ involved. Rarely, in a postoperative patient, does a prosthetic element need to be replaced if it is a nidus of infection.

Pericarditis

Inflammation of the pericardium is an illness occasionally seen in childhood. The etiology may be various types of infectious organisms (viral, bacterial, or fungal), malignancies, or postpericardiotomy syndrome seen after open heart surgery.

CLINICAL MANIFESTATIONS. The cardinal signs and symptoms are acute chest pain, a pericardial friction rub, and elevated ST segments on the ECG.

The pain is typically precordial in location and may be referred to the shoulder. It is usually sharp in nature and relieved by sitting up or leaning forward. With a significant effusion, the degree of pain becomes less pronounced.

A pericardial friction rub is a very characteristic sound usually having two components. It is often evanescent, varying several times during the course of the day. Its nature is that of two semi-rough surfaces being rubbed together.

The ECG typically shows elevation of the ST segments. During the course of the disease the ST segments become flat and T waves become inverted in the same leads. An echocardiogram helps to determine the presence of a significant pericardial effusion and possibly pericardial tamponade.

DIAGNOSIS. In the setting of chest pain, a pericardial friction rub, and typical electrocardiographic findings, pericarditis can be diagnosed. At that point one looks at the cause which may be a bacterial or viral infection, tuberculosis, collagen vascular disease, or postpericardiotomy syndrome.

Septic pericarditis is an acute illness of young infants associated with high fever, a marked leukocytosis, and rapidly progressive course. *S. aureus* accounts for the majority of cases followed by *Streptococcus pneumoniae, Hemophilus influenzae,* and *Neisseria meningitidis.* A pericardiocentesis with identification of the infecting organism may be necessary before the institution of antibiotic therapy.

In rheumatic pericarditis there is evidence of pancarditis associated with pericardial involvement. Noncardiac findings are frequently present.

In juvenile rheumatoid arthritis and other collagen vascular diseases, pericarditis may be the first manifestation of the disease. The exact diagnosis may not be made until the clinical picture has fully developed.

In viral pericarditis, the patient is often not acutely ill except for the presence of chest pain. Fever is not very high and there is little in terms of a leukocytosis. Coxsackie B virus is the most common organism causing this disease. Treatment is usually with antiinflammatory drugs and bed rest.

Postpericardiotomy syndrome is an autoimmune phenomenon that may occur after opening of the pericardial sac. Chief clinical findings are those of pericarditis with a low grade fever and mild leukocytosis. Treatment is usually with mild antiinflammatory agents.

Constrictive Pericarditis

Constrictive pericarditis is rarely encountered in childhood and adolescence. The cause is often unknown and may have occurred several years earlier. *H. influenzae* or tuberculous pericarditis may result in constrictive pericarditis within the course of several weeks or months. Clinically the diagnosis is suggested by the presence of right-sided heart failure with only a slight to moderate enlargement of the heart on the chest x ray. Echocardiography may show a thickened pericardium, and cardiac catheterization may reveal equalization of the atrial, ventricular, and pulmonary diastolic pressures. The treatment is pericardiectomy.

Kawasaki Syndrome

This illness, first described in Japan in 1967, has become a major cause of acquired heart disease in childhood. Once the diagnosis is confirmed, the cardiovascular system is the major system investigated for involvement. This is due to the fact that the most serious consequences may result if the heart is affected. Even with a full recovery, damage to the coronary arteries may add a risk factor to the development of atherosclerotic coronary disease in adulthood.

Kawasaki syndrome is a generalized inflammatory illness of unknown etiology. Due to the protean nature of the signs and symptoms, the illness may go undiagnosed for days or even weeks. The clinical picture is that of a high fever (unresponsive to antibiotics) for 5 or more days, conjunctival inflammation, stomatitis, erythema and induration of the distal extremities, periungual desquamation, nonsuppurative cervical lymphadenopathy, and a nonspecific erythematous exanthem. Hydrops of the gallbladder is frequently detected by ultrasound even in the absence of abdominal symptoms. Sterile pyuria, aseptic meningitis, and diarrhea represent other nonspecific inflammatory reactions. Early in the course of the illness, the differential diagnosis may include scarlet fever, rubella, rubeola, Stevens-Johnson syndrome, and other acute viral exanthems.

Involvement of the heart may include myocarditis and pericarditis. Coronary artery aneurysms may occur in the subacute phase of the illness. Approximately 20% of patients with this syndrome have some type of cardiac involvement. Cardiac examination is helpful in the presence of congestive heart failure or pericarditis. The electrocardiographic abnormalities include a prolonged PR interval, nonspecific ST-T wave changes, and, possibly, evidence of a myocardial infarction. Two-dimensional echocardiography provides a safe, repeatable, and reproducible means by which one can evaluate the coronary arteries for aneurysm formation. If an aneurysm is detected, cardiac catheterization with angiography may be considered because it can provide more detailed anatomic confirmation. Complications of aneurysm formation may cause death related to myocardial infarction in 1 to 2% of the children with Kawasaki syndrome.

Prevention of cardiac involvement is a cornerstone of therapy for Kawasaki syndrome in its early stages. Intravenous gamma globulin and aspirin in antiinflammatory doses is the recommended regimen. The aspirin should be continued until the acute phase is over. Then low-dose aspirin should be considered until the acute phase reactants have normalized and thrombocytosis is no longer present. If cardiac involvement is demonstrated, antithrombotic therapy should continue as long as coronary aneurysms are present or even longer thereafter. In cases where thrombosis and subsequent myocardial infarction have occurred, a coronary bypass has been performed.

Seymour I. Hepner, Mohamed K. Mardini, and Donald C. Fyler

References

Adams, F. H., and Emmanouilides, G. C. (Eds.). *Moss' Heart Disease in Infants, Children, and Adolescents* (3rd ed.). Baltimore: Williams & Wilkins, 1983.

Engle, M. A., and Perloff, J. K. *Congenital Heart Disease After Surgery*. New York: Yorke, 1983.

Goldberg, S. J., et al. *Doppler Echocardiography*. Philadelphia: Lea and Febiger, 1985.

Nadas A. S., and Flyer, D. C. *Pediatric Cardiology* (4th ed.). Philadelphia: Saunders, 1972.

Rudolph, A. M. *Congenital Diseases of the Heart*. Chicago: Year Book, 1974.

12

The Abdomen and the Gastrointestinal Tract

Abdominal Wall: Congenital Abnormalities

Omphalocele

In the sixth week of intrauterine development, the intestines enter the coelom of the umbilical cord and leave the abdomen. Failure to return in the tenth week results in an omphalocele, in which intestine covered by the amniotic membrane remains outside the underdeveloped abdominal cavity. Malrotation frequently occurs (Fig. 12-1A). Surgical repair requires a staged procedure allowing for gradual expansion of the abdominal cavity and wall.

Gastroschisis

When a defect (Fig 12-1B) is present in the abdominal wall usually on the right lateral side of the umbilicus, the intestine may escape and lie free in the amniotic fluid. No covering membrane is present. Malrotation is frequent; other associated anomalies include hydronephrosis (in up to 30% of patients) and various intestinal atresias. Surgical repair is difficult and requires a staged procedure.

Congenital Absence of the Abdominal Musculature (Prune Belly, Triad Syndrome)

This condition occurs almost exclusively in males. The thin, lax abdominal wall, the extraordinary wrinkled character of which gives the syndrome the sobriquet of "prune belly," and the peculiar scarlike appearance of the abdominal wall skin are so characteristic that the diagnosis is made at a glance. Instead of the normal muscles, only scattered fragments of the various muscular layers of the abdominal wall are found (Fig. 12-1C). The children have cryptorchidism with abdominal testes, megacystica, megaureter, and hydronephrosis. The condition may be so far advanced at birth as to be incompatible with life. The principal problem is the urinary disorder. There is no clear agreement on its nature; only rarely is it a mechanical one. These children have recently been surviving long enough so that reconstructive surgery on the abdominal wall has been undertaken with some success.

Umbilical Hernia

Small defects in closure of the linea alba result in umbilical hernias. Common in black infants, they are considered be-

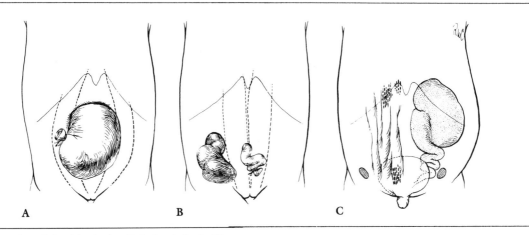

Fig. 12-1. Defects of the abdominal wall. A. Omphalocele. The intestines have not returned to the abdomen in the ninth and tenth weeks of intrauterine life and remain in the exocoelom covered only by translucent amnion. B. In gastroschisis, there is a full-thickness defect of the abdominal wall away from the umbilicus, and loops of bowel protrude through this uncovered by any membrane. C. Congenital absence of the abdominal musculature.

nign as most close spontaneously before age 3. Strangulation or obstruction is extremely rare. Treatment consists of reassuring the parents, preventing the taping or strapping of the defect, and simple observation. Surgical closure is performed for unusually large hernias or if no recession is noted by ages 3 or 4.

Inguinal Hernia

The most common abdominal wall defect, inguinal hernia usually presents as a bulge or swelling noticed when the child is crying. Inguinal hernias can strangulate and obstruct so surgical repair is performed soon after diagnosis. Incidence of inguinal hernias is higher in boys and premature infants. Bilaterality is common, and debate over routine bilateral exploration persists.

Umbilicus

Umbilical Granuloma

The major abnormality of the umbilicus in the newborn infant is umbilical granuloma, which is a tuft of granulation tissue in the umbilical cicatrix. It may be quite large and

persist for many weeks, with annoying discharge. The simplest treatment is excision and cauterization of the stump. The excised granuloma should be sent for histological section and study; occasionally it indicates persistence of an omphalomesenteric duct.

Persistent Omphalomesenteric Duct

The omphalomesenteric duct may be completely patent and open at the umbilicus (Fig. 12-2F), communicating by an intestinelike tube to the midileum. On the other hand, it may consist of a mere tuft of epithelium in the umbilical cicatrix or, at the intestinal end, in Meckel's diverticulum. A moist and discharging umbilicus should be probed. When there is only a small tuft of epithelium on the surface of the umbilicus, it may be merely excised. More commonly, there is communication by a sinus to a small pocket beneath the abdominal wall, which can be entered with a probe and, at times, be outlined by injection of radiopaque contrast material. In such instances, the entire umbilicus must be excised with the remnant of the omphalomesenteric duct. Care must be taken in the course of the operation not to injure the bladder, which in the newborn infant is quite close to the umbilicus. A continuous tract connecting the umbilicus to the intestine is excised in toto and the intestine closed.

Meckel's Diverticulum

Failure of the proximal end of the omphalomesenteric duct to close results in an ileal diverticulum known as Meckel's diverticulum (Fig. 12-2C). Autopsies have revealed this in up to 2% of the population. Located in the ileum, usually

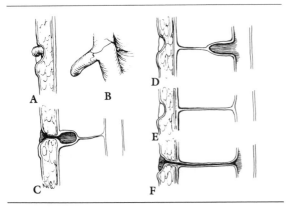

Fig. 12-2. Manifestations of omphalomesenteric duct remnants.

A. Mucosal tuft in the umbilicus without any deeply buried elements, often mistaken for an umbilical "granuloma."

B. Mucosal tuft in the umbilicus communicating with a small cyst cavity within the abdominal wall, extraperitoneal, and at times with a fibrous strand connecting to the ileum and representing the obliterated omphalomesenteric vessels.

C. The classic Meckel's diverticulum. If it is vermiform, as represented here, it is subject to a disease indistinguishable from appendicitis.

D. A Meckel's diverticulum associated with a strand of obliterated vessels passing to the umbilicus. This strand, either with a Meckel's diverticulum as shown here or without it as in (E), may serve as the mechanism for the development of a volvulus or as a band under which another loop of intestine may be caught.

F. Complete patency of the omphalomesenteric duct, with fecal discharge through the umbilicus.

within 2 m of the cecum, 40% may be lined with ectopic mucosa of either gastric or pancreatic origin. Those lined with gastric mucosa produce acid and may cause ulceration of surrounding intestinal mucosa.

CLINICAL MANIFESTATIONS. The passage of bright red blood in the rectum without associated stool in an otherwise healthy child is suggestive of Meckel's diverticulum. Though most common in the preschool age group, Meckel's diverticulum may produce bleeding at any age. The blood loss may be significant: therefore, the effect on hemodynamics should be considered. Diarrhea, abdominal pain, fever, or constipation are not symptoms. The diagnostic test of choice is a technetium-labeled isotope scan which is sensitive for gastric mucosa and which illuminates a lined diverticulum. Treatment requires surgical excision of the diverticulum.

Duplication Cysts

Duplication cysts, also known as enteric cysts are mucosal lined cysts that share a muscular wall with a bowel segment and may occur throughout the gastrointestinal tract. While true duplications of the stomach, colon, and esophagus do occur, most cysts are small with only minor bowel segments involved.

CLINICAL MANIFESTATIONS. Symptoms result from a gradual increase in size and the resultant mass effect on the adjacent bowel. Alternatively gastric mucosa lining cysts may produce acid and cause rectal bleeding. Intussusception with cysts as a lead point has also been reported. Diagnosis may be suggested if a mass is felt on examination but usually requires sonographic, CT-scan, or barium–x-ray studies. Treatment is surgical with varying degrees of difficulty from simple excision of small uncomplicated cysts to major, technically demanding surgery for a true double colon.

Persistent Urachus

A thin, shiny secretion at the umbilicus may suggest that the umbilical remnant, rather than being omphalomesenteric in origin, consists of urachal remnants (Fig. 12-3). In

Fig. 12-3. Urachal remnants. A. Patent urachus communicating with the bladder and permitting discharge of urine through the umbilicus. B. An umbilical sinus discharging mucus and lined by uroepithelium. C. Urachal cyst, which may present as a large, tense, midline extraperitoneal mass containing a large volume of fluid, but more commonly is smaller and subject to an insidiously developing infection. D. Urachal remnant communicating with the bladder. Diligent search and routine autopsies will demonstrate microscopical communications of this kind with considerable frequency; clinically significant communications occasionally occur.

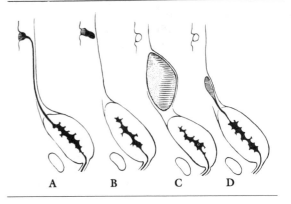

rare cases, this communicates with the bladder, and urine may discharge from the umbilicus; treatment consists of excision of the tract and closure of the bladder. More commonly, there is no connection with the bladder, but a sac is found beneath the abdominal wall (Fig. 12-3B). Operative relief requires excision of the umbilicus and the urachal remnant.

The urachal remnant may be blind in the anterior extraperitoneal space above the bladder, not communicating with either the bladder or the umbilicus (Fig. 12-3C). In this case a cyst forms which may occasionally reach very large proportions or may become the seat of acute or chronic smoldering infection. Treatment is by excision of the uninfected mass or by incision and drainage of the infected mass followed by secondary excision.

Liver and Biliary Tract

Jaundice is an important symptom at all ages. The differential diagnosis is thoroughly discussed in Appendix A, Section 14. Jaundice appearing in the first 24 hours of life is usually due to hemolytic disease from maternal-fetal blood group incompatibility; later, in the first week, it may be physiologic jaundice, less severe hemolytic disease, neonatal sepsis, or congenital infection. When obstructive jaundice appears after the first 2 weeks of life and before 3 months of age, the physician is faced with the difficult task of differentiating between the rare case of extrahepatic biliary atresia, which may be surgically treated, and the much more common intrahepatic diseases: so-called intrahepatic biliary atresia (Alagille's syndrome) neonatal hepatitis, or an inborn error of metabolism such as cystic fibrosis, alpha-1–antitrypsin deficiency, galactosemia, or tyrosinosis. After about 6 to 9 months of age, the development of nonhemolytic jaundice most often indicates viral hepatitis. Some of the disorders that must be considered in the differential diagnosis of chronic liver disease in children are listed on Table 12-1.

Hepatitis

ACUTE VIRAL HEPATITIS. See Chapter 20.

CHRONIC HEPATITIS. Hepatic inflammation that persists beyond 3 months after the initial episode may represent chronic hepatitis. This form of hepatitis is broadly divided into two categories, chronic persistent hepatitis (CPH) and chronic active hepatitis (CAH). The etiologies of the two differ dramatically. CPH is generally considered a benign condition. Patients may occasionally be symptomatic with fatigue, weight loss, and vague pain, but this condition rarely progresses. CPH is a post-viral condition, with mildly elevated transaminase levels (usually 200 I.U.) and minimal to absent fibrosis on biopsy.

CAH may be subdivided into infectious and noninfectious causes. While up to 10% of hepatitis B patients may eventually have the chronic disease, they make up only 20% of CAH cases. Forty-five percent of cases are idiopathic although many of these are of non-A, non-B hepatitis. Twenty percent are autoimmune, 5% are due to drug hypersensitivity reactions, and 10% are secondary to metabolic disorders (alpha-1-antitrypsin deficiency, Wilson's disease, cystic fibrosis, tyrosinemia). Hepatitis A almost never causes chronic hepatitis.

Clinical Manifestations. While adults frequently have asymptomatic abnormalities discovered on laboratory tests, children may present with fever, abdominal pain, jaundice, menstrual irregularities, joint pain, anorexia, and weight loss. Hepatitis B with CAH is predominantly a male condition (75% of patients), while autoimmune CAH is a disorder of adolescent females. Laboratory results include transaminase levels at least 5 times normal, IgG 2 times normal, and variable increases in bilirubin. Autoimmune CAH has a variety of coincident immunologic markers including antinuclear antibodies, antismooth muscle antibodies, and antimitochondrial antibodies.

Liver biopsy is required for diagnosis as well as for differentiating CPH from CAH. Histology of CAH may show a range from minimal portal inflammation and random necrosis to overt cirrhosis with bridging necrosis and fibrosis. Liver biopsy also allows diagnosis of Wilson's disease for which therapy is available.

Chronic hepatitis of viral origin may lead to cirrhosis in 10 to 30% of patients. Poor prognostic signs include the presence of HBeAg, non-A, non-B infection, and the presence of Delta hepatitis (HDV). HDV superinfection is now recognized as a common cause of cirrhosis and mortality. The treatment of CAH in HBsAg+ patients remains controversial, as the risk of any treatment must be evaluated against a high rate of spontaneous remissions (25%) and frequent mild disease courses. Attempts to treat hepatitis B and CAH have centered on immunosuppression with prednisone and azathioprine. While initial studies suggested a detrimental effect, a recent retrospective Italian study has suggested a more optimistic outcome in children treated with Prednisone. More promising may be the adult studies on alpha-interferon, a leukocyte derived protein, now created by recombinant techniques. Several studies have shown increased viral clearance with interferon therapy, but more work will be required prior to its general use.

The etiology of autoimmune CAH is unknown. By virtue

Table 12-1. *Causes of Childhood Cirrhosis*

Condition	Incidence	Defect	Clinical features	Laboratory studies	Treatment
Alpha$_1$-antitrypsin deficiency	1 : 2000 live births	Hepatocellular destruction; indistinguishable from neonatal hepatitis	Three forms: (1) fulminant hepatic failure in infants; (2) neonatal hepatitis progressing slowly to cirrhosis; (3) insidious presentation of cirrhosis in late childhood	As in viral hepatitis measure alpha-1-antitrypsin in blood	Supportive; Liver transplant
Budd-Chiari syndrome	Very rare	Obstruction at junction of hepatic veins with inferior vena cava or within liver substance	Often starts acutely with sudden vomiting, hepatomegaly, ascites, and mild icterus; if child survives, a picture resembling cardiac cirrhosis may develop	Difficult to diagnose; venography helpful; ultrasound with Doppler	Side-to-side portacaval anastomosis; symptomatic treatment
Cardiac cirrhosis	Rare	Chronic or recurrent congestive cardiac failure secondary to congenital or acquired heart disease	Signs and symptoms of heart disease, with firm, enlarged heart	Liver biopsy, venous pressure measurement, and other studies to rule out constrictive pericarditis. Ultrasonography of hepatic veins.	Treatemment of heart disease
Chronic active hepatitis	Not rare	Autoimmune reaction; following hepatitis, B, non-A non-B, or idiopathic	Occurs in children and adults of both sexes, but often in young females with amenorrhea, arthralgia, and febrile episodes	Hypergammaglobulinemia; hepatitis B studies; antinuclear antibody SGOT[a] and SGPT[b] ++; 2 anti-SM[c] and anti-LKM[d]; liver biopsy specimen shows periportal necrosis and fibrosis; may progress to cirrhosis; some patients LE cell — and HB,AG +	Steroids for the autoimmune chronic hepatitis; interferon (alpha) may be useful in infectious cases

Disease	Frequency	Pathology/Etiology	Signs and symptoms	Diagnostic findings	Treatment
"Congenital" atresia of bile ducts	(See App. A, Section 14)				
Congenital hepatic fibrosis	Very rare	Bands of fibrous tissue encircling normal hepatic lobules	Firm liver without failure until very late; portal hypertension; associated with microcystic disease of liver and kidneys	Liver biopsy (surgical)	Blood transfusion and portacaval anastomosis if severe hemorrhage; liver transplantation
Congenital syphilis	Not rare	Fetal infection with *Treponema pallidum*	Other signs of congenital syphilis; large, firm liver but no jaundice	Positive serological test for syphilis	Penicillin
Congestive splenomegaly	(See p. 219, Portal Hypertension)				
Cruveilhier-Baumgarten syndrome	Very rare	Failure of obliteration of umbilical vein	Cirrhosis with prominent paraumbilical veins, venous hum, and thrill	Splenoportal venography shows dilated umbilical vein	Symptomatic
Cryptogenic cirrhosis in infants	Not very rare	Signs and symptoms as in any cirrhosis	Firm, hard liver; splenomegaly	SGOT[a] and SGPT[b] ++, liver biopsy	Symptomatic
Cystic fibrosis of pancreas	1 : 2000 live births	Inspissation of bile	Cirrhosis in later childhood with minimal jaundice; firm liver	High sweat sodium, chloride; high alkaline phosphatase	No specific treatment; portacaval anastomosis; liver transplant
Cystinosis	(See Chap. 13)				
Galactosemia	(See Chaps. 7, 9)				
Glycogen storage disease	(See Chap. 7)				
Hemochromatosis	Very rare	Increased intestinal absorption of iron	Hepatomegaly, hyperpigmentation, peripheral neuritis, diabetes, gonadal atrophy	Positive urinary ferrocyanide test and biopsy of liver and skin	Repeated venisections; chelating agents
Hemosiderosis	Not rare	Fe deposition due to multiple transfusions for chronic anemia	Liver and spleen enlarged and firm; increased pigmentation of skin	Serum Fe increased	Removal of Fe by chelation
Hepatolenticular degeneration (Wilson's disease)	Rare	Inability to excrete Cu normally in bile	Signs of hepatitis or cirrhosis; Kayser-Fleischer rings; acute hemolytic crisis; neurological findings	Low ceruloplasmin or Cu oxidase; high Cu in urine and liver; slit-lamp examination	Reduction of Cu intake; removal of Cu by chelation with penicillamine Symptomatic

Table 12-1. (Continued)

Condition	Incidence	Defect	Clinical features	Laboratory studies	Treatment
Hereditary hermorrhagic telangiectasia	Very rare	Liver has congenital telangiectasia	Signs of cirrhosis	Splenoportal venography	Symptomatic
Malnutrition and chronic infection, e.g., malaria, tuberculosis, schistosomiasis, kala-azar	Not rare in some parts of world	Depends on etiology	Depends on etiology	Tests for chronic infections and hypoproteinemia; liver biopsy	Good diet with specific therapy for the infection
Neonatal cirrhosis of liver	(See App. A, Jaundice)				
Sideric cirrhosis of South Africa	Rare	Diet rich in acidic food cooked in iron pots	Malnutrition, hemochromatosis	Liver biopsy	Correction of diet; portacaval shunt
Tyrosinosis	(See Chap. 7)				
Ulcerative colitis with cirrhosis	(See p. 235)	Sclerosing cholangitis	May be asymptomatic	Elevated enzymes ERCP	Treatment of colitis
Venoocclusive disease of Jamaica	Common in Jamaica; rare in Africa and Europe	Toxins of plant origin acting on liver of malnourished children ("bush tea" containing senecio and/or crotolaria alkaloid which is a hepatotoxin)	Clinical picture may be acute, subacute, or chronic; death usually due to repeated hematemesis and hepatic coma	Liver biopsy	Symptomatic; often spontaneous cure after elimination of toxins from diet; portacaval anastomosis for cirrhosis with portal hypertension
Viral hepatitis including neonatal hepatitis	(See Chap. 20)				

[a] Serum glutamic oxaloacetic transaminase.
[b] Serum glutamic pyruvic transaminase.
[c] Anti–smooth muscle antibody.
[d] Anti–liver-kidney microsomal antibody.

of differing autoantibodies, this group is presently being subdivided. What all the groups have in common is a pathologic picture similar to viral CAH, an association with a variety of other autoimmune disorders (Sjögren's syndrome, Hashimoto's thyroiditis, systemic lupus erythematosus, and a clinical picture of hepatomegaly, abdominal pain, fevers, rashes, and joint pains. Treatment of patients with these conditions is more accepted and far more successful. Prednisone in a dosage of 1 to 2 mg/kg/day is initiated. Serial evaluation of transaminases and immunoglobulins usually reveals biochemical remission in 6 to 12 months. Azathioprine is often employed to lower the Prednisone dosage, though it is of little use as a single agent. Remission should be confirmed histologically, and Prednisone may be weaned. Patients usually require steroids for 1 to 2 years, but over 80% enter remission. Adult relapse rates of 50% at 6 months are much higher than the limited childhood experience. Long-term outcome remains unclear and may differ depending on which variants of autoantibodies are present.

Complications. All forms of CAH can progress to cirrhosis and portal hypertension. Accordingly, children must be monitored frequently for development of coagulation abnormalities, hypoalbuminemia, hyperbilirubinemia, ascites, and gastrointestinal bleeding. Clinical evidence of progression or histologic evidence of extensive necrosis, fibrosis, or nodular cirrhosis suggests a poor prognosis. Many patients with such conditions may now be considered transplant candidates.

Cirrhosis of the Liver

Hepatic cirrhosis in infants and children is an uncommon disorder all over the world except in some tropical and subtropical regions such as India, the West Indies, Egypt, and the Middle East, where it is a relatively common condition.

This chronic disorder of liver is manifested clinically by a firm liver, often with splenomegaly, portal hypertension, and evidence of hepatic failure. Pathologically, thick bands of fibrous tissue are found encircling part or the whole of many lobules, distorting the normal hepatic architecture (pseudolobulation). Signs of degeneration and regeneration of parenchymal cells are also present. Cases that do not satisfy all these criteria but have some of the features may be called early or developing cirrhosis. Many diverse conditions, congenital or acquired or both, terminate in cirrhosis. Table 12-1 summarizes their important features.

PORTAL HYPERTENSION. Portal hypertension results when there is intrahepatic or extrahepatic obstruction to portal venous flow; better therapeutic results are obtained

when the obstruction is extrahepatic than in the presence of cirrhosis. In adults, most cases are associated with alcoholic cirrhosis and impaired liver function; in children, many cases are due to extrahepatic occlusion of the portal vein, and thus liver function is normal. Some patients with extrahepatic portal vein obstruction have an established history of neonatal umbilical infection, with presumed ascending thrombophlebitis involving the umbilical vein and the portal vein.

Thrombosis of the portal vein results in many small, high-resistance vessels providing the portal circulation. This is called cavernous transformation of the portal vein and can usually be diagnosed with sonography. In addition many of the diseases in Table 12-1 can progress to cirrhosis in children. If a child survives long enough, secondary portal hypertension results. Clinically, portal hypertension produces a large spleen with signs of hypersplenism (thrombocytopenia, anemia) and evidence of systemic collateral venous circulation including esophageal varices, hemorrhoids, and superficial abdominal vessels (caput medusa). In cirrhotics, evidence of liver disease may include hepatomegaly, ascites, jaundice and multiple laboratory abnormalities.

Treatment. Treatment remains controversial. Acute variceal bleeding requires transfusions, intravenous vasopressin, and occasionally injection sclerotherapy. Nonselective beta-blockers may lessen the risk of bleeding as will prophylactic sclerosis of known varices. Liver transplant in cirrhotic patients may be curative. If the patient is not a transplant candidate or in cases of portal cavernous transformation a decompressive shunt may be indicated. The greatest experience has been with the splenorenal shunt or end-to-end portacaval shunt. In children under the age of 3 years, the splenic vein is too small to allow for a satisfactory anastomosis to a systemic vein, and it is clear that the older the patient at the time of operation, the greater the likelihood of success in preventing further hemorrhage. Successes are few below the age of 3 years and fairly common above the age of 9. If the spleen has been removed, or if, at the time of operation, the splenic vein is still too small, satisfactory portacaval shunts can be formed or the superior mesenteric vein and the central end of the divided inferior vena cava can be joined (the so-called mesocaval shunt). Nevertheless, in a certain number of patients with radiographically patent anastomoses, bleeding resumes.

Other Diseases of the Biliary Tract

Several congenital malformations of the gallbladder and the ducts are described, but only a few of them occur with any degree of frequency.

BILIARY ATRESIA. Extrahepatic biliary atresia usually presents at 4 to 6 weeks of age with jaundice, acholic stools, dark urine, and an elevated direct bilirubin. Originally thought to be congenital, it is now felt to result from an intrauterine injury or infection and be progressive. The gallbladder is absent in 25% of cases. Hepatic scintiscan is useful diagnostically with absent isotope excretion in true atresias. Confirmatory diagnostic tests are liver biopsy and cholangiogram. Biopsy reveals a proliferation of intrahepatic ducts and pooling of the bile. Cholangiogram reveals no outflow tract.

Treatment. Palliative surgery with a Kasai procedure (hepatojejunostomy) is effective in patients under 2 months of age. Most of these patients eventually require liver transplantation.

CHOLEDOCHAL CYST. Infants or young children presenting with jaundice, pain, and a right upper quadrant mass have the classic clinical triad of choledochal cyst. These are segmental dilatation, diffuse dilatation, and diverticulum or choledochocele where the intraduodenal portion of the common bile duct is dilated. As symptoms may be mild and intermittent, this diagnosis can be missed for long periods. Diagnosis is made with ultrasonography, computed tomography (CT) scan, or cholangiogram.

Treatment. Surgical excision of the cystic area and revision of the drainage system is effective. Occasionally, choledochojejunostomy is required.

CONGENITAL ANOMALIES OF GALLBLADDER. The following congenital anomalies of the gallbladder may occur:

1. Absence of the gallbladder is a very rare anomaly, and the signs and symptoms are indistinguishable from those of congenital absence of the bile ducts. Diagnosis is confirmed by operative cholangiography.
2. Double gallbladder is uncommon. The accessory organ may often be the seat of acute and chronic cholecystitis. Diagnosis is made by cholecystography. Treatment is surgical.
3. Intrahepatic gallbladder is very rare. The gallbladder is often diseased as it cannot contract adequately, resulting in stasis, infection, and often cholelithiasis. Diagnosis is made by cholecystography. Treatment is usually by cholecystectomy.
4. Floating gallbladder is a rare congenital anomaly. The gallbladder is freely movable below the lower edge of the liver because of a longer peritoneal fold surrounding the organ. This sometimes produces torsion of the gallbladder, which brings severe pain, vomiting, and collapse. Cholecystectomy is the treatment of choice.
5. Adenomyomatosis of the gallbladder is rare and is characterized by hyperplasia of the muscular layers and mucosa of the gallbladder. There are usually no symptoms; however, biliary tract symptoms may be present in the absence of stones. Cholecystectomy is recommended.

ACQUIRED DISEASES OF THE GALLBLADDER. Cholecystitis is infrequent in childhood. It is characterized by fever, nausea, vomiting, distention of the abdomen, and colicky abdominal pain in the right upper quadrant, often associated with guarding and tenderness. In chronic cholecystitis such episodes recur over a time and are usually associated with gallstones.

The etiology of gallbladder disease is often obscure. The main predisposing factors to be considered in children include congenital malformation of the cystic duct leading to obstruction, parenteral nutrition, and chronic hemolytic disorders, with the formation of pigment stones. Diagnosis is confirmed by ultrasonography or radioisotope scan. Stones without cholecystitis can frequently be handled conservatively, but older patients or patients with other symptoms require cholecystectomy.

Pancreas

ACUTE PANCREATITIS. Mumps is the most common cause of acute pancreatitis, of a nonsuppurative variety, in childhood. Symptoms are vomiting, fever (elevation of temperature for 3 to 5 days), epigastric pain with deep tenderness in the left upper quadrant, and diarrhea. There is a marked rise in serum amylase (higher than usually produced by salivary gland involvement). At least one other locus of mumps infection — generally parotitis, but sometimes meningoencephalitis, orchitis, or oophoritis — may precede or follow the episode of pancreatic involvement. This is a self-limited disease requiring no treatment.

Acute fulminant pancreatitis, with release of pancreatic enzymes, chemical peritonitis, fat necrosis, and serosanguineous peritoneal fluid, seldom occurs in children; it may be a manifestation of generalized infection, or the result of trauma. It must be suspected in any individual with prostration, severe upper abdominal pains, and deep tenderness in the epigastrium. It may be diagnosed by a high serum and urinary amylase level and usually may require surgical intervention in the presence of hemorrhagic pancreatitis or pancreatic abscess.

DIFFERENTIAL DIAGNOSIS OF PANCREATIC INSUFFICIENCY. Though cystic fibrosis is the primary consideration in children with pancreatic insufficiency, other causes include inflammatory pancreatitis, familial recurrent pancreatitis, Schwachman syndrome, and congenital aplasia. Pancreatitis is usually viral and self-limited, with mumps the most likely etiologic agent identified. Schwachman syndrome is a rare disorder with chest wall abnormalities, neutropenia, pancreatic insufficiency, and growth retardation. Recurrent familial pancreatitis usually presents in adolescence and with the advent of enterohepatic retrograde cholangiopancreatography (ERCP) is frequently found to be secondary to anatomic abnormalities. Work-up of pancreatic insufficiency of any cause should include 72-hour stool fat, stool trypsin, sweat chloride test, abdominal sonogram, and fat-soluble vitamin levels. Further investigation may include chest x ray, enterohepatic cholangiopancreatography, pancreatic stimulation tests, and viral serology.

Cystic Fibrosis

Cystic fibrosis (CF) is the most common inborn error of metabolism in Caucasians and the most frequent cause of pancreatic insufficiency. It is a multisystem disease affecting the pancreas, lungs, sweat glands and liver with manifestations in the nasopharynx and reproductive organs as well. Almost 80% of affected children now live beyond their 20th birthday.

GENETICS. CF is transmitted as an autosomal recessive disorder located on the long arm of chromosome seven. Incidence in Caucasians is about $\frac{1}{1600}$ with a carrier frequency of $\frac{1}{25}$. It has been reported in all races, though it is most common in whites of European descent. In affected families, the chance of a child being born with CF is $\frac{1}{4}$. No test is available to identify the carrier who is phenotypically normal.

PATHOPHYSIOLOGY. The exact primary defect of CF is unknown. Evidence suggests abnormal regulation of chloride transport in exocrine glands. As these glands depend on chloride secretion to carry water into the lumen, failure to do so causes dehydrated, hyperviscous secretions and obstruction.

MANIFESTATIONS. *Pancreas.* The initial lesion is the presence of eosinophilic, inspissated plugs in the pancreatic ductules. As these become obstructed, tissue damage from enzyme release ensues. Progressive fibrosis and fatty infiltration follows. The end stage is a small, fibrotic organ with loss of both acinar and islet cell function.

Pancreatic insufficiency is present in 80 to 85% of CF patients. Their exocrine function is less than 2% of normal, and the consequence is malabsorption. Steatorrhea with large, bulky, greasy stools, chronic constipation, failure to thrive, or rectal prolapse all suggest CF. Recurrent pancreatitis may predate the diagnosis in 10% of patients. Infants usually have excellent appetites but exhibit poor weight gain.

Intestines. A variety of intestinal conditions may result from CF and should prompt evaluation. These begin in utero with meconium ileus (MI) and meconium peritonitis (MP). Meconium ileus presents as neonatal intestinal obstruction secondary to abnormally viscid meconium obstructing the area of the ileocecal valve. Proximally, the small bowel dilates; distally, the colon never receives stool and remains a microcolon. Complications include mid-gut volvulus, intussusception, and perforation with MP. MI occurs in 10 to 15% of CF patients. Intestinal atresias may warrant evaluation for CF as well because 20% of patients with small bowel atresias are found to have CF. Diagnosis of MI is made with gastrograffin enema which may be therapeutic as well if the plug is dislodged. Surgery is required when the infant is stabilized.

In older patients, MI equivalent or distal intestinal obstruction syndrome refers to partial obstructions with abdominal pain, obstipation, and a palpable mass. Treatment is supportive and rarely is surgery required.

Lungs. Viscid mucus in the bronchi and bronchioles leads to bronchiectasis, recurrent infections, and chronic obstructive lung disease. Histologic changes include emphysematous blebs, atelectasis, consolidation, and tubular bronchiectasis with a predilection for the upper lobes. Progressive respiratory disease is the major factor in limiting life expectancy. Recurrent pneumonia with *Pseudomonas* is common. Cor pulmonale may be the end result.

Hepatobiliary System. Most hepatic complications of CF are of minor clinical concern. Occasionally, infants present with direct hyperbilirubinemia from bile ducts obstructed with plugs. Focal biliary fibrosis is more common, occurring in 25% of CF patients. Most of these patients are asymptomatic but must be watched for progression to biliary cirrhosis. Biliary stones occur in 5 to 10% of patients and may relate to abnormal lithogenic bile production. More serious is the rare development of biliary cirrhosis with portal hypertension and esophageal varices.

Sweat Glands. These provide material for the diagnostic sweat test for CF because of their excessive output of sodium and chloride. The inability to regulate this output puts patients in hot climates at risk for heat prostration from electrolytes loss.

DIAGNOSIS. Evaluation of patients with any of the previously mentioned conditions should include a pilocarpine iontophoresis sweat test. This requires collection of 100 mg of sweat after stimulation with pilocarpine. In children, values over 60 mEq/L of chloride are considered positive for CF. False positives occur in malnutrition, hypothyroidism, several skin conditions, and a variety of rare metabolic disorders (Table 12-2). Stool trypsin activity can be mea-

Table 12-2. Conditions in Which False Positive Sweat Tests for Cystic Fibrosis Occur

Malnutrition
Hypothyroidism
Nephrotic syndrome
Ectodermal dysplasia
Adrenal insufficiency
Dehydration
Mucopolysaccharidosis
Glycogen storage type I

sured and is low in CF patients with pancreatic insufficiency. Immunoreactive trypsinogen is now being tested to screen newborns and young infants. Elevated valves resulting from pancreatic obstruction and dumping of acinar contents into plasma occur early in infancy.

Treatment. In childhood the major factors in treatment center on nutrition and respiratory disease. Inhaled mucolytic agents, postural drainage, routine chest physiotherapy, and bronchodilators are used to minimize the pulmonary obstructive component. Aggressive treatment of infection with antibiotics and monitoring of sputum production are indicated. Eventually, progressive disease may require oxygen support.

Nutritional Support. Eighty-five percent of patients have pancreatic insufficiency and require enzyme supplementation. In young infants, hydrolyzed formulas may bypass the defect and provide adequate calories for growth. Medium chain triglycerides or glucose polymers can provide additional calories. A variety of pancreatic supplements are now available, with minor differences in enzyme composition. These are given with meals in amounts sufficient to limit steatorrhea.

Fat malabsorption is complicated by the increased caloric needs of older children with CF. These increases result from chronic lung disease, decreased intake from generalized anorexia, and inadequate digestion. Aggressive nutritional support involving nighttime nasogastric feedings, total parenteral nutrition, or gastrostomy tubes have been used to meet caloric goals.

Fat soluble vitamin supplementation may be required and vitamin E is usually given to all CF patients. Multivitamin tablets in double dosage are recommended as well.

Gastrointestinal Disorders

Achalasia

Achalasia is an uncommon disease of childhood characterized by a functional obstruction at the lower esophageal sphincter. Normal swallowing involves propulsive waves coordinated with a relaxing lower esophageal sphincter to move food down the esophagus and into the stomach. Patients with achalasia have an absence of these normal peristaltic waves combined with a lower esophageal sphincter that fails to relax, resulting in functional obstruction, dilatation of the esophagus, and the clinical symptoms. The etiology is unclear, though speculation centers around functional abnormalities in the myenteric plexus.

CLINICAL MANIFESTATIONS. An inherited form of achalasia has been reported in infants, but most patients are adolescents. Symptoms usually have been present for at least 1 to 2 years prior to the diagnosis. These include difficulty swallowing, nocturnal cough, wheezing, orthopnea, frequent regurgitation, recurrent pneumonias, weight loss, and decreased exercise tolerance. The diagnosis is usually made by barium swallow, though air fluid levels in the esophagus can occasionally be seen on chext x ray. Confirmation involves esophageal manometry with four classic findings: (1) absent peristaltic waves, (2) high resting lower esophageal sphincter pressures, (3) failure of the lower esophageal sphincter to relax with swallowing, and (4) an exaggerated response to methocholine stimulation. Treatment of choice is dilatation via endoscopic placement of an inflatable balloon at the level of the lower esophageal sphincter and stretching of the sphincter by inflation of the balloon. Repeat dilatation for recurrence of symptoms may be required, but is usually limited to two to three attempts. The Heller myotomy provides surgical correction if dilatation fails.

Gastroesophageal Reflux

Gastroesophageal reflux (GER) refers to the presence of gastric contents in the esophagus. This condition is now the subject of extensive investigation and has been implicated as a factor in asthma, sudden infant death syndrome, aspiration pneumonia, and Sandifers syndrome. Gastric obstruction, esophageal anatomic abnormalities, and motility disorders should all be ruled out prior to making the diagnosis of GER.

CLINICAL MANIFESTATIONS. Spitting or vomiting small amounts are common in infancy. Persistence beyond 9 months is not. The development of severe vomiting, failure to thrive, hematemesis, guaiac-positive stools, wheezing, or recurrent respiratory infections are all indications for investigating the degree of reflux in infants. In older children, dysphagia, heartburn, asthma, persistent vomiting, recurrent pneumonia, and nocturnal cough may be symptoms of GER.

EVALUATION. A careful history attending to degree of symptoms, secondary effects (i.e., bleeding, failure to thrive), and exacerbating factors (i.e., medications, respiratory disease, developmental delay) is critical. Radiologic evaluation (upper gastrointestinal series) is useful to rule out anatomic abnormalities but is a relatively insensitive exam for reflux. Nuclear medicine isotope scans are far more sensitive for GER and quantify gastric emptying as well. The gold standard remains the 24-hour pH probe which allows prolonged evaluation as well as temporal correlation with recorded events (such as apnea). The definition of pathologic reflux based on pH probe data varies among centers but is based on the number of reflux episodes, the percent of time esophageal pH is below 4, and the duration of episodes. Adjunctive tests include endoscopy for esophageal biopsies to evaluate esophagitis and motility studies if underlying neurologic dysfunction is suspected.

TREATMENT. Traditional conservative therapy, though unproved by studies, remains the universal starting point. For mild uncomplicated reflux, inclining the head of the bed, frequent, smaller feeds, and thickening feeds with rice cereal may suffice. In more severe, complicated cases, medications are added to treat the acid injury and the cause. Antacids, cimetidine, or ranitidine are used to protect the esophagus from acid injury. In cases where apnea or asthma are involved, treatment of the esophagitis may be as important as treating the reflux. Bethanecol and metaclopromide have been used to increase lower esophageal sphincter pressure and speed gastric emptying (metaclopromide). Newer prokinetic drugs like Cisapride and Domperidone may soon be available as well.

If medical therapy is ineffective and complications are present, surgical therapy utilizing a Nissen fundoplication can be done.

Hypertrophic Pyloric Stenosis

Previously considered congenital, pyloric stenosis is now viewed as a developmental sequence initiated in utero and completed in the early neonatal period. The result is a hypertrophied pyloric muscle with gastric outlet obstruction and vomiting.

CLINICAL MANIFESTATIONS. Symptoms begin between the second and fourth week of life. Projectile vomiting, frequently occurring immediately after or even during feeding is usually the presenting complaint. If symptoms are prolonged the child may exhibit failure to thrive or actual weight loss.

Physical examination is directed toward palpation of the hypertrophied pylorus, described as an olive-like mass in the upper right quadrant. Examination may be more successful if the patient is prone on the examiner's hand and kept quiet to keep the abdomen soft. With an appropriate clinical history the finding of the "olive" is sufficient to recommend surgery. If questions remain after examination, sonographic evidence of an enlarged pyloric muscle or an upper gastrointestinal series revealing a "string sign" confirms the diagnosis.

TREATMENT. Surgical correction utilizing a pyloromyotomy is simple and safe in a well-prepared patient (Fig. 12-4). With gastric outlet obstruction hyperchloremic, hypokalemic metabolic alkalosis may complicate the presenting picture and should be corrected with intravenous fluids prior to surgery. As the operation does not invade the stomach, feedings may begin almost immediately postoperatively, and hospitalization is usually short.

Peptic Ulcer

Concepts regarding pediatric ulcer disease have undergone radical change recently. The advent of endoscopy has provided a diagnostic tool far more sensitive than radiology and, combined with increased clinical suspicion, has provided a marked increase in the diagnosis of peptic ulcers in children. The discovery of *Campylobacter pylori* and its association with gastritis and ulcer disease has provided a new factor in the pathogenesis.

Pathophysiology. A peptic ulcer is a loss of mucosal tissue in the duodenum or stomach. This injury occurs in the

Fig. 12-4. Congenital hypertrophic pyloric stenosis. A. The heavy, muscular, fleshy ovoid tumor is shown. The lumen is constricted to the point of near obliteration. Note the recess that appears in the lumen at the duodenal end. In this area perforation of the mucosa is most likely to occur during operation. B. Linear division of the tumor down to submucosa from well on the stomach to well on the duodenum allows the muscle to pull apart and the mucosa and submucosa to herniate out, establishing an adequate passageway.

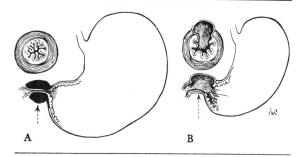

presence of acid, pepsin, and possibly infectious agents. Primary peptic ulcer disease is rare in achlorhydric patients, suggesting the critical role of gastric acid. Acid secretion studies in children with peptic ulcers will generally show an increase in maximal acid output after stimulation. This finding alone, however, does not explain ulcers as some normal patients have high acid output and never develop peptic conditions, suggesting the multifactorial nature of this condition. Other hypotheses suggest that local breakdowns in mucosal protection contribute, and this may be a factor in drug induced ulcerations.

Campylobacter pylori is a spiral bacteria recently described in the gastric antral mucosa. With endoscopic biopsies now standard, up to 70% of adult patients with gastritis and from 70 to 90% of adult patients with duodenal ulcer have *campylobacter* in the antral mucosa. Exactly how these organisms contribute to ulcer development is unclear, but it is probably related to breakdown in local defense mechanisms. At present, no clear causative role can be ascribed to these organisms but research continues.

CLINICAL MANIFESTATIONS. The signs and symptoms of childhood ulcer disease vary greatly with age. While primary ulcers may occur in the newborn, the most neonatal ulcers are stress related and gastric in location. These usually present as bleeding or perforation. While older infants may show poor feeding or vomiting, hematemesis or guaiac-positive stools remain the likely presentation. The predominance of gastric ulcer continues through the preschool age. Abdominal pain becomes a frequent complaint but may be atypical and not the classic burning epigastric pain of adult ulcer disease. Up to 50% of children with ulcers present with a major complication, usually hemorrhage.

Older children and adolescents have a clinical picture similar to adults with localized burning epigastric pain, nocturnal pain, and pain if meals are missed. They also predominantly have duodenal ulcers.

DIAGNOSIS. Endoscopy locates 90 to 95% of peptic ulcers. Radiography localizes 75% of ulcer disease in adults, but studies in children are less successful. Gastric ulcers are frequently superficial may be diagnosed only 25 to 50% of the time and duodenal ulcer disease approximately 50%. Clearly, in the seriously ill child, endoscopy offers the advantage of accuracy and biopsies. In outpatients with milder symptoms many physicians may begin the work-up radiologically and utilize endoscopy if x-ray studies are negative and suspicion is high.

TREATMENT. Decreasing the acidic pH of the stomach remains the mainstay of therapy. Antacids and H_2 histamine-receptor blockers are utilized to keep the luminal pH greater than 4.5. Newer blocking agents provide once or twice daily dosages and are more potent. Sucrolfate is a mucosal protective agent and is equally effective in promoting ulcer healing. Misoprostal is a new drug specifically designed for protection from drug-induced injury of the nonsteroidal antiinflammatory agents. Treatment courses are usually 4 to 6 weeks. This is adequate for gastric ulcers and frequently duodenal ulcers as well. Recurrence may suggest evaluation of serum gastric levels to look for hypergastronomia states (Zollinger-Ellison syndrome) or gastric acid analysis to find hypersecretion in children. Both groups can be treated with prolonged, higher dose H_2 blockers.

Diarrhea

Diarrhea is one of the most common pediatric illnesses and is the major cause of infant mortality in the underdeveloped world (Table 12-3). It can be defined as an increase in stool volume which is predominantly an increase in the water content of the stool. Acute diarrheal episodes result from one of three alterations in colonic function. The first, and clinically most significant, is a decrease in the water absorptive capacity of the bowel. Second is decreased intestinal surface area may be important in postinfectious states in which the small bowel villi have been flattened. Changes in intestinal transit time occur most commonly in short-bowel postoperative cases. Clinically, regardless of cause, acute diarrheal episodes are characterized by multiple loose, watery stools, with or without blood and mucus. There is a frequent association of abdominal pain, vomiting, fever, and occasionally, extraintestinal symptoms. These symptoms tend to be most severe in infants or chronically ill children who are most often compromised by dehydration and nutritional limitations.

General treatment principles apply to virtually all cases of acute diarrheal episodes. Out-patient management can be attempted for all but the most severe episodes of diarrhea in any immunocompetent patient outside of infancy. Rehydration is the key with the utilization of preprepared rehydration solutions or electrolyte containing liquids, such as GatorAde and Pedialyte (Table 12-4). Secretory diarrhea does not cease simply with the stoppage of oral alimentation; however, absorption in the face of secretory diarrhea is not necessarily impaired, and, consequently, oral alimentation may be maintained in the face of massive stool output. In the severest of cases, and in young infants where dehydration is a great risk, hospitalization and intravenous hydration may be required. In these patients attention to sodium and potassium balance is critical because of the predilection for infants to have significant sodium shifts, depending on the mechanism of their dehydration. Once

Table 12-3. Infectious Causes of Diarrheal Illness

Organism	Disease type	Incubation	Characteristics
Staphylococcus	Toxin	2–6 hours	Preformed toxin in meats and pastries
Clostridium difficile	Pseudomembra-nous colitis	?	Heat-resistant spores—toxin formed in gut. Associated with antibiotic usage.
Shigella	Dysentery	1–5 days	Human source, fecal spread—fever, seizures
Salmonella	Enteritis	12–48 hours	Animal reservoir—common source outbreak—occasional enteric fever
Campylobacter	Colitis	2–5 days	Bloody diarrhea, colicky abdominal pain, fever. Often resolves spontaneously within a few days
E. coli	EPEC	2–14 days	Nursery epidemics—occasional dysentery
	Toxin	12 hours–? days	Choleralike toxin—organism "normal flora"
Cholera	Toxin	12–48 hours	Clear stools with mucus, no fever—profound fluid loss
Viral	Enteritis	16–48 hours	Rotavirus and Norwalk agent most common etiologies—Vomiting may be worse than diarrhea
Entamoeba histolytica	Dysentery	Days to weeks	Chronic bloody dysentery—may be acute or asymptomatic, excreting only cysts
Giardia	Duodenitis and malabsorption	Weeks to months	May cause acute diarrhea and malabsorption especially in dysgammaglobulinemia

EPEC = enteropathic *E. coli.*

the diarrhea has slowed a gradual increase toward a normal diet may be attempted. There remains considerable debate over the institution of lactose containing formulas and foods. In severe cases lactose can be withheld for 7 to 10 days after the acute diarrheal episode to allow the lactase in the brush border to regenerate.

VIRAL AGENTS. Viruses cause 80% of acute diarrhea. Viral gastroenteritis is characterized histologically by patchy villus flattening and intraepithelial lymphocytic invasion. The clinical illnesses are self-limited, yet remain the most common cause of hospitalization in infancy. Stools are frequent, watery, and without blood or mucus. Treatment requires maintenance of hydration and nutrition.

Table 12-4. Composition of Oral Glucose-Electrolyte Solution for Therapy of Diarrhea

Ingredient	Amount[a]		Concentration[b]	
Glucose	25.0	2 tablespoons	Glucose	140
KCl	1.35	¼ teaspoon	K	20
NaCl	3.0	½ teaspoon	Cl	70
NaHCO$_3$	2.5	½ teaspoon	Na	80
			HCO$_3$	28

[a] In grams per liter or level spoons per liter.
[b] In millimoles per liter of solution.

Rotavirus. Rotavirus is now recognized as the most common cause of viral gastroenteritis in children. Rotavirus is a RNA virus, 70 nm in size, and is shed in the feces in high concentrations. The clinical illness is most common among infants and children under 2 years of age. It consists of initial fever and vomiting followed by profuse watery diarrhea. The illness usually lasts between 5 and 10 days and can easily be diagnosed by serologic stool studies, which are available in most hospitals. Most adults and older children have immunologic protection from rotaviral infections. Rotavirus is a frequent cause of small bowel injury and secondary lactose intolerance. Accordingly, it is frequently recommended that lactose containing products be avoided in the immediate postinfectious state. Rotaviral vaccines are in the investigational stage and should soon be available.

Norwalk Virus. Norwalk agents were the first viruses to be identified in epidemic gastroenteritis. In 1968, in an elementary school epidemic in Norwalk, Connecticut, the Norwalk agent, a small 27 nm virus was isolated from the stool of many children. When introduced into volunteers, the symptomatology was reproduced. Norwalk viruses are now felt to cause much of the epidemic gastroenteritis occurring in children (over 5 years of age) and adults. The illness is usually short-lived, with vomiting, diarrhea, and abdominal cramps lasting 1 to 2 days. There is no generally available diagnostic tool as Norwalk viruses are shed in small amounts in the stool. Treatment requires attention to hydration, and only occasionally is hospitalization required.

Other Viral Agents. Enteric adenovirus is being identified more frequently as a gastroenteritis pathogen. It is now reported in 6 to 8% of viral diarrheal episodes. The clinical illness resembles that of rotavirus, and diagnostic tests are not easily available. Viral culture and electronmicroscopy are still required, and because treatment varies little from rotaviral illness, little attention is usually placed to confirming an adenoviral infection. Calcivirus, astrovirus, and echovirus have all been implicated as diarrhea-producing agents in children.

BACTERIAL AGENTS. Salmonella. *Salmonella enteritidis* (see also Chapter 20) produces diarrhea by direct penetration of intestinal epithelium and production of an inflammatory response in the lamina propria. There is only minimal tissue destruction and only 5 to 10% of patients become bacteremic. It is usually acquired through contaminated food or drink or directly from house pets. The incubation period is between 8 and 48 hours with the initial illness consisting of nausea, vomiting, fever, and abdominal pain. Diarrhea begins shortly after exposure and stools may contain both blood and mucus. The spectrum of clinical illness runs from very mild with diarrhea alone to septicemia with fever, seizures, and dehydration. The diagnosis is made with positive stool cultures. Though treatment has not been shown to alter the course of the illness, it may prevent bacteremia and so is indicated in those patients at higher risk of becoming septicemic. This would include infants under 6 months of age, children with chronic illnesses or hemoglobinopathies, or immunocompromised patients. Development of a carrier state is extremely unlikely in nontyphoid *salmonella* infections. Treatment is with ampicillin or third-generation cephalosporins.

Shigella. *Shigella sonnei* and *Shigella flexneri* are the main pathogenic organisms in North America. Man is the only host for *Shigella* organisms. They produce diarrhea by invasion of the mucosa and cellular damage, generally in the distal colon and rectum. Blood stream invasion is extremely rare. Clinical illness is characterized by fever, crampy abdominal pain, tenesmus, and bloody mucoid stools lasting 6 to 8 days. Patients with *Shigella* may be extremely sick, and seizures have been reported secondary to a convulsive neurotoxin produced in approximately 10% of infections. Diagnosis is by stool culture, and treatment may be ampicillin or other appropriate antibiotics. As opposed to *Salmonella* infection, antibiotic treatment does shorten the course and severity of *Shigella* illness; however, it is usually a self-limiting disease and only severely ill or compromised patients receive antibiotics.

Campylobacter. *Campylobacter jejuni* has been described as an etiologic agent in infectious diarrhea since 1977. It makes up 6 to 14% of diagnosed diarrheal episodes and is most frequently acquired from contaminated poultry products. *Campylobacter* infects predominantly the distal small bowel and colon with an incubation period of 2 to 5 days. Abdominal pain, low grade fever, and diarrhea, frequently with blood and mucus, make up the clinical picture. Severe illness leading to dehydration and hospitalization is unusual. Diagnosis is made using an aqueous fuchsin stain of a stool sample and identification of a spiral bacteria. Sigmoidoscopy demonstrates inflammatory changes identical to that of ulcerative colitis. Most patients have a moderate course which resolves spontaneously. For more acutely ill patients or persistent infections, erythromycin or an aminoglycoside may be helpful if taken during the first few days of infection.

Yersinia Enterocolitica. *Yersinia* enterocolitis is a disease predominantly of the distal small bowel and, as such, may mimic appendicitis or Crohn's disease. The clinical picture is of profuse bloody diarrhea with right lower quadrant pain and high fevers. In older children extraintestinal manifestations, such as seronegative polyarthritis and erythema nodosum, may be present and may persist several months after the acute diarrhea illness. Diagnosis is by identification on stool culture. Treatment of *Yersinia* infection utilizing Bactrim or tetracycline has been shown to decrease bacterial shedding in stool, but it is unclear of the impact on symptoms. It is not unusual for patients with *Yersinia* enterocolitis to be taken to surgery for presumed appendicitis, and up to 5% of appendectomies in some studies have involved *Yersinia* infection.

Escherichia Coli. The incidence of *E. coli* as an agent in infectious diarrhea is unclear because of its presence in normal bowel flora and the relative infrequency with which serotyping is performed. It is well known that it may cause diarrhea by four separate mechanisms. Enterotoxigenic *E. coli* produces both heat labile and heat stable toxins that produce a secretory diarrhea by its effect on the cyclic-AMP and cyclic-GMP modulated pumps in the intestine. Enteroinvasive *E. coli* produces diarrhea through direct invasion and destruction of the mucosa similar to *Shigella* infection. Enteropathogenic *E. coli* produces diarrhea by disruption of the micro villi secondary to its adhesive properties. Lastly, enterohemorrhagic *E. coli* reportedly produces a cytotoxin with resultant cellular destruction and bloody diarrhea. Pathogenic *E. coli* is usually acquired through contaminated food and water sources. Traveler's diarrhea, the best known of the *E. coli* infections, is usually produced by enterotoxic *E. coli*. The illness produced by *E. coli* usually runs 3 to 5 days and is self-limited. Diagnosis requires stool culture and serotyping. Treatment is predominantly supportive and hydration, although ampicillin and trimethoprim-sulfamethoxazole may be taken for enteroinvasive infections. Enteropathogenic *E. coli* has a predilection for young infants under 6 months of age and may cause a more severe illness in this age group.

OTHER BACTERIA. Aeromonas hydrophilia and Vibrio parahemolyticus. These cause a small percentage of bacterial gastroenteritis in children. They should be looked for in the appropriate clinical setting, in which a patient is immunocompromised or has been hospitalized with a chronic illness.

Clostridium difficile. Antibiotic related colitis, or pseudomembranous colitis is caused by bacterial overgrowth with *Clostridium difficile* after eradication of normal bowel flora with antibiotics. The illness may begin from days to weeks after completion of a course of antibiotics, and it is now clear that virtually any antibiotic may be the cause. The clinical picture consists of diarrhea, with or without blood, and abdominal pain. Diagnosis is made by identifying the *C. difficile* toxin in the stool. Sigmoidoscopy reveals white plaque-like pseudomembranes coating the large bowel with underlying mucosal ulceration. Treatment, if required, consists of either vancomycin or metronidazole or, in milder cases, cholestyramine.

PARASITIC AGENTS. Giardia lamblia. This is the most common parasitic agent (also see Chapter 20) causing diarrhea in children. Endemic in areas of the United States, it may be water or food borne, and can be spread by person to person contact, especially among homosexuals. Clinical illness is usually insidious in onset, with abdominal pain, cramping, bloating, and diarrhea. If prolonged, malabsorption and failure to thrive may ensue. Patients who are at high risk for *Giardia* infection include the immunocompromised, especially those with IgA deficiency, patients with blood group A, the poor or those living in poor sanitary conditions, and institutionalized patients. *Giardia* colonizes the duodenum, and diagnosis by stool studies alone may miss 10 to 50% of cases. Examination of duodenal fluid via aspiration or string test is more sensitive. Treatment, if medically indicated, involves furazolidone, quinacrine, or metronidazole.

Entamoeba histolytica. Amebiasis occurs predominantly in those living in the southwest, in low socioeconomic areas, in mental institutions, and in tourists returning from developing countries. Acute infection consists of bloody mucoid diarrhea with abdominal pain and tenesmus. More chronic colonization may cause hepatic abscesses and hepatomegaly in 1 to 3% of patients. Diagnosis is by examination for trophozoites in a fresh stool within 2 hours of excretion. Treatment is usually with metronidazole.

Cryptosporidia. *Cryptosporidia* is a small protozoan of recently growing importance in diarrheal illness. Diarrhea is usually watery, nonbloody, and large in volume. It is more prevalent in immunocompromised patients, AIDS patients, and those in day care. It follows a self-limited, but frequently prolonged course, especially in young patients. Diagnosis is by stool stain for oocysts. There is no effective medication for eliminating *Cryptosporidia* and treatment is supportive.

CHRONIC DIARRHEA AND MALABSORPTION: DIAGNOSIS AND MANAGEMENT. Chronic diarrhea is often difficult to define. Significant malabsorption can occur in children with two to three bulky stools per day, whereas breast-fed infants have six or more "normal" loose, seedy stools per day. A high-bulk diet, excessive amounts of formula, predigested formulas, large amounts of liquids, or perhaps even diets low in fat may cause frequent loose stools in otherwise healthy children. Toddler's diarrhea (the childhood irritable colon syndrome) or chronic nonspecific diarrhea is seen in children 6 months to 4 years of age and is characterized by the passage of three to five stools per day with the first stool of the day being the best formed. Most stools are passed in the morning, and most contain mucus with occasional undigested food. Often the parents have had irritable colon syndrome. There is no associated failure to thrive.

It is important to recognize normal entities that cause "chronic diarrhea" in order to avoid extensive diagnostic workup and to institute appropriate therapy if required.

The hallmarks of pathological chronic diarrhea of significant etiology are:

1. Associated failure to thrive
2. Persistence of diarrhea for more than 3 weeks in spite of appropriate dietary changes (temporary elimination of lactose-containing foods and avoidance of fatty foods)
3. Persistence of blood in the stool for longer than 1 week without finding an infectious cause
4. Associated systemic illness, e.g., persistent fever, rash, pulmonary disease, or abdominal pain
5. Persistent fecal soiling in a previously toilet-trained child
6. Significant interference in a child's day-to-day routine, including school performance and peer relationships

Symptoms and signs of malabsorption (Table 12-5) result from pathophysiological defects in either the lipolytic, micellar, mucosal, or delivery phase of intestinal absorption (Table 12-6).

History. The *age of onset* is important since certain diarrheal diseases characteristically begin at birth (glucose-galactose

Table 12-5. *Pathophysiological Basis for Symptoms and Signs in Chronic Diarrhea with Malabsorption*

Clinical features	Pathophysiology
Generalized malnutrition and weight loss	Malabsorption of fat, carbohydrate, and protein → loss of calories
Diarrhea	Impaired absorption of sodium and water (esp. colon), irritant effect of unabsorbed fatty acids, bile salts
Nocturia	Delayed absorption of water
Anemia	Impaired absorption of iron, vitamin B_{12}, and/or folic acid
Glossitis, cheilosis	Deficiency of iron and other vitamins
Peripheral neuritis	Deficiency of vitamin B_{12} and/or other B vitamins
Edema	Impaired absorption of amino acids → protein depletion → hypoproteinemia
Amenorrhea	Protein depletion → secondary hypopituitarism
Bone pain	Protein depletion → impaired bone formation → osteoporosis
	Calcium malabsorption → demineralization of bone → osteomalacia
Tetany, paresthesias	Calcium malabsorption → hypocalcemia; magnesium malabsorption → hypomagnesemia
Hemorrhagic phenomena	Vitamin K malabsorption → hypoprothrombinemia
Weakness	Anemia; electrolyte depletion (hypokalemia)

Table 12-6. *Classification of Malabsorption*

Intraluminal maldigestion
  Enzyme abnormalities (lipolytic phase)
    Pancreatic insufficiency
      Protein-energy malnutrition
      Cystic fibrosis
      Shwachman-Diamond syndrome
      Chronic pancreatitis
      Enterokinase deficiency
    Acid hypersecretion
      Zollinger-Ellison syndrome
    Gastric resection
  Altered bile salt metabolism (micellar phase)
    Bacterial overgrowth
      Protein-energy malnutrition
      Blind-loop syndrome
      Malrotation
      Immune deficiency
    Hepatic and biliary tract disease
      Neonatal liver disease
      Biliary atresia
      Cirrhosis
    Ileal resection (or disease)
      Bile salt–induced diarrhea
  Abnormal mucosal cell (mucosal phase)
    Nonspecific defects
      Protein-energy malnutrition
      Gluten-induced enteropathy (celiac sprue)
      Tropical sprue, giardiasis
      Lymphoma, immune deficiency
      Regional enteritis
      Short small bowel
      Radiation
      Protracted diarrhea of infancy
    Specific defects
      Disaccharidase deficiency
      Abetalipoproteinemia
      Glucose-galactose malabsorption
      Hartnup disease, oathouse disease, "blue diaper," cystinuria
  Altered intestinal lymphatic function (delivery phase)
    Malrotation
    Lymphangiectasia
    Lymphoma
    Constrictive pericarditis
    Chronic congestive heart failure

malabsorption, familial enteropathy, cystic fibrosis), whereas others are unusual until adolescence (Crohn's disease and ulcerative colitis). Obviously 2 years of mild diarrhea with malabsorption has greater consequences than 2 weeks of diarrhea; hence, *duration* is of major importance.

Associated symptoms such as fevers, arthritis, or rash may be a clue to a particular diagnosis. Although the *character of stools* is important (for example, oily, floating, foul-smelling stools may be associated with pancreatic insufficiency), this may be misleading because significant fat malabsorption may take place with two to three bulky stools per day. The *presence of blood or mucus* in the stools and its *color and location* in the stool may be helpful. Colitis is frequently associated with bright red blood and mucus. Melena (black, tarry stool) usually indicates bleeding proximal to the transverse colon. *Location of pain* in the right lower quadrant may indicate *versinia* or Crohn's disease; most infectious diarrheas are usually associated with periumbilical or poorly localized pain.

Physical Examination. Physical examination should involve careful examination of the skin for the presence of reduced skin turgor which signifies a loss of at least 5% of body weight. Rashes such as erythema nodosum, which occurs in Crohn's disease or with *yersinia,* may be helpful in making a specific etiological diagnosis. Dry mouth, sunken eyes and fontanel, washerwomen's hands, and hoarseness or aphonia occur with 10% dehydration. Weak pulse, tachycardia, acrocyanosis with cold extremities and oliguria are reflections of a dangerous reduction in intravascular volume and impending shock and suggest an acute process rather than chronic malabsorption.

Abdominal examination should include liver size determination because liver disease such as cirrhosis may be an etiological factor in diarrhea secondary to bile salt depletion. A sausage-shaped, firm but doughy mass in the left lower quadrant usually indicates fecal impaction with overflow diarrhea. Abdominal neuroblastoma may be associated with diarrhea in 10 to 25% of cases and may present as an abdominal mass. A choledochal cyst, palpable in the right upper quadrant, may obstruct bile flow and lead to steatorrhea and diarrhea.

Because children and their parents often do not give a history of preceding constipation, the importance of *rectal examination* in the child with diarrhea cannot be overemphasized.

Rectal tone may be diminished in neurological lesions involving peripheral nerves or spinal cord, in *Shigella* infection, and in psychogenic fecal impaction. The presence of a fecal mass in the rectal ampulla with a history of diarrhea indicates overflow diarrhea. The absence of an anal wink is another clue that neurological disease may be the cause of constipation with overflow diarrhea. Overflow diarrhea is fairly common and only becomes worse if antidiarrheal agents are administered. A consistently empty ampulla in the presence of constipation is a clue to the diagnosis of Hirschsprung's disease.

For chronic diarrhea, a growth chart is essential for determining the presence of failure to thrive and also to determine at what point in time the child's diarrhea had a significant impact on weight and growth. Weight usually begins to fall into a lower percentile within weeks of the onset of chronic diarrhea, whereas the impact of diarrhea on growth may take months to years.

Diagnostic Studies. After an appropriate history, physical examination, and a few simple laboratory tests indicate that a pediatric patient has chronic diarrhea, one should approach the differential diagnosis on a physiological basis and choose the appropriate laboratory tests. Certain laboratory tests are essential in every patient with chronic diarrhea; others may be called upon under special circumstances. The following gastrointestinal tests are important to understand.

Determination of Stool pH and Reducing Substances. This test is for the presence of monosaccharides and disaccharides in the stool, which indicates carbohydrate malabsorption. Stool pH is normally greater than 6. If sugars are malabsorbed, they are fermented by colonic bacteria into organic acids, which lower stool pH.

Microscopic Stool Examination for Fatty Acids and Neutral Fats. Isolated spot fat examination is useful only as a screening test. A large amount of neutral fat indicates pancreatic or bile salt deficiency. A large amount of fatty acids may indicate a mucosal epithelial lesion or the presence of colonic bacteria that hydrolyze neutral fat.

Stool Examination for Polymorphonuclear Leukocytes. The presence of these cells indicates enteritis or colitis of infectious or noninfectious etiology.

Stool Examination for an Occult Blood. When one suspects gastrointestinal blood loss from any source, including ulcers, polyps, or colitis, this test is important.

72-Hour Stool Fat. This is a very sensitive but nonspecific test for malabsorption because it may be abnormal with mucosal, pancreatic, intraluminal, or bile salt deficiency. No more than 5% of ingested fat per day should appear in the stool in children older than 2 years of age. Full-term infants should absorb 80 to 85% of their ingested fat. Performance of this test requires a normal diet including at least 35% of calories as fat. This test also gives the total volume of stool per day to indicate whether it is excessive.

Hydrogen Breath Test. Bacterial metabolism of carbohydrate reaching the colon produces hydrogen. Elevation beyond 10 to 20 ppm occurs in lactose or sucrose malabsorption, decreased intestinal transit time, and bacterial overgrowth conditions.

D-Xylose Test. This tests the absorption of an orally administered sugar that is passively transported across the intestinal mucosa. In diseases that cause damage to the surface epithelium of the mucosa, the increase is less than 20 mg/100 ml in the 1-hour serum D-xylose.

Small Intestinal Biopsy. This can be done by guided capsule (Crosby capsule) or directly on endoscopy. Duodenal fluid can be obtained for *Giardia* examination. Histologic examination of villous structure. Inflammation can be assessed with enzyme assays if necessary.

Sigmoidoscopy and Colonoscopy. These tests may be helpful in the diagnosis of ulcerative colitis, Crohn's disease, polyposis, arteriovenous malformations, and pseudomembranous colitis.

Chronic Diarrhea During the Neonatal Period. There are relatively few noninfectious causes of chronic diarrhea in the neonate, but because of the enormous growth requirements at this time, it becomes important to make the diagnosis rapidly. Because of pancreatic insufficiency, diarrhea in the neonatal period may be the presenting feature of cystic fibrosis. Sucrase-isomaltase deficiency is the most common genetic disaccharidase deficiency. Infants with this deficiency have watery acid diarrhea when given a sucrose-containing formula. Diagnosis is suspected on clinical basis and with a positive sucrose breath test but a negative hydrogen breath test. Confirmation of the diagnosis is made by demonstration of normal histology but decreased sucrase levels in the small-bowel biopsy specimen. Congenital short gut or malrotation with potential associated bacterial overgrowth is easily diagnosed with an upper gastrointestinal tract examination with small-bowel follow-through.

Hepatobiliary disease decreases intraluminal bile salt concentration. This results in decreased micellar function and impaired fat absorption. Biliary atresia, neonatal hepatitis, cirrhosis and choledochal cyst may interrupt bile flow. Dietary supplements include medium chain triglycerides (not micellar dependent) and large doses of water soluble forms of vitamins A, D, E, and K.

Familial enteropathy is a rare cause of diarrhea in the neonate. Diagnosis is made from the family history and small-bowel biopsy specimen, which demonstrates villus atrophy without crypt hyperplasia. These infants generally die without long-term parenteral nutrition.

Celiac Disease

Celiac disease, or gluten sensitive enteropathy, is defined as a nonallergic sensitivity to gliadin, a wheat storage protein, which results in villous atrophy of the small intestine and malabsorption. Gliadins are storage proteins found in rye, barley, oats, and wheat. Celiac disease is most common in the British Isles where prevalence rates reach 1/300. In affected patients, the disease is life long and requires strict adherence to a gluten-free diet.

CLINICAL MANIFESTATIONS. The classic presentation is a young toddler, irritable and anorectic with failure to thrive and diarrhea. Stools are foul-smelling, large, frothy, and floating. In patients with long courses prior to diagnosis, malnutrition evidenced by a distended abdomen, wasted limbs and buttocks, peripheral edema, long eye lashes, and delayed development may be present. The clinical presentation, may vary greatly to include constipation, iron deficiency anemia, rickets, osteoporosis, and vitamin K deficiency.

DIAGNOSIS. Initial evaluation includes a complete blood count, serum albumin, total protein liver function tests, vitamin B_{12} level, folate levels, and stool studies for fat and carbohydrate malabsorption. Stool examination to rule out Giardia Lamblia should be performed. Screening immunologic tests include IgG and IgA antigliadin antibodies. IgG antibodies are nonspecific and may be elevated in any disease causing small bowel injury. These include severe milk protein sensitivity, regional enteritis, allergic enteropathy, and transient gluten sensitivity. IgA antibodies are less sensitive but more specific. Antireticulin and IgA endomysial antibody tests are being proposed as even more specific immunologic tests for celiac disease.

Despite these immunologic advances, definitive diagnosis requires a stringent sequence of gluten challenges, withdrawals, and small bowel biopsies.

Initial biopsy is performed while the child is on a gluten-containing diet. If pathology reveals villous atrophy, elongated crypts, and increased plasma cells, the patient is placed on a gluten-free diet. Clinical improvement usually begins within 3 to 6 weeks. After 6 to 12 months, repeat biopsy should document normal villous histology. Present recommendations call for a rechallenge with gluten for 3 weeks with biopsy proved villous injury prior to making a definitive diagnosis.

TREATMENT. Adherence to a lifelong gluten-free diet relieves the symptoms and allows growth. Extensive dietary counseling, regarding the use of grains as fillers, in commercial products, and in processed foods is required. At initial diagnosis vitamin deficiencies should be replenished and lactose removed from the diet. Though dietary therapy alleviates much celiac disease, it is unproved whether the late gastrointestinal malignancies known to occur in celiacs can be prevented.

Other Diarrheal Conditions

Milk protein allergy is an important cause of diarrhea during the first year of life. Infants may have diarrhea, gastrointestinal blood loss, and hypoalbuminemia. Disorders found in milk-protein allergy may be gastritis or enteritis with some patients even having milk-induced colitis. Withdrawal of cow's milk and possibly soy protein results in the recovery of the colon; however, about 10% of patients will also have a soy protein allergy. By the age of 3 years these children can usually tolerate milk protein without diarrhea.

Abetalipoproteinemia is an autosomal recessive disorder that presents in infancy with steatorrhea, failure to thrive, subsequent ataxia, and acanthocytosis. These infants do not produce apolipoproteins B-100 and B-48; therefore, chylomicrons cannot be formed to transport fat out of the enterocytes. As a result the infants develop steatorrhea, and a characteristic small-bowel biopsy demonstrates lipid-laden enterocytes. The diagnosis is confirmed by absence of beta-lipoprotein on serum protein analysis. Medium-chain triglycerides are nutritionally therapeutic because they do not require lipoprotein for transport. Vitamin E therapy is necessary.

Intestinal lymphangiectasia is a disorder of the intestinal lymphatics, and frequently the peripheral lymphatics, that results from a blockage of the main lymphatics draining the intestine. Besides steatorrhea and protein loss, patients with this rare disease may have peripheral manifestations of lymphatic obstructions such as edema of the face, scrotum, or extremities. Losses of immunoglobulin producing lymphocytes may account for the increased incidence of infection and alterations of delayed hypersensitivity in a minority of these patients. Diagnosis is based on a small-bowel biopsy showing dilated lymphatics and a typical clinical picture. Therapy with a low-fat diet and medium-chain triglycerides results in a decrease in steatorrhea and improvement in ascites and edema.

Immunodeficiency Disorders

Immunodeficiency disorders are commonly associated with gastrointestinal manifestations. On a global basis, the most common cause of immunodeficiency is malnutrition, predisposing not only to enteric disease but also to numerous disorders of the respiratory tract. It has been clearly demonstrated, however, that the abnormalities in immune regulation induced by chronic malnutrition are rapidly corrected by nutritional rehabilitation. In the clinical setting, therefore, it is important to do immune function tests only in patients whose nutritional status is known to be normal or nearly normal.

If one divides the immunodeficiency disorders into those involving B cells and those involving T cells, it becomes apparent that gastrointestinal abnormalities are uncommon in patients with B-cell deficiencies other than common variable agammaglobulinemia and selective I_gA deficiency. In common variable agammaglobulinemia, 20 to 50% of patients develop gastrointestinal manifestations including malabsorption, giardiasis, protein losing enteropathy, and lymphonodular hyperplasia. I_gA deficiency is the most common B-cell defect occurring in 1/700 people. I_gA secreting plasma cells are decreased throughout the gastrointestinal tract. Steatorrhea, food intolerances, and chronic diarrhea are common symptoms. Increased incidence of giardiasis, celiac disease, and inflammatory bowel disease occurs.

Patients with T-cell deficiencies almost invariably develop some form of diarrhea, often intractable watery diarrhea caused by *Salmonella, Shigella,* enteropathogenic *E. coli,* or *Giardia lamblia.* Patients whose disorders due to T-cell deficiency have been corrected by bone marrow transplantation have had prompt diminution or cessation of diarrhea.

Acquired immunodeficiency syndrome (AIDS) is caused by an RNA retrovirus capable of causing gastrointestinal manifestations though the gastrointestinal tract is not a main target organ. Chronic diarrhea, weight loss, and malabsorption are clinical manifestations though weight loss can occur without diarrhea. Oral candidiasis, candidal or viral esophagitis, and increased incidence of malignancy are upper tract complications. Opportunistic infectious organisms include *Giardia, Cryprosporidia,* gram-negative bacteria, herpes, and cytomegalovirus.

The differential diagnosis of the immunodeficiencies associated with gastrointestinal disease is listed in Table 12-7. In the evaluation of chronic diarrhea, it is important always to obtain quantitative levels of serum immunoglobulins. Sophisticated tests of immune function can be postponed until nutritional status is assessed and malnutrition is treated. Treatment of diarrhea consists of elimination of an underlying secondary cause (disaccharide intolerance, infection), supportive care with nutrition and electrolyte replacement, and, ultimately, treatment of the primary disorder.

Tumors of the Gastrointestinal Tract

Malignant diseases of the gastrointestinal tract are uncommon in childhood and adolescence, with the most common tumor being lymphoma. Associated symptoms may be obstructive in nature or may mimic celiac sprue. Adenocarcinoma of the esophagus, stomach, and colon is rarely reported. Patients with familial polyosis syndromes are at significantly higher risk for malignancy.

Of particular interest in the pediatric population are tumors of the gastrointestinal tract that produce secretory diarrhea. Profuse watery diarrhea is the main complaint in these patients, leading to electrolyte depletion, dehydration, acidosis, and severe debility with malnutrition. This syndrome has been noted in association with neuroblastoma, ganglioneuroma, tumors of the organ of Zuckerkandl, carcinoid, pheochromocytoma, villous adenoma, and tumors associated with the secretion of high levels of vasoactive intestinal polypeptide.

The stools are similar to those found in cholera, with copious secretions of nearly isotonic fecal water and variable amounts of mucus. The diagnosis must be made by radio-

Table 12-7. Immunodeficiencies and Gastrointestinal Diseases

Immunodeficiency disorder	Gastrointestinal involvement
AIDS	Diarrhea, weight loss. Opportunistic infections, unexplained malabsorption
Common variable agammaglobulinemia	Giardiasis (most common); lymphoid nodular hyperplasia; atrophic gastritis leading to pernicious anemia; bacterial overgrowth; disaccharidase deficiency; "flat villus" lesion (not gluten sensitive)
Transient hypogammaglobulinemia of infancy	Diarrhea (giardiasis, chronic enteritis)
Selective IgA deficiency	Giardiasis (common) gluten-sensitive enteropathy; isolated reports of inflammatory bowel disease; nonspecific diarrhea.
Secretory IgA deficiency	Intestinal candidiasis
X-linked agammaglobulinemia	Unusual, PLE, giardiasis
X-linked immunodeficiency with increased IgM	Gastrointestinal malignant disease
Severe combined immunodeficiency	Chronic diarrhea; usually idiopathic, occasionally salmonella or E. coli
Ataxia-telangiectasia	IgA deficiency; rare gastrointestinal manifestations; malignant reticuloendothelial disease
Wiskott-Aldrich syndrome	Increased incidence of malignant disease
Thymic hypoplasia	Candidiasis

PLE = protein losing enteropathy

graphic studies, ultrasound, computed axial tomography (CAT scan), angiography, or selective catheterization of various venous sites by venacavography to identify the level of the secretory tumor.

Permanent cure can be achieved only by surgery. When the tumor is a diffuse adenoma of the pancreas, subtotal pancreatectomy has been recommended. Long-term prognosis is guarded.

Chronic Diarrhea During Childhood and Adolescence

Development of chronic diarrhea during childhood and adolescence is relatively infrequent except for a few disor-ders, the most common being constitutional lactase deficiency.

LACTASE DEFICIENCY. Onset of lactase deficiency is genetically related with presentation at approximately 5 years of age in White American children but as early as 3 years in Black children (Table 12-8). Small bowel histology is normal, but measured enzyme activity levels are low. The clinical symptoms range from mild discomfort and loose stools after several glasses of milk to severe diarrhea, cramps, bloating, and flatulence after small exposures. Most adolescents avoid the full-blown symptoms by intuitive knowlege of their tolerance level. Lactose intolerance should be suspected in thriving children or adolescents with chronic diarrhea or abdominal pain.

Secondary lactase deficiency (Table 12-9) follows injury to small-bowel mucosa with loss of mature enzymes in the brush border. Commonly associated with infections, especially viral gastroenteritis in infants, it may follow any inflammatory process, and resolves with recovery of villous brush border epithelium.

Diagnosis is suspected clinically and confirmed by hydrogen breath test or lactose tolerance test. The presence of reducing sugars and an acid pH of stool are associated findings. Institution of a lactose-free diet results in resolution of symptoms.

Inflammatory Bowel Disease

Diarrhea often heralds the onset of ulcerative colitis (see Ulcerative Colitis, below). The stools are commonly bloody, loose, and associated with tenesmus. Crohn's disease may affect both the large and small intestine with ulcerations, fistulas, and stenosis.

Protein-Losing Enteropathy

The gastrointestinal tract plays a significant role in regulating the synthesis and degradation of plasma proteins. Most plasma proteins are synthesized by the liver and plasma cells of the lymphoid system. The intestinal mucosa synthesizes beta-lipoprotein for long-chain triglyceride transport during dietary fat ingestion and very low density lipoprotein for endogenous lipid absorption during fasting. Protein synthesis in these organs is regulated in part by the intestinal absorption of amino acids. Normally serum proteins secreted into the intestinal lumen are rapidly broken down into their constituent amino acids, which are reabsorbed and reenter the synthetic pool of amino acids. Excessive protein loss into the gastrointestinal tract can be a cause of hypoproteinemia seen in association with many disorders.

Table 12-8. Prevalence of Genetic Late-Onset Lactose Malabsorption Among Ethnic and Racial Groups

Group	No. in study	Age	No. with LM	Prevalence of LM (%)
Alaskan Eskimos	36	Adults	34	94
Oklahoma native Americans	20	Adults	19	95
Children in Ghana	100	2–6	73	73
Bantu	52	Adults	51	98
Orientals in U.S.	11	Adults	11	100
Danes	670	Adults	16	2
"Anglo-American" whites	142	Adults	21	15
American blacks	25	4–5	6	24
American blacks	98	Adults	79	81
Mexican Americans	75	10–14	42	56
Indians in Bombay	100	Adults	64	64

Source: Adapted from F. Simoons, *Am. J. Dig. Dis.* 23:963, 1978.

Hypoproteinemia occurs when the rate of protein catabolism exceeds the body's capacity to synthesize protein.

PHYSIOLOGY. The dynamics of gastrointestinal protein loss in normal individuals are not completely understood, and the mechanism, site of loss, and precise magnitude are unknown. Current studies suggest that the normal albumin turnover is about 0.2 g/kg/L of which only 10% is lost in stool.

In patients with disease affecting the gastrointestinal tract, however, loss of serum proteins may increase markedly. The mechanisms involved in such a process may be (1) obstruction of the gastrointestinal lymphatics with loss of lymph into the intestinal lumen, (2) exudation through an inflamed or ulcerated mucosa, or (3) a disorder of mucosal cell metabolism or turnover. In normal subjects, 5 to 10% of the intravascular pool of albumin or ceruloplasmin is catabolized each day. In patients with intestinal protein loss, 45%

Table 12-9. Causes of Secondary Lactase Deficiency

Viral enteritis
Celiac disease
Bacterial enteritis
Giardiasis
Inflammatory bowel disease
Cow-milk and soy protein intolerance
Bacterial overgrowth
Radiation enteritis
Immunodeficiency disorders

of the plasma pool of these proteins may be catabolized each day, and presumably the excess is lost into the gastrointestinal tract, hence the hypoproteinemia. The reduction in serum protein concentration affects most severely the proteins that have the longest survival (albumin, gamma globulins) and spares those proteins with a relatively short survival (alpha$_2$-macroglobulins, fibrinogen).

DISEASES ASSOCIATED WITH GASTROINTESTINAL PROTEIN LOSS. Clinically, findings vary from mild peripheral or dependent edema to failure to thrive. In some patients, the symptoms associated with the underlying disorder may predominate. Hypoproteinemia, specifically hypoalbuminemia results in low colloid oncotic pressure, hyperaldosteronism, and excess fluid in the intestinal space. Losses of other plasma proteins (immunoglobulins, ceruloplasmin) may not be apparent.

The diagnosis of protein-losing enteropathy is established by the use of the alpha$_1$-antitrypsin clearance test, tagged albumin excretion scans or stool protein collection, and elimination of renal or dermal sites of excessive loss. Identification of the primary disease leading to excessive protein loss depends upon absorptive, radiologic, endoscopic, and histologic studies.

In the pediatric age group, the gastrointestinal diseases that are commonly associated with excessive protein loss are celiac sprue, Crohn's disease, ulcerative colitis, allergic gastroenteropathy, bacterial or parasitic enteritis, lymphoma, radiation enteritis, intestinal lymphangiectasia, eosinophilic gastroenteritis, Ménétrier's disease, and dysgammaglobulinemia. Protein loss is also seen occasionally in aganglionic megacolon. Renal and cardiac diseases should be excluded as possible causes of excessive protein losses.

TREATMENT. Excessive gastrointestinal protein loss must be regarded as the intestinal correlate of albuminuria. It is a symptom and not a disease. Therapy depends upon identification of the underlying disease process. Surgical extirpation of inflammatory or diseased portions of the stomach or bowel has been curative in a limited number of cases. In the majority of patients with small-bowel disease, however, the disorder is too diffuse for surgical therapy.

In patients with gluten enteropathy a gluten-free diet usually results in a complete remission. In patients with allergic gastroenteropathy a milk-free diet or steroids have been efficacious. Patients with intestinal lymphangiectasia are benefited by lowering the fat intake and by substituting medium-chain triglycerides for long-chain triglycerides in the diet. Corticosteroid therapy must be considered for regional enteritis, ulcerative colitis, eosinophilic gastroenteritis, and allergic gastroenteritis. Appropriate antimicrobial or antiparasitic drugs should be administered in acute enteric infections. Surgical resection, radiotherapy, chemotherapy or a combination of these is indicated in lymphoma.

CROHN'S DISEASE. Crohn's disease (granulomatous colitis, regional ileitis, regional enteritis) is a chronic inflammatory disease of the gastrointestinal tract characterized by exacerbations and remissions. The incidence of disease is rising; 20% of new diagnoses are in the pediatric age group. Its prevalence is increased in the Jewish population. Age of presentation is bimodal with peaks in the second and sixth decades. The incidence of disease is increased among first-degree relatives, but the mode of genetic transmission has not been established.

Etiology and Pathophysiology. The etiology of Crohn's disease is unknown. Suspected infectious causes have included viruses, atypical mycobacteria, and cell-wall deficient *Pseudomonas*. Present research is focused on breakdowns in the regulatory mechanisms of the gut immune system and the impact of a multitude of mediators.

Crohn's disease may affect any portion of the gastrointestinal tract from mouth to anus, but 60% of children have ileocolitis, 10 to 15% isolated small bowel disease, and 10 to 15% isolated colonic disease. All layers of the bowel wall may be involved, leading to fistula formation, and the lesions are often discontinuous. Microscopically, the bowel wall may show variable degrees of edema, increased lymphoid aggregates, fissures, ulceration, and fibrosis. Non-caseating granuloma, present in only 15% of endoscopic biopsies and 60% of surgical resections strongly supports a diagnosis of Crohn's disease.

Clinical Manifestations. The onset of disease is usually insidious; the most common presenting features in children are abdominal pain, diarrhea, weight loss, fever, and rectal bleeding. Extraintestinal symptoms, including arthritis, iritis, erythema nodosum, and malnutrition, may be present. Growth failure is present in 30% of newly diagnosed children and adolescents. Subnormal growth velocity may be even more common. Delayed sexual maturation accompanies growth retardation. With such protean manifestations, the differential diagnosis may be extensive. Infectious diseases must be excluded, and small-bowel tuberculosis and lymphoma must be considered.

Physical examination may be normal, but signs of weight loss, pallor, delayed maturation, digital clubbing, and aphthous stomatitis may be noted. Abdominal tenderness, distention, mass, and anal ulcerations are suggestive of Crohn's disease.

Diagnostic Studies. There is no specific laboratory test for Crohn's disease. Anemia; an elevated sedimentation rate; hypoalbuminemia; depressed serum folate, B_{12}, iron, and zinc levels may be present. These abnormalities reflect dietary inadequacies or excessive fecal losses due to mucosal injury, bacterial overgrowth, or bile salt deficiency. Sigmoidoscopic findings may be normal, or examination may show a patchy, inflamed mucosa, with spontaneous friability. Results of rectal biopsy may be entirely normal, or there may be abnormal histological findings, such as submucosal inflammation and granulomas, even if the rectum appears grossly normal. Radiological examination of the gastrointestinal tract is essential. Barium studies of affected colon demonstrate loss of haustral folds, ulcerations, and segmental involvement. Small-bowel examinations may demonstrate abnormalities of the terminal ileum, such as mucosal hypertrophy (cobblestone appearance) or overall narrowing and rigidity (string sign) and separation of intestinal loops. Fistula formation is characteristic of Crohn's disease.

Treatment. Treatment for this disorder of unclear etiology is empiric, with goals of achieving and maintaining remissions. In acute exacerbations, steroids are the mainstay of therapy. Sulfasalazine and newer 5-ASA drugs are effective especially in maintenance therapies. Azathioprine, 6-mercaptopurine, and cyclosporine are efficacious but employed mostly for intractable cases, complex fistulae, or partial obstructions. Metronidazole is indicated for perianal disease and fistulae.

Nutrition is the critical factor in growth failure where caloric sufficiency has reversed the delay. Elemental diets have been shown to decrease disease activity as well as improved nutrition. Caloric intake goals may be as high as 150% of average for age. Supplemental vitamins, B_{12}, folic acid, and iron may be required.

Surgical treatment should be avoided unless the patient has an acute form of the disease (obstruction, perforation) or fails to resond to medical management. Up to 90% of patients with ileocolitis may eventually require surgery. Primary resection of the involved bowel is the procedure of choice. Recurrence in other areas of the intestinal tract is common, and the incidence of repeated resection increases with each subsequent operation. The risk of small-bowel and colonic cancer is greater than that in the normal population but is not significant enough to warrant prophylactic resection.

ULCERATIVE COLITIS. Ulcerative colitis is a chronic inflammatory disease of the colon characterized by its course of intermittent relapses followed by long symptom-free periods; in a small number of patients the activity of the disease is continuous, whereas a few patients experience a single attack with no subsequent recurrence. The incidence of disease varies from 3.9 to 7.3 per 100,000. The incidence is increased among whites, and in some populations, i.e., those of Jewish descent. Males are affected slightly more often than females. Onset of disease is bimodal, with a peak in the second and third decades of life, and later in the fifth and sixth; 20 to 30% of patients are under the age of 21 years at onset. The incidence of disease increases tenfold with a positive family history.

Etiology and Pathophysiology. The etiology of ulcerative colitis is unknown. Current research involves disordered immunoregulation of the gut response to antigenic stimulation. A genetic predisposition is suspected. The exact defect has not been elucidated.

Ulcerative colitis is a mucosal lesion limited to the colon and characterized by diffuse ulcerations, erythema, and edema of the luminal surface. Histologically, an acute and chronic inflammatory process is present, with an increase in polymorphonuclear leukocytes and with crypt abscesses in the mucosal and submucosal layers. A decrease in mucus in epithelial goblet cells reflects regenerated activity. Thickened bowel wall and fibrosis are not seen, but focal strictures are seen in long-standing disease.

Clinical Manifestations. The onset of disease may be acute or, more commonly, insidious. Diarrhea, rectal bleeding, and weight loss are the most common presenting symptoms. With increasing severity, foul bloody diarrhea with mucous shreds involving 6 to 20 stools per day, abdominal cramps, stool urgency, fever, weight loss, anemia, and hypoalbuminemia may be seen. Extraintestinal manifestations include arthritis, iritis, pyoderma gangrenosum, sto-

matitis, liver disease, and growth failure, all of which may precede the onset of intestinal symptoms.

The differential diagnosis is extensive; however, enteric infections, Crohn's disease, Meckel's diverticulosis, ischemia, and carcinoma should be excluded.

Physical findings tend to be minimal with the exception of diffuse abdominal tenderness. Peritoneal signs are absent unless toxic dilatation of the colon (or megacolon) is present. Pallor, skin lesions, joint swelling, digital clubbing, eye changes, or growth failure may be identified.

Diagnostic Studies. Anemia, leukocytosis, and increase in the erythrocyte sedimentation rate, reticulocyte, and platelet counts are found in moderate and severe cases. There may be depression of serum iron, total protein, and albumin. Occult or gross blood is found in stools. Stool culture for *Yersinia* and *Campylobacter* and examination for amebae should be negative.

Sigmoidoscopic examination with rectal biopsy and radiological studies are fundamental to diagnosis and management of ulcerative colitis. In active disease, hyperemic mucosa, friability, edema, and ulceration are seen. In inactive disease, the mucosa appears granular and the vascular pattern is more prominent, reflecting mucosal atrophy. Rectal biopsy demonstrates acute and chronic inflammation. Barium studies of the colon in acute cases characteristically show spasm, ulcerations, and loss of haustral markings, with the most severe abnormalities seen in the distal portion of the colon. In long-standing disease, barium studies demonstrate a foreshortened, tubular, and featureless colon, with or without pseudo-polyps and strictures. Dilatation of the terminal ileum and loss of mucosal pattern without ulceration (backwash ileitis) may be present but is of no known clinical significance.

Treatment. The treatment of ulcerative colitis in children is directed toward early control of symptoms, prevention of relapse, and maintenance of remission. Remission is maintained by means of daily doses of sulfasalazine and well-balanced diets.

In acute disease the severity of the attack governs the therapeutic approach. Limited disease may be controlled with sulfasalazine or the newer 5-ASA preparations above or if needed combined with steroid enemas.

More extensive (pancolonic) or more severe disease usually requires steroids either orally or parenterally. Hospitalization may be required for bowel rest and intravenous alimentation. Bleeding rarely necessitates transfusion. Most patients respond to intravenous steroids and bowel rest; however, a small number with either intractable symptoms or acute complications (Toxic Megacolon) require surgery.

Children are more likely than adults (35% versus 20%) to

require a colectomy for ulcerative colitis. Surgical alternatives have been developed to make this more tolerable. Ileoanal anastomoses with construction of a reservoir pouch provide reasonable continence and no ostomy. Continent ileostomy avoids the ostomy bag. Regardless of the procedure, colectomy is essentially curative for ulcerative colitis.

Prognosis. At present, more than 80% of pediatric patients should have a normal life span. The risk of colonic cancer in a patient whose disease begins before the age of 10 years is highest in patients with pancolonic disease and increases approximately 1%/year after 10 years of disease. Annual colonoscopic examination with multiple biopsies are recommended in patients who have had ulcerative colitis for more than 10 years. Cure of the disease is assumed after total colectomy and ileostomy.

Neonatal Intestinal Obstruction

Intestinal atresia, malrotation of the intestine, meconium peritonitis, meconium ileus (see Cystic Fibrosis), and Hirschsprung's disease may all present as neonatal intestinal obstruction (see Chapter 9 and Fig. 12-5). The cardinal symptom in all cases is vomiting. Newborn infants may normally regurgitate, but they do not usually vomit; any vomiting should be treated with suspicion and considered an indication for x-ray examination of the infant. The appearance of bile in the vomitus should be tantamount to a diagnosis of intestinal obstruction. In all of these conditions, except probably Hirschsprung's disease, it is common to find polyhydramnios. If gastric aspiration of the infant is done at the time of birth, the recovery of more than 25 to 33 ml of fluid from the stomach should also suggest the probability of some form of congenital intestinal obstruction.

The lower the obstruction, the more serious are the consequences of intestinal atresia. Overdistention of the proximal bowel may lead to gangrene, secondary volvulus, or perforation.

DUODENAL ATRESIA. With duodenal atresia, distention of the abdomen obviously cannot occur, but the duodenum enlarges enormously; a plain film of the abdomen shows the characteristic double-bubble sign, with a fluid level in the gastric fundus and another one in the duodenum (Fig. 12-5A). The obstruction may be due to a mucosal diaphragm, to actual absence of a segment, or to replacement of a segment by a fibrous strand. The obstruction is usually distal to the ampulla of Vater. An actual mucosal diaphragm may be excised and the bowel repaired.

For most intrinsic duodenal obstructions, the treatment is

either duodenoduodenostomy around the obstruction or else duodenojejunostomy.

ANNULAR PANCREAS. Annular pancreas results in duodenal obstruction from an embryonic persistence of the dorsal anlage of the pancreas; this is not infrequently associated with an intrinsic duodenal obstruction as well. In any case, division of the pancreatic ring is not recommended because (1) some of the pancreatic tissue is actually intramural in the duodenum; (2) pancreatic fistula or pancreatitis may result; and (3) even in the absence of these complications, enough local inflammation may arise to cause a secondary obstruction. Treatment is, therefore, either duodenoduodenostomy or duodenojejunostomy.

MALROTATION OF THE INTESTINE. This condition usually presents as duodenal obstruction because of anomalous peritoneal bands. In addition, there may be volvulus of the entire small bowel, the mesentery of which is not fixed; the bowel hangs like a bunch of grapes on the stalk of the superior mesenteric vessels. Distention does not result in either case; whether caused by bands or volvulus, the obstruction is extremely high, and the fluid proximal to the obstruction is evacuated by vomiting. In volvulus, by the time the signs of significant distress appear, the entire small bowel is likely to be already necrotic. The possibility of a midgut volvulus is, therefore, one of the most specific reasons for immediate x-ray filming of any child whose vomiting is in any way suspected of being due to intestinal obstruction. Exploratory operation is needed when a good possibility of intestinal obstruction exists in the neonate. Occasionally a malrotation with intermittent obstruction goes uncorrected for some years, allowing the child to survive, with episodic vomiting until the diagnosis is made.

MECONIUM PERITONITIS. Meconium peritonitis (see also p. 221) usually presents as neonatal intestinal obstruction. The diagnosis is frequently made on the basis of x-ray findings; x-ray films show not only dilated loops but an area of the abdomen free of intestine, opacified with spotty, or sometimes quite extensive, calcification (see Fig. 12-5D). At times the peritoneal inflammatory process is spread into the sac of an inguinal hernia, and calcification may be seen there. This type of calcification is pathognomonic of meconium peritonitis.

Meconium peritonitis is produced by an intrauterine rupture of the fetal intestine, with leaking of the intestinal contents into the fetal peritoneal cavity. The cause of the rupture is commonly either an atresia distal to it or else meconium ileus. The latter condition is associated with cystic fibrosis of the pancreas, in which the meconium becomes so thick, tarry, and glutinous that it cannot pass beyond the terminal ileum and, therefore, obstructs the

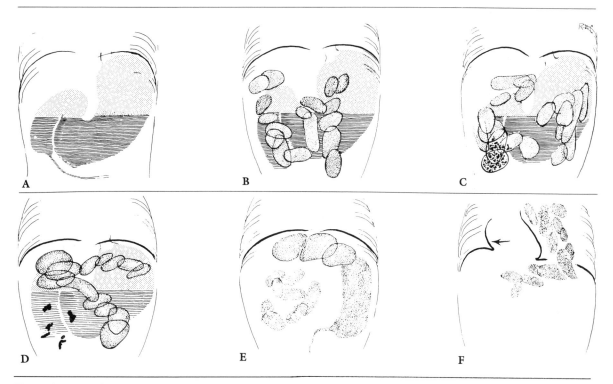

Fig. 12-5. Neonatal intestinal obstruction

A. *Duodenal atresia. Vomiting is early; distention is absent. The vomitus contains bile except in rare instances of preampullary obstruction. The plain film shows the typical double-bubble sign, and contrast films are not required.*

B. *Ileal and jejunal atresia. No air is recognizable in the colon, and numerous distended loops of small bowel, some with fluid levels, are present. Distention does occur. Volvulus of the small bowel may occur in association with atresia or in association with incomplete rotation of the bowel and twisting of the unfixed mesentery. In atresia, distention is early; in malrotation and volvulus distention may be late. The associated peritoneal bands crossing over the duodenum in patients with incomplete rotation may produce the picture of duodenal obstruction.*

C. *Meconium ileus as part of the picture of cystic fibrosis of the pancreas. The x-ray film shows an appearance identical with that of ileal atresia except that several loops of ileum are*

seen to be filled with stippled material, which is the meconium partly honeycombed by air bubbles.

D. *Meconium peritonitis — the picture of intestinal atresia with the addition of pathognomonic spots of calcification, usually in the portion of the abdomen that does not contain distended loops. The rupture of the bowel that produced this extravasation and calcification may have been due to atresia or to obstruction in association with meconium ileus. The latter occurs occasionally.*

E. *Hirschsprung's disease. The classic x-ray picture is of the narrowed distal segment and dilated proximal segment. This may be indistinct in the newborn infant, and a rectal biopsy may be required for the definitive diagnosis.*

F. *Diaphragmatic hernia. The presenting symptom is usually respiratory distress from the collapse of the ipsilateral lung and the immaturity of both lungs, but intestinal obstruction usually supervenes and may be prominent early.*

bowel completely. In any event the perforation, having allowed the escape of intestinal contents, frequently closes and is no longer to be found at birth. Operation is directed at correcting the initial cause of the obstruction. In rare cases, no original cause of the obstruction can be found, and

the obstructions that occur appear to be due to meconium peritonitis itself.

In a variant of meconium peritonitis, instead of a diffuse peritoneal process, the meconium is encysted in a discrete mass that may have to be removed en bloc together with the segment of intestine which gave rise to it. At first appearance the affected babies seem to be beyond salvage; the dense peritoneal adhesions superimposed on a primary lesion are in themselves dangerous. Actually, however, an appreciable number of these infants can be saved.

MECONIUM PLUG. Meconium plug is mentioned here only because of possible confusion arising from the similarity of the term to meconium peritonitis or meconium ileus. In this condition there is an apparent colonic inertia at birth which is relieved without much trouble — perhaps after gentle rectal manipulation. Explosive passage of a large plug of meconium is expected, after which the child is free of symptoms. Exactly the same phenomenon may occur in children who have neonatal obstruction on the basis of Hirschsprung's disease. In such children the intestine may deflate quite strikingly after the expulsion of a meconium plug, but it will become obstructed again.

CONGENITAL AGANGLIONIC MEGACOLON (HIRSCHSPRUNG'S DISEASE). Aganglionic megacolon (AM) results from a congenital absence of ganglion cells in the submucosal and myenteric plexus. Incidence is 1/5000 live births with a 4:1 male preponderance. The exact cause of the neurologic defect is unknown. In 75% of cases, the defect is limited to the rectosigmoid colon, but any length of bowel may be involved (Fig. 12-5E).

Clinical Manifestations. Neonatal intestinal obstruction with failure to stool is due to AM in 20 to 50% of cases. Over half of the cases are diagnosed in the first month of life, many before leaving the nursery. The history of difficulty passing stool from birth with a distended abdomen and an empty ampulla suggests the diagnosis. In later childhood the diagnosis may be more evasive. Again, the history usually dates back to infancy, incontinence is rare, and the ampulla is empty. In severe cases, malnutrition and wasting may be present.

Diagnosis. An unprepped barium enema is the radiologic exam of choice. The classic findings include a distal narrowed segment and a dilated, stool-filled proximal bowel. Rectal biopsy either by suction tube or surgically obtained should reveal the absence of ganglion cells (Fig. 12-6).

Treatment. Surgical correction involves either a Soave endorectal pull through or a Duhamel transanal pull through. In stable infants either procedure can allow resection of the diseased bowel with anastomosis of normal bowel to distal rectum. Frequently, a colostomy is done initially and a two-stage correction performed.

Complications. Untreated, AM can lead to major complications secondary to obstruction, perforation, or enterocolitis. Enterocolitis may develop rapidly in infants and manifest with shock, massive fluid shifts, and electrolyte

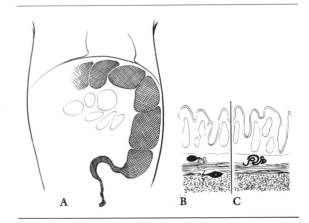

Fig. 12-6. Hirschsprung's disease. A. The pathognomonic x-ray finding of a narrowed distal segment extending down to the anus, with dilated and hypertrophic bowel above. The narrow segment may involve only a few centimeters of rectum or may involve the entire colon; at times, in hopeless cases, the entire bowel may be affected. B. The normal appearance of ganglion cells and nerve fibers in the submucosal and intermuscular (Meissner's and Auerbach's) plexuses. C. The appearance of the narrow segment in Hirschsprung's disease. There are no ganglion cells, and the nerve fibers are unusually prominent.

abnormalities. Treatment is supportive with fluids, antibiotics, and immediate colostomy when stable.

NECROTIZING ENTEROCOLITIS. The most common cause of intestinal perforation in the neonate, necrotizing enterocolitis (NEC) is a multifactorial disorder resulting in the characteristic development of air in the bowel wall, or pneumatosis intestinalis. Though 90% of cases occur in premature infants, NEC may occur in infants of any gestational age. The exact sequence of injury is uncertain but involves a combination of hypoxic insult with mucosal injury, bacterial proliferation, and microvascular thrombosis.

Clinically, infants present with abdominal distension, blood in the stool, vomiting, thrombocytopenia, and anemia. The diagnosis is confirmed by documenting intramural air or air in the portal venous system. Treatment prior to perforation is conservative with antibiotics, intravenous alimentation, and careful observation. Twenty-five percent of cases require surgery for perforation or gangrenous bowel. Mortality remains high.

IMPERFORATE ANUS. In the most common form of imperforate anus, anorectal agenesis, the anus, anal canal, and lower rectum are absent, there is no true internal sphincter (which is a specially developed portion of the circular muscle of the intestine), but the striated muscle fibers of the external sphincter are present and usually recognizable. The site of the anus is marked by a dimple or by a thickened perineal raphe.

Associated anomalies of the genitourinary tract are common. In practically every case in the male, there is a fistula connecting posteriorly with the urethra or with the vesical trigone — at least it is safest to assume that there is such a fistula. In the female, there is almost always a fistula into the vagina (rarely, into the bladder). Whereas male infants usually show signs of intestinal obstruction immediately because the fistula is inadequate for evacuation of the rectum, females frequently evacuate fairly effectively through the fistula. In females, close inspection of the external genitalia and perineum usually leads to a precise diagnosis of the nature of the anatomical anomaly, which will be one of the following:

1. One orifice. There is a single opening into the vestibule representing the outlet of the cloaca. By endoscopy and contrast radiography, one can demonstrate three orifices opening into the cranial end of the canal, i.e., the urethra, the vagina, and the rectal fistula.
2. Two orifices. There is the urethra anteriorly and the vagina posteriorly. This finding signifies an anorectal agenesis with rectovaginal fistula; the fistula is found on the posterior wall of the vagina above the hymen and is sometimes so high as to be located with difficulty.
3. Three orifices. This finding excludes anorectal agenesis and signifies either a vestibular ectopic anus or a covered anus with an anovulvar fistula.

Treatment. The most important anatomical factor, from the standpoint of reconstruction, is the level at which the rectum terminates and the position of the fistula that usually accompanies it. It has recently been shown that rectal continence after operation depends on the rectum's being brought down within the sling of the puborectalis portion of the levator ani muscle. The position of the terminal portion of the rectum is best demonstrated by lateral x-ray film in the head-down position. The pubococcygeal line, drawn between the body of the pubis and the lower border of the last sacral segment, is the important landmark in the roentgenogram. If the rectum is above this level, it has not reached the levator ani, and a combined perineal or abdominosacroperineal operation must be done to pull it through the ring of the puborectalis. If the rectum is substantially below this, it may be assumed to be through the puborectalis, and a perineal operation may be possible.

Because of the necessity for preserving the delicate levator

fibers and leading the rectum down through their loop in the high anomalies, it is preferable to perform a colostomy in the neonatal period for the one-orifice but not for the two-orifice type. The definitive operation is postponed until the infant has reached a weight of 8 to 10 kg or more. In females with fistulas in the distal vagina or at the fourchette, evacuation through the fistula, particularly if it is dilated, may be so satisfactory that further operative procedure can be postponed. In any case, the operation for imperforate anus is not one urgently undertaken within hours of birth, and if precise information is not available as to the operation that should be performed, a colostomy is preferable to a less-than-expert attack on the perineal structures. The surgeon usually has only one operative opportunity for an optimal result.

Intestinal Obstruction in Older Children

Acute mechanical obstruction in the older child, whether it occurs as a result of some congenital anomaly such as malrotation or is due to adhesions from a previous operative procedure, is a life-threatening complication that requires prompt decision and treatment. The commonly quoted quartet of symptoms is pain, vomiting, distention, and obstipation. Obviously obstipation requires long-continued obstruction before it can be determined to exist, and it is valid only as a late sign of intestinal obstruction. Distention does not occur at all in high-intestinal obstruction, because most of the material proximal to the obstruction is vomited, and occurs relatively late in low-intestinal obstruction. Vomiting usually occurs almost at once, and is at first reflex, then reflux. The single cardinal symptom of acute mechanical intestinal obstruction is cramplike abdominal pain. The situation here is much like that in the diagnosis of appendicitis. If the child comes in with a history of acute abdominal cramplike pain and there are no inconsistent features in the history, physical examination, and laboratory findings, operation should be undertaken essentially on suspicion. With volvulus or with a knuckle of bowel caught under an adhesion, a few hours' delay may be the difference between reducing viable bowel or resecting necrotic bowel, and perhaps a massive resection. There is no place for temporizing treatment in suspected acute mechanical obstruction; tube decompression does not cure or relieve it.

INTUSSUSCEPTION. Intussusception is the telescoping of one loop of bowel into the next (Fig. 12-7). In 95% or more of cases in infants and children, intussusception begins at or near the ileocecal valve. When the process begins well proximal to this point, it presents as a nonspecific acute intestinal obstruction and not as a true intussusception; when it be-

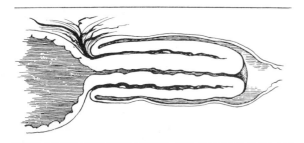

Fig. 12-7. Intussusception. The proximal bowel is to the left, the distal bowel to the right. Note that as soon as intussusception occurs the proximal bowel is obstructed, and the vessels drawn between the layers of the intussusception are similarly obstructed.

gins in the colon alone, the disease is significantly more benign. Incidence is 2.3/1000 live births with 63% occurring before age 2.

Pathogenesis. As the bowel inverts into itself, its lumen is compromised, and intestinal obstruction begins. Almost immediately, vascular embarrassment causes edema and increased pressure between the loops of bowel. These factors lead to progressively greater venous distention and transudation of fluid into the tissues between the loops. Finally the venous outflow and then the arterial inflow are completely obstructed, and gangrene occurs. At this point, histological studies show that all the cells of the mucous membrane of the intussusceptum become goblet cells which drip mucus into the lumen of the bowel. This mucus is mixed with bloody fluid leaking from the engorged bowel to form the so-called currant-jelly stool, a late finding in intussusception.

Clinical Manifestations. Intussusception in the infant characteristically attacks a husky male 5 to 9 months of age. The first symptom is likely to be a sudden cry or scream, with passage of the contents of the colon distal to the intussusception; thereafter, usually no stool or only a currant-jelly stool is passed. Recurrent episodes of severe pain, screaming, and pulling up his knees alternate with remarkably calm recovery periods. Examination generally shows a flat, relaxed abdomen and the palpable, characteristic, sausage-shaped mass, except when the intussusception is at the hepatic flexure and the mass is hidden by the right lobe of the liver.

Treatment. Although some surgeons still advocate operative intervention in all cases of intussusception, we believe that this is in most cases unnecessary. We favor an initial attempt at reduction with the barium-enema technique, which is a combination of two procedures, diagnostic and therapeutic. Barium reduction is not attempted in children with signs of shock, peritonitis, or perforation.

On suspicion of the diagnosis of intussusception, the operation should be formally planned. A tube is passed into the child's stomach and placed on suction. As in any potential intestinal obstruction, intravenous fluids are started. An unlubricated balloon catheter is inserted into the rectum, the balloon is inflated and pulled down against the levators, and the buttocks are then strapped together. Barium is let into the rectum from a height of 90 cm (3 feet) but no more than 100 cm (3½ feet), and the progress of the barium is observed fluoroscopically. The intussusception can be recognized by the negative shadow it imparts to the advancing head of the barium column, much as if it were the cervix and the barium were placed in the vagina. In 65% to 70% of cases, the barium enema reduces the intussusception completely. Total reduction of the intussusception is manifested by (1) free passage of barium into many loops of small bowel; (2) disappearance of the mass; (3) passage of feces or flatus per rectum; and (4) a changed condition of the child. The remaining patients are found to have had the intussusception reduced as far as the cecum, so that the intraabdominal manipulation can be confined to the right lower quadrant. Barium enema must always be undertaken under the direction of a surgeon, in a hospital, and with the operating room in formal readiness.

Errors in the diagnosis of intussusception are attributable to failure either to realize that a mass may not be palpable because it is behind the liver or to appreciate that some children continue to pass small amounts of stool. One of the greatest advantages of the barium enema is that it allows for accurate diagnosis without operation when even the slightest suspicion of intussusception exists. It must be emphasized that fluoroscopic examination should be kept at a minimum in order to avoid unnecessary x-ray exposure. Furthermore, one must *never* increase the height of the barium and hydrostatic pressure to more than 1 meter. Occurrence of intussusception in older children suggests the presence of a mechanical lesion acting as a lead point. Lead points occur in less than 10% of children under 2 but up to 75% of children over 5. Meckel's diverticulum, polyps, and hematomas are the most common.

Recurrent intussusceptions appear to be no more common after hydrostatic-pressure reduction than after operative reduction. One hazard of operative reduction which does not accompany hydrostatic-pressure reduction is the subsequent occurrence months or years later of mechanical intestinal obstruction due to adhesions caused by the operation and by the manipulation of the bowel.

Appendicitis

The classic history of appendicitis in a child old enough to give an accurate account is that of vague epigastric pain, followed by nausea and vomiting, and the migration of the pain to the right lower quadrant as it becomes cramplike. Violent pain, vomiting appearing before pain, high fever, and chills may rarely be seen. Occasionally a child does not vomit and even continues to eat. Pain is worsened by coughing, sneezing, or riding in the car.

In infants no subjective history is available. There may be fretfulness, vomiting, or persistent flexion of the hip.

DIAGNOSIS. Examination of the child with appendicitis, or any acute abdominal condition, should be a formal and leisurely procedure. Sitting by the right side of the bed, feeling the right pulse with the fingers of the left hand, the physician begins to palpate the abdomen, keeping his attention on the child's face and maintaining a reassuring conversation. With suspicion that the lesion is in the right lower quadrant, palpation should begin in the left lower quadrant; the first palpation, proceeding counterclockwise, should be so gentle as almost to be a caress, with slightly firmer palpation each time around until tenderness is elicited or muscle spasm and guarding are felt. Rebound tenderness — that is, the elicitation of pain in one part of the abdomen on release in another — is an excellent sign of peritoneal irritation, and tenderness referred to the right lower quadrant on release anywhere else is highly suggestive of appendicitis. This rather painful sign should not be elicited until the end of the examination in order to avoid losing the child's cooperation.

Digital rectal examination requires that the gloved finger be well lubricated and be very slowly inserted and withdrawn to avoid pain from the dilatation of the sphincter alone. Once the finger has been inserted fully in the rectum, one should pause for several moments until the child has become accustomed to the discomfort, then feel to the left, in the midline, and then to the right, feeling for possible mass and seeking to elicit tenderness.

A mild elevation of temperature is common early in the disease, as is a moderate degree of leukocytosis. In fact, in children suspected of having appendicitis the temperature and the white cell count are useful principally for their negative value.

In the child complaining of abdominal pain, the differential diagnosis is frequently between appendicitis and abdominal cramps from gastroenteritis, constipation, or dietary indiscretion. If the temperature or white cell count is significantly elevated, one cannot dismiss a child as not having a significant lesion, although the disease may be something other than appendicitis.

The mortality of appendectomy if the appendix is unruptured, whether acutely inflamed or not, is a small fraction of 1%. On the other hand, once the appendix has ruptured, a much higher mortality is risked, together with a very substantial morbidity and serious prolongation of hospitalization. It is incumbent upon the physician to take every precaution to make certain that no child with appendicitis suffer a delay in operation. One must accept the attitude that the unpardonable sin is not operating for what proves to be a normal appendix, but failure to operate for any period of time for what ultimately proves to have been acute appendicitis. Prompt operation for children with abdominal pain who have abdominal tenderness, preferably localized to the right lower quadrant, and in whom there is no inconsistent or incompatible feature in the history, physical examination, or laboratory studies is, therefore, strongly recommended. A history of pain of several weeks' duration in a child who is not particularly ill, a history that the pain recurs on a given day of the week, a child who appears quite well and is contentedly munching a candy bar — all these are inconsistent with appendicitis. Similarly, a purulent vaginal discharge, pus in the urine, a sore throat with red tonsils or rapid respirations, and dullness in the right side of the chest are inconsistent with the diagnosis of acute appendicitis.

In infants there is usually very little muscle spasm or resistance, and the only physical sign may be grimacing or restlessness or acute flexion of the hip each time the right lower quadrant is palpated or rectal examination is performed.

From time to time the question of appendicitis arises in patients with diseases that may mimic appendicitis, for example, sickle cell anemia, pneumonia, and measles. Appendicitis is a sufficiently common disease so that such coincidence is inevitable, even if there is not necessarily a causal relationship. If the signs and symptoms of appendicitis are convincing, appendectomy should be undertaken.

TREATMENT. Surgery is indicated for suspected appendicitis whether believed to be early or after rupture. In profoundly ill children, delay of several hours to restore intravascular volume and initate antibiotics may be indicated.

Between 27% to 60% of children have ruptured appendixes, prior to surgery. Studies show delay over 36 hours after onset of pain correlate with highest rate of perforation. Much of this delay is after contact with medical personnel is initiated. Advent of new ultrasound techniques (e.g., graded compression sonography) may provide diagnostic help, but a high index of suspicion remains the key.

Any child with a ruptured appendix should be treated postoperatively as if paralytic ileus already is present rather than waiting to see whether or not it develops. This treatment consists of nasogastric suction, preferably the passage of a long, indwelling, single-lumen tube, total intravenous alimentation, and so forth. The child who has had a ruptured appendix must be observed carefully from day to day for the development of an abscess, which, in order of frequency, may be in the right lower quadrant under the wound; in the pelvis, palpable on rectal examination; subphrenic on the right side; or intraabdominal on the left side, having passed up along the left border of the mesenteric root. The abscess usually does not resolve with antibiotic therapy; as soon as it can be approached without passing through the peritoneal cavity, it should be drained.

Miscellaneous Conditions

POLYPS. Juvenile polyps (retention polyps, inflammatory polyps) are the most common cause of painless rectal bleeding after age 1. They are differentiated pathologically from adenomatous polyps of familial polyposis coli, or the hamartomatous polyps of Peutz-Jegher's syndrome. Histologically, they are characterized by a dense inflammatory infiltrate of neutrophils and eosinophils within the myxomatous stroma and large dilated glandular spaces.

Ninety percent of polyps in childhood are juvenile polyps, and 90% are solitary. Usually less than 2 cm in size and pedunculated they never undergo malignant transformation. While most frequent in the rectosigmoid, polyps can occur throughout the colon. Symptoms include rectal bleeding, prolapse, and, occasionally, intussusception with the polyp as lead point. If the polyps do not slough spontanously, they are removed endoscopically.

Familial polyposis coli is a genetically determined disease (autosomal dominant) with childhood onset of multiple polypoid adenomas. These have a high rate of malignant transformation and patients require colectomy. Onset can be between ages 2 and 10, with risk of cancer increasing after age 20.

Peutz-Jegher's syndrome involves scattered hamartomatous polyps throughout the gastrointestinal tract associated with pigment spots on the lips, mucous membranes, palms, and soles. These polyps have no malignant potential but can bleed or function as lead points.

IRRITABLE BOWEL SYNDROME. Irritable bowel syndrome (IBS), also known as spastic colon, mucous colitis, or functional bowel disease consists of a variable combination of abdominal pain and altered bowel habits. Patients with IBS make up 20% of out-patient gastrointestinal consultations, yet, the disorder has no diagnostic test, etiologic cause, accepted definition, or reliable treatment. It does have

a reproducible list of symptoms including, alternate periods of diarrhea and constipation, abdominal pain relieved by defecation, more frequent, looser stools with onset of pain, sensation of incomplete rectal evacuation, abdominal distention and mucus in the stool. Most studies delineating IBS have been done on adults, and characteristics of IBS in children may vary. Pain predominates over bowel irregularity in children. It is frequently severe, persistent, located anywhere in the abdomen, and may not relate to stool passage.

The diagnosis of IBS is dependent on normal laboratory studies. Those performed depend on the clinical picture, but may include stool studies, upper and lower gastrointestinal radiologic exams, amylase, chemistry profile, blood count, sedimentation rate, abdominal and pelvic ultrasound, and even endoscopy. Physical examination is usually normal though excessively palpable and tender colon has been described as has excessive pain on rectal examination. Most physicians suspect IBS from the completion of the history. How extensive the investigations required frequently depends on the parental and patient anxiety. The impact of psychosocial stresses in exacerbations of abdominal pain cannot be underestimated. In studies on healthy populations, almost 30% of people had enough of the above symptoms to be classified as IBS patients. Yet, these people never saw a physician for their complaints, nor did they consider themselves ill. Interpretation and coping with these symptoms may explain much of the difference in IBS patients and coping in children is a complex psychosocial issue.

Treatment. Possible explanations of the pathophysiology of IBS center on intestinal motility and bowel contraction patterns. Though no clear acceptable explanation is available, many physicians explain IBS as decreased luminal filling allowing increased smooth muscle contraction. Others implicate altered motility causing trapping of pockets of gas, especially in the flexures with the resultant distention causing pain. Treatments have been aimed at relieving the muscle spasm, regulating transit time and increasing luminal bulk. Supplemental fiber, either dietary or medicinal is useful especially in patients with constipation. Antispasmodics like hyoscyamine or propanthaline are helpful to some though not scientifically proved. Antidiarrheal agents like Loperamide are useful in selected patients. The role of dietary factors, food allergies, and intolerances remains unclear. Clearly, a great deal more is to be learned before reliable treatment regimens are found. Psychologic counseling in children may be the most reliably useful tool and should be instituted early.

CONSTIPATION. Complaints relating to constipation and encopresis constitute 3% of outpatient pediatric visits. Evaluation of these symptoms in a child requires consideration of a range of rare disorders and physical abnormalities, understanding of normal pediatric bowel habits, and time to discuss psychologic issues with patient and family.

Defecation involves a coordinated process of autonomic and voluntary neuromuscular functions. Distention of the rectum stimulates the sensory pathways that provide conscious awareness or the need to evacuate. Internal anal sphincter relaxation, widening of the anorectal angle, and increased abdominal pressure provide for expulsion of feces. The external sphincter is not required for continence except in cases of diarrhea.

Clinical Manifestations. Twenty-five percent of constipation presents in the first year of life. While many autonomic problems can cause constipation, predominant concern should be to rule out anorectal deformities, neurologic abnormality, and Hirschsprung's disease. Hypothyroidism and hypercalcemia can present with constipation as the initial complaint. More common in infants are dietary problems (excessive milk product ingestion) and misinterpretation of acceptable stooling patterns.

Most constipation presents between ages 2 to 4. This period coincides with the physiologic maturation leading to external anal sphincter control and toilet training. Ninety-five percent of children 1 to 4 years of age have stools from every other day to 3 times daily. Constipation may reflect a primary failure to establish bowel control, an active retention process in an upset child, or an intermittent response to external events.

Chronic constipation in older children and adolescents is frequently complicated by encopresis. History may date back to early childhood with infrequent, large stools, difficulty or pain with passage, and soiling. These patients with megarectum and megacolon have large stool masses on exam and require long-term treatment protocols. Older patients may have constipation due to slowed transit time or incomplete evacuation. Neurologically impaired patients of all ages have increased incidence of constipation and, in severely impaired patients, early institution of protocols to ensure reasonable stool frequency and avoid impactions are helpful.

Encopresis. Initially used in 1926 by Weissenberg referring to passage of whole bowel movement in an abnormal place, it has come to encompass all degrees of fecal incontinence. Incidence ranges from 1 to 7% of school-age children. Excluding children with neurologic abnormalities (spina bifida) and neurodevelopmental delay, most encopretic patients have constipation and secondary overflow soiling. The constipation may be unrecognized. Children may exhibit denial even in the face of extensive soiling and obvious odor. Extensive conflicts may develop in the family relating to encopresis. Behavioral efforts involving both child and parent help remove blame and promote successful therapy. Avoidance of well-identified risk factors during toilet training may prevent some problems. These include overly coercive discipline, painful defecation secondary to fissures, parental overreaction, and excessive medical intervention.

Treatment. After eliminating suspected physical causes (e.g., barium enema rules out Hirschsprung's), a combined modality approach based on age of the patient, complications, and severity of condition should be established. Careful, patient explanation by the physician is required as constipation and encopresis can be a prolonged, frustrating problem. Occasional patients require psychiatric evaluation and psychotherapy. In infancy, constipation usually warrants minimal intervention. Parental education, reassurance, and stool softeners or osmotic agents like Karo syrup usually suffice. Milk formulas may be avoided, but reliance on formula switching may be counterproductive. Intermittent use of glycerine suppository in short-term situations can be helpful.

In older children with established retentive constipation and encopresis, treatment is aimed at catharsis, maintenance of regularity, and psychologic support. Manual disimpaction, enemas, and suppositories are avoided when possible; however, in cases of prolonged constipation with megarectum, they may be required to fully evacuate and allow reestablishment of rectal muscle tone.

Catharsis may require several days of enemas or suppositories (Biscodyl) and should be accompanied by the initiation of patient participation. Children are asked to sit-down on the toilet 2 to 3 times per day, preferably after meals. There should be no stress placed on these "sit-downs," but positive reinforcement is appropriate if the child stools. A chart kept by the patient is helpful in keeping young children involved.

Following catharsis, a maintenance protocol utilizing laxatives and a continuation of the behavioral regimens is initiated. Lubricants (mineral oil), stimulants (senna), osmotics (lactulose), or fiber may all play a role. High roughage diets or avoidance of milk products help in specific cases. Most important may be the time the physician spends with the patient and family. Issues surrounding blame, guilt, responsibility, family stress, school performance, and punishment may surface. Time alone with the child for exploration of these issues and support is required. Follow-up care of 6 months to 2 years may be necessary. In some centers biofeedback is offered as a form of retraining or behavior modification.

ANAL FISSURE. Cracks in the mucocutaneous line of the anus are common during infancy. Whether they are best termed anal abrasions or anal fissures is perhaps academic because the symptoms and natural history seem identical.

In infants several months of age, anal abrasions usually cause painful defecation, stool retention, and blood around the stool. If the anal lesion is not associated with perianal atopic dermatitis or *Candida* infection, the best treatment is protective creams and scrupulous hygiene following bowel evacuation. If the stools are persistently hard, a stool softener such as dioctyl sodium sulfosuccinate is likely to be helpful.

Toddlers with pruritus ani, perianal excoriations, and anal abrasions should be suspected of having pinworms. Older children with persistent anal fissure should be examined for inflammatory diseases of the colon or small bowel.

COLIC. Almost all small infants cry sometimes during the day. At one end of the crying spectrum is a group of infants who display fussiness and crying to a far greater degree than most. Various descriptive terms have been used, such as *colic* or *paroxysmal fussing of infancy,* but none quite conveys the overt crisis that this symptom can cause in a home.

The onset of symptoms occurs in the second or third week of life, affects 20 to 30% of infants, and lasts for about 3 months. The infant may be hypertonic, bright, healthy appearing, and respond in an exaggerated manner to auditory stimuli and rapid changes in body position. The period of fussiness is most likely to occur in the evening hours after feeding and is characterized by forceful crying, abdominal distention, borborygmus, flexion of the knees, and the passage of flatus. The infant is inconsolable and gives the appearance of having abdominal pain. A vicious cycle is set in motion; the screaming infant, the harried new mother, and the helpless father all fervently wish they were someone or somewhere else. The parental anxiety reinforces the symptom, and by the time the physician is consulted there is an array of distraught and disheveled human beings.

There are several etiological factors associated with colic. A detailed history is indispensable in the evaluation of pertinent factors. Family tension of a degree beyond the usual postpartum domiciliary disorganization is often an associated finding. Food intolerance to carbohydrate and cow's milk has also been implicated in a number of cases. Faulty feeding techniques and air swallowing were formerly said to

be contributing factors, but current opinion does not favor this view. Needless to say, organic factors such as inguinal hernia or intestinal stenosis must be considered.

Treatment. The successful management of colic requires consideration of the entire family unit. After reassuring the parents that there is no organic cause for the symptom, the physician can play a supportive and directive role by predicting the termination of the symptom by the third month. Reduction in the sugar or fat content of the formula is seldom successful; changing formulas buys time but offers little else unless there are signs of hypersensitivity to food such as eczema or sniffles; then alterations in the diet should be considered. An orderly plan must be pursued, the parents being cautioned that immediate results following diet changes are not often to be expected. The use of sedative-antispasmodic combination drugs before feeding has proved useful. Commonly used drugs include antispasmodics (hyoscyamine, Donnatal) and antiflatulents (simethicone). The age-old techniques, such as use of a pacifier, rocking, walking, patting, and the application of warmth to the abdomen, are recommended in severe cases. Creative solutions include rockers, rides in the car, and auditory relaxation tapes. Most important is the supportive role the physician plays in helping the young, first-time parents cope.

Ian Leibowitz, Richard J. Grand, and Mohsen Ziai

References

Alvarez, F., et al. Portal obstruction in children. I. Clinical Investigation and hemorrhage risk. *J. Pediatr.* 103:696, 1983.

Auricchio, S., et al. Gluten-sensitive enteropathy in childhood. *Pediatr. Clin. N. Am.* 35:157, 1988.

Berguist, W. E., et al. Achalasia: Diagnosis, management and clinical course in sixteen children. *Pediatrics* 71:798, 1983.

Bindee, H. J. The pathophysiology of diarrhea. *Hosp. Pract.* 107:1984.

Brendee, J. D., et al. Childhood appendicitis: Factors associated with perforation. *Pediatrics* 76:301, 1985.

Harty, R. F., and Leibach, J. R. Immune disorders of the gastrointestinal tract and liver. *Med. Clin. North Am.* 69:685, 1985.

Hutch, T. F. Encopresis and constipation in children. *Pediatr. Clin. N. Am.* 35:257, 1988.

Herbst, J. J. Diagnosis and treatment of gastroesophageal reflux in children. *Pediatr. Review* 5:75, 1983.

Hoofnagle, J. H., and Alter, H. J. Chronic Viral Hepatitis. In A. Vyas, J. L. Dienstag, and J. H. Hoofnagle (Eds.) *Viral Hepatitis and Liver Disease*. New York: Grune and Stratton, 1984.

Kirscher, B. S. Inflammatory bowel disease in children. *Pediatr. Clin. N. Am.* 35:189, 1988.

Kopelman, H. Gastrointestinal manifestations of cystic fibrosis. *Med. Clin. N. Am.* 20:3854, 1988.

Motil, K. J. and Grand, R. S. Ulcerative colitis and Crohn's disease in children. *Pediatr. Review* 9:109, 1987.

Nord, K. S. Peptic ulcer disease in the pediatric population *Pediatr. Clin. N. A.* 35:117, 1988.

Ryckman, F. C., and Noseworthy, J. Neonatal cholestatic conditions requiring surgical reconstruction. *Semin.* Liver Dis. 7:134, 1987.

Trier, J. S. Intestinal malabsorption: Differentiation of cause. *Hosp. Pract.* May:195, 1988.

Silverman, A., and Roy, C. C. *Pediatric Clinical Gastroenterology*. St. Louis: Mosby, 1983.

13

The Genitourinary System

Kidneys and Urinary Tract

Evaluation of Clinical Clues in Children

Clinical features of diseases of the kidney and the collecting system may be quite specific, but they are frequently vague, nonspecific, and may be overlooked. The younger the child, the more elusive are the symptoms and signs. When renal function is significantly reduced, the function of other organ systems may be secondarily disturbed, and clinical features relative to these systems may predominate.

In the newborn and young infant, poor feeding, vomiting, and failure to thrive may be the only features demonstrated. When these findings are persistent, and particularly if they are associated with recurrent dehydration or acidosis, appropriate studies to investigate a renal cause are justified. Growth failure at any age, with or without other findings, should make one question the presence of renal disease.

The presence of other congenital abnormalities should always make one suspect associated anomalies of the urinary system. Some abnormalities are so commonly associated with renal anomalies that they deserve special mention:

presence of a single umbilical artery, abnormalities of the external genitalia (hypospadias, epispadias), low-set or malformed ears, imperforate anus, absence of abdominal musculature, spina bifida, aniridia, cataracts, congenital aganglionic megacolon, and both atrial and ventricular septal defects.

Examination of the urine is an extension of the patient evaluation and is a sensitive and broadly useful method for the screening and study of patients with renal and systemic illnesses. For satisfactory results, the urine specimen should be freshly voided, clean, and concentrated and should be examined promptly by a competent examiner. When abnormalities are detected, the examination should be repeated at least once in order to assure the accuracy and persistence of the aberration.

POLYURIA. Polyuria is a relatively frequent clinical sign of renal disease and must be distinguished from urinary frequency. True polyuria is usually associated with polydipsia. If the volume of urine is actually increased, it should be subcategorized on the basis of concentration of the urine and compared with the extracellular fluid (ECF).

Polyuria with dilute urine (hyposthenuria) is seen in conditions such as: (1) absence of antidiuretic hormone (primary diabetes insipidus), (2) lack of tubular responsiveness to antidiuretic hormone (e.g., congenital nephrogenic diabetes insipidus, chronic potassium deficiency, hypercalcemia, some cases of cystic renal disease), or (3) absence of a stimulus for release of antidiuretic hormone (chronic water overloading or psychogenetic polydipsia). In any of these, the urine specific gravity rarely exceeds 1.005 or the urine osmolality 200 mOsm/kg.

Polyuria with either isotonic or slightly hypertonic urine (isosthenuria) is seen in patients with partial antidiuretic hormone (ADH) responsiveness (such as those with sickle-cell disease) or in those in whom the kidney is subjected to an osmotic diuresis, characterized by an increase in both urine flow rate and solute excretion. The osmolality of the urine is never lower than 300 mOsm/kg and may be as high as 450 to 500 mOsm/kg. The urine specific gravity is, however, quite variable, ranging from levels of 1.008 to 1.010, in situations in which the solute is predominantly electrolytes and urea (renal failure, diuretic administration), to levels as high as 1.034 to 1.045 when the solute mass is large (glucose in diabetes mellitus, contrast media following excretory urograms).

The workup of the child with polyuria should first confirm the presence of increased urine volume. It is also necessary to identify any associated symptoms or signs (e.g., growth failure may suggest either congenital or acquired nephrogenic diabetes insipidus; abdominal masses may suggest cystic disease or hydronephrosis). After an appropriate period of water deprivation, the first morning voidings are obtained for measurements of concentration. In general, the urine specific gravity of older children should reach a value of 1.026 (approximately 1000 mOsm/kg) and that of infants a value of 1.016 (approximately 500 mOsm/kg). In cases showing deviations from these norms, more specific tests are needed, and the physician should obtain appropriate consultation.

OLIGURIA. Oliguria signifies a marked reduction in urine flow rate, whereas anuria indicates complete cessation of urine flow. Oliguria commonly occurs in infants and children, but only rarely does it signify serious disease of the urinary system.

Primary among causes of oliguria in infants and children are those associated with reduction of ECF volume and prerenal causes of oliguria should always be considered first. Appropriate measures to ensure that adequate ECF volume is present should be the first diagnostic-therapeutic modality employed.

Almost any disease of the renal parenchyma or the urinary collecting system can produce oliguria. In addition, certain drugs may either decrease glomerular filtration rate (GFR) or increase ADH secretion, resulting in transient oliguria. Among these are barbiturates, opiates, and some antihistamines, anticonvulsants, and antimicrobials.

URGENCY OR FREQUENCY OF URINATION. The symptoms of urgency and frequency, when occurring together, are usually associated with small or normal urine volumes and are manifestations of disease of the lower urinary tract or external genitalia. Vaginitis, both infectious and irritative (secondary to bubble baths, local trauma, or foreign bodies), is a common cause of these symptoms. In the male, meatal stenosis or meatal ulceration should be suspected. Urinary tract infections and idiopathic hypercalciuria are among other causes.

ENURESIS. Enuresis is inappropriate urination by a child who has reached an age when bladder control is expected. Enuresis may be nocturnal (bed wetting), diurnal (daytime), or both. Nocturnal enuresis is more common, but approximately 10% of those with bed wetting have diurnal enuresis. Primary enuresis is the term applied to children who have never had an extended time of dryness. Enuresis that recurs after a period of 1 or more years of dryness is termed secondary enuresis.

Enuresis is common and is dependent on development of bladder control. Some children are dry at night by the age of 1 year, but it is not until about 3 years that 75% of children are consistently dry. This figure reaches about 90% by the age of 5 years. Between 5 and 19 years, the annual spontaneous cure rate of enuresis averages about 15%.

In the counseling of children and their parents, there are several epidemiological and etiological factors to be considered:

1. Most children with enuresis have neither an organic nor a psychiatric illness
2. Enuresis has a strong familial occurrence; 74% of boys and 58% of girls having one or both parents with a history of enuresis
3. It is most common in the first born
4. It is twice as common in males as in females under the age of 12 years, but occurs equally thereafter
5. It is more common in children who have experienced psychosocial problems during early childhood
6. It may occur during any stage of sleep except the first stage
7. It is usually associated with a structurally normal-sized bladder but one that is functionally smaller
8. The likelihood of demonstrating a significant anatomical

abnormality appears to be very slight, even in those who have associated urinary tract infections

Enuresis is the presenting symptom in 15 to 20% of children with urinary tract infection (UTI) and may be the only symptom in girls with "asymptomatic" bacteriuria.

In evaluation of enuresis, a thorough history is the most rewarding examination, particularly as it explores those epidemiological and etiological factors alluded to earlier. The usual evaluation should include a urinalysis and one or more urine cultures. Imaging studies are not indicated unless there is infection or findings suggestive of a more serious problem.

The high spontaneous cure rate should be presented to the child and parents along with a sympathetic and understanding attitude. Various specific measures are difficult to evaluate because of the high rate of spontaneous cure. These include fluid restriction prior to bed, awakening and encouraging toilet voiding, and enuresis alarms. The only medications to have demonstrated a beneficial effect are the tricyclic antidepressants with which a desirable effect is produced in about 50% of cases. Response is usually within 1 to 2 weeks, and late benefits have rarely been observed. Upon discontinuance of the drug, the relapse rate is very high. The significant side-effects of these drugs should temper the physician's use of such agents.

HEMATURIA. Hematuria is a common clinical feature of urinary tract disease. It may be gross, microscopic, transient, intermittent, or persistent. Hematuria may be painless or accompanied by dysuria. The urine may be uniformly mixed with blood or blood may be present only during one segment of the voiding pattern. Microscopic hematuria that is not accompanied by other clinical features is called primary or asymptomatic hematuria. A careful and detailed history often leads directly to the etiology, but the cause may be elusive.

In consideration of this problem, several questions must be posed and appropriate answers sought:

1. What qualifies as hematuria?
2. What is the magnitude of the problem?
3. What is the natural history of children who have asymptomatic hematuria?
4. With what urgency should one begin a workup?
5. Once begun, what constitutes an appropriate evaluation and follow-up?

If asymptomatic microhematuria is detected, the initial step should be to confirm its existence on two or three occasions. Even when confirmed, it usually resolves within 1 year (about 30% persist). By the end of a 5-year follow-up, about 20% of those originally found to have hematuria still have an abnormal urine. In the absence of coexistent proteinuria, there is little urgency for elaborate investigations. Periodic clinical evaluation and urinalysis appear sufficient for the first 2 to 3 years. At that time, an appropriate battery of tests might include serum creatinine, C_3-complement determination, and a renal ultrasound. Emergence of abnormal symptoms or signs, or demonstrated abnormalities on screening evaluations, would dictate earlier or more detailed evaluation.

One examination which may be of help in directing the subsequent evaluation is a detailed examination of the morphology of the urinary red blood cells (RBCs). Red cells that are of glomerular origin are usually distorted in their configuration while postglomerular RBCs appear much the same as those in the peripheral blood.

One of the more common causes of both gross and microscopic hematuria is hypercalciuria. There is often a family history of nephrolithiasis. A random urine sample analyzed for calcium and creatinine is a good screening test. Once hypercalciuria has been documented, the etiology of increased calcium excretion must be sought.

Acute glomerulonephritis, or one of the so-called benign, recurrent hematurias, must always be considered. Recurrent, usually asymptomatic (but occasionally with abdominal or flank pain), gross hematuria occurring in conjunction with a respiratory infection suggests the possibility of either IgA nephropathy or a benign, recurrent hematuria. In the absence of such history, gross hematuria might suggest trauma (history, clots, other injury), urolithiasis (past and family history, pain), hemorrhagic cystitis (urgency, frequency, dysuria), bleeding defects or coagulopathies (bleeding elsewhere), hemoglobinopathies (history, race), congenital abnormalities (pain, abdominal mass, or asymptomatic), or, rarely, a tumor (Wilms' or adenocarcinoma). Fortunately, tumors are very uncommon causes of isolated hematuria in children, and this removes some of the urgency from evaluation. In addition to the above, various drugs and chemicals can produce hematuria, and, in this age of physical fitness, one should not overlook extreme exercise, particularly jogging, as an occasional cause of gross hematuria.

PROTEINURIA. If the proteinuria is associated with definitive signs or symptoms of clinical disease (e.g., edema, hypertension, growth failure, significant hematuria), then specific evaluations usually lead to a final diagnosis. Problems arise most commonly, however, in establishing a plan of investigation in those proteinuric children who are asymptomatic. Proteinuria may be transient, orthostatic, or persistent.

Transient proteinuria is most common and is usually inconsequential. It has been observed in association with changes in posture, exercise, exposure to cold, fever, and emotional stress although frequently it is impossible to define a specific cause.

Orthostatic or postural proteinuria is also common. Orthostatic proteinuria which is transient, disappearing after 1 or more years, does not appear to be of clinical significance. Orthostatic proteinuria may also be fixed, or of prolonged persistence. Although there are no prospective studies in children, isolated biopsies performed in some have generally been normal. Most retrospective studies and the only notable prospective evaluation in adults have suggested a favorable prognosis without increased incidence of renal failure. Although some investigators are concerned that fixed orthostatic proteinuria may represent an early manifestation of renal disease, additional testing other than continued observation is not warranted.

Persistent proteinuria should be evaluated. If the serum creatinine is normal for age, the quantitative protein excretion is less than 1 g/24 hr/m^2, and the C$_3$-complement is within the normal range, then only follow-up is recommended at 6- to 12-month intervals. With significant change, a more extensive evaluation including possible renal biopsy may be indicated.

EDEMA. Edema (see also Appendix A, Section 17) is generalized but may be apparent only in those areas where tissue resistance is low. The pathophysiology of the edema can be broadly grouped into two categories: (1) the primary event is a reduced GFR associated with exaggerated tubular reabsorption of sodium and water (as in glomerulonephritis); and (2) there is heavy proteinuria with associated hypoproteinemia, decreased oncotic pressure, contraction of plasma volume, secondary hyperaldosteronism, and increased tubular reabsorption of sodium and water (as seen in the nephrotic syndrome). In the former, there is usually celluria (RBCs or white blood cells [WBCs] or both) in association with small amounts of proteinuria.

HYPERTENSION. Hypertension (see also Appendix A, Section 19) is discussed elsewhere, and only the evaluation of the renal causes will be considered here. In most adolescents, there is no defined cause, and they are thus considered to have essential hypertension. Secondary hypertension should be considered if: (1) the child is less than 10 years of age at onset, (2) the hypertension is severe (greater than 2 standard deviations above the mean for age), (3) the hypertension is nonlabile, and (4) the child demonstrates abnormalities on laboratory examinations. Most children with secondary hypertension have some form of renal disease.

There may be clues in the history that point toward the kidney as a potential cause. Some of these clues are: recurrent urinary tract infections, periodic unexplained fevers (? pyelonephritis), abdominal or flank trauma, occurrence of gross hematuria, presence of edema, and use of an umbilical arterial catheter during the newborn period. Physical findings suggesting a renal origin include edema, flank or costovertebral angle tenderness, flank mass, and an abdominal bruit.

Laboratory investigations are useful in helping define the cause and direct further evaluations. Hematuria, proteinuria, or both provide evidence of an intrinsic renal or renovascular lesion. The finding of decreased renal function is a useful indicator of intrinsic renal disease.

The radiographic evaluation should include a renal ultrasound and, perhaps, either a computed tomography (CT) scan with contrast or a rapid sequence intravenous pyelogram to define kidney size, surface contour, the caliceal system, and pelvic and ureteral anatomy. This study may suggest the origin of the hypertension: obstructive uropathy, renal scarring from chronic infection, cystic disease, or hypoplasia. Other studies may prove useful in defining an arterial lesion. One such, relatively noninvasive study is the renal uptake and excretion of iodohippurate sodium ^{131}I (Hippuran). The radiographic study that most clearly demonstrates an abnormality of the renal artery is angiography, but this invasive procedure should be performed only when a vascular lesion is strongly suspected.

Urinary Tract Infections

Urinary tract infections (UTIs) are defined as a group of conditions that have in common the presence of significant numbers of bacteria in the urine. The bacterial concentration is estimated by quantitative urine culture, and the term significant bacteriuria is defined as over 100,000 colonies/ml of urine on midstream voided collections. The accuracy of diagnosis of UTI is 80% when one clean-catch urine specimen has this number of the same organism. With two positive cultures, the accuracy of diagnosis increases to 95%.

Incidence

There is a varying incidence of UTI during infancy and childhood. Full-term neonates have an incidence of less than 1%, while prematures have higher reported rates of around 2.4%. Males seem to predominate, but after the neonatal period, females are more commonly infected. Infants and toddlers have an incidence of approximately 3%, while a number of studies in school children have shown that approximately 1.2% of girls and 0.04% of boys have bacteriuria. It is estimated that 5 to 6% of girls have one or more episodes of bacteriuria between the ages of 6 and 18 years.

Etiology

Gram-negative enteric organisms are the most common cause of urinary tract infection, with *Escherichia coli* being detected most often (i.e., 80% of first infections and 75% of recurrent infections). Other common gram-negative organisms causing infection include *Klebsiella, Proteus, Enterobacter,* and *Pseudomonas*. Gram-positive organisms may also cause infection, with *Staphylococcus epidermidis, Staphylococcus aureus,* and *Enterococcus* being the most common. In patients with associated urinary tract abnormalities, one of the less common organisms is more likely to result in infection. Mycobacteria and fungi may also result in UTI and these are usually secondary to hematogenous spread. The role of viruses in UTI is still unclear although they have been implicated in cases of hemorrhagic cystitis.

Pathogenesis

Two primary routes for development of infection have been described. The hematogenous route seems to be primary in neonatal infections and may occasionally be the route in older children and adults; however, the ascending route is more common outside the neonatal period. The bacteria responsible for the infection are usually part of the host's endogenous flora, and the reservoir for these organisms is felt to be the lower intestinal tract. These organisms gain access to the urethra and ascend into the bladder. Here, if the local milieu supports bacterial multiplication or the number of bacteria is very high, infection results.

Most patients with UTI have no anatomical abnormalities that can account for the UTI. The short female urethra has been implicated as a predisposing factor. Local conditions favoring or inhibiting bacterial colonization of the periurethral cells are implicated. Bacterial adherence to uroepithelial cells is increased in some patients with recurrent UTIs as compared with normal persons. In addition, certain strains of bacteria seem to have particular virulence for the urinary tract. Increased adherence by certain strains of *E. coli* associated with pyelonephritis has been shown, as compared with strains causing asymptomatic bacteriuria having little adherence and those causing cystitis with intermediate adherence. The amount of K (capsular) antigen of *E. coli* strains is also regarded as a virulence factor.

Predisposing factors for UTIs include obstruction of urinary flow with urinary stasis. Obstruction may be from anatomical abnormalities or it may be functional as seen in neurogenic bladder, with spina bifida, or with the prune-belly syndrome and adynamic ureters. Vesicoureteral reflux may also result in sufficient stasis to predispose to infection. Mechanical factors include bladder catheterization and surgical instrumentation.

Clinical Features

The signs and symptoms of UTI vary with age. Infected neonates usually have few symptoms referable to the urinary tract but may demonstrate feeding problems, failure to thrive, central nervous system symptoms including seizures, vomiting, diarrhea, unexplained fever, or hypothermia. Other signs of sepsis may be present as well, including sluggishness, irritability, and jaundice. The infant or toddler often demonstrates fever and may also exhibit other nonspecific symptoms such as failure to thrive, vomiting, diarrhea, irritability, and abdominal pain. Older children may be asymptomatic but usually have symptoms attributable to the urinary tract, including urgency, frequency, dysuria, and either abdominal or flank pain. They may or may not exhibit fever and up to 30% have enuresis.

Diagnosis

A urine culture is mandatory for the diagnosis of UTI. Most commonly urine is collected in midstream after cleansing of the external genitalia. One such culture containing 50,000 to 100,000 colonies of a single organism is essentially diagnostic in the symptomatic child, whereas two or three cultures in excess of 100,000 colonies might be needed to validate an infection in the asymptomatic person. Alternatives to the clean-catch specimen include suprapubic puncture of the bladder and urethral catheterization. Both are useful procedures in selected instances, but potential complications of both make them less desirable.

Urinalysis may be helpful in the diagnosis, but may be normal even in the presence of infection. One bacterium or more per high power field of freshly voided, uncentrifuged urine is usually equated with a colony count of greater than 10^5 organisms/ml of urine. White blood cells are present in increased amounts with most infections, but pyuria may be present in the absence of infection. Additionally, pyuria does not always occur with overt infection.

Both direct and indirect methods have been used in an attempt to differentiate upper from lower urinary tract infection. Because clinical signs and symptoms alone are not always reliable indicators of the location of infection and because indirect methods are noninvasive, it has been suggested by some that all patients with culture-proved UTI be screened; however, because the tests are variable in their ability to distinguish between upper and lower tract infections and since most nephrologists feel that all patients should have an ultrasound of the kidney and a voiding cystogram, there appears little reason to perform extensive testing for localization.

Treatment and Follow-up

Antibiotic therapy should be instituted as soon as the diagnosis has been confirmed. In some cases, as in the neonate or in the child who appears to be in a toxic state, culture material should be obtained and antibiotic therapy instituted prior to knowledge of final culture results. Therapy can be modified later when sensitivity results are available. The selection of either oral or parenteral therapy depends primarily on the degree of illness of the patient; most can usually be treated orally with one of several drugs. Because *E. coli* is most commonly the infecting organism, the use of one of the sulfonamides is most appropriate. In patients unable to tolerate sulfonamides or when there is a resistant organism, other drugs are available such as ampicillin, nitrofurantoin, trimethoprim-sulfa combination, and cephalosporins. Organisms isolated from patients with recurrent infections or from those with structural abnormalities may be resistant to sulfonamides. If the patient is not ill, it is advisable to await the sensitivity results prior to the institution of therapy. Patients with clinical signs and symptoms of acute pyelonephritis may initially require hospitalization and parenteral antibiotics. Ampicillin, with or without an aminoglycoside, is frequently used in these patients until culture results are known. Neonates with suspected infection should be hospitalized and treated parenterally.

The length of antimicrobial treatment is controversial. Ten days of therapy has been shown to be effective in eradicating lower tract infections in almost 100% of patients. Recent studies have reported recovery with the administration of only one large oral dose of an appropriate drug in patients with lower tract involvement. Even 10 days of therapy, however, may not be adequate for patients with upper tract involvement because as many as 50% relapse within 1 week of stopping therapy. For this reason, most experts recommend 2 to 6 weeks of therapy in known cases of upper tract infection. Because, in most cases, lower and upper tract infections are not easily differentiated, it would seem prudent to treat all patients for at least 10 days until further studies are available regarding one-dose therapy.

In certain patients with recurrent infections, after the initial therapy has been completed, smaller doses of anti-biotics are used for prolonged periods as prophylaxis. Patients in whom prophylaxis may be helpful include those with repeated infections over a short interval, patients with grade 3 to 5 vesicoureteral reflux, and those who have residual urine after voiding. Nitrofurantoin has commonly been used for prophylaxis, its advantage being that it does not alter gastrointestinal flora. Other useful prophylactic agents include trimethoprim-sulfa, methenamine mandelate, and nalidixic acid. Treatment has been recommended for periods of 3 to 12 months initially. If there is rapid recurrence after the antimicrobials are stopped, more prolonged periods of treatment are indicated.

All patients with UTI should have follow-up cultures to ensure that the infection has been eradicated. Symptoms of illness may disappear while bacteriuria is still present. As many as 80% of girls with asymptomatic bacteriuria have a recurrent infection within the first 2 years. A culture should be obtained within the first week after completion of therapy, again at 6 weeks, and then at 3-month intervals for the first year. The miniculture method seems to be one of the better screening methods in following these patients, being inexpensive and easy to use. If it is positive, colonies can be subcultured from the dipslide for identification and determination of sensitivity.

Although the incidence of radiological abnormalities of the urinary tract is relatively low, the consequences of such abnormalities may be severe. All persons with a single documented UTI should have a renal ultrasound and a voiding cystourethrogram, the latter most commonly being performed 6 to 8 weeks after the infection has subsided. Some disagreement still exists about when girls with UTI should be studied radiographically, but most prefer to perform these studies after the first infection because of the high rate of recurrence.

The majority of patients with uncomplicated UTI have at least one recurrence. In long-term follow-up of patients with UTI, the incidence of renal failure is extremely low; however, in those with recurrent infections morbidity may be very high. These patients in particular seem to have an increased number of recurrences when they become sexually active and during pregnancy. Bacteriuria in pregnancy has been associated with an increased incidence of acute pyelonephritis as well as an increase in stillbirths, perinatal deaths, and amnionitis.

Nephrotic Syndrome

The nephrotic syndrome, or nephrosis, is characterized by massive proteinuria, hypoalbuminemia, generalized edema, and hyperlipidemia. The syndrome may be produced by a number of diseases or conditions for which the management and course are quite different. In most, there is altered glomerular function with a marked increase in the filtration of albumin. In approximately 80% of children with nephrosis, a glomerular abnormality cannot be detected by light microscopy of renal biopsy tissue, but relatively typical ultrastructural changes (e.g., fusion of foot podocytes) can be seen by electron microscopy. This entity is known as minimal lesion nephrotic syndrome. Most of the remaining 20% of children with nephrosis have membranoproliferative glomerulonephritis, focal global or focal segmental glomerulosclerosis, or membranous nephropathy.

Minimal Lesion Nephrotic Syndrome

DEMOGRAPHIC FEATURES. Minimal lesion nephrotic syndrome (MLNS, idiopathic nephrosis, minimal change nephrotic syndrome) is predominantly a disease of preschool children with over one-half of all new cases occurring in children under 6 years of age. It rarely has its onset prior to 6 months of age, and it is relatively unusual to start in teenagers. Males are affected almost twice as frequently as females. Although unusual, the disease is occasionally seen in siblings.

ETIOLOGY AND PATHOGENESIS. The etiology of MLNS is unknown. A history of a viral infection a few days to a few weeks prior to onset is often obtained, but the relationship to etiology is not certain. Associated and, perhaps, etiologically related are environmental allergies such as those from insects, drugs, and food. Various factors have led some to consider a primary T-cell abnormality but studies designed to identify such have been inconclusive.

Proteinuria results from electrostatic and ultrastructural changes in the glomerular capillary wall, which normally functions as a filter via two mechanisms. First, it is a physical barrier with a specific minimum pore diameter, allowing molecules below a certain size to pass through without difficulty while hindering or preventing filtration of larger molecules (partly dependent on the molecular configuration or "shape"). Second, all three layers of the glomerular capillary wall — the endothelium, basement membrane, and epithelium — contain negatively charged components, collectively known as glomerular polyanion. These repel other negatively charged molecules in the plasma and prevent their filtration. Albumin is anionic and is, therefore, normally filtered in insignificant amounts. In MLNS there is loss of glomerular polyanion resulting in massive albuminuria.

Hypoproteinemia is largely secondary to the albuminuria; however, there is also some evidence for decreased synthesis. Catabolism of filtered albumin is increased. The hypoalbuminemia results in lowering of plasma oncotic pressure and reversal of Starling's forces. Movement of fluid from the vascular compartment to the interstitium results in reduction of plasma volume and accumulation of edema. Renal reabsorption of sodium and water increases as a result of several factors, including hyperaldosteronism, reduction in GFR, and physical factors concerned with oncotic pressure differences between the proximal tubule and the peritubular capillaries. Edema increases until a balance is achieved between the low plasma oncotic pressure and the increased interstitial fluid pressure.

Serum cholesterol and low-density lipoproteins are increased. Although the mechanism has not been completely defined, there is evidence of both increased synthesis and decreased catabolism of cholesterol. Increased hepatic synthesis of lipoproteins is evident, and both serum triglycerides and very low density lipoproteins may also be increased.

RENAL HISTOPATHOLOGY. Typically, normal glomerular architecture is seen by light microscopy, although a minimal increase in mesangial cellularity is occasionally present. Protein casts are seen in the tubular lumen, and lipid accumulations may be seen within tubular cells. Immunofluorescent microscopy does not usually show immunoglobulins or complement components. Electron microscopy reveals widespread fusion of the epithelial foot processes, with no electron-dense deposits suggestive of immune complexes.

In a minority of patients the mesangial hypercellularity is more prominent, and electron-dense deposits may be present. In these there is IgM deposition without complement in the mesangium. The pathogenetic and prognostic significance of these findings is not clear but such patients tend to have a recurrent course.

CLINICAL FEATURES. Edema is the usual presenting symptom and may be the singular finding. Occasionally anorexia and irritability may be present. The edema is usually first noted around the eyes and increases progressively in degree over a period of days or weeks. Occasionally, a history of transient edema in the preceding months may be obtained. With progressive disease the edema may become generalized, and fluid may collect in pleural and peritoneal cavities. Severe ascites and pleural effusions may result in respiratory difficulty. Occasionally, massive swelling of the scrotum, penis, or labia may be particularly distressing. The edema is, classically, dependent in nature and usually pits with pressure. Diarrhea is not uncommon at the height of edema, presumably because of involvement of the intestinal wall.

On physical examination, the presence of edema predominates. The child usually appears pale. Blood pressure is generally normal but is elevated above the ninety-fifth percentile in about 25% of children. Infections, such as otitis media or peritonitis, may be present.

LABORATORY FEATURES. The most impressive abnormality is the presence of proteinuria (albuminuria), which is always in excess of 1 g/m^2/24 h (40 mg/m^2/hr), usually above 4 g/m^2/24 h and may be in the range of 12 to 15 g/m^2/24 h. As a consequence, the concentration of albumin in the serum is less than 2.5 g/100 ml. Often there is a partial compensatory increase in the serum concentrations of alpha$_2$- and beta-globulins, moderating the reduction in total protein concentration.

In 20% of children with MLNS, there is microscopic hematuria, while gross hematuria occurs in about 4% of such patients. Red cell casts may occur, but normally the urine contains waxy, hyaline, and granular casts. Oval fat bodies and cholesterol crystals (demonstrated as "maltese crosses" under polarized light) predominate.

The hemoglobin concentration and hematocrit are usually increased because of reduction in the plasma volume (hemoconcentration). On the other hand, concentrations of serum electrolytes, particularly sodium, may be decreased because of the relatively higher concentration of plasma solids (elevations in lipids). The blood urea nitrogen and creatinine concentrations are normal in most instances, but elevation above the ninety-fifth centile occurs in about 20% of such children. The concentration of complement components is usually normal.

DIFFERENTIAL DIAGNOSIS. Because of the presence of massive proteinuria, the nephrotic syndrome is usually differentiated with ease from other conditions that produce edema. In its classic form, MLNS can be readily distinguished from other glomerular causes of the nephrotic syndrome. The presence of significant hematuria, hypertension, or azotemia would more likely suggest other causes. A normal C$_3$-complement concentration eliminates about 50% of the cases of membranoproliferative glomerulonephritis (MPGN). Renal biopsy, if studied by all three techniques, usually distinguishes other forms, but perhaps the best test is a therapeutic trial of steroids.

COMPLICATIONS. Patients with the nephrotic syndrome, not only MLNS, have increased susceptibility to bacterial infection, with defective opsonization and loss of IgG in the urine being among the probable causes. Septicemia, peritonitis, and cellulitis are not uncommon. *Streptococcus pneumoniae* still appears commonly, but *E. coli, Pseudomonas,* and *Serratia* have also been implicated.

A hypercoagulable state exists in nephrosis partially as a result of the decreased plasma volume, and thromboembolic phenomena can occur, particularly if there are associated episodes of dehydration. Renal vein thrombosis, pulmonary arterial and venous occlusion, and peripheral venous thrombosis have all been described. Steroids may increase the potential for thrombosis.

Growth failure is common among children with a frequently relapsing course, and glucocorticoid therapy is felt to be a major factor; however, the urinary protein loss, anorexia, and impaired absorption from an edematous gut may also be partly responsible. Osteomalacia, osteoporosis, and hypocalcemia secondary to urinary loss of a vitamin-D transport protein have been described. A similar mechanism has been reported for the occasional "iron-deficiency" anemias that are seen in proteinuric children.

MANAGEMENT. The child should be allowed to function as normally as possible, and activity need not be restricted. The diet should be relatively normal, but moderate salt restriction is advisable during edematous episodes. Fluid restriction is generally not necessary, and diuretic therapy is advisable only in the presence of significant edema. Massive hydrothorax, ascites, or scrotal edema occasionally necessitate rapid diuresis. The safest and most effective therapy is intravenous administration of albumin followed by furosemide. Potent diuretics should not be given intravenously without prior expansion of the plasma volume with albumin. Infections, if present, need to be actively treated.

An occasional patient with MLNS will have a spontaneous remission, but most require specific therapy (a remission is defined as complete clearing of proteinuria). Corticosteroids, administered almost universally as prednisone, will induce a remission in approximately 90% of patients with MLNS. It is usually administered in a dosage of 60 mg/m^2/day (2 mg/kg) in divided doses for 4 weeks. This is then followed by a maintenance dosage of prednisone of 45 mg/m^2/day (1.5 mg/kg) on alternate days *in the morning*. This dose is progressively tapered over 4 to 6 months. Of those children who respond to such therapy and whose urine remains clear during the maintenance therapy, remission appears to be permanent in approximately 30%. The remaining children will experience one or more relapses per year. If the relapses are infrequent (no more than two in 6 months or three in 1 year), each episode is best treated with a daily course of steroids until remission, followed by a brief period of alternate morning therapy. A frequently relapsing course, however, often dictates repeated courses of prednisone therapy. Some children will become nonresponders, and may demonstrate focal global glomerulosclerosis. The major problem with these frequent-relapsers, however, is the development of steroid complications: growth failure, obesity, cataracts, steroid diabetes, gastric or duodenal ulceration, hypertension, nephrolithiasis, behavioral abnormalities, or combinations of these.

In children who either fail to respond to prednisone or who have a frequently exacerbating course associated with steroid complications, an alternative course of therapy should be considered. Alkylating agents such as cyclophosphamide, chlorambucil, and nitrogen mustard have been used successfully in such patients. Cyclosporine A has been successful in some. Such therapy can induce prolonged remissions but should be undertaken only after consultation with a pediatric nephrologist and, in the opinion of many, after an assessment of the renal histology.

Other Causes of Childhood Nephrotic Syndrome

Table 13-1 summarizes some of the characteristics of the other causes of childhood nephrosis and are compared to those of MLNS. Some of these can be diagnosed on the basis of their clinical characteristics, but most are separated from MLNS by their poor response to steroid management. Definitive diagnosis is made by renal biopsy.

Management protocols for these forms of nephrotic syndrome are not often effective, and all should have benefit of referral to a pediatric nephrologist.

Glomerulonephritis

The name glomerulonephritis per se implies an inflammatory alteration of the glomerulus. Histologically, in each of the instances to be discussed here, there is proliferation of cells within the glomerular tuft, and this is associated with varying degrees of other inflammatory changes. Glomerulonephritis has been associated with a number of bacterial, viral, and protozoal infections as well as with a number of drugs and toxic agents.

Acute Glomerulonephritis

Acute glomerulonephritis (AGN), mostly postinfectious, is still among the most common of the nonsuppurative renal diseases of childhood. Group A, beta-hemolytic streptococci have been linked with AGN in the majority of cases and the following will concentrate on poststreptococcal AGN (PSAGN). Criteria necessary for the diagnosis of PSAGN include evidence of acute nephritis in previously normal kidneys, serological evidence of recent streptococcal infection, and decrease in serum complement.

INCIDENCE. The true incidence is unknown, but is likely higher than suspected on the basis of those requiring intervention because the majority of cases are mild or asymptomatic and the ratio of subclinical to clinical cases is estimated at about 3 : 1. The highest incidence occurs in early school years, with a 2 : 1 male predominance.

Certain strains of streptococci have been found to be nephritogenic; the more important of these include M-protein types 1, 4, and 12, commonly producing pharyngitis, and types 2, 49, 55, 67, and 60, frequently associated with pyoderma.

PATHOGENESIS. Although the precise mechanism of injury is still unknown, evidence that immunological mechanisms are involved in the pathogenesis have been derived from both morphological and serological studies. Circulating immune complexes occur in over 60% of patients, and transient decreases in both classic and alternative complement pathway components occur in almost all cases. The third component of complement (C3) is decreased in 90 to 100% of cases during the first week, returning to normal levels in over 90% of cases within 2 months. Renal biopsy specimens show granular subepithelial deposits of IgG and C3, and less often of C4, C2, and properdin, along the glomerular basement membrane and in the mesangium of the glomerulus. Some have postulated an increased affinity of some streptococcal M proteins for fibrin, suggesting that the mesangial deposits may be fibrinogen-M-protein complexes, or that the streptococcus produces alterations in the properties of IgG, rendering it antigenic.

PATHOLOGICAL FINDINGS. Even though the degree of severity varies from patient to patient, the findings of renal histological evaluation are consistent. Glomerular tufts are increased in size, often filling Bowman's space. The increased size of the tufts is produced by proliferation of both mesangial and epithelial cells. With the consequent edema, the capillary lumina may appear closed and bloodless. Early in the course of disease there may be an increase in nonglomerular cells, in particular polymorphonuclear cells and macrophages. With extensive inflammatory changes, epithelial cells of Bowman's space proliferate, producing crescents. In general, the severity of lesions seen histologically correlates well with clinical severity.

CLINICAL MANIFESTATIONS. Many of the symptoms and signs in PSAGN can be attributed to a decrease in excretion of water and sodium, partially due to a decrease in GFR, resulting in ECF volume expansion. The increase in ECF is a major cause for the resultant hypertension, anemia, and circulatory congestion.

Presentations at onset vary from those that are discovered incidentally and are asymptomatic to those with severe

Table 13-1. Nephrotic Syndrome in Children

Classification	Frequency (%)	Age of onset	Hematuria (%)	Hypertension (%)	Azotemia (%)	C3	Steroids response (%)	Progression to ESRD (%)
Minimal lesion	80 95 90 50	Overall < 2 yr < 6 yr >10 yr	20 (micro); 4 (gross)	20	20	Normal	>90	>2
Focal segmental glomerulosclerosis	8–10	Similar to MLNS or slightly older	50–60	30	20–30	Normal	<20	>50
Mesangiocapillary, or membranoproliferative glomerulonephritis (all types)	7–9	>7 yr; 10–20 yrs (peak)	>75	30–40	30–40	70% below normal; 30% normal	<10 (?)	>70
Membranous	1–2	>10 yr	~90	~40	~20	Normal	Poor	>30
Others (including proliferative glomerulonephritis)	2–4	Variable	Variable	Variable	Variable	Normal	Poor (?)	Variable

edema, marked oliguria, gross hematuria, or hypertensive encephalopathy. There is regularly a latent period of approximately 10 days after pharyngitis and 15 to 21 days after skin infection. In symptomatic patients, the three cardinal features are the abrupt onset of edema, hematuria, and hypertension. The severity of edema depends on several factors including degree of glomerular involvement, amount of fluid intake, and degree of proteinuria. Virtually all patients have microscopic hematuria, but gross hematuria occurs in 30 to 50% of patients classified as severe.

Hypertension is multifactorial in etiology and overload of the ECF is the only well-recognized contributor, but studies have suggested an overactivity of the renin angiotensin system. The most serious early consequences of PSAGN is hypertensive encephalopathy, where the hypertension is severe and accompanied by one or more signs of central nervous system dysfunction (headache, vomiting, decreased sensorium, confusion, seizures, visual disturbances, memory loss, coma).

Circulatory congestion, although common, is rarely severe enough to result in congestive heart failure. Pallor is common and is mostly related to skin edema and compression of skin capillaries. Mild to moderate anemia is also common and is largely dilutional. Uncommonly, proteinuria is severe enough for the patient to have the nephrotic syndrome as the initial feature.

LABORATORY FINDINGS. Urinalysis characteristically shows hematuria with the degree of proteinuria usually in direct proportion to the amount of blood present. Increased numbers of WBCs are frequently present. Casts (hyaline, granular, and cellular) are often present, and RBC casts can be seen in 60 to 85% of patients hospitalized. Serological evidence of a recent streptococcal infection is present in approximately 98% of patients. The antistreptolysin-O (ASO) titer becomes elevated in most patients with pharyngeal infections but is increased in only 50% of those with pyoderma, in which anti-DNase B and antihyaluronidase titers are more likely to be elevated. The C3 level is decreased in the majority of patients.

Nonspecific findings include an increased sedimentation rate, mild normochromic anemia, leukocytosis, an increase in kidney size demonstrated by ultrasonography and pulmonary congestion in the hilar areas. The blood urea nitrogen and serum creatinine concentrations may be normal to moderately increased.

DIFFERENTIAL DIAGNOSIS. Other causes for postinfectious glomerulonephritis must be considered, particularly if there is no evidence of recent streptococcal infection. An acute exacerbation of chronic glomerulonephritis may be difficult to distinguish from PSAGN, particularly if the exacerbation is provoked by a streptococcal illness. Failure of expected improvement in a reasonable time, evidence of growth failure, or failure of the C3 level to return to normal may be helpful in distinguishing between the two. Other glomerular diseases such as anaphylactoid purpura nephritis, IgA nephropathy, familial nephritis, and hemolytic uremic syndrome can usually be differentiated on the basis of historical, clinical, and laboratory findings.

TREATMENT. The morbidity and mortality associated with PSAGN are influenced by appropriate supportive care, and, therefore, such care is extremely important. Hypertension is the most common problem demanding attention. Mild elevations in blood pressure frequently respond to bed rest and fluid and salt restriction; however, moderate to severe hypertension requires immediate therapy.

Upon admission, the patient should be considered as having potential renal failure; thus, fluid administration should be limited and diuretics administered. Occasionally, severe oliguria persists, and the resulting renal failure should be managed with supportive care, including dialysis if needed. The majority of these patients will have return of renal function within several weeks.

COURSE AND PROGNOSIS. All patients with PSAGN should be observed on a long-term basis. The frequency of development of chronic renal disease is not completely clear. Studies of children during epidemic PSAGN have reported a 100% recovery. Sporadic cases of PSAGN may have a higher incidence of long-term complications, with approximately 5 to 10% of children and 15 to 30% of adults progressing to chronic renal disease.

Anaphylactoid Purpura with Nephritis

The full spectrum of anaphylactoid purpura with nephritis (APN) includes purpuric skin lesions, abdominal pain, and arthritis, but all three may not be seen in every patient. Approximately 50% of cases occur in children between 6 months and 5 years of age. Symptoms are usually preceded by an upper respiratory infection; however, no specific organism has been consistently implicated. Renal involvement has been reported in 20 to 50% of patients and is more common in children older than 5 years.

Renal involvement accounts for most of the long-term morbidity and mortality, and symptoms or signs of renal involvement usually occur within the first 4 weeks. Signs and symptoms are similar to those of PSAGN. In the more severe cases, either an acute nephritic syndrome or a severe nephrotic syndrome occurs. Rarely, there is a rapidly progressive course leading to a diagnosis of rapidly progressive glomerulonephritis (RPGN).

Treatment is usually supportive. No specific therapy has been found to affect the overall course of the disease, although gastrointestinal symptoms may improve with the use of steroids, azathioprine, or both. These drugs do not affect the course of the renal disease. Some investigators have reported success in using cyclophosphamide in those patients with severe renal involvement.

Postinfectious Glomerulonephritis

Glomerulonephritis has been associated with a number of bacterial, viral, and protozoan infections. Glomerulonephritis occurring with subacute bacterial endocarditis (SBE) or with ventriculoatrial shunt infections (shunt nephropathy) has been most commonly described. Other infectious causes of an immune complex nephritis include syphilis, malaria, hepatitis B antigen, and infectious mononucleosis.

IgA Nephropathy

IgA nephropathy (Berger's disease), the most common cause of recurrent gross hematuria in childhood, is commonly seen in the second decade of life. Overall the disease in children appears to have a chronic, benign course even though a small number of cases (approximately 10%) may demonstrate slowly progressive renal failure. The disease appears more ominous when it presents in late adolescence or adult life.

Characteristically there is symptomless gross hematuria, without other renal symptoms or signs, during or immediately following an upper respiratory tract illness. Proteinuria may occur along with red blood cell casts. There is no evidence of streptococcal infection, and the level of C3 is characteristically normal. Serum IgA levels may be elevated. The gross hematuria subsides after 2 to 5 days, as does the proteinuria. Microscopical hematuria may persist, or the urine sediment may become normal. The hematuria tends to recur with subsequent upper respiratory tract illnesses or, on occasion, extreme physical exercise. The only symptom that is occasionally associated is flank or abdominal pain in association with gross hematuria. The recurrent hematuria may persist over several years.

The similarity of the clinical picture and the histopathology to anaphylactoid purpura with nephritis has been previously mentioned. Renal biopsy specimens show a focal glomerulonephritis with IgA deposits in the mesangium.

Similar IgA deposits are seen in the small blood vessels of the skin.

Familial Nephritis

There are a variety of familial forms of nephropathy, two of which will be discussed here.

Familial nephritis with nerve deafness (Alport's syndrome) is the most frequently diagnosed familial nephritis syndrome. Clinical disease is more common in males and has a serious prognosis, often culminating in renal failure in the second to fourth decade of life. In females the disease rarely results in renal failure.

Characteristically the syndrome makes its appearance in early childhood with persistent hematuria, either gross or microscopic. The hematuria is often initially noticed during a respiratory illness or following exercise. Hypertension is a late finding as are edema and azotemia. The disease is usually suspected on the basis of a family history of renal disease, hearing deficits (sensorineural), or ocular defects (most notably spherophakia). On the other hand, some cases are sporadic while others appear to be inherited.

Familial nephritis with nerve deafness is believed by most to be an autosomal dominant trait with male predominance, but there are still questions of sex linkage. A separate form inherited as an autosomal recessive trait has been described. Pathologically this condition appears to represent a defect in basement membrane synthesis whereby the glomerular basement membrane (GBM) is regenerated at an accelerated rate, ultimately producing glomerulosclerosis. In the early stages, the definitive diagnosis can be made by renal biopsy if the tissue is studied by electron microscopy. The basement membrane appears to be split longitudinally, there appearing to be layers of basement membrane-like material.

Familial nephritis occurs in several other noted syndromes, many of which have a prognosis similar to that of Alport's syndrome. Among these are thoracolumbar dysplasia (Jeune's syndrome), nail-patella syndrome, and carpal-lysis syndrome.

Familial hematuria (benign hematuria) may be a variant of familial nephritis but is nonprogressive. Histologically the GBM is thinned in segmental areas, suggesting a defect in synthesis. The condition must be distinguished from the more serious familial nephritis, and only family history and renal biopsy are helpful in accomplishing this.

Familial juvenile nephronophthisis (medullary cystic disease) is, strictly speaking, not a glomerulonephritis but is one of the cystic dysplasias. It is one of the more frequent causes of end-stage renal disease in teenagers and young adults. The final stages consist of glomerulosclerosis, extensive interstitial fibrosis, and small, contracted kidneys. The mode of inheritance remains controversial, with some data suggesting an autosomal dominant mode while others suggest it to be autosomal recessive in character.

The earliest and most consistent symptom is polyuria; this is occasionally noted, often in retrospect, as early as infancy. The polyuria is rarely severe enough to suggest diabetes insipidus and is most often overlooked as a normal variant. A fall-off from the normal growth curve occurs around 4 to 6 years of age and often is marked by the age of 10 years. A common presenting symptom consists of progressive malaise and pallor in the early to mid teens. Moderate to severe anemia, detected either on routine examination or in response to the malaise and pallor, is often the finding that eventually leads to diagnosis.

Part of the difficulty in making an earlier diagnosis is the relatively normal urinalysis. Hyposthenuria is present, as is excessive urinary sodium loss, but the usual abnormalities expected with a serious renal illness are absent. Proteinuria and cylindruria are late manifestations, and hematuria rarely is present at all. Hypertension and edema are not seen until extensive renal damage has occurred, primarily because of the diuresis and natriuresis. By the time the disease is suspected, there is usually moderate azotemia, and there may already be evidence of significant renal osteodystrophy.

Rapidly Progressive Glomerulonephritis

Rapidly progressive glomerulonephritis (RPGN) is a disease of acute onset and rapid progression leading to renal failure in weeks or months and characterized histologically by the formation of "crescents" in at least 50% of the glomeruli. As described here, RPGN is an idiopathic condition and should be distinguished from the rapid deterioration in renal function accompanied by crescent formation that sometimes occurs in diseases such as acute glomerulonephritis, MPGN, systemic lupus erythematosus, APN, and polyarteritis nodosa. These five illnesses probably account for 75 to 85% of the cases seen during childhood. Consequently their presence should be excluded as an initial step in diagnosis.

Urinalysis reveals microhematuria and proteinuria. Serum creatinine and blood urea nitrogen values are markedly elevated, and the C3 level is usually normal. Circulating antiglomerular basement membrane antibodies can often be demonstrated. Histologically there is focal glomerular involvement with cellular proliferation in Bowman's space, resulting in formation of crescents that may be partial or circumferential. Crescents are often replaced by fibrous tissue, and the glomerulus may undergo global sclerosis. The presence of circumferential crescents in more than 70% of the glomeruli generally indicates a bad prognosis, with rapid onset of renal failure; however, on occasion, spontaneous remissions do occur in patients with crescents in 100% of the glomeruli. No therapeutic method as yet has been unequivocally demonstrated to favorably alter the course of the disease. Immunosuppressive agents, anticoagulants, and plasmapheresis have been used in various combinations in small series of patients, often with good results. Because of the potential toxicity of these regimens, it is obligatory that they be used only in centers equipped to handle the complications.

The Kidney in Systemic Disease

Systemic Lupus Erythematosus Nephritis

Systemic lupus erythematosus (SLE) is a disease with a wide range of presentations. The basic lesion is a diffuse vasculitis probably mediated by antigen-antibody complexes and the complement system. The incidence of renal involvement based on clinical findings such as proteinuria, abnormal urinary sediment, and abnormal renal function is variously estimated to be 35 to 95%, whereas if altered renal histology is the criterion the incidence increases to 85 to 100%.

Nephritis, manifest by hematuria, proteinuria, and casts, is the most common clinical presentation of renal involvement. Occasionally the proteinuria may be severe and result in the nephrotic syndrome. Hypertension occurs in 15 to 50% of patients. Four different categories of renal histologic involvement are described: (1) mesangial, (2) focal proliferative, (3) diffuse proliferative, and (4) membranous. The clinical course and prognosis are correlated with the nature of the renal lesion. In diffuse proliferative glomerulonephritis (DPLN), the prognosis is worst, whereas in those with the other lesions, prognosis is relatively good.

Evidence that SLE is an immune complex disease is abundant. Serum complement is decreased in most cases and correlates with activity of disease. The immunoglobulins present in glomeruli demonstrate antinuclear activity. Antibodies against a large number of nuclear and cytoplasmic antigens are present in the sera of these patients. Antibodies to native or double-standard DNA correlate best with the degree of activity of the disease.

Untreated DPLN is progressive, accounting for 50% of mortality. For this reason, therapy is now aimed at control of the glomerulopathy. To obtain a baseline for evaluation, biopsy should be done in all patients soon after diagnosis, even if no clinical evidence of renal disease is present. Several studies have described progression of renal disease from normal, mesangial, or focal proliferative glomerulonephritis to diffuse proliferative in serologically active cases.

Patients with DPLN should be treated with high-dose steroids. This is often initiated with intravenous bolus infusions of methylprednisolone followed by oral prednisone. With adequate therapy, complement levels and anti-DNA antibody titers usually become normal within this time. Prednisone dosage can then be gradually reduced to a smaller daily dose or an alternate-day regimen can be instituted. Some recommend combined therapy with either azathioprine or cyclophosphamide from the beginning.

Patients with all forms of SLE-nephritis require long-term follow-up, as many have episodes of increased activity of disease, each of which requires prompt intervention. With aggressive steroid and immunosuppressive therapy, mortality figures for children with SLE have markedly improved, 5- to 10-year survivals of 65 to 85% being reported.

Hemolytic Uremic Syndrome

Hemolytic uremic syndrome (HUS), characterized by microangiopathic hemolytic anemia, thrombocytopenia, and acute renal failure, was first described in children in 1955; a similar picture was recognized in adults in 1977. Although uncommon, HUS is a frequent cause of acute renal failure in infants and children.

Infants and young children are most often affected, the highest incidence being in those between the ages of 2 months and 8 years (mean age of 12 months). Endemic areas have been described but, in this country, most cases occur sporadically. An infectious etiology is suspected and several possible pathogens have been identified in sporadic cases. Current evidence supports either a viral cause or *E. coli* as responsible agents. Studies have demonstrated occurrence of HUS in families, with symptoms occurring either within days or weeks or separated by more than 1 year. Multiple recurrences have been described.

Clinically a prodromal period of 3 to 16 days occurs during which time vomiting and diarrhea occur in 80 to 100% of patients, occasionally with hematemesis or melena or both. A small percentage have symptoms of an upper respiratory tract infection. This phase is followed by a second phase manifest by pallor, hematuria, oliguria or anuria, and possibly neurological dysfunction. On physical examination the patient appears pale and weak with signs of dehydration secondary to vomiting and diarrhea. The blood pressure is elevated in 30 to 60%, hepatosplenomegaly occurs in 30 to 50%, petechiae in approximately 30%, and CNS dysfunction in 30 to 50%. The major prognostic determinant is the severity of renal involvement, although CNS dysfunction may occasionally be severe and lead to permanent neurological sequelae or death. Anuria occurs in 30% of patients; oliguria in almost all others. The reduction in urine volume may last from 4 days to several weeks; it averages approximately 10 days. Neurological signs include seizures, severe alterations in consciousness, and, less frequently, decerebrate posturing and hemiparesis.

Patients with HUS characteristically have a microangiopathic hemolytic anemia with fragmented RBCs and burr cells on the peripheral blood smear. Reticulocytosis is almost always present in spite of severe degrees of renal failure. Thrombocytopenia lasting 7 to 14 days is detected in 90%. Results of other coagulation studies are usually normal except for the thrombin time and serum fibrin degradation products, which may be abnormal. Urinalysis shows microscopic or gross hematuria and proteinuria. Azotemia is usually present, as are other metabolic derangements associated with acute renal failure, including metabolic acidosis, hyperkalemia, hypocalcemia, and hyperphosphatemia. The primary pathogenetic feature in the majority of cases is damage to vascular endothelial cells, which is thought to be confined primarily to the glomerular capillaries and renal arterioles. Similar findings have also been demonstrated in the brain as well as other tissues in some cases with severe neurological dysfunction.

In early reports, mortality ranged from 40 to 50%. Primarily because of aggressive supportive care, early insertion of a peritoneal catheter and early initiation of dialysis if symptoms or signs warrant its use, the mortality today has been reduced to around 5 to 20%. Prevention of hypervolemia is most important. If the child is not dehydrated initially, management consists only of replacement of insensible fluid losses. Anemia often requires transfusion, which should be given as fresh, packed RBCs. Hypertension should be controlled and seizures managed by standard therapy. As noted, the importance of early dialysis has been clearly demonstrated.

Therapy aimed at reversing the altered coagulation state has been attempted. At present, heparinization and fibrinolytic therapy cannot be recommended because there is little evidence of an overall beneficial effect. Recently, exchange transfusion and plasmapheresis were reported to produce dramatic improvement in anemia, thrombocytopenia, and neurological symptoms. Infusions of plasma, particularly in those with severe central nervous system dysfunction and continuing severe anemia and thrombocytopenia, have been reported as effective. Improvement has occurred in most cases in 24 to 48 hours, but the infusions may be required for several weeks to maintain improvement.

Long-term prognosis is good in the majority of patients with adequate supportive care. In 10 to 30% of patients, however, there will be progression to chronic renal insufficiency, or they will develop significant hypertension, or both will occur.

Diabetes Nephropathy

It is estimated that 5% of the population in the United States has diabetes mellitus (DM). This disease is listed as the third most frequent cause of death. One of the major complications contributing to the high mortality is microvascular disease of the kidney. Approximately 25 to 40% of persons with type I diabetes (insulin-dependent or IDDM) develop renal failure within 25 years of onset. Clinically, nephropathy is usually first manifest by proteinuria, and once persistent proteinuria occurs, renal failure develops in one-half of these patients within 5 years and in 80% by 10 years. Even though clinical renal disease rarely occurs during childhood, evidence suggests that the cause begins early in the life of those with IDDM. Management, therefore, should be begun during childhood.

Early in the course of IDDM there is an increase in kidney size; this consists of both glomerular and tubular enlargement. Associated with these changes is an increase in glomerular plasma flow and transcapillary hydraulic pressure, in filtering area, in glomerular filtration rate, and in filtration fraction. The resultant hyperfiltration is presumed to be a major determinant of progression of renal disease. With strict control of diabetes these changes can be reversed. The GBM thickening and increased excretion of albumin, not detectable by routine methods, have also been demonstrated within 2 to 3 years after onset of IDDM. Evidence suggests that these changes may be reversal by normalization of blood glucose.

How should diabetic patients be managed in an attempt to prevent nephropathy or to stabilize the nephropathy once it exists? The evidence cited supports attempts at good control, and this implies normalization of blood glucose. In the future this goal may become more feasible with precise glucose regulation by the artificial beta cell or with islet cell transplantation. Vigorous control of elevated blood pressure is essential as hypertension has clearly been shown to accelerate the progression of nephropathy.

Renal Failure

Acute Renal Failure

Acute renal failure (ARF) denotes rapid deterioration in the ability of the kidney to maintain homeostasis, resulting in retention of nitrogenous end products of metabolism and in abnormalities in water, electrolyte, and acid-base balance. It is generally, but not invariably, accompanied by oliguria.

PATHOGENESIS. Based on the pathophysiology, ARF can be divided into three categories.

Prerenal. Reduction in renal blood flow and perfusion pressure of a magnitude sufficient to depress the GFR results in azotemia and metabolic imbalances in the presence of normal kidneys. Gastroenteritis with severe dehydration is the most common situation in which this phenomenon occurs; it can also be seen in any condition that results in hypovolemia and hypotension such as septic shock, burns, and severe congestive cardiac failure. Prerenal azotemia is completely reversible if the circulatory insufficiency is corrected before structural renal damage has occurred.

Renal. Prolonged renal hypoperfusion results in acute tubular necrosis (ATN). Scattered areas of renal tubular epithelial cells undergo necrosis and may be "shed," leaving denuded areas of tubular basement membrane. The debris plugs the tubules, raises intratubular pressure, and further depresses glomerular filtration. There is a severe and simultaneous renal arteriolar constriction, and some studies suggest this renin-angiotensin–mediated phenomenon as the primary contributor to ARF. ATN appears reversible as long as the glomeruli are not destroyed. Prolongation of renal ischemia results in glomerular damage and renal cortical necrosis with permanent loss of renal function.

ARF can also be caused by drugs and toxins such as the aminoglycoside antibiotics, mercury, and ethylene glycol, which damage the tubular epithelium, and by massive hemolysis or rhabdomyolysis, resulting in tubular obstruction by hemoglobin or myoglobin casts. Each also produces a vasoactive response. Radiopaque dyes used in angiography and intravenous pyelography are being increasingly implicated in ARF: the risk appears to be higher in the presence of dehydration, congestive cardiac failure, diabetes, and multiple myeloma.

ARF may occur in the course of primary glomerular diseases such as MPGN and acute poststreptococcal glomerulonephritis, from renal involvement in systemic diseases like the hemolytic uremic syndrome or SLE, and from acute interstitial nephritis. These conditions are discussed elsewhere.

Postrenal. Acute bilateral obstruction to the flow of urine by blood clots, stones, or crystals raises renal tubular and interstitial pressure, resulting in diminished glomerular filtration. Obstructive causes are uncommon in children.

ACUTE TUBULAR NECROSIS. *Clinical Features.* In most patients, the first clinical sign of ATN is diminution in the urine output, but anuria is rare. In some patients, urine volume remains normal in spite of compromised renal function, so-called nonoliguric or high-output renal failure. Hypertension is not a feature of ATN; its presence indicates secondary hypervolemia. Tachypnea and hyperpnea may result from severe metabolic acidosis. Central nervous system manifestations depend on the degree of azotemia and electrolyte imbalance and may range from a normal sensorium to drowsiness, irritability, and seizures.

Urine volume is less than 180 ml/m²/24 h (6 ml/kg/24 hr). The urine contains protein and abundant hyaline and granular casts. Urine osmolality is typically less than 350 mOsm/kg with a sodium content in excess of 40 mEq/L. In prerenal azotemia, on the other hand, urine osmolality exceeds 500 mOsm/kg and the sodium content is less than 20 mEq/L, indicating better preservation of nephron function.

Blood urea nitrogen and creatinine levels are elevated, the rate of increase depending on the degree of catabolism. An increase of 10 to 20 mg/100 ml/day in blood urea nitrogen and 0.5 to 1.0 mg/100 ml/day in serum creatinine are typical; the presence of fever, infection, or damaged tissue can easily double this rate. The serum level of potassium is elevated and that of serum bicarbonate is depressed. After the first few days the serum calcium level gradually falls and the serum phosphorus level rises. Mild anemia is common, as is leukocytosis.

Management. Because ATN is generally a reversible condition, management is directed toward maintenance of homeostasis until renal function recovers; this may take from a few days to 4 to 6 weeks. The clinical course of ATN consists of an oliguric phase followed by a recovery phase and requires management of fluid and electrolyte balance, azotemia, and infections.

Hypovolemia with hypotensive shock is the most common cause of ATN in children, and restoration of circulating fluid volume is the first priority. Isoosmotic fluids such as isotonic sodium chloride, dextran, plasma, or whole blood (the selection of which depends on the underlying cause) should be administered rapidly. Unless cardiac disease is suspected, severely dehydrated oliguric patients should receive at least 20 ml/kg of fluid in the first hour; this rate of administration should be continued until approximately half the dehydration is corrected; then rehydration should be more gradual. If oliguria persists despite correction of dehydration and restoration of normal blood pressure, ATN has occurred. Fluid administration should then be curtailed and consist only of replacement. A loss of 0.5% of body weight a day indicates appropriate fluid therapy.

In ATN, release of intracellular potassium during catabolic processes can result in hyperkalemia, especially in the presence of tissue injury or hemolysis. Hyperkalemia is exaggerated by the acidosis that frequently accompanies it. In most patients, restriction of dietary potassium is adequate to prevent hyperkalemia, but regular monitoring of serum potassium is essential; a level exceeding 6 mEq/L is an indication for obtaining an electrocardiogram (ECG).

Serum potassium concentrations should be kept below 6 mEq/L. Minor elevations can be managed by administration of Kayexalate (sodium polystyrene sulfonate). If ECF changes are present, the intravenous infusion of 25 to 50% glucose (0.5–1.0 g/kg), together with insulin (0.05–0.1 I.U./kg) and sodium bicarbonate (2–3 mEq/kg) can be given while preparations are made for dialysis. Serum potassium concentrations above 7 mEq/L with advanced ECG changes require administration of 10% calcium gluconate.

Acidosis does not require treatment unless the serum level of bicarbonate falls below 15 mEq/L. Small doses of sodium citrate or bicarbonate can be used but may result in fluid overload or hypernatremia. Phosphate binders such as aluminum hydroxide or calcium carbonate may help in partially correcting both the hyperphosphatemia and the hypocalcemia.

A high-calorie, high-carbohydrate diet (70–100 g/m²/day) with approximately 0.5 g/kg of high-quality protein helps suppress endogenous catabolism and prevent a rapid increase in the azotemia.

Uremic patients are overly susceptible to infection. Invasive procedures such as catheterization, placement of indwelling venous cannulas, and dialysis-related surgery serve as portals for bacterial invasion. In addition, prolonged recumbency promotes pneumonia. Infection is the most common cause of mortality in ATN, and avoidance of nonessential surgery, meticulous asepsis, early ambulation, a high index of suspicion for infection, and early and vigorous antibiotic therapy after obtaining appropriate cultures are essential.

Peritoneal dialysis is a safe procedure and should be used before life-threatening clinical or biochemical abnormalities occur. The indications for dialysis are: (1) fluid overload with severe hypertension or congestive cardiac failure, (2) severe, persistent, or recurring hyperkalemia, acidosis, or other electrolyte abnormalities such as hyponatremia, and (3) blood serum urea nitrogen approaching 100 mg/dl or a change in sensorium such as drowsiness or irritability.

The recovery from ATN is heralded by a marked increase in urinary output. All aspects of nephron function do not recover simultaneously, however, and improvement in the biochemical abnormalities may not commence until a few days later. In fact, initially, there may be worsening of the azotemia in the presence of increasing urinary output. The magnitude of the diuresis steadily increases, and in some patients it may reach several liters per day. Large amounts of electrolytes may be lost in the diuretic phase, and frequent monitoring of serum is imperative. The diuresis results partly from continuing inability to concentrate the urine (in which case the losses should, ideally, be replaced) and partly from excretion of accumulated water, salt, and nitrogenous waste products (in which case the losses are appropriate and do not need to be replaced). The relative contribution of the two mechanisms to the diuresis may be ascertained by not replacing a part of the previous day's loss. If urine volume decreases appropriately, the second mechanism is operative; at this stage the best way to regulate fluid balance is to allow the patient free access to fluids. Urine volume eventually returns to normal.

Chronic Renal Failure

Chronic renal failure (CRF) is an irreversible, often progressive, loss in the number of functioning nephrons until homeostasis can no longer be maintained, resulting in clinical and biochemical abnormalities.

ETIOLOGY. The common causes of CRF in children are: (1) congenital abnormalities of the kidneys and urinary tract (dysplastic kidneys, ureteral reflux, atonic bladder), (2) glomerular diseases (MPGN, focal segmental sclerosis), (3) renal involvement in systemic diseases (SLE, hemolytic-uremic syndrome), and (4) hereditary disorders (familial nephritis, medullary cystic disease).

PATHOPHYSIOLOGY. With progressive renal damage, the surviving nephrons undergo hypertrophy, and tubular transport processes are augmented in an effort to maintain homeostasis. With continuity nephron loss, compensation is no longer possible, and the clinical and biochemical features of CRF develop.

As renal function diminishes, serum concentrations of urea, creatinine, and other nitrogenous end products of metabolism increase. Metabolic acidosis develops from inability to reabsorb bicarbonate and to secrete ammonia. Phosphorus retention results in hyperphosphatemia and depression of serum calcium concentration. The serum parathormone level rises, and the hyperparathyroidism, hypocalcemia, and acidosis lead to the combination of osteomalacia (defective bone mineralization) and osteitis fibrosa cystica (bone reabsorption) known as renal osteodystrophy. Anemia results from decreased erythropoietin production, suppression of erythropoiesis by uremia, and a decrease in RBC life span.

CLINICAL AND LABORATORY FEATURES. In some patients the onset is insidious, with lethargy, anorexia, headaches, and pallor; in others, edema, hypertension with congestive cardiac failure, or seizures may be the presenting features. Growth failure is common in preadolescent and adolescent patients. Clinical rickets may result from renal osteodystrophy. Absence of tendon reflexes indicates the presence of peripheral neuropathy. A bleeding tendency may be present, resulting in easy bruisability. In uremia there is increased susceptibility to infection.

The GFR is low; blood urea nitrogen and serum creatinine concentrations are elevated. Serum parathormone level is high, and alkaline phosphatase is increased. A normochromic anemia is common with the hemoglobin concentration being as low as 5 to 7 g/100 ml. Hyperuricemia occurs but is rarely severe. The urine specific gravity is fixed around 1.010. Radiological evidence of hyperparathyroidism, and renal rickets may be present.

MANAGEMENT. *Diet.* The ideal diet would supply adequate calories for growth, suppress endogenous protein catabolism, and be low in phosphorus and potassium. These objectives are best served by a high-calorie, high-carbohydrate diet containing 0.5 to 1.0 g/kg of body weight of high quality protein to supply the essential amino acids (and to make the diet more palatable). Anorexia is common in CRF, and most children have to be constantly reminded to eat adequately. The effort is justified, because an adequate caloric intake is associated with increased linear growth.

Fluid and Electrolytes. Neither water nor salt should be restricted in the polyuric phase of CRF. With the development of oliguria, hypertension, or edema, dietary salt should be restricted and fluid intake limited. Serum bicarbonate should be corrected to at least 20 mEq/L with a sodium bicarbonate or citrate solution given orally. The ability to excrete potassium is well retained even in late CRF, but hyperkalemia can occur with a sudden increase in catabolism or dietary intake.

Hypertension. Chronic hypertension may accelerate the progression of CRF, and treatment is mandatory. Some patients respond to salt and water restriction, which may be combined with diuretic therapy. In others, the use of other antihypertensives is indicated.

Anemia. The hemoglobin level should be maintained at or around 10 g/100 ml. If this cannot be accomplished with traditional means, then the administration of recombinant erythropoietin should be given.

Calcium, Phosphorus, and Osteodystrophy. Derangements in calcium and phosphorus metabolism are a major cause of growth retardation in CRF. Hyperphosphatemia responds to reduction in dietary phosphorus and the use of phosphate binders such as calcium carbonate or gluconate. The hypocalcemia can be corrected either with the combined use of oral calcium (10–20 mg/kg/day of elemental calcium) and 1,25-dihydroxy-D3 (Calcitriol).

Dialysis is indicated when CRF has progressed to the extent that conservative management is no longer effective. Significant advances have been made in both hemodialysis and peritoneal dialysis of pediatric patients in the last decade. Normal growth, however, does not occur in children undergoing dialysis, and renal transplantation has to be the ultimate goal for young children with end-stage renal disease. With rapid improvements in the long-term prognosis of renal transplantation, this goal is being achieved in more and more patients.

Luther B. Travis, Alok Kalia, and José Luis Enriquez

Renal Tubular Disorders

Anatomy and Physiology

Renal tubules begin at the glomeruli and end at the renal papillae. The main divisions (proximal, intermediate, and distal collecting tubules) have been further subdivided into fourteen individual tubule segments according to their cell types and functional anatomy. Specific information from tedious in vivo and in vitro studies has resulted in a more comprehensive understanding of individual renal transport processes as well as an integrated appreciation for axial heterogeneity, glomerular-tubular, and tubulo-tubular relationships. Functionally, the tubule portion of the nephron may be divided into two groups of tubule segments: the proximal tubule system and the distal tubule system. The proximal system, 10 to 12 mm in length, reabsorbs essential nutrients, filtered salts and water, and secretes unessential waste products. The distal system, 3 to 4 mm in length, is composed of the thick ascending limb of Henle, distal convoluted tubule, and collecting segments. Their main function is to dilute the tubular fluid by reabsorbing sodium in excess of water so that subsequent dilute or concentrated urine may be excreted depending on the absence or presence of vasopressin (antidiuretic hormone [ADH]). There are short- and long-looped nephrons, the length of the long loops being very important to urine concentration.

In brief, the tubules receive the glomerular ultrafiltrate (120 ml/min/1.73 m^2 of body surface area at maturity) and process this enormous volume of fluid and solutes with great precision so as to homeostatically control the volume, osmolality, composition, and acidity of the intra- and extracellular fluid compartments.

The basic mechanisms of transport in epithelia directly apply to the renal tubules. The structural polarization of the cell membrane into apical and basolateral membranes with consistent cellular orientation maintained by the junctional complexes, together with the polarization of transport mechanisms by localization of sodium-potassium-ATPase to the basolateral surface and diffusional and carrier-mediated mechanisms to the apical surface, creates two separate membranes facing different fluid compartments (lumen vs. renal interstitium) and allows for transepithelial transport to occur. The energy-dependent extrusion of intracellular Na into the lateral intercellular and basolateral spaces by the Na^+-K^+-ATPase pump provides the electrochemical gradient for most of the other transport processes across the apical membrane. Most transport processes are energy dependent and use the transcellular pathway. In addition, permeability-dependent paracellular transport across the junctional complexes occurs for bulk movement of solutes and water (particularly in the proximal system). The transport capabilities of the tubule are segment specific and segregate along the nephron. Among the broad array of important tubular functions, the transport of electrolytes, the reabsorption of organic nutrients, the secretion of organic cations and anions, urine concentration and dilution, urinary acidification, and clearance of urea are most notable. In addition, the tubules are important endocrine organs via their secretion of 1,25-$(OH)_2$ vitamin D, renal prostaglandins, catecholamines (dopamine), and kinins.

TRANSPORT OF ELECTROLYTES AND WATER. *Sodium.* The proximal system reabsorbs 60 to 70% of the filtered NaCl. Much of this Na^+ reabsorption results from active cotransport with amino acids and glucose; however, some NaCl is reabsorbed as a result of Na^+-H^+ exchange via brush border membrane-bound antiporter with subsequent passive Cl^- diffusion. NaCl absorption in the thick ascending limb may account for 20 to 30% of the filtered load. As in the proximal segments, NaCl reabsorption is a secondary active Na^+ process (basolateral Na^+-K^+-ATPase pump is primary). In the thick ascending limb, however, a Na^+, K^+, and $2Cl^-$ symporter (carrier) located in the luminal membrane working in parallel with a K^+ diffusion pathway results in the net reabsorption of one Na^+ and two Cl^- ions. The Cl^- diffuses out the basolateral side with the Na^+ actively extruded by the Na^+-K^+-ATPase pump. This segment is impermeable to water, and fluid, therefore, becomes dilute as salt is selectively removed. The distal convoluted tubule also continues this dilution process by active Na$^+$ reabsorption. Finally, the principal (light) cells of the collecting tubule are responsible for Na$^+$ reabsorption and in establishing the final urinary concentration for Na$^+$. In the cortical segment of the collecting tubule, the NaCl reabsorption is partly mineralocorticoid dependent (aldosterone increases Na$^+$ reabsorption).

Water. Water moves according to the intrinsic permeability of the tubular epithelium in a given segment and the osmotic gradient existing across the cell membranes. Some segments are very permeable to water (proximal), while others are strictly impermeable (thick ascending limb) or permeable only in the presence of ADH (collecting tubule).

Potassium. Ninety to ninety-five percent of filtered K$^+$ is reabsorbed before the tubule fluid reaches the collecting tubules, which are, therefore, the source of K$^+$ in the urine. Depending on the potassium balance, the collecting tubule is capable of both active K$^+$ secretion (by the principal cells) and reabsorption (by the intercalated or dark cells). Potassium secretion is dependent on dietary intake, Na$^+$ and fluid delivery rates to the collecting tubule, and mineralocorticoid activity.

Phosphorus(P), Calcium(Ca), and Magnesium(Mg). The renal handling of these three ions is a complex interdependent process. Many hormones (parathyroid hormone [PTH], prostaglandins), acid-base homeostasis, ECF volume, and other modulators affect their mutual regulation. Ninety percent of plasma inorganic P$^+$ is filtered by the glomeruli with 70 to 75% reabsorbed in the proximal tubule and an additional 5 to 10% reabsorbed in the distal tubule (in part PTH dependent). Because albumin-bound Ca$^+$ is not ultrafilterable, only 65 to 70% of total plasma Ca$^+$ is filtered. Fifty to sixty percent of the filtered load is reabsorbed in the proximal segments, 20% in the thick ascending limb, and 10% in the distal tubule (role of PTH). The fractional excretion of Ca$^+$ is normally less than 1 to 2%. Finally, 70 to 80% of plasma Mg$^+$ is filtered at the glomerulus, 25 to 30% of which is complexed to oxalate, citrate, and P$^+$. Ninety percent of the filtered Mg$^+$ is reabsorbed, primarily in the thick ascending limb of Henle.

REABSORPTION OF ORGANIC NUTRIENTS. *Glucose*. Following nearly complete glomerular filtration, 98% of the filtered glucose is reabsorbed in the proximal tubule, primarily by active cotransport with Na$^+$. The glucose transport carrier in the luminal brush border appears to be specific for D-glucose. There exists a maximal tubular transport rate for glucose such that filtered loads of glucose may exceed transport capacity and glycosuria result.

Amino acids. For each class of amino acid (AA), there is active, carrier-mediated transport from the tubular lumen across the brush border membrane of the proximal segments, which is dependent on Na$^+$ cotransport. D-isomers are transported at a much lower rate than L-isomers. Normally, only 1% of the freely filtered AA is excreted in the final urine, although mild generalized aminoaciduria is commonly seen in neonates, particularly premature neonates, and even apparently normal infants.

SECRETION OF ORGANIC CATIONS AND ANIONS. Organic waste products, both cations (e.g., creatinine, choline, catecholamines) and anions (e.g., bile salts, hippurates, osalate, urate), many produced by the liver, as well as drugs (e.g., antibiotics, furosemide, salicylate, cimetidine, morphine, atropine) cannot be excreted in the urine by filtration alone given their degree of plasma protein binding. These organic molecules require active carrier-mediated transport into the proximal tubular cells from the peritubular plasma across the basolateral membrane and passive organic ion diffusion into the tubule fluid. Essentially all organic ions and drugs are removed from plasma in one passage through the renal cortex.

URINE CONCENTRATION AND DILUTION. The arrangement of tubule segments and medullary blood vessels (vasa recta) allows for the two fundamental processes of the countercurrent mechanism to occur, countercurrent multiplication and countercurrent exchange, thus, establishing and preserving the high osmolality of the medullary interstitium. In order to maintain water balance, the volume and osmolality of the urine must be controlled by the interaction of ADH and the collecting tubules whose permeability to water depends on the presence of ADH. Given establishment of medullary hypertonicity, ADH renders the otherwise impermeable collecting duct principal cells permeable to water and a concentrated urine is formed. The absence of ADH allows for the excretion of the diluted urine formed via the active solute reabsorption of the thick ascending limb and distal tubule.

URINARY ACIDIFICATION. The major tubular contribution to renal net acid excretion revolves around hydrogen ion (H$^+$) secretion (generated by cytosolic carbonic anhydrase) by many nephron segments. The reaction of H$^+$ with tubular fluid bicarbonate, phosphate, and ammonia permits the kidney to both reclaim 99% of filtered bicarbonate and excrete large acid loads without developing a steep pH gradient between blood and tubular fluid. The principal method (80 to 90%) of proximal H$^+$ secretion involves a neutral Na$^+$-H$^+$ antiporter in the luminal membrane working in conjunction with brush border carbonic anhydrase to form reabsorbable CO$_2$ and water from filtered bicarbonate reacting with secreted H$^+$. In the distal tubule the remaining bicarbonate is reabsorbed by H$^+$ secretion and additional H$^+$ secretion is titrated by urinary buffers, ammonia (produced from glutamine primarily in the proximal segments), and filtered phosphates, with consequent generation of new bicarbonate and restoration of the bicarbonate consumed by metabolic acid production in the body. The intercalated cells of the collecting tubule segments are particularly important to this final regulation of renal H$^+$ secretion. Mineralocorticoids, hypokalemia, and conditions of metabolic acidosis may increase H$^+$ secretion.

UREA CLEARANCE. Although urea excretion is the primary means to remove excess nitrogen from the body, it also plays a major role in facilitating a number of renal tubular functions, including the operation of the medullary countercurrent multiplication system, water abstraction from the thin descending limb, passive NaCl reabsorption from the thin ascending limb, and active secondary Cl$^-$ reabsorption from the thick ascending limb through its contribution to medullary hypertonicity. Urea is passively reabsorbed in the proximal convoluted tubule (increased reabsorption in states of decreased effective circulating volume) and passively enters the lumen of the thin limb of Henle. Both the cortical and medullary collecting tubules are impermeable to urea while the papillary collecting tubule is highly permeable and enables the recycling of urea into the medullary interstitium where it facilitates the concentrating function of the thin limbs of Henle. Under conditions of water conservation the urea concentration in the urine may reach 50 times the plasma concentration.

Tubular Injury

Tubular defects may result from cystic disorders (Table 13-2), specific transport functional disorders (Table 13-3), and many tubulointerstitial diseases (with or without underlying urologic disorders). Selective loss of tubule function may result from inherited or acquired diseases affecting tubules of the interstitium to a greater extent than the glomeruli. Because tubular functions are clustered in nephron segments, injury often affects groups of functions, causing natural syndromes (see Table 13-3). Hereditary diseases, in particular, tend to damage individual nephron segments and spare others. Some inborn errors of metabolism such as galactosemia, hereditary fructose intolerance, glycogen storage disease type I, xanthinuria, cystinosis, Wilson's disease, Lowe syndrome, Zellweger syndrome (cerebro-hepatorenal), and oxalosis are associated with renal tubular functional defects in addition to physical cellular injury. Pyelonephritis is a relatively common disorder also associated with transient or even residual tubular defects depending on the magnitude of tubular injury.

Characteristic manifestations of tubular disease include: salt wasting (Na$^+$, Cl$^-$); renal tubular acidoses (hyperchloremic or nonanion gap acidosis) from either proximal bicarbonate loss, failure of the distal tubule to acidify the urine normally, or both; reduced principal cell responsiveness to ADH (polyuria, nocturia); renal glycosuria, phosphaturia, aminoaciduria, uricosuria, potassium wasting alone or in combination; and tubule proteinuria. The evaluation of these disparate disorders includes careful documentation of the tubular defects (urinalysis, timed urine collections for quantitative analysis), appropriate serum chemistries and radiologic imaging (e.g., ultrasound, nuclear medicine, magnetic resonance, computed tomography) as directed by the presenting symptoms/signs and family history. The application of molecular biology to the prenatal diagnosis of many of these disorders is either currently available or expected shortly.

Robert Fildes

Congenital Anomalies of the Genitourinary Tract

Congenital anomalies of the genitourinary system are among the most frequent and important encountered in clinical practice. Early diagnosis and treatment can result in preservation of renal tissue and function.

Clinical Forms of Congenital Renal Anomalies

Renal anomalies can be categorized into those of abnormal formation, position, or number. Renal agenesis is the failure of a kidney to develop. If only a single kidney develops, it may show hypertrophy, making it more easily palpable. Renal dysplasia is an accompaniment of other malformations of the urinary tract, and the dysplastic kidney may contain other abnormal tissues within the renal substance. It may be a source of discomfort, vague abdominal pain, and hypertension. The ureter may be obliterated or patent. A hypoplastic (miniature) kidney may be present during early childhood and adolescence without symptoms. It may fail later and cause hypertension.

Simple malrotation may also be found when the kidney pelvis is directed anteriorly instead of medially; this usually produces no symptoms. Horseshoe kidney may result if the metanephric tissue fuses early in gestation. The two lower poles of the kidney are joined by an isthmus of renal tissue in front of the aorta, the kidney lies lower in the pelvis, and the

266

Table 13-2. *Clinical and Laboratory Presentation of Renal Cystic Disorders*[a]

Disorder	Inheritance	Clinical findings					Serum				Urine		
		General	Tubule segment	NaCl Wasting	K⁺ Wasting	Polyuria	Cl⁻/K⁺	Low CO_2	Ca	P	Ca	TRP	Amino acids
Polycystic kidneys (adult)[b]	AD	H, HTN, CRF (late), abdominal mass, US(+)	All	−	−	−	N	+	N	N	N	N	−
Polycystic kidneys (infantile)	AR	Abdominal mass, US(+), pulmonary hypoplasia, CRF (early)	All; gross distortion	−	−	−	N	+	N	N	N	N	−
Medullary cystic disease	AD	A, CRF	Tubulointerstitial disease ± cysts	+	−	−	N	+	N	N	Inc	N	−
Familial juvenile nephronophthisis	AR	Ophthalmologic, CNS, hepatic, and skeletal anomalies	Tubulointerstitial disease ± cysts	+	−	+	N	+	N	N	Inc	N	−
Medullary sponge	AR (?)	H, lithiasis, CT imaging	Collecting duct, medulla papilla	−	−	±	N	+	N	N	N	N	−
Single/multiple renal cysts	?	H, US(+)	?	−	−	−	N	−	N	N	N	N	−

[a] Excludes cystic dysplasias.
[b] Findings prior to onset of chronic renal failure.
AD = autosomal dominant; AR = autosomal recessive; ? = unknown; H = hematuria; HTN = hypertension; CRF = chronic renal failure; N = normal; + = presence of; − = absence of; Inc = increased; TRP = tubular reabsorption of phosphate; US = ultrasound; CT = computed tomography; CNS = central nervous system.

Table 13-3. Clinical and Laboratory Presentation of Major Renal Tubule Defects in Functional Tubular Disorders

		Clinical findings					Low	Serum			Urine		
	Tubule segment	NaCl	K+ wasting	Polyuria	General	Cl⁻/K+	CO₂	Ca	P	PTH	Ca	TRP	Amino acids
RTA													
Type I[a]	D	–	+	–	FTT, NL, H	Inc/Dec	+	N	N	N or Inc	N	N	–
Type II[a]	P	+	+	+	FTT, OM	Inc/Dec	+	N	N	Inc	Inc	Dec	±
Type IV[a]	D	±	–	–	FTT	±/Inc	+	N	N	N?	N	N	–
Fanconi syndrome[b]	P	±	–	+	OM, G	Inc/Dec	+	Dec	Dec	N or Inc	Inc	Dec	+
Cystinuria[c]	P	–	–	–	NL, H	N/N	–	N	N		N	N	+
Nephrogenic DI	D	–	+	+	Primary and secondary	N/N	–	N	N		N	N	–
Bartter's syndrome	TALH	+	+	+	Severity variable	Dec/Dec	–	±Dec	N	N	N/Inc	N	–
Renal glycosuria	P	–	–	–	Benign	N/N	–	N	N		N	N	–
Familial hypocalciuric hypercalcemia	TALH?	–	–	–		N/N	–	Inc	N	Inc	Dec		–
Renal idiopathic hypercalciuria	?	–	–	–	NL	N/N	–	N	N	N or Inc	Inc	N or Dec	–
Liddle's syndrome	D	–	+	–		N/Dec	–	N	N		N	N	–
Familial X-linked hypophosphatemic rickets	P	–	–	–	OM	N/N	–	N	Dec	N or Inc	N	Dec	–
Pseudohypoparathyroidism													
Type I	?P	–	–	–		N/N	–	Dec	Inc	Inc	N	Inc	–
Type II	?P	–	–	–		N/N	–	Dec	Inc	Inc	N	Inc	–

[a] Can be acquired as well as hereditary; secondary or acquired Type I, IV often related to obstructive uropathy with or without pyelonephritis or drugs; also postrenal transplantation.

[b] Coma causes include: cystinosis, Wilson's disease, Lowe's syndrome, hereditary fructose intolerance, tyrosinemia, vitamin D-dependent rickets, vitamin D deficiency, pseudovitamin D deficiency, lead or cadmium poisoning, renal transplantation.

[c] Loss of dibasic amino acids (cystine, arginine, ornithine, lysine).

P = proximal; D = distal; TALH = thick ascending limb of Henle; FTT = failure to thrive; NL = nephrolithiasis; H = hematuria; OM = osteomalacia; blank space for an entry indicates lack of data; G = glucosuria; TRP = tubule reabsorption of phosphates; PTH = parathyroid hormone; + = present; – = absence of; inc = increased; dec = decreased.

renal pelvis faces ventrally instead of medially. The kidneys are also found in many ectopic locations (pelvis, chest).

CYSTIC DISEASE. The secretory and collecting tubules may not effect a perfect juncture, and cystic disease, an uncommon affliction, may then develop and be evident in a variety of forms. Infantile polycystic disease is an autosomal recessive condition and manifests itself with bilateral flank masses. Renal insufficiency soon ensues. Nephrosonography is helpful in establishing the diagnosis. The adult form of the disease is inherited as an autosomal dominant disease. As a rule it does not cause symptoms until 40 to 50 years of age, but it may occur in childhood. It is usually bilateral.

Multicystic dysplastic kidneys are generally unilateral. The loose conglomeration of cysts resembles a bunch of grapes. The ureter is atretic, and renal arteries are poorly developed. Most patients have renal enlargement during infancy. Observations of nonfunction of the kidney by renal scan and a cystic mass with septa by ultrasound make the diagnosis relatively certain. Nephrectomy is indicated as the contralateral kidney is usually normal.

Solitary cysts are also found usually arising from the renal cortex. They present as abdominal masses or urinary infection. Destruction of the renal parenchyma may take place on account of pressure. Unroofing of the cyst is sometimes necessary. Multilocular cysts (cystadenomas) are found mostly in adults, although they have been reported in children and are confused with Wilms' tumors.

ABNORMALITIES OF THE COLLECTING SYSTEMS AND URETERS. Not infrequently the collecting systems, calices, pelves, and ureters are duplicated; at times, the entire kidney is a double structure with ureters that may empty into the urethra, vagina, or bladder at some abnormal site. The ureter may develop behind the vena cava, and a retrocaval ureter may be the result. Stenosis and strictures of these tubular structures are found with greatest frequency at the points of junction.

The malfunction of these embryonic deviations usually produces obstruction to urine flow, with infection that is hard to eradicate. Pain in the loins may result from obstruction. Incontinence may occur with ectopic ureters opening into the vagina or urethra distal to the sphincter mechanism. Ureteroceles cause urinary infection and flank pain and may diagnostically appear as a cobra-head or bubble within the bladder on imaging studies.

Ureterovesicular obstruction with accompanying hydronephrosis and hydroureter may be improved by surgical reconstruction and reimplantation of the ureter in the bladder.

CONGENITAL HYDRONEPHROSIS. The age at which congenital hydronephrosis is diagnosed has changed dramatically since fetal ultrasound has come into widespread use. Renal anomalies can be detected by 20 weeks gestation. Few situations for antinatal intervention are indicated except for obstruction with severe bilateral hydroureteronephrosis that results in diminished volume of amnionic fluid. Fetal shunting from a point proximal to the obstruction into the amnionic fluid cavity has been performed. Early diagnosis and surgical correction of obstruction is possible and results in improved renal function.

Urinary tract infections in infants should be viewed with suspicion. Cultures should be taken to identify the organism. Ultrasonography, voiding cystography, radionuclide scan, and intravenous pyelography may be performed to rule out an anatomical defect. If none is found, instrumentation should be avoided, and careful, long-term antibiotic therapy administered. In general, cystoscopy is unnecessary and unproductive in children unless an anatomic abnormality has been demonstrated.

Exstrophy of the Bladder. Exstrophy of the bladder usually results from failure of the anterior portion of the cloacal membrane to develop. In this condition, babies are born with the bladder open on the abdominal wall and associated complete epispadias. In males this may proceed to a completely bifid phallus and in females a bifid clitoris. Vesicoureteral reflux is usually present. Invariably associated with the deformity is wide separation of the symphysis pubis, but other anomalies may also coexist.

When infants are encountered with typical exstrophy of the bladder at birth, the moist bladder mucosa should be covered with either a Silastic membrane or moist sterile dressing. The infant should be operated upon as soon as possible. Closure within the first 72 hours after delivery often eliminates the need for sacroiliac osteotomies. Staged repair should initially consist of bladder closure, reapproximation of the pubis, and reconstruction of the abdominal wall. At approximately 1½ years of age, sphincter reconstruction, ureteral reimplantation, and genital reconstruction is performed.

Gratifying results have been achieved in selected medical centers that have been prepared to undertake the multidisciplinary, long-term care of such patients.

Bifid Kidneys with Double Ureters. This anomaly is of particular interest. The ureter draining the upper half of the kidney inserts lower in the bladder than the ureter draining the lower half. This ureter may be obstructed, producing infection and hydronephrosis in one-half of the kidney. Often the ureter from the upper half inserts into the urethra beyond the sphincter mechanism or into the vagina, leading in either case to constant dribbling of urine. In addition to this dribbling, the patient also voids normally and adequately at intervals. This history is characteristic and should lead to the diagnosis. Treatment is by surgical correction as well as by elimination of infections with antibiotics.

Urethral Obstruction and Bladder Neck Obstruction. These conditions may be manifested by urinary retention with a large palpable bladder, difficulty of micturition, urgency, incontinence, infection, and secondary renal damage. The etiologies include urethral valves, strictures of the urethra, urethral polyps, diverticula of the urethra, or meatal stenosis. Many of these conditions have been detected by micturition urethrocystography and cystoscopy.

Surgical procedures on children with lower urinary tract infections secondary to bladder neck dysfunction have fallen from favor. The neuromuscular control of micturition is an extremely delicate matter; and the patient's condition may indeed be made much worse by operation. These patients are usually managed by clean intermittent catheterization. In contrast, resection of the obstructive tissue and reconstruction of the hydroureters in newborns with anatomic lesions give gratifying results.

Vesicoureteral Reflux. Damage to the kidney is debatable with sterile vesicoureteral reflux, but if the reflux is associated with infection, the risk is considerable. Low grades of reflux usually resolve spontaneously. Severe degrees of reflux and recurrent episodes of pyelonephritis often require surgical correction with ureteral reimplantation. Diagnosis of reflux is made by cystography (radioisotope or x ray). Control of infection with antibiotics and close follow-up are required.

Neurogenic Bladder. A neurogenic bladder is one that cannot store or cannot empty urine. Patients with this condition are usually managed pharmacologically and with clean intermittent catheterization. Surgery is rarely needed.

Hypospadias. Hypospadias is the condition in which the urethral opening is not on the tip of the penis. It is often associated with ventral chordae. When anything more than mild hypospadias is seen in newborn infants, it is essential to consider the possibility of renal anomalies. Circumcision should not be performed as the prepuce is used later for surgical reconstruction of the urethra.

MISCELLANEOUS CONDITIONS OF THE GENITOURINARY TRACT. *Phimosis.* In this condition, retraction of the prepuce over the glans penis is limited and the preputial opening narrowed. This finding is physiological and normal in the newly born infant. The American Academy of Pediatrics, endorsed by the American College of Obstetrics and Gynecology, has taken the position that circumcision of the newly born infant should not be performed routinely, although recent studies leave this in question. Older infants and children with phimosis-balanitis usually require circumcision.

Torsion of the Testis. This is a very dangerous condition in which gangrene and loss of the testis rapidly occur from strangulation. The anatomic abnormality which predisposes this condition is usually bilateral, and once it happens on one side there is an increased chance that it will happen on the other. Noninvasive Doppler ultrasound, radionuclide testicular scan, and the presence or absence of the cremaster reflex have aided in the prompt diagnosis of this condition. Surgical exploration, however, is still required in equivocal situations.

Hydrocele. This is an accumulation of fluid in the tunica vaginalis testes or processus vaginalis of the spermatic cord. Hydrocele may be present in the newborn as a soft, fluid-filled scrotal swelling that transilluminates. It resolves over a period of months and requires no treatment. Hydrocele may also appear during childhood and adolescence. Pawnbroker's sign — three balls — is present. Transillumination distinguishes it from tumor.

Varicocele. This varicose condition is a result of incompetent valves in the spermatic veins which cause elongation, dilatation, and tortuosity of the pampiniform plexus. It usually occurs in adolescents. During palpation of the spermatic cord, the scrotum feels like a bag of worms. Varicocele may be accompanied by a vague pulling, dragging pain that is relieved by reclining or scrotal support. Surgery may be required.

Hydrometrocolpos. In this condition either an imperforate hymen or, more commonly, atresia of the upper part of the vagina results in massive dilatation of the proximal vagina and the uterus by retained fluid. This may occur in infancy or may be deferred until the onset of menses. The large abdominal mass created by the fluid-distended uterus is frequently mistaken for a large bladder or some type of intraabdominal tumor. Incision of the obstructing membrane and maintenance of the patency of the new channel by catheter for a time are curative.

Testicular Tumors. These are uncommon in children, but when they occur they are usually during the first year of life. Early diagnosis and treatment are essential. They are not found unless one takes time to inspect and palpate the testes. There is an increased risk of tumors with undescended testes.

Ovarian Tumors. Tumors of the ovaries occur in a considerable number of children. The teratomas and dermoid cysts are more common than other types. An ovarian tumor may give rise to symptoms either as an abdominal mass, if it comes up out of the pelvis, or as an obstruction to the rectum, to the urethra, or to the ureters. Calcification within the tumor, particularly if it is just bone or tooth, suggests that it is probably a dermoid cyst. Any of these cysts or

270

tumors may produce symptoms because of torsion of their vascular pedicles, producing gangrene and severe abdominal signs.

All the tumors should be removed on diagnosis because teratomas are likely to be or to become malignant. Endocrinologically active tumors are rare, and of these, granulosa cell tumors are the most striking. They secrete estrogens in amounts sufficient to cause precocious puberty even in infants. Dermoid cysts may be bilateral; in the treatment of such cases, any normal portion of one or both ovaries should be preserved if possible.

Undescended Testes. See page 80.

Abnormal Sexual Development. See Appendix A, Section 25.

Robert M. Berger and Mohsen Ziai

References

Brenner, B. M., and Stein, J. H. (Eds.). *Pediatric Nephrology, Contemporary Issues in Nephrology.* New York: Churchill Livingstone, 1984. Vol. 12.

Feld, L. G., et al. Urinary Tract Infection in Infants and Children. In *Pediatrics in Review,* September, 1989. Vol. 11, No. 3.

Feld, L. G., et al. Acute renal failure. I. Pathophysiology and diagnosis. *J. Pediatr.* 109:401, 1986.

Fildes, R. D., et al. Acute renal failure. II. Management of suspected and established disease. *J. Pediatr.* 109:567, 1986.

Gruskin, A. B. (Ed.). *Pediatric Clinics of North America.* Philadelphia: Saunders, 1987. Vol. 34, No. 3.

Kaufman, D. B., et al. Systemic lupus erythematosus in children. *Curr. Probl. Pediatr.* 18:4, 1988.

Makker, S. P., et al. Nephrotic syndrome in childhood and adolescence. *Curr. Probl. Pediatr.* 16:10, 1986.

Edelmann, C. M., Jr. (Ed.). Nephrology. *Pediatr. Ann.* 19:9, 1988.

14

The Nervous System

Neurological History and Physical and Laboratory Examination

The first step in establishing a diagnosis is to determine the site of the lesion. This principle is well illustrated in neurology, which lends itself easily to logical reasoning. If one keeps in mind the bare essentials of the functional anatomy of the nervous system, the question, Where is the lesion?, can be answered in a vast majority of patients after a good history and physical examination. These must be thorough and, above all, systematic. Following a set routine often saves a great deal of time.

History

In all children, history begins with the state of health of the parents and with previous pregnancies and births. There follows an inquiry into pregnancy, labor, delivery, birth, and the developmental milestones. The specific complaint is then elucidated in full and pertinent questions are asked. Some of them, relating to epilepsy, disturbance of con-

sciousness, mental deficiency, and familial disorders, are discussed in the appropriate sections of this text.

Physical Examination

Physical examination starts with observation of the child as a whole; behavior, pattern of movement, and evidence of asymmetry or malformation being noted. Intelligence is assessed by observation of the general behavior and the child's ability to perform tasks expected at a particular age. A fairly accurate estimation can usually be made in the clinic. This may be complemented, in the older child, by psychological testing. An attempt is made to establish handedness and, hence, cerebral dominance. If the child is old enough to talk, speech is examined for disturbance of symbolism (dysphasia) or articulation (dysarthria).

The skull is examined for size and shape, palpated for masses, bulging of fontanels, or abnormal closure of sutures, and, finally, percussed and auscultated for abnormal sounds. General examination including the skin and spine is quite important.

Systematic examination of each of the twelve cranial nerves, the motor and sensory systems, reflexes, stance, and gait is next. A complete examination is often impossible in infants and difficult in young or uncooperative children, but the basic scheme is not altered; ingenuity helps.

CRANIAL NERVES. In the examination of the cranial nerves, the following functions should be tested:

I. One seldom finds a child with significant abnormality of the sense of smell. Bilateral anosmia is most often due to upper respiratory tract infection or allergy; however, head injury or tumor may damage one or both olfactory bulbs. In older children, coffee or mint may be used to assess the sense of smell.

II. Examination of the second cranial nerve includes assessment of visual acuity and visual fields and ophthalmoscopy.

III, IV, and VI. Extraocular movements, nystagmus, and size, shape, and equality of pupils, as well as their reaction to light and accommodation, are assessed.

V. The motor division of the fifth nerve supplies muscles of mastication; the sensory division, facial sensation. These may be difficult to test in children, but the corneal reflex can be evaluated objectively at any age.

VII. The seventh nerve is the motor supply of all the muscles of the face. Eye closure, facial expression, and symmetry help in the evaluation of its function. Upper motor neuron weakness may be differentiated from lower motor neuron weakness by the fact that the forehead and emotional movement are not affected in the former. The chorda tympani division of this nerve serves the sensation of taste in the anterior two-thirds of the tongue.

VIII. Deafness may be conductive, related to middle ear disease, or of neurological origin. In nerve deafness, bone conduction as well as air conduction is impaired. In infants and young children, a toy bell or whistle may be used to determine if attention can be attracted toward the unseen source of the sound.

IX and X. Palatal movement, the gag reflex, swallowing, and vocal cord movements are served by these nerves. The ninth nerve also supplies the posterior third of the tongue for taste.

XI. The sternocleidomastoid and trapezius muscles are supplied by this nerve. They are tested together with the rest of the motor system.

XII. The tongue should be examined for atrophy, fasciculation, and movement.

MOTOR SYSTEM. In the examination of the motor system each of the following is assessed in turn:

1. Appearance of muscles for bulk and abnormal movement (Is there any wasting?)
2. Tone, or resistance to passive movement (Is it increased [spastic], decreased [flaccid], or normal?)
3. Power (Is there any weakness? If so, how severe?)
4. Coordination (Are the movements smooth or do they show tremor?)

Reflexes. Sudden stretching of any voluntary muscle provokes a reflex contraction. The tendon jerks traditionally employed are the biceps, triceps, and brachioradialis in the upper extremity and the knee and ankle in the lower. Quality and force of the response should be noted. The most informative observation is the asymmetry of tendon reflexes rather than a vague notion of what the normal should be. The plantar response (Babinski) and the superficial abdominal and cremasteric reflexes complete this part of the examination.

Sensory Examination. The sensory examination of the child is often incomplete or unreliable because of lack of cooperation. At times it is confined to observation of the child's emotional or motor response to painful stimuli at various sites. When possible, the following modalities should be tested: touch, pain, or pinprick sensation, temperature, vibration (using a tuning fork), and position sense in the fingers and toes.

Stance and Gait. The stance (including Romberg's sign) and gait of the walking child should be examined and any abnormality described in detail.

INTERPRETATION OF PHYSICAL EXAMINATION. The aspects of functional anatomy essential for diagnosis are simple and easy to remember. Increased intracranial pressure, disturbance of consciousness, and cranial nerve involvement obviously point to disease within the cranium. Epilepsy and intellectual deterioration also suggest cerebral dysfunction. Dysarthria, nystagmus, incoordination of voluntary movements, and ataxia are signs of cerebellar dysfunction. Tremor at rest, choreoathetosis, muscular rigidity, and economy of expression localize the lesion to the extrapyramidal system.

Muscular weakness is conveniently divided into two categories: upper and lower motor neuron paralysis. The section of the motor system from its origin in the precentral or motor area of the frontal cortex through the internal capsule, brain stem, decussation in the medulla, and pyramidal tracts in the spinal cord constitutes the upper motor neuron. The remainder, comprising the anterior horn cells, motor roots, and peripheral nerves, is designated the lower motor neuron. An upper motor neuron paralysis has one or more of the following features: increased tone or spasticity, hyperactive tendon reflexes, extensor plantar response, clonus. The lower motor neuron variety is characterized by wasting (by far the most important sign), decreased tone, hypoactive tendon jerks, and sometimes fasciculation. It should be emphasized that not all the signs need be present to categorize a muscular paralysis.

In the sensory system, the posterior columns of the spinal cord serve vibration and position senses, decussating in the medulla oblongata before continuing their path to the sensory cortex. Pain and temperature are conveyed through the spinothalamic tract of the cord, crossing over almost immediately in the cord on their way to the thalamus and cortex. Diagrams showing the dermatomes and the sensory distribution of peripheral nerves assist in pinpointing the site of the lesion.

Laboratory Studies

Once the anatomical diagnosis is established, the next step is to determine the pathology of the lesion. History, examination, and finally laboratory studies help in answering the question, What is the lesion?

Laboratory investigations may lead one to a proper diagnosis. X-ray films of the skull may show erosion, calcification, or signs of increased intracranial pressure. The electroencephalogram is helpful in evaluating seizure disorders and localizing brain lesions, and in a few instances it may suggest a specific diagnosis. Cranial computed tomography (CCT) and nuclear magnetic resonance (MRI), when available, are by far the best studies to show a brain tumor, hydroencephalus, abscess, subdural collections, hemorrhage, or brain atrophy. A brain scan or arteriography, air-contrast studies, and myelography may be required.

SPECIAL DIAGNOSTIC PROCEDURES. *Lumbar Puncture.* If properly carried out, lumbar puncture is a safe procedure. It is important to have the patient correctly positioned and securely held by a good assistant. The best site for the needle is the interspace between the fourth and fifth lumbar vertebrae. The spinal cord ends at about the first lumbar vertebra in older children, but it may extend down as far as the fourth lumbar vertebra in newborn infants. Spinal puncture is dangerous when there is increased intracranial pressure due to a space-occupying lesion because herniation of the brain through the tentorium or the foramen magnum may occur. If available, CCT or MRI should be done before lumbar puncture if a space-occupying lesion is suspected. Spinal fluid should always be tested for cells and protein content. Bacteriological examination and measurement of sugar content are also indicated when an inflammatory process is suspected.

Subdural Puncture. A short-beveled needle with a stylet is used for this procedure. It is inserted through the coronal suture at least 2 cm from the midline perpendicular to the surface. Care must be exercised not to go deeper than 10 to 12 mm. The stylet is removed, and if no fluid is obtained, the needle is slowly withdrawn. The stylet is then replaced; it will push out a small amount of spinal fluid if the subdural space has been traversed.

Disorders of the Cranium

Microcephaly

When the head circumference is considerably below the third percentile in a child whose height is more nearly average, the diagnosis of microcephaly can safely be made. This is a heterogeneous condition, however, the term *microcephaly* merely referring to the size of the head. Almost any condition that causes serious brain injury early in life may result in a small head. Some familial cases have been referred to as true microcephaly.

The head circumference may be within normal limits at birth but fail to keep up with normal growth. Intelligence is usually severely impaired. Roentgenographic studies of the skull must be made to rule out craniostenosis. Other investigations to identify the possible etiology include a search for toxoplasmosis and cytomegalic inclusion disease.

Macrocephaly

Macrocephaly refers to enlargement of the head. It has many causes, including hydrocephalus, subdural hematoma, megalencephaly, tumors, and cerebral degenerative diseases. Megalencephaly is a congenital anomaly of the brain and may be familial. The neurons are abnormal and diminished in number, while glial elements are present in great excess. This diagnosis is established by demonstration of ventricles of normal size in the presence of a large head.

There are rare congenital tumors that result in a large head without hydrocephalus because of their enormous size. Some cerebral degenerative diseases, including the globoid and metachromatic types of leukodystrophy and the lipid storage diseases, may cause mild enlargement of the head.

Craniostenosis or Craniosynostosis

Cranial sutures may close prematurely, causing an abnormally shaped head, increased intracranial pressure, and brain damage. Usually, but not always, the abnormal closure occurs before birth. The head shape depends on the pattern of suture closure (Fig. 14-1). Early sagittal closure results in scaphocephaly (i.e., a long, narrow head). A similar head shape, however, is seen in some premature infants because of the position maintained postnatally and not because of suture abnormality. Closure of both coronal sutures limits the anteroposterior growth and results in a short, flat head, or brachycephaly. Unilateral closure of a coronal suture produces an asymmetrical head, plagiocephaly, and may be associated with hypertelorism and duplication of the nasal septum. Premature closure of all sutures results in accelerated upward growth and a small circumference of the skull, oxycephaly, or tower skull. Craniofacial dysostosis (Crouzon's disease) refers to oxycephaly, hypertelorism, small maxilla, beaklike nose, external strabismus, and exophthalmos. Involvement of the frontal (metopic) suture alone produces a narrow forehead, or trigonocephaly.

In some cases, increased intracranial pressure, brain damage, and optic atrophy may ensue. Therapy is primarily helpful when there is evidence of increased intracranial pressure and consists of creating artificial sutures and covering the edges with plastic to retard bone regrowth.

Congenital Malformation

Failure of closure of the neural tube or its covering may lead to a variety of congenital malformations along the neural axis.

Neural Herniations

Encephalocele and cranial meningocele signify protrusion of the meninges and frequently brain tissue out of the cranial cavity into a sac covered by skin or a thin membrane. Simple meningeal sacs may cause no symptoms, but encephaloceles (which include brain tissue) are often associated with brain damage. Associated malformations of the brain are common. Air-contrast studies are indicated to determine the extent of the malformation and the amount of brain tissue within the sac and decide about possible surgical intervention. CCT may provide all the information needed.

Meningocele and meningomyelocele refer to external projections of the meninges along the spine. They are most common in the lumbar area. Nervous tissue usually accompanies the sac and causes varying degrees of paralysis, sensory loss, and sphincter disturbance below the lesion. In newborn infants the sensory level sometimes may be determined by the level of sweating.

Many cases are complicated by the Arnold-Chiari malformation (herniation of the cerebellar tonsils and elongation and kinking of the brain stem) and hydrocephalus. Treatment by surgical intervention in selected cases may be successful.

Spina bifida occulta is frequently an incidental radiographic finding. It consists of one or more bifid spines, which are usually in the lumbosacral region. A tuft of hair may cover the overlying skin and may need to be investigated.

Spinal rachischisis is a severe form of meningomyelocele with no membrane covering the spinal defect.

Myelodysplasia

The spinal cord may be abnormal without gross superficial defects. Frequently there is an associated bony malformation of the vertebral column. Lipoma, hydromyelia, dermoid cysts, diastematomyelia (bony or cartilaginous septum bisecting the cord), and a tight filum terminale are among the pathological conditions seen. Minor superficial abnormalities such as hemangioma, lipoma, a tuft of hair, or a dermal sinus may be seen overlying the dysplastic cord. If the cord symptoms are progressive, exploration of the spinal canal should be attempted to search for a treatable lesion. All dermal sinuses above the coccyx should be removed surgically. The first sign of a dermoid cyst in neural tissue with a sinus tract leading to a midline dimple may be an attack of meningitis due to an unusual saprophytic organism.

Hydrocephalus

Hydrocephalus (see Appendix A) means an increased amount of fluid in the head; most authors, however, restrict the term to those with concomitant increased intracranial

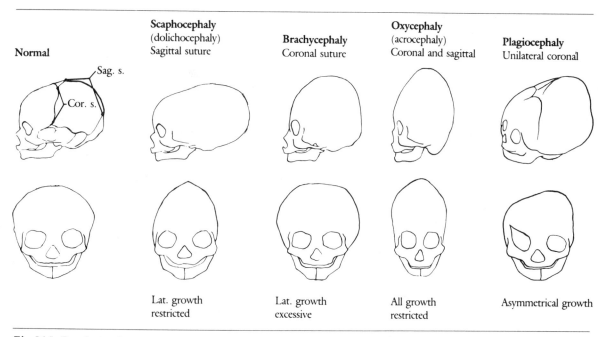

Normal	Scaphocephaly (dolichocephaly) Sagittal suture	Brachycephaly Coronal suture	Oxycephaly (acrocephaly) Coronal and sagittal	Plagiocephaly Unilateral coronal
	Lat. growth restricted	Lat. growth excessive	All growth restricted	Asymmetrical growth

Fig. 14-1. Craniostenosis.

pressure. Hydrocephalus may be due to increased production, a block in the flow, or decreased absorption of cerebrospinal fluid (CSF). When there is no block between the lateral ventricles and the subarachnoid space, the hydrocephalus is said to be communicating.

Papilloma of the choroid plexus constitutes the sole cause of hydrocephalus due to increased production of CSF. This tumor is situated in the lateral ventricles and may be demonstrated with MRI or computerized axial tomography (CAT) scans. Diagnosis is important because removal of the tumor may afford a cure.

A block in the normal flow of CSF may occur at almost any point in its pathway and lead to hydrocephalus. A tumor of the lateral ventricle can cause partial dilatation of that ventricle. Tumors of the third ventricle or midbrain may block the aqueduct of Sylvius. The aqueduct may be too small because of either a developmental anomaly (atresia or forking) or an acquired stricture caused by inflammation (gliosis). Tumors of the posterior fossa may block the fourth ventricle or its foramina. Congenital absence of the foramina of Luschka and Magendie leads to ballooning of the fourth ventricle into a large cyst (Dandy-Walker syndrome).

Communicating hydrocephalus may be due to obliteration of the subarachnoid spaces on the outer surface of the brain, which interferes with absorption of cerebrospinal fluid through the arachnoid villi. In a few cases hypoplasia of the villi has been found with apparent congenital failure of absorption. *Hydrocephalus ex vacuo* is the term used when the increased amount of fluid replaces atrophic brain without an increase in intracranial pressure.

The most extreme form of hydrocephalus ex vacuo is hydranencephaly. Patients with this anomaly have no cerebral hemispheres, except perhaps the tips of the frontal, temporal, or occipital lobes. The resulting empty space is filled with CSF. No physical signs may be present in early infancy, but within a few months it becomes apparent that the child is severely defective. Cyanotic spells and subnormal temperature are common.

DIAGNOSIS. An important bedside examination in any suspected case of hydrocephalus is transillumination of the head. A very bright flashlight, with a lightproof adapter to fit snugly to the head, should be used, and the examination must be carried out in a dark room. The enlarged posterior fossa in Dandy-Walker syndrome and the unusual findings of hydranencephaly are examples of interesting diagnoses that a clinician can make.

The diagnosis of hydrocephalus should be made as early as possible. The best clinical indication is simply the head circumference, measured at frequent intervals. An abrupt deviation from the expected growth curve, indicative of an abnormally enlarging head, may represent either hydrocephalus or subdural hematoma. Unfortunately, a few cases of hydrocephalus progress without enlargement of the head; when the fontanel is open, it may be tense and bulging. X-ray films of the skull are helpful in showing a small posterior fossa with stricture of the aqueduct, or calcification in some tumors. CCT or MRI are by far the best and safest tests to evaluate hydrocephalus and the need for a surgical shunt. Ultrasound may help, but if these are not available, the older contrast studies may be carried out.

These should be performed with caution because an arrested (compensated) hydrocephalus may be activated. They should be carried out only when there is clear evidence that the hydrocephalus is progressive.

TREATMENT. When progression of the hydrocephalus is established, surgical intervention should be considered. This consists in shunting the CSF past the obstruction. The best results are currently obtained by a ventriculoperitoneal shunt with a pump and one-way valve. Complications include blocking of the tubes and infection.

Pseudotumor Cerebri

This nontumorous condition signifies increased intracranial pressure of unknown origin without enlarged ventricles. Papilledema may be severe and leads to secondary optic atrophy and blindness if the pressure is not relieved. The disease is self-limited, and fatalities are rare. Decompression by repeated lumbar puncture or removal of a subtemporal bone flap may be necessary.

Infants with temporary bulging of the fontanel may possibly represent a related condition. It has been reported in association with viral infections, excessive intake of vitamin A, and treatment with tetracycline and cortisone. The pressure usually subsides within a few days, either spontaneously or after the offending agent is removed.

Cerebral Palsy

Cerebral palsy denotes a motor disorder due to a fixed and nonprogressive lesion of the brain. The cerebral damage may be acquired prenatally, during delivery, or early in life. The severity of the disease is variable, ranging from minor neurological deficits to total incapacity. Mental retardation, although a frequent associated feature, is not always present. There are two main types of cerebral palsy: spastic and extrapyramidal.

Spastic cerebral palsy implies injury to the pyramidal system within the cranium. It is manifested by increased muscle tone of the clasp-knife type, brisk reflexes, extensor plantar

responses, and, at times, scissoring of the legs. Depending on the site of the lesion, the paralysis may be unilateral (hemiplegia), bilateral (tetraplegia), worse in the lower extremities (diplegia), or, rarely, affecting only one limb (monoplegia). While the lesion may be present at birth, symptoms may not be recognized until the delay in function becomes apparent, perhaps as late as 1 year of age.

The signs and symptoms in extrapyramidal cerebral palsy include athetosis, chorea, rigidity, and, less often, dystonia and tremor. Athetosis is marked by slow writhing movements, whereas chorea consists of irregular and rather fast jerking of the extremities or face. These symptoms are usually brought on by attempts to move voluntarily or to maintain posture; they disappear during rest or sleep. Tone is often increased and is of a plastic (lead-pipe) quality. Dystonia is an involuntary assumption of abnormal posture that is maintained for many seconds or minutes. Extrapyramidal tremor is present at rest and disappears on movement, in contrast to cerebellar tremor, which is maximal on intention.

ETIOLOGY. The causes of cerebral palsy are numerous. Prematurity is the most common associated condition and is usually associated with spastic diplegia. Cortical inflammation or vasculitis as well as vascular accidents may also lead to this clinical picture. Kernicterus is the best-known cause of extrapyramidal cerebral palsy, although with proper prevention it is becoming less common. Other conditions that may primarily injure the basal ganglia are anoxia and encephalitis.

TREATMENT. The most important aspect of therapy is social. The patient should be helped to live with his handicap. Occupational therapy and rehabilitation are helpful. Ultimate success depends to a large extent on the patient's intelligence. Physical therapy and orthopedic procedures are effective in combating contractures.

ATTENTION DEFICIT DISORDERS. See Ch. 23.

Intracranial Hemorrhage

Epidural Hematoma

Epidural (extradural) hematoma is an acute complication of head injury. It is usually caused by a transverse fracture of the parietal bone and a tear of the middle meningeal artery, which bleeds into the space between the calvarium and the dura mater. The classic picture is one of head injury with a short period of unconsciousness, then a lucid interval followed by deepening coma. The explanation is obvious: The patient is recovering from the head injury when increased intracranial pressure due to the expanding hematoma causes unconsciousness again. CCT or MRI are usually diagnostic.

TREATMENT. If treatment is not received promptly, death may occur within 24 to 48 hours. Treatment consists in surgical evacuation of the blood and clipping of the torn artery; when it is accomplished expeditiously, complete recovery may be expected.

Subdural Hematoma

Subdural hematoma is fairly common in infants under the age of 1 year. There is usually a history of birth injury or head trauma. Bleeding from torn veins traversing the subdural space from cortex to the superior sagittal sinus may be the result of shifting of the brain in head trauma. The venous oozing is stopped by tamponade effect, but this may cause irritation of the meninges. A fibrous membrane may be formed around the hematoma, with serum exudation slowly adding to the volume of the collection.

Presenting symptoms are irritability, vomiting, poor weight gain, enlarged head, or a bulging fontanel. Parietal bossing and hemorrhages in the fundi may be seen on examination. CCT or MRI may show a collection of fluid with increased density early or decreased density later. The diagnosis is usually made with needle puncture of the subdural space through the lateral part of the anterior fontanel or the coronal suture. Bloody or xanthochromic fluid is found, with a high total protein content (500 to 3500 mg/100 ml). Although the lumbar spinal fluid may show xanthochromia and elevated protein, it is much closer to normal. (In subarachnoid hemorrhage, fluid obtained from the subarachnoid space, the ventricles, and the spinal canal is identical.) Treatment consists in daily punctures for a week or 2, no more than 30 ml being removed on each occasion. Should fluid collection persist longer, surgical intervention for excision of possible subdural membrane must be considered. Prognosis depends upon the degree of brain injury resulting from the original trauma and upon the delay in starting therapy.

In patients with subdural hematoma a thorough search must be made for other evidence of trauma such as fractured bones. These infants are frequently the innocent victims of mistreatment and injury inflicted by adults, including their own parents (the battered-child syndrome).

Subdural Effusion

Subdural effusions may follow meningitis or pneumoencephalography. Symptoms are similar to those of subdural hematoma, but the diagnosis is usually made earlier since one is aware of the preexisting condition. Prolonged convalescence with excessive fever, vomiting, irritability, or enlarging head is an indication for MRI, CAT scan, or subdural taps. Small effusions are usually absorbed without therapy, although larger ones may require the same treatment as that outlined for subdural hematoma.

Subarachnoid Hemorrhage

In newborn infants, especially those who are premature, hemorrhage into the ventricles is not rare. This may be fatal, or the infant may survive with or without neurological sequelae. One complication is hydrocephalus, presumably due to plugging of the arachnoid villi with red blood cells. There is a high rate of spontaneous "arrest" in these cases, and some physicians believe that repeated lumbar punctures to reduce the pressure may speed the arrest of the hydrocephalus and minimize brain injury.

In older children, subarachnoid bleeding (into the CSF) is accompanied by headache, fever, stiffness of the neck, and sudden prostration progressing to coma. If intracerebral or cerebellar hemorrhage occurs, localizing neurological signs may be present. A saccular aneurysm or an arteriovenous malformation may be found in some cases; arteriography is indicated when the patient has recovered from the acute stage, as some of these lesions may be amenable to surgery.

Epilepsy

Epilepsy is defined as a recurrent paroxysmal disorder due to abnormal electrical discharges from the brain. With secondary or organic epilepsy a demonstrable brain lesion is known or strongly suspected. Cryptogenic or idiopathic epilepsy, on the other hand, means that no definite brain lesion is suggested by history, physical examination, or laboratory studies. Because of its serious social implications, great care should be taken in making the diagnosis of epilepsy.

The causes of epilepsy are numerous. Almost any disease of the brain can lead to seizures. Degenerative disorders may be manifested by epileptic attacks for a long period before other features become apparent. Brain tumors are seldom a cause of seizures in children because most of them do not involve the cerebral cortex. Electroencephalography, MRI, or CAT scan and measurement of serum calcium and phosphorus, blood urea nitrogen, and blood sugar may help unmask the underlying cause.

In addition to the usual history, attention must be paid to certain specific questions in any patient suspected of having seizures. Age at onset, frequency and uniformity of attacks, diurnal variation, and known precipitating factors are sought. It is then best to obtain a detailed description of a typical attack, preferably from a reliable eyewitness. This should include the type of warning, color changes, eye movements, convulsions, tongue biting, incontinence, injuries that may have resulted from accidents during the unconscious state, postictal phenomena, and duration of each phase. The effect of any medication should be checked, and it may be valuable to ask patients or parents to record details of each attack for future visits. Convulsive disorders and the drugs used to control them are discussed in the following pages.

Generalized (Grand Mal) Seizures

The most common type of epilepsy is the generalized or major seizure. It can occur at any time during day or night. There may be a short warning or aura, like nausea, dizziness, faintness, or tingling. The patient loses consciousness suddenly and may fall and be injured. The color, initially pale, usually becomes blue on account of anoxia; the pupils dilate, and the eyes roll up. The muscles go into spasm and become rigid, and the tongue may be caught between the teeth and badly lacerated. This tonic phase lasts a few seconds and is followed by clonic movements or twitching of muscles. The whole episode lasts less than 5 minutes (seldom any longer). There may be foaming at the mouth and incontinence of urine or, rarely, feces.

Afterward the patient may remain unconscious for some time, be confused, or sleep for some hours. On waking there is often severe headache. The electroencephalogram may show generalized paroxysmal slowing or a diffusely disorganized pattern. Occasionally a patient with seizures has a normal tracing.

TREATMENT. Therapy is directed to the underlying cause. In the idiopathic variety or in the absence of specific therapy, anticonvulsants should be used. Phenobarbital, phenytoin (Dilantin), valproic acid (Depakene), primidone (Mysoline), and carbamazepine (Tegretol) are the most effective of these agents.

Absence (Petit Mal) Seizures

The term *absence* or *petit mal* has come to be used for a particular type of seizure that is accompanied by a very specific electroencephalographic abnormality. The seizures are brief, lasting less than 10 seconds; they involve a transient loss of consciousness, staring, and occasionally smacking of the lips. Patients do not fall and usually do not realize that a spell has occurred. They may have as many as 50 or 100 seizures per day. The electroencephalogram shows a three- to four-per-second spike-wave pattern, synchronous in all leads, occurring in bursts of a few seconds or longer. If

a clinical seizure occurs, the electroencephalographic abnormality will be detectable for at least 5 or 6 seconds. Hyperventilation for 2 minutes is helpful both in bringing out the electroencephalographic abnormality and in producing a clinical seizure.

TREATMENT. Ethosuximide (Zarontin) and valproic acid (Depakene) are the most effective drugs.

Minor Motor Seizures (Infantile Spasms)

Massive myoclonic jerks, head-drop seizures (salaam type), sudden akinetic spells, and other momentary motor seizures may occur in infants and young children. Quite often this type of convulsion disappears in about 4 to 6 years, but the majority of children are left mentally defective and have other types of seizures. The electroencephalogram is usually abnormal and may show hypsarrhythmia (very irregular high-voltage spikes and waves).

TREATMENT. Therapy is usually disappointing. Phenobarbital, phenytoin, and a number of other drugs have been tried without much success. Diazepam (Valium), valproic acid (Depakene), or the ketogenic diet may help. Steroids (especially ACTH) are recommended for those infants thought to be neurologically normal before the onset of seizures.

Simple Partial (Focal) Seizures

Focal or jacksonian epilepsy is characterized by seizures involving only one part of the body. Usually they are clonic movements of one side of the body. There may be no loss of consciousness. Carbamazepine (Tegretol) is probably the most effective drug. Because such attacks are usually due to a focal lesion of the cortex that may be amenable to surgical removal, thorough investigation including contrast studies is indicated in cases refractory to medication.

Complex Partial (Temporal Lobe, Psychomotor) Seizures

Seizures due to discharges from the temporal lobe are manifested by periods of confusion or automatic behavior. Motor phenomena may be absent or limited to staring, smacking of lips, posturing, or quasi-purposive movements of the extremities. Such episodes may continue for up to 10 minutes and may even terminate in a major seizure. Patients frequently have rather peculiar behavior or personality problems between seizures. The electroencephalogram usually shows a temporal lobe spike focus, particularly when the tracing is made with the patient asleep.

TREATMENT. Phenobarbital, phenytoin, and primidone are effective, and carbamazepine (Tegretol) is probably most effective but regardless of what treatment is used, psychomotor seizures are frequently difficult to control.

Simple Febrile Convulsions

Many infants who have a convulsion with high fever do not subsequently develop epilepsy. The outlook is best in "simple febrile convulsions." These occur between 6 months and 3 years of age, are generalized and brief (less than 2 minutes), and are associated with high fever. They do not recur with the same illness and show no electroencephalographic abnormalities. It is probably safe to allow one or possibly two such seizures to occur before instituting anticonvulsant therapy. Any deviation from these criteria, however, greatly increases the likelihood of recurrent seizures, and continuous anticonvulsant medication should be given.

Reflex Epilepsy

A rare group of seizures, precipitated by a variety of stimuli — for example, flashing light (including television viewing), music, certain movements, micturition, startle, or a tap on the head — is known. The attacks vary from grand mal to myoclonus or akinesia. Anticonvulsants give disappointing results.

Breath-Holding Spells

Anger, fright, pain, or minor head bumps in infants and young children may precipitate a brief spell of apnea and cyanosis leading to unconsciousness. The child becomes stiff for a short period and subsequently limp. Recovery is rapid. The breath is always held after expiration, and the next inspiration occurs shortly before the episode is terminated. These are not considered true convulsions. Some patients can be shown to have excessive sensitivity to vagal stimulation. Rarely the attacks precipitate grand mal seizures, and only in such cases are anticonvulsants indicated. This condition may occur as early as a few months of age; it tends to disappear before the age of 6 years.

Miscellaneous Seizures

Rarely, abdominal pain or headaches may be episodic and associated with a seizure pattern on the electroencephalogram. If such symptoms disappear with anticonvulsants, it is fair to consider them convulsive manifestations of an unusual nature.

Status Epilepticus

A patient is considered to have status epilepticus when seizures succeed one another before consciousness is regained. This state may last several hours and constitutes a major emergency in pediatric practice. For treatment see Appendix B.

Drug Therapy for Convulsions

Many drugs are used in the management of epilepsy; however, the majority of seizures can be controlled by the use of one or two preparations. It is advisable to start with one drug and gradually increase the amount until seizures are stopped or symptoms of overdosage appear. If accurate blood levels can be determined then these should be used, of course. If this regimen is not successful, another drug is added. If allergy or idiosyncrasy is noted, the drug should be stopped and never given again. Care must be taken to shake a liquid suspension well, as sedimentation may cause great variation in drug concentration. When the dose is calculated on the basis of the patient's weight, a somewhat larger dose may be used in infants as compared to older children.

PHENOBARBITAL. This drug is used because of its effectiveness and very low frequency of complications. The beginning daily dose is 5 mg/kg of body weight in infants to 2 mg/kg in older children. If necessary, the dose can be increased until seizures are controlled or toxic levels are reached. Overdosage results in drowsiness and occasionally unsteadiness. Other reactions, such as skin eruptions, are rare. Children who are already hyperactive may become more so when receiving any form of barbiturate therapy.

PHENYTOIN. This is a very effective drug, but it has a higher incidence of toxicity than phenobarbital. The starting dose is about 5 mg/kg of body weight, adequate levels being maintained when given twice a day. Overdosage results in ataxia, diplopia, nystagmus, vomiting, and drowsiness. These symptoms usually disappear rapidly when the dose is reduced, but occasionally the unsteadiness may persist for long periods. Swelling of the gums and hirsutism are quite common, particularly with large doses, and may not subside completely when the medication is stopped. About 5% of patients are found to be hypersensitive to this drug. The reactions usually occur between the fifth and the fifteenth day of treatment and include skin rash, fever, cervical glandular enlargement, leukocytosis with increased eosinophils, and splenomegaly. The drug must be stopped immediately; otherwise it may lead to exfoliative dermatitis. Leukopenia is also a rare complication. Blood level testing should be mandatory in small infants because ataxia and other toxic symptoms are difficult to evaluate.

PRIMIDONE (MYSOLINE). The initial daily dose of this drug is 10 mg/kg of body weight. Overdosage may result in drowsiness and ataxia. Idiosyncrasy is not common, but skin eruptions and fever have been reported. This drug is seldom used in infants. Doses should be gradually instituted over a week or 2.

ETHOSUXIMIDE (ZARONTIN). This drug is used for the control of petit mal seizures. The initial daily dose is 10 to 20 mg/kg of body weight. Vomiting or drowsiness may indicate an overdose. Rarely, skin rash or leukopenia may develop as a reaction to this drug.

CARBAMAZEPINE (TEGRETOL). This is a very effective drug in treating grand mal, focal, and temporal lobe seizures. The initial dose is about 10 mg/kg started gradually over a week or 2 and increased if necessary to 15 to 20 ml/kg. Leukocyte counts and liver function studies should be done periodically. Overdosage may cause drowsiness or vomiting. Skin rash may occur.

VALPROIC ACID (DEPAKENE). This drug is effective in both petit mal and grand mal seizures. The initial dose is 10 to 20 mg/kg and it may be increased to 30 ml/kg if necessary. It can affect liver function, and increased appetite and alopecia are among the side-effects.

Hereditary and Degenerative Diseases of the Neuromuscular System

The heredodegenerative diseases of the neuromuscular system comprise a large and varied group of disorders. They have in common a tendency to occur in families and a degenerative pathological process. Even though no cure is yet available in the vast majority of cases, it is important to make the diagnosis for prognostic and counseling purposes. In addition to the signs and symptoms, the mode of inheritance, course of the illness, associated clinical features, and ancillary investigations assist in reaching the diagnosis.

Muscular Dystrophy

Muscular dystrophy includes progressive weakness of varied rates and patterns, but all with the apparent primary defect in the muscle itself. At this time, these dystrophies are separated by clinical manifestations such as age of onset, distribution of muscles affected, rapidity of progression, and hereditary pattern. Serum enzymes, electrical studies, and muscle biopsies help confirm the presence of dystrophy.

Dystrophy leads to progressive weakness that is most often proximal. There are a few exceptions to this including myotonic dystrophy (see below). Sensation should be normal, reflexes should be normal or reduced, but absent only when muscle weakness is severe. Spinal fluid protein and nerve conduction studies should be normal, while electromyography (EMG) may show a myopathic pattern and the biopsy shows variation in fiber size and increased endomesial fibrosis.

Pseudohypertrophic or Duchenne's muscular dystrophy appears to be the most common progressive muscle disorder. It is inherited as an X-linked recessive disease and, therefore, confined to males. It starts early in life, usually before the age of 6 years, and rapidly progresses to incapacity by the tenth or twelfth year and death usually before the twentieth. Proximal muscle weakness with muscle hypertrophy in the calves is seen relatively early. Enzyme studies such as creatine phosphokinase (CPK) have been found to be very high, even in infancy, before clinical manifestations.

A condition that is clinically identical, but slower in progression, is termed Becker's muscular dystrophy. This, too, has X-linked inheritance, hypertrophic calves, high CPK levels, but they tend to be ambulatory through late teenage or into the twenties. Both Becker's and pseudohypertrophic dystrophy may have cardiac muscle involvement with heart failure.

Dystrophin, a muscle protein found in small quantities on the sarcolemmal membrane, appears to be significant for prevention of most cases of muscular dystrophy. Dystrophin is virtually absent in most cases of pseudohypertrophic dystrophy and either reduced or of abnormal molecular weight in the Becker's variety. A number of other unclassifiable dystrophies may have intermediate values. The gene responsible for dystrophin has been located at Xp21. This discovery may eventually lead to better diagnosis, carrier recognition, intrauterine diagnosis, and possibly treatment. Some of the "outliers" are patients with nonspecific clinical pattern, such as females with what strongly resembles Duchenne's dystrophy.

Fascioscapulohumeral muscular dystrophy is inherited as an autosomal dominant trait affecting both sexes and multiple generations. These patients do not appear to have abnormal dystrophin. The onset is in the first or second decade with slow progression, although there may be temporary acceleration during adolescence. There is striking weakness of muscles of the face, and usually prominent weakness and wasting of the muscles of the upper torso proximally. Although the disease may be a handicap, patients usually remain ambulatory and able to compete in the marketplace.

There are a number of other clinical syndromes that are clearly muscular dystrophy, but not typical of any of the above patterns. The *limb-girdle dystrophy* title has been used for these in the past. "Outliers" to the Duchenne-Becker group of dystrophies have been mentioned above. Other cases have the electrical and biopsy studies confirming a dystrophy but do not fall into a specific pattern. Ocular myopathy with slow progression of extraocular muscles and sometimes with pharyngeal involvement may be seen in late childhood or adolescence but usually begin later.

Myotonic dystrophy is characterized by myotonia (difficulty in relaxation), masklike facies, and atrophy and weakness of the sternomastoid and distal muscles of the extremities. The myotonia tends to improve with repeated movement. Onset is extremely variable and may be as late as the fourth decade, with slow progression. The mode of inheritance is autosomal dominant. Associated features include cataracts, gonadal atrophy, frontal baldness, and intellectual impairment.

A benign variety (myotonia congenita or Thomsen's disease) is usually congenital with no weakness or associated stigmas. It may be self-limiting. Quinine sulfate is useful in reducing the myotonia.

Congenital Myopathies

There are a number of muscle disorders leading to weakness that are present at birth or recognized in childhood that are nonprogressive or very slowly progressive. These are uncommon and usually turn up in the course of studying a child for muscular dystrophy. One of the earlier described conditions is that of *central core disease* in which an oxidative enzyme defect can be demonstrated in the central part of the muscle fibers throughout their length. This and most of the congenital myopathies are thought to be hereditary, but almost all are autosomal recessive and many single cases occur.

Another condition in which a coiled worm-like inclusion is found is called *nemaline myopathy*. When part of each coil is seen on the thin sections, it appears like parallel bars, and this is sometimes referred to as rod body disease.

A striking myopathy called *myotubular disease* has muscle fibers that resemble early fetal muscle cells (a uniform smallness of fibers with abnormal staining and central placing of the muscle nuclei along what is thought to be the primitive myotubule). This condition may be mild or extremely severe with death in infancy. Many of these patients have an extraocular muscle palsy, not common with the other congenital myopathies.

Other conditions causing weakness may be associated with an abnormal ratio of Type I and II fibers, excessive numbers of mitochondria, excessively enlarged mitochondria, or other rare changes. It should be remembered that muscle weakness and wasting may be seen with various systemic diseases such as glycogen storage disease, viral and parasitic infections, and polymyositis.

Hereditary Neurogenic Syndromes

WERDNIG-HOFFMANN SYNDROME. Best known of the hereditary neurogenic muscular atrophies is the Werdnig-Hoffmann syndrome. Its mode of inheritance is autosomal recessive. Wasting, flaccidity, and weakness of trunk and limb muscles appear early in infancy and rapidly progress to a fatal termination within 2 or 3 years. The tendon reflexes are usually absent. Fasciculation of the tongue is often an additional finding. The bulbar muscles are affected late in the disease, and death is the result of respiratory infection. The CSF is normal. Electromyography and muscle biopsy reveal neurogenic atrophy. The pathological process consists of degeneration of the anterior horn cells.

The Kugelberg-Welander syndrome is a more benign form of neurogenic muscular atrophy of much longer duration and characterized by proximal muscle weakness.

PERONEAL MUSCULAR ATROPHY (CHARCOT-MARIE-TOOTH DISEASE). Inherited as an autosomal dominant trait, peroneal muscular atrophy is primarily a degeneration of the peripheral nerves. Symmetrical wasting and weakness begin most commonly in the second decade, affecting the peroneal and other distal muscles of the lower extremities, spreading to the rest of the leg and later to the hands. The extremely slow rate of progress makes this condition compatible with a normal life span. The tendon reflexes are lost early. Sensory impairment is variable. The CSF is normal, and muscle biopsy usually shows neurogenic atrophy. Peripheral nerve conduction velocities are abnormally slow, even in the preclinical state.

Spinocerebellar Degenerations

A group of progressive diseases characterized clinically by incoordination and ataxia and pathologically by degeneration of the structures concerned with control of smooth movement are designated by the general term *spinocerebellar degenerations*. They have been variously classified according to the age of onset, mode of inheritance, predominance of certain signs, or course of the illness.

FRIEDREICH'S ATAXIA. By far the most common type encountered in pediatric practice is Friedreich's ataxia. It is inherited as an autosomal recessive trait. An autosomal dominant variety has also been described, but this may well be a different disorder.

Clinical Manifestations. Friedreich's ataxia usually begins in late childhood. Ataxia of gait due to both cerebellar dysfunction and impairment of position sense is an early sign. The incoordination soon spreads to the arms and is followed by dysarthria. Examination reveals, in addition, pes cavus and frequently kyphoscoliosis. The deep tendon reflexes are absent or diminished, and the plantar responses are extensor. Nystagmus is frequently present, and there may be optic atrophy. Diminution of vibration and position sense due to involvement of the posterior columns of the spinal cord is a constant finding.

A cardiopathy is commonly associated with Friedreich's ataxia, and death may be due to heart failure. The duration of the disease is 10 to 20 years.

OTHER SPINOCEREBELLAR DEGENERATIVE DISORDERS. Many other familial disorders involving degeneration of parts of the spinal cord or the cerebellum (or both) are known. Those with predominantly cerebellar signs such as Marie's ataxia and olivopontocerebellar degeneration occur in adult life. Hereditary spastic paraplegia is sometimes included in this group, in spite of the fact that cerebellar signs are either absent or minimal. This disorder commonly starts in the second decade and runs a prolonged and benign course. There is marked spasticity of the lower limbs in the absence of any sensory loss of sphincter disturbance.

Phakomatoses

A number of distinct clinical entities with major neurocutaneous manifestations are often grouped together under the general title phakomatoses. Von Recklinghausen's disease, tuberous sclerosis, von Hippel-Lindau disease, Sturge-Weber syndrome, and ataxia-telangiectasia are included in this group.

VON RECKLINGHAUSEN'S DISEASE (NEUROFIBROMATO-SIS). The manifestations of this disease are multiple tumors (neurofibromas) of the skin and peripheral nerves, café au lait spots, cysts or erosions of bones, and tumors of other organs including the brain. When it is familial, the mode of inheritance is autosomal dominant.

Pheochromocytoma has been described in some cases, and all patients with neurofibromatosis should have periodic blood pressure determinations. Treatment is empirical. Tumors should not be removed unless they are symptomatic or for cosmetic reasons.

TUBEROUS SCLEROSIS. Tuberous sclerosis is an uncommon disorder that produces mental retardation, convulsions, skin lesions, and tumors of many organs. It is inherited as a dominant trait. Sporadic cases are common; some patients may have only mild symptoms. The skin lesion is adenoma sebaceum (pinkish yellow papules on the face); it may not be evident until the tenth year or later.

X-ray films of the skull or CCT may show areas of calcification. Small cysts in the bones of the hands or feet are sometimes found. The electroencephalogram is usually abnormal and in infants may show hypsarrhythmia. Treatment is symptomatic and includes the use of anticonvulsant drugs.

VON HIPPEL-LINDAU DISEASE. This disease is characterized by tumors, classified as hemangioblastomas, in the retina, cerebellum, brain stem, or spinal cord. The disorder is usually inherited as a dominant trait. The retina lesions may lead to blindness. Neurological symptoms result from compression or hemorrhage. Retinal lesions may be treated with coagulation and cerebellar tumors by surgical removal.

STURGE-WEBER SYNDROME. Sturge-Weber syndrome consists of facial nevus flammeus, peculiar calcification in the brain, hemiplegia of the opposite side, convulsions, and often mental defect. The facial nevus is flat, but it may have an underlying cavernous component. It is generally unilateral and over the distribution of the trigeminal nerve. Nevi in the choroid may cause buphthalmos and congenital glaucoma over the affected side. Management calls for controlling the convulsions. Aspirin has been recommended for prevention of the damaging recurrent cortical vein thromboses.

ATAXIA-TELANGIECTASIA (LOUIS-BAR SYNDROME). Ataxia-telangiectasia is manifested by progressive cerebellar ataxia, telangiectasia, and unusual susceptibility to infections. It is recessively inherited. Ataxia, intention tremor, and other cerebellar signs may begin in the first 2 years of life, while the telangiectasia may be delayed for several years. The vascular malformations are usually found on the bulbar conjunctiva, ears, the butterfly area of the face, and the eyelids, as well as the antecubital and popliteal fossae. Acute and chronic respiratory infections are common, and bronchiectasis frequently develops. This seems to be related to a deficiency of the immune system (see Chapter 19). Treatment is symptomatic, but prognosis is poor. Most patients die in the second decade.

Lipidoses

The lipidoses constitute a rare familial group of diseases characterized by deposits of lipids in various tissues.

TAY-SACHS DISEASE (AMAUROTIC FAMILY IDIOCY). Tay-Sachs disease is a recessively inherited cerebral degeneration, primarily of Jewish infants. Abnormal quantities of gangliosides are stored within the neurons secondary to a deficiency of hexosaminidase A enzyme. There is no visceral involvement. Symptoms begin in the first few months of life, and death usually occurs within 2 to 4 years. Early signs are lethargy, impaired motor development, hyperacusis, and poor visual responses. The patient subsequently becomes blind and severely defective. There may be spasticity or flaccidity and seizures, both myoclonic and grand mal. Examination of the fundi shows pale optic nerves and a typical cherry-red spot at the macula surrounded by a grayish retina.

There is no effective therapy.

JUVENILE AMAUROTIC FAMILY IDIOCIES. There are degenerative cerebral diseases with excessive storage of ceroid and lipo fusin in neurons that manifest themselves after infancy, at different ages according to the specific type. They are recessively inherited and occur mostly in non-Jews. No enzyme defect has been found.

Symptoms may begin any time in the first decade after the first or second year. Convulsions, mental deterioration, extrapyramidal or pyramidal signs, and gradual blindness are apparent. Funduscopic examination reveals macular dystrophy, optic atrophy with very small retinal vessels, and pigmentary changes in the periphery.

There is no therapy. Death occurs after a few years.

There are many other rarer forms of familial lipid storage diseases that the reader is referred elsewhere for information.

Leukodystrophies

The leukodystrophies are degenerative diseases of the nervous system showing abnormal metabolism of sphingolipids. These diseases are characterized by diffuse demyelination and the accumulation of abnormal chemical substances in the white matter.

METACHROMATIC LEUKODYSTROPHY. Metachromatic leukodystrophy is now thought to be the most common childhood form of diffuse cerebral sclerosis. It is inherited as an autosomal recessive trait. Demyelination occurs in the brain, spinal cord, and peripheral nerves, with excessive deposits of metachromatic material (sulfatides).

The onset of symptoms is usually at 18 months to 3 years of age but may come as late as the third decade. Ataxia is an early sign; tendon reflexes may be diminished because of polyneuropathy. Mental deterioration and upper motor neuron involvement are evident later, and convulsions occasionally occur. The enzyme arylsulfatase A is decreased. Nerve conduction velocity is reduced. There is gradual deterioration leading to death within a few years. No effective therapy is yet available.

DIFFUSE INFANTILE FAMILIAL CEREBRAL SCLEROSIS (KRABBE'S DISEASE). In Krabbe's disease, a hereditary form of leukodystrophy, large globoid bodies filled with cerebroside are seen throughout the white matter. This disorder occurs most often in infants and usually has a short course. The clinical picture is one of apathy, stupor, generalized ridigity, and convulsions. The enzyme, β-galactosidase is decreased.

Subacute Sclerosing Panencephalitis

Subacute sclerosing panencephalitis is similar to the leukodystrophies but can be distinguished by neuronal inclusions and distinct clinical features. A virus quite similar to the measles (rubeola) virus has been recovered from the brains of a number of patients. The disease usually occurs sporadically, although minor epidemics have been reported.

The onset of the disease is commonly between 5 and 20 years of age, and the course may last a few weeks to several years. Apathy, mental deterioration, and spasticity occur, but the characteristic feature is periodic (every 15 to 30 seconds) myoclonic jerks of large amplitude, associated with repetitive spike-and-wave bursts on the electroencephalogram. The CSF shows an elevation of total protein (mostly gamma globulin) and perhaps a few cells. Measles titers are elevated in blood and CSF. The disease is fatal, and no treatment is available, but, fortunately, it has virtually disappeared lately.

Hepatolenticular Degeneration (Wilson's Disease)

Hepatolenticular degeneration is a recessively inherited disorder of copper metabolism and manifests itself by progressive cirrhosis of the liver and extrapyramidal dysfunction. Free copper is deposited in the liver, brain, and corneas. The copper in the cornea results in a greenish-brown ring on the outer edge of the cornea (Kayser-Fleischer ring). Symptoms seldom begin before the age of 6 years, although ceruloplasmin levels are probably deficient from infancy. When the disease appears in the first decade, liver symptoms usually precede those of the central nervous system. In patients with a later onset, neurological manifestations predominate, and frequently there is little defect in liver function. Neurological symptoms include tremor, rigidity, a fixed facial expression, mild dystonia or athetosis, difficulty in speech and swallowing, and emotional lability.

All children with extrapyramidal syndromes or evidence of cirrhosis of the liver should have examination of the cornea by slit lamp and, if possible, determination of serum ceruloplasmin levels. The relatives at risk of developing Wilson's disease should also be studied because early treatment may prevent the symptoms. The administration of penicillamine is effective in most cases.

Huntington's Chorea

Huntington's chorea, while more commonly appearing in adult life, may begin or even run its course in childhood. It is inherited as a dominant trait. Degeneration occurs in the basal ganglia, especially the caudate nucleus, and the cortex. Symptoms include involuntary movements, usually chorea, and mental deterioration. There is no therapy; total disability leads to death within 10 to 20 years.

Polyneuropathy

As the name implies, polyneuropathy (or polyneuritis) involves affection of many peripheral nerves. Symmetrical involvement of all four limbs is the rule, but in certain diseases (e.g., leprosy) multiple single nerves may be affected (mononeuritis multiplex).

As might be expected, the signs and symptoms of a polyneuropathy are paresthesia and muscle weakness, more marked in the periphery, absence of or diminished tendon jerks, and impairment of sensation of all modalities in a glove-and-stocking distribution.

The causes of polyneuropathy are numerous, but in general the condition is rare in childhood. Some cases may be familial (e.g., metachromatic leukodystrophy). In heredopathia atactica polyneuritiformis (Refsum's syndrome), polyneuritis is associated with cerebellar ataxia, retinitis pigmentosa, hemeralopia, paresthesia, deafness, and sometimes ichthyosis; the protein content in the CSF is increased. Progressive hypertrophic interstitial neuropathy (Dejerine-Sottas disease) is a dominantly inherited disease, with thickened nerves and very slow progression. Postdiphtheritic polyneuritis used to be common. It differs from other types by early involvement of the soft palate and other bulbar structures. Polyneuritis may be a complication of certain infections, vaccinations, and porphyria. Most often seen is the Guillain-Barré syndrome, which is described in more detail.

Acute Infectious Polyneuritis (Guillain-Barré Syndrome)

Frequently there is history of an antecedent respiratory infection. The onset of weakness may be relatively sudden, causing paralysis in a day or two or even in a few hours. The proximal muscles are often more severely affected. Bilateral facial weakness is common; the bulbar and respiratory muscles may also be involved. The tendon reflexes are diminished or absent. Loss of sensation is variable and may be minimal. The CSF findings are characteristic: elevation of protein content (sometimes as high as 1 or 2 g/100 ml) without any increase in the number of cells.

Commonly the weakness progresses for a few days and then gradually improves over a period of 6 to 10 weeks; however, the course of this illness is highly variable, and the condition may last for several months. Treatment is symptomatic; the patient's vital functions are maintained in the hope of eventual recovery. Respiratory failure may result from paralysis of muscles of respiration. Tracheotomy may be indicated, and a mechanical respirator should always be at hand. With proper management, prognosis is very good in a large majority of children.

Polymyositis

Polymyositis is an inflammatory disease of muscle that may mimic the clinical picture of muscular dystrophy. It may be a manifestation of a collagen disease (see Chap. 18). In addition to muscular weakness, tenderness, low-grade fever, leukocytosis, and eosinophilia may be present. Sedimentation rate and CPK are usually elevated. Muscle biopsy showing inflammatory changes and lymphocytic infiltration usually establishes the diagnosis. Treatment with corticosteroids has proved quite effective in polymyositis. Whereas some patients show partial or even full recovery, others continue on a relentless downhill course.

Other causes of muscle inflammation include trichinosis and certain bacterial or viral infections.

Myasthenia Gravis

Myasthenia gravis is a disease of neuromuscular transmission characterized by easy fatigability and muscle weakness. It may be (1) acquired, (2) congenital (frequently familial), or (3) transient neonatal in infants born to a myasthenic mother.

The onset of myasthenia gravis may be gradual or fairly sudden and is often precipitated by a mild respiratory infection. The eye muscles are commonly affected, causing diplopia or ptosis; general weakness may then follow. Characteristically the weakness is least marked on waking and increases with activity.

DIAGNOSIS. Electromyography shows rapid diminution in size of muscle potentials with sustained contraction. Muscle biopsy findings are not helpful. Antibodies to the acetylcholine receptor are elevated in "acquired" cases. Administration of a small dose of an anticholinesterase drug is a most useful diagnostic aid. Because of its rapid and short action, edrophonium chloride (Tensilon) is preferred. An intravenous injection of 1 or 2 mg causes marked increase in muscular strength of the myasthenic patient within 1 minute, the effect lasting no more than 10 minutes.

COURSE AND PROGNOSIS. The course of myasthenia gravis is marked by remissions and exacerbations, with a tendency toward general aggravation. Patients in whom the disease is confined to the ocular muscles have a better prognosis. In the newborn infant, especially if vigorous therapy is not instituted quickly, death is likely.

TREATMENT. Treatment consists in control of the weakness with an anticholinesterase preparation such as neostigmine (Prostigmin) or pyridostigmine (Mestinon). Dosage varies with each patient, depending on the response to the initial amount. Overdosage may cause toxic effects or a cholinergic crisis. The latter, presenting with sudden weakness, should not be confused with inadequate therapy. The antidote is atropine, which should always be at hand when such drugs are given parenterally. Thymectomy may be beneficial in some patients; however, there are no clear-cut criteria for predicting its value. Plasmapheresis is a valuable adjunct to treatment in some instances.

Infantile Hypotonia

Floppy baby is a descriptive term referring to excessive hypotonia in infants and children. Depending on the severity, the child may be unable to hold the head erect or sit unsupported, or may merely appear slow in motor development. It must be emphasized that this condition is not a specific entity but a common sign in a large number of disorders. Any myopathy, neuropathy, or other lower motor neuron disease may occur with severe hypotonia. Prematurity and certain conditions associated with mental defect often show a similar clinical picture. Floppiness is a universal finding in infants born with Down's syndrome. It is helpful to divide children with infantile hypotonia into two broad categories: those who in addition to the floppiness show muscular weakness, and those who do not. This differentiation is usually possible even among infants. By far the most common entity in the first group is the Werdnig-Hoffmann syndrome, accounting for about 90% of the total. The remaining 10% have "congenital myopathies" and such conditions as poliomyelitis, vascular or developmental lesions of the spinal cord, polymyositis, myasthenia gravis, polyneuropathy, and some very rare diseases. Ancillary investigations, including electromyography and muscle biopsy, are necessary to establish the diagnosis in this category. In the second group, with marked hypotonia in the absence of muscle weakness, a large number of conditions must be considered, including prematurity, Down's syndrome, mental defect, acute fevers, metabolic disorders, connective tissue disorders, and benign congenital hypotonia (the terms *amyotonia congenita* and *Oppenheim's disease*

are best discarded in favor of *benign congenital hypotonia*). As the name implies, the hypotonia in this condition is not progressive and may even improve with age. The current thinking is that this is not just one entity but a heterogeneous group of disorders with similar clinical manifestations.

Tumors

Intracranial tumors (see also Chapter 17, Neoplastic Diseases) are not uncommon in the pediatric age group. They are rare in the first year of life, increase in frequency up to the age of 8 years, and fall off as adolescence is approached. Males and females are equally affected.

The intracranial mass most often seen in children used to be tuberculoma. Although still not uncommon in certain parts of the world, tuberculoma is very rarely encountered in the more advanced countries. Gliomas account for about 75% of all intracranial tumors in this age group, of which 60% to 75% are located in the posterior fossa. There is a tendency for these tumors to arise from the central neural axis, in or near the third or fourth ventricles and the brain stem.

Clinical Manifestations

Signs and symptoms of intracranial tumors in children are due primarily to occupation of space within the cranium or to obstruction of the free flow of cerebrospinal fluid (which gives rise to increased intracranial pressure and hydrocephalus) and secondarily to the local effects of the tumor.

Because the skull of the infant can expand, clinical signs of increased intracranial pressure may not be evident early in the disease. Additional difficulties causing delay in diagnosis include the young child's inability to communicate and the paucity of other neurological signs when the lesion is situated in the central neural axis. Such delay is unfortunate because many tumors are amenable to effective therapy when detected early; therefore, careful and frequent examination of patients is essential in the prompt establishment of diagnosis.

The cardinal manifestations of increased intracranial pressure are (1) headache, which is usually generalized, intermittent, and worse on waking — in the young child, irritability may be the only sign; (2) vomiting, which is often forceful rather than projectile; and (3) papilledema, necessitating careful ophthalmoscopy, especially because children tend not to complain of visual difficulties until nearly blind. Other signs include a cracked-pot sound on percussion of the skull when hydrocephalus is present and, occasionally, a sixth nerve palsy due to increased pressure rather than to local compression by the tumor.

Any patient with the above features or hydrocephalus should be investigated thoroughly with CAT or MRI scans, especially because local signs may not be evident until much later. The local signs depend on the site of the lesion and are discussed under separate headings.

Tumors of the Posterior Fossa

Tumors of the posterior fossa tend to have the same clinical manifestations independent of their type. Increased intracranial pressure usually dominates the picture, with local signs appearing much later. Hydrocephalus or headache, vomiting, and papilledema are the initial features. Later, unsteadiness of gait with frequent falling, easy fatigability, general weakness, and nystagmus become apparent.

To determine the location of the mass, CCT or MRI are the most helpful; however, only surgical exploration can establish the definitive diagnosis.

The two common tumors at this site are cerebellar astrocytoma and medulloblastoma. The former is usually insidious in onset, has a longer course, and is often amenable to surgical removal. In contrast, medulloblastoma is a rapidly growing tumor with a relentlessly progressive course. Although it is highly sensitive to irradiation with roentgen rays, the eventual prognosis is poor; rarely is there a 5-year survival.

EPENDYMOMA. Ependymoma arising from the floor of the fourth ventricle is a less common tumor in this area. The clinical manifestations are similar in this and the other types, but often they are restricted to those of increased intracranial pressure. Because of its adherence to the floor of the fourth ventricle, surgical removal is hazardous and, at best, only partial. More favorable results have been claimed for surgery followed by x-irradiation.

GLIOMA OF THE BRAIN STEM. Brain stem gliomas are infiltrative lesions and thus usually do not produce increased intracranial pressure. The signs and symptoms are due only to the local effect of the tumor and consist of multiple cranial nerve palsies, pyramidal signs, and progressive ataxia. The tumor is frequently mistaken for encephalomyelitis, cerebral palsy, or poliomyelitis. Results of cerebrospinal fluid studies are usually normal. CAT scan, and especially MRI, and posterior fossa angiography frequently confirm the diagnosis. This tumor tends to advance rapidly, leading to death within a few months. X-irradiation is said to be helpful in some cases.

Supratentorial Tumors

CRANIOPHARYNGIOMA. Craniopharyngioma arises from cells of pharyngeal origin that migrate into the base of the skull during embryonic life and form the anterior pituitary body. It is a fairly common supratentorial mass in the first and second decades of life.

As may be expected from the location of the tumor, the clinical manifestations include (1) increased intracranial pressure, with headache and vomiting as frequent initial symptoms; (2) compression of the optic chiasm resulting in temporal-field defects; (3) pituitary gland dysfunctions causing retardation of growth, arrested skeletal development, or infantilism; and (4) when it extends to the hypothalamic area, listlessness, subnormal temperature, and polyuria.

Plain x-ray films of the skull show calcification in the tumor in a majority of patients. CAT scan or MRI can define the tumor even if it is very small.

Because, as a rule, the tumor cannot be completely removed, the prognosis is usually not favorable, although operation may improve vision and prolong life. Because of its intimate relation to the hypothalamus and pituitary, removal of the tumor necessitates intensive medical supervision during the postoperative period.

GLIOMAS OF THE CEREBRAL HEMISPHERES. These tumors are uncommon in children, constituting no more than 15% of the total, in contrast to adults. The diagnosis is often delayed because of the patient's inability to cooperate in assessment of such cortical functions as aphasia, apraxia, memory loss, or visual field defects. Headache may be the initial symptom, and papilledema may be discovered on ophthalmoscopy. Later, upper motor neuron weakness, evidenced by a disturbance of gait, appears. Epileptic seizures are rare. X-ray studies, especially CAT scan or MRI, are very helpful in establishing the diagnosis. Treatment consists in surgical removal of the tumor, but the results are disappointing.

Tumors of the Choroid Plexus

These uncommon tumors arise from the choroid plexus in the lateral ventricles, or that in the fourth ventricle. Because there is no invasion of the nervous tissue, the clinical manifestations are confined to hydrocephalus and increased intracranial pressure. CAT scan and MRI are useful in establishing the diagnosis. Treatment consists of surgical removal of the tumor. If total excision can be accomplished, the prognosis is good.

Intraspinal Tumors

Intraspinal tumors are rare in childhood, fortunately, because children seldom complain of sensory disturbance, and the diagnosis usually is delayed until the appearance of frank motor disability. Cerebrospinal fluid studies and roentgenography, including myelography, help to establish the diagnosis. The results of surgical intervention depend upon the type of tumor, but in general the prognosis is poor.

Brain Abscess

Brain abscess is uncommon except with certain predisposing conditions: pericranial infections (sinusitis, otitis media, mastoiditis, cranial osteomyelitis), penetrating head injuries, and cyanotic heart disease. The early stage of cerebritis is seldom recognized, especially with the widespread use of antibiotics.

Clinical Manifestations

The usual clinical picture is one of increased intracranial pressure due to an encapsulated abscess, presenting as a space-occupying lesion. Headache is common; papilledema, retinal hemorrhage, and separation of the cranial sutures indicate a critical stage. Localizing signs such as hemiplegia or cerebellar deficit may be present, but convulsions are seldom seen. Fever, leukocytosis, and other evidence of infection are often absent and should not be relied upon as a lead for diagnosis of cerebral abscess. The CSF may show some increase in cells and protein. Rupture of the abscess results in coma, shock, stiff neck, purulent CSF, and usually rapid death.

The electroencephalogram may localize the abscess or at least point to the involved hemisphere. CCT, MRI, or radionuclide brain scans are very efficient in the diagnosis, and contrast studies (arteriography or ventriculography) are not usually necessary. A needle puncture through a properly placed bur hole are both diagnostic and therapeutic.

Treatment

Treatment consists of immediate drainage. Delay of days, or even hours, can result in fatality. Block resection of the abscess may be indicated. Antibiotics are given systematically and may be instilled directly into the abscess cavity.

Epidural Abscess

Recognition of acute transection of the spinal cord, with paralysis and hypesthesia below the level of transection, is always a surgical emergency, because restoration of function depends on the rapidity with which pressure can be relieved. Epidural abscess should be suspected in any child with signs of infection (particularly staphylococcal), evidence of spinal cord transection, and local tenderness over the spine.

William T. McLean, Jr., and Mohsen Ziai

References

Adams, R. D., and Lyon, G. *Neurology of Hereditary Metabolic Diseases of Children*. Washington, DC: Hemisphere, 1982.

Aicardi, J. *Epilepsy in Children — International Review of Child Neurology*. New York: Raven, 1986.

Bell, W. E., and McCormick, W. F. *Neurologic Infections in Children — Major Problems in Clinical Pediatrics* (2nd ed.). Philadelphia: Saunders, 1981. Vol. 12.

Brooke, M. *A Clinician's View of Neuromuscular Disease* (2nd ed.). Baltimore: Williams & Wilkins, 1986.

Cohen, M. E., and Duffner, P. K. *Brain Tumors in Children — International Review of Child Neurology*. New York: Raven, 1984.

Dreifuss, F. E. *Pediatric Epileptology*. Boston: John Wright–PSG, 1983.

Engel, A. G., and Banker, B. Q. *Myology*. New York: McGraw Hill, 1986.

Menkes, J. H. *Textbook of Child Neurology* (3rd ed.). Philadelphia: Lea & Febiger, 1985.

Roach, E. S., and Riela, A. R. *Pediatric Cerebrovascular Disorders*. Mt. Kisco, NY: Futura, 1988.

Swaiman, K. F. *Pediatrics Neurology — Principles and Practice*. St. Louis: Mosby, 1989.

Volpe, J. J. *Neurology of the Newborn — Major Problems in Clinical Pediatrics* (2nd ed.). Philadelphia: Saunders, 1987. Vol. 22.

15

The Skeletal System

The kinship between pediatrics and orthopedics is as significant as their etymological derivation suggests. The pediatrician's function is largely that of prevention and diagnosis. Awareness and utilization of developing medical knowledge results in a substantial reduction of disabling conditions.

There remain, however, many conditions that demand the combined attention of pediatrician and orthopedist. This requires the knowledge to participate in a decision, to advocate restraint, or to endorse vigorous surgical procedures — in essence, to be child oriented, not system oriented.

One cannot overemphasize the importance of completely undressing the child for a discriminating survey of the musculoskeletal system.

Many of the major orthopedic deformities can be diagnosed in the neonatal period and their treatment started in the nursery.

In study of the musculoskeletal system a few general clinical concepts must be emphasized. In the first place, no other group of diseases exhibits such extreme variability. It is common to study a single disease entity with three constant features and ten inconstant features. Second, musculoskeletal disorders exemplify the concept of overlapping clinical entities: Systemic bone diseases do not stop and start at well-defined clinical signposts; they merge into one another along a spectral band, very much like the collagen vascular diseases. It is, therefore, essential that one not be frustrated by the refusal of some patients and their problems to fit snugly into a textbook description of a specific entity. Third, the pediatrician should always examine the radiographs and not rely completely on their interpretation by the radiologist. Fourth, children with bone diseases must be evaluated as individuals, and their individual needs must be met. Fifth, because many of these disorders are familial, one should make a complete and exhaustive analysis of the ancestry of each patient. An understanding of the principles of genetics, together with an appreciation of the place of genetic counseling and chromosome analysis in clinical pediatrics, is essential. Finally, the presence of a single congenital anomaly should start the clinician on a careful search for other abnormalities.

Congenital Abnormalities

One of the main elements in examining the newborn infant is the assessment of musculoskeletal integrity. The physician must estimate all of its parts and recognize whether they are augmented, reduced, distorted, or weakened and must be alert to the clues that suggest concurrent involvement of other systems.

Deformities of the Chest Wall

A variety of deformities of the ribs and sternum occur, many of which are symptomatic and amenable to operative correction. This must, however, be decided upon with considerable scrutiny after ample observation of the patient, preferably with serial photographs.

STERNAL CLEFTS. Complete cleft of the sternum is extremely rare, as is congenital absence of the sternum. There may be true ectopia cordis in which the heart, sometimes not covered by either skin or pericardium, lies well anterior to the chest wall. In this event the heart is usually grossly abnormal, and the infant rarely survives, though surgery is advisable.

Superior Clefts of the Sternum. These clefts have often been considered examples of cervical thoracic ectopia cordis because of the abnormal prominence and pulsation of the heart in what seems to be the neck. In fact, the heart is not displaced cephalad. In the neonatal period, the halves of the sternum can be directly brought together in the midline. In later childhood, relaxing chondrotomies may be required. If operation is delayed still longer, prosthetic reconstruction of the defects is all that is possible.

Distal Clefts of the Sternum. These clefts occur either alone or as a part of a pentalogy of defects — sternal cleft, ventral abdominal omphalocelelike defect, diaphragmatic defect, pericardial defect, and cardiac malformation, usually a ventricular septal defect. The sternal and abdominal defects should be corrected as early as possible. The cardiac defect may be corrected according to the specific indications for the given lesion.

DEPRESSION DEFORMITIES OF THE STERNUM. These are the most commonly seen deformities of the chest wall. Pectus excavatum (funnel chest) is an incurvation of the costal cartilages with a depression of the sternum. The incurvation of the sternum usually begins at the second or third interspace, and the depth and breadth of the deformity vary markedly. The deformity is usually asymptomatic. In older children, some decrease in exercise tolerance occurs. The associated postural deformity — kyphosis, rounded shoulders, and forward-thrust head — is conspicuous. This,

together with the sternal deformity itself, renders these children self-conscious and frequently interferes with their social activities. Surgical intervention satisfactorily corrects the sternal defect.

PROTRUSION DEFORMITIES OF THE STERNUM. Protrusion deformities (pectus carinatum, pigeon breast, chicken breast) are less stereotyped than the depression deformities. There is an abnormal prominence of the sternum, much of which is caused by depression of the costal cartilages on either side. The sternum itself may be somewhat more prominent than usual and arched forward; equally commonly, the distal end may tip backward. The deformity may be quite grotesque, requiring correction for this reason alone. The correction consists in elevating the depressed costal cartilages to either side of the sternum.

Absence of the pectoralis major and minor muscles; absence of the costal cartilages of the second, third, and fourth ribs; and deformity of the sternum — this association of deformities is the only one of the large variety of congenital deformities of the ribs that occurs with some regularity. Increase in the deformity with age, conspicuous paradoxical motion of the chest wall, and exposure of the thoracic viscera, particularly the heart, all indicate the advisability of operative correction, which is accomplished by a combination of prosthetic coverage and rib-strut implantations.

Deformities of the Extremities

Certain incapacitating conditions affecting the extremities, described below, usually occur in association with rather severe congenital malformation affecting other parts of the body and are, therefore, likely to be incompatible with life. Some of them have been observed in patients whose mothers ingested thalidomide during gestation.

Brachydactyly is shortness of hands and fingers, sometimes due to missing phalanges. Brachydactyly may be seen in association with pseudohypoparathyroidism. It may also be inherited as an autosomal dominant trait. There is no treatment.

Amelia is complete absence of all extremities, while ectromelia is absence of one limb. In hemimelia the distal portions of the limb are defective; this is the characteristic anomaly produced by the prenatal maternal ingestion of thalidomide. Rhizomelia refers to shortness of proximal portions of limbs, and mesomelia is shortness of distal portions of limbs. Early fitting of prosthetic devices and supportive care by a team of experts have made rehabilitation and a reasonably happy life possible.

Syndactyly — that is, fusion of digits, usually by soft tissue bridges — may be found as an isolated benign affection in certain sibships or be associated with severe congenital malformations. Surgical treatment of the isolated defect usually produces good results. Both sides of the digit can be released at one stage. Recently an association between syndactyly and learning disabilities has been noted.

Polydactyly (supernumerary digits) may be seen as an isolated finding or in association with other deformities (e.g., Laurence-Moon-Biedl syndrome or chondroectodermal dysplasia). It may also be inherited as a dominant trait. Operative removal of the extra digit may be carried out.

Absence of the radii, one of the more common anomalies, may be found as an isolated anomaly of the skeletal system or be associated with other systemic problems (e.g., thrombocytopenia and congenital hypoplastic anemia). The Holt-Oram and the Vater syndromes include radial anomalies.

SPRENGEL'S DEFORMITY. In this condition the scapula fails to descend normally. Usually the displacement occurs on one side and is associated with an omovertebral connection of bony or fibrous nature. Surgical repair, involving the removal of the omovertebral connection, is generally successful and is done for cosmetic reasons and improvement of motion.

KLIPPEL-FEIL SYNDROME. This anomaly involves the vertebral column, occurring with fusion or absence of cervical vertebrae, or both. Fortunately, in the majority of cases only two to three cervical vertebrae are involved, but in severe forms all of the cervical and many of the thoracic vertebrae may be deformed. Most of the patients with more extensive involvement have other associated deformities: hemivertebrae, vertebral arch, clefts, spina bifida, and rib malformations. Motion of the neck is usually limited, and the patient often has a low hairline. Some patients have Sprengel's deformity. Certain neurological symptoms may also appear. Webbing of the neck can be deceptive and may simulate that seen in Turner's syndrome. There is no effective treatment except for correction of the webbing of the neck for cosmetic reasons.

Generalized Diseases of Bone

Osteogenesis Imperfecta

Insignificant trauma as is caused by hand shaking or diaper changing may lead to fractures in the pathetic group of children who have osteogenesis imperfecta. Blue sclerae and otosclerosis, the latter resulting in deafness, may be associated findings. The disease may be so severe in its congenital form as to cause death. Milder forms are compatible with long life.

X-ray studies of the skeleton show the cortex of the bones

to be thin and discontinuous and the mineral content reduced. Fractures heal well, and serious deformities can be avoided by appropriate treatment.

These children are small but not necessarily confined to the limited life of a wheelchair. Intelligence is normal. Most cases are inherited according to an autosomal dominant pattern. The treatment is supportive, consisting in rehabilitative measures. Magnesium oxide has been tried as a method of therapy. This therapy is still experimental as is the use of calcitonin.

Polyostotic Fibrous Dysplasia

This rare bone disease is characterized by thinning of the cortex and replacement of bone by fibrous tissue. Some patients may have the lesion confined to one area, while others have several lesions, usually restricted to one side of the body. Those who also suffer from precocious puberty and skin pigmentation are said to have McCune-Albright disease, a condition that is more common in girls than in boys. If the osseous lesion is large and either causing or potentially causing a pathological fracture, it may be excised and treated with a bone graft. The cause of this condition is unknown.

Pseudohypoparathyroidism

See Chapter 6, The Endocrine Glands.

Chronic Glomerular and Tubular Diseases

See Chapter 13, The Genitourinary System.

Idiopathic Hypercalcemia

Idiopathic hypercalcemia may be benign and evanescent or protracted and serious. The only stable features of the syndrome are failure to thrive and an elevated serum calcium level. In addition, one may find osteopetrosis, craniostenosis, supravalvular aortic stenosis, nephrocalcinosis, and tissue deposits of calcium salts. Many of the infants have a typical facies, labeled elfin, with puckered lips, small nose, pointed chin, and widely spaced eyes. Developmental delay is common as is an outgoing friendly personality. This is now known as the Williams syndrome. Aortic valvulotomy should be considered.

Scurvy

The dramatic symptom complex appearing in sailors whose diets for many weeks were entirely devoid of fresh fruit and vegetables was one of the first deficiency diseases to be widely recognized and successfully prevented. In adults the typical clinical findings are swollen, bleeding gums, hemorrhage into the skin and other sites, weakness, listlessness, and shortness of breath; anemia of varying degrees may be present.

Infantile scurvy is most commonly due to the exclusive consumption of milk diets that have lost their ascorbic acid in processing; it is frequently misdiagnosed because the symptoms and signs mentioned above seldom are present.

CLINICAL MANIFESTATIONS. The chief early manifestation in infantile scurvy is the development of large subperiosteal hemorrhages. Scurvy is generally seen between the ages of 6 and 18 months. Because breast milk contains a fairly adequate supply of vitamin C, the condition is usually not seen in breast-fed infants. It most frequently involves the distal end of the femur and the proximal end of the humerus, causing excruciating pain, a great deal of screaming, and characteristic immobility in the frog-leg position.

X-RAY STUDIES. The subperiosteal hemorrhages described above are not obvious on roentgenograms until they become calcified, but other characteristic radiological signs can be found (Fig. 15-1).

The most useful diagnostic aids are the marked increase in capillary fragility and the very low concentration of ascorbic acid in the blood. Response to treatment with vitamin C is prompt and dramatic.

Rickets

Rickets (see also Chap. 8, Nutrition) is due to failure of calcification of growing bone in infancy and childhood and is seen most frequently in the temperate zones. The unavailability of calcium for ossification can be caused by inadequate intake or by failure of absorption due to chronic diarrhea, steatorrhea, an inappropriate intestinal calcium-phosphate ratio, or, most important, a deficiency of vitamin D due to inadequate exposure to sunlight or failure of hydroxylation by the liver or kidneys. Decreased serum calcium and inorganic phosphate levels are characteristically present, but marked elevation of serum alkaline phosphatase activity is the most valuable biochemical evidence of active rickets.

CLINICAL MANIFESTATIONS. When the concentration of ionized serum calcium is very low in infants, tetany may develop, with spasms of the hands and feet and of the vocal cords, the last resulting in a high-pitched, distressing cry and difficulty in breathing. Although osseous manifestations are most important, others may be present: restlessness, pallor, flabby muscles, and excessive sweating.

In infancy, craniotabes is frequently seen as the result of unossified areas in the membranous bones of the skull that yield to the pressure of the examining finger. After 6 months of age, it is more common to see "bossing" of the frontal and parietal bones and delayed closure of the fontanels. Exten-

Fig. 15-1. Scurvy and rickets. In scurvy (left), the epiphysis is heavily ringed with calcium and the periosteum is elevated, calcium being deposited subsequently; the location of fracture, usually incomplete, is at the thinned subepiphyseal zone. In rickets (right) there is lateral spread of diaphysis, with a wide zone of provisional calcification, a small epiphysis, and characteristic cupping.

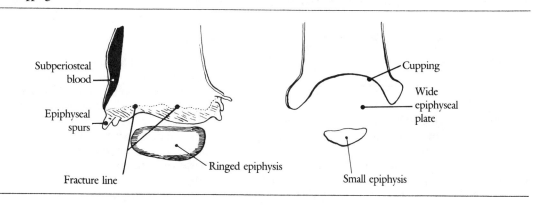

sion and widening of the epiphyses are clinically most obvious at the distal end of the radius and at the costochondral rib junctions, the latter causing the beading of the rachitic rosary. Abnormal ossification at the epiphyseal line is seen radiologically as a wide and irregular cartilage zone (see Fig. 15-1).

In later infancy and childhood the softness of bones results in chest deformities such as pigeon chest (pectus carinatum), Harrison's sulcus, kyphosis, enlargement of the lower ends of the femur, tibia, and fibula, deformities of the shafts with knock knees and bow legs, and pelvic deformities.

TREATMENT. Although appropriate treatment with supplementary dietary calcium and a single massive dose or prolonged moderate doses of vitamin D brings prompt correction of the biochemical abnormality and the epiphyseal widening, the skeletal deformities may persist; in some cases these deformities are amenable to corrective surgery.

Refractory Rickets (Resistant Rickets)

This is a hereditary disorder of varied etiology in which x-ray and physical findings of vitamin D–deficient rickets are found, including craniotabes, rachitic rosary, and prominent epiphyses at the wrists and ankles. The serum phosphorus concentration is low, the serum calcium is usually normal, and the alkaline phosphatase activity is elevated (see also Chap. 13). X-ray findings consist of increased width of uncalcified bone at the epiphyses, frayed epiphyses, cupping of epiphyses, and double contour along lateral edges of long bones.

TREATMENT. Patients may require as much as 100,000 to 300,000 units of vitamin D daily to bring about satisfactory healing of the rickets. Care must be taken to avoid producing hypercalcemia. With early treatment the epiphyseal lesions will heal. In those who are treated late and who have serious deformities, surgical correction may be instituted.

Infantile Cortical Hyperostosis (Caffey's Disease)

This disease has disappeared.

Hypervitaminosis A

The administration of 50,000 units or more of vitamin A daily for at least 3 months may result in clinical and radiographic evidences of toxicity. Eating excessive amounts of liver or carrots may also be toxic. The patients are irritable and move poorly. They have tender, hard lumps over the affected bones. Loss of hair is common. The serum level of vitamin A is elevated. Infants given large doses of vitamin A may have increased intracranial pressure and a bulging fontanel (see Appendix A, Section 2). The foolish use of vitamin A to treat adolescent acne must alert the physician to the occurrence of this syndrome in the teenage group.

X-RAY STUDIES. Roentgenography reveals hyperplasia of subperiosteal bone, with the ulna and the long and the metatarsal bones being primarily involved.

TREATMENT. These children respond readily to the cessation of vitamin A administration.

Hypophosphatasia

The nature of this severe bone disease is poorly understood. Severe forms produce neonatal death. Mild forms are associated with spontaneous improvement and are compatible with long life. Inheritance is X-linked dominant.

CLINICAL MANIFESTATIONS. The presenting clinical features may be related to a wide variety of complaints, including rachitic bone changes, craniosynostosis, failure to thrive, premature loss of deciduous teeth, and dimpling or bowing of the extremities.

X-RAY FINDINGS. The x-ray films show changes identical with those of rickets. There is generalized reduction of mineralization. The x-ray examination of the newborn infant with severe hypophosphatasia shows the extraordinary picture of the whole infant with practically no calcium visible. A few scattered flecks may be seen at the base of the skull.

LABORATORY STUDIES. The serum alkaline phosphatase concentration is low, the calcium level is normal or high, and the phosphate level is normal. The excretion of phosphorylethanolamine in the urine is increased. Presumably this is related to the lack of utilization of a phosphorylated substrate by osteoblasts in the formation of bone because of the absence of alkaline phosphatases.

TREATMENT. Steroid therapy may be of benefit.

Osteopetrosis

Osteopetrosis (Albers-Schönberg disease) is characterized by a defect that causes bone formation to proceed more rapidly than bone resorption. It results in very dense bones radiologically and is characterized clinically by the development of increased intracranial pressure, anemia, and splenomegaly due to extramedullary hematopoiesis. Thrombocytopenia is also present in most cases. Children with osteopetrosis seek medical help because of shortness of stature (not dwarfism), fractures, signs related to poor hematopoiesis due to inadequate quantities of bone marrow, deafness, cataracts, optic atrophy, or osteomyelitis. The teeth tend to be abnormal. Success in treatment of this condition by bone marrow transplantation has been encouraging.

Osteoporosis is a condition in which the bone matrix is defective. It occurs in protein-calorie malnutrition.

Osteomalacia is a term used to characterize bone disorders in which mineralization of the osteoid in diaphyseal bone is defective. This condition is not to be confused with other metabolic bone diseases in which there is failure of production of bone matrix. Osteomalacia is similar to rickets in its pathological and pathophysiological picture except that the latter occurs in children before epiphyseal closure.

Arachnodactyly (Marfan's Syndrome)

Arachnodactyly is characterized by long, slender extremities (Fig. 15-2B), usually associated with kyphoscoliosis, dislocation of lenses, and medial necrosis of the aorta and occasionally with septal and valvular cardiac defects, most commonly mitral valve prolapse and spontaneous pneumothorax. Treatment is directed to the specific anomaly involved. A relative's early death from ruptured aneurysm should alert the physician to a diagnosis of this disorder. Some patients reach adult life, and, therefore, the prognosis is not always grim. Inheritance is autosomal dominant.

Chondrodystrophy

Chondrodystrophy (see also Chapter 9, The Newborn Infant) is a hereditary disorder characterized by abnormal body proportions. Affected children achieve a median height of 96 cm (37.8 in.) as adults. Endochondral bone formation is defective all over the body, and the patient may have nasal and eustachian tube obstruction; hydrocephalus also occurs, but mentality is normal.

X-RAY FEATURES. Bones are short, with normal caliber, cupped metaphyses, and frayed epiphyses (Fig. 15-2A). The mineral content of the bones is normal. The fibula is longer than the tibia, the acetabular roof is flat, and the intervertebral disks are often herniated.

Mucopolysaccharidoses

The mucopolysaccharidoses constitute a group of familial disorders characterized by abnormal metabolism of mucopolysaccharides, with their accumulation in many cells. Six types have so far been described, including Hurler's (gargoylism), Hunter's, and Morquio's syndromes. Some affect the nervous system, causing progressive mental deteriora-

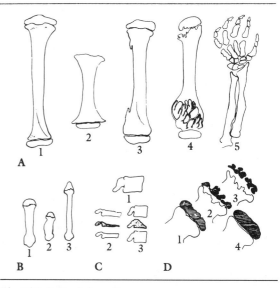

Fig. 15-2. Systemic bone diseases.
  A. 1, Normal tibia; 2, chondrodystrophy — short cylindrical bones of normal caliber, and with unimpaired periosteal osteogenesis; 3, exostoses — starting at epiphysis and receding with the growth of bone (occasionally much larger disfigurement); 4, Ollier's disease — abnormal proliferation of disorganized cartilage cells; and 5, Hurler's disease (gargoylism) — misshapen radius and ulna with angulation of distal ends (clawhand).
  B. 1, Normal metacarpal; 2, misshapen, tapering metacarpal of Hurler's disease; and 3, arachnodactyly (Marfan's syndrome) — elongated, slender bone (spider finger).
  C. 1, Normal vertebra; 2, Morquio's disease (eccentro-osteochondrodysplasia) — flattened vertebra; and 3, Hurler's disease — shortened vertebra, often with concavities anterior and posterior (collapsed vertebra producing kyphosis depicted).
  D. Osteochondrosis of the hip (Legg-Calvé-Perthes disease) showing 1, early stage; 2, fragmentation, flattening clearly visible; 3, advanced stage, and 4, restoration with flattened head — acetabulum adjusts to this alteration.

tion. Other manifestations include dwarfism, misshapen skull, neck, and spine, stiff joints, clouding of the cornea, deafness, and hepatosplenomegaly. Recently mitral valve abnormalities have been reported. They are all recessively inherited. The diagnosis is established by detecting excessive mucopolysaccharides in the urine. More refined methods are used to differentiate the various types.

In Morquio's disease (eccentro-osteochondrodysplasia) the children are dwarfed. The trunk is short, and the sternum bulges anteriorly. They have knock knees and severe kyphosis. The teeth are defective, and corneal opacities may be present. Mentality is normal. X-ray studies reveal wedge-shaped vertebral bodies (Fig. 15-2C) and bizarre bone shapes, with changes similar to those of healed rickets. Surgical treatment is possible.

In Hurler's disease (gargoylism) the child characteristically is short, ugly, and mentally retarded. The liver and spleen are enlarged. The tongue is large and thick. The skin is also thick, presumably because of the storage of excessive amounts of mucopolysaccharides. The corneas are cloudy and the hands wide and spadelike. Some leukocytes may have diagnostic changes, especially those in the bone marrow. Abnormal granulations (Reilly bodies) of certain leukocytes can be demonstrated. Excretion of specific mucopolysaccharides in the urine is increased. X-ray studies reveal short vertebral bodies with concavities anteriorly and posteriorly (see Fig. 15-2C), cylindrical phalanges, tapering metaphyses with a thick cortex (see Fig. 15-2B), irregular epiphyses, elongated sella turcica, and concave mandibular condyles. There is no specific therapy, but recent advances in genetic engineering may soon provide us with a practical way to provide the child with the missing enzyme.

Chondrodystrophia Calcificans Congenita (Conradi's Disease)

In this condition, also called dysplasia epiphysialis punctata, the children are short and have a saddle nose, cataracts, and skin problems. The karyotype is normal. Optic atrophy and a wide variety of other inconstant anomalies may also be present. On x-ray study the wrist and ankle bones are seen to be represented by scattered flecks that represent calcium in malacic cartilage. Tracheal cartilages are calcified sometimes producing respiratory embarrassment. Epiphyses are stippled as in hypothyroidism. There is no effective treatment.

Chondroectodermal Dysplasia (Ellis-Van Creveld Syndrome)

Children with this condition are short and have polydactyly, chondrodystrophy, and ectodermal anomalies. Congenital cardiac anomalies are common. X-ray study reveals short, thick long bones with primary involvement of the distal end of the long bones. Prognosis depends on associated malformations. Congenital heart disease may be treated medically and surgically. Significant hand deformities can be treated by surgery.

Dyschondroplasia (Ollier's Disease)

Ollier's disease (see Fig. 15-2A) is manifested by failure of ossification at the ends of long bones. The patient has unequal bone growth or pathological fracture. The bones are broad and short. Bony swellings, which are multiple and often unilateral, are internal proliferations of cartilage considered the equivalent of the external proliferations seen in multiple hereditary exostosis. On x-ray study, islands of nonmineralized cartilage give the appearance of defective cortex with areas of rarefaction that tend to be unilateral. Corrective orthopedic surgery may be helpful. Inheritance is dominant.

Neoplasms

The two common malignant bone tumors of childhood are Ewing's tumor and osteogenic sarcoma. Both usually occur as swellings, although pathological fracture may be the first reason for consulting the physician. Ewing's tumor may mimic osteomyelitis with fever and even moderate leukocytosis. With the combination of surgery, radiation therapy, and chemotherapy, the prognosis for osteogenic sarcoma as well as Ewing's tumor is improving. (See also Chap. 17)

The common benign bone tumors include bone cysts, giant-cell tumor, and osteoid osteoma. The last lesion tends to be painful. These tumors also occur as swellings or pathological fractures. They are usually treated by excision and packing with bone chips.

Positional Deformities

Positional deformities are usually congenital, but a few occur after birth. They are produced by the compactly folded position of the fetus in utero. The newborn infant may be found to have torticollis, a long total curve of the spine, adduction deformity of one hip, abduction deformity of the other hip, or internal tibial torsion with calcaneovalgus on the other side. Positional deformities usually respond well to simple exercises, which may be taught to the mother.

CONGENITAL TORTICOLLIS. Congenital torticollis is a contracture of obscure etiology involving one of the two sternocleidomastoid muscles. The infant's head is laterally flexed to the side of the contracture and rotated to the opposite side. Movements of the head in the reverse direction are restricted. A mass is often present in the center of the involved muscle at birth, although it may not be apparent for 10 to 14 days. Biopsy specimens from these masses prove them to be hematomas. Congenital torticollis may be associated with congenital dislocation of the hip as well as clubfoot.

Treatment. Early diagnosis and treatment often lead to rapid correction of the deformity (sometimes within 3 months); delay encourages the likelihood of persistent facial and skull asymmetry. Conservative treatment consists of exercises handled by the mother in the direction opposite to the deformity. Most children respond to this conservative management, and it usually averts any operative correction. Surgical correction is needed when proper treatment is delayed or unsuccessful. Its object is to lengthen the sternocleidomastoid muscle at one or both ends, depending on the severity of the deformity. The result is not successful unless an adequate program of postoperative exercise and bracing is used to maintain the correction and prevent recurrence.

BRACHIAL PALSY. See Chapter 9.

SPINA BIFIDA AND MENINGOCELE. See Chapter 14.

CONGENITAL DISLOCATION OF THE HIP. This serious malformation affects females more commonly than males. The diagnosis should be made at birth, well before weight bearing begins and secondary adaptive changes in the femoral head and acetabulum appear. There are predispositions to dislocation in children of American Indians.

Clinical Manifestations. The classic signs can be elicited in the nursery or at least in the first examination after discharge home. If one hip is involved, that extremity appears shorter than the other. There is asymmetry of the buttock and thigh folds. On the affected side, the trochanter appears more prominent and the thigh shorter. The femoral head is not felt under the femoral artery. If both limbs are placed in the frog position, abduction is restricted on the involved side. Furthermore, the examiner's hand may be able to reduce and dislocate the hip in this position, and a distinct click (Ortolani maneuver) may be felt (Fig. 15-3). On a push-pull motion of the extremities in flexion as well as extension, there may be more mobility on the involved side. If both hips are involved, most of these signs are bilateral, and the perineum seems wider and the thighs shorter than normal. These clinical findings are particularly helpful in the newborn infant when the radiological abnormalities may not yet be characteristic. Ultrasound examination is now preferred to x-ray examination for diagnosis.

Treatment. Treatment must be started without delay. The purpose of treatment is to restore the femoral head to a normal relationship with the acetabulum and thereby stimulate both to develop normally. The earlier this reduction is achieved, the better the prognosis.

In the infant, the position of abduction and external rotation, achieved by various splints, may be all that is

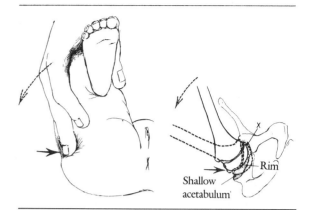

Fig. 15-3. Congenital dislocation of the hip. External abduction of the flexed thigh is limited. A click can occasionally be elicited as the femoral head slides over the rim of the acetabulum at X (Ortolani maneuver).

necessary. At the age of 1 month or older, closed reduction is carried out under anesthesia with x-ray control. The reduction should be maintained by plaster splints in the frog-leg position until there is radiological evidence that the hip is adequately developed; this may require 9 to 12 months of immobilization. When closed reduction cannot be achieved, open reduction, usually preceded by traction, is indicated.

Foot Deformities Present at Birth

The most common positional foot distortions (Fig. 15-4) — equinovarus, forefoot adduction, and calcaneovalgus — are differentiated from the classic fixed deformities by their ease of correction.

TALIPES EQUINOVARUS. The classic equinovarus (clubfoot) deformity present at birth is distinguishable from its positional counterpart by the incomplete correctability of the former with passive maneuvers. A thorough examination is essential to rule out other congenital deformities (torticollis and congenital dislocation of the hip) and associated problems (e.g., spina bifida) that may affect treatment.

Treatment. In the classic equinovarus deformity, the treatment of choice is manipulative correction followed by the application of plaster of paris. This must not be deferred until the child is "old enough to stand treatment." If the proper treatment is begun on the first day of life, good results can be anticipated.

Application of plaster casts needs to be repeated until the foot rests in a neutral position and x-ray films show satisfac-

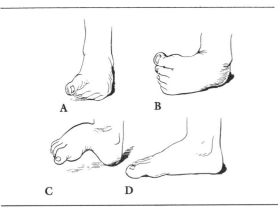

Fig. 15-4. A. Anteroposterior view of pes equinovarus. B. Lateral view of pes equinovarus; the entire foot is supinated, with torsion and generally with tight Achilles tendon pulling in equinus position. C. Pes cavus. D. Pes planus — normal for infants and small children and often painless, functional, and heritable.

tory bone alignment. When these goals are achieved, however, treatment must not be discontinued. When the child is ambulatory, special shoes are recommended to maintain correction. Various surgical procedures are available to correct those aspects of the deformity that do not respond to conservative measures.

Forefoot adduction in most cases responds well to stretching exercises and the application of valgus-reverse baby shoes. Casts may be required in severe cases.

Foot Deformities Developing After Birth

Most children pronate their feet as they first stand and walk. A 3-mm wedge applied to the inner side of each heel may be recommended at this time. If within 6 to 12 months the child's feet do not improve spontaneously, accessory support with longitudinal arch pads is advisable. Such support may be required throughout the period of growth to prevent ligamentous stretch and strain and to allow normal development of bones and joints.

Some children with apparently good feet assume a toe-out position and pronate their feet as they walk. Application of inner heel wedges when the pronation is mild, and long arch pads when it is significant, is beneficial in these cases. In many children, the pes planus (Fig. 15-4D) or pronation resists all treatment. Their deformities are often of a constitutional and familial nature and permit good function with-

out pain. Congenital heel-cord contractures cause flatfeet. Often mature heel-cord stretching and temporary heel raising are necessary. Genu valgum or genu varum exaggerates the tendency to heel valgus. The cavus foot (Fig. 15-4C) may be familial or caused by a neurological disorder. Treatment is by metatarsal support and stretching of the plantar fascia. Normal children do not need shoes. Low sneakers are entirely adequate.

TOEING IN (PIGEON TOE). Among the many reasons for the tendency to toe in are forefoot adduction, pronation (as a protective mechanism), internal torsion of the tibia, and internal-rotation contracture of the hip. Most cases of internal torsion of the tibia are corrected with adequate foot support and growth. When the deformity is significant, it is helpful to apply a night shoe splint with a short bar between the shoes. When the genu valgum (knock knees), ligamentous relaxation, and foot pronation are significant, such night support should be deferred, as it tends to aggravate genu valgum and pronation. Surgery is rarely needed for correction.

TOEING OUT. The toe-out position may be secondary to pronation, external torsion of the tibia, external-rotation contracture of the hip, congenital dislocation of the hip, and even slipped femoral capital epiphysis.

External tibial torsion is usually corrected with arch supports, 3-mm inner heel wedges, gait training, and growth. Surgical correction by osteotomy is rarely indicated. The management of slipped femoral capital epiphysis is described on page 300.

GENU VALGUM (KNOCK KNEES). Genu valgum may be familial or may be associated with pronated feet, ligamentous relaxation, and obesity. Severe degrees of genu valgum require osteotomy of the distal portion of the femur or proximal part of the tibia after the age of 6 or 7 years.

GENU VARUM (BOWLEGS). Bowlegs may be congenital, familial, positional, or rachitic in origin. In some cases osteochondrosis of the medial aspect of the proximal tibial epiphysis (Blount's disease) may be present. Mild degrees of genu varum and tibia vara are treated with an outer sole wedge, 3 mm thick. Operative correction by osteotomy is reserved for severe degrees of deformity that do not respond to conservative treatment. This approach should not be considered before the patient is 6 or 7 years of age.

Postural Deformities

The child first stands with a wide base and with the trunk forward. By 2 years of age, the usual compensatory curves are developed: As seen on side view, these curvatures are

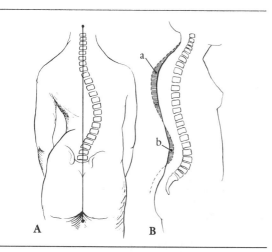

Fig. 15-5. A. Marked scoliosis of the spine showing primary curve; there is usually a secondary curve above and below (note rotation of body and drop of the shoulder that usually accompany the primary condition). B. a, Kyphosis; b, lordosis with broad zone of normal variation.

cervical lordosis, thoracic kyphosis, and lumbar lordosis (Fig. 15-5). Lumbar lordosis may persist longer in young girls than in boys. If by 8 years of age good posture is not achieved, a search must be made for possible causes.

Persistent lordosis may be due to a hip flexion deformity or spondylolisthesis. Significant thoracic kyphosis may be caused by epiphysitis.

SCOLIOSIS. There are two types of scoliosis, functional and structural. Functional scoliosis is related to poor posture or a discrepancy between the lengths of the two legs; there is no structural change or rotation of the spine. Postural exercises and correction of the leg-length discrepancy are sufficient for the treatment of this condition.

In structural scoliosis there are structural changes in the vertebrae. There are two or more curves, including a primary deforming curve and a compensatory one (Fig. 15-5A). The primary curve may decrease on recumbency but does not disappear unless it is minimal. This is a distinguishing feature between the functional and structural types of scoliosis.

In structural scoliosis there is rotation as well as lateral deviation of the spine. The rotation is often seen in the thoracic area on forward flexion of the spine. The ribs adapt to this, creating the classic "razor back" deformity. The

parents may note that one shoulder is held higher than the other and that one hip is more prominent.

It is striking that severe degrees of scoliosis may go unrecognized by parents for long periods. The physician, by regular assessments of the patient, is in a favorable position to identify structural scoliosis early and to refer patients for further treatment. X-ray studies are important. They testify to the extent, flexibility, and correctability of the curves. They may also help to identify some etiological factors such as congenital anomalies or neurofibromatosis. The majority of cases of structural scoliosis, however, have no identifiable underlying cause and are characterized as idiopathic. Girls are more commonly affected than boys. The spinal deformity may not be obvious until the age of puberty.

Treatment. In planning treatment, one must remember that the deformity progresses during the entire period of growth, and particularly during adolescence, when growth may be especially rapid. Treatment consists in attempts to produce good posture and maintenance of the flexibility of the curves as well as of the strength of the spinal musculature. All existing muscular contractures or discrepancy in the lengths of the two legs require treatment.

Removable jackets or braces, such as the Milwaukee brace, are used for support to prevent slumping and to maintain good posture. When a curve is cosmetically deforming, progressive in spite of treatment, and endangering cardiorespiratory function, surgical correction is ordinarily necessary.

Infections of the Skeletal System

Osteomyelitis

Osteomyelitis is seen at all ages, but most frequently in children. The hematogenous spread of infection from a distant focus, such as skin or respiratory tract, leads to localization in the bone. Although any bacterial organism can produce this pathological process, *Staphylococcus aureus* is the chief causative agent. Pathologically, an abscess forms in the metaphysis of a long bone and subsequently ruptures into the subperiosteal space. This subperiosteal abscess may totally denude the diaphysis of its periosteal blood supply; the whole shaft may die and become a sequestrum. The goal is to recognize this disease early, to identify the causative organism with its antibiotic sensitivity, and to begin prompt and massive antimicrobial therapy. By early treatment, the full evolution of this pathological process can be prevented, and the illness can be controlled.

CLINICAL MANIFESTATIONS. The child with osteomyelitis is systemically ill. There are high fever, local pain, swelling, and a tendency to guard the affected limb. Local tenderness and swelling are found over the metaphyseal lesion. There may be a confusing "sympathetic" sterile effusion of the neighboring joint. Due to the anatomic differences in an infant's blood supply, the infection may extend to the adjacent joint through the growth plate and present as septic arthritis.

DIAGNOSIS. Evidence of infection includes polymorphonuclear leukocytosis and elevation of the erythrocyte sedimentation rate. Repeated blood cultures constitute the most important laboratory test, but needle aspiration at the point of maximum tenderness and culture of the original focus when identifiable may also yield the causative organism. X-ray films taken in the early stages may show no bony defect and only soft tissue changes indicative of underlying infection. Radioisotope scanning is helpful in early stages.

TREATMENT. One should not wait for radiological confirmation before beginning treatment. Once the clinical diagnosis has been made and appropriate cultures have been obtained, vigorous antibiotic therapy with bactericidal agents must be started without delay. Patients with sickle-cell disease are especially susceptible to salmonella osteomyelitis. The recovery of uncommon bacterial agents may require modification of the drug problem. With early diagnosis and treatment, changes in the x-ray pictures may be absent or minimal.

Surgical drainage may be needed in children with osteomyelitis that does not rapidly respond to conservative treatment. Systemic chemotherapy is continued for at least 6 weeks. Recently oral therapy has been used following intravenous antibacterial therapy. After the initial intravenous antibiotic therapy, well-monitored oral treatment can be continued successfully.

Tuberculosis

In the initial dissemination from a primary tuberculous focus, bacilli may lodge in bones of the skeleton. In infants and young children dactylitis is the most common lesion. The carpals or the phalanges are involved with spindlelike swelling and tenderness. A single bone or several bones may be affected.

In older children the bodies of vertebrae are attacked, resulting in kyphotic deformity (Pott's disease). An abscess may form and may burrow and appear at the inguinal ligament. The joint usually involved is the hip joint, the disease commencing in the epiphysis of the head of the femur and erupting into the joint capsule.

These lesions are potentially disabling but cause initial symptoms that are mild and intermittent. Early suspicion and identification of tuberculous disease by roentgenography and tuberculin testing can avert prolonged incapacity and fixed disabling deformity.

See also Bacterial Infections in Chapter 20.

Congenital Syphilis

Syphilitic (Parrot's) pseudoparalysis may be confused with brachial plexus injury. This condition occurs as a result of osteochondritis and subepiphyseal fractures. Other signs of congenital syphilis, changes on x-ray films, and a positive serological test for syphilis permit the diagnosis of the condition.

See also Spirachetal Infections in Chapter 20.

Joint Sepsis

The usual sources of septic arthritis are hematogenous dissemination and spread from another focus, such as osteomyelitis. The most commonly involved joints are the hip and the knee, but other large joints may also be frequently affected. As in the case of osteomyelitis, all pathogenic bacteria can cause this infection, but *S. aureus,* hemolytic streptococcus, *Hemophilus influenzae,* pneumococcus, and salmonella are the most common organisms.

CLINICAL MANIFESTATIONS. Children with a septic joint are usually very ill and have a high fever. Their dislike of moving the affected limb may in infants produce pseudoparalysis. When superficial joints are involved, they are exquisitely painful and swollen. There is effusion and synovial thickening; all motions are extremely painful. A deep-seated joint such as the hip shows little superficial swelling in the early stages of the disease.

DIAGNOSIS AND TREATMENT. It is imperative to identify the organism and to begin vigorous and appropriate chemotherapy. Various bacteriological cultures, especially of blood, are helpful. Aspiration of the affected joint with meticulous surgical technique — in the operating room — is the most accurate way to establish a bacteriological diagnosis and provide drainage. *S. aureus* arthritis requires early surgical drainage because of cartilage destruction. The septic hip joint is considered a surgical emergency. Adequate drainage is essential as soon as the diagnosis is made to prevent destruction of the joint and an irreparable dislocation. Radioisotope scanning with technetium or gallium is useful when joint sepsis is suspected.

Aseptic Arthritis

Nonbacterial arthritis such as rheumatoid arthritis often requires orthopedic treatment to prevent deformity of the affected extremities (see also Chap. 18). Part-time application of removable casts and exercises should be recommended, while weight bearing on the affected extremity is deferred until complete resolution of the process.

Children with rheumatoid arthritis may have the fully developed clinical picture or involvement of a single joint. In the latter situation, adequate care may bring complete restoration of function. Failure to include orthopedic care in the management of the patient may result in fixed deformity of the involved joints. The adequate management of systemic arthritis, therefore, calls for the talents of both the pediatrician and the orthopedic surgeon.

Synovitis of the Hip

Toxic synovitis of the hip is a condition seen frequently by the pediatrician. Its benign nature and swift response to bedrest may reduce alertness to the important systemic conditions that often simulate it — for example, monarticular arthritis, tuberculosis, and coxa plana.

Nonspecific synovitis, identified by limitation of hip motion, is treated by the prevention of weight bearing until the synovial reaction in the affected hip joint subsides. Mild cases respond to strict bedrest for 3 to 7 days with nonsteroidal antiinflammatory drugs. In severe, persistent, or recurrent cases it is obligatory to complete a thorough investigation. The patients may require hospitalization and the application of traction. The clinical features may represent the early signs of aseptic necrosis of the head of the femur (Legg-Calvé-Perthes disease). Reexamination of the hip and repeat x-ray examination are advisable after full hip motion has been achieved.

Osteochondrosis

Osteochondrosis (aseptic necrosis) represents a group of disorders of unknown etiology. Although they are studied collectively, they may stem from different basic processes: They seem to be related to periods of growth, with involvement of many different bones (Fig. 15-6). Eponyms have been attached according to each of the bones involved, the more common ones being Legg-Calvé-Perthes disease (femoral capital epiphysis), Osgood-Schlatter disease (tibial tuberosity), Köhler's disease (tarsal scaphoid), Blount's disease (proximal shaft of the tibia), and Scheuermann's disease

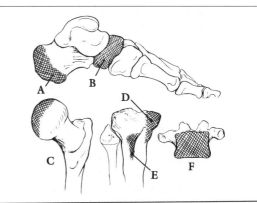

Fig. 15-6. Osteochondrosis. A. Calcaneus. B. Navicular (scaphoid). C. Head of femur. D. Proximal shaft of tibia (Blount's disease). E. Tibial tuberosity. F. Vertebra.

(vertebral body). Calcaneal apophysitis is also common but is usually not given an eponym.

The entire process ranges from distention of the joint capsule through focal necrosis, diffuse necrosis, compression, sclerosis, and healing. Recovery is spontaneous and generally seems to be unrelated to therapy. In Legg-Calvé-Perthes disease elimination of weight bearing is stressed from the point of view of trying to prevent adult problems with osteoarthritis of the hip. Understanding Scheuermann's disease is important because of its confusion with tuberculous osteomyelitis (Pott's disease) and discitis. These disorders are noted for the gradual onset of pain, spasm, and limitation of motion preceding any radiographic changes. It is important to remember that children with Legg-Calvé-Perthes disease often complain first of knee pain. In any black child with aseptic necrosis of bone the presence of hemoglobin S disease should be suspected. X-ray findings consist of patches of bone destruction, increasing areas of necrosis, sclerosis, and healing (see Fig. 15-2D).

OSTEOCHONDROSIS OF THE HIP (LEGG-CALVÉ-PERTHES DISEASE, CAVA PLANA). Osteochondrosis of the hip is a self-limited condition in which the femoral head is revascularized over a period of 2 to 4 years. The main principles in management are early diagnosis and prevention of the deformity of the femoral head. Traction for 2 or 3 weeks may be needed to decrease the synovial reaction.

The principle of treatment is to maintain the femoral head in the acetabulum. This is generally done by an apparatus that provides abduction and internal rotation.

When it is not possible to maintain the femoral head in the acetabulum because of deformity and overgrowth, it may be necessary to do a subtrochanteric osteotomy, providing varus and less anteversion to properly seat the femoral head in the acetabulum.

OSTEOCHONDROSIS OF TIBIAL TUBEROSITY (OSGOOD-SCHLATTER DISEASE). Much more frequently involved in osteochondrosis is the epiphysis of the anterior tibial tuberosity. This involvement is recognized by complaint of localized pain that is markedly aggravated by any strong quadriceps contraction. The condition is associated with swelling and tenderness; x-ray study reveals fragmentation or separation. Activities requiring knee bending should be reduced, and motion of knee restricted by use of elastic bandage. The duration of disability is 6 to 15 months.

CALCANEAL APOPHYSITIS. Quite frequently, fragmentation of the epiphyseal shelf occurs. It is usually assumed to be the result of a direct blow to the area, but possibly an abrupt pull of the Achilles tendon may be a factor. A pad in the shoe heel to protect and to reduce stretching of the tendon is useful to reduce pain until healing occurs.

Slipped Capital Femoral Epiphysis (Epiphysiolysis)

Mild dislocation of the femoral capital epiphysis is the main cause of hip difficulties in the adolescent. It is associated with periods of rapid growth and is more common in heavy boys than in girls. There is usually trivial pain and a minimal limp associated with mild limitation of motion and spasm on physical examination. Early physical signs are protective hip spasm, external-rotation restriction, and hyperextension of the hip. A high index of suspicion leads to radiographic examination and prompt confirmation of the diagnosis. The successful management of this condition depends on its early recognition and prompt institution of therapy before the process is advanced.

TREATMENT. The type of treatment depends upon the severity of the condition. Surgery is ordinarily the treatment of choice unless the epiphyseal plate is closed and the slip is minimal. If the slip is more than 1 cm, either an intraarticular or an extraarticular surgical procedure is necessary to realign the hip joint.

Trauma

An adequate discussion of traumatic injuries is beyond the scope of this pediatric textbook. Children lead a physically vigorous existence, and their ligamentous structures, awkwardness of movement, and intrepidity subject them to a high incidence of musculoskeletal disabilities. The practicing physician is, therefore, regularly confronted with sprains, fractures, and dislocations. Generally the physician sees these problems soon after the incident and is able to make significant observation before hemorrhage, edema, and muscle spasm obscure the basic findings. Distinction must be made between minor or simple conditions that the pediatrician can handle adequately and the major or more intricate ones that should be referred promptly for specialized orthopedic management.

Moderately disabling injuries require x-ray examination to ascertain the presence of fracture, either isolated or combined with sprains. Children, with bone structures more pliable and periosteum more abundant, are subject to incomplete or greenstick fractures. Moreover, their open growth lines are susceptible to displacement by stress, or transection by fracture. Either of these can distort later growth. Anyone who assumes the responsibility for management must be fully aware of the normal appearances of the sesamoid and supernumerary bones and the variations of epiphyseal configuration.

Even those injuries presumed to be uncomplicated must be checked in 7 to 10 days for satisfactory improvement. Lacking this, a reevaluation must be undertaken. X-ray films, originally normal, may now disclose unexpected callus formation or periosteal elevation, or the injury may have produced a ligamentous disruption more severe than that initially presumed.

All severe injuries, after first-aid care to ease pain and to prevent extension of the process, should be referred for immediate orthopedic attention.

One condition that the pediatrician treats more often than the orthopedist is subluxation of the head of the radius. It occurs in toddlers who are walking with arm held high by an accompanying adult. They stumble and are immediately jerked up by the arm in a position of extension. Pain in the elbow or referred to the wrist, restriction of use of the hand, and refusal to lift the arm above shoulder level are characteristic signs. With firm finger pressure applied to the head of the radius, supination and flexion of the forearm results in a return to a normal position in the annular ligament. This is accompanied by a distinct, palpable click. Recovery is swift and restoration of function dramatic. Recurrences are common.

Miscellaneous

TIETZE'S SYNDROME. This benign condition occurs with chest pain and swelling of the cartilaginous portions of the anterior ribs. Radiographs are normal. No treatment is necessary. It is important to know of this clinical entity whose cause is unknown simply to avoid putting the children through unnecessary diagnostic and therapeutic procedures.

Solomon J. Cohen and Mohsen Ziai

References

Harrison, H. E., and Harrison, H. C. *Disorders of Calcium and Phosphate Metabolism in Childhood and Adolescence.* Philadelphia: Saunders, 1979.

Lovell, W. W., and Winter, R. B. (Eds.). *Pediatric Orthopedics* (2nd ed.). Philadelphia: Lippincott, 1985.

Maroteaux, P., Beighton, P., Poznanski, A. K., et al. International nomenclature of constitutional diseases of bone with bibliography. *Birth Defects* 22:1, 1986.

16

The Blood

Anemia

Anemias of childhood can be classified into two broad categories: (1) those due to inadequate production of hemoglobin or erythrocytes or both, and (2) those due to an increased loss of erythrocytes. The reticulocyte count is low in the first and elevated in the second type. It is, therefore, a most helpful differentiating test. There are, of course, exceptions — when anemia results from a combination of circumstances, such as iron-deficiency anemia associated with chronic hemorrhage or aplastic crisis associated with chronic hemolytic anemia. Anemias of inadequate erythropoiesis are due to nutritional deficiencies or dependencies, to impairment of bone marrow function by infection, neoplasm, renal insufficiency, debilitating illness, or certain drugs, and to aplastic or hypoplastic bone marrow. Increased loss of erythrocytes may be caused by acute and chronic hemorrhage or by the various hemolytic anemias. An outline of the anemias follows:

I. Anemias due to inadequate production
   A. Iron-deficiency anemia
   B. Folic acid–deficiency anemia
   C. Vitamin B_{12}–deficiency anemia
   D. Vitamin dependency
      1. Pyridoxine-responsive anemia
      2. Thiamine-responsive anemia
   E. Aplastic anemia
      1. Congenital aplastic anemia (Fanconi's anemia)
      2. Acquired aplastic anemia
         a. Idiopathic aplastic anemia
         b. Aplastic anemia caused by toxins
         c. Aplastic anemia caused by malignant disease
   F. Hypoplastic anemia
   G. Other forms of anemia associated with inadequate erythropoiesis
II. Anemias due to excessive loss of erythrocytes
   A. Hemorrhage
   B. Idiopathic pulmonary hemosiderosis
   C. Hemolytic anemias
      1. Acute acquired hemolytic anemia
      2. Paroxysmal cold hemoglobinuria
      3. Infection
      4. Hypersplenism
      5. Toxins

6. Enzymatic defects of red blood cells
   a. Glucose 6-phosphate dehydrogenase deficiency
      (1) Primaquine-sensitive hemolytic anemia
      (2) Favism
      (3) Congenital nonspherocytic hemolytic anemia
   b. Pyruvate kinase deficiency (congenital nonspherocytic hemolytic anemia)
   c. Other red blood cell enzyme deficiencies
7. Other diseases associated with hemolytic anemia
   a. Collagen vascular diseases
   b. Microangiopathic hemolytic anemia
   c. Congenital hereditary spherocytosis
   d. Elliptocytosis
   e. Hereditary stomatocytosis
   f. Hemoglobinopathies

Anemias Due to Inadequate Production

IRON-DEFICIENCY ANEMIA. Iron deficiency is undoubtedly the most common cause of anemia during childhood. As a general rule, this should be the first diagnostic consideration in any anemic child until proved otherwise. Needless to say, the physician should not treat patients indiscriminately with iron over long periods without entertaining the possibility of other diagnoses. Iron is an integral part of the heme moiety of hemoglobin, and deficiency of this mineral results in inadequate hemoglobin synthesis.

Causes of Iron Deficiency. Iron deficiency can result from inadequate intake, inadequate absorption, inadequate utilization, or increased loss. It may also be due to insufficient iron stores of the infant, resulting from multiple births and especially prematurity. The incidence of iron-deficiency anemia is greatest between 6 months and 2 years. This is a period of rapid growth; the child's blood volume must be proportionately expanded; therefore, the requirement for iron is proportionately higher. The dietary intake of iron during this period is also most likely to be minimal because milk contains little iron. Failure of iron absorption may be the result of a malabsorption syndrome. A decreased concentration of transferrin in the patient's plasma may be associated with inadequate utilization of iron. This beta$_1$-globulin binds iron and transports it to the sites of erythropoiesis. Decreased concentrations of transferrin can occur with chronic infection or with hypoproteinemia from any cause. Increased loss of iron is ordinarily associated with chronic gastrointestinal hemorrhage in children. Sensitivity to cow's milk can result in an exudative enteropathy with the loss of red cells and protein. Iron deficiency per se can result

in the same type of enteropathy, which, of course, worsens the deficiency.

Clinical Manifestations. The infant with iron-deficiency anemia is usually on a diet consisting primarily of milk. Clinical symptoms related to the anemia are minimal as a rule, and the child tolerates a profound anemia with little difficulty unless infection occurs. A milk-fed infant is likely to be fat, pale, and sallow. There is usually anorexia and irritability, and there may be a history of pica in the older infant. A hemic murmur is often present, and if the anemia has been of long duration, some degree of cardiomegaly is also detected. Congestive cardiac failure due to anemia may occur, but it is quite rare unless some complication such as pneumonia develops. Significant hepatosplenomegaly, unrelated to cardiac failure, is also occasionally seen as is papilledema.

Laboratory Findings. The degree of anemia is variable, depending upon the severity of the deficiency. A smear of peripheral blood shows the red cells to be microcytic and hypochromic. There is some variation in the size and shape of the erythrocytes, but most are small, with only a rim of hemoglobin apparent around the periphery. Target cells and nucleated red blood cells may also be present. The white cells are usually normal, but the platelets may be increased or decreased in number. The reticulocyte count is probably decreased but may be normal. It is well to remember that reticulocytes are reported as a percentage of the total red cell count, and although the percentage may be reported as high as 4 to 5, the absolute number of reticulocytes is not increased. Examination of the bone marrow reveals erythroid hyperplasia with a predominance of normoblasts and absence of iron. The myeloid series is normal, as are the number and the morphology of the megakaryocytes. The serum iron is reduced below 60 μg/100 ml. The latent iron-binding capacity of the serum is usually as high as 450 μg/100 ml, and the serum ferritin concentration is less than 12 μg/ml.

In most situations, the diagnosis of iron-deficiency anemia can be made on the basis of the peripheral blood smear alone, if the characteristic hypochromia and microcytosis of the erythrocytes are present. Any anemia, however, that is characterized by inadequate hemoglobin synthesis, such as thalassemia or lead poisoning, is characterized by hypochromic microcytic erythrocytes.

Treatment. Therapy consists of the administration of iron. This is most conveniently given as an oral preparation in doses ranging between 4 and 6 mg/kg of elemental iron per day. Ferrous salts are absorbed better than ferric salts. The corresponding doses of ferrous sulfate are about 0.3 to 0.4 g/day in three divided doses. Iron should be administered between meals and not in conjunction with any other food. Therapy is generally continued for 2 or 3 months after restoration of the hemoglobin concentration to normal. Parenteral iron therapy can be used, but it is seldom necessary unless poor absorption is expected. If commercial preparations of iron are used, it is important to avoid combinations that contain various unnecessary compounds, such as vitamins. They make the treatment more expensive and confuse the picture, sometimes masking the basic process.

The first signs of recovery are loss of irritability and acceptance of solid food. The reticulocyte value begins to rise about the third day after the start of oral iron treatment, reaching a peak on the ninth day of therapy. The best test of the diagnosis of iron-deficiency anemia is an adequate hematological response to iron therapy.

Blood transfusions are seldom indicated in iron-deficiency anemia. Remarkable degrees of anemia are tolerated by children; unless there are some other complications, such as a serious infection, they can be easily and readily treated with oral iron. Anemia due to chronic infection or hypoproteinemia requires other specific measures. In chronic infection, there is an additional abnormality affecting the utilization of iron, and a hematological response is not observed until the infection has been properly treated.

FOLIC ACID–DEFICIENCY ANEMIA. Megaloblastic anemia of infancy is now a rarity, probably because ascorbic acid is included in most milk formulas. In parts of the world where malnutrition is uncommon, folic acid deficiency is usually associated with some type of malabsorption syndrome. The anemia associated with protein malnutrition or kwashiorkor is at least partially responsive to folic acid therapy; this anemia is complex and probably results from a deficiency of iron, folic acid, and protein itself. There are other conditions associated with folic acid deficiency. Children treated with folic acid antagonists such as methotrexate may show signs of folic acid deficiency. Rarely, the administration of phenytoin (Dilantin) or primidone (Mysoline) has resulted in the development of a megaloblastic anemia that responded to folic acid therapy. In certain cases of aplastic crises connected with chronic hemolytic anemias, particularly sickle-cell disease, relative folic acid deficiency has been reported to be of etiological importance.

Laboratory Findings. Folic acid deficiency is characterized by a macrocytic anemia, and sometimes moderate leukopenia and thrombocytopenia. The peripheral blood smear shows macrocytosis, anisocytosis, and poikilocytosis. The polymorphonuclear neutrophils are often large and hypersegmented; occasionally giant band cells are seen. Examination of the bone marrow reveals erythroid hyperplasia with megaloblastic erythropoiesis. The erythroid cells are large and have the characteristic cytoplasmic nuclear disassociation; there is also abnormal chromatin clumping of the nucleus. Giant myelocytes, metamyelocytes, and band forms are also seen.

Treatment. Treatment consists of oral or parenteral folic acid administration. If the cause of the folic acid deficiency is a malabsorption syndrome, therapy is best given by intramuscular injection of 5 mg/day of folic acid over a period of approximately 2 weeks. A hematological response to folic acid is necessary to confirm the diagnosis.

VITAMIN B_{12}–DEFICIENCY ANEMIA. Deficiency of vitamin B_{12} can result from malabsorption or juvenile pernicious anemia. Megaloblastic anemia responsive to vitamin B_{12} administration has also been found in patients with various intestinal lesions such as strictures, fistulas, anastomoses, and the so-called blind-loop syndrome. The clinical symptomatology of vitamin B_{12} deficiency is related primarily to the anemia but can also be complicated by subacute combined degeneration of the spinal cord. Glossitis and a beefy red tongue with papillary atrophy may also be seen.

The hematological findings are indistinguishable from those of folic acid deficiency. The peripheral blood smear as well as the findings in the bone marrow can be identical. There are three types of so-called juvenile pernicious anemia: congenital intrinsic factor deficiency with normal gastric mucosa and HCl excretion; a congenital selective abnormality in vitamin B_{12} absorption with normal intrinsic factor, gastric mucosa, and gastric HCl secretion; and true pernicious anemia.

Treatment. Therapy consists of parenteral administration of about 25 μg/day of vitamin B_{12} over a period of 2 weeks to a month, followed by injection of 100 μg of the vitamin every month. Megaloblastic anemia is rare in children. It is important to differentiate between folic acid and vitamin B_{12} deficiency because of the neurological complications of the latter. A hematological response in vitamin B_{12} deficiency can be obtained with large doses of folic acid, but, of course, folic acid has no effect on the development of the neurological complications. Blind therapy of undiagnosed anemia with iron preparations containing folic acid can, therefore, be very harmful.

VITAMIN DEPENDENCY ANEMIAS. *Pyridoxine-Responsive Anemia.* This rare disorder is characterized by early onset; hypochromic, microcytic anemia; and increased serum iron and iron stores with numerous sideroblasts, some of which may be ringed, in the bone marrow. The patients respond to superphysiological amounts of pyridoxine. Isonicotinic acid hydrazide (INH) is an antagonist of pyridoxine, and its administration to patients with tuberculosis may rarely be associated with a pyridoxine-responsive anemia.

Thiamine-Responsive Anemia. There have been some reports of children with severe megaloblastic anemia responsive to superphysiological amounts of thiamine.

APLASTIC ANEMIA. *Congenital Aplastic Anemia (Fanconi's Anemia).* This is a rare congenital disease characterized by the association of aplastic anemia with a variety of other abnormalities such as a bronze pigmentation of the skin, dwarfism, mental retardation, abnormalities of the skeletal system, renal abnormalities, and cardiac malformations. It is apparently transmitted as an autosomal recessive. The onset of anemia can come anywhere from 1 to 20 years of age, but it is most frequently seen around 4 to 6 years.

The hematological examination shows a normocytic, normochromic anemia, leukopenia, and thrombocytopenia. The reticulocyte count is low, and the bone marrow is usually quite hypocellular, but some areas of erythropoiesis can be seen. Congenital aplastic anemia is also characterized by a number of chromosomal defects, particularly chromosomal breakages. Surviving patients also have an increased risk of developing a malignant disease. The treatment of this disease is discussed below under the general topic of aplastic anemia.

Acquired Aplastic Anemia. Acquired aplastic anemia is usually classified as follows:

1. Idiopathic. Anemia of unknown etiology, occurring at any age. The hematological findings are essentially the same as with any aplastic anemia with a peripheral pancytopenia, a normochromic anemia, leukopenia, thrombocytopenia, and hypocellular bone marrow.
2. Toxic. Anemia caused by a variety of toxins. The most important of these are chloramphenicol and benzene derivatives. Various antineoplastic drugs such as methotrexate, 6-mercaptopurine, and nitrogen mustard, as well as radiation, are also known bone marrow depressants. Infectious hepatitis has been associated with a particularly severe form of aplastic anemia.
3. Malignant. Aplastic anemia caused by invasion of the bone marrow by malignant cells, as in leukemia and lymphosarcoma.

Treatment of Aplastic Anemia. Aplastic anemia is a severe disease associated with significant mortality. Before the final diagnosis is made, it must be confirmed beyond reasonable doubt. When looking at a bone marrow aspirate, it is difficult to tell whether the hypocellularity observed reflects the true state of the marrow or is a result of a technically poor aspirate. For this reason, to confirm the diagnosis of any aplastic anemia, a needle biopsy specimen of the bone marrow should be obtained.

Androgens and corticosteroids have been recommended as specific therapy for aplastic anemia. Corticosteroids have been given in the form of prednisone, 2.2 mg/kg of body weight with the total daily dose not to exceed 60 mg. Androgens have been given in the form of methyltestosterone, sublingual Linguets, 2.2 mg/kg of body weight with the total daily dose not to exceed 20 mg. The androgen oxymetholone has also been recommended. Several reports have indicated a 50% response rate to this form of therapy in patients with acquired aplastic anemia; however, studies have been presented that question the efficacy of the treatment. A group of patients were treated with only supportive therapy, and they had a 50% recovery rate. In addition, long-term follow-up of a relatively large number of such patients showed a 70% mortality with little evidence that androgen therapy influenced the outcome. In severely affected patients, the best prognosis is probably offered by bone marrow transplant if a suitable sibling donor is available. In congenital aplastic anemia the efficacy of androgens is more convincing, although the patients usually require continual drug therapy. Death usually results from either hemorrhage or an overwhelming infection. Supportive therapy is given to combat these complications — blood transfusions when necessary, platelet transfusions during periods of hemorrhage, and antibiotic therapy for infections.

HYPOPLASTIC ANEMIA. Hypoplastic anemia is a congenital disease characterized by failure of erythropoiesis. The cause is unknown, the onset of symptoms usually occurring between 2 and 3 months of age, when the infant is found to be pale and anemic. The anemia is chronic and persistent. Clinical features are related to the severity of anemia. The hematological findings reveal a normocytic, normochromic anemia with a normal number of platelets and white blood cells; the reticulocyte count is low. Bone marrow aspiration reveals decreased or virtually absent erythropoiesis with normal myelopoiesis and thrombopoiesis.

Hypoplastic anemia can also be acquired as an autoimmune disorder, a reaction to toxins or infections, or an idiopathic disorder that is transitory.

Treatment and Prognosis. Treatment consists of blood transfusions and administration of steroids. Prednisone, 2.2 mg/kg of body weight per day, may be used. If a hematological remission is achieved, the steroids are gradually decreased to the lowest level that maintains a normal hemoglobin level. Sometimes this can be an almost physiological dose of steroids. Approximately 50% of the children with the disease respond to steroids, and there is some evidence that the younger the patient is when therapy is instituted, the better the chance of a response. Patients who fail to respond to this treatment can be given repetitive transfusions, but they have a guarded prognosis, though spontaneous remissions do occur.

Other Forms of Anemia Associated with Inadequate Erythropoiesis

A variety of other diseases are associated with anemia as a result of inadequate production of red cells.

INFECTION. The anemia associated with infection is often complicated by concurrent iron deficiency; however, a depression of erythropoiesis and a moderate decrease in red cell survival are etiological factors as well. Some infections such as malaria can be associated with severe hemolysis.

JUVENILE RHEUMATOID ARTHRITIS. Some children with rheumatoid arthritis develop an anemia characterized by hypochromic, microcytic erythrocytes, low serum iron, normal or moderately decreased total iron-binding capacity, and increased iron stores in the bone marrow. Iron therapy is not effective, and the anemia responds only with control of the rheumatoid arthritis.

UREMIA. Children with chronic azotemia characteristically manifest anemia and growth retardation. The cause of the anemia observed in uremia is complex; it probably results from a combination of decreased erythropoiesis and decreased red cell survival.

LEAD POISONING. Children with lead poisoning typically manifest mild to moderate anemia. Lead interferes with the incorporation of iron into protoporphyrin to form heme; it may also interfere with the synthesis of protoporphyrin. As with any disease characterized by inadequate hemoglobin synthesis, the red cells are hypochromic and microcytic. Also present are the distinctive deep basophilic stippling of the red cells and an increase in the number of target cells. The reticulocyte count may be normal or slightly elevated. The platelets and white cells are unaffected.

It is well to remember that iron deficiency often occurs with lead poisoning.

OROTIC ACIDURIA. This is a hereditary disorder of pyrimidine metabolism characterized by megaloblastic anemia, growth retardation, mental retardation, and the excretion of large amounts of orotic acid in the urine. The patients have reduced activity of orotidylic pyrophosphorylase and orotidylic decarboxylase in their red cells and other tissues. They respond to the oral administration of uridine, which bypasses the metabolic block.

HYPOTHYROIDISM. Untreated hypothyroidism is often associated with a mild normocytic or slightly macrocytic anemia. The white cells and platelets are normal, and the reticulocyte count is low or normal. The bone marrow may be somewhat hypocellular or normal. The anemia is responsive to thyroid therapy.

Anemias Due to Excessive Loss of Erythrocytes

Erythrocytes may be lost by hemorrhage or by destruction. When the destruction is in excess of normal, a condition known as a hemolytic anemia results. Acute hemorrhage rarely constitutes a hematological problem unless it is associated with a hemorrhagic diathesis.

The anemia associated with chronic hemorrhage is normocytic and normochromic and is characterized by an elevated reticulocyte count. If the chronic hemorrhage is within an enclosed body cavity, as is the case with subdural or intraperitoneal hemorrhage, the bilirubin level, especially in young infants, may be found to be elevated. Chronic hemorrhage usually becomes complicated by iron deficiency; these factors cannot be differentiated except by history and the discovery of a bleeding source. Thus, in any child with iron-deficiency anemia it is advisable to make at least one stool examination for occult blood. If the child's dietary history is not typical of iron deficiency, or the age is atypical for this condition, a rigorous search for a site of chronic hemorrhage should be undertaken. In severe iron-deficiency states, however, small amounts of occult blood may be found in the stools.

IDIOPATHIC PULMONARY HEMOSIDEROSIS. This condition is characterized by the extravasation of blood into the lungs. Signs of pulmonary involvement develop with a severe hypochromic anemia. The reticulocyte count is not always elevated, as the disease is frequently complicated by iron deficiency.

Hemolytic Anemias

ACUTE ACQUIRED HEMOLYTIC ANEMIA. In some patients one cannot discover the underlying condition causing this disorder, but it is sometimes associated with infection, infectious mononucleosis, lupus erythematosus, or lymphoid neoplasms. The anemia is characterized by the presence of an autoantibody to the patient's red cells. This antibody is usually an IgG or IgM. The disease can occur at any time in childhood; it has even been reported in infants. The onset is usually abrupt, and the severity of symptoms is related to the degree of anemia. Clinical jaundice is often present, and splenomegaly is an almost invariable finding.

Laboratory Findings. The hematological picture is that of any hemolytic anemia. The severity can be of any degree. The reticulocyte count is elevated, and erythroid precursors can be seen in the peripheral blood. During the acute stage, the white cell count can also be markedly elevated, with a shift to the left; even metamyelocytes may be present in the peripheral blood. The platelet count is frequently elevated. The serum bilirubin and stool urobilinogen are increased. The characteristic finding in this disease is a positive direct Coomb's test. The indirect Coomb's test may also be positive. Erythrocytes often show some degree of spherocytosis and increased osmotic fragility; autohemolysis may be increased. Examination of the bone marrow reveals marked erythroid hyperplasia.

Treatment. The treatment of this disease depends in large measure on its severity. There are certain cases in which the hemolytic anemia is well compensated and no therapy is necessary. In most cases, however, some type of therapeutic measure must be undertaken — transfusion, steroid therapy, immunosuppressive agents, or splenectomy. It must be remembered in considering transfusion that the transfused cells are destroyed just as rapidly as the patient's own cells if the disease is due to a panagglutinin. If it is due to an antibody to a specific blood group factor, cells not containing this factor can be used for transfusion. Steroids in the form of prednisone, 2.2 mg/kg of body weight (1 mg/pound) per day, usually bring the disease under control. Before steroids were available, splenectomy was the only specific treatment, but at present this procedure is seldom indicated. If the steroid therapy must be prolonged or steroids must be given in such doses that toxic manifestations of the drug become a problem, immunosuppressants may then be considered. If, with the institution of steroid therapy, there is a hematological response, the drug is continued until the hemoglobin reaches its maximal level. The dose is then gradually tapered off and either finally discontinued or reduced to the level necessary for maintenance of a normal hemoglobin. The positive direct Coomb's test may remain positive for 1 to 1½ years; in some cases intermittent steroid therapy is required during this time.

PAROXYSMAL COLD HEMOGLOBINURIA. This acute hemolytic anemia is characterized by intravascular hemolysis, hemoglobinemia, and hemoglobinuria. The hemolysis is the result of an autoantibody that, in the presence of complement, combines with red cells in the cold and hemolyzes them on rewarming of the blood. This phenomenon is the basis of the Donath-Landsteiner test that is used to diagnose the disease. Paroxysmal cold hemoglobinuria occurs in association with a variety of infectious diseases. Symptoms are related to the hemolytic anemia; patients often give a history of exposure to the cold and subsequent warming. It is usually followed by the excretion of dark red urine.

Laboratory Findings. The hematological findings are those of any hemolytic anemia. Free hemoglobin may be found in the plasma as well as in the urine, depending upon the severity of the attack. Leukopenia may also occur during the height of an attack. Platelets are usually unaffected. The direct Coomb's test may be positive at the height of an attack but is usually negative. The diagnosis is made by the characteristic history of hemoglobinuria following exposure to cold and subsequent warming, a positive Donath-Landsteiner test, and the general evidence of a hemolytic anemia.

Treatment. There is no specific treatment except when the cause is known. The patient must be advised against exposure to cold.

HEMOLYTIC ANEMIA ASSOCIATED WITH INFECTION. Hemolytic anemia is often associated with a variety of infections, particularly those due to gram-negative bacteria, certain viral diseases such as infectious mononucleosis and primary atypical pneumonia, malaria, toxoplasmosis, giant-cell hepatitis, and cytomegalic inclusion disease. Some degree of hemolytic anemia has also been described in other infections. As a rule the symptoms are related to the infection itself, and the hemolytic anemia is of secondary importance. The hematological findings are those characteristic of any hemolytic anemia along with those characteristic of the infection. Treatment is directed primarily against the causative disease.

HEMOLYTIC ANEMIA ASSOCIATED WITH HYPERSPLENISM. Hypersplenism may be associated with any disease in which the spleen is enlarged; however, it is most frequently seen with portal hypertension resulting from cirrhosis of the liver or extrahepatic portal obstruction. The enlarged spleen sequesters peripheral blood elements. The clinical features are often primarily related to the underlying condition, unless anemia or thrombocytopenia is severe. The hematological findings show varying degrees of anemia, thrombocytopenia, and leukopenia, and the bone marrow is normal or slightly hyperplastic. The reticulocyte count is moderately elevated.

Treatment. Splenectomy would seem to be the treatment of choice; however, with the recognition of the increased risk of sudden overwhelming infection in splenectomized children, the operation is less frequently performed. Hypersplenism can often be ameliorated in the patient with portal hypertension by some type of shunt procedure. When the severity of the clinical situation warrants a splenectomy, the patient should be put on prophylactic antibiotics and immunized with pneumococcal vaccine. Also, the parents must be advised to seek immediate medical attention if their child develops fever.

HEMOLYTIC ANEMIA CAUSED BY TOXINS. Sufficient exposure to a variety of toxins can result in a hemolytic anemia. Examples are such compounds as benzene, trinitrotoluene, and nitrobenzene. Other toxic factors that cause hemolysis include certain snake venoms, the bite of the brown recluse spider, and severe third-degree burns.

HEMOLYTIC ANEMIA ASSOCIATED WITH ENZYMATIC DEFECTS OF RED CELLS. To maintain the ion concentration gradients and the hemoglobin in reduced form, the red cells require a source of energy and, therefore, the ability to utilize glucose. Prior to metabolism by the red cells, glucose must be phosphorylated to glucose phosphate. This process is accomplished by the transfer of high-energy phosphate from adenosine triphosphate (ATP) to glucose in the hexokinase reaction. The hexokinase activity appears to be the rate-limiting step to the utilization of glucose by the red cells and is relatively low compared to the activity of enzymes involved in later stages of glucose metabolism. Following phosphorylation, glucose may be metabolized either anaerobically or aerobically, although under normal conditions anaerobic glycolysis predominates. In this pathway, glucose metabolism involves several steps and results in the production of lactic acid. The derived energy is stored in the form of high-energy phosphate bonds by phosphorylation of adenosine diphosphate (ADP) to form ATP.

The oxidative pathway of glucose metabolism is the pentose phosphate pathway or hexose monophosphate shunt (see Fig. 7-1). Under normal conditions this pathway accounts for about 10% of the glucose utilized by the red cells.

Methylene blue and a number of other dyes, drugs such as acetylphenylhydrazine and primaquine, and certain physiological substances readily activate this route of metabolism. In this pathway glucose is taken through another route by glucose 6-phosphate dehydrogenase and is oxidized to 6-phosphogluconic acid. During the same step, nicotinamide-adenine dinucleotide (NADP) is reduced to NADPH. Subsequently, 6-phosphogluconic acid undergoes further oxidation through the action of 6-phosphogluconic dehydrogenase, which results in further reduction of NADP. The NADPH thus produced serves to maintain glutathione in the reduced form through the glutathione reductase system. Reduced glutathione (GSH) has major functions in the erythrocytes — namely, to protect the red cells from oxidative agents and to serve as coenzyme for several erythrocytic enzymes.

It is now recognized that certain drug-induced anemias as well as some chronic hemolytic anemias are associated with deficiency of one or more of the enzymes in the glycolytic pathway or pentose phosphate shunt.

Glucose 6-Phosphate Dehydrogenase Deficiency. The inheritance of glucose 6-phosphate dehydrogenase (G-6-PD) deficiency is X linked. The hemizygote males exhibit marked deficiency of this enzyme, with associated clinical features, while female heterozygotes may show only mild reduction of the activity of the enzyme, with no clinical manifestations. This widespread enzyme deficiency is associated with three main clinical manifestations, which are classified under three groups: (1) primaquine–sensitive hemolytic anemia; (2) favism; and (3) congenital nonspherocytic hemolytic anemia.

Primaquine–Sensitive Hemolytic Anemia. In affected persons a hemolytic anemia develops with the administration of a variety of drugs or chemicals. At least 40 such compounds — for example, primaquine, various sulfonamides, nitrofurantoin (Furadantin), aspirin (acetylsalicylic acid), phenacetin, synthetic vitamin K compounds, and naphthalene — have been incriminated. The disease occurs in blacks and certain peoples of Mediterranean origin and is a genetic disorder, being transmitted by a sex-linked gene. Males are fully affected and heterozygous females are asymptomatic or moderately affected. Red cells from affected individuals have a decreased concentration of G-6-PD. This enzyme is involved in the generation of NADPH in the pentose-phosphate pathway. NADPH functions with glutathione reductase to reduce oxidized glutathione. The primaquine–sensitive red cells, therefore, have a decreased concentration of reduced glutathione, and when these red cells are exposed to a drug such as acetylphenylhydrazine in vitro, the reduced glutathione concentration falls precipitously.

These persons are asymptomatic as long as they do not come into contact with one of the drugs or chemicals to which they are sensitive. With exposure to such compounds, a brisk hemolytic anemia ensues within 24 to 72 hours. Hemoglobinuria and icterus may develop. If the drug is continued, the hemolytic process goes on for 1 to 1½ weeks. After this period, however, even with continued administration of the drug, the hemoglobin starts to increase, and the hemolytic anemia becomes compensated. The reason is that with hemolytic anemia there is an outpouring of reticulocytes, and the population of circulating erythrocytes becomes quite young. The young erythrocytes are less susceptible to the effects of the drug because of a higher concentration of G-6-PD. If the drug is stopped, it takes several weeks before the patient is again susceptible to hemolytic anemia from further drug administration.

The hematological findings are those of any severe hemolytic anemia, with falling hemoglobin, rising reticulocyte count, icterus, hemoglobinemia, and sometimes hemoglobinuria. The presence of Heinz bodies is of diagnostic importance; these are observed by staining a wet preparation of the patient's blood with a supravital stain such as gentian violet. The diagnosis is made by one of a variety of screening tests available or actual assay of the enzyme, G-6-PD, in the patient's erythrocytes. Treatment consists in withdrawal of the offending drug. When the acute hemolytic reaction is severe, the patient may require immediate care, including blood transfusions.

Favism. Favism is mostly encountered among people of Mediterranean origin. The contact with fava bean or its pollens causes a severe hemolytic anemia in these persons, who often require multiple blood transfusions. The patients are also susceptible to drugs known to induce hemolysis in blacks with G-6-PD deficiency. In favism, the deficiency of erythrocyte G-6-PD is a necessary, but not a sufficient, factor in production of hemolysis; another factor, which seems to be of genetic origin, is involved. Furthermore, blacks with G-6-PD deficiency do not develop hemolytic anemia after the ingestion of fava beans.

Congenital Nonspherocytic Hemolytic Anemia. Unlike the more prevalent forms of G-6-PD deficiency, chronic hemolysis is seen in some persons without drug ingestion. Because the red cells are not spherocytic and the hemolysis can often be traced back to infancy or to the neonatal period, this condition is referred to as congenital nonspherocytic hemolytic anemia. The hemolytic process is usually mild, and the anemia is normochromic, normocytic, and of moderate degree; reticulocytosis is an expected finding. The osmotic fragility of the fresh blood is within normal range. The rate of autohemolysis is generally increased, but it is occasionally normal, in contrast to congenital spherocytosis. Splenectomy is of no help. The study of partially purified G-6-PD from the erythrocytes of patients with the above clinical manifestations has revealed great physiochemical variations, which may explain the heterogeneity of the clinical manifestations. There have now been 35 variants of G-6-PD described that are associated with chronic hemolytic anemia.

Erythrocyte Pyruvate Kinase Deficiency. Pyruvate kinase, an enzyme of the glycolytic pathway, is responsible for the interconversion of phosphoenolpyruvic acid to pyruvic acid. It is an important enzyme because through its action ATP is regenerated. Deficiency of this enzyme would result in inadequate synthesis of ATP and, in consequence, an inadequate source of energy for the red cells. In some patients with congenital nonspherocytic hemolytic anemia the erythrocytes have pyruvate kinase deficiency. This condition seems to be inherited as a mendelian recessive. The heterozygotes have about half of the normal enzyme levels in their erythrocytes. In the homozygotes the enzyme activity is almost absent. As expected, the level of ATP is below normal. Fourteen other separate deficiencies of erythrocytic enzymes have been described in patients with congenital hemolytic anemia. They are associated with either decreased production of the enzyme or an abnormal enzyme and are inherited as an autosomal recessive or sex-linked trait.

Other Causes of Red Cell Loss

Other causes of red cell loss include the following conditions: the collagen vascular diseases, thrombotic thrombocytopenic purpura, hemolytic uremic syndrome (see p. 259), congenital hereditary spherocytosis, elliptocytosis, and the hemoglobinopathies.

COLLAGEN VASCULAR DISEASES. Hemolytic anemia is often associated with the various collagen vascular diseases, particularly disseminated lupus erythematosus; it can often be the presenting symptom of this condition. There may be an associated positive direct Coomb's test.

MICROANGIOPATHIC HEMOLYTIC ANEMIA. Mechanical disruption of red cells is seen in hemolytic uremic syndrome, thrombotic thrombocytopenic purpura, disseminated intravascular coagulation, and the so-called Waring blender syndrome associated with cardiac prostheses. It is characterized by the presence of red cell fragments in the peripheral blood and hemolysis.

CONGENITAL HEREDITARY SPHEROCYTOSIS. This disease is transmitted as a simple mendelian dominant trait. It is characterized by the presence of spherocytic red cells in the peripheral blood that are selectively removed by the spleen at an increased rate.

Clinical Manifestations. The clinical symptoms are variable and may differ considerably from case to case. The onset can occur in infancy and result in icterus neonatorum. More often, however, the disease is not apparent until the child is somewhat older. There is generally a mild, well-compensated hemolytic anemia, but periods of increased anemia occur, often in association with infection. These episodes are referred to as crises. Splenomegaly develops after infancy. Because of the chronic hemolytic anemia, the incidence of gallstones is increased; symptoms referable to this complication may appear even in childhood.

Laboratory Findings. Hematological findings are those of any hemolytic anemia. Depending on the severity of the disease, the hemoglobin may range from normal to very low levels during periods of crisis. The reticulocyte count is elevated commensurate with the degree of hemolysis. The peripheral blood smear reveals the presence of numerous spherocytes as well as macrocytic, polychromatophilic erythrocytes, and normoblasts during periods of crisis. The specific finding in this disorder is marked increase in the osmotic fragility of the red blood cells. Occasionally it is possible to show this only after incubation. The bilirubin level is usually elevated, depending upon the severity of hemolysis.

Treatment. Since the spherocytes are selectively removed in the spleen, splenectomy relieves the patient of symptoms, although the surgery does not alter the abnormality of the red cells.

ELLIPTOCYTOSIS. In this genetic disorder, which is transmitted as a mendelian dominant trait, the erythrocytes are oval. Although usually asymptomatic, in certain individuals the disease may be symptomatic and produce a chronic hemolytic anemia. The onset of hemolysis may occur shortly after birth, resulting in icterus neonatorum. Splenomegaly is usually present.

Laboratory Findings. The hematological findings are characterized by the presence of numbers of elliptocytic erythrocytes in the peripheral blood. Polychromatophilia and even some normoblasts can be seen. The degree of anemia varies considerably from case to case but is usually compensated at only a moderate severity. In the neonatal period, the appearance of the peripheral blood can be very bizarre, with the red cells showing extreme anisocytosis, poikilocytosis, and fragmentation without many identifiable elliptocytes. As the child grows older, however, the morphology of the red cells becomes more characteristic of the disorder.

Treatment. The treatment is primarily symptomatic, but reports of beneficial effects of splenectomy are found in the medical literature.

HEREDITARY STOMATOCYTOSIS. This is a rare hereditary hemolytic anemia in which the red cells are cup shaped and the central area appears as a slit or mouth on the smear.

Hemoglobinopathies

There are a number of hereditary abnormalities of either hemoglobin structure or synthesis that result in anemia. Though a great number have been described, sickle cell disease and its variants and the thalassemia syndromes are clinically the most important.

SICKLE-CELL DISEASE. Sickle-cell disease is a congenital hemolytic anemia characterized by an abnormal hemoglobin. The trait is transmitted as a mendelian dominant, and the disease is a mendelian recessive. The abnormal hemoglobin has an abnormal electrophoretic migration and decreased solubility at lowered oxygen tension and lowered pH; it is the result of the substitution of valine for glutamic acid in the sixth residue of the beta chains of the hemoglobin molecule. This disease is found primarily in blacks. In the United States approximately 8.5% of blacks have the abnormal hemoglobin (sickle-cell trait), but only about 0.3 to 1.3% of these have the anemia.

Clinical Manifestations. In sickle-cell anemia the symptoms are related to the decreased life span of the red cells and to the formation of thrombi in the small blood vessels of various organs because of the abnormal biology of the affected cells. One of the features of these red cells is their tendency to sickle when exposed to low oxygen concentrations.

The onset of clinical symptoms can come as early as 7 weeks of age but more often does not appear until 6 months. The manifestations of the disease are protean and are characterized by a chronic hemolytic anemia and various types of "crises." These may be thrombotic, hypersequestration, aplastic, or a combination of all three. Although any organ system can be involved, the most commonly affected are the bones, abdominal organs, lungs, brain, and kidneys.

The first sign of the disease may be that the baby is colicky and fails to thrive. The mother may seek the advice of a physician because she has palpated the enlarged spleen in the upper left quadrant. Often the disease is first diagnosed somewhat incidentally in infants brought to the physician because of a severe infection such as pneumonia or meningitis. If this is not the case, the children start having painful crises in one anatomical area or another. One of the main types of crisis in young children with sickle-cell disease is the "hand-foot" syndrome — that is, involvement of the small bones of the hands and feet with swelling, tenderness, and redness. Cerebral vascular accidents may occur in sickle-cell disease and are sometimes the presenting symptom. The renal involvement is usually characterized by hematuria and an inability to concentrate urine. These children seem to have more frequent infections in general, often associated with crises, and are definitely more susceptible to severe infections with encapsulated organisms and *Salmonella.* Although the spleen is palpable in young children, at the end of childhood this organ is no longer palpable. The reason for the disappearance of the spleen is the recurrence of infarcts followed by fibrosis and shrinkage, a process known as autosplenectomy.

The major problem in sickle-cell disease, because of the variety of symptoms, is differentiating it from other diseases — for example, differentiating an acute abdominal crisis from appendicitis, or bone involvement of sickle-cell disease from osteomyelitis and rheumatic fever. In a black child, therefore, any bizarre symptoms associated with any degree of anemia should be considered sickle-cell disease until proved otherwise.

Laboratory Findings. Hematological study reveals a hemolytic anemia, with a hemoglobin concentration of around 7 g/100 ml, although with crisis this can be considerably lower. The anemia is normocytic and normochromic, and there is an elevated reticulocyte count. On smear of the peripheral blood, the red cells are characterized by anisocytosis and poikilocytosis, with some targeting and the appearance of sickle forms. Large polychromatophilic cells can also be seen, and normoblasts are almost invariably in evidence. Ordinarily the white cell count and platelet count are normal; during a crisis, however, leukocytosis is usually present. The serum bilirubin level is elevated, and the sickle-cell preparation is positive. The diagnosis is confirmed by the characteristic electrophoretic mobility of the patient's hemoglobin.

Treatment. The treatment is primarily symptomatic. If infection is present, it should be treated vigorously. A variety of specific therapeutic agents have been suggested, but none has yet proved to be of real benefit. If anemia is severe, transfusion should be employed, but there is nothing to be gained by raising the hemoglobin above the patient's normal level except under exceptional circumstances such as preoperatively or with severe cerebral vascular episodes. Oxygen and hydration are sometimes helpful. The use of prophylactic penicillin and immunization against the pneumococcus and *H. influenza* may reduce the incidence of these severe infections.

SICKLE-CELL TRAIT. This is the heterozygous form of sickle-cell disease and is essentially asymptomatic. Persons with sickle-cell trait are not anemic and are without the stigmas of sickle-cell disease, but the sickle-cell preparation is positive. The ability to concentrate urine is impaired and, occasionally they have hematuria. Under extreme conditions of hypoxia, such as being at high altitudes, they can have difficulty such as splenic infarction.

SICKLE-CELL–C DISEASE. This disease stems from the interaction of two abnormal hemoglobins — hemoglobin S and hemoglobin C. Hemoglobin C is a result of replacement of glutamic acid by lysine in the sixth residue of the beta chain of hemoglobin. The symptoms of SC disease are essentially those of sickle-cell disease except that they are usually milder. The crises are generally less severe, and the patients maintain higher hemoglobin levels, usually around 10 g/100 ml. The peripheral blood smear is characterized by numerous target cells. The distinguishing feature of the

disease, in contradistinction to sickle-cell disease, is its milder course, persistent splenomegaly, and typical demonstration of hemoglobins S and C by electrophoresis. When anemia is severe, blood transfusions may be required.

SICKLE-CELL–THALASSEMIA DISEASE. This disease, another variant of sickle-cell disease, occurs through the interaction of hemoglobin S with the thalassemia gene. The disorder is differentiated clinically by milder anemia, persistent splenomegaly, the presence of numerous target cells, and hypochromic, microcytic erythrocytes in the peripheral blood. The diagnosis is suggested by the presence of hemoglobin A, elevated levels of hemoglobin A_2, or increased concentrations of hemoglobin F on hemoglobin electrophoresis. It is confirmed by appropriate family studies of hemoglobin polypeptide synthesis.

THALASSEMIA MAJOR (COOLEY'S ANEMIA). Thalassemia is a congenital disorder characterized by the presence of increased concentrations of hemoglobin F or hemoglobin A_2 (or both), a decreased life span of red cells, ineffective erythropoiesis, and abnormal red cell formation. It occurs primarily in people of Mediterranean origin, although it has been described in black Americans. Thalassemia major represents the homozygous state and thalassemia minor the heterozygous form of thalassemia. The former is, therefore, the more severe.

Clinical Manifestations. The symptoms are related to progressive and unremitting anemia, expansion of the marrow cavities of the bones, and development of hemosiderosis, in part as a result of repetitive transfusions. The disease has an onset early in life and is clinically evidenced by the signs of anemia, gigantic splenomegaly, and the characteristic mongoloid facies, the result of marrow hypertrophy affecting the anatomy of facial bones. Patients are usually of small stature, pale, and somewhat icteric. The abdomen is protuberant because of the large spleen. X-ray films show the effects of the expanded bone marrow cavity, typically seen in the skull with the well-known "hair on end" appearance.

Laboratory Findings. Hematological studies reveal pronounced anemia. The reticulocyte count is elevated, but not tremendously. On a smear of the peripheral blood, red cells are predominantly microcytic and hypochromic, targeting is marked, and nucleated red cells are almost invariably found. Basophilic stippling can also be seen, and there are polychromatophilic cells as well as anisocytosis and poikilocytosis. The leukocytes and platelets are usually normal. Fetal hemoglobin values are notably elevated. The level of hemoglobin A_2 in thalassemia major is not high. The serum bilirubin may be slightly increased. The bone marrow reveals marked erythroid hyperplasia. The serum iron level is elevated, and the iron-binding protein is usually saturated.

Treatment. Because the anemia is progressive, most authorities agree that a program of hypertransfusion is the treatment of choice. The hemoglobin is maintained at around 10 g/100 ml by repetitive transfusions. Such programs prevent most of the complications associated with this disease. Hemosiderosis remains a problem, and no truly satisfactory chelating agent has been found, though the use of desferrioxamine on a regular basis has been reported to be of value. Most patients with thalassemia eventually undergo splenectomy, either because of the large size of the spleen or because of increasing transfusion requirements.

THALASSEMIA MINOR. Thalassemia minor is generally considered to be the heterozygous form of thalassemia. The clinical spectrum of thalassemia minor can run from extremely mild to moderately severe anemia. A smear of the peripheral blood shows the erythrocytes to be hypochromic and microcytic. Anisocytosis, poikilocytosis, targeting, elliptocytes, and normoblasts may also be present. The concentration of hemoglobin F may be normal or only slightly elevated, whereas that of hemoglobin A_2 is more often elevated. Splenomegaly is seldom seen, and transfusions are seldom required. The diagnosis of this disease is suggested in a patient with a mild anemia that is unresponsive to iron therapy and unassociated with iron deficiency; it is confirmed by discovery of some of the characteristic features of the abnormal erythrocyte morphology and by the finding of an increase of either hemoglobin F or hemoglobin A_2. Persons who are asymptomatic carriers of thalassemia can be identified by the presence of increased levels of hemoglobin A_2.

METHEMOGLOBINEMIA. Methemoglobinemia can be either congenital or acquired. This disease should be considered when there is cyanosis without any obvious explanation. Further evidence can be gained by taking a sample of venous blood and shaking it in the air; it does not become pink but retains a characteristic brown color.

Congenital methemoglobinemia may result either from the deficiency of an enzyme necessary to reduce methemoglobin when it is formed or from the presence of an abnormal hemoglobin, hemoglobin M. Acquired methemoglobinemia occurs as the result of ingestion of drugs or chemicals that oxidize the hemoglobin; most important of these are nitrites. Young infants are particularly susceptible to exposure to these toxic agents. Treatment of acquired methemoglobinemia is by intravenous administration of parenteral methylene blue, 1 to 2 mg/kg of body weight.

APLASTIC CRISIS. Aplastic crisis can occur in association with any chronic hemolytic anemia. It is particularly likely to occur in congenital hereditary spherocytosis and sickle-cell disease. It has also been reported in thalassemia major. The cause of aplastic crisis is not completely understood, but there is some evidence that it may be connected to a relative deficiency of folic acid. Recently an association with parvovirus infection has been described. For whatever reasons, during the course of the hemolytic anemia patients may develop a failure of erythropoiesis with a marked decrease or virtual absence of reticulocytes in the peripheral blood. Leukopenia and thrombocytopenia may occur as well. The bone marrow shows virtual absence of erythropoiesis, although occasionally large proerythroblasts are seen. Myelopoiesis may also be decreased, and there is often a shift to the left in the white cell series. The number of megakaryocytes may also be decreased. The failure of erythropoiesis in association with a hemolytic anemia represents a life-threatening situation. It is, therefore, important to obtain a reticulocyte count in patients with hemolytic anemias who are having a crisis, to determine that the erythroid response is adequate and an aplastic crisis is not developing.

Treatment. The treatment of aplastic crisis is primarily symptomatic, although folic acid therapy can be tried. The aplasia generally lasts from a week to 10 days, at which time the bone marrow spontaneously recovers.

F. Stanley Porter

Disorders of White Blood Cells

Leukopenia

Leukopenia may result from an increased rate of destruction or a decreased rate of production of white blood cells or a combination of both mechanisms.

ISOIMMUNE NEUTROPENIA. In the newborn infant the most common cause of leukopenia is infection; however, in some cases, isoimmunization with a mechanism resembling that of erythroblastosis may cause a transitory leukopenia immediately after birth. As in Rh sensitization, maternal antibodies are formed against the infant's leukocytes. They cross the placental barrier into the infant's circulation and produce leukopenia, which lasts from a few weeks to a few months after birth. In most instances, maternal antibodies may be demonstrated not only against the infant's leukocytes but also against the white blood cells from the father and other siblings, while no antibody is demonstrable against the mother's own white blood cells. The neutrophil specific antigens involved are NA1, NA2, NC1 and NB1. The treatment of autoimmune neutropenia is generally symptomatic using antibiotics appropriate for the infection. In severe neutropenia associated with life-threatening infection, plasma exchange is indicated. This could be followed by transfusion of granulocytes from the mother.

CYCLIC LEUKOPENIA. This condition is characterized by cyclic or periodic leukopenia associated with malaise, fever, headache, mouth ulcers, and furunculosis. Severe infections, however, are unusual. During the period of well-being the white cell count is normal and the patient is asymptomatic. The leukopenia precedes the clinical symptoms and lasts about 7 to 10 days, following which the white cell count returns to normal for 3 or 4 weeks. During the periods of illness, the bone marrow shows arrest of maturation at the level of myelocytes and promyelocytes.

A variety of investigations have revealed that cyclic neutropenia is the result of a regulatory abnormality involving early hemopoietic progenitor cells. Such a hypothesis is supported by observation of cyclic neutropenia that occurs as an inherited disease in collie dogs. In these animals the cyclic length is 12 days. Transplantation studies transferring marrow from normal dogs to affected animals abolishes the cyclic blood count fluctuation. Inversely, the disease can be transferred from affected to normal animals by marrow cell infusion.

LAZY LEUKOCYTE SYNDROME. This is a defect in neutrophil motility associated with recurrent stomatitis, gingivitis, otitis, and low-grade fever. The neutrophil count is low ($100-200/mm^3$). The bone marrow reveals adequate numbers of myeloid element with normal maturation. The peripheral blood and bone marrow morphology of neutrophils and phagocytic and bactericidal capacities are normal. The ability of the patient's neutrophils to accumulate in skin abrasion and to respond to endotoxin administration is abnormal. There are also abnormalities in both chemotactic ability and in random mobility of neutrophils. Thus the clinical manifestations are the result of both severe neutropenia and functional abnormalities.

SHWACHMAN SYNDROME. This is a combination of exocrine pancreatic insufficiency and neutropenia. Occasionally the patient may exhibit pancytopenia and bone marrow hypoplasia. This disorder seems to be inherited by an autosomal recessive gene. Approximately one-third of the patients also have metaphysical dysostosis.

It should be pointed out that neutropenia can occur as a prodromal sign of leukemia and acquired and constitutional aplastic anemia.

CHRONIC BENIGN GRANULOCYTOPENIA. A chronic course associated with repeated infections and diminished number of granulocytes in the peripheral blood is the major finding in this condition. The bone marrow reveals arrest of maturation. During infections there is usually transient leukocytosis with a shift to the left.

INFANTILE GENETIC AGRANULOCYTOSIS. Severe skin infection is the usual manifestation of this condition and is associated with granulocytopenia, leukopenia, and often eosinophilia and monocytosis. The mortality is high. This disease, which was described by Kostman, is transmitted as an autosomal recessive inheritance. Granulopoiesis is markedly reduced in the bone marrow. There is usually a decreased number of myeloid colonies. The colonies formed contain macrophages or eosinophils and not neutrophils. It has recently been found that the administration of granulocyte colony stimulating factor (GCSF) to these children can result in a substantial increase in the number of neutrophils and a significant decrease in the number of infectious episodes.

Leukocytosis

An increased rate of production of white blood cells, with entry into the blood stream, seems to be the usual mechanism for leukocytosis. The chief cause of leukocytosis in children is bacterial infection. Most of the infections produce granulocytosis, although some (e.g., pertussis) produce lymphocytosis, while others such as *Toxocara canis* infestations cause severe eosinophilia. There are also some noninfectious conditions that may lead to leukocytosis — for example, diabetic acidosis, serum sickness, convulsive seizures, paroxysmal tachycardia, burns, salicylate or hydrocarbon poisoning, ether anesthesia, postoperative states, and immunizations.

Leukemoid reaction is a benign increase in the number of granulocytes up to $30,000/mm^3$ or higher, with the appearance of mature myeloid cells in the blood. The usual cause of this condition is infection; occasionally, rheumatoid arthritis may lead to this phenomenon in infants.

INFECTIOUS LYMPHOCYTOSIS. This self-limited and benign disease is thought to be of infectious origin. The symptoms of a mild upper respiratory tract infection are usually seen early in the course. Fever, if present, is low grade; some patients may complain of abdominal pain or diarrhea. Occasionally a morbilliform rash is seen; there is no lymphadenopathy or hepatosplenomegaly. The white cell count is striking, ranging between 15,000 and $150,000/mm^3$, with the mature lymphocytes comprising more than 60% of the total count. There are no characteristic hematological abnormalities, and the number of platelets and the hemoglobin level are within normal range. The condition does not require any therapy.

INFECTIOUS MONONUCLEOSIS. See Section on Viral Diseases in Chapter 20.

Congenital Anomalies of Leukocytes

PELGER-HÜET ANOMALY. In this benign familial condition, none of the granulocyte nuclei has more than two lobes, a fact that may suggest a shift to the left. The findings persist, however, and are unrelated to infection.

CONGENITAL HYPERSEGMENTATION OF NEUTROPHILS. In this condition 1 or 2% of the neutrophils have nuclei with more than six lobes and are twice the size of normal neutrophils. The only possible confusion is with the hypersegmentation seen in megaloblastic anemias.

REILLY BODIES. Reilly bodies are coarse and fine granules, which, upon staining with Wright's stain, take various shades of color such as blue, purple, and red. The granules are usually seen in about 60% of the neutrophils of patients with Hurler's syndrome. The granules are the same as those noted by Alder as a hereditary anomaly.

DÖHLE BODIES. Döhle bodies are round or oval bluish bodies in the cytoplasm of polymorphonuclear neutrophils. This leukocyte anomaly appears particularly in patients with scarlet fever.

CHÉDIAK-HIGASHI ANOMALY. This anomaly consists in green-grayish, peroxidase-positive inclusion bodies in the cytoplasm of polymorphonuclear leukocytes; large, dark granules in the cytoplasm of lymphocytes; and eosinophils with giant granules. These findings may be present in the blood of patients with malignant lymphomas or may be associated with certain clinical manifestations, including nystagmus, photophobia, lymphadenopathy, and partial albinism. Hepatosplenomegaly may be present and is usually a terminal sign. The large granules seen within the leukocytes are giant lysosomes. Microscopic examination of the hair and skin reveals giant melanosomes, suggesting that the partial albinism is due to abnormal clumping of pigment rather than to decreased pigmentation. The phagocytosis is usually normal in these patients, but lysosomal degranulation into phagocytic vacuoles is impaired, and there is delayed bactericidal activity, particularly against staphylococcus. Recent studies have suggested that the basic abnormality in this disorder may be a defect in microtubular assembly associated with high intracellular cyclic adenosine monophosphate levels.

Nasrollah T. Shahidi

Hemostasis and Its Disorders

The cessation of bleeding and the transformation of blood from a liquid to a solid phase are triumphs of evolutionary protein interaction. The mechanisms are different, and thus there are diseases that primarily affect one function or the other. The *bleeding disorders* involve failure to stop bleeding when a blood vessel has been severed, generally due to qualitative or quantitative abnormalities of the platelets. For the practicing pediatrician these are by far the more common situations encountered in practice. The *clotting disorders* involve failure to make the transition from the liquid phase to the solid clot due to qualitative or quantitative abnormalities of the soluble clotting factors. There is also an interplay between platelets and clotting factors, and hence there are diseases involving both systems. As the clinical manifestations, investigation, and treatment of all these diseases are different, it is very important to have a clear understanding of the basic physiological principles.

Termination of Bleeding

There is a dynamic interplay between circulating platelets and blood vessel endothelial cells. The presence of platelets enhances the continuity of the endothelial lining, and a decrease in platelets predisposes to loss of vascular integrity — thence petechiae. Under normal circumstances platelets are produced by megakaryocytes in the bone marrow to survive for 8 days in the peripheral blood, and to be present in a concentration of 200,000 to 400,000/mm^3. When trauma exposes subendothelial tissue, platelets adhere to the site of damage. This adhesion is mediated by a high molecular weight protein, von Willebrand's factor (vWF), which itself is closely related to, but distinct from, the antihemophilic factor (factor VIII). Following adhesion, the platelets undergo a phase of primary aggregation in which there is a physical transformation from a discoid to spheroid shape, plus an extension of pseudopods. This occurs in response to collagen and ADP released from damaged subendothelial cells. These same stimuli cause endogenous ADP, which is stored in cytoplasmic platelet granules, to be released via canaliculi that connect with the platelet surface. This, in turn, enlarges the platelet plug by causing nearby platelets to aggregate and undergo a release reaction. Activation of the platelet begins when the membrane binding sites for collagen, ADP, or epinephrine are saturated. The critical mediator in this is arachidonic acid, which is normally present in the platelet membrane. This is released internally and undergoes conversion by the enzyme cyclooxygenase to a nonprostaglandin, thromboxane A$_2$. Thromboxane A$_2$ is a potent stimulant of endogenous ADP release and is also a powerful vasoconstrictor. As in all physiological systems, however, there is a delicate system of checks and balances that prevents an unending autocatalytic reaction. Intermediaries in the production of thromboxane A_2 enhance the release from vascular endothelial cells of prostaglandin I_2, which is an inhibitor of platelet aggregation and a powerful vasodilator.

The platelet plug takes only minutes to form and is stable for several hours. At that time, however, it undergoes dissolution, and the continuance of hemostasis thereafter depends upon the interim formation of the fibrin clot.

Disorders of Platelets and Blood Vessels

QUANTITATIVE PLATELET DISORDERS — THE THROMBOCYTOPENIAS. A decreased platelet count occurs when there is increased destruction of platelets, decreased production, abnormal distribution, or dilutional loss. Although the platelet count may be very low for any of these reasons, there is much less morbidity or mortality when the underlying problem is increased platelet destruction. This is due to the fact that the bone marrow is able to produce normal platelets that, though diminished in number, are young and metabolically active. Thus, a platelet count of $5000/mm^3$ in a child with idiopathic thrombocytopenic purpura does not have the worrisome significance it would have in a marrow failure syndrome such as leukemia or aplastic anemia. The exception to this rule is disseminated intravascular coagulation in which platelet function is abnormal and the soluble clotting factors are partially depleted as well.

Increased Destruction of Platelets. Idiopathic Thrombocytopenic Purpura (ITP). This is the most common acquired disorder of hemostasis in pediatric practice, one that a pediatrician is certain to encounter with some regularity. It is most commonly seen in children ages 2 to 8, but it may be seen at any age. The onset is usually sudden, often 1 to 3 weeks after a viral infection. Presumably this triggers an immune response in which the platelet is coated with antibody, and the complex is removed from the circulation within minutes or hours by the reticuloendothelial system. Transfused platelets suffer the same fate, so they are of no therapeutic value. A variety of tests for antiplatelet antibodies have been developed but are still rather imprecise and of little practical value in directing therapy.

Petechiae are extensive, especially on the legs and ankles, and frequently about the face and eyes if the child has been crying. There is no splenomegaly. The platelet count is usually below $40,000/mm^3$ and often below $5000/mm^3$. The white cell count is normal, as is the hemoglobin, unless there has been significant blood loss. In the peripheral smear the only abnormality is the number of platelets, 0 to 1 per oil immersion field instead of the usual 10 to 20. The few platelets present are larger than normal, because they are very young.

Bone marrow aspiration is advisable to exclude acute leukemia, especially if corticosteroids are to be administered. There are abundant megakaryocytes that are easily recognized under low power, and there is no monotonous infiltrate of blasts. It is well within the scope of the general pediatrician to perform the bone marrow procedure and interpret the findings when the diagnosis of ITP seems likely. When leukemia seems likely, because of hepatosplenomegaly, circulating blasts, or other criteria, immediate referral to a specialized center for cell marker studies of the marrow is essential.

Serious bleeding occurs in less than 1% of patients. Spontaneous recovery occurs within 3 weeks in about two of three patients whether they receive corticosteroids or not, and within 6 months in nine of ten patients. Whether or not to use corticosteroids is largely a matter of judgement. With children under 2 years and those over 12 it is probably wise to do so as the risk of bleeding is somewhat greater. The same is true for children with active bleeding, semiconfluent petechiae, and retinal hemorrhages. The dosage of prednisone is 60 mg/m^2/day, but this should not be continued beyond 3 weeks lest the treatment be more hazardous than the disease. Teenagers with extensive petechiae and younger children with active bleeding should receive intravenous gamma globulin 400 mg/kg for 5 days or 1.0 g/kg for 2 days. The response is very prompt, often within 24 hours. The main argument against routine use is cost; there is no risk of transmitting human immunodeficiency virus (HIV).

The pediatrician should not be frightened by ITP and should try to impart a sense of optimism to the family. Even in cases that extend beyond 6 months, spontaneous resolution can occur, although thought should be given to splenectomy. If the platelet count remains below $40,000/mm^3$ 2 years after diagnosis, and booster doses of intravenous gamma globulin are ineffective, splenectomy should be performed. The likelihood of success is 85%, although preoperative pneumococcal and *H. influenzae* vaccination and postoperative penicillin prophylaxis are necessary. Immunological suppression with vincristine, cyclophosphamide, or azathioprine can be used in the 1 to 2% of all patients in whom there is failure to respond to standard treatment.

Recurrence with minor viral infections is not rare, but it is usually not as severe as the primary episode. Underlying collagen diseases may be present in a small percentage of patients. A mother with chronic ITP has a significant chance of giving birth to an infant with transient thrombocytopenia. These infants should receive intravenous gamma globulin or steroids until the platelet count exceeds $20,000/mm^3$.

Neonatal Alloimmune Thrombocytopenia. This occurs in one in 3000 births, so it is a predictable occurrence in pediatric practice. Correct management is of great importance. These newborns have extensive petechiae at birth or shortly thereafter and a platelet count below $20,000/mm^3$. The etiology is analogous to that in erythroblastosis fetalis: the fetus and mother are of differing platelet types, the mother PL^{A1} negative, the fetus PL^{A1} positive. The mother develops an anti-PL^{A1} antibody that crosses the placenta to destroy the fetus's platelets. Fetal mortality may be 15% and morbidity an additional 15%. Treatment is a pediatric emergency, washed maternal platelets being given to the neonate as soon as possible. Steroids, random blood bank platelets, and intravenous gamma globulin are appropriate temporizing measures pending the preparation of maternal platelets.

Drug-Induced Thrombocytopenia. Even though rare in pediatrics, thrombocytopenia may be associated with almost any drug. It is most commonly seen with the following:

1. *Antibiotics, sulfonamides, and sulfonamide derivatives:* penicillin, ampicillin, nafcillin, cephalothin, rifampicin, INH, PAS, sulfisoxazole, trimethoprim-sulfamethoxazole, thiazides, acetazolamide, diazoxide, chlorpropamide, furosemide.
2. *Analgesics:* acetylsalicylic acid, acetaminophen, phenylbutazone
3. *Anticonvulsants:* phenytoin, barbiturates, sodium valproate, benzodiazepines
4. *Miscellaneous:* quinidine, alpha-methyldopa, chlorpheniramine, digoxin, gold salts, heparin, propylthiouracil, penicillamine, spironolactone

Various diagnostic tests are available but are not wholly reliable. Removal of likely drug offenders results in a rise in platelet count within a few days. Corticosteroids are of little or no value, but intravenous gamma globulin may hasten recovery.

Bacterial Sepsis. The presence of circulating bacteria, especially in neonates, often causes thrombocytopenia. This is probably a combination of shortened platelet survival plus marrow suppression. The platelet count is rarely below $20,000/mm^3$, and treatment need be directed only at the sepsis itself.

Disseminated Intravascular Coagulation. See page 321.

Hemolytic Uremic Syndrome. The renal vasculature is the target organ in a process of accelerated coagulation with entrapment and deposition of platelets. A platelet count less that $80,000/mm^3$ is present in nearly all patients, though bleeding is rarely a problem. This is a process of localized intravascular coagulation that is largely uninfluenced by anticoagulants or antiplatelet drugs. Treatment should be directed at sustaining kidney function until the process expends itself.

Thrombotic Thrombocytopenic Purpura. This is a much rarer though much more devastating disease of localized intravascular coagulation in which the target organ is the central nervous system. The etiology is unknown; the onset is fulminant in teenagers and young adults. Thrombocytopenia and hemolytic anemia occur together with bizarre and variable neurological signs. Treatment is plasma exchange transfusion or massive plasma infusion.

Cyanotic Congenital Heart Disease. Platelet counts of 60,000 to $100,000/mm^3$ with mild prolongations of prothrombin time (PT) and partial thromboplastin time (PTT) are very common in secondary polycythemia. The etiology is multifactorial — some shortening of platelet survival and clotting factor half-life and some suppression of synthesis. Bleeding is rarely, if ever, a problem. It is important to decrease the volume of anticoagulant in blood collection tubes in proportion to the increased hemoglobin concentration (and hence decreased plasma volume).

Indwelling Prostheses. Arterial catheters, arteriovenous fistulas, and prosthetic heart valves may absorb platelets or cause activation with shortened survival. This rarely causes any clinical problem.

Giant Hemangioma (Kasabach-Merritt Syndrome). The result of localized intravascular coagulation, this is rarely a cause of bleeding; it should be treated expectantly pending spontaneous resolution.

Phototherapy. Phototherapy may cause mild thrombocytopenia in the icteric neonate. It is clinically unimportant, but other causes of thrombocytopenia must be given proper consideration.

Decreased Production of Platelets. Thrombocytopenia is the most common abnormal laboratory finding in children with leukemia. Thus it is very unlikely that a child has leukemia if there is not concomitant thrombocytopenia. Because the risk of bleeding is much greater than in ITP the decision to use prophylactic platelet transfusions must be individualized. In the presence of sepsis, it is wise to transfuse platelets to keep the platelet count above $20,000/mm^3$.

Metastatic cancer, e.g., neuroblastoma or rhabdomyosarcoma, myelofibrosis, or miliary tuberculosis may also result in bone marrow failure. In the neonate, the TORCH (*T*oxoplasmosis, *r*ubella, *c*ytomegalic inclusion disease, *h*erpes simplex) infections may cause decreased platelet production.

Radiation Therapy, Chemotherapy, or Both. Moderate thrombocytopenia may result, but the platelet count rarely falls below 60,000/mm³. CCNU is probably the most potent long-acting marrow suppressor.

Aplastic Anemia. There may be isolated thrombocytopenia in the initial stages (see also p. 305) The use of platelet transfusions when the platelet count is below 20,000/mm³ must be individualized according to the clinical situation.

Thrombocytopenia-Absent Radius Syndrome. Apparent at birth, this syndrome is very uncommon. There is a lifelong moderate decrease in platelet count that is due to a decrease in megakaryocytes.

May-Hegglin Anomaly. A rare, dominantly inherited syndrome, this disorder is characterized by giant platelets and cytoplasmic Döhle's bodies in granulocytes.

Bernard-Soulier Syndrome. Variable thrombocytopenia is present in association with platelet dysfunction and giant platelets.

Wiskott-Aldrich Syndrome. Only males are affected by this syndrome. It is part of a complex immunodeficiency state involving helper T cells and is associated with eczema and decreased IgM production. Bone marrow transplantation is the definitive treatment.

Megaloblastic Anemias. Characterized by vitamin B_{12} or folic acid deficiency, these anemias are associated with marrow underproduction that can involve megakaryocytes as well as the red cell and white cell lines.

Abnormal Platelet Distribution. Any condition causing giant splenomegaly, e.g., Gaucher's disease, portal hypertension, and thalassemia major, can result in sequestration of large numbers of platelets. These are unavailable for hemostasis and may be removed prematurely by the reticuloendothelial system.

Dilution of Circulating Platelets. Extensive blood loss followed by replacement with nonplatelet-containing blood products results in dilution of a normal platelet pool. It is frequently seen postoperatively and is correctable by platelet transfusion.

QUALITATIVE PLATELET DISORDERS — THE THROMBO-CYTOPATHIAS. Abnormal platelet function may be acquired or congenital. There may be increased bruisability and postoperative or mucous membrane bleeding but rarely petechiae. The platelet count is normal, but the bleeding time is invariably prolonged. There are specific disorders for each of the three phases of the process that leads to the formation of the platelet plug: adhesion, primary aggregation, and secondary aggregation.

Disorders of Adhesion. von Willebrand's Disease. Strictly speaking the platelets are normal but are unable to adhere to the subendothelium because the bridging protein, von Willebrand's factor, (vWF), is missing. This is discussed further on page 320.

Disorders of Primary Aggregation. Glanzmann's Thrombasthenia. In this rare disorder the membrane receptor sites for ADP, collagen, and epinephrine are absent. Platelets adhere to subendothelium but do not aggregate to form a plug. Clinical bleeding is a serious problem, and treatment is platelet transfusion. Inheritance is autosomal recessive.

Milder variants with only partial dysfunction of the receptor sites may be more common than realized and the reason for some children's easy bruisability or postoperative bleeding.

Disorders of Secondary Aggregation. Aspirin Effect. Aspirin inhibits the enzyme cyclooxygenase that mediates the release of endogenous ADP. This in turn retards the formation of the definitive platelet plug. Aspirin affects some patients more than others, but the effect is universal. All platelets are affected by a single ingestion of as little as 60 mg, and the inhibition is irreversible for the lifetime of the platelet. Thus some prolongation of the bleeding time can be expected for 8 to 10 days following ingestion. All families should be advised to avoid aspirin for 10 full days prior to elective surgery, especially tonsillectomy and adenoidectomy.

Storage Pool Diseases. There are a variety of inherited diseases in which secondary aggregation cannot occur because of a lack of intracellular ADP. There may be an isolated platelet defect, or there may be additional clinical findings as in oculocutaneous albinism, Wiskott-Aldrich syndrome, or Chédiak-Higashi syndrome.

Miscellaneous Disorders of Platelet Function. There are a wide variety of conditions in which abnormal platelet function may be encountered. Bleeding may or may not be a problem, but when it is, the bleeding time is always prolonged. The precise effect on the platelets may not be clear, or the effect may be at several sites. Platelet transfusion is of temporary benefit. These conditions include:

1. The Neonate
2. Uremia
3. Liver disease
4. Cyanotic congenital heart disease, with or without thrombocytopenia
5. Myeloproliferative syndrome, acute and chronic myelocytic leukemia, myelofibrosis, polycythemia vera
6. Intake of various drugs:
   Indomethacin
   Sulfinpyrazone
   Dipyridamole (Persantine)
   Naproxen

Penicillin, ampicillin, carbenicillin, ticarcillin
Tricyclic antidepressants
Phenothiazines
Antihistamines
Guaifenesin (Robitussin)
Nitrofurantoin
Sodium valproate
Ethyl alcohol

VASCULAR PURPURAS. This is a broad category of diseases in which the platelet count and platelet function are normal, but the vascular integrity is decreased. Petechiae and purpura are present, but the bleeding time may or may not be prolonged.

Henoch-Schönlein Purpura (Allergic Vasculitis). Henoch-Schönlein purpura may be trivial or very severe. It is a multisystem disorder in which petechiae are the most prominent manifestation. These tend to cluster in the buttocks, along the lower limbs, or on the arms below the elbows. In children under 2 years they may be generalized. Often the petechiae are raised and thus palpable. Later they become brownish. Polyarthralgia and arthritis are seen in two of three patients, and abdominal pain in one of two. Renal involvement with gross or microscopic hematuria is seen in one of three children. This may persist for months or years with or without functional impairment.

The disorder often follows a minor infection, viral or streptococcal, and appears to result from the deposition of antigen-antibody complexes. It usually runs its course spontaneously in 1 to 3 weeks but has a frustrating tendency to wax and wane. There is no specific treatment, although prednisone should be considered for severe abdominal pain to avoid intussusception. Prednisone should be given for as short a period as possible and should not be given for rash or joint involvement alone.

Miscellaneous Causes of Vascular Purpura
1. Gram-negative sepsis; Rocky Mountain spotted fever
2. Ehlers-Danlos syndrome
3. Scurvy
4. Heredity hemorrhagic telangiectasia

THROMBOCYTOSIS. Platelet counts greater than 400,000/mm^3 are quite common. The usual causes are iron deficiency, recent blood loss, chronic inflammation, splenectomy, and vitamin E deficiency in the premature infant. Often no cause can be found. In the prepubertal child there is virtually no risk of hypercoagulability so no treatment need be considered. In the pubertal child, platelet counts greater than 1,000,000/mm^3 could possibly trigger patho-

logical thrombus formation, though data are scanty. It is recommended that 60 mg of acetylsalicylic acid be given twice weekly, enough to inhibit cyclooxygenase but not enough to stimulate prostaglandin I$_2$.

Clot Formation

At the same time that damaged subendothelial tissue activates platelets, nonspecific activating factors are released that initiate the process of converting soluble clotting factors to an insoluble protein clot. This takes longer than platelet plug formation but is more durable and acts as the infrastructure upon which tissue repair can occur. Limiting reactions are also initiated that prevent the clot from extending too far and lead to its ultimate dissolution. This delicate balance can be upset by the absence of any of the necessary factors, by abnormalities in their structure, by inhibitors of their activity, or by excesses in their functional capacities.

The clotting factors (Table 16-1) act as either enzymes or cofactors. In their resting state the enzymes are present as inactive enzyme precursors, or zymogens. When activated they undergo conformational alteration or peptide cleavage to become proteases that act on the zymogen substrate of

Table 16-1. Nomenclature and Function of Clotting Factors

Usual designation	Synonym	Function
Fibrinogen	Factor I	Substrate
Prothrombin	Factor II	Zymogen
Tissue factor	Factor III; thromboplastin	Cofactor
Ca^{2+}	Factor IV	Divalent cation in enzymatic reaction
Factor V (Factor VI does not exist)	Labile factor	Cofactor
Factor VII	Stable factor	Zymogen
Factor VIII	Antihemophilic factor	Cofactor
Factor IX	Christmas factor	Zymogen
Factor X	Stuart factor	Zymogen
Factor XI		Zymogen
Factor XII	Hageman factor	Zymogen
Factor XIII	Fibrin-stabilizing factor	Zymogen

the next clotting factor in the clotting sequence. As enzymes they are not consumed in the process but can move on to other zymogen substrates in a process of amplification or cascading. The clotting factors that act as cofactors are consumed in the process (Fig. 16-1).

There are two independently activated systems that link together with the activation of factor X. Events beyond that point are common to both systems and hence known as the common pathway.

The faster of the two systems is initiated by the release of subendothelial tissue factor, often as profound external trauma. This is the extrinsic system. Factor VII becomes activated and in turn binds to factor X. The events in the extrinsic system and common pathway are measured by the PT.

The slower system is activated by the exposure of collagen or a variety of intracellular factors that activate circulating factor XII. This is the intrinsic system. Activated XII initiates three reactions: (1) activation of factor XI, (2) activation of kallikrein, which is chemotactic for the cellular repair system, and (3) activation of plasminogen to prevent the clot from overextension. Factor XI then activates factor IX, which interacts with factor VIII to bind to factor X. The events in the intrinsic system and common pathway are measured by the PTT.

Activated X, with factor V as a cofactor, then cleaves prothrombin at several sites to form a distinct protein, thrombin. This in turn cleaves fibrinogen into a slightly smaller molecule, fibrin, which interacts with neighboring fibrin molecules to form a loose fibrin clot. A transpeptidation reaction mediated by factor XIII converts this to a stable fibrin clot.

The parallel system of clot limitation is mediated by plasmin, which diffuses into the fibrin network and breaks it down into smaller nonclottable proteins, the fibrin split products.

A further limiting reaction is that of antithrombin III (AT III), which slowly neutralizes thrombin by forming a complex with it. This effect is markedly enhanced by heparin, which also binds to factor IX. Its effect is detected most sensitively by the PTT.

Structural homology exists among prothrombin, VII, and X at one point on each molecule. This is mediated by vitamin K, inhibited by coumarin anticoagulants, and detected most sensitively by the PT.

Disorders of Clot Formation

CONGENITAL. *The Hemophilias.* Factor VIII Deficiency (Hemophilia A). Though not a common disease, hemophilia A occurs frequently enough that a pediatrician should be adept in both diagnosis and treatment. Factor VIII is present in an antigenically normal amount but is functionally deficient in its measurable activity as a clot-promoting cofactor. The carrier female may have a normal amount of clot-promoting VIII activity, but has roughly twice as much antigenically measurable VIII protein. This is the basis of carrier testing. Antenatal diagnosis can be made by gene probes on fibroblasts or chorionic villi.

Neonatal diagnosis can easily be made on cord blood if there is a positive family history; however, it is more often made because of easy bruising when the child is learning to walk. Hemarthroses, mucous membrane bleeding, deep hematomas, and abdominal pain mimicking appendicitis are the other major problems of childhood.

The PTT is prolonged, the PT normal, and the VIII level constant throughout life. Clinical severity is related to the VIII concentration:

Severe: less than 1%
 Spontaneous bleeding may occur; bleeding always follows trauma; average 20 to 100 infusions annually
Moderate: 1–5%
 No spontaneous bleeding; usually bleeding after trauma; average few to 40 infusions annually

Fig. 16-1. The coagulation cascade. The factors in parentheses (tissue factor, factor VIII, factor V) act as cofactors. All other factors act as enzymes on the subsequent step in the cascade.

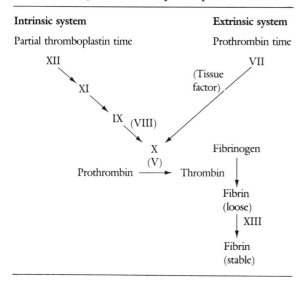

Intrinsic system	Extrinsic system
Partial thromboplastin time	Prothrombin time

Mild: 5–20%
   Bleeding after trauma unpredictable; none or few infusions per year
Subclinical: 20–50%
   PTT may be normal; bleeding only after major trauma if ever

As this is a lifelong disorder with many unique characteristics, referral to the nearest chapter of the National Hemophilia Society is in order. It provides a wealth of educational materials for both the family and physician. Counseling of the family can now be very positive. The outlook for hemophiliacs is excellent, joint deformities are rare, fatalities anecdotal. Children are at school full time and lead happy, productive lives.

Treatment is not easy, but the deficiency is manageable. The focus is on early and vigorous factor replacement when bleeding is even suspected, let alone proved. Factor VIII is available in two forms:

1. Purified, commercially available factor VIII concentrate. This is easily stored, transported, and administered; each bottle contains 200 to 1000 units and is accurately labeled. It also may contain hepatitis antigen, although this is not a problem for hemophiliacs with moderate or severe disease. The potential transmittability of HIV via these concentrates is an unlikely but worrisome possibility. This should not deter their use in severe hemophiliacs with significant need.
2. Cryoprecipitate. This must be kept frozen. It is more difficult to administer. Each bag contains 60 to 100 units, but the precise amount is usually not known. There is much less risk of hepatitis, so it is preferable for hemophiliacs with mild disease. The potential risk of HIV transmission is the same as in blood transfusion.

For both forms of factor VIII, one unit per kilogram of body weight increases the circulating VIII level by 2%. For hemarthrosis and soft-tissue bleeding, 20 units/kg give a 40% level, with a half-life of only 6 to 8 hours; this is repeated in 24 hours. For central nervous system bleeding, 50 units/kg gives a 100% level; this is repeated at 8-hour intervals.

Mucous membrane bleeding may be treated by blocking salivary plasmin activity with epsilon-aminocaproic acid (EACA). The initial dose is 200 mg/kg followed by 100 mg/kg every 4 to 6 hours around the clock. This should be continued for 8 to 10 days, as rebleeding is common. It must never be given for genitourinary bleeding lest insoluble clots form.

The major problem in hemophilia is the formation of factor VIII inhibitors. This appears to be inevitable in 10 to 15% of patients regardless of how many infusions they receive. Thus, the fear of inducing an inhibitor should never be a reason for delaying a necessary VIII infusion. An inhibitor can be suspected when an infusion fails to arrest bleeding or correct the PTT. Specific assays are available. Low-titer inhibitors can be treated by high VIII infusions. High-titer infusions require factor IX concentrates, which appear to contain small quantities of thrombin. This bypasses the inhibitor.

Home infusion has been a great advance in the management of hemophilia. Parents readily learn how to give intravenous concentrates to children 3 years old, and 12-year-old children may learn self-administration. Careful records must be kept, and there must be close supervision of possible joint, dental, and psychosocial problems.

For patients with moderate or mild hemophilia, DDAVP increases the baseline VIII level 2 to 4-fold. The dosage is 0.3 µg/kg IV every 12 to 24 hours. Aspirin and other platelet-inhibiting drugs should be avoided. An excessively protective environment should also be avoided to prevent development of psychological abnormalities.

von Willebrand's Disease. This is a deficiency of the vWF multimer that binds platelets to subendothelial tissue and also acts as carrier of factor VIII. Patients, therefore, have both a prolonged bleeding time and a prolonged PTT, although there is considerable variability of expression within families and within the same person from time to time. The incidence is not clearly established, but with its variants it is probably more common than hemophilia. Inheritance is usually autosomal dominant but can be recessive.

Clinically there is a greater tendency for bruising and postoperative or postpartum bleeding, consistent with the platelet function defect. There is a lesser tendency, however, for hemarthroses or intraabdominal bleeding because the VIII coagulant activity is usually greater than 1%.

Confirmation of diagnosis requires the demonstration of absence of vWF or the failure of platelet aggregation in response to ristocetin. Differentiation from the hemophilia carrier can be made by demonstrating an equimolar concentration of VIII coagulant and VIII antigen in von Willebrand's disease.

Treatment consists of factor replacement with cryoprecipitate rather than factor VIII concentrate, which does not contain vWF. DDAVP may also be useful in increasing the baseline vWF level.

Factor IX Deficiency (Christmas Disease, Hemophilia B). Factor IX deficiency is much less common than factor VIII deficiency but is clinically indistinguishable from it. Inheritance is sex linked. Factor IX replacement in mild cases is most safely given as fresh frozen plasma 10 ml/kg every 6 to 8 hours. In moderate or severe cases, commercially available concentrates provide a reliable source of high-potency factor IX. An infusion of 1 unit/kg gives an increment of only 1%, but the half-life is 30 hours; thus, more must be given initially in severe bleeding, but the dose is repeated less frequently.

Factor XI Deficiency (Hemophilia C). A rare, autosomal recessive disorder with carriers having a prolonged PTT, factor XI deficiency is seen in females as well as males. Bleeding is rarely a problem, but should it occur, fresh frozen plasma 10 ml/kg is required every 6 to 8 hours.

Factor XII Deficiency. PTT is prolonged, but there is no clinical bleeding whatever, hence no treatment is necessary. Variants known as Fletcher factor deficiency and high-molecular-weight kininogen deficiency are of laboratory interest only.

Factor XIII Deficiency. Poor wound healing, easy bruisability, and late umbilical stump bleeding characterize this disorder. The PT, PTT, and bleeding time are normal. Diagnosis is by specific assay of clot solubility in 5M area. Treatment is administration of fresh frozen plasma.

Miscellaneous Deficiencies. Fibrinogen, prothrombin, V, and X deficiencies have a prolonged PT and PTT. Factor VII deficiency has a prolonged PT but normal PTT. All are exceedingly rare.

ACQUIRED. *Disseminated Intravascular Coagulation (DIC).* DIC is a very common acute problem in pediatric medicine. Virtually any pathological process can trigger the activation of factor XII and thence the entire coagulation cascade. In its most malignant form, purpura fulminans, the resultant fibrin clots can occlude peripheral arterioles, resulting in gangrene of fingers, toes, nose, and skin. More commonly, the clinical manifestation is bleeding because of consumption of fibrinogen, prothrombin, factors V and VIII, and platelets in the uncontrolled clotting sequence. Conditions that may trigger DIC are:

1. Infections
   a. Any gram-negative or gram-positive sepsis
   b. Any viremic process
   c. Malaria, kala-azar
   d. Histoplasmosis, aspergillosis
   e. Rocky Mountain spotted fever
2. Liberation of tissue factor
   a. Intravascular hemolysis
   b. Malignant disease, especially acute promyelocytic leukemia

   c. Abruptio placentae, amniotic fluid embolus, toxemia
   d. Respiratory distress syndrome
   e. Fat embolism
3. Endothelial damage
   a. Shock
   b. Heat stroke
   c. Acute glomerulonephritis
   d. Giant hemangioma (Kasabach-Merritt syndrome)

In its full-blown form the PT and PTT are prolonged, the platelet count and fibrinogen concentration are decreased, and fibrin split products are increased. Often the laboratory findings are more erratic. The platelet count is most frequently involved, and if two additional tests are abnormal the diagnosis is almost certain.

Treatment is the replacement of consumed clotting factors with fresh frozen plasma, 10 ml/kg every 6 to 8 hours, and platelets, 4 to 8 units every 6 to 8 hours. If active bleeding continues, cryoprecipitate should be added as an additional source of fibrinogen and factor VIII.

Purpura fulminans presents a special problem because of direct tissue necrosis. As soon as the diagnosis is made, heparinization should be started to arrest fibrin deposition.

Acute Liver Failure. In its initial stages it may be difficult to differentiate acute liver failure from DIC, although the platelet count is usually normal. Treatment of the coagulopathy is the same, with supportive infusions of fresh frozen plasma.

Vitamin K Deficiency. Usually a dietary deficiency most commonly seen in infants who fail to receive a prophylactic vitamin K injection, vitamin K deficiency is also seen with biliary atresia, cystic fibrosis, chronic diarrhea, and long-term antibiotic administration. Often there is concomitant dietary deficiency. Prothrombin, VII, IX, and X fail to develop their homologous Ca^{2+} binding sites, and hence the PT is selectively prolonged. Intramuscular administration of 5 mg of vitamin K corrects the PT within hours.

Circulating Anticoagulants. Circulating anticoagulants occasionally develop with lupus erythematosus or in the postpartum state. Bleeding is uncommon in spite of marked derangements of PTT or PT.

Nephrotic Syndrome. Factors IX and XII may be lost in the general proteinuria of the nephrotic syndrome. Factor IX must be replaced prior to renal biopsy.

HYPERCOAGULABILITY. A much greater problem in adult than in pediatric medicine, hypercoagulability remains poorly understood. Spontaneous arterial or venous thromboses may occur. The criteria used in adults must be used in treatment of children. The patient with deep venous thromboses should receive heparin for 1 week followed by coumarin for 8 to 12 weeks. Underlying associations should be sought and corrected when possible:

1. Estrogen-containing oral contraceptives
2. Pregnancy
3. Cigarette smoking
4. Diabetes mellitus
5. Early stages of DIC
6. Nephrotic syndrome
7. Thrombocytosis in adolescents
8. Kawasaki syndrome
9. Malignancy
10. Familial antithrombin III deficiency
11. Protein C, and protein S deficiency
12. Hyperbetalipoproteinemia type II
13. Hypercholesterolemia
14. Homocystinuria
15. Prosthetic devices in circulation

John T. Truman

References

Colman, R. W., Hirsch, J., Marder, V. J., and Salzman, E. W. *Hemostasis and Thrombosis* (2nd ed.). Philadelphia: Lippincott, 1987.

Miller, D. R. *Blood Diseases of Infancy and Childhood* (6th ed.). St. Louis: Mosby, 1989.

Nathan, D. G., and Oski, F. A. *Hematology of Infancy and Childhood* (3rd ed.). Philadelphia: Saunders, 1987.

Smith, P. S., Keyes, N. C., and Forman, E. N. Socioeconomic evaluation of a state-funded comprehensive hemophilia-care program. *N. Engl. J. Med.* 306:575, 1982.

17

Neoplastic Diseases

Advances in pediatric oncology during the past decade have resulted in significant improvement in survival and cure rates in children with cancer (Fig. 17-1). These improvements were achieved by (1) multidisciplinary approach to therapy by utilizing the skills of the pediatric oncologists, radiotherapists, surgeons, and the other specialists, (2) clinical research by multiinstitutional cooperative study groups, (3) advances in supportive care such as blood banking, total parenteral nutrition, and newer antibiotics, (4) advances in diagnostic imaging techniques, and (5) advances in immunobiology, immunogenetics, and other areas of basic sciences.

Cancer, although rare in pediatric practice, nevertheless ranks as the leading cause of nonaccidental death. Table 17-1 shows the order of frequency and the rate of the most common childhood malignancies. Between 6000 to 7000 children under the age of 16 develop cancer in the United States every year. Annual incidence is 12 per 100,000 for white children and 9.3 per 100,000 for black children.

Some subgroups of children carry a much higher risk for malignancy than the general population. These subgroups include individuals with certain chromosome abnormali-

ties, hereditary cutaneous and neurocutaneous syndromes, immunodeficiency syndromes, hereditary or acquired gastrointestinal syndromes, congenital malformations, and individuals with a sibling with malignancy or survivors of prior cancer.

Children with cancer differ from adults in the way they react to treatment and in the types of malignant disease with which they are afflicted. They are on the whole better able to tolerate radical surgery and chemotherapy per unit of body weight than adults. Radiation therapy, however, has more adverse effects on children than adults.

Diagnosis of Malignant Neoplasms

Malignant diseases should be diagnosed at the earliest possible stage, therefore, the primary physician should be able to recognize the early symptoms and signs of a neoplastic disease.

A complete history and physical examination is essential. Symptomatology, age, sex, race, and the family history should be recorded. After these, the likelihood of malig-

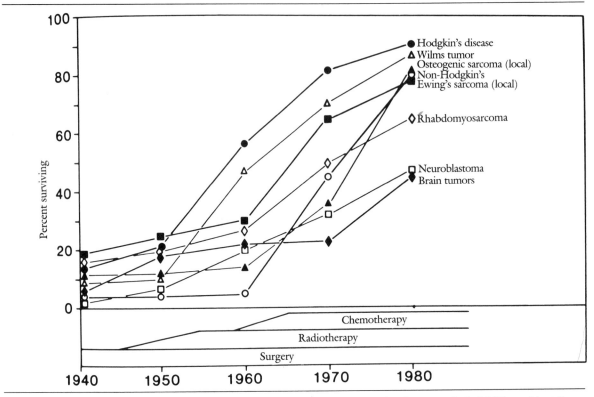

Fig. 17-1. Improving 2-year survival of children with malignant tumors during the decades when surgery, radiation therapy, and chemotherapy were developed as combined modality therapy (1940–1980). (From G. D. Hammond. The cure of childhood cancers. Cancer 58:407, 1986.)

nancy and the type can generally be determined with a high degree of accuracy.

A child suspected of having malignancy should immediately be referred to a center where a specialty team for diagnosis and management is available. Diagnostic evaluation should be tailored for the individual patient.

Hematological studies include a complete blood count (CBC) with platelets and differential. Bone marrow biopsy and aspiration is essential in diagnosis of hematological malignancies and useful in assessing the extent of disease in most of the solid tumors.

Biochemical tumor markers, such as vanillylmandelic acid (VMA), homovanillic acid (HVA), alpha-fetoprotein (AFP), neuron specific enolase (NSE), lipid associated sialic acid (LASA), carcinoembryogenic antigen (CEA), serum ferritin and copper, and chorionic gonadotropic hormone (CGH), are used in certain malignancies with variable sensitivity and specificity. Biochemical tests should include the liver and renal functions, electrolyte levels, and coagulation screening.

Imaging examinations including x-rays, ultrasonograms, computerized tomography (CT), magnetic resonance imaging (MRI), and nuclear scanning should be utilized for localization and the extent of the disease.

The final step in diagnosis is the biopsy of the mass. When major surgery, such as laparotomy is involved, complete removal of the tumor should be attempted without radical destruction of anatomy or function.

Once the diagnosis and the extent of disease are established, treatment then should be carried out by an oncology team which consists of a pediatric oncologist, oncology nurse specialists, social workers, counselors, and other support team members.

Carefully coordinated counseling by the oncology social worker and the physician will sustain the family through the

Table 17-1. The Relative Frequency and the Rate of Various Childhood Malignancies

Rank	Malignancy	Rate (per 1,000,000)
1	Leukemia	37.8
2	CNS tumors	24.1
3	Lymphomas	15.5
4	Neuroblastoma	10.4
5	Renal tumors	8.2
6	Soft tissue sarcomas	7.9
7	Bone tumors	6.1
8	Retinoblastoma	3.4
9	Liver tumors	1.4
10	Others	11.5

inevitable frustrating situations and help them to make the adjustments for living with the disease appropriately and toward coping with their grief and recovering from it if death ensues.

Treatment of Malignant Disease

Surgery

Total removal of the neoplastic mass remains the best treatment for solid tumors; however, very often, this is not possible and some gross or microscopic tumor is left behind. Microscopic tumor often is not detectable by current methods; therefore, if not treated, the tumor recurs either locally or as a distant metastasis. Debulking of solid tumors should be carried out without compromising patient's life or organ function whenever possible. With the advances in multimodality approach, the surgery often does not need to be as aggressive as it was before. Non-Hodgkin's lymphomas, rhabdomyosarcoma of the orbit or other vital organs, and osteogenic sarcoma are typical examples for which less radical surgery is practiced. On the other hand, improvements in supportive care allow the surgeons to be more aggressive when necessary.

Radiation

Radiation therapy continues to be an important part of the multimodality approach. Nevertheless, because of the adverse effects of radiation on the growing tissues of a child, clinical studies are being designed to eliminate or reduce the dose of radiation. As a result, the use of radiation in pediatric

patients has been in a continuous decline during the past few years. For example, it is no longer used in stage I and II Wilms' tumors, it has been eliminated from central nervous system (CNS) prophylaxis in most leukemia patients, and its use has decreased significantly in non-Hodgkin's lymphomas. Lungs are almost never irradiated anymore, and the use of radiation in Hodgkin's disease is also in decline.

Radiation is still the most important therapy for unresectable brain tumors, and also widely used for soft tissue sarcomas and retinoblastomas for curative or palliation purposes.

Chemotherapy

The role of chemotherapy has been increasing during the past two decades. Chemotherapy is no longer considered a palliation treatment, but it is used for curative purpose either as a single mode of therapy or part of multimodality approach.

New strategies that promoted chemotherapy to its current place during the last few years include (1) the Goldie-Coldman hypothesis, which indicates that drug resistance can be prevented and the total cell kill can be achieved by "front loaded," first-line treatment strategy when as many effective agents as possible are used in the highest doses possible, (2) new methods of drug delivery by central catheters, (3) reducing toxicity with prolonged intravenous infusions and other supportive therapies, (4) discovery of new chemotherapeutic agents, and (5) multiinstitutional clinical trials of treatment protocols.

The general classes of chemotherapeutic agents are antimetabolites, alkylating agents, antibiotics, steroids, vinca alkaloids, nitrosureas, and other miscellaneous agents (Table 17-2).

The antimetabolites interfere with the synthesis of nucleic acids or their incorporation into the nucleic acid chain. The alkylating agents attach themselves to at least two or more points in the DNA molecule, thus rendering DNA inactive. Their action is considered to be similar to irradiation, which inhibits mitosis, causes chromosome breakage, and prevents DNA-dependent RNA synthesis. Antibiotics produce their tumoricidal effect by forming stable complexes with DNA, thereby inhibiting DNA, RNA synthesis, or both. Modes of action of adrenocorticosteroids are not fully known, but it seems mainly to be via DNA binding. The plant alkaloids vincristine and vinblastine arrest mitosis in metaphase by an unclear mechanism. Nitrosureas have alkylating activity and also are capable of carbamylating the proteins.

There is a long list of new agents which are continuously tested through phase I, II, and III research trials.

Table 17-2. Common Antineoplastic Agents in Pediatric Oncology, Route of Administration, and Toxicities

Agent	Route of administration*	Common toxicities	Uncommon toxicities
Antimetabolites			
Methotrexate	PO; IM; IV; IT	Myelosuppression; mucositis; dermatitis	Nephrotoxicity; neurotoxicities; osteoporosis; pneumonitis; cirrhosis; GI ulceration; hepatitis
ARA-C	SC; IM; IV; IT	Myelosuppression; nausea and vomiting; fever	Mucositis; hepatitis; neurotoxicity with IT administration
6-TG	PO; (IV)	Myelosuppression	Nausea and vomiting
6-MP	PO; (IV)	Myelosuppression; nausea, vomiting and abdominal pain; hepatitis	Mucositis
5-FU	IV; PO unreliable	Myelosuppression; anorexia; nausea and vomiting; mucositis	Dermatitis; alopecia; hyperpigmentation; cerebellar ataxia
Alkylating agents			
Cyclophosphamide	PO; IV	Myelosuppression; hemorrhagic cystitis; nausea and vomiting; alopecia	Mucositis; hyperpigmentation; hypoosmolarity; infertility
Nitrogen mustard	IV; IC; avoid extravasation	Nausea and vomiting; myelosuppression; vein sclerosis	Mucositis; alopecia
Chlorambucil	PO	Myelosuppression	Nausea and vomiting; hepatitis
Melphalan	PO; (IV); avoid extravasation	Myelosuppression	Anorexia; nausea and vomiting
Busulfan	PO	Myelosuppression	Nausea and vomiting; alopecia; hyperpigmentation; pneumonitis
Antibiotics			
Adriamycin/ Daunomycin	IV; avoid extravasation	Myelosuppression; nausea and vomiting; alopecia; mucositis	Cardiomyopathy
Actinomycin D	IV; avoid extravasation	Myelosuppression; nausea and vomiting; mucositis; alopecia	Dermatitis; hyperpigmentation; radiation recall
Bleomycin	SC; IM; IV; IC	Nausea and vomiting; dermatitis; hyperpigmentation; alopecia	Pulmonary fibrosis; mucositis; hypersensitivity resections
Steroids		Cushing's syndrome; diabetes; hypertension; growth delay; irritability	Hypokalemia; myopathy; osteoporosis; psychosis; adrenal insufficiency
Prednisone	P.O.		
Prednisolone	I.V.		
Dexamethasone	I.V.; P.O.		
Vinca alkaloids			
Vincristine	IV; avoid extravasation	Peripheral neuropathy; jaw pain; constipation; alopecia	Obstipation; cranial nerve palsies; seizures; myelosuppression; hemolysis
Vinblastine	IV; avoid extravasation	Myelosuppression; nausea and vomiting; mucositis	Peripheral neuropathy; alopecia

Table 17-2. (Continued)

Agent	Route of administration*	Common toxicities	Uncommon toxicities
Nitrosureas			
CCNU/BCNU	PO/IV; avoid extravasation	Nausea and vomiting; delayed myelosuppression; immunosuppression; vein sclerosis	Hepatitis; stomatitis
Miscellaneous agents			
Epipodophyllotoxins			
VM-26 (tenoposide)	IV; avoid extravasation	Myelosuppression	Nausea and vomiting; alopecia; hypersensitivity reactions
VP 16-213 (etoposide)	IV; avoid extravasation	Myelosuppression; nausea and vomiting	Hypersensitivity reactions; hypotension
DTIC	IV; avoid extravasation	Myelosuppression; nausea and vomiting; stomatitis	Hepatitis; alopecia; flu-like syndrome
Procarbazine	PO; (IV)	Nausea and vomiting; myelosuppression; lethargy; dermatitis	Stomatitis; peripheral neuropathy; seizures; myopathy/myalgias
L-asparaginase	IM; IV	Hypersensitivity reactions; coagulopathy; hyperglycemia; hepatic dysfunction	Encephalopathy; pancreatitis; abdominal pain
Cisplatin	IV	Nausea and vomiting; nephrotoxicity; ototoxicity	Myelosuppression; seizures; peripheral and autonomic neuropathy
Hydroxyurea	PO; (IV)	Myelosuppression	Nausea and vomiting; mucositis; dermatitis; alopecia

*PO = oral. IM = intramuscular. SC = subcutaneous. IV = intravenous. IT = intrathecal. IC = intracavitary. () = investigational.

Chemotherapy should be administered by people who are trained to handle these drugs under the close supervision of an oncologist.

Follow-up Examinations

Meticulous follow-up after the initial treatment is important. Metastases occurring in the early and treatable stages are usually asymptomatic. Frequent and regular physical and imaging examinations should be carried out even in the asymptomatic child. With tumors that are prone to metastasize to lungs, a chest x-ray film should be taken every 1 to 2 months for the first year and every 3 months for the second year. X-ray examination of the skeleton should be carried out at regular intervals if the tumor is prone to metastasize to bones.

Terminal Care

Total care of a dying child includes providing medical and emotional support for the patient and the family. Although the death of a child seems unbearable, it can be endured if the child is comfortable and is provided with appropriate psychological support. Narcotic analgesics should be used to the point of effectiveness without the fear of addiction.

Leukemias

Leukemias are a heterogenous group of hematologic malignancies that appear to result from the malignant transformation of a single abnormal progenitor cell that possesses the ability for an unrestrained proliferation. Significant improvements have been achieved in the understanding and the treatment of this group of diseases during the past decade. The nomenclature of leukemias is based on the type of the proliferating cells.

Acute Lymphoblastic Leukemia

Acute lymphoblastic leukemia (ALL) is the commonest childhood malignancy in which most of the bone marrow cells are lymphoblasts. Annual incidence in children is 22.3 per million for males and 15.7 per million for females. Peak age of diagnosis is 3 to 5 years for white children. There is no peak age for the nonwhite race. Eighty to 85% of leukemias are ALL.

Currently, 60 to 70% of children with ALL are expected to have greater than 5 years survival, and most of these patients are likely to be cured. This progress is achieved by discovery of effective drugs, use of multiagent therapy, understanding the importance of induction, consolidation and maintenance chemotherapy, preventive therapy for CNS, adjustments in therapy for different prognostic groups, multiinstitutional trials, and the advances in the supportive care.

The disease develops from malignant transformation and clonal expansion of a single cell. The cause for malignant transformation is unknown but it is assumed to have multifactorial etiology, involving environmental, genetic, and infectious causes. There are some risk factors for developing leukemia; however, these factors do not exist for most of the cases (Table 17-3).

CLASSIFICATION OF ALL. Lymphoblasts in ALL are heterogenous and currently are classified according to their cell surface markers, using monoclonal antibodies and flow cytometry. Another method depends on the morphological appearance described by the French-American-British (FAB) international group. Predominance of different cell surface markers and morphological appearances has prognostic and therapeutic implications that are currently studied by various research groups (Table 17-4).

CLINICAL MANIFESTATIONS. The most common initial complaints are fatigue, bone pain, fever, and weight loss. The symptoms and signs of ALL are caused by anemia, neutropenia, and thrombocytopenia, which result from replacement of the bone marrow by the leukemic cells, and hepatosplenomegaly and adenopathy, secondary to diffuse infiltration of those tissues. Lack of erythropoiesis and thrombocytopenic hemorrhage produces the anemia and results in pallor, lethargy, and weakness. Petechiae and bruising are frequently the first signs noted by the parents. Occasionally, epistaxis, hematuria, or scleral hemorrhage may herald the presence of the disease. Fever is sometimes quite profound and, with only minimal erythema of the pharyngeal tissues and no other prominent abnormalities, a viral infection of the upper respiratory tract may be erroneously diagnosed and the patient treated accordingly for several days before the correct condition is suspected and its presence established. Bone and joint pain, especially in a youngster with fever, may lead the physician to suspect rheumatic fever. The differential diagnosis of unexplained pain or a limp in a child should certainly include leukemia, which should be excluded by appropriate studies. Enlargement of liver, spleen, and lymph nodes is not invariably found in leukemia, so absence of any of these abnormalities does not preclude its presence.

PROGNOSTIC FACTORS. Certain clinical and laboratory findings have prognostic value in ALL (Table 17-5). Most treatment centers group patients under different prognostic categories and try to tailor treatments accordingly. Patients

---

Table 17-3. Risk Factors for ALL

Ionizing radiation (therapeutic or diagnostic)
  Nuclear bombs
  Nuclear industry leaks
Twin of a leukemic patient (1 : 4 concordance)
Sibling of a leukemic patient (1 : 720 concordance)
Down syndrome (1 : 95)
Fanconi's anemia
Schwachman's syndrome
Ataxia telangiectasia
Neurofibromatosis
Klinefelter's syndrome
Bloom syndrome

Table 17-4. Classification of ALL

A. Immunophenotypic classification
  1. B-cell leukemia
  2. T-cell leukemia
  3. Null cell leukemia
    a. Pre-B cell
    b. Pre-T cell
    c. Common ALL antigen (CALLA)
B. Morphologic classification (FAB)
  L1. No correlation with immunophenotype
  L2.
  L3. Mostly B surface markers

Table 17-5. Prognostic Factors in ALL

Factor	Good	Bad
Initial WBC count	Low	High
Sex	Female	Male
Mediastinal Mass	Absent	Present
Age	2–10 years	< 2 and > 10 years
Platelet count	High	Low
Organomegaly	Absent	Present
FAB morphology	L1	L2 and L3
CNS involvement	Absent	Present
Surface markers	Null	T or B
Cytogenetics	Normal	Abnormal
Immunoglobulins	Normal	Low
Hb level	< 10 g/100 ml	> 10 g/100 ml

with poor risk features receive more intensive therapy. No single method of prognostic classification has been accepted universally yet. Clinical significance of cell surface markers and chromosomal abnormalities are surpassing the other criteria in prognostic classification.

LABORATORY DIAGNOSIS OF ALL. The CBC is the most important initial test. Hemoglobin (Hb) is less than 7 g/100 ml in 40% and less than 11 g/100 ml in 85% of the patients. Seventy-five percent have platelet counts less than 100,000/mm^3. Only 50% have leukocyte count less than 10,000/mm^3, and leukocytosis over 50,000/mm^3 occurs in 17% of the patients. Lymphoblasts on a peripheral blood smear may be seen in 85 to 90% of the patients.

Bone marrow examination is mandatory for definitive diagnosis. Further characterization of the cells is done by special stains, cell surface markers, and gene rearrangement studies. Extent of the disease is examined by routine chemistries, cerebrospinal fluid (CSF) examination, and imaging studies.

TREATMENT AND PROGNOSIS. For patients with good prognosis, induction with vincristine, prednisone and L-asparaginase results in 95 to 98% remission rate. Disease of the CNS can be prevented by intrathecal methotrexate in this group. Maintenance therapy consists of daily oral 6-mercaptopurine (6-MP) and weekly oral methotrexate. Five-year survival for this group is close to 90%.

For the high-risk patients, in addition to the above treatment, multiagent chemotherapy is given at various intervals as consolidation and intensification of the therapy. Cranial irradiation is added for CNS prophylaxis. Four years of event-free survival reaches to 55 to 60% in this group of

patients. Survival for infants is less than 45% at the present time.

These increased survival rates have made the oncologists more aware of the late complications of therapy, and efforts are being made to minimize the late effects. These delayed complications include second malignancies, CNS toxicities, damage to kidneys, pituitary, liver, gastrointestinal tract, lungs, immune systems, and the gonads.

Acute Nonlymphocytic Leukemia

Acute nonlymphocytic leukemia (ANLL) is a heterogenous group of hematologic malignancies involving the bone marrow cells other than the cells of lymphoid origin. It includes 15 to 20% of childhood leukemias.

Genetic conditions with increased risk of ANLL include Down syndrome, Fanconi's anemia, Bloom syndrome, neurofibromatosis, Kostmann's agranulocytosis, and Diamond-Blackfan anemia. Exposure to alkylating agents and radiation also increase the risk for ANLL.

CLINICAL MANIFESTATIONS. Symptoms and signs of ANLL result from either bone marrow failure or infiltration of extramedullary sites by leukemic cells. Symptoms are pallor and fatigue from anemia, infection due to granulocytopenia, and hemorrhagic findings as a result of thrombocytopenia. These may be preceded by prolonged low-grade fever, irritability, weakness, and bone pain. Mild liver enlargement and marked splenomegaly is common. Except in monocytic and myelomonocytic variants, generalized lymphadenopathy is not a striking feature. Meningeal and testicular involvement is rare. Unusual but distinctive findings include chloramas (greenish granulocytic masses in orbits, spinal cord, peripheral nerves, skin, or other areas), gum hyperplasia (mostly in monocytic or myelomonocytic variants), and disseminated intravascular coagulation (DIC) (mostly in promyelocytic type).

DIAGNOSIS AND CLASSIFICATION. Diagnostic evaluation is similar to ALL. Definitive diagnosis and classification is done by bone marrow aspiration and study of cells by morphologic and histochemical studies.

Most widely used morphological classification of ANLL is developed by the FAB cooperative group, and it is based on the differentiation of leukemic cells along a particular cell line and the degree of maturation (Table 17-6).

TREATMENT AND PROGNOSIS. Although different FAB morphologies imply different prognoses in ANLL, these have not been defined as accurately as in ALL; therefore, currently all subtypes receive the same therapy. The objective of therapy in ANLL is to induce remission with maximum cell kill, as suggested by the Goldie-Coldman hypoth-

Table 17-6. FAB Classification of ANLL

Type	Name
M1	Undifferential myeloblastic
M2	Myeloblastic
M3	Promyelocytic
M4	Myelomonocytic
M5a	Monoblastic
M5b	Differential monocytic
M6	Erythroleukemia
M7	Megakaryocytic

esis. This approach requires a skilled team approach, with optimum supportive care, including infection management, transfusions, and emotional support.

Effective agents include cytosine arabinoside, anthracyclines, 6-thioquanine, vincristine, prednisone, cyclophosphamide, VP-16, and intrathecal therapy with cytosine arabinoside and hydrocortisone.

Once remission is achieved, bone marrow transplantation is recommended, if there is a suitable donor. Chemotherapy continues for those without a marrow donor. The role of maintenance therapy in ANLL is not clear.

Currently, 3-year survival in ANLL is around 40%. Further improvements depend on introduction of new drugs, improvements in bone marrow transplantation technology, and development of sensitive methods for detecting residual disease.

Chronic Leukemia

CLINICAL MANIFESTATIONS. Chronic leukemia is exceedingly rare in young children; it is seen somewhat more commonly in teenagers. The leukemia seen in newborn infants or very young babies and referred to as congenital leukemia is usually of the chronic-appearing type, and in both age groups is of the granulocytic type. The term *chronic* applies to the signs, symptoms, and hematological blood and marrow picture rather than to any expectation of longevity. As a rule, the spleen is markedly enlarged, the liver less so. Adenopathy may be a prominent physical finding. Bruising and petechiae are seldom of significant extent.

LABORATORY MANIFESTATIONS. There are two forms of chronic granulocytic leukemia (CGL), the juvenile and the adult. They are distinguished on the basis of laboratory studies rather than age, although the younger the child, the greater the likelihood of having the juvenile type. Each type shows hyperleukocytosis with granulocytic predominance, a "shift to the left" in both blood and marrow, and a relatively small number of very immature cells and blasts compared with acute leukemia. The leukocyte count is usually not as high in the juvenile as in the adult type, and thrombocytopenia is more frequent and more profound in the juvenile type. The latter is also characterized by greater adenopathy, less splenomegaly, and a tendency to run a shorter course than the adult type. The adult type is distinguished by the presence of a specific abnormality of chromosome 22, which has lost about half of its long arm. This is called the Philadelphia or Ph^1 chromosome. It is not detectable in the juvenile type of CGL. In addition, the juvenile type has a very high level of fetal hemoglobin, whereas in the adult type the fetal hemoglobin level averages less than 7%.

TREATMENT. The initial drug of choice is busulfan (Myleran), 0.06 mg/kg of body weight per day until the white blood cell (WBC) count falls below 20,000/mm^3. Then the dose is adjusted to maintain the WBC count between 10,000 and 20,000/mm^3 and the platelet count above 100,000/mm^3. Although 6-mercaptopurine is less effective, it serves as a second drug after busulfan is no longer effective. In children, irradiation or surgical removal of the enlarged spleen has rarely been necessary except in those cases in which its size has become so gross as to cause distress to the child or when splenic rupture has occurred. Irradiation of the spleen sometimes lowers the WBC count in patients with hyperleukocytosis not responsive to chemotherapy.

Eventually the picture resembles that of acute leukemia with increasing peripheral blood and bone marrow blasts and progressive anemia and thrombocytopenia. At that time the chemotherapeutic agents used for acute leukemia are utilized. The effect of these drugs is usually short-lived, and death ensues from hemorrhage, sepsis, or leukemic infiltration of vital organs. Currently, bone marrow transplantation is the only modality that offers cure in CGL.

Non-Hodgkin's Lymphoma

Non-Hodgkin's lymphomas (NHL) are neoplasms of the different cell types that constitute the immune system. Various classification systems have been developed based on the histologic appearance (Table 17-7).

While therapies are designed according to the histology, immunologic characteristics are gaining importance in the classification of NHL. Clinical presentation is characteristic for the cell type in the majority of the cases. Lymphoblastic lymphoma most commonly presents with mediastinal mass. There may be pain, dysphagia, dyspnea, and edema of the face and neck due to superior vena cava obstruction. Bone

Table 17-7. Most Commonly Used Classification Systems for Childhood NHL

Classification system	Indistinguishable from ALL	Small cell undifferentiated	Large lymphoid cell
Rappaport	Lymphoblastic Convoluted Nonconvoluted	Undifferentiated Burkitt's non-Burkitt's	Histiocytic
World Health Organization	Diffuse lymphosarcoma-lymphoblastic	Diffuse lymphosarcoma-Burkitt's	Diffuse immunoblastic reticulosarcoma
Working formulation	Lymphoblastic Convoluted Nonconvoluted (mostly T cells)	Small noncleaved cell lymphoma (B cells)	Large cell lymphoma Immunoblastic (Mostly B cells)

marrow involvement is common in these patients, designating them into a "lymphoma-leukemia" syndrome by some study groups. Lymphadenopathy, if present, is usually above the diaphragm.

Most patients with undifferentiated (small noncleaved cell type) and large cell lymphomas present with abdominal tumor. Exception to this is the Burkitt's lymphoma of the jaw, common in some parts of Africa where annual rainfall is over 20 inches and the mean temperature is above 60°F. Ninety-five percent of the African Burkitt's lymphoma cases have Epstein-Barr virus (EBV) genomes in the tumor cells. The EBV association is present in 10 to 15% of the North American Burkitt cases.

Abdominal tumors may present with asymptomatic mass or may cause pain, nausea, vomiting, or changing bowel habits. There may be intussusception, intestinal obstruction, or, rarely, perforation. Lymphadenopathy in these patients usually involves inguinal, iliac, or para-aortic nodes.

Other presentations of NHL of any cell type are bone marrow involvement, CNS disease, skin involvement, bone lesions, pharyngeal disease, and testicular involvement.

Diagnosis must be confirmed with biopsy. The extent of disease is determined by CBC, blood chemistries, lactic dehydrogenase (LDH), uric acid, bone marrow aspiration and biopsy, and spinal fluid examination. Imaging studies include chest x ray, CT scan, MRI, and abdominal ultrasound. Callium scan and bone scan can be used as needed.

Staging does not seem to be too significant, except the advanced disease with bone marrow or CNS involvement.

TREATMENT AND PROGNOSIS. Primary therapeutic modality for all forms of NHL is chemotherapy. Patients with bulky abdominal tumors should have surgery in an effort to remove the entire tumor or for debulking. The role of radiation therapy has been decreasing in recent years, and it probably should be limited to acute superior vena cava syndrome and CNS prophylaxis or selected cases of intestinal obstruction.

By using intensive multiagent chemotherapy protocols, known as LSA_2-L_2 or Berlin-Frankfurt-Munster (BFM), patients with extensive lymphoblastic lymphoma have long-term survival rate approaching to 80%. Patients with limited disease have a 90% long-term survival rate. Nonlymphoblastic types are better treated with a protocol including cyclophosphamide, vincristine, methotrexate, and prednisone. In spite of these good results, CNS involvement still carries a very poor prognosis, and bone marrow involvement has a less favorable outcome.

Hodgkin's Disease

Hodgkin's disease is the malignancy of unknown cell origin involving the lymph nodes. Reed-Sternberg cell, once thought to be pathognomonic, can be found in various other benign conditions. Pathological classification includes lymphocyte predominant (LP), nodular sclerosing (NS), mixed cellularity (MC), and lymphocyte depletion (LD) types which represents the progression pattern of the disease except the NS histology.

An epidemiological pattern has been observed, and described as: type I pattern, which implies a poor prognosis and seen in developing countries; type III, which has the best prognosis and is seen in wealthy urbanized countries; and type II, which has an intermediate prognosis and is seen in rural areas of developed countries.

Hodgkin's disease is rare in the Orient. The incidence in

childhood is probably less than 5% of all malignant diseases, with the disease being quite rare under the age of 8 years. As in the adult, a male preponderance does exist. In contrast to the non-Hodgkin's lymphoma, two-thirds of the affected children have only involvement of peripheral lymph nodes, the vast majority of these occurring above the diaphragm.

CLINICAL MANIFESTATIONS. Hodgkin's disease in children presents with painless enlargement of lower cervical lymph nodes in over 60% of the cases. Extranodal primary site involvement is rare.

Anorexia, malaise, and lassitude are common symptoms. Fever is found in 30% of the cases. Autocannibalism, resulting loss of muscle protein and weight and a negative nitrogen balance may be present. Spleen is palpable in about half of the patients, and liver enlargement may imply disease below the diaphragm.

Diagnosis is established by surgical biopsy of the painlessly enlarged involved nodes. Presence of fever may mislead one to suspect an infectious disorder. If, in such cases, antibiotic therapy does not result in significant decrease in size or development of fluctuation of the node, it should be removed for pathological examination without delay. The majority of cases in children and youth is of either the nodular sclerosis or the mixed cellularity type.

Prognosis seems best for the lymphocytic predominance type, next best for nodular sclerosis, less favorable for mixed cellularity, and considerably worse for the lymphocytic depletion type. Prognosis also is related to the extent, or staging, of the disease.

Staging of Hodgkin's disease is done by imaging techniques such as chest x ray, CT or MRI of the chest and abdomen, and ultrasound of the abdomen for younger children. Lymphangiogram is a difficult and cumbersome procedure, but is very valuable in assessing the iliac and paravertebral node sizes and architectures. Furthermore, dye remains in the nodes for several months allowing the follow-up by plain abdominal x rays. Performing a staging laparotomy is controversial and probably should be reserved when the planned therapy is different for stages II and III disease. Bone marrow biopsy from more than one site should be done, especially in patients with symptoms of fever, weight loss, and night sweating.

Clinical staging is defined as follows:

Stage I Involvement of a single lymph node region (I) or of a single extralymphatic organ or site (I_E)

Stage II Involvement of two or more lymph node regions on the same side of the diaphragm (II). An optional recommendation is that the number of node regions involved be indicated by a subscript, e.g., II_3

Stage III Involvement of lymph node regions on both sides of the diaphragm (III); this may also be accompanied by localized involvement of extralymphatic organ or site (III_E) or by involvement of the spleen (III_{S+}) or both (III_{S+E+})

Stage IV Diffuse or disseminated involvement of one or more extralymphatic organs or tissues

Each stage is subdivided into A and B categories. The B classification is assigned to patients with (1) unexplained loss of more than 10% of the body weight in the previous 6 months, (2) unexplained fever, with temperature above 30°C, and (3) night sweats. Patients without these symptoms are placed in the A category.

Laboratory findings may include anemia, neutrophilia, eosinophilia, elevated sedimentation rate, increased serum copper, and alkaline phosphate. Tests for delayed type of hypersensitivity may be impaired.

THERAPY. Treatment of Hodgkin's disease consists of chemotherapy, radiotherapy, or both.

Radiation therapy might be adequate treatment for stages I and II diseases. Stages III and IV diseases are usually treated by chemotherapy with or without irradiation of the involved nodes. Various treatment protocols are being tried to achieve the best survival with minimum side effects.

The most effective multiagent chemotherapy protocols consist of: nitrogen mustard, vincristine, prednisone, and procarbazine (MOPP); and adriamycin, bleomycin, vinblastine, and actinomycin-D (ABVD). In some other protocols, nitrogen mustard is replaced by CCNV, cyclophosphamide, or chlorambucil, and vincristine may be replaced by vinblastine.

Long-term survival currently is about 90% for Stage I, 80% for Stage II, 65% for Stage III, and 40% for Stage IV disease.

The late complications of therapy include growth disturbances, infertility, secondary malignancies, and hypothyroidism.

Neuroblastoma

Neuroblastoma is a malignant neoplasm of the sympathetic nervous system. It may arise from the adrenal gland or at any site along the sympathetic chain, occurring in the retroperitoneum, posterior mediastinum, or cervical ganglia. Rarely the primary tumor may occur in the olfactory mucous membrane high in the nasal fossa. Three-fourths of all cases occur before age 5. About one-fourth are diagnosed in the first year of life with an occasional case noted at the time of birth. Metastases are present at the time of diagnosis in 50 to 70% of the patients, and frequently the presenting sign or symptom is caused by metastatic involvement.

Amplification of an oncogene (n-myc) may be significant in the etiology and prognosis of neuroblastoma.

Diagnosis

The most common site of onset is in the abdomen, with most lesions arising in the adrenal medulla. The presenting complaint is most often that an abdominal mass has been detected by a parent. The mass is usually hard upon palpation and irregular in outline, and it crosses the midline, in contrast to Wilms tumor, which is usually less hard, is smooth and regular in contour, and seldom crosses the midline. Masses arising in the cervical, thoracic, or pelvic area cause signs or symptoms related to the anatomy of the area, e.g., Horner's syndrome, cough, and dyspnea. Persistent fever and bone or joint pain related to skeletal metastases may simulate rheumatoid arthritis or rheumatoid fever.

When this diagnosis is suspected, investigation usually includes ultrasound or CT of the abdomen, skeletal survey by radioisotope scanning, x-ray studies of the chest and other suspected areas, intravenous pyelography, a complete hemogram including a platelet count, and urine collection for determination of the levels of excretion of catecholamines and their metabolic by-products, especially vanillylmandelic acid (VMA) and homovanilic acid (HVA). A positive LaBrosse spot test for VMA distinguishes between a neuroblastoma and Wilms tumor in just a few minutes on a random urine specimen, but quantitative levels should also be obtained for serial comparison in long-term follow-up care.

Neuron specific enolase (NSE) and ferritin may be elevated, especially in advanced disease. Degree of NSE elevation has prognostic significance.

Examination of a bone marrow aspirate may reveal characteristic clumps of metastatic tumor cells that are not roentgenographically detectable as bone lesions. The imaging studies with CT and MRI or intravenous pyelogram (IVP) frequently show downward and lateral displacement of the kidney by a suprarenal mass and may also reveal calcification in the tumor, displacement of the ureter by a mid-line or paravertebral mass, or a soft-tissue shadow in the paravertebral region sometimes extending through the diaphragm.

Clinical Staging

Staging proposed by Evans et al., currently is the most widely used system.

Stage I   Tumor confined to the organ or structure of origin

Stage II   Tumor extending in continuity beyond the organ or structure of origin but not crossing the midline
Regional lymph nodes on the homolateral side may be involved

Stage III   Tumor extending in continuity beyond the midline.
Regional lymph nodes may be involved bilaterally

Stage IV   Remote disease involving skeleton, organs, soft tissues, or distant lymph node groups

Stage IV-S   Patients who would otherwise be at stage I or II but who have remote disease confined only to one or more of the following sites: liver, skin, or bone marrow (without radiographic evidence of bone metastases on complete skeletal survey)

Treatment

When the initial evaluation is complete, the choice of treatment depends on the stage of the disease. There are well-documented cases of complete spontaneous regression of neuroblastoma. Isolated tumors, even when they are large, should be removed surgically if possible. Even partial excision sometimes results in long-term survival and, rarely, complete regression of the remaining tumor. If there are widespread metastases, removal of the primary lesion is probably not indicated except for relief of symptoms. The prognosis is good in the young child whose primary neuroblastoma was completely removed, and further therapy may not be needed. Those with stage IV-S tumors often do very well with minimal therapy, the tumor sometimes regressing completely after nothing more than a simple biopsy to establish the diagnosis. About three-fourths of the IV-S group are less than 1 year of age, and up to 90% of that subgroup can be expected to survive for at least 2 years. This contrasts with only about 25% survival for patients under 1 year of age who have stage IV disease initially.

Although metastatic neuroblastoma is often very responsive to chemotherapy, there has been no significant improvement in the survival rate as a result of these modes of treatment. Numerous chemotherapeutic agents have shown activity against this tumor, in particular those combinations that incorporate vincristine or cyclophosphamide or both producing up to 80% response rates. Duration of response is dismally short for the vast majority of the cases.

Intensive chemotherapy and irradiation followed by autologous bone marrow transplantation is currently being evaluated in the advanced stage disease.

The overall survival is approximately 25%, but it is 50% or greater in those with no evidence of metastasis when tumor was diagnosed.

Wilms Tumor (Embryoma of the Kidney)

Embryoma of the kidney is the most common malignant abdominal tumor in infancy and childhood. Congenital in origin, it ordinarily makes its appearance between the ages of 4 months and 6 years (median 3 years).

Some cases of Wilms tumor have a genetic origin. Incidence is uniform around the world with about 7.6 cases per million children per year.

Clinical Manifestations

The most common presentation is the discovery of an asymptomatic mass by the parent or the primary physician. The mass is usually firm, occasionally lobulated, and generally confined to one side of the abdomen. Hypertension may be present in 30% of the cases. Abdominal pain, vomiting, hemihypertrophy, and aniridia are less frequent manifestations. Gross hematuria is rare.

The method of spread is along the renal vein so metastases are first seen in the lungs.

Imaging studies such as IVP, CT scan, or MRI and ultrasound usually show a mass involving the kidney with distortion of the collecting system.

Treatment and Prognosis

There has been a remarkable improvement in the prognosis of Wilms tumor over the past few decades. This improvement is the result of multimodality approach by multi-institutional study groups. In the United States, National Wilms' Tumor Study Group (NWTS) contributed not only the prognosis but also defined new pathological subgroups with unfavorable histologies. These are "anaplastic" (4%), "clear cell sarcoma" (6%), and "rhabdoid" (2%).

Approximately 90% of these tumors occur unilaterally; therefore, the histological diagnosis should be made by removal of the whole tumor through a transperitoneal incision after the presence of a normally functioning opposite

kidney is confirmed with an IVP. Biopsy for diagnosis should be done only in those bilateral cases in which it is impossible or inappropriate to remove the more severely affected kidney. The opposite kidney should always be examined during surgery, even if it is apparently normal preoperatively.

Staging for extent of disease according to the criteria of the NWTS is

Stage I   Tumor limited to kidney and completely resected

Stage II   Tumor extending beyond the kidney but completely resected

Stage III   Residual nonhematogenous tumor confined to the abdomen

Stage IV   Hematogenous metastases

Stage V   Bilateral renal involvement either initially or subsequently

Through the NWTS investigations 1 through 3, the treatment modalities have been refined for different stages of the disease. The latest designed study, NWTS-4, can be summarized as: Stages I and II — surgery with vincristine and actinomycin-D and testing different duration and drug delivery methods; Stages III and IV — surgery, radiation, vincristine, actinomycin-D, and adriamycin with and without cyclophosphamide. Cyclophosphamide will be tested for the unfavorable histology group along with different doses of radiotherapy trials.

The most recent results suggest 88% long-term survival for all stages of disease in Wilms tumor.

Central Nervous System Tumors

Brain tumors are the most common solid tumors in children. The peak age of diagnosis is 5 to 10 years, but this varies with histologic type. Table 17-8 shows the relative frequency and the site of different histologic types.

There is no sex difference, and whites and blacks are equally affected in the United States. It is rare in African blacks, which suggests an environmental factor in the etiology.

Symptoms and Signs

Clinical manifestations are largely due to increased intracranial pressure as a result of obstruction of CSF circulation and space occupying effects in an unexpandable calvarium. Table 17-9 shows the common symptoms and signs of the brain tumors.

Table 17-8. Relative Frequency of Childhood Brain Tumors

Type	Percentage
Infratentorial	66 (total)
Astrocytoma	20
Medulloblastoma	18
Brain stem glioma	10
Ependymoma	8
Miscellaneous	10
Supratentorial	33 (total)
Astrocytoma	8
Ependymoma	6
High grade astrocytoma	6
Craniopharyngioma	5
Miscellaneous	8

Diagnosis

Computed tomography and MRI have replaced other imaging techniques such as pneumoencephalography and radioisotope scanning. Angiography, now rarely used, may give additional information about the blood supply. Myelography is useful in staging, especially in medulloblastoma, ependymoma, and germinomas which tend to disseminate along the neuroaxis. With paramagnetic enhancement agents, MRI may detect dissemination within the CNS. Bone marrow aspiration and bone scan are also used to assess the extent of disease. Definitive diagnosis is made by biopsy with a possible exception of brain stem glioma in which biopsy is not necessary.

Table 17-9. Common Presenting Manifestations in Childhood Brain Tumors

Manifestation	Percent
Increased intracranial pressure	85
Morning headache	70
Morning vomiting	75
Amblyopic episodes	10
Gait disturbance	40
Behavior change	35
Diplopia	25
Vertigo	25
Hemiparesis	15
Seizures	10
Head tilt	10

Treatment

Progress in the management of brain tumors has been slow as compared to other childhood malignancies. Until recently, progress has been due to improvements in surgical and radiation therapy techniques. Controlled cooperative studies by Children's Cancer Study Group (CCSG) and International Society of Pediatric Oncology (ISOP) have been evaluating the role of chemotherapy. The results of these studies have been encouraging, and there have been significant improvements in survival in medulloblastomas and possibly also in high-grade astrocytomas and ependymomas by including chemotherapy in treatment. Cooperative groups are currently trying multiple agents with different characteristics in the same therapy as an adjuvant to surgery and radiation.

Bone Tumors

Bone tumors arise from the bone-producing cells, the endothelial components, the reticulum cells, the cartilage, and fibrous tissue. The most common malignant bone tumors are osteogenic sarcoma and Ewing's sarcoma. Other tumors, such as chondrosarcoma and fibrosarcoma are extremely rare in childhood.

Osteosarcoma

It is a rare and highly malignant tumor of the bone. Five hundred to 900 new cases are diagnosed each year in the United States. Peak incidence is in adolescents and young adults when there is rapid bone growth. Male to female ratio is 1.3 : 1. Etiology is not known. Patients with hereditary retinoblastoma have an increased risk for developing osteosarcoma. It is most commonly seen in the metaphyses of long bones, especially of the distal femur. Clinical presentation usually is swelling with or without pain. Other signs and symptoms are rare, and they are related to metastasis. Diagnosis is established by biopsy. Evaluation for the extent of disease should include CT of the chest for lung metastasis and radionuclide bone scanning for bone metastasis.

X-ray findings of "sunburst" pattern are characteristic. Alkaline phosphatase is elevated in about half of the patients and may be used in assessment of disease activity.

Survival has improved significantly by using multimodality approach. Over 50% of the patients are expected to be long survivors and possibly cured. The goal of surgery is the removal of tumor with a wide margin of safety. Surgery alone is curative only for 15 to 20% of the patients without apparent metastasis, which means most patients have subclinical metastasis at the time of diagnosis. The most effective treatment currently is preoperative chemotherapy, followed by definitive surgery, followed by additional chemotherapy. Osteogenic sarcoma is highly resistant to radiation therapy; however, unresectable primary tumors, such as of the vertebral body or skull, should be managed by local radiation and chemotherapy. Lung metastasis should be removed surgically when possible. Limb-sparing surgery is increasingly used as experience with the procedure increases.

Effective chemotherapeutic agents are doxorubicin, cisplatin, high-dose methotrexate, bleomycin, cyclophosphamide, actinomycin-D, and ifosfamide.

Ewing's Sarcoma

Ewing's sarcoma is the second most malignant bone tumor, occurring in 2 per million white children per year. It is extremely rare in blacks and uncommon over the age of 30 years.

The most common presentation is pain at the involved area. There may be local swelling and heat. Fever, malaise, and anorexia are common, and as a result, misdiagnosis of osteomyelitis is often made. Other signs and symptoms depend on the location of the tumor.

X-ray appearance of "moth eaten" pattern and "onion skin" appearance may further confuse the diagnosis with osteomyelitis. Other diagnostic evaluations are similar to osteogenic sarcoma.

Treatment consists of surgery, radiation therapy, and chemotherapy. Surgical resection is carried out for lesions of the expendable bones, such as ribs, clavicle, scapula, ulna, fibula, and forefoot. Limb amputation should be considered for young children when growth arrest and nerve damage due to irradiation is unacceptable. Radiation should include the entire involved bone and surrounding soft tissues. Effective chemotherapeutic agents are vincristine, actinomycin-D, cyclophosphamide, and doxorubicin. Using this multimodality approach, over 50% of the children with Ewing's sarcoma are expected to survive their disease.

Soft Tissue Sarcomas

The soft tissue sarcomas are considered as a group because of the similarity of their clinical course. The group includes tumors arising in blood vessels, muscles, fibrous tissue, and fat. Sometimes it is not possible to decide the tissue layer of origin, and a pathological diagnosis of embryonal or undifferentiated sarcoma is made. In children the majority of these tumors are rhabdomyosarcomas. These tumors can

arise at any site in the body but do so more frequently in some areas than in others. The chief sites for the primary tumor are the region of the orbit, nasopharynx, vagina, pelvic structures, and limbs. The tumors tend to infiltrate widely and spread to lungs and regional lymph nodes.

The presentation depends upon the primary site. In young girls the tumor frequently presents in the vagina as a mass. When the bladder is involved, urinary symptoms are sometimes the first clue to disease; or in the region of the orbit, a squint or proptosis may be noticed first. Whatever the site, the definitive diagnosis must be made by biopsy.

Treatment of soft tissue sarcomas is a multimodality approach with surgery, radiation therapy, and chemotherapy. Therapy should be tailored for the individual patient, considering the histology, organ of involvement, and the degree of involvement. Optimum surgery removes as much tumor as possible without causing organ dysfunction. This is followed by a radiation therapy using the same principle. Chemotherapy principle is delivering the highest possible doses with multiple effective agents. Most active chemotherapy agents are vincristine, actinomycin-D, cyclophosphamide, cisplatin, and doxorubicin. Survival has improved significantly using the multimodal strategy.

Liver Tumors

Primary tumors of the liver, or hepatomas, are not common in childhood. More often a tumor in this region is secondary to a neuroblastoma or a Wilms tumor. Large hemangiomas, teratomas, and hamartomas may occur in this area. Primary liver tumors should be removed if surgically feasible or, if not, treated with irradiation. Use of the combination of actinomycin-D, cyclophosphamide, and vincristine with radiation therapy is sometimes beneficial in controlling or causing regression of the primary hepatoblastoma.

Langerhans' Cell Histiocytosis

Langerhans' cell histiocytosis (LCH), formerly known as "histiocytosis X" is a poorly understood disease characterized by the proliferation of Langerhans' cells. It can affect almost every organ in the body. Commonly used classification of eosinophilic granuloma, Letterer-Siwe, and Hand-Schuller-Christian disease is inadequate in describing the spectrum of this disease, and it is rarely possible to fit a patient into a single category.

Clinical presentation includes demarcated bone lesions without pain, endocrinopathies such as diabetes insipidus, growth failure, hypothyroidism and hypogonadism, skin lesions with seborrhealike appearance or vesiculo-pustules with hemorrhagic crusting. Pulmonary lesions are caused by interstitial histiocytic proliferation which results in restricted ventilation. Chronic otitis is common. Liver involvement leads to cholestasis and fibrosis. Diarrhea and malabsorption are frequently seen. Lymphadenopathy is common.

Bone marrow involvement most often occurs in young infants and is characterized by infiltration by histiocytes. Thrombocytopenia represents the worst prognostic sign and almost invariably is associated with a fatal outcome. Neutropenia can occur, commonly causing severe infections. Erythrophagocytosis can be seen in most of the patients with bone marrow involvement.

Prognosis depends on the extent of the disease at the time of diagnosis, the age of the patient, and the rapidity of the appearance of new lesions.

Definitive diagnosis is by biopsy of the suspected lesions. When diagnosis is made, a complete evaluation of the other organ systems is mandatory, including the immune system with special attention to T-cell abnormalities.

Treatment includes the curettage, local irradiation, or both of bone lesions. The aggressiveness of chemotherapy should be correlated to the severity of disease. Active agents include prednisone, vinblastine, nitrogen mustard, methotrexate, and VP-16.

Bone Marrow Transplantation in Pediatric Neoplastic Diseases

Bone marrow transplantation (BMT) is increasingly used for many immunologic, hematologic, and neoplastic diseases in children. (Table 17-10).

Primary reason for BMT in neoplastic diseases is to treat the iatrogenic bone marrow aplasia. BMT permits the administration of higher and curative chemotherapy and rescues the host by the transplanted marrow cells.

There are four types of BMT. *Autologous* BMT involves infusion of the patient's own previously harvested marrow. *Synergic* transplantation is when a genetically identical twin is the donor. The most common type is *allogeneic* transplant, a genetically nonidentical, but HLA-MLC compatible, donor, usually a sibling. The most recent and potentially most useful type is *partially or non-HLA* matching transplantation, which is at an experimental stage.

BMT provides healthy pluripotent stem cells from the donor, which proliferate and differentiate in the recipient's marrow microenvironment. After BMT, the recipient becomes a "chimera," whose hematopoetic system is of donor origin.

Major histocompatibility complex for tissue type is located on chromosome 6. Because one chromosome 6 is

Table 17-10. Conditions in Which Bone Marrow Transplantation May Offer Cure

Neoplastic diseases
  Leukemias
  Lymphomas
  Solid tumors
Hematologic diseases
  Bone marrow failure syndromes
  Severe hemoglobinopathies
Immunodeficiency diseases
  Wiskott-Aldrich
  Chédiak-Higashi
  DiGeorge
  Cartilage hair hypoplasia
  Severe combined immunodeficiency
  Reticular dysgenesis
Miscellaneous Inherited Diseases
  Osteopetrosis
  Storage diseases
  Metachromatic leukodystrophy
  Lesch-Nyhan

inherited from each parent, the chance of matching among siblings is 25%.

Procedure

When a donor is selected, the patient goes through a "conditioning" procedure. The purpose of "conditioning" is to create space in recipient's marrow for engraftment, to suppress the immune resistance to prevent the graft rejection, and to eradicate the malignant cells. Various conditioning regimens are being used, including total body irradiation, cyclophosphamide, busulfan, Ara-C, and BCNU. The risk to the donor is minimal.

Approximately 3×10^8 nucleated marrow cells are collected from the donor under general anesthesia by aspirating the marrow from multiple sites. Collected marrow is filtered and processed to remove the incompatible red cells and the T cells, in an effort to decrease the chance of immunologically competent T cells' rejection of the donor tissues (graft versus host disease [GVHD]). Chemical treatment may be needed for autologous BMT to "purge" the malignant cells. For autologous BMT, marrow is preserved in liquid nitrogen for later infusion. For other types of BMT, it is infused intravenously soon after harvesting.

Complications of BMT

INFECTIONS. Gram-negative and gram-positive bacterial infections are common until the engraftment takes place and neutrophil production is adequate. Complete recovery of the immune system may take several months or years, during which opportunistic infections with organisms such as *Pneumocystis carinii* and cytomegalovirus are common and life threatening. Prevention and treatment of infections are important in a successful BMT.

GRAFT VERSUS HOST DISEASE (GVHD). The most significant cause of morbidity and mortality, GVHD is mediated by the donor's immunocompetent T cells.

Acute GVHD develops in 30 to 50% of patients, with a mortality of 20 to 40%. Manifestations include maculopapular, later "burnlike" rash, jaundice, abdominal pain, liver failure, and diarrhea. Biopsy confirms the diagnosis.

Chronic GVHD resembles collagen vascular disease and usually develops 100 to 500 days after the BMT. It develops in 15 to 40% of patients and has a high mortality. Manifestations include dry skin, hyper- or hypopigmented skin lesions, which may progress to sclerosis and contractures. Esophagitis, sicca-like syndrome of lacrimal and salivary glands, biliary cirrhosis, myositis, polyserositis, and chronic obstructive bronchiolitis may develop. Prevention and treatment include use of cyclosporin-A, methotrexate, topical or systemic steroids, and supportive therapy.

HEPATIC VENOOCCLUSIVE DISEASE. Nonthrombotic narrowing and fibrous obliteration of hepatic venules and sublobular veins occur in 10 to 20% of the cases with 50% mortality. It usually develops within 30 days of BMT. Clinical manifestations include jaundice, right upper quadrant pain with hepatomegaly, and ascites.

OTHER COMPLICATIONS OF BMT. These include graft rejection, relapse on the donor or recipient marrow, and interstitial pneumonitis. Late complications are cataracts, restrictive and obstructive lung disease, hypothyroidism, sterility, growth failure encephalopathy, and second malignancies.

Future challenges in BMT technology are improving partially or non-HLA matching transplants, better malignant and T-cell purging, effective treatment for GVHD, enhancement of immune reconstitution, better "conditioning" techniques, and prevention of early and late complications.

Timur Sumer

References

Pizzo, A. P., Poplack, D. G. (Eds.). *Principles and Practice of Pediatric Oncology,* Philadelphia: Lippincott, 1989.

Pochedly, C. (Ed.). Cancer in children. *Hematol. Oncol. Clin. North Am.* 1(4), 1987.

Poplack, D. G. (Ed.). The leukemias. *Pediatr. Clin. North Am.* 35(4), 1988.

Sutow, W. W., Fernbach, D. J., and Vietti, T. J. (Eds.). *Clinical Pediatric Oncology.* St. Louis: Mosby, 1984.

18

Connective Tissue Diseases

Connective tissue diseases represent one of the major unsolved problems of pediatrics, and they are of far greater importance to child health than their frequency would suggest because of their chronicity and the permanent disability that they may cause.

The original term *collagen diseases* was introduced by Klemperer to describe those diseases in which he considered the primary lesion to be fibrinoid necrosis of collagen, the main structural protein of connective tissue. Since the effect on collagen is secondary and we find inflammation in the connective tissue itself, a better and more descriptive term is *connective tissue diseases*.

Rheumatic Fever

Rheumatic fever is one of the most important childhood illnesses because of the chronic disability that it may produce by damage to the heart. It is found in most parts of the world, in warm as well as cold climates.

Pathogenesis

It is now clearly established that rheumatic fever is a complication of group A beta-hemolytic streptococcal infection.

Approximately 2 to 3 weeks or longer after the streptococcal infection, which almost always involves the respiratory tract, the disease appears in about 1 or 2% of individuals. The factors making for susceptibility to rheumatic fever are poorly understood. Both genetic and environmental factors seem to be operative; that is, the disease tends to have a familial incidence but is also associated with crowding and social conditions. It is only indirectly caused by streptococcal organisms, as the evidence for active infection in the lesions is lacking. The immunological evidence, however, that beta-hemolytic streptococcal infection has preceded an attack of active rheumatic fever can almost always be established by testing for different antistreptococcal antibodies; of these, antistreptolysin-O titer is the most commonly measured. Adequate and timely treatment of streptococcal infections can prevent rheumatic fever.

Incidence

Although the apparent decrease in incidence and severity of rheumatic fever in the United States and Europe is in part due to the availability of effective drugs in the treatment of streptococcal infections, it is clear that this disease had already been declining in frequency before such treatments were available. Because rheumatic fever seems to occur more often among lower socioeconomic groups in which crowded housing and poor hygienic conditions predispose them to a higher incidence of streptococcal disease, the apparent fall in the incidence of rheumatic fever may be partially attributable to such factors as general improvement in the standard of living. This decrease in the incidence and severity of rheumatic fever in the United States and Europe was seen through 1985.

Although the fall in frequency of rheumatic fever preceded the use of antibacterial agents, the mild resurgence of cases in the United States since 1985 has suggested other possibilities for the fall and resurgence. Genetic susceptibility is an old theory and has been joined by the consideration that certain strains of *Streptococcus* are more likely to result in acute rheumatic fever.

The new epidemics have been reported from widely separated geographic areas such as Utah, two separate areas of Ohio, Pennsylvania, and several outbreaks among military trainees in Missouri and California.

This resurgence should signal a heightened degree of suspicion and viligance among pediatricians seeing children with sore throats.

Rheumatic fever is almost unknown below the age of 2 and rare before 5 years. The incidence falls after 10 years of age, and the disease becomes rare after the age of 20, except in those who suffer from recurrences. It has a predilection for certain families and tends to recur, with a greater chance of permanent cardiac damage with each recurrence.

Clinical Manifestations

The so-called major and minor manifestations of rheumatic fever are listed in Table 18-1 under the Jones criteria for diagnosis. Of these, carditis is the critical one because it may lead to the irreversible lesions of the heart valves of rheumatic heart disease. The major manifestations are discussed briefly below.

CARDITIS. As a rule, the younger the child, the greater are the chances of cardiac involvement. Pericarditis, myocarditis, and endocarditis may be seen, but endocardial involvement is of the greatest concern to the physician because of the permanent scarring of the valves that may follow. Of the four heart valves, the mitral is the most commonly affected. Next in frequency is the aortic valve; disease of the pulmonic or tricuspid valve is rare. In many young children carditis may be the only initial evidence of rheumatic fever.

Table 18-1. The Modified Jones Criteria for Acute Rheumatic Fever

Major manifestations	Minor manifestations	Others
Carditis	Fever	Family history
Migratory polyarthritis	Arthritis	Epistaxis
Chorea	Prolonged PR interval	Weight loss
Subcutaneous nodules	Positive C-reactive protein	Anemia
Erythema marginatum	Leukocytosis (over 10,000/mm^3)	
	Evidence of prior streptococcal infection (antistreptolysin titer)	
	Elevated sedimentation rate	
	Prior history of rheumatic fever	
	Presence of inactive rheumatic heart disease	

MIGRATORY POLYARTHRITIS. Arthralgia is to be differentiated from true arthritis, which produces objective signs of redness, swelling, pain, and limitation of motion. The joints usually affected are the large joints — the knee, elbow, and ankle. Pain is generally severe, and there is a tendency for the arthritis to be migratory and leave the involved joints after a few days. The response to salicylate or steroid therapy is usually dramatic, and therapeutic trial of these drugs sometimes constitutes an important aid in the differential diagnosis. Once the arthritis passes the acute stages, there is no residual permanent joint damage. Frequent recurrent episodes in the hands may produce loosening of periarticular structures (e.g., the joint capsule) and lead to reducible deformities (Jaccoud's arthritis) without evidence of joint damage.

SYDENHAM'S CHOREA. This self-limited disorder is typically marked by involuntary movements, emotional lability, and apparent muscle weakness. It is considered a major manifestation of rheumatic fever, although other evidence for that disease may be lacking. The reason may be that there is a latent period, up to several months long, between streptococcal infection and chorea, and that the antistreptolysin-O titer has already fallen to normal by the time the chorea appears. No consistent pathological changes in the central nervous system have been found.

The onset is gradual over a few days or weeks. Handwriting is poor, and speech is dysarthric; both may be lost for a time. Many patients are completely bedridden during the height of the illness. Inappropriate laughing or crying may occur, and rarely a frank psychosis appears. All symptoms subside gradually after several weeks. Occasionally the condition recurs. Death is rare and is usually the result of carditis, although exhaustion from chorea has been described. When chorea occurs alone as a rheumatic manifestation, carditis is rare, but such a case may be followed years later by evidence of mitral stenosis.

SUBCUTANEOUS NODULES. These painless nodules, varying in size from a few millimeters to more than a centimeter, are demonstrable under a good light on the extensor surface of the joints, including the spine; they can also occur over the scalp and the occiput. Subcutaneous nodules may be seen in conditions other than rheumatic fever, particularly polyarticular juvenile arthritis, and usually occur in patients with severe and chronic rheumatic activity. They may also appear as benign lesions (pseudorheumatoid nodules).

ERYTHEMA MARGINATUM. This rash, consisting of erythematous elevated or marginated eruptions, is usually of transient nature and occurs in a small percentage of patients with rheumatic fever. Few clinicians, therefore, have sufficient experience to distinguish it clearly from some other nonspecific eruptions such as those caused by drugs.

Diagnosis

Most discussions of rheumatic fever stress the need of accurate categorization of each suspected case as definitely rheumatic or definitely nonrheumatic. The psychic trauma of prolonged periods of bedrest, the necessity for prolonged penicillin prophylaxis, and the stigma associated with the label "rheumatic" are given as reasons for this strict categorization. The sensitive physician should be able to minimize these in the management of the patient. Because there is no specific diagnostic test for acute rheumatic fever, many patients inevitably fall into a third category, "possibly rheumatic."

Table 18-1 lists the Jones criteria for the diagnosis of acute rheumatic fever. The application of these criteria to specific clinical situations is one of the most challenging responsibilities in the practice of pediatrics. Attention should be directed primarily to the diagnosis of carditis. In the absence of carditis, the patient may receive therapeutic and prophylactic courses of antistreptococcal therapy, be sent back to normal activities, and be carefully followed. The

presence of two major criteria or one major and two minor criteria suggests with a high degree of probability that the patient has acute rheumatic fever.

A newly appearing murmur, a pericardial friction rub, pericardial effusion, or congestive heart failure is definite diagnostic evidence in favor of carditis. Radiological finding of definite cardiac enlargement is added confirmatory evidence. It was formerly assumed that the presence of subcutaneous nodules was a fairly good indication of the coexisting presence of carditis, but this theorem must be dropped. Tachycardia out of proportion to the degree of fever, changing poor quality of heart sounds associated with a newly appearing systolic murmur, gallop rhythm, and fluctuating systolic murmurs are all suggestive of rheumatic carditis. The astute physician is also the humble one who will not make the diagnosis of rheumatic carditis unless the auscultatory findings are confirmed by an objective consultant. In the absence of other obvious causes, a child with definite carditis is assumed to have acute rheumatic fever and, after recovery, is given prophylactic antistreptococcal medication.

Children suspected of having Sydenham's chorea should be investigated for other possible causes — for example, drugs (such as the promazine derivatives), familial neurological disease (Huntington's chorea or Wilson's disease), and tics, which usually cause the greatest problem in differential diagnosis. A carefully taken history and observation generally make the diagnosis obvious; in that event the child may reasonably be assumed to have acute rheumatic fever and should be given long-term prophylactic antistreptococcal therapy.

Erythema marginatum is a notoriously difficult clinical diagnosis to make with absolute certainty. Very few observers can readily and unequivocally distinguish this rheumatic rash from the other erythemas. It seems more reasonable that this be relegated to the category of minor manifestation.

One should remember that the erythrocyte sedimentation rate (ESR) may not be elevated in some of the sickest children with acute rheumatic fever. This is especially the case in children with congestive heart failure.

There are so many spurious causes for a leukocytosis over 10,000/mm^3 that this should be eliminated from the list of minor manifestations. A negative C-reactive protein test may be interpreted as good evidence against the presence of the acute rheumatic state, but a positive test occurs in many unrelated conditions.

Also, many of the features of acute rheumatic fever may overlap some of those of other diseases. For example, children with rheumatic fever may have hematuria suggesting acute hemorrhagic nephritis, polyarteritis, or lupus erythematosus.

Treatment of Acute Rheumatic Fever without Carditis

Corticosteroids are not used, although this issue is still not completely resolved. The existence of streptococci must be assumed and a 10-day course of full doses of penicillin therapy instituted. Antiinflammatory therapy with aspirin (maximum dose, 120 mg/kg body weight/24 hours in four divided doses) should be given until there is no fever, arthritis, or arthralgia, and until the ESR has returned to normal values. Bedrest for 2 weeks is indicated; gradual mobilization over the next 2 weeks is reasonable if no evidence of carditis is observed. Oral penicillin prophylaxis for a period of 5 to 10 years is probably mandatory.

Treatment of Acute Rheumatic Fever with Carditis

Careful and frequent observation is in order. In addition to receiving antistreptococcal therapy, the patient is kept in bed until the cardiac inflammation has subsided. Aspirin in doses of up to 120 mg/kg/day, close to the level of toxicity, is the generally accepted form of antiinflammatory therapy, although most experienced observers are convinced that large doses of corticosteroids (60 mg of prednisone per day) are more effective in severe carditis and may be lifesaving in persons with severe congestive heart failure. All the techniques useful in the treatment of cardiac failure should be employed; the judicious combination of two or all of them may make a great difference in the outcome in the child with a severely decompensated heart. Oxygen therapy, digitalization, diuretics, and a low-salt diet must be used as in other forms of cardiac decompensation. The electrolytes must be watched carefully, especially when corticosteroids are given and when the child is receiving intravenous fluids because of poor oral intake. Adequate nutrition should be maintained. Rotating extremity tourniquets and phlebotomy are useful but often forgotten measures in severe emergency. Transfusion of packed red cells may also be helpful in anemic patients.

The patient must be kept under careful, frequent observation. The absence of fever, tachycardia, or peripheral venous congestion, the presence of heart sounds of good quality, and a normal electrocardiogram and erythrocyte sedimentation rate are all good signs and can be taken as an indication for gradual tapering of antiinflammatory therapy. As the dose of corticosteroids is gradually lowered, evidence for increased rheumatic activity should be sought.Then aspirin therapy should also be eliminated little by little and the child

observed for signs of rebound rheumatic activity. In the severe case this entire process usually consumes several months, and it should not be hurried.

Prognosis

The best sign is good morale, a vigorous appetite, and weight gain. The cheerful, smiling patient is likely to have the best prognosis.

Follow-up Period

Children with rheumatic fever should be followed regularly and must continue antistreptococcal prophylaxis, probably for the remainder of their lives; this is best accomplished by monthly administration of 1,200,000 units of benzathine penicillin. Oral penicillin, 200,000 units twice daily on an empty stomach, or oral sulfadiazine (0.5 g for children weighing less than 30 kg and 1.0 g for those weighing more) once daily is also satisfactory but less reliable. Patients who are sensitive to these drugs may receive erythromycin orally. Management of their physical activities depends on the presence or absence of damaged heart valves and the evidence for cardiac enlargement or failure.

Juvenile Arthritis

In adults rheumatoid arthritis is one of the most chronic of all diseases. Recent studies in juvenile arthritis have been able to establish subtypes that show features different from those in the adult form of the disease. The term *juvenile rheumatoid arthritis* should be retained only for patients who are seropositive for rheumatoid factor. These children are more frequently females and have an older age of onset. In general, they appear to have adult rheumatoid arthritis beginning at a younger age. A general classification is given in Table 18-2.

Etiology and Pathological Findings

Attempts to demonstrate a specific infectious agent as the cause of rheumatoid arthritis have all ended in failure. Focal infections of the teeth or colon, hemolytic and viridans streptococci, pleuropneumonialike organisms (PPLO), and now viruses have each had their day, but proof of their relationship to juvenile arthritis has not been established. In recent years the discovery of rheumatoid factor — classically a macroglobulin with specific affinity for immunoglobulin G — in the serum of patients and some of their relatives has

Table 18-2. Classification of Juvenile Arthritis

1. Systemic onset (about 20%). This group can go into remission but usually develops into seronegative polyarticular disease.
2. Polyarticular (about 30%). Equal incidence in males and females with the development of seronegative disease in younger groups; more females in teenage development of seropositive disease. This can be a more destructive disease.
3. Pauciarticular (about 50%). The most characteristic type in the childhood years. In younger girls, 20% are positive for ANA. In older boys, there is an association with HLA-B27. About 20% may develop ankylosing spondylitis as adults.

ANA = antinuclear antibody.

aroused interest in host susceptibility or an autoimmune mechanism for the production of the disease process. This serological abnormality, however, has not been established as central to the disease and indeed is rare in juvenile arthritis (about 20%, mostly in the group starting in older girls).

The unifying pathological feature of the rheumatoid process appears to be the inflammatory lesion of the synovium, with fibrinoid necrosis, predominantly lymphocytic infiltration, and ultimate fibrosis. Destruction of the cartilage and fusion of joints occurs if the process continues long enough. This inflammatory process is reflected in the joint fluid by an increase in cells, usually both polymorphonuclear and mononuclear leukocytes, and by breakdown by inflammatory products of the hyaluronic acid with resultant lowering of viscosity of the synovial fluid.

Clinical Manifestations

The most important feature of juvenile arthritis is its chronic course. Serious and potentially deforming joint manifestations may supervene in children with persistent polyarthritis, although they may be absent during the initial phases of systemic involvement. Involvement of other organs is common, but the exact nature of the involvement varies from case to case, appearing most frequently in those children with systemic onset.

Arthritis is the major clinical problem, particularly when the disease has assumed chronicity. The commonly involved joints are the knees, ankles, feet, wrists, hands, elbows, temporomandibular joints, and spine, especially in the cervical region. There is pain, swelling, heat, and limitation of motion. In the fingers the swelling is characteristically fusiform in appearance. Inflammatory changes in the joints may involve the tendons and bones. These changes result in

marked limitation of locomotion in the early stages of the disease, and without physical therapy contractures and serious deformities can develop.

The manifestations of juvenile arthritis may take several different clinical forms, all of which are seen in adults with the disease but in differing proportions. These common clinical patterns in childhood are, first, the acute systemic form of the disease, which is much more frequent in childhood; second, the more insidious type of chronic polyarthritis, which is most common in adults; and third, the milder pauciarticular or monoarticular form. There are now described subtypes such as the pauciarticular HLA-B27–positive form seen in adolescent males.

The systemic form is characterized by high, spiking fevers, ranging from 35.5 to 41.7°C in extreme cases; marked leukocytosis up to 30,000 to 50,000/mm³; lymphadenopathy; splenomegaly; and an evanescent but very characteristic erythematous, usually nonpruritic rash. The child often does not seem as sick as he should be for the degree and duration of fever, although he may be irritable and drowsy during periods of hyperpyrexia. Joints may not be involved initially or at all. When they begin to be, there is often a recession of the systemic manifestations. The rash comes and goes, often appearing only at times of fever; it is a salmon-pink, faint, polymorphous, macular erythema with occasional iris lesions as well as some linear streaks suggesting urticaria. It is usually confined to the trunk and extremities and may easily be missed at morning rounds when the temperature is normal or subnormal. There may be cardiac involvement with pericarditis, a pericardial friction rub or massive pericardial effusion, and even cardiac failure, confusing the disease with acute rheumatic fever. In some cases, pleural effusions with pleuritic pain and friction rub are also found. In children, a preceding episode of beta-hemolytic streptococcal infection may have triggered the disease in as many as one-third of the cases, so that a high antistreptolysin titer may further confuse the diagnosis. The disease runs a variable course. Fever usually lasts from 3 to 12 weeks with occasional remissions and may prove very resistant to treatment. It has recently been determined that a response of the fever and rash can be obtained in about 50% of the patients using tolmetin sodium (Tolectin) at a dose up to 50 mg/kg. Antibiotics are totally useless. Both salicylates and corticosteroids, given to the point of causing toxic side-effects, may be ineffective, although usually the latter drugs, which should be administered only when pericarditis or hyperpyrexia is alarming, are more efficacious in suppressing symptoms and generally bring the temperature down promptly. Ultimately the fever subsides and there may be no more attacks, or there may be a repetition of the same clinical picture after months or years of good health, or, as fever declines, joint involvement may gradually become the predominant manifestation of the disease.

The polyarthritic form of juvenile arthritis appears in 30% of involved children, as it does in adults, with the insidious onset of fairly symmetrical involvement, predominantly of the smaller, more distal joints. Fever, when it occurs, is low-grade, but anemia, lethargy, and irritability characterize the chronic course, in which, though there are remissions and exacerbations, there tends to be progression in the number of joints involved and in the extent of synovial destruction, scarring, and deformity. A subgroup of rheumatoid factor–positive girls have the worst prognosis for destructive disease.

The pauciarticular or monoarticular form of the disease, appearing in 50% at onset, tends to be most benign in terms of its systemic effects. An otherwise healthy child presents with a somewhat painful, swollen large joint (knee or ankle). There may be a history of injury, but the aspirated joint fluid is usually characteristic of inflammatory arthritis with high white cell counts, predominantly polymorphonuclear leukocytes. Over a period of months or even a few years several other joints may be involved, but systemic symptoms are generally absent. The joint involvement, four joints or less, is usually asymmetrical and most often confined to joints of the lower extremity. This otherwise benign disease, however, is the form of juvenile arthritis in which uveitis occurs most frequently (up to 20% of cases), so that the child should be examined by an ophthalmologist at 6-month intervals for early signs of this serious complication.

Multiple nodules, ordinarily appearing at points of trauma or pressure and as a rule considerably larger than those in rheumatic fever, may be a prominent manifestation in a few children, generally those with low-grade but progressive disease. They must be distinguished from the nodules seen in lipogranulomatosis or infantile Gaucher's disease, both of which usually occur in younger children.

Laboratory Findings

No specific laboratory test for juvenile arthritis is available. There is usually a moderate anemia, either of the type seen in chronic infections or rarely with some hemolysis. Leukocytosis is generally present during the early stages, particularly in younger patients with systemic onset. C-reactive protein, elevation of other acute-phase reactants, and an elevated ESR are often found. On electrophoresis the most common abnormality is a marked increase in alpha$_2$ globulins. As noted above, the finding of rheumatoid factor is a bad prognostic sign. Antinuclear factors are most often found in pauciarticular disease and frequently in children in whom uveitis develops. HLA-DR5 is frequent in pauciarticular diseases in males.

X-ray Studies

Widening of the joint spaces is the first radiological manifestation. Rarefaction and surface irregularities of the bones are followed by fusion and narrowing of the joint spaces. There may also be premature closure of the epiphyses and disturbances of bone growth. Monoarticular disease of the knee causes local hyperemia and subsequent stimulation of growth on the side of the affected joint; therefore the arthritic knee is accompanied by the longer limb.

Differential Diagnosis

Distinction between juvenile arthritis and acute rheumatic fever may be difficult during the initial stages, particularly when there is evidence of pericarditis as well as joint manifestations. A negative antistreptolysin-O titer rules out acute rheumatic fever, but a positive test does not necessarily exclude the possibility of rheumatoid arthritis. Other connective tissue diseases, tuberculous and pyogenic arthritides, psoriasis, inflammatory bowel disease, and malignant neoplasms also pose problems in differential diagnosis (see App. A, Sec. 10). Early stages of systemic-onset disease before the development of joint manifestations closely resemble an acute infectious process.

Course and Prognosis

The overall survival rate in juvenile arthritis is excellent, and the disease seems to burn itself out after varying periods. About 1% of cases have a fatal outcome either directly or indirectly resulting from the disease. Death is mostly due to complications of treatment and infection in the United States and to secondary amyloidosis in some European countries. Orthopedic deformities such as growth abnormalities, contractures, and to a lesser extent bony fractures are among the other complications, but the final prognosis can be strongly influenced by expert management, particularly by good orthopedic care and physical therapy.

Treatment

The main objective in the management of a patient with juvenile arthritis is to prevent irreversible psychological damage and physical deformities that may occur during the active phase of the disease, so that when the process comes to a standstill the child is able to continue a reasonably normal life. To this end the cooperation of the pediatrician, orthopedist, ophthalmologist, physical and occupational therapists, public health nurse, teacher, and family is required.

Continuation of physical activity that brings the involved part into full motion is to be encouraged whenever the patient's condition permits. Splinting of wrists and hands may help to decrease acute inflammation and maintain good position. The use of lightweight plastic leg splints may permit normal ambulation, especially when the subtalar joint is involved. Psychological and nursing care is as important as medical therapy; home care and provision for a normal existence, whenever possible, are the best safeguards against future emotional handicaps.

Drug therapy is primarily aimed at the reduction of inflammation and alleviation of pain and discomfort rather than reversal of the basic pathological process. Corticosteroids have no influence on the basic condition and are hazardous when used over long periods. They are to be avoided except in the management of serious systemic or eye manifestations and when the disease appears to be refractory to other forms of therapy. The smallest effective dose should then be given for the shortest possible period. Even then the discontinuation of therapy is often followed by a rebound of symptoms that makes the reinstitution of therapy necessary. Aspirin in doses from 80 to 100 mg/kg is useful for the relief of pain and for the antiinflammatory effect. Because the margin between effective and toxic doses is usually narrow, however, careful monitoring of the blood salicylate levels is necessary. Therapeutic levels are between 20 and 30 mg/100 ml; levels above 30 mg/100 ml are likely to induce toxicity without increasing the effectiveness of the aspirin.

The threat of the development of Reye's syndrome, though rare, has proved to be a major deterrent to the use of aspirin in the long-term therapy of juvenile arthritis. Studies of other nonsteroidal antiinflammatory drugs such as naproxen, piroxicam, ibuprofen, and tolmetin, have shown them to be as effective as aspirin with the advantage of fewer gastrointestinal side effects and the opportunity to cut down on dosage intervals. Some are available as liquid preparations and are more easily used by young children.

Dosages can be pushed beyond recommended levels if higher doses are felt to be needed for control of symptoms.

Injectable gold compounds such as sodium aurothiomalate have been shown to be effective in the treatment of polyarticular juvenile arthritis. Recently an oral compound, auranofin, has been successfully used in therapy. It was better than the placebo and probably has fewer side effects and is of course easier to give than the injectable form of gold. Another double-blind study of hydroxychloroquine and *d*-penicillamine did not show any difference from placebo therapy in children.

Systemic Lupus Erythematosus

Systemic lupus erythematosus (SLE) is a relatively rare but serious illness during childhood. The pathological process involves multiple organs and tends to occur much more frequently in females than in males, with a ratio of approximately 10:1. The disease may be seen at any age during childhood and even in infancy but most frequently occurs in adolescence.

Etiology

The cause of SLE remains unknown, but certain factors seem to contribute to its occurrence. Some patients give a history of prolonged exposure to sunlight, and others with known disease trace exacerbations of their clinical manifestations to such exposure. Drug hypersensitivity is also thought to be contributory. Another important factor is familial incidence. The family members of patients with SLE have a higher incidence of the disease and show a generally higher level of serum gamma globulin. Antinuclear antibodies and especially antibodies to double-stranded (native) DNA are the hallmark of SLE. These points and the fact that patients with the disease are capable of producing antibodies to a variety of antigenic stimuli more readily than normal persons suggest a combination of factors as well as inherent susceptibility.

Clinical Manifestations

The onset of SLE is usually more acute and the disease more rapidly progressive in children than in adults. The widespread degenerative changes, with fibrinoid formation, involve many organs and tissues. The first manifestation is variable, and the disease may mimic numerous other conditions. The most frequent presenting complaints in children include arthritis, arthralgias, rash, and fever. Bouts of thrombocytopenic purpura, pleural effusion, or unexplained febrile episodes may herald the onset or precede the disease by several months or years.

The most characteristic feature of the disease is a photosensitive erythematous skin rash that covers the butterfly region of the face. It occurs in three-quarters of all cases. Other skin manifestations, particularly punctate erythematous lesions over the fingers and palms of the hands as well as capillary tortuosities and hemorrhages in the nail beds, may also be evident.

Generalized lymphadenopathy, splenomegaly, hepatomegaly, irregular fever, polyserositis, and arthralgia are common. Cardiac manifestations include transient pericardial friction rubs, cardiac murmurs, and electrocardiographic changes. Verrucous endocarditis, known as Libman-Sacks syndrome, is found in some cases, usually at autopsy. Renal involvement, a poor prognostic sign, occurs in up to two-thirds of the patients. It is likely to be progressive and constitutes the main cause of mortality in this disease. Infection is the second most frequent cause of death. Central nervous system involvement has a bad prognosis.

Diagnosis

The distinction of SLE from other diseases involving joints and blood vessels is relatively easier in children and adolescents than in adults because in the former group the course is more rapid and evidence for multiple-organ manifestation is usually clear in the early stages. Renal involvement is commonly found from the beginning of the illness and is progressive, giving rise to abnormal urinary findings and an elevated blood urea nitrogen level. Percutaneous renal biopsy provides positive evidence for the presence of lupus nephritis, most often showing a diffuse proliferative nephritis.

The SLE cell test is now of historical interest only. It is difficult to do properly, and the titered fluorescent antinuclear antibody (ANA) test is about 10 times more sensitive. Eventually all patients have a positive test. The titer shows a significant positive correlation with disease activity. The ANA test is positive in about 20% of patients with pauciarticular juvenile arthritis but in low titer; thus the titer has important diagnostic and prognostic value. Measurement of complement, either CH_{50} or C3 and C4, is valuable because low levels also have some correlation with disease activity. High levels of circulating immune complexes as measured by C1q (solid-phase assay is the best) correlate with heightened disease activity. Other common laboratory findings include anemia, leukopenia, thrombocytopenia, positive direct Coombs' test, and false-positive serological tests for syphilis. The ESR is expected to be elevated in SLE although the test for C-reactive protein is usually negative — a point that is important in differentiating the illness from some of the other connective tissue diseases (e.g., rheumatic fever and juvenile arthritis).

Drug-induced lupus erythematosus must be identified by careful scrutiny, because in this situation the pathological process can be reversed. A suggestive history of drug intake, the absence of a positive Coombs' test, leukopenia, thrombocytopenia, and an increased blood urea nitrogen level are helpful diagnostic points.

Treatment and Prognosis

Although the prognosis of SLE was once poor, the use of corticosteroids and the increasing knowledge of the disease have made it possible to suppress its acute manifestations, to reverse the renal disease responsible for a fatal outcome, and to keep patients active for long periods, with eventual recovery in some patients. Corticosteroids must be given in large doses (1 to 2 mg/kg/day) at times of crises (fever, cerebral symptoms, or renal involvement), with gradual reduction in the dose until the lowest dose compatible with maintenance of the remission is found; this maintenance dose is continued over a long period. Administration of double the daily dose every other morning has been found to diminish the metabolic effects of the steroids. This must be done carefully and usually cannot be used until the patient is well controlled on a steady daily morning dose. "Immunosuppression" therapy may also be needed at times. It is ordinarily reserved for patients with renal or central nervous system disease who are not responding to the high-dose corticosteroids. The patients, usually adolescent girls, require close supervision over a period of years by someone familiar with the disease for best results, because multiple complications tend to occur.

Dermatomyositis

Dermatomyositis, a rare systemic disease, is characterized by relatively nonspecific but acute inflammatory perivascular lesions that are found primarily in the skeletal muscles and their overlying skin. The cause is unknown; the occasional association of this illness in adults with malignant neoplasms is not observed in the pediatric age group.

Clinical Manifestations

The cardinal clinical manifestations of dermatomyositis are weakness, soreness, and stiffness in the involved striated muscles. The disease characteristically attacks proximal muscle groups around the hip and shoulder girdle. Thickening and induration of the affected areas of skin and muscle are best detected in the extremities. A violaceous hue around the eyes, occasionally in conjunction with periorbital edema, especially involving the upper lids, is pathognomonic. An erythematous, indurated rash over the butterfly area of the face and atrophic, erythematous skin lesions over the knuckles, elbows, and knees are common. As the disease progresses, there may be marked muscle atrophy with contractures. In subsequent years, after the inflammatory component has subsided, calcinosis universalis may appear. Systemic manifestations, with the involvement of the kidneys, heart, gastrointestinal tract, and mucous membranes, may rarely occur. Hepatosplenomegaly and lymphadenopathy are not unusual, and low-grade fever is common.

Diagnosis

There is no specific diagnostic test for dermatomyositis except muscle biopsy, which shows an inflammatory myopathy. The increase in serum enzymes derived from muscle, especially creatine phosphokinase, and urinary creatine level as well as abnormalities in the electromyogram serve as supportive evidence in diagnosis and may be used to follow the progress of the disease. The absence of ANA and rheumatoid factor in the serum helps differentiate this illness from the other connective tissue diseases. Polymyositis, with muscle pain, weakness, and fever but without skin manifestations, appears in a few patients.

Prognosis and Treatment

Although the disease is characterized by remissions and exacerbations, it is ultimately self-limited and may leave the patient with relatively few permanent deformities if properly treated. Death can occur through involvement of the muscles of deglutition and respiration in the acute phase and gastrointestinal involvement with multiple perforations in a later phase.

Treatment is primarily supportive and makes use of early ambulation, physical therapy, and rehabilitation measures. Corticosteroids given for short or long periods, as well as methotrexate as an immunosuppressive, are symptomatically useful. Recent studies have shown that early high-dose therapy can improve the prognosis. Pulse therapy (250–1000 mg of IV prednisone for 3 days) can produce striking short-term remission. This must be followed up by continuous oral corticosteroids.

In general if the initial involvement is mild then it is appropriate to start therapy with low-dose prednisone (3–10 mg/day). If the symptoms do not resolve then the corticosteroid can be increased for symptomatic control. The creatinine phosphokinase levels and the erythrocyte sedimentation rate may lag behind the clinical improvement but will usually respond in time.

Scleroderma

Scleroderma (progressive systemic sclerosis) is a rare disease of unknown cause. There is a perivascular inflammation of the affected area, usually the skin and subcutaneous tissues, sometimes the adjacent muscles, and less frequently the heart, esophagus, and lungs. Raynaud's phenomenon is a frequent early symptom. With the progression of the disease fibrotic changes occur, leading to contractures and cosmetic deformities. There are usually remissions and exacerbations, but the disease may be self-limited. High-dose corticosteroids (even pulse therapy) appears to be ineffective during the early edematous phase. The early use of penicillamine (250–500 mg/day) may reduce or deter the development of the thickened skin collagen.

Localized Scleroderma (Morphea)

This rare disease is differentiated from progressive systemic sclerosis in its limitation to certain areas of the skin and subcutaneous tissues. The lesions are erythematous at first, but they gradually assume a whitish, waxy consistency and are surrounded by a violaceous border. These patchy areas may eventually coalesce and fibrose, producing a larger deformity. The prognosis for survival is good, although the residual deformities can cause serious handicaps if large areas (e.g., hemi-involvement) are affected. Penicillamine can also be used in this condition.

Acute Glomerulonephritis

See Chapter 13.

Erythema Nodosum

See Chapter 22.

Vasculitides

The conditions included under the heading of vasculitis — namely, polyarteritis (periarteritis nodosa, including Kawasaki's disease), hypersensitivity vasculitis (including Henoch-Schönlein purpura), allergic granulomatous angiitis (including Wegener's granulomatosis), giant-cell arteritis (including Takayasu's disease), and vasculitis in the connective tissue disease — are all characterized by perivasculitis. Although relatively distinct clinical entities, they nevertheless have certain clinical features in common.

Henoch-Schönlein Syndrome

See Chapter 13, The Genitourinary System. Henoch-Schönlein syndrome is a systemic disease with a purpuric skin eruption and joint involvement, as well as gastrointestinal and renal manifestations. The cause is unknown, although preceding acute infections, particularly with beta-hemolytic streptococci, are considered important as precipitating factors, and historical data attesting to their role can be obtained in about 90% of cases. The disease is seen primarily in the colder months when respiratory infections are common. Allergy to certain foods and drugs has also been considered an etiological factor in some patients. Pathologically, infiltrates of round cells are found surrounding small blood vessels in affected skin.

CLINICAL MANIFESTATIONS. The order and combination of the following features of the disease vary from case to case. A recurrent type of nonthrombocytopenic purpura is the cardinal manifestation of the disease and is essential for making the diagnosis. It is characteristically found over the lower part of the trunk and lower extremities but may occur elsewhere. The lesions are urticarial at the beginning, but they later become maculopapular and erythematous with a hemorrhagic center and finally assume an ecchymotic appearance. A painful, brawny edema localized over the scalp and dorsum of the feet and hands is concomitantly present in some patients, particularly those under 3 years of age.

Joint involvement manifested by periarticular pain, and less often swelling, is the second most common feature of the disease. This is usually a transient, nonmigratory arthritis that mainly affects the knees and ankles; it leaves no residual deformity.

Renal involvement tends to occur early in the course, chiefly in older children. It constitutes the most important prognostic feature of the disease, although its frequency and severity vary considerably, according to different reports. The principal sign of renal involvement is hematuria, but albuminuria, hypertension, and, rarely, elevation of blood urea nitrogen may occur. The renal histology, however, is different from that seen in acute glomerulonephritis, and the incidence of subsequent chronic nephritis is substantially higher in this condition.

Gastrointestinal manifestations are commonly found in patients with this disease and include nausea, vomiting, and crises of severe abdominal pain associated either with gross melena or with the presence of occult blood in stools. Bleeding may be severe enough to require blood transfusions. Hemorrhagic sites in the bowel may serve to induce an intussusception that is characteristically resistant to reduction by hydrostatic pressure. Any child with Henoch-Schönlein purpura who complains of abdominal pain must therefore be watched and followed carefully.

DIAGNOSIS. The diagnosis is primarily clinical. The white blood count may be elevated. Coagulation studies are characteristically normal, and platelet counts are either normal or elevated. The tourniquet test is negative. Repeated examinations of the urine show hematuria, proteinuria, and red cell casts. In contrast to acute glomerulonephritis due to beta-hemolytic streptococcal infection, progressive glomerulonephritis, or active lupus nephritis, in which serum complement levels are low, serum complement (or beta$_1$-C globulin) is high in this nephritis. Frequent determinations of hematocrit discloses the presence of massive gastrointestinal bleeding.

TREATMENT. Treatment is supportive. Corticosteroids, although often effective for symptomatic relief, prevention of intussusception, and perhaps shortening the course of illness, do not seem to affect the prognosis of renal involvement. The prognosis, however, even with renal involvement is excellent.

Kawasaki Disease

This syndrome, first described by Kawasaki in Japan in 1967, has recently been reported from a number of centers (Hawaii, Los Angeles, New York, Rochester [N.Y.], etc.) in the United States. In Hawaii there is still a disproportionate number of children of Japanese descent with this disease. There are three stages to the disease. The acute state presents with fever, enlargement of lymph nodes (usually cervical), rash (erythema multiforme), and involvement of the hands and feet. The tongue becomes discolored (strawberry tongue). The hands initially show palmar erythema, but with the fever they become indurated and swollen. This stage lasts for 1 to 10 days. The second or subacute stage lasts for 10 to 25 days. All children show thrombocytosis and desquamation of the hands and feet. There is often arthritis and occasionally myocarditis with coronary aneurysms, which may be detected by ultrasonography. An arteritis can be demonstrated. Other features may include aseptic meningitis, sterile pyuria, and hydrops of the gallbladder. The recovery phase can last up to 45 days. The ESR is elevated, but ANA and rheumatoid factor are not found. Although the disease is self-limited, long-term cardiac damage due to arterial inflammation can be found in a few patients.

The major threat to life in Kawasaki disease is from the development of aneurysms of the coronary arteries. This is fatal in about 2% of the patients. Using various diagnostic modalities (two-dimensional echocardiography and coronary angiography), these aneurysms can be identified early. Many resolve, but 20% can develop cardiovascular sequelae.

Therapy has been successful in reducing the long-term problems when the lesion has been identified. Treatment consists of aspirin 80 to 100 mg/kg/day for up to 8 weeks plus intravenous gamma-globulin 400 mg/kg/day for 4 days.

Polyarteritis (Periarteritis Nodosa)

Polyarteritis is a serious, rare systemic disease of uncertain cause. Males are more often affected than females. The onset of this condition is not uncommonly traced back to episodes of upper respiratory infections, again presumably incriminating streptococci.

CLINICAL MANIFESTATIONS. The children present with fever and small red painful nodules (smaller than the lesions of erythema nodosum) on the feet (including the soles) and legs. They have an elevated ESR and a high white cell count. Nervous system involvement may cause a variety of symptoms including convulsions, hemiplegia, and polyneuritis. Cardiac failure, progressive renal disease, with proteinuria, hematuria, cylindruria, hypertension, and azotemia, and an asthmatic type of pulmonary affection are common. Ischemia of the extremities may lead to gangrenous changes. Abdominal pain and skin eruptions are among other usual manifestations. The exclusion of an infectious cause for the illness, multiple organ involvement, urinary findings, and the presence of anemia, leukocytosis, eosinophilia, and increased ESR should suggest the diagnosis. Confirmation of the diagnosis is by histological examination, usually of muscle tissue obtained by biopsy.

TREATMENT AND PROGNOSIS. Treatment with corticosteroids or cyclophosphamide or both gives an improved prognosis, but the ultimate prognosis is guarded.

Lyme Disease

Lyme disease, since its definition in 1977, has developed into a major cause of arthritis in children in endemic areas. From the first cases reported in children in Old Lyme, Connecticut, there has been an explosion both in the geographic spread of the disease and the realization of its importance as a well-defined form of infectious arthritis in children. It now rivals in some parts of the East Coast the frequency of presentation of pauciarticular juvenile arthritis.

The organism, a spirochete *(Borrelia burgdorferi)*, is carried by all phases of the life cycle of the deer tick, *Ixodes dammini*. Children are most susceptible to bites and transmission of the spirochete in the nymphal stage. These are carried by small mammals and have been found not only in the woods, but even on well-manicured lawns immediately surrounding houses.

Because this problem is now reported from much of the Northeast, the upper Midwest, and the West, tests for the presence of the infection (antibody levels) should be performed if a child presents in a known endemic area with any of the manifestations of the disease besides arthritis. The initial bite and transmission of the organism can produce an erythema migrans. It can also result in a febrile illness with a number of constitutional symptoms including central nervous symptoms.

Therapy with penicillin and other antispirochetal agents is usually successful.

John Baum and Mohsen Ziai

References

Samter, M., et al. (Eds.). *Immunological Diseases* (4th ed.). Boston. Little, Brown, 1988.

Steere, A. C., et al., Longitudinal assessment of the clinical and epidemiological feature of Lyme disease in a defined population. *J. Inf. Dis.* 154:295, 1986.

Stiehm, E. R. *Immunological Disorders in Infants and Children* (3rd ed.). Philadelphia. Saunders, 1989.

19

Immunity and Immunization

The Immune System

The immune system recognizes and distinguishes self from foreign insults such as infectious microorganisms, tumor cells, or allogeneic tissue grafts. Recognition is followed by a response to eliminate the foreign substance and an immunological memory of the foreign substance that produces an accelerated and enhanced response upon reexposure to the same antigens. The body has both specific and nonspecific recognition, or afferent effector mechanisms. The specific components of the immune system include lymphocytes and immunoglobulins, and the nonspecific components include complement and polymorphonuclear and mononuclear leukocytes.

Ontogeny of the Immune System and Neonatal Immunity

Lymphocytes arise from pluripotent stem cells that are found originally in the fetal yolk sac. At about 2 months'

gestation the fetal liver is the main site of lymphoid development. By 4 months' gestation the bone marrow has replaced the liver as the major repository of early lymphocyte development; it retains this role throughout life.

The earliest B lymphocyte, or bone marrow–derived lymphocyte, detectable is a large proliferating cell that synthesizes the IgM heavy chain, which can be detected only in the cytoplasm of the cell and not on the cell surface. Pre-B cells are found in the fetal liver and later in the bone marrow, where they can be detected in adults. The pre-B cell differentiates to become a mature B cell independent of antigenic stimulation. An orderly set of rearrangement of immunoglobulin gene segments occurs to give rise to antigen-specific B cells that collectively express a diverse repertoire of antibody receptors. The immunoglobulin heavy chain genes are located on chromosome 14, kappa–light chain genes on chromosome 2, and lambda–light chain genes on chromosome 22. Each gene family consists of multiple members of separate gene segments, which are located on separate exons. The heavy chain gene segments include several hundred variable-region (V_H) genes, 20 or more diversity (D) genes, and six joining (J_H) genes that are located 5' of the constant (C_H) region genes. The light chain gene loci are also composed of variable-region and joining-region genes in addition to light chain constant-region genes. The pre-B cell first transposes one of the D_H genes next to one of the J_H genes, and the DNA between the two transposed genes is deleted. This is followed by rearrangement of one of the V_H genes next to the D_H-J_H rearrangement to form a complete VDJ rearrangement. This rearrangement process brings a promoter sequence 5' of the transposed V_H under the influence of a transcriptional enhancer located on the intron between J_H and the Cu gene. If the rearrangement process has been productive, a VDJ-Cu transcript is generated that is spliced to remove introns, and the processed transcript is translated and a u heavy-chain protein expressed in the cytoplasm of the pre-B cell. Next, gene rearrangement occurs at the kappa chain locus with switching to rearrangement to the lambda–light chain locus if a nonproductive rearrangement has occurred at the kappa locus.

With further differentiation the B cell acquires surface IgD. According to some evidence, a cell that has expressed IgD and other differentiation antigens is more mature and less susceptible to the development of tolerance than are immature B cells. IgD remains a major surface and a minor serum immunoglobulin throughout life. Upon further differentiation the cell acquires surface IgG and later IgA. Although exact steps in differentiation have not been elucidated, there is evidence that multiple isotypes are expressed on the surface of cells expressing IgG or IgA in the fetus and newborn.

Whereas morphologically typical B cells exist by 3 months' gestation, only minimal immunoglobulin synthesis occurs in utero. The normal fetus produces IgM by about 30 weeks' gestation reaching levels in the cord blood of 10% of the adult concentration. The antigenic specificity of the IgM is unknown. The fetus is capable, however, of mounting a specific antibody response by about 4 to 5 months' gestation with antigenic stimulation. This most commonly occurs with in utero congenital infection. The antibody response of the fetus is unlike that of the adult. Only IgM (minimal or no IgG or IgA) antibody is produced after antigenic stimulation. The lack of production of IgG and IgA in utero is due to immaturity of the B cells producing these isotypes and possibly a lack of T-cell help and increased suppressor activity for their production. Even neonatal cells continue to show poor production of IgG with good production of IgM. This relative decrease of IgG production by B cells can be demonstrated in vitro until the infant is 2 years of age.

With the antigenic stimulus of a congenital infection, B cells differentiate in utero to become plasma cells that secrete primarily IgM. Most, but not all, infants with congenital infection show elevated levels of cord IgM (greater than 20 mg/dl) and specific IgM antibodies to the pathogen. Newborns with congenital rubella, however, may have low levels of total IgM although specific antibody to rubella is detectable. The level of IgM with congenital infection is related to the type and severity of infection and to the newborn's maturity. In addition to congenital infection, elevated cord IgM may reflect a placental leak of maternal blood. This possibility can be distinguished from congenital infection by the fact that with a placental leak, the serum IgA level is elevated and the IgM quickly decreases from catabolism. One exception to this rule is that infants with congenital cytomegalovirus may have elevated cord IgA levels.

The newborn is provided with some passive protection against pathogens that are prevalent in the environment. Maternal IgG begins to cross the placenta as early as 40 days' gestation but remains at low levels in the fetus until the third trimester, when it starts to increase markedly. Premature infants have cord IgG levels directly related to the length of their gestation. IgG is the only immunoglobulin isotype that passes across the placenta. The IgG_1 subclass crosses the placenta better than the IgG_2 subclass. Transport occurs by an active transport mechanism that depends on recognition of the Fc portion of the gamma heavy chain. The lack of maternal IgM in the newborn leaves infants susceptible to some gram-negative bacteria.

After delivery, IgG levels decrease (Fig. 19-1) because its half-life is only 20 to 30 days and, to some extent, because of the increase in the infant's body mass. The duration of specific antibody protection from maternal passive antibody depends on the height of the initial antibody titer and the titer required for protection. Passive immunity to pyogenic bacteria may last only 1 to 3 months, whereas against measles and hepatitis immunity may last up to 1 year of age. A nadir of the infant's IgG level occurs at about 3 to 4 months of age when the majority of maternal IgG has been catabolized and the infant's antibody production is still low. This level is even lower in premature infants because of the lower levels of maternal antibody acquired by the time of birth. Infants tend to have greater susceptibility to infections at the time of this lower IgG level.

After delivery, the newborn is quickly colonized by microbes on the skin, in the nasopharynx, and in the gastrointestinal tract. Lymph nodes and plasma cells become evident, and active antibody synthesis and immunoglobulin formation rapidly ensue. IgM synthesis begins in the first week of life, and IgG synthesis quickly follows thereafter. IgA synthesis is delayed until late in the first month or the

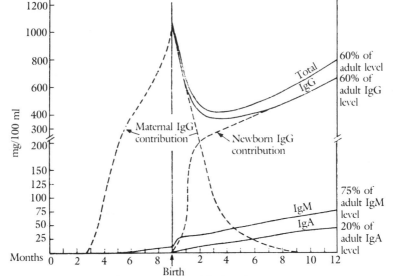

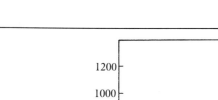

Fig. 19-1. Immunoglobulin (IgG, IgM, and IgA) levels in the fetus and infant in the first year of life. The IgG of the fetus and newborn infant is solely of maternal origin. The small amount of IgM of the newborn is synthesized by the fetus. The maternal IgG decreases after birth, at which time IgM and IgG endogenous synthesis accelerates. The nadir of the infant's IgG level occurs at 3 to 5 months of age. (From Stiehm, E. R. The B lymphocyte system. In E. R. Stiehm [Ed.], Immunologic Disorders in Infants and Children (3rd ed.). Philadelphia: Saunders, 1988.)

second month of life. Age-related immunoglobulin levels are found throughout childhood (Table 19-1). Adult levels of IgG and IgA are not reached until about age 10 and 15 years respectively.

Specific antibody responses to immunization in newborns are not comparable to those in older infants. First, maternal antibodies can exert an immunosuppressive effect on the infant's active antibody response. This is one reason for delaying immunization for diphtheria, pertussis, and tetanus until the infant is 1 month old and with measles until after 1 year of age. Antibody responses increase in later infancy due to not only a decrease in maternal antibody levels but to maturation of the cells participating in the response. The antibody response of newborns and young infants is predominantly IgM and shows a slow switch to IgG antibody synthesis. Poor antibody responses to some antigens can persist through 2 years of age. Infants do not produce protective levels of antibody to the polysaccharide capsules of *Hemophilus influenzae* b and of some pneumococci until this age. Hence, very young infants can be susceptible to recurrent bouts of *H. influenzae* disease. This age-related maturational delay in responding to some polysaccharides can be overcome by immunizing with vaccines in which the polysaccharide has been covalently linked to a protein carrier. Such vaccines are termed *conjugate*

vaccines. The protein carrier is able to recruit T lymphocyte help that stimulates proliferation and differentiation of the polysaccharide-specific B cell.

Infants who are breast-fed receive additional passive immunity against infections. Colostrum and breast milk have antibodies of the IgA isotype bound to secretory component. The antigenic specificity of these antibodies can differ from that found in sera. There is a common mucosal IgA immune system that produces antibody synthesis at mucosal sites distant from the site of antigen challenge. Thus, bacterial challenge in the small intestine induces antibody synthesis in the breast and in salivary glands. The mechanism of this generalized mucosal immune response is that B cells sensitized in lymphoid tissue in the small intestine travel specifically to distant mucosal sites, where they can produce IgA antibodies. The breast-fed newborn is,

Table 19-1. Levels of Immune Globulins in Normal Subjects at Different Ages

Age	No. of subjects	Level of γG*		Level of γM*		Level of γA*		Level of total γ-globulin*	
		mg/100 ml (range)	% of adult level	mg/100 ml (range)	% of adult level	mg/100 ml (range)	% of adult level	mg/100 ml (range)	% of adult level
Newborn	22	1031 ± 200 (645–1244)	89 ± 17	11 ± 5 (5–30)	11 ± 5	2 ± 3 (0–11)	1 ± 2	1044 ± 201 (660–1439)	67 ± 13
1–3 mo	29	430 ± 119 272–762)	37 ± 10	30 ± 11 (16–67)	30 ± 11	21 ± 13 (6–56)	11 ± 7	481 ± 127 (324–699)	31 ± 9
4–6 mo	33	427 ± 186 (206–1125)	37 ± 16	43 ± 17 (10–83)	43 ± 17	28 ± 18 (8–93)	14 ± 9	498 ± 204 (228–1232)	32 ± 13
7–12 mo	56	661 ± 219 (279–1533)	58 ± 19	54 ± 23 (22–147)	55 ± 23	37 ± 18 (16–98)	19 ± 9	752 ± 242 (327–1687)	48 ± 15
13–24 mo	59	762 ± 209 (258–1393)	66 ± 18	58 ± 23 (14–114)	59 ± 23	50 ± 24 (19–119)	25 ± 12	870 ± 258 (398–1586)	56 ± 16
25–36 mo	33	892 ± 183 (419–1274)	77 ± 16	61 ± 19 (28–113)	62 ± 19	71 ± 37 (19–235)	36 ± 19	1024 ± 205 (499–1418)	65 ± 14
3–5 yr	28	929 ± 228 (569–1597)	80 ± 20	56 ± 18 (22–100)	57 ± 18	93 ± 27 (55–152)	47 ± 14	1078 ± 245 (730–1771)	69 ± 17
6–8 yr	18	923 ± 256 (559–1492)	80 ± 22	65 ± 25 (27–118)	66 ± 25	124 ± 45 (54–221)	62 ± 23	1112 ± 293 (640–1725)	71 ± 20
9–11 yr	9	1124 ± 235 (779–1456)	97 ± 20	79 ± 33 (35–132)	80 ± 33	131 ± 60 (12–208)	66 ± 30	1334 ± 254 (966–1639)	85 ± 17
12–16 yr	9	946 ± 124 (726–1085)	82 ± 11	59 ± 20 (35–72)	60 ± 20	148 ± 63 (70–229)	74 ± 32	1153 ± 169 (833–1284)	74 ± 12
Adults	30	1158 ± 305 (569–1919)	100 ± 26	99 ± 27 (47–147)	100 ± 27	200 ± 61 (61–330)	100 ± 31	1457 ± 353 (730–2365)	100 ± 24

* Mean is ± 1 S.D.

Source: E. R. Stiehm and H. H. Fudenberg, Serum levels of immune globulins in health and disease: A survey. *Pediatrics* 37:717, 1966. Copyright © 1966 by the American Academy of Pediatrics.

therefore, passively fed a solution of IgA antibodies directed against prevalent enteric pathogens. Infants who are breast-fed have a lower incidence of gastroenteritis. Other factors in addition to IgA antibody contribute to this protection. The bacterial enteric flora of newborn infants is predominantly *Lactobacillus bifidus*, which resists growth of *Escherichia coli* and *Shigella*. Several nonimmunological antimicrobial factors in breast milk such as lysozyme and lactoferrin also contribute to protection. Lastly, there are macrophages and lymphocytes in breast milk that may be important protective factors for some pathogens.

T-cell, or thymus-derived lymphocyte, development occurs in the thymus. The epithelial lining of the third and fourth pharyngeal pouches gives rise to the thymus. At about the seventh week of gestation, stem cells are attracted to and enter the thymus by a process that is not well ex-

plained. The precursor cells rapidly divide under the capsule of the thymus in the outer cortex. Associated with cell division are acquisition and loss of cellular membrane antigens termed differentiation antigens. Monoclonal antibodies have been generated that allow recognition of discrete stages of T-cell development. In severe combined immunodeficiency disease, the few T cells that are detectable in the peripheral blood may express a surface phenotype found only on immature thymocytes.

Associated with T-cell division and differentiation in the thymus is a large amount of cell death. Only a small proportion of mature thymocytes enter the medulla and emigrate to the blood stream to circulate as mature helper/inducer and cytotoxic/suppressor T cells. In the thymus several processes occur before T cell or its descendents are allowed to egress from the thymus as a mature T cell. These include elimination of self-reactive T cells by immunological tolerance induction, cell death, or clonal deletion and active selection of cells because their receptors are likely to recognize antigen with self-MHC in the periphery. The exact mechanisms of positive and negative thymic selection is under active investigation.

Just as B cells have an antigen-binding receptor, T cells have a two-chain receptor that recognizes antigen when it is associated with membrane-bound products of the major histocompatibility complex (MHC). This dual recognition of both antigen and MHC is required for both activation of both the CD4 or helper/inducer immunoregulatory subset as well as the CD8 cytotoxic/suppressor subset. The MHC antigen recognized by CD4-bearing T cells is usually class ii antigen while the CD8-positive T cells usually respond to antigen presented with class i MHC antigens. The majority of T cells express a multichain receptor complex composed of a 90-kd alpha-beta heterodimer bound to the T3 complex. The alpha-beta heterodimer engages antigen and the MHC complex and the T3 subunits serve to transduce signals into the cell after the receptor is engaged. Like the immunoglobulin genes the T-cell receptor is encoded by genes that need to rearrange to be expressed. This rearrangement process occurs during T-cell development in the thymus. A minor subset of T cells in the peripheral blood and a major population of T cells in the intestine use a different T-cell receptor composed of a gamma-delta heterodimer that uses different gene elements than the alpha-beta–bearing T cells. The function of gamma-delta T cells has not been elucidated.

Fetal thymocytes acquire function by the third month of gestation. In general, fetal T cells have poor helper/inducer activity and better suppressor/cytotoxic activity than adult cells. It has been suggested that the enhanced suppressor activity may be an important mechanism in maintaining a pregnancy. During pregnancy, maternal lymphocytes cross the placenta and could potentially mount a response against the fetus. Fetal lymphocytes can specifically prevent maternal lymphocytes from responding in this manner.

Neonatal T cells have normal in vitro proliferative responses to plant lectins and allogeneic cells. Lymphokine production, however, is decreased. A decrease in helper and an increase in suppressor T-cell activity are also found in the newborn period. Delayed hypersensitivity skin tests are absent in newborns because of a poor inflammatory response and not solely because of immunological immaturity.

Newborns have decreased levels of components of the classical and alternative complement pathways. These deficiencies, in addition to the lack of specific antibody, have been implicated in the predisposition of the neonate to

bacterial sepsis with gram-negative bacteria and group B streptococci.

Immunodeficiency Disorders

Defects of the immune system may involve antibody-mediated immunity, T-cell-mediated immunity, both B- and T-cell immunity, the phagocytic system, which includes circulating neutrophils, monocytes, and tissue-fixed macrophages, or the complement system. Either a primary specific deficiency or a secondary deficiency may occur. The incidence of symptomatic primary immunodeficiency is approximately 1/10,000. Onset occurs within the first year of life in less than 10% of cases. Congenital disease may be of autosomal recessive or X-linked inheritance (Table 19-2). Secondary immunodeficiency disease is far more common. One of the most common causes of immunodeficiency in children during the next decade will be the acquired immunodeficiency syndrome (AIDS) due to infection with the HIV-1 virus (see Chapter 20, Infectious Diseases). Secondary defects in immunity may be caused by protein-calorie malnutrition, steroids and cytotoxic drugs, viral infection (Epstein-Barr virus, congenital rubella), parasitic infection, uremia, malignancy, burns, cirrhosis, and diabetes mellitus.

An immunodeficiency should be suspected if a child has an increased frequency, unusual severity, prolonged duration, or unusual complication of infections; however, normal infants can have numerous infections each year for the

Table 19-2. Genetic Basis of Human Immunodeficiency Diseases

Immunodeficiency disease	Chromosomal location
X-linked agammaglobulinemia	Xq21.3-22
Immunodeficiency with hyper-IgM	Xq24-26
Agammaglobulinemia following EBV infection	Xq24-q27
X-linked severe combined immunodeficiency	Xq13
Adenosine deaminase deficiency	20q13-ter
Ataxia-telangiectasia	11q22.3
Wiskott-Aldrich syndrome	Xp11
Purine nucleoside phosphorylase deficiency	14q13.1
X-linked chronic granulomatous disease	Xp21.1

first 4 to 5 years of life. Most of these infections do not occur until the level of transplacentally acquired maternal antibody declines during the latter half of the first year of life. Although one-third of children remain infection-free during the first year of life, approximately 40% of children have one cold and 10% have two colds during this period. Otitis media occurs in about the same frequency as colds in the first year of life, and 10 to 20% of normal infants experience more than one episode of otitis. By the age of 6 years, 10% of presumably normal children have sustained six episodes of otitis media. In the normal older children recurrent tonsillitis is not uncommon because of recrudescence of the original infection or new infections secondary to repetitive exposure to family members and school mates who are carriers of group A β-hemolytic streptococci. An increased frequency of infections in the early years of life can be caused by frequent exposure to other children. This commonly occurs in day care and nursery centers as well as in larger families, especially where there are school-age siblings or crowded sleeping conditions. The rate of infection may increase during the winter months because of increased close contacts and the drying effects on mucous membranes of winter heating.

In contrast to the normal child, the child with an immunodeficiency has more prolonged and severe infections, and between acute infections the child may not completely recover. Chronic moniliasis, draining ears, diarrhea, or bronchiectasis may be a presenting symptom. As a rule, recurrent infections of varying types and in more than one anatomical location occur. Unusual or opportunistic organisms such as *Pneumocystis carinii, Serratia, Pseudomonas,* or *Aspergillus* may cause infections.

The type of infection varies among the primary immunodeficiency states. Recurrent pyogenic infections — otitis media, pneumonia, meningitis, arthritis, osteomyelitis, conjunctivitis, sinusitis, pyoderma, and sepsis caused by encapsulated bacteria such as *Streptococcus pneumoniae, H. influenzae, Neisseria meningitidis,* and *Staphylococcus aureus* — should suggest a deficiency of antibody or less commonly a polymorphonuclear leukocyte or complement abnormality. Immunity to encapsulated bacteria is mediated by antibody that binds to the bacterial surface and activates complement. Either lysis of the bacteria, which occurs for only gram-negative bacteria, or adherence and phagocytosis of the bacteria by polymorphonuclear leukocytes or tissue macrophages ensues. A deficiency of any of these mechanisms allows encapsulated bacteria to persist and cause invasive systemic disease. The infection may involve an organism to which the child should have developed immunity from a previous infection. Antibody deficiency should be initially

suspected and investigated because it occurs at a greater frequency than complement deficiency — C3, C3b inactivator, or C5 deficiency — or white blood cell abnormalities, which may produce the same clinical picture. Polymorphonuclear leukocyte abnormalities are usually also associated with recurrent abscess formation and infections with nonencapsulated bacteria. Isolated antibody deficiency is not likely to predispose to infections until the latter half of the first year of life because of passive protection provided by maternal antibody. Infections occurring at an earlier age should suggest one of the other immunodeficiencies or a localized anatomical or physiological defect.

Recurrent pyoderma, abscesses of the lungs, liver, or peritoneal cavity, chronic lymphadenitis, draining lymph nodes, and osteomyelitis should suggest an abnormality of circulating polymorphonuclear leukocytes. The common bacteria causing these infections are *S. aureus, Staphylococcus albus, Streptococcus pyogenes,* and the gram-negative bacteria *Klebsiella, Escherichia, Serratia, Pseudomonas,* and *Salmonella.* Many of these bacteria constitute nonpathogenic normal flora that reside at the skin and mucosal surfaces. Resistance to these microorganisms is maintained by the integrity of these barriers. When the barriers are breached, circulating white blood cells migrate into the area and phagocytize and kill the invading bacteria. A deficiency of number, movement, phagocytosis, or killing by leukocytes allows persistence and multiplication of bacteria and leads to chronic infection and abscess formation.

Immunity to viruses and fungi is provided by T lymphocytes. Chronic moniliasis with thrush and skin rashes unresponsive to appropriate therapy is typical of T-cell deficiency in childhood. The infant with a T-cell or combined T and B-cell deficiency may suffer from chronic respiratory and gastrointestinal infections and fail to thrive. Severe varicella or rubeola with pneumonitis is suggestive of T-cell deficiency. Because the infant with a T-cell deficiency has no maternal protection, symptoms often begin during the first 3 months of life.

Antibody Deficiency Disorders

Patients with antibody deficiency sustain recurrent pyogenic infections. The defect may be due to an absence or a dysfunction of B cells or may be secondary to a lack of T-cell help or an increased T-cell suppressor effect.

Congenital X-linked hypogammaglobulinemia is usually characterized by absence of peripheral blood B cells and absence of lymphoid follicles in the nodes, with marked deficiency of plasma cells. Low levels of IgG (< 100 mg/dl) are detected, and patients with this disease are unable to form detectable antibodies. T-cell number and function are normal. The absence of B cells is due to a block in differentiation of pre-B cells, which exist in normal numbers in the bone marrow, to develop into mature B cells. In addition to suffering from recurrent pyogenic infections, the patients may present clinically with arthritis of the larger joints with effusion. Absent or only very small tonsils are detected on physical examination and should suggest the diagnosis. Occasionally this disorder is associated with a chronic enterovirus central nervous system infection.

Hypogammaglobulinemia with increased IgM and decreased IgG and IgA can occur as an X-linked or acquired disorder. Clinically, the patients often have large lymph nodes and tonsils and are prone to autoimmune manifestations (hemolytic anemia, thrombocytopenia, neutropenia). Malignant lymphomas involving the gastrointestinal tract have been described. In this disorder the B cells cannot differentiate to become IgG- or IgA-producing cells.

Selective deficiency of serum IgA is observed at about 5 per 1000 population, but most such individuals remain asymptomatic. In some, with absent IgA, recurrent sinopulmonary infections, chronic diarrhea-malabsorption, or autoimmune disease (rheumatoid arthritis or systemic lupus erythematosus) occurs. These disorders are secondary to the lack of the protective effect of IgA at mucosal surfaces, which results in an increased number of mucosal surface infections and increased systemic absorption of antigens from these sites. Patients with IgA deficiency with recurrent infection of mucosal surfaces not uncommonly have concomitant deficiency of the IgG_2 and for IgG_4 subclasses, which have a major role in the predisposition to infection. Food antigens — such as milk — are readily absorbed systemically by the patients, and promote antibody production. Patients with IgA deficiency may have circulating antibodies to IgA that can cause an anaphylactic reaction to transfusion with blood products or to the administration of the trace amounts of IgA found in some preparations of immunoglobulin used in the therapy of patients with IgG deficiency. Patients with isolated IgA deficiency should not be routinely treated with immunoglobulin replacement because of the risk of anaphylaxis and because the IgA is unable to enter mucosal surfaces and, therefore, cannot provide protection. Most individuals with selective IgA deficiency have circulating B cells with surface IgA. Probably multiple defects, some that are reversible, account for the lack of terminal differentiation of these B cells. T-cell and intrinsic B-cell abnormalities have been implicated.

In some infants a temporary delay in immunoglobulin synthesis causes the nadir of the IgG level that occurs in normal infants at 3 to 4 months of age to be prolonged.

Transient hypogammaglobulinemia in infants may be accompanied by otitis media, bronchiolitis, wheezing, diarrhea, or unexplained fevers. In contrast to patients with X-linked hypogammaglobulinemia, circulating B cells are detected, the IgG level is higher, IgA and IgM are found, and normal antibody responses to immunization with tetanus toxoid occur. The immunoglobulin abnormalities disappear by about 2 to 3 years of age in many of these patients.

Common variable immunodeficiency usually presents later in childhood or in adult life. The hypogammaglobulinemia is not as profound as in the X-linked form and may involve some immunoglobulin classes more than others. The defect is commonly associated with recurrent sinopulmonary infections that may result in bronchiectasis. A frequent complication is a diarrhea-malabsorption syndrome due to bacterial overgrowth or *Giardia lamblia* infection in the gastrointestinal tract. Most of the patients have B cells, but the B cell fails to either differentiate to a cell that synthesizes immunoglobulin or secrete the immunoglobulin produced. Some patients have a deficiency of helper T cells and others have activated T-cell suppression of B-cell function.

T-Cell Deficiency Disorders

Congenital thymic aplasia (DiGeorge syndrome) is a developmental abnormality involving abnormal embryogenesis of the third and fourth pharyngeal pouches that occurs prior to 8 weeks of gestation. The etiology is unknown but the defect is thought to be a sporadic event in morphogenesis. The thymus and parathyroid glands fail to develop or are hypoplastic. Clinical symptoms are related to the severity of aplasia. Affected infants often suffer with neonatal tetany from hypocalcemia caused by hypoparathyroidism. Persistent thrush, recurrent infections, rhinitis, and rashes begin in early infancy with the rare child who has complete thymic aplasia. The aortic arch and facial structures, which also develop from these involved tissues, may be deformed. Cyanosis and heart murmurs from truncus arteriosus, interrupted aortic arch, or tetralogy of Fallot constitute another mode of presentation. T-cell function is abnormal, but defects of varying severity occur because most patients have remaining remnants of thymic tissue. In fact, spontaneous acquisition of T-cell function over a period of several years usually occurs. Rarely, some patients, however, may require a fetal thymus transplant to correct the defect; recovery after transplantation is usually rapid.

Absence of the enzyme *nucleoside phosphorylase,* an enzyme of purine metabolism, causes T-cell deficiency. This rare disorder is associated with recurrent infections and at times hematological abnormalities. The pathogenetic basis of the disease is thought to be the lack of metabolism of the deoxynucleoside, deoxyguanosine, in T cells. Deoxyguanosine is converted to dGTP, which accumulates in the cell, and inhibits the enzyme ribonucleotide reductase, which is required for DNA synthesis. T-cell proliferation, and therefore, function, is inhibited.

Chronic mucocutaneous candidiasis is characterized by chronic *Candida* infection of the mucous membranes, skin, and nails. The disease often begins in infancy with intractable thrush that spreads to involve the skin and nails. About one-half of the patients with this disorder have an associated endocrinopathy, most commonly hypoparathyroidism, or adrenal insufficiency. T-cell function is normal except for impaired in vitro responses and delayed hypersensitivity skin tests to *Candida*.

Combined Deficiency Disorders

Severe combined immunodeficiency (SCID) is a heterogeneous disorder affecting both T- and B-cell function. Autosomal recessive and X-linked forms of the disease occur. The patients have marked susceptibility to all types of infections, which begin in the early months of life. Chronic moniliasis, chronic pneumonitis, diarrhea, marked wasting, and failure to thrive usually occur. The clinical course inexorably progresses until death ensues by about 2 years of age unless immunity is reconstituted. Chest roentgenographs reveal absence of a thymus and commonly pulmonary infiltrates. An interstitial pneumonitis caused by *P. carinii* may occur. Tonsillar tissue and lymph nodes are absent or scanty. The normally benign childhood infections of measles and chickenpox may be lethal in these patients.

A decrease in the absolute small lymphocyte count is at times present. The absolute T-cell number is usually decreased, and the B-cell number may be decreased, normal, or increased. Antibody responses are defective because of lack of T helper cell function, and immunoglobulin levels are usually decreased. In vitro T-cell function is markedly abnormal.

Graft-versus-host (GVH) disease may complicate the clinical picture. If a patient with severe combined immunodeficiency receives viable foreign lymphoid cells from a transfusion or from the mother either in utero or at delivery, these lymphoid cells mount a cytotoxic response to the patient's MHC antigens on several organs. Rashes, hepatosplenomegaly, jaundice, diarrhea, and failure to thrive occur with GVH disease. Diagnosis of suspected GVH disease can be confirmed by a skin biopsy or by demonstration of lymphoid chimerism.

Several forms of the SCID occur. In most cases the basis

of the defect in unknown. In about a quarter of patients with the autosomal recessive form of the disease, an enzyme of purine metabolism, adenosine deaminase, is absent or nonfunctional. Loss of this enzymatic activity causes accumulation of deoxyadenosine and dATP, which inhibits ribonucleotide reductase and prevents DNA synthesis. This is thought to be the pathogenetic basis fo the disease. Another explanation is that deoxyadenosine accumulation inactivates *S*-adenosyl homocysteine hydrolase so that *S*-adenosyl homocysteine accumulates and blocks methylation reactions. Whatever the exact mechanism of the disease, T-cell development is more sensitive to these inhibitory effects, and both proliferating and nondividing cells are killed. Clinically, it is not usually possible to distinguish this subgroup without performing enzyme assays on the patient's erythrocytes. Some patients, however, have a delayed onset of symptoms compared to that observed in other forms of the disease, and some have bony abnormalities detected by roentgenographs. Bone marrow transplantation is required to correct the lymphoid abnormality permanently, but some patients have received transient benefit from enzyme replacement therapy as described below.

Mixed partial T- and B-cell deficiency occurs in the immunodeficiency of *ataxia-telangiectasia* and the *Wiskott-Aldrich syndrome*. The former, an autosomal recessive disorder, begins early in life with progressive ataxia. Telangiectasia of the bulbar conjuctiva and skin occurs by 5 years of age, and recurrent sinopulmonary infections occur in later childhood. Death from lymphoreticular malignancy is not uncommon in late childhood or early adulthood. Variable degrees of in vitro T-cell dysfunction and anergy are observed. Progressive attrition of T-cell function is likely. Deficiency of IgA and IgE is quite common. Elevated serum levels of alpha-fetoprotein are found and possibly reflect an immaturity of development found also in other organs. The thymus in this disease appears embryonic rather than atrophic, and abnormal differentiation of the gonads also occurs. Chromosomal aberrations and increased sensitivity to x radiation with abnormal DNA repair are demonstrable in cells from these patients. Chromosomal rearrangements involving the T-cell receptor genes on chromosome 14 are commonly found.

The *Wiskott-Aldrich syndrome* is an X-linked disorder characterized by thrombocytopenia, eczema, and recurrent infections. Otitis media and chronic otorrhea are classically found. The patients have low levels of serum IgM, absent isohemagglutinins, and poor antibody responses to polysaccharides and eventually to proteins. A high incidence of lymphoma occurs in later childhood.

Deficiency of Nonspecific Components

Congenital deficiency of the third component of complement resembles antibody deficiency because of the predisposition to recurrent pyogenic infections. C3b inactivator deficiency causes consumption and depletion of C3 that mimics congenital absence of C3. C5 deficiency has also been associated with recurrent pyogenic infections due to loss of the chemotactic activity provided by C5a. Recurrent *Neisseria* infections occur with absence of complement components C6, C7, or C8. Protection against these bacteria requires complement-mediated lysis, which is dependent on terminal complement components.

Splenic absence or dysfunction predisposes to fatal sepsis with pyogenic bacteria, most commonly pneumococci. The spleen and liver normally clear the blood of microorganisms. In nonimmune states, the spleen assumes a larger role. Its absence predisposes to overwhelming infection, meningitis, and shock with disseminated intravascular coagulation. Congenital asplenia is associated with partial situs inversus and heart abnormalities. Functional hyposplenia occurs in sickle-cell anemia during the first 2 to 3 years of life and gradually progresses to anatomical asplenia from repeated thrombotic episodes and fibrosis. Surgical splenectomy can put children at risk for infection. At greatest risk of sepsis are children less than 5 years of age, children with an underlying disorder that involves the reticuloendothelial system or predisposes to infections, and children within 2 years of splenectomy.

Defects of polymorphonuclear leukocyte number or function can predispose to infection. Qualitative disorders of leukocyte chemotaxis, phagocytosis, and killing have been described. One well-characterized disorder of oxidative metabolic responses is *chronic granulomatous disease*. The defect is due to an absent respiratory burst that normally occurs after phagocytosis because of an abnormal cytochrome-dependent NADPH oxidase. Patients with such a condition lack or have low amounts of phagocyte-specific cytochrome b. In the X-linked form, the 95 kd chain of the protein is defective. With phagocytosis there is a lack of the normal production of increased oxygen uptake, superoxide, and hydrogen peroxide. Phagocytized bacteria remain viable in the polymorphonuclear leukocyte and infections persist with development of chronic infected abscesses and granulomas. Clinically, the patients suffer from recurrent pyogenic infections of the skin, lymph nodes, lungs, and bones. Lymphadenopathy from purulent adenitis that requires surgical drainage is a common symptom. Hepatosplenomegaly, staphylococcal liver abscesses, recurrent pyoderma, lung abscesses, perianal abscesses, and osteomy-

elitis are frequent symptoms. The diagnosis can be confirmed with the nitroblue tetrazolium test. The lack of formation of superoxide anion following phagocytosis does not promote reduction of the yellow, water-soluble electron receptor to insoluble blue formazan.

Laboratory Evaluation of Immunodeficiency

Laboratory studies should be selected on the basis of the history and physical examination to confirm a diagnosis of immunodeficiency. If severe combined immunodeficiency disease is suspected, early referral to a medical center is indicated. Live viral immunization, such as oral poliovirus vaccine, should be avoided in any child with suspected immunodeficiency until the diagnosis is disproved because of the risk of inducing a chronic persistent viral infection. Unnecessary transfusion with all blood products should be avoided in patients with suspected immunodeficiency because of the risk of inducing graft-versus-host (GVH) disease in patients with a T-cell deficiency. If blood products must be provided, they should be irradiated to avoid this complication.

Judgment in ordering laboratory tests avoids unnecessary costs. If only an antibody deficiency is suspected, quantitation of immunoglobulins (IgG, IgA, IgM) should be initially performed (Table 19-3). There is a wide range of normal values, and the level varies according to the age of the patient, so that age-matched normal values must be compared to the results (see Table 19-1). X-linked hypogammaglobulinemia is characterized by extremely low levels of IgG (< 100 mg/dl), while patients with transient hypogammaglobulinemia have higher but still low levels of IgG. Borderline low levels of IgG should not be overinterpreted. Confirmation of an antibody deficiency requires measurement of specific antibody levels. There are some disorders with combined T- and B-cell deficiency in which normal immunoglobulin levels occur although no specific antibodies are induced by immunization. Antibodies to blood group substances (isohemagglutinins) are easily measured and are produced by all normal children without blood group AB by 12 months of age. Antibodies prior to and following immunization with killed antigens such as tetanus or diphtheria toxoid or the *H. influenzae* b polysaccharide vaccine can be quantified. More extensive studies, including quantitation of B cell number and examination of in vitro B-cell function, can be performed to determine whether the defect is due to absence or dysfunction of B or T cells. The former occurs in X-linked hypogammaglobulinemia; the latter usually in common variable immunodeficiency.

T-cell deficiency should be assessed initially by quantitat-

Table 19-3. Laboratory Evaluation

General
Complete blood count
Sedimentation rate
Chest x ray (note for chronic disease and presence of thymus)
Antibody deficiency
Initial: Quantitative immunoglobulins
       Isohemagglutinin titer
   : Tetanus and diphtheria toxoids and *H. influenzae* b
       capsular polysaccharide antibody before and after
       immunization
Later: B-cell number and in vitro function
   : secretory IgA, IgG subclasses
T-Lymphocyte deficiency
Initial: Skin tests — *Monilia*, streptokinase-streptodornase,
       mumps
       Absolute lymphocyte number; quantitation of total and
        subsets of T cells
       Chest x ray for thymus
Later: Lymphocyte proliferation, lymphokine production, and
       cytotoxicity
Other: Enzyme levels — adenosine deaminase, nucleoside
       phosphorylase
       Calcium level
       Antilymphocyte antibody
Complement deficiency
Initial: Total hemolytic complement (CH_{50})
Later: C3, C5, C6, C7, C8 levels and function
Polymorphonuclear leukocyte and macrophage deficiency
Initial: Counts and morphology
       Howell-Jolly bodies
       IgE level
       Nitroblue tetrazolium reduction test
Later: Rebuck skin window
       Chemotactic, random migration, phagocytosis, killing,
        and oxidative metabolism assays
       Spleen scan

Source: Modified from R. A. Insel, The Child with Recurrent Infections. In
M. Ziai (Ed.), *Bedside Pediatrics.* Boston: Little, Brown, 1983.

ing total lymphocytes, the total number of T cells and of the
T-cell subsets, performing delayed hypersensitivity skin
tests, and examining for a thymus on chest roentgenograph.
An absolute lymphopenia ($< 1500/mm^3$) is a common but
not an invariable occurrence with T-cell deficiency. The
absolute number of T cells and of the helper/inducer (CD_4)
and suppressor/cytotoxic (CD_8) T-cell subsets can be quan-
titated using monoclonal antibodies. Delayed hypersensitivity skin tests are performed to evaluate cellular immunity.
Most children have positive responses by 1 year of age to

Candida antigens. A positive delayed hypersensitivity skin
test to mumps is found in more than 90% of children who
have received mumps immunization. The major value of
skin tests is that they attest to a relatively normal T-cell
system if reactions to skin testing are normal.

T-cell function can be assayed by quantitating T-cell proliferation after culturing the cells in vitro with plant lectins
or with specific antigens. Poor responses to the plant lectins
concanavalin A and phytohemagglutinin reflect a major
impairment of T-cell function. Antigens commonly used to
stimulate lymphocyte proliferation include *Monilia*, tetanus
toxoid, and streptococcal antigens. In some T-cell disorders
responses to antigens are lost although responses to plant
lectins are preserved.

Suspected white blood cell dysfunction should be assessed initially by determination of white blood cell number
and morphology. Further studies that may be useful include
a nitroblue tetrazolium assay to diagnose chronic granulomatous disease and assays to study chemotaxis, phagocytosis, and killing.

The total hemolytic complement (CH_{50}) is abnormal
with a deficiency of C3, C5, C6, C7, and C8 that predisposes to infection. Levels of individual components
should be measured if the CH_{50} is abnormal.

Therapy of Immunodeficiency

Antibody deficiency can be corrected with immunoglobulin
replacement therapy administered by the intramuscular or
intravenous route. Patients who have clinical disease and
low levels of IgG or lack specific antibody responses will
benefit from IgG replacement. The normal half-life of IgG is
about 20 to 30 days but is shortened in some patients and
especially in the presence of an ongoing infection. Patients,
especially those who require large doses of immunoglobulin, can be spared painful intramuscular injections with the
intravenous preparations.

In severe combined immunodeficiency, transplantation of
histocompatible bone marrow can restore immunocompe-
tence. A donor is selected on the basis of HLA and mixed
lymphocyte culture typing. New techniques that remove or
kill T cells from partially matched bone marrow, such as
haploidentical bone marrow from a parent, without altering
the stem cells allow bone marrow transplantation to be
employed more widely without risk of severe GVH disease.
The infant is maintained in a sterile environment to prevent
infections and decrease the risk of GVH disease. One experimental treatment approach for severe combined immunodeficiency disease with adenosine deaminase deficiency is
enzyme replacement therapy by treatment with the purified

bovine enzyme coupled to polyethylene glycol, which increases the circulating half-life of the enzyme and prevents development of antibodies to the enzyme. Red cell transfusions have also been experimentally administered as a form of enzyme replacement. Fetal thymus transplants can completely restore the immunodeficiency of the rare child with complete thymic aplasia and persistent symptomatic T-cell deficiency in the DiGeorge syndrome.

Aggressive and immediate antibiotic treatment should be instituted for infection to prevent organ damage such as bronchiectasis. If bronchiectasis occurs, physical therapy, postural drainage, and antibiotics are required. Hearing loss secondary to chronic otitis should be prevented with antibiotics. Malabsorption and diarrhea should be treated with dietary restriction and parenteral alimentation. If *Giardia* infestation is demonstrated by duodenal aspirate, the patient should be treated with metronidazole. Multiple organisms may be responsible for clinical diseases. Abscesses may need to be surgically drained in patients with chronic granulomatous disease. Lung infiltrates in patients with immunodeficiency disease may be secondary to *Pneumocystis* infection, which requires antibiotic treatment. Increased amounts of immunoglobulin should be administered during infections, and immunoglobulin prophylaxis is indicated for viral exposures.

Prophylactic antibiotics have been used to prevent infection in patients with immunodeficiency diseases, chronic granulomatous disease, and splenic dysfunction. Patients with T-cell deficiency are treated with antibiotics to prevent *P. carinii* pneumonia. It is important to educate parents to the risk of sepsis and the necessity of seeking immediate medical attention at the first sign of infection in patients with splenic absence or dysfunction. Immunization with pneumococcal, *H. influenzae,* and meningococcal polysaccharide vaccines is recommended to prevent infections.

Siblings of children affected with severe combined immunodeficiency should be isolated and screened at birth, and family members of patients with immunodeficiency disease should be screened for inherited immunodeficiency disorders. The carrier state for X-linked agammaglobulinemia, X-linked severe combined immunodeficiency, or the Wiskott-Aldrich syndrome can sometimes be detected by demonstrating nonrandom X chromosome inactivation in peripheral blood lymphocytes or by studying restriction fragment length polymorphisms using disease-specific gene probes in a family with an affected member. In normal females either of the two X chromosomes is used randomly as the active X chromosome in different cells. In female carriers of immunodeficiency diseases that affect lymphocyte development, cells using only the normal X chromosome as the active X develop. The B cells in X-linked agammaglobulinemia, T cells in X-linked severe combined immunodeficiency, and both T and B cells in the Wiskott-Aldrich syndrome show nonrandom inactivation patterns in female carriers. Prenatal detection of SCID is possible by demonstrating low numbers of T cells and poor in vitro T-cell function in fetal blood collected during the second trimester. The prenatal diagnosis of adenosine deaminase deficiency and chronic granulomatous disease is also possible with amniocentesis.

Richard A. Insel

Immunization

Immunization is a cornerstone of disease prevention. Through the immunizing process, one attempts to confer protection on the host against a specific infection. Protection may be achieved by specific circulating humoral antibody (IgM and IgG), by cell-mediated immunity, or at the mucosal surface by local antibody (secretory IgA).

Active Immunization

Currently available vaccines include both bacterial and viral products. There are several categories of immunizing agents: (1) killed whole organisms, e.g., pertussis and influenza vaccine; (2) attenuated live organisms, e.g., measles, mumps, rubella, and poliomyelitis vaccines; (3) toxoids, e.g., diphtheria and tetanus vaccines. Attenuated live organism vaccines are superior because the immunity after administration is more like that after natural infection and the duration of immunity is longer. Inactivated vaccines and toxoids generally require several doses to achieve protective antibody levels and periodic booster injections to maintain immunity.

Bacterial Vaccines

DIPHTHERIA AND TETANUS TOXOIDS AND PERTUSSIS VACCINE. Routine immunization against diphtheria, tetanus (lockjaw), and pertussis (whooping cough) has been widely practiced in the United States for 40 years. The efficacy of this triple vaccine is reflected in the remarkable reduction in disease incidence for each of these three diseases. Several combinations and concentrations are available for administration: (1) diphtheria and tetanus toxoids with pertussis vaccine (DTP), (2) diphtheria and tetanus toxoids

(DT) infant type, (3) diphtheria and tetanus toxoids (dT) adult type, (4) tetanus toxoid (T).

The DTP preparation is the standard vaccine in infancy. Reactions to DTP administration are common. Pertussis vaccine is the most reactogenic component. Reactions may include a febrile response, acute behavior changes ranging from irritability to screaming fits, and local reactions consisting of redness, pain, and swelling. If severe reactions to vaccination with DTP occur, such as convulsions, screaming fits, marked somnolence, high fever (>40.5°C), or thrombocytopenia, or if there is a preexisting neurological condition, the pertussis vaccine should be eliminated and DT vaccine substituted. After the age of 6 years increasing reactogenicity to a full dose of diphtheria toxoid (5–25 Lf [flocculating units]) mandates a reduced dose (<2 Lf) of antigen. The availability of the dT vaccine fulfills this need. Some physicians prefer to administer only tetanus toxoid (T) boosting immunizations to adults.

New purified, acellular vaccines, first developed in Japan are under investigation for use in the United States. It is hoped that acellular pertussis vaccines will provide improved efficacy and safety over that achieved with the currently available whole-cell vaccine.

BCG. In the United States BCG vaccine has been used primarily for children who have an unavoidable risk of exposure to tuberculosis, e.g., children of migrant workers. The bacillus of Calmette and Guérin (BCG) was originally derived from a strain of *Mycobacterium bovis* and since has been further attenuated many times over. After BCG vaccination it is very difficult to distinguish between a mildly positive delayed hypersensitivity response to tuberculin caused by virulent tuberculosis and persistent post-BCG vaccination sensitivity.

MENINGOCOCCUS. A vaccine consisting of the purified polysaccharide capsule of *Neisseria meningitidis* serogroups A and C produces serogroup-specific immunity, probably of lasting duration. Side-effects are limited to local reactions at the site of vaccination. Unfortunately, the most prevalent serotype of meningococcal disease is group B, for which there is currently no vaccine available. Thus, administration of meningococcal A and C vaccines is not recommended for the general population. Instead, vaccination is at present used as an adjunct to antibiotic chemoprophylaxis for household contacts of meningococcal disease cases, for travelers planning to visit countries with endemic meningococcal disease, and in epidemics. The vaccines are not effective in children less than 2 years of age.

PNEUMOCOCCUS. *Streptococcus pneumoniae* is a significant cause of meningitis, pneumonia, and otitis media in children. For those with sickle-cell disease, chronic liver disease,

nephrotic syndrome, malignancy, or primary immunodeficiency, pneumococcal infection is an even more serious problem. The 23-valent polysaccharide vaccine contains purified capsular material of pneumococci extracted separately from the types of organisms to be combined in the final vaccine; the 23 particular types of pneumococci cause more than 88% of all bacteremic pneumococcal disease. Immunity is provided only against the pneumococcal types in the vaccine. The duration of protection is at least 10 years. Side-effects of vaccine administration consisting only of mild local pain and swelling occur in about half of the recipients. Children less than 2 years old respond poorly to several of the serotypes in the vaccine, and, therefore, vaccination in children should be deferred until at least age 2.

HEMOPHILUS INFLUENZAE TYPE B. *Hemophilus influenzae* type b (Hib) is the most common cause of bacterial meningitis in children. A vaccine prepared from the purified capsule of this organism (polyribosylribitolphosphate [PRP] conjugated to a protein carrier, diphtheria toxin [PRP-D]) has been developed and shown to be effective in preventing Hib disease in children over 18 months of age. Because children less than 18 months of age constitute the group at highest risk for invasive Hib disease, recommendations for use of PRP-D and similar conjugate Hib vaccines for this younger age group should be forthcoming soon.

Virus Vaccines

POLIOMYELITIS. In 1955 Salk's inactivated poliovirus (IPV) vaccine was put to widespread use in the United States. This resulted in a marked decrease in the incidence of poliomyelitis; however, immunity was not sustained so booster doses every 4 years were required. Epidemics still occurred, sometimes involving "adequately" immunized patients. Then in 1962 Sabin's live oral poliovirus vaccine (OPV) gained acceptance over the inactivated vaccine. OPV was easier to administer and it produced both a local and a systemic immune response similar to that induced by natural infection. The result was durable immunity. The only known side-effect is the very rare development of poliovaccine-induced paralysis, which occurs in 0.06/1,000,000 doses. Nevertheless, concern over this potential side-effect combined with the development of improved IPVs has recently led to consideration of switching back to IPV.

A primary series of three adequately spaced doses of trivalent OPV (TOPV), consisting of a mixture of attenuated poliovirus types 1, 2, and 3, produces immunity in approximately 95% of recipients. Infection of the gastrointestinal tract with TOPV is a necessary prerequisite to the establishment of immunity. Subsequent shedding of the virus can produce dissemination of vaccine virus into the community with resultant herd immunity. Possible interference with this "infectious" process can be caused by a subclinical or ongoing wild enterovirus infection. The recommendation for several doses of poliovirus vaccine at spaced intervals is aimed at overcoming this problem.

MEASLES (10-DAY MEASLES). Measles can be a severe disease complicated by suppurative otitis media, bronchopneumonia, or encephalitis. Death from respiratory and neurological causes occurs in one out of 1000 reported cases. The measles vaccine is a live, attenuated strain of measles virus. Measles antibodies are induced in 95% of children vaccinated at about 15 months of age. With time, immunity may wane. Booster doses at school entry (age 5) or at age 12 are currently recommended.

Replication of the vaccine virus may be inhibited by preexisting serum antibody; therefore, immunization in infancy should be delayed until after the disappearance of passively acquired maternal antibody. Maternal antibody may interfere with measles vaccination efficacy. The current recommendation is for administration after 12 months of age and preferably at approximately 15 months of age. Immunization, however, should not be delayed if there is an epidemic of measles in the community. In this event, children 6 months old and older should be vaccinated. Such children should be revaccinated after 15 months of age.

Measles vaccine produces a mild, noncommunicable infection in 15% of recipients. Symptoms occur 7 to 10 days after immunization and may include fever, malaise, and a measleslike exanthem. Subacute sclerosing panencephalitis (SSPE) is a "slow virus" infection of the central nervous system associated with measles virus. Five to ten cases of SSPE result per million cases of natural measles infection. Measles vaccination is associated with the development of SSPE in one out of 1,000,000 cases.

RUBELLA. Rubella (3-day measles, German measles) is a relatively mild viral illness. When infection is acquired by a woman in the first trimester of pregnancy, however, the concomitant infection in the fetus can produce a variety of congenital anomalies. Rubella immunization was developed to prevent this congenital rubella syndrome. Rubella vaccine is live and attenuated; antibodies develop in 95% of the recipients, and immunity is sustained.

Joint pain, usually in the small peripheral joints, is the most common complaint following rubella vaccination. It usually occurs 2 to 8 weeks after immunization. The incidence is about 5 to 10%. A rash or lymphadenopathy (or both) occasionally occurs.

Live rubella virus vaccine should not be given during pregnancy because of the theoretical risk to the developing fetus. Inadvertent administration during pregnancy, however, may not mandate a therapeutic abortion because reports indicate that the real risk to the fetus may be nil.

MUMPS. Mumps is generally a self-limited illness of young school children. Serious sequelae such as nerve deafness are uncommon. Mumps occurring in postpubertal males may result in orchitis, with subsequent sterility. Live mumps virus vaccine produces protective antibodies in 95% of persons vaccinated; immunity is durable. There are no side-effects from mumps vaccination.

INFLUENZA. Efforts to vaccinate against influenza have been aimed at protecting persons at highest risk for morbidity and mortality. Bivalent influenza A vaccine is a killed vaccine product. The composition of influenza A vaccine may be changed yearly, depending on the antigenic makeup of the anticipated prevalent strain. Vaccination is targeted for patients with chronic health problems such as those with heart disease, pulmonary disease, renal failure, diabetes, or collagen vascular disease. General use of this vaccine is not recommended because of its limited duration of protection, the low attack rate of disease in most yearly outbreaks, and lack of serious complications from disease. Side-effects from vaccination may include local reaction at the injection site or a mild systemic reaction such as low-grade fever, chills, and malaise. Influenza vaccine should not be given to egg-sensitive patients nor should it be administered with DTP vaccine because of the possibility for an enhanced febrile response to this combination of vaccine products.

RABIES. Rabies vaccine, composed of inactivated virus, is given as 5 doses (on day 1, 3, 7, 14, and 28) following a suspected rabid bite. Carnivorous animals such as skunks, foxes, rats, coyotes, raccoons, dogs, and cats may carry rabies. The risk varies in different geographic areas. The circumstances surrounding the occurrence of the bite, the availability of the animal for confinement, and the local rabies experience dictate the need for vaccination.

HEPATITIS B. The current vaccines are prepared from purified concentrate of plasma containing a high titer of hepatitis B surface antigen (HBsAg) or from a genetically engineered product. The vaccines induce anti-HBsAg antibody in 75 to 90% of adults after two doses, and more than 90% acquire antibody after a third dose. Children mount a more vigorous antibody response than adults when given half the adult dose (10 μg). Side-effects are predominantly local soreness at the injection site (15%) and transient low-grade fever (3%). HBV should be given to individuals at high risk for exposure to hepatitis B (e.g., health professionals), infants born to HBsAg-positive mothers, and others in close, prolonged, or intimate contact with a known HBsAg-positive person (e.g., family members). It should be given in the deltoid muscle rather than the gluteus.

Passive Immunization

Passive immunization provides temporary immunity when active immunization is unavailable or has not been given prior to exposure.

Intramuscular Immune Serum Globulin

Human immune serum globulin (ISG) is an antibody-rich fraction of pooled plasma obtained from normal healthy donors. It is commonly referred to as gamma globulin and consists primarily of IgG immunoglobulin though trace amounts of IgA, IgM, and other serum proteins may be present. ISG is a concentrated antibody solution that can be given intramuscularly. It does not contain transmissible viruses (e.g., hepatitis virus and/or AIDS virus) and is stable for many months if stored at 4°C.

Maximal serum antibody levels may not be achieved for 24 to 48 hours following the intramuscular injection of ISG; therefore, it is essential that it be administered as soon after exposure as possible in order to achieve maximal benefit. The half-life of ISG in the circulation is about 3 weeks.

The disadvantages of ISG include the following: (1) the protective effect is temporary, (2) the antibody content against specific agents may vary as much as tenfold between preparations, (3) administration is painful, and (4) inadvertent intravenous injections may result in anaphylaxis as a consequence of complement activation by immunoglobulin aggregates.

ISG is used in the following infections.

HEPATITIS A VIRUS (HAV) INFECTION. High titers of HAV antibody are found in nearly all ISG preparations. Administration modifies rather than prevents infection in susceptible individuals. That is, though clinical infection may not be observed, serum transaminase usually rises. ISG should be given only to patients intimately exposed to HAV-infected persons, e.g., household contacts. A dose of 0.02 ml/kg is recommended.

ISG is also useful in prophylaxis against HAV infection for people who travel or work in areas of endemic disease. A standard dose of 0.02 ml/kg is effective for about a month. If residence in such areas is extended for several months, larger doses should be given.

HEPATITIS B VIRUS (HBV) INFECTION. ISG should be given only when hyperimmune HBV globulin is not available.

MEASLES (RUBEOLA). It is well established that ISG is effective in preventing or modifying measles. Passive immunization for measles is currently used when unvaccinated children (usually less than 1 year of age) are exposed to measles or reside in a community in which a measles epidemic is ongoing. The recommended dose is 0.25 ml/kg for prevention and 0.05 ml/kg for modification.

OTHERS. There are several other circumstances in which ISG may be useful such as in the prevention of rubella in the first trimester of pregnancy and in the prevention or modification of varicella in immunocompromised patients when hyperimmune globulin is unavailable.

Hyperimmune Serum Globulin

Hyperimmune globulin products are prepared from plasma of individuals who have high titers of antibody against a specific organism or antigen. It is derived from artificially hyperimmunized donors or from persons convalescing from natural infection.

HEPATITIS B IMMUNE GLOBULIN. Hepatitis B immune globulin is effective in reducing the incidence of hepatitis if given soon after exposure to those experiencing an HBV-contaminated needlestick. It has also been shown to decrease the incidence of hepatitis in hospital personnel, patients in renal dialysis units, and in individuals exposed by the oral-fecal route (e.g., institutionalized children).

RABIES IMMUNE GLOBULIN. Rabies immune globulin should be given as soon as possible after a strongly suspected or proved rabid bite. Half the dose is infiltrated around the wound and the remainder given intramuscularly.

TETANUS IMMUNE GLOBULIN. Tetanus immune globulin is used in the treatment of tetanus and in prophylaxis when patients who are inadequately immunized have incurred a tetanus-prone wound. A total dose of 5 units/kg should be administered with a portion infiltrated around the wound.

ZOSTER IMMUNE GLOBULIN (ZIG). Because herpes zoster and varicella are different manifestations of the same virus infection, ZIG can be given to prevent or modify these infections. Because of its limited supply, ZIG is used only in immunocompromised patients (those with malignancy or collagen vascular diseases, renal transplant recipients on immunosuppressive therapy, and persons with congenital immune deficiencies) and in infants born to mothers who develop varicella just prior to delivery.

INTRAVENOUS IMMUNE GLOBULIN (IVIG). IVIG has been recently developed to allow for larger and repeated doses of gamma globulin. Administration is painless (following establishment of intravenous access) and generally free of side effects. IVIG has become the product of choice in the therapy and prophylaxis of severe bacterial and viral infections. IVIG use has been suggested as *adjunct* therapy for prevention and treatment of septicemia in premature and low-birth-weight infants, treatment of bacterial meningitis, treatment of children with Kawasaki syndrome, treatment of idiopathic thrombocytopenia purpura (ITP), and treatment of children with AIDS. Other indications for IVIG are under study.

General Recommendations Concerning Active Immunization Procedures

These recommendations are taken from the American Academy of Pediatrics (AAP) publication *Red Book* and represent present practices in the Americas. The reader must become informed about the required immunization procedures in his or her particular area of the world.

Recommended Schedule for Active Immunization*

The schedule for active immunization given in Table 19-4 is recommended for healthy infants and children in the Americas.

Parents (and patients of responsible age) should give written informed consent about the immunizations proposed. They should know the antigens to be administered, the reasons for their use, and the associated reactions which might occur. They should be encouraged to report any response of a severe or unusual nature to their physician. Any severe or unusual reactions should be carefully evaluated, documented, and reported to local or state health officials.

AGE TO COMMENCE ACTIVE IMMUNIZATIONS. The generally recommended age for beginning routine immunization of normal infants is 6 to 8 weeks, and the first vaccines given are DTP (diphtheria and tetanus toxoids combined with pertussis vaccine) and trivalent OPV (oral poliovirus vaccine).

DOSAGE AND TECHNIQUES OF ADMINISTRATION. Depot antigens should be injected deep into the muscle, preferably into the mid lateral thigh or the deltoid. The manufacturer's package insert should be consulted regarding the volume of individual doses of immunizing agents.

GENERAL PRECAUTIONS AND CONTRAINDICATIONS TO ROUTINE ACTIVE IMMUNIZATIONS. An acute febrile illness may be reason to defer immunization until a subsequent

* Adapted from the *Red Book* (Report of the Committee on Infectious Diseases). Chicago: American Academy of Pediatrics, 1988.

Table 19-4. Recommended Schedule for Active Immunization of Normal Infants and Children

Recommended age	Vaccine(s)	Comments
2 mo	DTP,[1] OPV[2]	Can be initiated earlier in areas of high endemicity
4 mo	DTP, OPV	2-mo interval desired for OPV to avoid interference
6 mo	DTP	OPV optional for areas where polio might be imported (e.g., some areas of southwest United States)
12 mo	Tuberculin test[3]	May be given simultaneously with MMR at 15 mo
15 mo	Measles, mumps, rubella (MMR)[4]	MMR preferred
18 mo	DTP, OPV, Hib[5]	Consider as part of primary series — DTP essential
4–6 yr[6]	DTP, OPV	
14–16 yr	Td[7]	Repeat every 10 yr for lifetime

[1] DTP — Diphtheria and tetanus toxoids with pertussis vaccine.
[2] OPV — Oral, attenuated poliovirus vaccine contains poliovirus types 1, 2, and 3.
[3] Tuberculin test. Frequency of tests depends on local epidemiology. For groups at high risk of acquiring tuberculosis the Committee recommends annual or biennial testing or testing at three times — in infancy, preschool, and adolescence — for low-risk groups.
[4] MMR — Live measles, mumps, and rubella viruses in a combined vaccine (see text for discussion of single vaccines versus combination).
[5] Hib (*Hemophilus influenzae* b) vaccine in a conjugated form, e.g., PRP-D may be administered at 18 months or thereafter.
[6] Up to the seventh birthday. MMR reimmunization should be accomplished at school entry or at age 12 to 14.
[7] Td — Adult tetanus toxoid (full dose) and diphtheria toxoid (reduced dose) in combination.
For all products used, consult manufacturer's brochure for instructions for storage, handling, and administration. Biologics prepared by different manufacturers may vary, and those of the same manufacturer may change from time to time. The package insert should be followed for a specific product.
Source: Modified from *Red Book* (Report of the Committee on Infectious Diseases). Chicago: American Academy of Pediatrics, 1988.

visit or until the infection is properly controlled. Minor infections, even if associated with low-grade fever (e.g., the common cold) are not contraindications. In considering this recommendation, one must weigh the risk that the child might not be brought back and therefore would be inadequately immunized.

Some vaccine products are produced in cell culture systems, and they may contain trace amounts of cell culture materials. No adverse, hypersensitivity effect has been reported from the administration of these vaccines in individuals able to eat products containing these foreign antigens, e.g., egg-"sensitive" patients able to eat eggs, bread, or cookies.

INTERRUPTION OF SCHEDULE. Interruption of the recommended schedule, with a delay between doses, does not interfere with the final immunity achieved; nor does it necessitate starting the series over again, regardless of the length of time elapsed.

IMMUNIZATION RECORDS. A personal immunization record of a child's history of immunizations should be maintained by the parent.

COMBINED LIVE VIRUS VACCINES AND SIMULTANEOUS ADMINISTRATION OF LIVE VIRUS VACCINES. Simultaneous administration of various vaccines offers obvious advantages, particularly when there is a threat of concomitant exposure or the possibility that the child will be inaccessible for further immunization. The simultaneous administration of DTP, trivalent OPV, and MMR is acceptable.

Special Circumstances

PRIMARY IMMUNIZATION OF CHILDREN NOT IMMUNIZED IN INFANCY. Some children may not have been immunized as outlined in Table 19-4. A schedule suggested for these children has been developed by the AAP, and their *Red Book* should be consulted for information. In brief, children less than 6 years of age may be immunized with depot triple antigen (DTP), using three doses intramuscularly at intervals of 4 to 8 weeks. For children more than 6 years of age, adult-type diphtheria-tetanus toxoid (dT) is preferred. Pertussis vaccine at this age is not regularly recommended, but it may be used in special circumstances. Live attenuated measles, mumps, and rubella vaccines may be used in persons of any age if no contraindication exists. Similarly, live poliovirus vaccines may be used for older children and adolescents.

IMMUNIZATION OF PREMATURELY BORN INFANTS. Since transplacental antibody acquisition is terminated at birth and since the newborn has the capacity to produce immunoglobulin in response to antigenic stimulation, immunization can be started at 2 months of age regardless of gestational age at birth. If the infant is 2 months old but still hospitalized, then DTP (or DT if there is a neurologic

disorder) should be given. TOPV should not be given to hospitalized prematures because of the potential spread of a live vaccine virus to other babies.

IMMUNIZATION OF CHILDREN WITH NEUROLOGIC DISEASE. Generally, static neurologic disorders in infants and children do not constitute a valid reason for deferring or withholding routine immunizations. Children with fluctuating or progressive neurologic disease should not receive immunization because of the risk of cerebral irritation until their condition has been stabilized for at least 1 year.

IMMUNIZATION OF IMMUNODEFICIENT OR IMMUNOSUPPRESSED CHILDREN. **Children with known or suspected immunodeficiency disease should not receive any live virus vaccines since this may initiate a severe or fatal infection.** Asplenic children are a special subset of immunodeficient patients who deserve special mention. All asplenic children have an increased risk of overwhelming bacteremia, usually due to *Streptococcus pneumoniae*, *Neisseria meningitidis*, or *Hemophilus influenzae* type b (Hib). Pneumococcal and Hib vaccines should be administered to these children at the earliest age when efficacy can be expected.

Children receiving immunosuppressant agents (corticosteroids, antimetabolites, alkylating compounds, irradiation) may have aberrant responses to active immunization procedures. Immunizations for patients on short-term therapy should be deferred until treatment has been discontinued. Children on long-term therapy should not be given live vaccines but may receive inactivated antigens such as DTP; 3 months or more after cessation of therapy, an additional dose of inactivated vaccine is recommended, and live vaccines may be started.

Children who require bone marrow transplantation should be considered unimmunized and reimmunized according to Table 19-4 or as recommended for older children by the AAP.

IMMUNIZATION OF CHILDREN WHO HAVE RECENTLY RECEIVED BLOOD, PLASMA, OR GAMMA GLOBULINS. Immunization with live attenuated virus vaccines should be delayed for 3 months following administration of blood, plasma, or immune serum globulin because of the potential for inhibition of the desired antibody response.

IMMUNIZATION OF CHILDREN WITH AIDS. Live virus and live-bacterial vaccines (e.g., MMR, OPV, BCG) generally should not be given to children who are immunosuppressed, as occurs in association with symptomatic AIDS. Immunization with inactivated vaccines (e.g., DTP, IPV, and Hib) is generally recommended, although immunization may be less effective than it would be in immunocompetent children. However, because of reports of severe measles in symptomatic human immunodeficiency virus (HIV) infected children, MMR vaccination is recommended as the potential benefits appear to outweigh the potential risks. IPV should be given in place of OPV. BCG remains contraindicated in these children.

Children without clinical or epidemiologic manifestations of HIV infection should be immunized in accordance with routine recommendation, with the exception of the use of OPV, where IPV should be substituted.

Michael E. Pichichero

References

Immunization

American Academy of Pediatrics. *Report of the Committee on Infectious Diseases* (21st ed.). Evanston, IL: American Academy of Pediatrics, 1988.

DeForest, A., et al. Simultaneous administration of measles-mumps-rubella vaccine with booster doses of diphtheria-tetanus-pertussis and poliovirus vaccines. *Pediatrics* 81:237, 1988.

Givner, L. B., and Anderson, D. C. Immunization. In R. D. Feigin, and J. D. Cherry (Eds.). *Textbook of Pediatric Infectious Diseases* (2nd ed.). Philadelphia: Saunders, 1987.

Katz, S. L. Controversies in immunization. *Pediatr. Infect. Dis.* 6:607, 1987.

Kimura, M., and Hikino, N. Results with a new DTP vaccine in Japan. *Dev. Biol. Stand.* 61:545, 1985.

Stiehm, E. R. Specific Human Immunoglobulins as Therapeutic Agents. In A. Morell, and U. E. Nydegger (Eds.). *Clinical Use of Intravenous Immunoglobulins.* Orlando, FL: Academic, 1986.

Ward, J. Newer *Haemophilus influenzae* type b vaccines and passive prophylaxis. *Pediatr. Infect. Dis.* 6:799, 1987.

The Immune System

G. L. Asherson, and A. D. B. Webster (Eds.). *Diagnosis and Treatment of Immunodeficiency Diseases.* Boston: Blackwell, 1980.

Buckley, R. H. Immunodeficiency diseases. *J.A.M.A.* 258:2841, 1987.

Insel, R. Recurrent Infections in Children. In M. Ziai (Ed.), *Bedside Pediatrics.* Boston: Little, Brown, 1983.

Lau, Y. L., and Levinsky, R. J. Prenatal diagnosis and carrier detection in primary immunodeficiency disorders. *Arch. Dis. Child* 63:758, 1988.

Lichtenstein, L. M., and Fauci, A. S. (Eds.). *Current Therapy in Allergy, Immunology and Rheumatology-3.* Philadelphia: Decker, 1988.

Primary Immunodeficiency Diseases. Report of a WHO sponsored meeting. *Immunodeficiency Rev.* 1:173, 1989.

Rosen, F. S., Cooper, M. D., and Wedgwood, R. J. The primary immunodeficiencies. *N. Engl. J. Med.* 311:235, 300, 1984.

Stiehm, E. R. (Ed.). *Immunologic Disorders of Infants and Children* (3rd ed.). Philadelphia: Saunders, 1989.

Soothill, J. F., Hayward, A. R., and Wood, C. B. S. (Eds.). *Pediatric Immunology.* Boston: Blackwell, 1983.

Waldman, T. A. Immunodeficiency Diseases: Primary and Acquired. In M. Samter, et al. (Eds.). *Immunological Diseases* (4th ed.). Boston: Little, Brown, 1988.

20

Infectious Diseases

Bacterial Infections

Sepsis and Meningitis

Septicemia and meningitis constitute medical emergencies. A high index of suspicion and complete familiarity with the diagnostic procedures and proper management of these conditions are necessary for the physician entrusted with the care of children.

Despite numerous advances in antimicrobial therapy and intensive care support, the morbidity and mortality remain high (3–10%), and permanent sequelae occur in a large number of survivors of meningitis.

Epidemiology

The true incidence of bacterial sepsis and meningitis is difficult to ascertain, but it is clearly age-related. In the United States, the incidence of neonatal sepsis varies from 1 to 8 per 1000 live births, and a fourth of these cases have associated meningitis. After the neonatal period, the incidence of men-

ingitis is highest during the first year of life (about 300 cases/100,000 population annually). The mortality and morbidity of all types of bacterial meningitis are higher for males than for females, and the incidence of sequelae is directly related to the age of the patient and the interval between onset of meningitis and the institution of appropriate treatment.

Etiology

Sepsis and acute bacterial meningitis are caused by a variety of pathogenic agents, some of which are more prevalent in certain age groups. In the premature infant and during the neonatal period, group B streptococci, *Escherichia coli, Listeria monocytogenes,* other gram-negative bacilli, and streptococci species are the most common pathogens.

In infants and toddlers (<2 years of age), *Haemophilus influenzae* type b (Hib), *Streptococcus pneumoniae,* and *Neisseria meningitidis* account for more than 90% of the cases. In the older child, *S. pneumoniae* and *N. meningitidis* prevail, but Hib remains a rare cause. *Staphylococcus aureus,* beta-hemolytic streptococci, and a variety of gram-negative bacteria or anaerobes can cause septicemia and, rarely, meningitis after trauma, surgery, or from dissemination from a local focus such as an oropharyngeal, musculoskeletal, urinary, or gastrointestinal infection.

Coagulase-negative *Staphylococcus* sp., *Candida* sp., and other saprophytic fungi that are usually nonpathogenic for healthy individuals are emerging as important pathogens in premature newborns and patients with immunosuppression and indwelling intravascular catheters.

Because some of these pyogenic organisms are important causes of morbidity and mortality, they deserve special emphasis.

In the neonate, group B *Streptococcus* is a significant pathogen. In early onset disease, usually acquired from the mother and following a premature and complicated delivery, shock and respiratory distress carry a 30 to 50% mortality. Late onset disease, usually presenting as meningitis and bacteremia, carries a better prognosis.

N. meningitidis is usually found in the high posterior nasopharynx and is spread by respiratory droplets and close contact. In the United States the main endemic type is group B, while groups A, C, and Y may be more epidemic.

The usual form of the disease is bacteremia with meningitis and associated sites of infection involving the skin, pericardium, myocardium, joints, and lungs. The exanthem is initially a morbilliform rash and then develops into petechial and purpuric lesions. When purpura is prominent, ulceration and necrosis may occur.

A serious complication of meningococcemia is purpura fulminans caused by disseminated intravascular coagulation, which may lead to ischemia and gangrene of the extremities. Associated with consumption coagulopathy is adrenal hemorrhage (Waterhouse-Friderichsen syndrome).

Streptococcus pneumoniae, an encapsulated organism, is a frequent constituent of the respiratory flora. Predisposing conditions can be categorized into anatomical and host defense abnormalities. The former is associated with rhinorrhea and otorrhea; the latter includes immunoglobulin deficiencies, sickle-cell disease, diabetes mellitus, and complement (C3) defects. In addition to sinusitis, otitis media, mastoiditis, and pneumonia, pneumococci may cause sepsis leading to meningitis and, very rarely, to endocarditis or arthritis. Pneumococcal peritonitis may develop either as a primary infection or as a result of bacteremia in patients with the nephrotic syndrome.

Haemophilus influenzae is seen most commonly in children under the age of 5 or 6 years. It has been estimated that 1 in 200 children in the United States will develop serious infection from Hib by 5 years of age. The encapsulated type B is the most common cause of severe infections. Specific antibodies usually are present after 6 to 8 years of age, thus accounting for the decreased incidence in older children. This pathogen is the main cause of purulent meningitis in children, and associated infections include sinusitis, mastoiditis, pneumonitis, and pyoarthrosis. Acute epiglottis causes rapid upper airway obstruction, making this one of the most serious medical emergencies.

Staphylococcus aureus remains an important pathogen in systemic childhood infection. The source of the organism is usually cutaneous or musculoskeletal. Metastatic infection (endocarditis, brain abscess, renal carbuncles, splenic abscesses) can develop in various organs.

Pathogenesis

While *bacteremia* refers to the mere invasion of the circulation by bacteria, the term *septicemia* is reserved for clinical disease associated with hypotension, vascular collapse, and variant degrees of end-organ failure due to inadequate tissue perfusion. These vasoactive phenomena are largely related to release of endotoxin into the circulation.

Bacteremia may be primary, or secondary, to a local infection. Then hematogenous spread of bacteria may localize in the meninges, and other organs. Anatomical defects contributing to meningitis include meningomyelocele, neuraxial dermal sinuses, postsurgical fistulas, and foreign bodies in the central nervous system (e.g., shunts for hydrocephalus). In skull fractures or other head trauma, the portal of entry is obvious. Parameningeal sites resulting from otitis, mastoiditis, sinusitis, and abscesses (cranial and epidural) are significant sources of infection. Finally, host defense alterations must be considered when unusual organisms or other underlying disease is associated with purulent meningitis. The lack of protective antibodies, or complement deficiencies (such as in meningococcal diseases), is the major host factor in childhood meningitis and septicemia.

The pathophysiology of bacterial meningitis complex involves bacterial products and many mediators of the inflammatory process (arachidonic acid, metabolites, complements, cachectin), which disrupt the blood-brain barrier, causing vasogenic and cellular edema and tissue necrosis.

Clinical Manifestations

Early signs of septicemia and meningitis are fever, fussiness, poor feeding, vomiting, and lethargy. Paradoxical response to holding, poor eye contact with the examiner, and refusal to sit or stand up may be early signs of meningeal or localized infection.

Later, septic shock presents with fever (or hypothermia in the neonate), tachycardia, tachypnea, hypotension, and mental obtundation. Inadequate tissue perfusion may lead to acute renal failure, cardiorespiratory insufficiency, and death.

The signs and symptoms of meningitis are due to meningeal irritation, increased intracranial pressure, vascular thrombosis, and the general effects of a severe systemic infection. In infants, tense or bulging anterior fontanel, irritability, poor feeding, fever, high-pitched cry, or vomiting may be the only presenting sign. The older child may have additional physical findings of headache and nuchal rigidity with positive Kernig's and Brudzinski's signs. Skin rashes, particularly petechial and purpuric lesions, may be of further aid in the diagnosis of meningococcal meningitis, although other organisms, including *H. influenzae* and *S. pneumoniae,* may at times produce similar skin manifestations. Children less than a year old who present with coma, seizure, and shock, and have a low cerebrospinal fluid (CSF) glucose and anemia have the worse prognosis. As the disease progresses, coma, convulsions, and opisthotonic posturing become apparent.

Initial and follow-up evaluations should focus on recognition of end-organ failure as well as identification of metastatic foci of infection, which can occur even with appropriate antibiotic treatment.

Diagnosis

Examination of the CSF of a patient with acute bacterial meningitis is mandatory and constitutes the only sure way of establishing a diagnosis of the disease. The characteristic findings are (1) a cloudy appearance of the fluid (although in patients who have received antimicrobial therapy before the first lumbar puncture, as in very early cases, the fluid may be clear and the other CSF findings modified); (2) an increased cell count with a predominance of polymorphonuclear cells; (3) a low sugar level (usually less than half that in the blood); and (4) an elevated concentration of protein. There is no pathognomonic sign or symptom that accurately identifies the causative agent in the case of sepsis or purulent meningitis. Identification of the offending organism, therefore, requires further studies — that is, a Gram's stain of the CSF and of smears made from petechiae and cultures of the CSF, blood, and urine.

Specific, rapid detection of bacterial antigens by latex agglutination can be useful when the patient has been partially treated with antibiotics. The presence of capsular antigen of *N. meningitidis, H. influenzae* type b, or *S. pneumoniae* in the CSF or of group B streptococci in the serum of a neonate can be established in the blood, CSF, or concentrated urine. The sensitivity of this test is presently best for *H. influenzae* b, but poorer for *S. pneumoniae* or *N. meningitidis* because of the multitude of serotypes and the lower antiserum titers against these two organisms in commercial assays.

In the differential diagnosis of pyogenic meningitis one must consider the possibility of tuberculous meningitis, aseptic meningitis, and brain or epidural abscess. In the neonate, Herpes simplex meningoencephalitis can also clinically mimic bacterial sepsis and meningitis. Whenever sufficient doubt exists, it is best to begin antimicrobial therapy promptly while awaiting the final diagnosis.

Identification of the bacteria whenever possible, prompt, specific antimicrobial therapy, and adequate supportive measures are fundamental to the optimal management of acute bacterial meningitis or sepsis. Any unnecessary delay in treatment may result in increased mortality and seriousness of complications. Table 20-1 lists the antimicrobial agents effective in acute bacterial meningitis and sepsis.

Treatment

In selecting the specific antibiotic, the physician must consider the particular age group of the patient. For infants less than 8 weeks old in whom unusual organisms are suspected, ampicillin plus an aminoglycoside or a third-generation cephalosporin plus ampicillin should be considered. In children older than 2 months with suspected meningitis, ampicillin and chloramphenicol or a third-generation cephalosporin (cefotaxime, ceftriaxone) should be administered until the causative agent is identified and its antimicrobial sensitivity determined. Persistent fever in a patient thus treated with appropriate dosage is usually related to complications of the primary illness, nosocomial infections, or drug reaction and not to antibiotic failure.

Initially, when the diagnosis of meningitis is made and after the correct cultures are obtained, the patient should receive the appropriate antimicrobial by an intravenous route. There is no established duration of treatment. The regimen usually recommended is treatment by the intravenous route for a minimum of 7 to 10 days of treatment.

Table 20-1. Antimicrobial Agents for Treatment of Sepsis and Meningitis

	Daily dose*		
	Neonates		
Regimen	0–7 days of age	8–28 days of age	Infants and children
Penicillin G	100,000–150,000 U/kg[a]	150,000–200,000 U/kg[b,c]	250,000 U/kg[c,d]
Ampicillin	100–150 mg/kg[a]	150–200 mg/kg[b,c]	200–300 mg/kg[c]
Kanamycin	15–20 mg[a]	20–30 mg[b]	
Gentamicin†	5 mg/kg[a]	7.5 mg/kg[b]	
Tobramycin†	4 mg/kg[a]	6 mg/kg[b]	
Amikacin†	15–20 mg/kg[a]	20–30 mg/kg[b]	
Chloramphenicol†	25 mg/kg	50 mg/kg[a]	75–100 mg/kg[c]
Cefotaxime	100 mg/kg[a]	150–200 mg/kg[b,c]	200 mg/kg[c]
Ticarcillin	150–225 mg/kg[a,b]	225–300 mg/kg[b,c]	
Methicillin	100–150 mg/kg[a,b]	150–200 mg/kg[b,c]	
Oxacillin	100–150 mg/kg[a,b]	150–200 mg/kg[b,c]	
Nafcillin	100–150 mg/kg[a,b]	150–200 mg/kg[b,c]	
Vancomycin	20 mg[a]	30 mg/kg[b]	40–60 mg/kg[c]
Ceftriaxone			100 mg/kg[a]
Ceftazidime	60 mg/kg[a]	90 mg/kg[b]	125–150 mg/kg[b]

* Dosage divided and given every: [a]12 hours, [b]8 hours, [c]6 hours, [d]4 hours.
† Serum concentrations should be monitored and dosages adjusted accordingly.
Source: J. O. Klein, R. D. Feigin, and G. H. McCracken, Jr. Report of the task force on diagnosis and treatment of meningitis. *Pediatrics* 78[Suppl. II.]: 959, 1986. Copyright American Academy of Pediatrics 1986.

Neonatal meningitis with group B streptococci or gram-negative bacilli should be treated for 14 and 21 days, respectively.

Fluid intake and serum electrolytes should be monitored to avoid water overload, inappropriate antidiuretic hormone (IADH) secretion syndrome, and cerebral edema. In case of shock, measurement of central venous pressure, blood pressure regulation, and administration of and volume expanders are necessary. Good supportive therapy should be provided for optimal care of the patient. Recently, the use of dexamethasone at 0.6 mg/kg/day every 6 hours for 4 days has been reported to decrease the sequelae of hearing loss following meningitis; the benefits of steroid therapy may be even greater if given early and before antibiotic administration. (See Table 20-1 for selection of antimicrobials.) A final lumbar puncture should be performed 24 to 48 hours after treatment of neonatal meningitis, but it is routinely not indicated in childhood meningitis, in which bacteriologic relapse is extremely uncommon (< 0.5%).

SEQUELAE AND FOLLOW-UP STUDY. Various neurological sequelae including hydrocephalus, cranial nerve involvement, deafness, blindness, mental retardation, epilepsy, and subdural effusions develop in about 30 to 40% of children who survive an attack of meningitis. They occur more frequently in patients who receive inadequate therapy, in young infants, and in those in whom therapy is not instituted early in the course of the disease. Repeated examination of the patient, including the measurement of the head circumference, is needed while the patient is in the hospital. With an enlarging head, undue irritability, poor feeding, vomiting, or recurrence of fever, computed axial tomography (CAT scan) or magnetic resonance imaging (MRI) must be performed. Subdural taps are usually not necessary unless the effusions cause significant neurological deficits.

Responsibility for the care of a patient with meningitis does not end with discharge from the hospital. Careful follow-up study for months and even years is needed in order to be certain about the outcome and to provide the proper rehabilitation for those who need it.

Prevention

All infants and children should be adequately immunized against *H. influenzae* type b with the conjugate vaccine (see Chapter 17). Pneumococcal and meningococcal vaccines are not routinely recommended for normal healthy children but can be used for selected immunocompromised patients or in the event of meningococcal outbreaks. In hospitalized patients, infection control measures should be followed to decrease the risk of nosocomial sepsis, especially from intravascular catheters.

Chinh T. Le

Brucellosis

Brucellosis is an infectious disease transmitted to human beings by (1) contact with the secretions or excretions of infected swine, goats, cows, sheepdogs, or horses, (2) consumption of raw milk or dairy products, and (3) accidental inoculation while working with the organisms in the laboratory. Brucellosis is caused by *Brucella melitensis* (goats), *B. suis* (hogs), *B. abortus* (cattle), and *B. canis* (dogs). Animals may be invaded by any of the three species; thus, cows and pigs may be infected by either *B. abortus* or *B. suis*. Children contract the disease most frequently after ingestion of unpasteurized milk or dairy products from infected animals.

B. melitensis causes the most severe disease (Malta or undulant fever), often characterized by a clinical picture resembling that of typhoid fever. A relatively mild illness follows infection with *B. abortus*. In general, illness occurs approximately 14 days after gross exposure to any of the *Brucella* organisms.

Clinical Manifestations

The clinical picture of brucellosis is very difficult to define because of the protean nature of the disease. There may be an acute onset, with spiking fevers, chills, sweats, pain in the extremities, backache and headache, anorexia, and weakness. Or the onset may be insidious, with a low-grade fever, weakness, somatic aches and pains, and mental depression. The outstanding features are the intensity of complaints and the toxic, disturbed appearance of the patient in contrast with the paucity of objective findings. In addition to fever, the following findings are observed in a descending order of frequency: splenomegaly, lymphadenopathy, hepatomegaly, abdominal tenderness, cardiac and neurological abnormalities, skin rashes, and jaundice. Suppurative complications may also occur. The disease may persist for weeks and rarely for months and years.

Diagnosis

Leukopenia and lymphocytosis are usual in brucellosis; atypical cells resembling those of infectious mononucleosis may be present. The diagnosis can be securely established only by determination of specific agglutinin titers (1 : 160 or above) and by isolation of the organisms from the blood, bone marrow, and liver. Because the organism may grow slowly, the blood cultures must not be discarded for at least 3 weeks. In performing agglutination tests, one must pay special attention to the prozone phenomenon as a cause of negative reactions. The brucellin skin test is of little value except that a negative reaction tends to rule out the diagnosis.

Physicians caring for patients in areas where consumption of unpasteurized milk or milk products is likely would do well to consider brucellosis in a child with obscure fever or toxic hepatosplenomegaly.

Prognosis and Treatment

In general, the prognosis in brucellosis is good; however, in severe infections, especially with *B. melitensis*, death may occur within 2 or 3 weeks of onset. Relapses are rare in children and are generally mild. Tetracycline, the antimicrobial agent of choice for most infections, may be given orally in a total dose of 40 to 50 mg/kg/day in four equally divided doses for a period of 21 days. This drug should not be administered in children less than 7 years of age. In severe infections, or in those not responding to tetracycline, the concomitant administration of streptomycin, 0.5 to 1.0 g in two divided doses every 12 hours for at least 2 weeks, is recommended. In children under 7 years of age, as well as older patients, the alternatives are chloramphenicol or rifampin. Relapses are treated in the same manner as the initial episode.

Prevention of brucellosis requires the pasteurization of all milk and milk products, eradication of infection in domestic animals, vaccination of persons working with animals, and education of the public regarding the hazards of consuming raw milk.

Diphtheria

Diphtheria is a highly infectious, potentially fatal disease acquired by contact with active cases or asymptomatic carriers. It may be prevented by immunization against the disease. The principal portal of entry for the diphtheria bacillus *(Corynebacterium diphtheriae)* is the upper respiratory tract, but the organism may also invade the skin, genital tract, eye, or middle ear. The incubation period is 2 to 6 days but may be as short as 1 day or as long as 9 days.

Clinical Manifestations

The systemic reactions in uncomplicated diphtheria are, as a rule, of only minor to moderate severity, and the fever is usually low-grade. When toxic manifestations are absent, patients feel quite well except for mild discomfort in the pharynx. In those in whom the toxin exerts its effects, pallor, listlessness, tachycardia, and weakness are striking. In the terminal stages of the disease, peripheral vascular collapse is common.

The very early pharyngeal exudate may be indistinguishable from that seen in the follicular pharyngitis or tonsillitis of streptococcal infections. As the disease progresses, a pseudomembrane forms over the tonsils or posterior pharyngeal wall, or both. Later, it becomes more dense, is white, gray, or black in color depending on the degree of hemorrhage, and is firmly attached to the underlying mucous membrane so that, when it is detached, bleeding spots are visible. There is usually a small area of inflammation about the periphery of the membrane. If there is mixed infection — for example, with beta-hemolytic streptococci — the pharynx is diffusely red and edematous. The leukocytosis is only moderate, usually not over 15,000 white cells/mm^3.

The membrane may spread to cover completely the fauces, tonsils, uvula, soft and hard palates, and posterior pharyngeal wall. It may also extend upward into the nares and cause a serosanguineous discharge that may have an offensive odor. In patients with severe disease there is marked enlargement of the cervical lymph nodes and striking edema of the submandibular areas and anterior aspect of the neck, producing the typical "bull neck." This severe infection is characterized by noisy breathing through an open mouth, foul breath, and thickened speech. The patient has a waxy pallor and is very weak. Occasionally, purpuric eruptions of the skin may appear, particularly in the region of the neck and the anterior chest wall. Varying degrees of drowsiness and delirium are not uncommon.

Complications

The complications of diphtheria are of two types: (1) those resulting from spread of the tonsillopharyngeal membrane into the lower respiratory tract and (2) those produced by the absorption of exotoxin. With extension of the pharyngeal exudate into the lower respiratory tract, there is gradual interference with breathing. Involvement of the trachea or larynx (or both) leads to occlusion of the airway and progressive respiratory difficulty, which may terminate fatally unless tracheostomy or intubation is carried out. Diphtheria may rarely be limited to the larynx or trachea without involvement of the pharynx. This possibility must always be kept in mind in the differential diagnosis of "croup."

On the basis of clinical findings alone, approximately 10% of patients have cardiac involvement with various forms of arrhythmia. Electrocardiographic tracings show other changes in many cases. Cardiac failure may develop during the course of diphtheria and is due to toxic myocarditis and the accompanying damage to the intrinsic conduction system. While cardiac failure may occur at any time, it is most common between the fifth and twelfth days.

Paralysis of a given muscle or group of muscles may occur as the result of a toxic peripheral neuritis, which is painless and may persist for several days or weeks. In severe cases, paralysis of the soft palate and posterior pharyngeal wall may develop very early because of direct action of the toxin on the pharyngeal motor nerve endings. More frequently neuritis develops later in the disease. The cranial nerves are the ones most often involved, but any of the peripheral nerves may be affected.

The mortality from diphtheria varies not only with the stage of the disease at which an adequate amount of antitoxin is administered but also with the degree of the electrocardiographic and physical changes. In young infants the mortality is higher (as high as 90%) because of the frequency of laryngeal involvement and bronchopneumonia.

Diagnosis

The presence of diphtheria should be suspected when a membrane having the features described above is observed in the pharynx. It must be emphasized, however, that the exudate in the pharynx is not always typical and that pseudomembranes which may easily be confused with diphtheria membranes appear in a number of other infections. Among these are infectious mononucleosis, streptococcal pharyngitis, viral exudative pharyngitis, fusospirochetal angina, acute moniliasis, and staphylococcal infections of the throat secondary to chemotherapy.

The only positive method of establishing the diagnosis of diphtheria is by demonstrating typical *C. diphtheriae* in stained smears and cultures of the membrane on special media.

Treatment

The only specific treatment for diphtheria is antitoxin, and this should be administered promptly on the basis of clinical diagnosis and before bacteriological confirmation. Delay in treatment increases the frequency of complications and death. Antitoxin must never be given until tests for sensitivity to horse serum have been carried out. The recommended dosage schedule varies, according to severity and location of the lesion, from 20,000 to 100,000 units. In severe cases at least one-half the dose is given intravenously.

Desensitization must be carried out in persons highly reactive to horse serum.

Penicillin (or erythromycin in persons sensitive to penicillin) is used as an accompaniment to serotherapy in order to eradicate the carrier state. Resistance to erythromycin is increasing.

In obstruction of the larynx due to diphtheria, intubation or tracheostomy may be necessary. The course of diphtheritic myocarditis cannot be influenced significantly by any specific measures. Strict bedrest is mandatory.

Diphtheria, in large measure, is a preventable disease (see Chapter 19 on immunization). Individuals exposed to a known case of diphtheria who have never been actively immunized should receive 5000 I.U. of antitoxin; such passive protection lasts for about 2 weeks. In those who have previously received toxoid, a booster dose of toxoid is usually sufficient to protect against development of the disease. Diphtheria antitoxin is recommended because (1) penicillin is not totally effective in eradicating the organism, (2) antibiotics do not appear to prevent progression of disease in symptomatic persons, and (3) the factors that make surveillance of contacts impractical may contribute to delay in receiving antitoxin after diphtheria develops. Toxoid in the *nonimmune* individual does not result in a protective level of antitoxic antibodies.

Salmonella Infections

Salmonellosis

There are three main species of *Salmonella* — *S. typhi* (one serotype), *S. choleraesuis* (one serotype), and *S. enteritidis* (more than 1700 serotypes). The peak incidence of *Salmonella* infection is in the summer and the lowest in winter; however, substantial numbers of infections occur in all months. The infections are more common in infants and children than in adults; the incidence is particularly high in the first year of life.

CLINICAL MANIFESTATIONS. There are four main groups of clinical manifestations, any of which may occur simultaneously, consecutively, or individually: (1) acute gastroenteritis, (2) septicemia with or without focal manifestations, (3) "typhoidal" symptoms, and (4) the carrier state.

The most common form of salmonellosis is acute gastroenteritis, because the organisms are frequently ingested in foods that have been contaminated by animal feces or by human carriers. This condition is discussed in Chapter 12.

Salmonella septicemia is most often due to *S. choleraesuis* and is the most serious of the infections produced by this group of organisms. Intestinal symptoms are usually absent. A high, often spiking fever with frequent chills is usual. The white cell count may be elevated or, more commonly, depressed. The main features of this syndrome result from the spread of the bacteria via the blood stream to different organs. Such metastatic infections may lead to the development of meningitis, osteomyelitis, and pneumonia. Other, less prevalent complications are endocarditis, purulent arthritis, pyelonephritis, and abscesses in the subdural space, spleen, muscles, and other soft tissues. The prognosis in this form of the disease is poor, accounting for most of the fatalities in *Salmonella* infections. The presence of hemoglobin in the patient's plasma may increase the chances of septic complications such as osteomyelitis.

The typhoidal form, frequently referred to as salmonella fever, is produced most often by the paratyphoid bacilli, the *S. paratyphi* (paratyphoid A) and *S. schottmülleri* (paratyphoid B). While the clinical picture resembles that of typhoid fever qualitatively, the disease is usually milder. The fever may be quite variable in degree and duration. As in typhoid fever (*S. typhi*), a leukopenia with a relative lymphocytosis is the rule. Gastrointestinal symptoms are mild when present; constipation is a frequent complaint. Bradycardia and splenomegaly are common, but rose spots are infrequent. Bronchitis or bronchial pneumonia may develop, and the causative organisms are present in the sputum. Salmonellae may not be demonstrable in the feces until many days or up to several weeks after the onset of infection; they may appear in the urine later in the course of the disease.

The carrier state may initiate or terminate every clinical form of salmonellosis. Antibiotics are disappointing in eradication of the carrier state.

DIAGNOSIS. The clinical diagnosis of salmonellosis is difficult. In the absence of diarrhea, the nature of the disease is often not apparent, and it is labeled fever of undetermined origin. The specific diagnosis can be established only by isolation of the organisms from the stool or blood and by demonstration of a significant increase in serum agglutinin titer. Serological studies are necessary when the organisms cannot be isolated. Serum samples obtained 12 to 14 days apart should be titrated for specific agglutinins.

TREATMENT AND PREVENTION. The treatment of *Salmonella* infections with antibiotics has been disappointing, particularly that of carriers of all types including *S. typhi*. In general, the use of antibiotics is to be avoided in the treatment of infections that are limited to the intestinal tract.

Antimicrobial treatment should be reserved for use in the septicemic and severe forms of salmonellosis and in neonates and young infants. There is general agreement that chloramphenicol, 50 to 100 mg/kg/day beyond the neonatal period, is the drug of choice under these circumstances; the antimicrobial may be given perorally or parenterally in four equally divided doses, for an average period of 2 weeks. Duration of treatment must be individualized, and hard-and-fast rules cannot be given. Ampicillin, in large doses, is particularly effective in severe septic and metastatic infections with salmonellae requiring therapy for more than 2 weeks. It is important to keep in mind that rapidly increasing antibiotic resistance of many strains of salmonellae has taken place in recent years. Trimethoprim and sulfamethoxazole have been used successfully in the treatment of *Salmonella* infections; they may be considered for a patient who fails to respond to the other agents or who is sensitive to one of them. Ceftriaxone is another alternative antibiotic. Surgical drainage of collections of pus is required if any antimicrobial is to be effective in eradicating the organism.

The prevention of *Salmonella* infections, as in *Shigella* infections, cannot be effected by the use of antimicrobial agents. The essentials of prophylaxis include proper sanitation control, quarantine of carriers from food handling, elimination of flies, and the boiling or cooking of potentially contaminated food or water. There is no effective immunization procedure for the prevention of infection by *Salmonella* species other than *S. typhi*.

Typhoid Fever

Typhoid fever, caused by *S. typhi*, is the most serious infection caused by *Salmonella* organisms. The clinical manifestations of typhoid fever are similar in the child more than 2 years old and in the adult, except that the disease is usually less severe in the child.

CLINICAL MANIFESTATIONS AND COURSE. The onset of the disease may be insidious or acute. During the initial stages it often resembles an acute upper respiratory tract infection. After an incubation period of 10 to 14 days (range, 3–40 days), the patient may present with low-grade fever and mild grippelike symptoms or, less commonly, with high fever, marked headache, chills, and constipation. Or symptoms suggestive of central nervous system involvement may predominate: delirium, mania, marked irritability, and severe headache. Or the presenting symptoms may be severe abdominal pain and vomiting, or fever, chills, cough, and signs of lower respiratory tract involvement.

The entire course of the disease is no longer than 2 or 3 weeks; in some children the whole course may not last more than a week. During the first week of illness, fever may increase gradually to 40 to 41°C, or it may continue low-grade; in children, it is ordinarily quite irregular. Generally, there is some degree of bradycardia, but the disparity between the height of the fever and the pulse is not as striking as in the adult; often there is a mild tenderness and slight distention of the abdomen. Constipation is the rule, although diarrhea may occasionally be present, especially in infants. Toward the end of the first week, enlargement of the spleen (in over two-thirds of the patients) and rose spots appear. The latter are irregular, blanching macules, 2 to 5 mm in diameter, which yield *S. typhi* on culture. The spots are few in number and are distributed on the anterior wall of the chest and abdomen. They may appear in successive crops but are likely to be less frequent in children than in adults. The course of the disease is modified with antimicrobial therapy and supportive measures. If the diagnosis is not made, the full course, as described below, may be observed.

All the manifestations of the illness tend to be aggravated during the second week. Fever is then sustained at a high level, the pulse becomes rapid, and the characteristic mental torpor, from which the disease derives its name, makes its appearance. Abdominal symptoms become marked, and there is a danger of hemorrhage or perforation of the bowel at this time. In mild cases the patient's condition may begin to improve by the end of the second week, but with a moderately severe illness, symptoms may persist into the third week, with increasing risk of complications. These must be suspected particularly when abdominal distention and pain are prominent. In most instances convalescence sets in by the end of the third week, but in some the disease may persist and death may occur.

COMPLICATIONS. In general, the disease is milder in infants than in older children, and milder in both groups than in adults. In infants and children it is usually of shorter duration, and complications are infrequent. The complications include intestinal perforation and hemorrhage, alopecia, parotid gland swelling with uveitis, spontaneous rupture of the spleen, and involvement of specific organs and tissues. Other complications include pneumonia, pleural effusion, and infarction of the lungs and evidences of pericarditis, myocarditis, or endocarditis. Multiple liver abscesses, cholecystitis, pyelonephritis, osteomyelitis, spondylitis, suppurative arthritis, neuritis, meningitis, cerebral vein thrombosis, and localized abscesses involving many organ systems including muscle and skin may also develop.

RELAPSES. Relapses are less frequent and less severe in children than in adults, but they may occur from 1 to 6 weeks after the fever comes down and on rare occasions may happen several times. The carrier state occurs less frequently in children than in adults, although during the initial stages of convalescence positive stool cultures are not infrequent.

DIAGNOSIS. The diagnosis of typhoid fever is difficult to make on clinical grounds, but the presence of fever, rose spots, splenomegaly, and constipation (or diarrhea) in addition to leukopenia should suggest the disease. The presence of the disease can be established only by bacteriological and serological methods. The typhoid bacillus can almost always be isolated from the blood during the first week of infection, and less frequently as the disease progresses. By the fourth week only about 10% of the patients show a bacteremia. In contrast, only 5 to 10% of the stool cultures may be positive during the first week and 50 to 75% in the fourth week of illness. Organisms do not appear in the urine until late in the disease. Thus, early in the disease, blood cultures are of greatest help in the diagnosis, whereas cultures of the stool and urine are most useful later. It must be realized, however, that the organism may grow slowly on blood culture.

TREATMENT. Although ampicillin is a useful agent when the organism is sensitive, chloramphenicol is the drug of choice for the specific treatment of the disease. The recommended dose beyond the neonatal period is 50 to 100 mg/kg/day in four divided doses orally or the succinate derivative intravenously. The dose should not exceed a total daily dose of 2 g. After defervescence, the drug may be administered at 8-hour intervals for 14 to 21 days. Therapy should not be discontinued too early because of the risk of relapse. Trimethoprim-sulfamethoxazole has been of therapeutic value, especially in patients infected with chloramphenicol-resistant strains. Other alternative drugs are Ceftriaxone and Cefotaxime.

All patients should be observed carefully for the development of any complications. In case of perforation, surgical intervention is usually the procedure of choice in children.

Isolation of the patient and proper handling of excreta to prevent spread of infection are essential.

Shigella Infections

See Chapter 12.

Staphylococcal Infections

See also specific organ systems.

Infections due to staphylococci appear to be increasing, and the increase has been related to the advent of modern antibiotic therapy. The prolongation of life of many patients with serious disease has created a group highly vulnerable to infection with either coagulase-positive (most frequently) or coagulase-negative staphylococci. Moreover, the use of steroids and antimetabolites is thought to alter host defense mechanisms. Advances in surgery and the increased use of cutdowns and catheters offer new portals for microorganisms such as staphylococci. In addition to the almost universal presence of pathogenic staphylococci in the nasopharynx and on the skin of normal human beings, certain other characteristics of staphylococci are responsible for the frequency with which infections due to these microorganisms are encountered: (1) their capacity to become resistant to almost every new antimicrobial agent; (2) a tendency for resistant staphylococci to sequester in closed areas, such as hospitals, where seriously ill patients are gathered; and (3) an avidity for producing disease in patients already seriously compromised with other illness. When infections develop in this last group, the mortality is high, and treatment is often unsatisfactory. The serious major infections that may be caused by staphylococci are (1) infections in newborn infants and their nursing mothers; (2) primary pneumonia and empyema in infancy and secondary pneumonia in childhood; (3) bacteremia, with or without involvement of the endocardium, but frequently with osteomyelitis; (4) wound infections, some with a scarlatiniform rash due to erythrogenic toxin, (5) enterocolitis; (6) staphylococcal scalded skin syndrome; and (7) toxic shock syndrome.

Over the last two decades severe neonatal staphylococcal infections and staphylococcal pneumonias and empyema in older infants and children have declined. Today, severe staphylococcal septicemia is being encountered primarily in association with serious underlying disease, intravenous drug abuse, or recent antibiotic use or in immunosuppressed persons. The occurrence of staphylococcal sepsis in the absence of such predisposing factors in older children is uncommon, even though staphylococcal osteomyelitis is relatively frequent in this age group.

Treatment

In considering specific therapy, one should bear in mind certain general characteristics of staphylococcal infections:

1. Staphylococci characteristically produce rapid necrosis and tissue death at local sites of infection. Thus, delay in treatment may permit an acute and readily reversible process to become well entrenched, suppurative, and chronic, responding slowly, if at all, to antibiotic treatment.
2. Abscess formation is the rule in staphylococcal infection, and surgical drainage plays an important role in management.
3. Staphylococci are eradicated slowly, and infections by these organisms tend to become chronic, with a high rate of relapse; thus, therapy must be prolonged.
4. In view of the tendency to abscess formation and slow killing rate of staphylococci, it is prudent to use "bactericidal" rather than "bacteriostatic" agents.
5. In toxic shock syndrome as well as other serious staphylococcal infections, supportive therapy with intravenous fluids and other measures constitutes the most essential aspect of management.

Because of the changing patterns of an antimicrobial sensitivity of the staphylococci, it is essential that in vitro sensitivity studies be carried out to determine optimal therapy.

It is generally agreed that penicillin G is the agent of choice in treating infections due to an organism known to be sensitive to this antibiotic. Administration of the crystalline aqueous form provides optimal blood and tissue levels. The dose depends on the severity of the infection and the age and size of the patient: in infants, 150,000 to 3,000,000 units/day; in small children, 300,000 to 5,000,000 units/day; and in older children, 600,000 to 12,000,000 units/day. The penicillin (aqueous crystalline penicillin G) may be administered by intermittent intramuscular injection or by the continuous or "push" intravenous route.

In older patients with impetigo or furuncles, oral treatment may be satisfactory; penicillin or erythromycin (15–20 mg of either drug/kg/day in four divided doses) may be used when the infecting organisms are sensitive to these agents. In infections caused by staphylococci resistant to penicillin G, a penicillinase-resistant (beta-lactamase-resistant) penicillin that is well absorbed when administered orally, such as cloxacillin or, preferably, dicloxacillin, should be given in a dose of 30 to 50 mg/kg/day in four divided doses. Topical therapy is not recommended inasmuch as the elimination of organisms is less certain and less rapid than with systemic therapy.

If the susceptibility of the organism is not known, as will often be the case at the beginning of treatment, we recommend that penicillin G be combined with one of the new semisynthetic penicillinase-resistant penicillins such as methicillin or nafcillin.

If the microorganism is shown to be resistant to penicillin, this antibiotic is discontinued and nafcillin is administered alone.

The cephalosporin group of antimicrobials are also resistant to penicillinase and may be used for infections caused by penicillin-resistant staphylococci or in patients who may be hypersensitive to penicillin.

Collections of pus in the skin or elsewhere may require surgical drainage, and this should always be done when indicated.

Staphylococcal Enterocolitis

Staphylococcal enterocolitis is an uncommon clinical syndrome characterized by nausea, vomiting, diarrhea, peripheral vascular collapse, and a high fatality rate. It may be recognized as a complication of several factors: (1) prolonged use of broad-spectrum antimicrobials, including a combination of a penicillin and an aminoglycoside; (2) abdominal surgery; (3) episodes of hypotension; and (4) poor oral food intake. In infancy, and especially in the neonate, a staphylococcal gastroenteritis may be encountered during a staphylococcal nursery epidemic. In such cases, gram-positive cocci are present in large numbers in smears of the stool and grow well on nonselective media. Blood cultures are usually sterile.

Staphylococcal Scalded Skin Syndrome (SSSS)

This is a syndrome characterized by dermatological reaction to infection with phage group II coagulase-positive staphylococci (to a lesser extent with phage group I) that elaborate an erythrogenic and exfoliative toxin. The generalized dermatitis associated with these organisms strikingly resembles that produced by scalding; hence the name. Bullous impetigo, a distinctive clinical entity within the larger group of impetiginous lesions, and staphylococcal scarlatiniform disease, resembling in many respects the streptococcal rash associated with scarlet fever, are characterized by a desquamative process and are associated with phage group II staphylococci producing an exfoliative toxin (ET). Their inclusion in an "expanded SSSS" appears reasonable and useful. Toxic epidermal necrolysis, which has many clinical similarities to SSSS and is usually due to hypersensitivity reaction, should be differentiated histologically and historically from it as their management is different.

Toxic Shock Syndrome

This syndrome is caused by toxin-1 and exotoxin produced by *Staphylococcus aureus*. It is now divided into menstrual- and nonmenstrual-associated categories. There has been a decline of the menstrual-associated subgroup since the recognition of the role played by the use of tampons in its pathogenesis. The nonmenstrual subgroup may be related to any staphylococcal infection including relatively minor skin infections.

The clinical manifestations consist of malaise, fever, myalgia, headache, weakness, abdominal pain, and vomiting. A scarlatiniform (sunburnlike) rash and infection of the mucous membrane, dizziness, confusion, and diarrhea follow, and on examination postural hypotension leading to shock is observed. The findings may be suggestive of gastroenteritis, scarlet fever, or Kawasaki's disease, but the dominant picture of postural hypotension and shock, unexplained by the degree of diarrhea, must arouse suspicion about this condition. There is leukocytosis with a left shift. Pyuria and some increase in blood urea nitrogen (BUN) may be observed. Because multiple organs are involved, there may be other changes in serum chemical composition and chest x ray. Blood cultures are negative, but culture of the site of original staphylococcal infection yields the toxin-producing organisms.

Unless the treatment is promptly instituted with antibiotics and fluids to combat shock, disseminated intravascular coagulation and death may ensue. The use of corticosteroids in conjunction with other measures is recommended by some authors. About a week or 10 days following onset, desquamation of the skin is seen, frequently accompanied by a pruritic rash and edema. There may also be changes in the nails and hair weeks later.

Streptococcal Infections

Streptococcal disease in humans is most frequently the result of infection by organisms belonging to Lancefield's group A. A small percentage of infections are caused by group B, C, D, and G strains. Beta-hemolytic streptococci commonly produce infections of the upper respiratory tract, usually of the pharynx and tonsils, with a tendency to spread to adjacent structures such as lymph nodes, middle ear, sinuses, and lungs; however, they may also produce surgical infections — cellulitis, lymphangitis, sepsis, and osteomyelitis. The important group B streptococcal infections encoun-

tered in the natal and neonatal periods of life are discussed in Chapter 9. For pharyngitis and tonsillitis see Chapter 10 for more detailed discussion.

Systemic symptoms such as fever, headache, malaise, and vomiting are common and frequently associated with local inflammatory signs. The age of the patient, in general, determines the type of clinical response to infection with group A streptococci. In infants under 6 months of age, respiratory infection is accompanied by fever and moderate inflammation of the mucosa of the nasopharynx. In the untreated infant the acute episode lasts about 1 week and is followed by a persistent nasal discharge and some indisposition for about 6 weeks. In children 6 months to 3 years of age, symptoms are often mild, with low-grade fever that may persist for 1 to 2 weeks.

A chronic form of streptococcal infection of the pharynx may occur in children less than 3 years of age; it is characterized by a subacute constitutional reaction and a mild nasopharyngitis with a slight serous discharge from the nose. The fever fluctuates and may persist for 4 to 8 weeks. The cervical lymph nodes may be enlarged, and there may be a complicating otitis media. The child with this kind of streptococcosis may be cranky, fretful, and "out of sorts," with poor appetite and pallor. This type of streptococcal infection, while not common, must be considered in any young child who presents with a history of sore throat and prolonged low-grade fever; convalescence is long and trying to both parents and child. While streptococcal infection of the pharynx at this age is generally not intense, spread to the middle ear and cervical lymph nodes is common. In children over 3 years of age, and in young adults, the disease tends to be more abrupt in onset, accompanied by more severe systemic manifestations, but often of shorter duration. Treatment is with penicillin or erythromycin for 10 days (see Chap. 10).

Streptococcal Pneumonia

See Chapter 10.

Complications

The complications of streptococcal infections are of two types: suppurative and nonsuppurative. The former result from direct spread of the organisms from the throat or from invasion of the blood stream. Extension of infection from the pharynx may result in parapharyngeal or peritonsillar abscess, otitis media, sinusitis, mastoiditis, meningitis, tracheobronchitis, or pneumonia. In infants and children who habitually place fingers in mouth a paronychia may develop, or streptococci may come in contact with the skin elsewhere, producing impetigo. This latter complication is frequently encountered about the lips and chest in patients with a profuse nasal discharge. Invasion of the blood stream may lead to distant foci of infection in any organ system of the body, localizing most commonly, however, in the bones, heart valves, and meninges. Particularly in infants between the ages of 6 months and 3 years, suppurative cervical lymphadenitis is likely to develop as a late complication of unrecognized or inadequately treated nasopharyngitis. The node or nodes become markedly firm and swollen and may be confused with lymphoma if the initial infection several weeks before was overlooked. The usual site is the tonsillar node at the angle of the jaw draining the tonsil, but drainage from infected adenoids may produce retropharyngeal lymphadenitis, which often is not detected until it forms a retropharyngeal abscess, producing respiratory obstruction and necessitating immediate drainage.

Although infection of the lungs and pleura by beta-hemolytic streptococci is uncommon, it may occur as either a primary infection or a secondary one following a viral infection.

Rheumatic fever and acute glomerulonephritis are the two chief nonsuppurative complications of streptococcal sore throat and usually appear after a latent period of 1 to 6 weeks after infection. While rheumatic fever is said to occur in about 2 or 3% of patients with streptococcal tonsillo-pharyngitis, recent studies in children indicate that the attack rate for rheumatic fever after a streptococcal infection is probably somewhat less than 1% but is much higher during epidemic periods than after sporadic infections. This complication is generally seen in children from 5 to 10 years of age, although primary attacks and recurrences may develop at any age. The streptococcal disease that initiates rheumatic fever may be mild and may not be detected by the patient or the physician. The disease may be produced by streptococci of all types.

Diffuse glomerulonephritis follows deep-seated or superficial streptococcal infections such as pharyngitis and eczema, erysipelas, cellulitis, and meningitis. This complication occurs in considerably fewer children than rheumatic fever does; however, the attack rate varies with the type and strain of the streptococci. Certain types (e.g., type 12) may frequently cause glomerulonephritis, whereas others may never produce nephritis.

Scarlet Fever

When the infecting streptococci produce erythrogenic toxin and the patient does not possess specific antibodies against this toxin, streptococcal disease may be manifested by an erythematous eruption in addition to the other, previously described features of the infection. The illness is then known as scarlet fever. It is unusual in children less than 3 years of age.

Clinically the disease may be mild and the rash relatively transient, or it may be very severe. In some cases the rash appears within the first 2 days of illness; occasionally, not until the third or fourth day. There is often one bout of vomiting at the onset, together with flushing of the cheeks, fever, and sore throat. The pulse rate is commonly higher than expected for the degree of fever (Trousseau's sign).

The rash appears on the border of the lower jaw, merging with the flush of the face, and on the base of the neck, the axilla, and the groin. The trunk and extremities are subsequently involved, but the palms and the soles are spared. Circumoral pallor and Pastia's sign (hyperemic lines on the flexor surfaces at the wrists, elbows, and groin) are characteristic. Petechiae are not infrequent in severe cases, and the Rumpel-Leede test is commonly positive. The rash, which is brightly erythematous and finely papular, and blanches on pressure, may last from less than 24 hours to 1 week. The conditions that most closely resemble it are Kawasaki's disease, early measles, German measles, infectious mononucleosis, drug eruptions, staphylococcal scarlatin-form rash, and toxic shock syndrome.

The tongue is coated on the first and second day, but the visible red papillae give it the name of "strawberry tongue." As the white coat desquamates, the "raspberry tongue" makes its appearance.

As the rash fades, the hypertrophy of the subcutaneous papillae gives the characteristic "sandpaper" feel. Within 10 days the skin starts to peel, as after a sunburn. This phenomenon begins around the neck and upper chest; it then becomes generalized, involving the hands and feet at last. At the roots of the nails one may observe tags of skin for some time during convalescence. The cervical lymphadenopathy and brilliant red appearance of the throat are typical of streptococcal infection. Albuminuria is commonly observed during the acute phase.

Erysipelas

Erysipelas is a severe acute infection of the skin caused by group A hemolytic streptococci. The portal of entry may be an abrasion of the skin or a minor surgical procedure. The infection spreads rapidly through the dermal lymphatics and causes painful erythematous swelling of the involved area, but the edema spares the areas where the skin is tight, as over the facial bony prominences or groin. There is a definite edge of tender induration to the involved area. Systemic manifestations include fever, malaise, vomiting, and diarrhea, but they vary depending on severity. The condition is particularly serious in the neonatal period.

Impetigo

Superficial infection of the skin may be caused by group A hemolytic streptococci, as well as by staphylococci. The lesions ooze serum, which dries and forms yellowish crusts, with wrinkling and redness of the adjacent skin. Streptococcal impetigo often develops in open or itching lesions from contamination and scratching; it is highly contagious and is often associated with acute glomerulonephritis, particularly in the tropics.

Surgical Infections

Virulent streptococci from the respiratory tract, skin, or wounds of infected individuals may be introduced after trauma such as burns or lacerations, or may penetrate breaks in the skin — for example, an area of epidermophytosis on the feet or hands. They produce a rapidly spreading cellulitis, with lymphangitis characterized by brilliant red, narrow, often tender streaks running up the extremity, chills, fever, and painful swelling of the regional lymph nodes. "Surgical" scarlet fever occasionally develops in infections of this type.

Tetanus (Lockjaw)

Tetanus is an acute, often fatal disease caused by the exotoxin produced by the anaerobic, spore-forming, grampositive bacillus *Clostridium tetani*. The disorder is characterized by painful, tonic muscular contractions, primarily involving the masseter and neck muscles and secondarily affecting the trunk.

Pathogenesis

C. tetani is a normal inhabitant of the intestinal tract of farm animals; therefore, spores are prevalent on manured soil in rural areas and may be carried by the wind, contaminating the soil and streets of cities. Tetanus bacilli are not invasive; they enter the body through areas of injury, usually a puncture wound, burn, or crushed area. At the site of entry, the proliferating bacilli produce a potent toxin (tetanospasmin) that affects the central nervous system. The toxin acts at the motor end-plate, causing muscular stiffness and a lowering of the threshold for reflex excitability.

Clinical Manifestations

The incubation period is ordinarily between 4 and 21 days. Usually, when tetanus develops within a few days after a wound, the disease proves fatal, while symptoms occurring 2 or more weeks later indicate a mild case. There is a general susceptibility to the action of the toxin in the nonimmune human host. Active immunization is induced by tetanus toxoid and passive immunity by tetanus antitoxin.

The disease usually begins with progressive stiffness and tenderness of the jaw and neck muscles, hence the term *lockjaw* (*trismus*). Spasm of the facial muscles produces the classic sardonic smile (risus sardonicus). Within 24 to 48 hours, tonic spasms involve the trunk and cause extreme arching of the back (opisthotonos) and a boardlike abdomen. The limbs become rigidly extended. The sensorium is usually unimpaired; mild stimuli such as bright lights, noise, feeding, or even physical examination can precipitate a generalized spasm. Death may result from exhaustion. Laryngospasm and tetany of the muscles of respiration and accumulation of secretions predispose to pneumonia and atelectasis.

Tetanus neonatorum, an almost invariably fatal form of the disease, usually occurs at the end of the first week of life. This preventable disease is a major cause of neonatal death in the developing countries. The major mode of entry of the organisms is by gross contamination of the umbilical cord. In the early stages the illness is characterized by convulsions, irritability, and feeding difficulties.

Treatment

Treatment is by the administration of tetanus antitoxin and penicillin to which most strains of the organism are sensitive. Sedation and supportive care in expert hands are the only possible solutions to the prospects of a favorable outcome. The details of therapy are beyond the scope of this text.

Mohsen Ziai and Charles V. Pryles

Tuberculosis

Tuberculosis is a mycobacterial disease that causes significant morbidity and mortality in many parts of the world. It is characterized by a lifelong "check and balance" between the host and the organism which can remain latent or reactivate years after the primary infection.

Etiology and Epidemiology

Tuberculosis is caused by acid-fast bacilli, commonly *Mycobacterium tuberculosis*. *M. bovis* and *M. africanum* rarely cause disease in the United States. Other mycobacterial species can cause localized adenopathy in young children but rarely cause pulmonary or disseminated disease in the normal host.

Transmission of *M. tuberculosis* is usually by inhalation of infectious droplets from an adult with active pulmonary disease, resulting in a 25 to 30% infection rate in the household contacts. The risk of infection is directly related to duration and intensity of exposure. Rarely, contaminated fomites have been implicated. Neonatal disease can also occur through transplacental transmission or via amniotic fluid from the infected mother.

Although all ages can be affected, the risk of developing active disease is highest among infants and pubertal children and among elderly individuals in whom the disease is generally a reactivation of earlier infection. Additional risk factors are suppression of cell-mediated immunity from other diseases or from chemotherapy, severe malnutrition, diabetes mellitus, gastric ulcer disease, silicosis, and sarcoidosis. In the United States, case rates have been highest among minority groups (i.e., first-generation immigrants from endemic countries and Hispanics, Blacks, American Indians, and Alaskan natives), and among the urban poor or homeless. Up to 80% of childhood tuberculosis cases are identified while still in the asymptomatic stage of the infection through contact investigation of recently diagnosed adults.

Pathogenesis

The incubation period from infection to development of a positive skin test is about 2 to 10 weeks. The risk of disease is about 1 to 2% within the first 2 years after infection, and the cumulative life-risk is about 5 to 10%.

Following inhalation of *M. tuberculosis* through the respiratory tract, infection, which is usually silent, starts in the lower or middle lung fields, then spreads to the hilar lymph nodes. It may enter the blood stream and can reach any organ in the body. Tuberculosis is characterized pathologically by the formation of granulomas made up of giant and epithelioid cells, caseation, which is a unique form of nonliquefying necrosis, and, finally, fibrosis. The primary lesion usually heals as a calcified Gohn's complex and may be the only marker of infection in the asymptomatic patient with latent infection. Depending on the host's susceptibility and immune functions, foci of infection may disseminate or remain dormant but viable and at risk of reactivation for many years.

Clinical Manifestations

The primary infection is usually asymptomatic and self-limiting, or causes only mild nonspecific systemic symptoms. Ninety percent of clinically apparent childhood pulmonary disease involves the lungs (with segmental or lobar consolidation, endobronchial lesion, pleural effusion or rarely a miliary pattern) and/or lymph nodes (usually hilar, mediastinal, or cervical). Other manifestations from lymphatic or hematogenous spread occurring usually weeks after the initial presentation include tuberculous meningitis and intracranial tuberculoma, pericarditis, peritonitis and enteritis, and miliary spread to the bone marrow, liver, spleen, and adrenal glands; but, they are rare in the United States. Later clinical disease presenting 7 to 12 months after the initial infection may involve bones, joints, and skin but may include any organ system. Renal and genital tuberculosis and reactivation of pulmonary disease usually present years after primary disease.

Nonspecific systemic symptoms include failure to thrive, fever, night sweats, and anemia of chronic disease.

A discussion of clinical manifestations of primary infection, meningeal and generalized tuberculosis, follows. The reader is referred to larger texts for a discussion of other complications.

COURSE OF THE PRIMARY COMPLEX. The end products of metabolism of tubercle bacilli, which are known as tuberculoproteins, sensitize the body tissues and are responsible for the positive skin reactions. The development of hypersensitivity generally coincides with the end of the incubation period — usually 3 to 5 weeks — and marks the clinical onset of tuberculosis. With the onset of hypersensitivity, the perifocal reaction around the primary focus may become larger and the regional lymph nodes may increase in size. The morphology of such perifocal reactions resembles that of any exudative tuberculous reaction. There is seldom any evidence of destruction of pulmonary tissue. The parenchymal perifocal reaction varies greatly in size and often is so slight as to cast no shadow on a roentgenogram. In most cases the reaction subsides slowly over a period of months or years, and the small tuberculous focus that caused it heals with fibrosis and calcification or occasionally disappears entirely. Sometimes the primary parenchymal focus does not behave in this benign manner. Local progression of the primary focus resulting in more severe pulmonary involvement, known as local progressive primary tuberculosis, is an example.

The nodal component of the primary complex shows less tendency to heal completely than the pulmonary component. Even when the infection is slight in extent, caseation may persist and tubercle bacilli may continue to live in partially calcified lymph nodes for long periods. Tuberculous disease is rarely limited to the first group of draining nodes but progresses to other lymph nodes. The tendency for massive lymphatic spread is most marked in very young children or in persons with little resistance. The pulmonary and mediastinal lymph nodes play an important part in the pathogenesis of tuberculosis in children. The enlarged, inflamed nodes become adherent to the walls of the bronchi; as the tuberculous disease progresses, it often eventually involves the mucosa and produces a chronic tuberculous bronchitis that may cause permanent scarring. In addition, it may interfere with the flow of air, causing obstruction in the early stage of the disease. Fibrosis or bronchiectasis may occur as a late sequel of the tuberculous bronchitis. Because the bronchi of infants and small children are soft and the nodes tend to be larger, endobronchial disease is more of a problem in this age group.

The lymph nodes furnish an avenue through which tubercle bacilli may reach the blood stream. In children there is good evidence that at least a few bacilli reach the blood in this manner and that this dissemination begins during the incubation period before hypersensitivity to tuberculin is established. Such sporadic dissemination is often called occult hematogenous tuberculosis.

Obviously not every tubercle bacillus that reaches the blood stream results in a tuberculous focus. Some bacilli die; others form tubercles in metastatic areas, which then regress and heal completely. Some bacilli fall on fertile soil and progress at varying rates, creating complications of primary tuberculosis. Other bacilli progress for a time, and then their development is checked by host forces although the bacilli contained within the foci remain alive but dormant. Such metastases may never become active disease, but they remain a menace and may be the site of active tuberculosis many years after the development of the primary complex if general or local resistance is lowered, as by disease, injury, or malnutrition.

There is great variation in organ susceptibility to the development of a tuberculous focus. The thyroid gland, the pancreas, and the stomach are rarely involved in progressive tuberculosis, but theirs is only a relative immunity, and if conditions are right any area of the body may become a site for metastasis. In metastatic areas the focus of tuberculosis may progress by invading an adjacent channel. Thus meningitis develops when a previously seeded focus in the menin-

ges or cortex invades the subarachnoid space; joint tuberculosis usually arises from a metastasis in an adjacent bone.

TUBERCULOUS MENINGITIS. Tuberculous meningitis, especially in infants, may have an abrupt onset with a convulsion. In most cases the onset is insidious, with fever and apathy or sometimes irritability. Many children also vomit. These general symptoms, common to so many diseases, make diagnosis difficult in the first stage unless the child is known to have a primary tuberculous infection, or to have been exposed recently to a person with tuberculosis. The diagnosis may also be made if a lumbar puncture is done because of convulsion. In the second stage of meningitis neurological signs develop. Ptosis, strabismus, or other evidence of cranial nerve involvement is among the first manifestations. Increasing apathy and periods of somnolence are often present, but the patient reacts to stimuli. A child first seen in the third stage of meningitis is usually unresponsive and has signs of marked neurological involvement in the form of decerebrate rigidity and highly irregular respirations.

During the second stage of the disease, the diagnosis of meningoencephalitis is clear, but the cause must be sought. In tuberculous children the tuberculin skin reaction is positive in at least 90% of cases. A strong reaction should help in the diagnosis even in a child who has been vaccinated with BCG. An x-ray film of the chest showing shadows compatible with those in tuberculosis serves as additional evidence. Only a small percentage of roentgenograms are negative in the presence of tuberculous meningitis. Microscopical examination of the CSF is essential, including bacteriological cultures if no organisms of any kind are seen on direct examination. Cryptococcosis (torulosis) may be ruled out by specific agglutination test and culture. The CSF in tuberculous meningitis is relatively clear, with cell counts ranging from 10 to 350/mm^3; usually at least 50% of the cells are lymphocytes, and this percentage continues to increase. In rapidly developing meningitis as many as 1000 cells/mm^3 are sometimes encountered, in which case the polymorphonuclear leukocytes may predominate on early examinations.

The protein content of the CSF is usually slightly higher than normal (40 mg/100 ml) on early examinations and continues to increase.

The sugar content is of greatest value in the differential diagnosis. In the initial stages of meningitis it is usually below normal. In advanced stages the sugar content of the CSF is usually very low or even absent.

GENERALIZED HEMATOGENOUS TUBERCULOSIS. A single dissemination of a large number of tubercle bacilli through the blood causes numerous tubercles of approximately the same size (miliary tuberculosis) and produces an acute illness usually characterized by persistent fever, often by enlargement of the spleen and superficial lymph nodes, and sometimes by pleurisy and involvement of the skeletal system. When varying numbers of bacilli are disseminated at repeated intervals, the resultant lesions are larger and of unequal size (protracted hematogenous tuberculosis), the illness may be acute or prolonged, there is marked spleno-megaly, massive panadenitis is seen, and often caseous polyserositis as well as skeletal involvement takes place.

Diagnosis and Evaluation

The tubercle bacilli can be isolated from any infected organ or body fluid. Children often do not produce sputum, so gastric washings are a useful alternative source for culture. While older routine culture techniques may take up to 8 weeks to grow and identify mycobacteria, these organisms may be recovered in 1 to 2 weeks by the Bactec method, or even faster by newer techniques of polymerase chain reaction, gas chromatography, or specific enzymatic assays. Antimicrobial susceptibility testing should be done in all *M. tuberculosis* isolates to guide therapy.

Acid-fast bacilli can also be demonstrated by the Ziehl-Neelsen stain, or fluorescent auramine-rhodamine stains. Histologic finding of caseating granulomas also suggests tuberculosis.

A *tuberculin skin test* is the most useful and cost-effective way to establish the diagnosis of tuberculosis. When positive in the right epidemiologic context and with the clinical picture compatible with tuberculosis, it is an adequate diagnostic tool to help in the decision of starting antituberculous therapy pending culture results. The standard test material is the purified protein derivative (PPD or Mantoux test), which contains 5 tuberculin units in 0.1 ml of solution. (Other dose strengths of 1 and 250 units have not been standardized and have little practical value.) A positive test is an area of induration (not erythema) of 10 mm or greater 48 to 72 hours after intradermal injection. Although a smaller reaction is often suggestive of infection with other cross-reacting mycobacteria or from the Bacillus Calmette-Guerin (BCG) vaccine years after its administration, it should be considered significant if the clinical and epidemiologic evaluation (such as close contact with an adult with active disease) suggests tuberculous infection. Severely ill or immunocompromised patients may not initially react with a positive skin test. Accordingly, a negative PPD does not exclude a diagnosis of tuberculosis.

The evaluation of a child with suspected or proved tuber-culosis should also include case finding of infected index case (usually an adult), and evaluation of other contacts in the household and day-care setting.

Treatment

If the patient's compliance can be insured, the treatment for tuberculosis can be very effective with a 95% cure rate. Relapse rarely occurs with development of drug resistance.

Antituberculous agents are listed in Table 20-2. For the treatment of drug-susceptible pulmonary (parenchymal or pleural) tuberculosis, as well as extrapulmonary infection, a 9-month regimen with isoniazid and rifampin is recommended. If the patient can be carefully supervised, then the combination therapy can be first administered on a daily basis for 4 to 8 weeks, then on a twice-weekly basis for the remainder of the therapy. For tuberculous and miliary tuberculosis, however, three or four drugs (isoniazid, rifampin, pyrazinamide, plus streptomycin or ethambutol) should be used, particularly for the first 2 months, then isoniazid and rifampin can be given for another 10 months.

If drug-resistant tuberculosis is suspected or proven (especially if imported from areas in the world with a high rate of drug resistance), then therapy should consist of isoniazid and at least two more drugs. Consultation with an expert should be obtained in these cases for optimal therapy.

Careful follow-up of the patient and close contacts during and after therapy are extremely important to insure compliance and to monitor drug side effects or bacteriological or clinical relapse.

Prevention and Control of Tuberculosis

Routine tuberculin skin testing is recommended in all children and adults. In populations of low tuberculous prevalence, this can be done during regular health appraisals, such as at 12 to 15 months of age (before or at the time of the measles immunization), before school entry (4–6 years), and in adolescence. For such routine screening, the use of multiple puncture devices (*Monovac, Tine test,* and others) is adequate, with positive results confirmed by the standardized 5–tuberculin unit (TU) PPD. In areas for populations at higher risk for developing tuberculosis (see above), annual testing with the 5 TU PPD is recommended.

A chest x ray, a complete physical examination, and contact evaluation should be obtained on all children with a positive PPD. Asymptomatic patients with a negative chest x ray should receive isoniazid prophylaxis for at least 6 months or preferably 9 to 12 months. For those with ab-

Table 20-2. Drugs for the Treatment of Tuberculosis in Infants, Children, and Adolescents

Drug	Dosage forms	Daily dose (mg/kg/day)	Twice weekly dosage (mg/kg/dose)	Maximum daily dosage	Adverse reactions
			Commonly Used		
Isoniazid*	Tablets: 50 mg, 100 mg, 300 mg Syrup: 50 mg/50 ml	10–20	20–40	Daily: 300 mg Twice weekly: 900 mg	Mild hepatic enzyme elevation, hepatitis, peripheral neuritis, allergic reactions
Rifampin*	Capsules: 150 mg, 300 mg Syrup: formulated in syrup from capsules, 10 mg/ml	10–20	10–20	600 mg	Orange discoloration of secretions/urine, nausea, vomiting, hepatitis, febrile reaction, thrombocytopenia
Pyrazinamide	Tablets: 500 mg	15–30	50–70	2 g	Hepatotoxicity, hyperuricemia
Streptomycin	Vials: 1 g, 4 g	20–40 (IM)	20–40 (IM)	1 g	Ototoxicity, nephrotoxicity
Ethambutol	Tablets: 100 mg, 400 mg	15–25	50	2.5 g	Optic neuritis (reversible), decreased visual acuity, decreased red-green color discrimination, gastrointestinal disturbance, allergic reaction
			Less Commonly Used		
Capreomycin	Vials: 1 g	15–30 (IM)		1 g	Ototoxicity, nephrotoxicity
Kanamycin	Vials: 75 mg/2 ml, 500 mg/2 ml, 1 g/3 ml	15–30 (IM)		1 g	Auditory toxicity, nephrotoxicity, vestibular toxicity
Ethionamide	Tablets: 250 mg	15–20		1 g	Gastrointestinal disturbance, hepatotoxicity, allergic reactions
Cycloserine	Capsules: 250 mg	10–20		1 g	Psychosis, personality changes, convulsions, rash

* Formulations for parenteral administration may be useful for the patient who is vomiting or obtunded. IM = Intramuscular.

normal chest x rays, gastric washings for acid-fast culture should be done and a two-drug regimen started pending culture results.

Children intimately exposed to an adult with active pulmonary tuberculosis (such as in household or day-care contact) should be evaluated and given isoniazid prophylaxis regardless of their initial skin test results. Once the adult has been adequately treated (with negative sputum smears), the chemoprophylaxis can be discontinued if the repeat skin test is negative. If the skin test is positive, appropriate evaluation for active disease should be done and the appropriate treatment prescribed.

For contacts of patients with isoniazid-resistant *M. tuberculosis*, a prophylactic regimen with rifampin (with or without isoniazid) should be considered. Consultation for expert advice is recommended.

The efficacy of the *BCG vaccine*, which is a live attenuated strain of *M. bovis*, is controversial, and varies from 0 to 80% in published studies. It may lower the risk of miliary and meningeal tuberculosis in young children. Its routine use is not recommended in the United States, but may be considered in countries or population groups with an excessive rate of new tuberculous infections. It is contraindicated in individuals with immunosuppression.

Diseases Caused by Atypical Mycobacteria

Nontuberculous mycobacteria are ubiquitous and found in soil, food, water, and animals. The species most frequently found in humans are *M. avium intercellulare*, *M. kansasii*, *M. scrofulaceum*, *M. marinum*, *M. fortuitum*, and *M. chelonei*. They usually cause asymptomatic infections, but may also cause disseminated and fatal diseases in immunocompromised hosts. In previously healthy children, the most common syndromes are localized lymphadenopathy (scrofula) or cutaneous infections. Diagnosis can be made by the clinical picture, a positive tuberculous skin test (usually smaller than for *M. tuberculosis*), and culture. Because most of these organisms are multiply-resistant to common antituberculous drugs, surgical excision of the infected nodes is the treatment of choice. The need for combination drug therapy must be individualized and is best made with an infectious disease consultation.

Chinh T. Le, Ali Akbar Velayati, and Mohsen Ziai

Tularemia

Tularemia is an infectious disease of rodents that is transmissible to humans. It is less frequently seen in children than in adults. The causative agent is *Francisella (Pasteurella) tularensis,* a gram-negative rod with bipolar-staining granules. Infection follows (1) contact with infected rabbits (most common), (2) bites by deerflies, dog or wood ticks, cats, coyotes, dogs, or skunks, (3) skinning or dressing of infected animals, and (4) ingestion of contaminated meat (uncommon).

Clinical Manifestations

Several clinical forms of tularemia have been described: ulceroglandular, oculoglandular, gastrointestinal and typhoidal, pulmonary, and oropharyngeal. The ulceroglandular form is the most common type of the disease. The incubation period may vary from 1 to 10 days (average, 2–5 days). The onset is abrupt, with headache, chills, generalized aching, weakness, and temperature as high as 40°C. Within 36 to 48 hours the site of inoculation of the organism becomes inflamed and tender. A papule then appears and is soon capped by a vesicle, which pustulates and becomes ulcerative; tenderness of regional lymph nodes, with suppuration, usually accompanies the skin lesion. The fully developed lesion is an ulcer covered by a black eschar; a scanty serous discharge is present. Papular, pustular, petechial, and vesicular rashes are observed in some cases. Splenomegaly is sometimes seen, but hepatomegaly is rare.

Pneumonia occurs in less than 10% of cases of ulceroglandular tularemia; it is usually patchy, confluent, and often migratory, and it is frequently accompanied by pleuritic pain and pleural effusion, which may be bloody. Sputum is scant and mucoid; hemoptysis may occur. X-ray films of the chest show a ground-glass appearance of the involved areas of the lungs and enlargement of the hilar nodes. The fatality rate is high in cases with pulmonary involvement. Leukopenia usually characterizes the acute phase, a polymorphonuclear leukocytosis is likely to be present from 1 month to 2 years after the onset of the disease. The organisms can be isolated from skin and eye lesions, from the blood, and, when pneumonia is present, from the sputum in most cases. Serological tests are confirmatory.

The oculoglandular type of tularemia results when the portal of entry is the conjunctival sac. The conjunctivae and eyelids are inflamed and swollen, and the periorbital area is reddened and edematous. Systemic manifestations of infection, including fever, are usually present. Tiny yellow papules appear on the conjunctiva and soon become ulcerated. If they develop on the cornea, perforation may occur. The preauricular, submaxillary, and anterior cervical lymph nodes may enlarge, become painful, and suppurate and drain. Leukocytosis is generally present.

Tularemia may occur as cryptogenic infection without a localized lesion and without symptoms or signs suggestive of involvement of a specific organ system. The only manifestation is fever, which may be high. This type presents itself as an obscure fever, and the diagnosis can then be established by blood culture and serological methods.

Treatment

F. tularensis is very sensitive to gentamicin and streptomycin; the fever declines to normal in 48 to 72 hours, and local lesions and lymphadenitis resolve rapidly. Treatment should be given as early in the course of the disease as possible and continued for 1 week. Tetracycline has also proved effective, but cessation of therapy is sometimes followed by relapse.

The prevention of tularemia requires precautions in contact with infected persons and animals, and avoiding ticks and flies. Rubber gloves and face masks should be worn by those dressing wild rabbits and handling infectious material in the laboratory. Thorough cooking of the meat of wild rabbits kills the organisms. Disinfection of discharges from patients is mandatory.

Whooping Cough (Pertussis)

Whooping cough is a common, acute, highly contagious bacterial infection caused by *Bordetella pertussis* (*Hemophilus pertussis*). It is characterized by paroxysms of coughing followed by respiratory whooping and vomiting.

Pathogenesis

The disease is transmitted by direct contact or droplet spread and has fastidious growth requirements. The incubation period of pertussis is usually about 7 days, with a range of 5 to 21 days. A nonimmune person is susceptible to pertussis at any age, but characteristically it is a disease of children under 7 years old. There is probably no transplacental immunity, and 40% of all deaths from pertussis occur among infants less than 5 months of age. The period of infectivity begins 7 days after exposure and extends for 3 weeks after onset of the paroxysms of coughing. After 6 weeks patients may be considered noninfectious.

The occasional second attacks do not represent true pertussis; they are usually caused by *B. parapertussis* or *B. bronchiseptica,* neither of which shares cross-immunity with *B. pertussis.* They are milder illnesses.

Clinical Manifestations

The clinical course of pertussis is usually divided into three stages: (1) catarrhal, (2) paroxysmal, and (3) convalescent. The catarrhal stage lasts about 1 or 2 weeks. It begins as a typical upper respiratory tract infection, with low-grade fever, coryza, sneezing, lacrimation, irritability, and a dry, poorly productive cough. The cough worsens and after a week begins to occur paroxysmally.

The paroxysmal stage lasts from 4 to 6 weeks (range, 1–10 weeks). There are explosive bursts of coughing in rapid succession during which the child cannot breathe. The coughing is followed by a sudden, long inspiration that rushes air into the emptied lung and produces the crowing, high-pitched whoop. One paroxysm of coughing may follow another until the child is able to cough up a thick, tenacious mucous plug. During the coughing spell the child appears cyanotic or livid, the tongue protrudes, and the eyes bulge. After the attack the child vomits, perspires profusely, and appears lethargic and exhausted. Periorbital edema, conjunctival hemorrhages and epistaxis may also be present. In infants under 6 months of age, the characteristic whoop may not be present.

The uncomplicated convalescent stage is marked by cessation of whooping and vomiting and an improvement in appetite and mood. The paroxysms are milder and occur less frequently, but coughing may persist for several weeks. If a secondary respiratory infection has developed, recurrent paroxysms of coughing and whoops may reappear repeatedly for many months.

Complications

The most frequent complication is pneumonia, usually caused by secondary bacterial invaders. Atelectasis and pneumonia predispose to the late development of bronchiectasis. Otitis media is commonly seen among infants. Convulsion is a serious complication of whooping cough; predisposing conditions are brain damage due to hypoxia or focal hemorrhage and alkalosis produced by repeated vomiting.

Diagnosis

The catarrhal stage cannot be easily differentiated from viral infection of the upper respiratory tract, although the increasing severity of the cough may suggest the disease. At this stage the diagnosis can be made only microbiologically. Fluorescent-antibody techniques are available for rapid diagnosis of the infection but should be used only as an adjunct to culture. Although complement-fixing and agglutinating antibodies appear, they do so late in the course of the disease and are of use mainly retrospectively.

The white cell count is often helpful; after the first week of infection, counts are in the range of 20,000 to 40,000/mm^3, with a preponderance of small lymphocytes (60–90%). There may be, however, an absolute polymorphonuclear leukocytosis (as high as 100,000) in young infants with pertussis pneumonia.

It is important to note that paroxysms of cough are not found exclusively in pertussis. Bronchiolitis, bronchitis, bronchopneumonia, pulmonary lesions of cystic fibrosis, compression by enlarged mediastinal lymph nodes (usually tuberculous), and foreign bodies must be considered. Usually these entities may be identified by appropriate clinical, laboratory, and x-ray studies. Infections caused by *B. parapertussis* and *B. bronchiseptica* can be differentiated only by bacterial culture. Adenoviruses have also been implicated in the production of pertussislike syndromes.

Treatment

The treatment of pertussis requires both specific and general measures. Erythromycin is ineffective in modifying the course of uncomplicated whooping cough. Late in the course of the disease it may still decrease the number of bacteria, possibly reducing communicability. The use of serotherapy in the form of hyperimmune gamma globulin is controversial. Apnea and encephalopathy are probably toxin-related complications of pertussis. These, as well as atelectasis and pneumonia, necessitate the availability of expert medical and nursing care for the sick patient with the disease.

Prophylaxis

The value of active immunization against pertussis is now well established (see p. 360). Although untreated patients may be contagious for approximately 4 weeks, antimicrobial therapy (erythromycin) reduces this period, even if coughing persists. Treatment of exposed family contacts with erythromycin estolate is recommended.

Campylobacter Enteritis

See Chapter 12.

Helicobacter Pylori Infections

This organism is implicated in the pathogenesis of gastritis and peptic ulcer in a considerable number of cases. The diagnosis is usually made by endoscopy and examination of the biopsy specimens obtained from the areas of the stomach which are involved. Even a better test is thought to be the serological titer to the organism which remains elevated even after treatment. The treatment of the infection helps to eradicate most of the organisms, but usually there are recurrences that would have to be treated repeatedly. In addition to the usual treatments for gastritis and peptic ulcerations with specific microbials against *H. pylori* Pepto-Bismol or tetracycline are recommended. The latter is to be avoided in young children.

Yersinia Enterocolitica Infections

See Chapter 12.

Chlamydial Infections

Chlamydia trachomatis is an important pathogen in infants and children as well as in adolescents and adults. It is the causative agent for trachoma, a nonsexually transmitted eye infection affecting about 400 million of the world population, almost all of them living in developing countries under poor sanitary conditions. It is the leading cause of blindness and serious eye disease in these areas.

In the industrialized world the main chlamydial infections are sexually transmitted and caused by a different serotype of the organism, causing nongonococcal urethritis in the male and genital infections that may result in serious complications of pelvic inflammatory disease in the female. These infections account for a large proportion of sexually transmitted diseases in the adolescent population. The reader is referred to larger references about these important medical and social problems. When a mother is infected by this organism she may transmit the disease to her infant during the birth process. The results are chlamydial conjunctivitis and chlamydial pneumonia. These diseases are briefly discussed in Chapter 9. The treatment of conjunctivitis is by topical erythromycin or tetracycline and for pneumonia, systemic erythromycin.

Chlamydia psittaci causes psittacosis, an atypical pneumonia. It is usually transmitted by parakeets or other birds. It is manifested by cough, fever, chills, and a severe headache. Arthralgia may be present, and there is a patchy pulmonary infiltration. There may be some eosinophilia but usually no leukocytosis is present. The diagnosis is made by the isolation of the organism from the blood or sputum and by a fourfold increase in complement-fixing antibodies. Treatment is by tetracycline for 8 weeks. In children under 8 years of age, erythromycin is recommended although the experience with this drug is limited.

Mohsen Ziai and Charles V. Pryles

Viral Infections

Viral infections occupy an increasingly prominent position in pediatric practice. This has come about not only as a result of the appearance of the acquired immunodeficiency syndrome (AIDS) and of improved control of bacterial infections but also because of the advances in medical practice that have permitted the extended support of critically ill patients, immunocompromised by disease or its therapy and thus susceptible to serious viral infections. These events have taken place coincident with a period of advancements in virology, especially in the areas of rapid viral diagnostic techniques and the development of effective antiviral agents. Together these changes have revolutionized our approach to the management of serious viral illness, bringing about a significant reduction in their associated morbidity and mortality. This section provides a brief overview of the most important viral infections of children without attempting comprehensive discussions, which are more appropriately covered in larger texts.

Virology

In order to understand the nature of viral infections and possible sites for intervention by therapeutic agents, a basic understanding of viral structure and replication is necessary. The mature virion, which varies greatly in size from one virus to the other, is composed of a structural protein envelope encasing an inner matrix of nucleic acid material, either ribonucleic acid (RNA) or deoxyribonucleic acid (DNA). Though viruses contain all the genetic material necessary to direct self-replication, they rely on the host cell machinery in order to complete the task. Viruses are obligate intracellular parasites and cannot replicate outside the living cell. The first step in the infective process is attachment of the virus to the cell. This is followed by cellular penetration and uncoating of the virus with release of its nucleic acid into the cell. The viral nucleic acids contain the information for the synthesis of new viral particles. Under appropriate conditions the parasitized cell ceases normal protein synthesis, producing instead the viral nucleic acids and proteins. New virions are assembled, released from the cell, and the cycle repeats itself. The viral nucleic acid of selected viruses can become integrated into the host cell genome where it can remain latent indefinitely and reactivate periodically.

Classification of Viruses

Several hundred species of viruses have been shown to be pathogenic to man. These viruses have been grouped into *families, genera,* and *species* based on physicochemical and biological properties. Table 20-3 summarizes the current classification scheme for the most important human viruses.

Rapid Viral Diagnosis

Rapid methods for the detection of viruses or the host's immune response to infection have become widely available. These techniques are gradually replacing older time- and labor-intensive procedures. Rapid viral diagnosis is helpful in allowing anticipation of management problems and disease complications, in permitting the early initiation of effective therapy for certain viral infections, and in decreasing unnecessary antibiotic use.

The laboratory diagnosis of most viral infections has traditionally been accomplished by the examination of clinical specimens for changes characteristic of a specific viral infection, by growth and identification of viruses in tissue cultures, by demonstration of a fourfold or greater rise in virus-specific IgG antibody titers, or by the detection of virus-specific IgM antibody.

Viruses present in sufficient numbers in clinical specimens (e.g., rotaviruses in stool specimens) can be directly visualized by *electron microscopy*. This method can only differentiate between major groups of viruses with characteristic morphologies (e.g., herpesviruses versus rotaviruses) but cannot distinguish between members of the same family (e.g., herpes simplex virus versus varicella-zoster virus). *Immunoelectron microscopy* enhances the sensitivity of the technique by adding virus-specific antibodies to the specimen before staining and examination. Viral antigens can be detected directly in clinical specimens by *immunofluorescent* or *immunoperoxidase* staining; these immunostaining techniques have been modified for use directly or indirectly on infected tissue cultures. A variety of immunoassays such as the *enzyme-linked immunosorbent assay* (ELISA) or the *radioimmunoassay* (RIA), utilizing either monoclonal or polyclonal antibodies, can be used for the detection of virus-specific antigens in tissues or body fluids, as well as virus-specific antibodies of the IgG, M, or A classes in serum. More recently, *nucleic acid hybridization* techniques have been used for the detection of nucleic acid fragments known to be specific for the virus of interest. A molecularly cloned, complementary DNA fragment serves as a probe that is applied to the clinical specimen to be examined. The recent introduction of the *polymerase chain reaction* allows the amplification of the number of viral genome copies in a given sample to levels detectable by hybridization techniques.

Antiviral Chemotherapy

The field of antiviral chemotherapy is undergoing a phase of rapid growth and development. It has not been long since the diagnosis of viral infection was often either presumptive, established late in the course of infection, or after its resolution at which stage specific therapy, even if available, would have been unhelpful. Advances in rapid viral diagnostic techniques together with the development of specific antiviral agents has revolutionized our approach to the management of serious viral infections and brought about significant reductions in the associated morbidity and mortality. An ever-growing number of agents are available for clinical use or are undergoing clinical evaluation (Table 20-4).

Amantadine and Rimantadine

These are symmetrical amines of similar structure which act by preventing viral penetration and uncoating of the virus. Used prophylactically and in the early treatment of influenza A, they are effective in reducing the incidence of clinical

Table 20-3. Viruses Infecting Humans

Family	Size and shape (nm)	Genus	Members	No. of types	Diseases
RNA Viruses					
Picornaviridae	24–30 Spherical (icosahedron)	*Enterovirus*	Poliovirus	3	Poliomyelitis
			Coxsackievirus A	24	Herpangina, aseptic meningitis, common cold
			Coxsackievirus B	6	Aseptic meningitis, Bornholm disease (pleurodynia), myocarditis (neonatal), URTI
			Echovirus	34	Mainly inapparent, fever, aseptic meningitis with rash, encephalitis
			Enteroviruses (68–72)	5	Aseptic meningitis, hemorrhagic conjunctivitis
			Hepatitis A	1	Infectious hepatitis
		Rhinovirus	Rhinovirus 1A-114	180+	Rhinitis, coryza
		Cardiovirus		1	Encephalomyocarditis
Caliciviridae	36–39 Spherical (icosahedron)	*Calicivirus*	Calicivirus	1	? Gastroenteritis
Reoviridae	60–80 Spherical (icosahedron)	*Reovirus*	Reovirus 1–3	3	Mainly inapparent, occas. resp. tract or gastrointestinal manifestations
		Rotavirus	Human rotavirus	4	Infantile diarrhea
		Orbivirus	Colorado tick fever	1	Colorado tick fever
			Kemerovo	20	Encephalitis
Togaviridae	40–70 Spherical (enveloped)	*Alphavirus* (group A arboviruses)	Many types, primarily mosquito-transmitted, including equine encephalitides, Sindbis, Ross River	26	Great variation in clinical disease from encephalitis to fever, rash, and joint pains; many inapparent infections
		Flavivirus (group B arboviruses)	*Mosquito-borne*		
			Yellow fever	1	Yellow fever
			Jap. B, MVE, St. Louis, West Nile	4	Encephalitis
			Dengue	4	Dengue, hemorrhagic fever/shock syndrome
			Tick-borne		
			Kyasanur forest Omsk hem. fever Encephalitis viruses	11	Encephalitis and hemorrhagic fevers
		Rubivirus	Rubella	1	Rubella, congenital abnormalities, SSPE

Table 20-3 (Continued)

Family	Size and shape (nm)	Genus	Members	No. of types	Diseases
Bunyaviridae	80–110 Spherical (icosahedron)	*Bunyavirus* (arboviruses)	Bunyamwera virus, California encephalitis virus, La Crosse virus; mostly mosquito-transmitted	13	Meningoencephalitis
		Phlebovirus	Phlebotomus (sandfly) fever virus, Rift Valley fever virus; predominantly transmitted by sandfly but also mosquito-borne.	30+	Influenza-like illness, meningoencephalitis
		Nairovirus	Many types, predominantly transmitted by ticks	19+	Crimean-Congo hemorrhagic fever
		Hantavirus	Hantaan virus	1	Korean hemorrhagic fever, epidemic nephropathy
Rhabdoviridae	L (130–300) D (60–80) Bullet-shaped (enveloped)	*Lyssavirus*	Rabies virus	1+	Rabies
		Vesiculovirus	Vesicular stomatitis virus	Several	Influenza-like illness
Orthomyxoviridae	80–120 Spherical or filamentous (enveloped)	*Influenzavirus*	Influenza virus A	Many	Influenza, upper and lower resp. tract infections
			Influenza virus B	Several	Influenza, upper and lower resp. tract infections
			Influenza virus C	1	Upper resp. tract infections
Paramyxoviridae	100–300 Spherical or filamentous (enveloped)	*Paramyxovirus*	Parainfluenza virus	4	URTI, laryngotracheobronchitis bronchiolitis (mainly types 1, 2, and 3)
			Mumps virus	1	Parotitis, pancreatitis, orchitis, meningoencephalitis
		Morbillivirus	Measles virus	1	Measles and its complications — bronchopneumonia, encephalitis, SSPE
		Pneumovirus	Respiratory syncytial virus	1	Obstructive bronchitis, bronchiolitis, bronchopneumonia, laryngotracheobronchitis

Table 20-3 (Continued)

Family	Size and shape (nm)	Genus	Members	No. of types	Diseases
Arenaviridae	50–300 Spherical (enveloped)	*Arenavirus*	Lymphocytic choriomeningitis virus	1	Lymphocytic choriomeningitis
			Lassa fever virus	1	Lassa fever
			Tacaribe complex (Junin, Machupo, Pichinde)	8	Hemorrhagic fevers
Coronaviridae	80–160 Spherical (pleomorphic and enveloped)	*Coronavirus*	Human coronavirus	1	Respiratory disease
			Human enteric coronavirus	1	Enteric infection
Retroviridae	80–100 Spherical	Type C oncovirus group	HTLV, HIV, sarcoma and leukemia viruses	15+	AIDS, T-cell leukemia, mycoses fungoides
DNA Viruses					
Parvoviridae	18–26 Spherical (icosahedral)	*Parvovirus*	Parvovirus B19	1	Erythema infectiosum, aplastic crisis, hydrops fetalis, arthritis
Papovaviridae	45–55 Spherical (icosahedral)	*Papillomavirus* *Polyomavirus*	Papillomavirus	40+	Common, genital, and plantar warts
			JC virus	1	Progressive multifocal leukoencephalopathy
			BK virus	1	Inapparent infection
			Simian virus 40	1	Inapparent infection
Adenoviridae	70–90 Spherical (icosahedral)	*Mastadenovirus*	Virus types 1–36	36	Pharyngoconjunctival fever, nasopharyngitis, conjunctivitis, rhinitis, broncho-pneumonia; types 1, 2, 3, 5, 7, and 11 primarily involved; hemorrhagic cystitis and pertussislike disease in children

Table 20-3 (Continued)

Family	Size and shape (nm)	Genus	Members	No. of types	Diseases
Herpesviridae	120–200 Spherical (enveloped)	*Simplexvirus*	Herpes simplex virus	2	Stomatitis, glossitis, cold sores, whitlows, genital herpes, encephalitis
			Varicella-zoster	1	Chickenpox, zoster, encephalitis
		Cytomegalovirus	Cytomegalovirus	1	Cytomegalic inclusion disease, neonatal jaundice, hepatospleno-megaly, congenital deformities
		Lymphocryptovirus	Epstein-Barr virus	1	Infectious mononucleosis
			? Human herpes virus 6	1	Roseola infantum
Poxviridae	230 to 300 × 190 to 280 Brick-shaped	*Orthopoxvirus*	Smallpox virus (variola)	1	Smallpox
			vaccinia virus	1	
			Monkeypox	1	Exanthemata
			Cowpox	1	
		Parapoxvirus	Pustular stomatitis virus	1	Orf
			Virus of milkers' nodes (paravaccinia)	1	Milkers' nodes
		Leporipox	Molluscum contagiosum virus	1	Molluscum contagiosum
			Tanapox virus	1	Similar to monkeypox
Hepadnaviridae*	40–50	*Hepadnavirus*	Hepatitis B	1	Hepatitis

* Hepatitis B 'S' antigen is 22 nm.

Table 20-4. Systemic Antiviral Agents

Agent	Spectrum of Activity	Indications	Side Effects
Amantadine/rimantadine	**Influenza A,*** influenza B, rubella	Prophylaxis of children at high risk of severe infection; early treatment of infection	Insomnia, jitteriness, decreased concentration, xerostomia
Ribavirin	**RSV, HIV,** parainfluenza, adeno-, entero-, arena-, bunya-viruses, vaccinia, HSV	RSV pneumonia and bronchiolitis; Lassa fever	Hemolytic anemia, may worsen respiratory status in ventilator-dependent patients
Vidarabine (Ara-A, adenine arabinoside)	**HSV, VZV,** EBV, CMV, vaccinia, some RNA viruses	Severe HSV infections; VZV in the immunocompromised host	Neurotoxicity, seizures, confusion, encephalopathy, hepatotoxicity, thrombocytopenia
Acyclovir	**HSV, VZV,** CMV, EBV	Severe HSV infections; VZV in the immunocompromised host	Phlebitis, nephrotoxicity
Ganciclovir	**CMV,** HSV, EBV, VZV	CMV retinitis, enteritis, ?CMV pneumonia (investigational)	Myelosuppression
Zidovudine	**HIV**	Symptomatic infection	Myelosuppression, nausea, headache, malaise
Dideoxycytidine	**HIV**	Symptomatic infection (investigational)	Rash, mouth sores, peripheral neuropathy
Dideoxyinosine	**HIV**	Symptomatic infection (investigational)	Unknown at present

* Clinically relevant activity is in bold.

infection and ameliorating its course. They are not active against influenza B. Dose-related side effects include insomnia, jitteriness, decrease in concentration ability, xerostomia, and lethargy. Side effects with rimantadine appear to be somewhat less than those associated with amantadine.

Ribavirin

Ribavirin, a synthetic nucleoside analogue, inhibits viral protein synthesis. It has a wide spectrum of activity against both DNA and RNA viruses. Its main clinical utility is related to its efficacy against the respiratory syncytial virus (RSV). It can be given either intravenously, orally, or by aerosolization. A reversible hemolytic anemia has developed in recipients of the oral or intravenous preparations, whereas aerosolization allows for high concentrations at the site of infection. It is not currently recommended for use in respirator-dependent children as mechanical problems secondary to drug precipitation within the ventilator tubing network may arise. Aerosol delivery has proven effective in the treatment of RSV bronchiolitis and pneumonia in chil-

dren, and the successful use of both the oral and intravenous forms for the treatment of Lassa fever has been reported.

Adenine Arabinoside (Ara-A, Vidarabine)

Vidarabine, a purine nucleoside, inhibits viral DNA synthesis. Its spectrum of activity includes a wide range of DNA viruses. Clinical utility is restricted to the treatment of severe herpes simplex virus (HSV) infections and varicella-zoster virus (VZV) in the immunocompromised host. Even within these areas it has now largely been replaced by acyclovir, an agent with equal or superior efficacy and less associated toxicity. Side effects of vidarabine include gastrointestinal, myelosuppressive, and neurotoxic adverse reactions. Tremors, seizures, and encephalopathic changes have all occurred in association with its use. Though the availability of acyclovir has decreased the use of vidarabine, it remains a potentially important agent. The superiority of either agent in the treatment of neonatal HSV infections remains to be determined. Furthermore, reports of the emergence of viral resistance to acyclovir remind us that it is too early to dismiss this drug from our armamentarium.

Acyclovir

This nucleoside analogue is a selective inhibitor of viral DNA polymerase, an enzyme critical for viral replication. This selective inhibition is a key factor accounting for the relative lack of toxicity associated with it use. While its spectrum of activity encompasses many of the DNA viruses, it is used clinically for the treatment of HSV 1 and 2 and VZV infections. As VZV is considerably less sensitive to its activity than HSV, and the bioavailability following oral administration is relatively poor, it must be given intravenously at a higher dose for the treatment of VZV compared to HSV infections. Nephrotoxicity is its main associated toxicity, which can be minimized or prevented if adequate hydration is maintained. Clinical indications for its use in pediatrics include severe HSV infections and VZV infections in the immunocompromised host. Use of this agent should be restricted to situations where it is clearly indicated as the emergence of viral resistance has been documented.

Ganciclovir (DHPG)

Ganciclovir is a nucleoside analogue of acyclovir with in vitro activity against many of the herpes family of viruses. Its importance lies in its specific activity against cytomegalovirus (CMV). Clinically useful in arresting the progression of CMV retinitis, it does not effect a cure, and disease recurs in the absence of a maintenance regime. Similarly beneficial in the control of CMV enteritis, results in the treatment of CMV pneumonia are disappointing. A significant improvement in outcome was found in patients receiving it in combination with high-dose intravenous gamma globulin. Treatment is often limited by the development of myelosuppression.

Dideoxynucleosides

These are a family of nucleoside analogues which have been shown to be capable of inhibiting the cytopathic effects of HIV infection in vitro. Three, zidovudine (AZT), dideoxycytidine (ddC), and dideoxyinosine (ddI) are currently under evaluation for the treatment of HIV-infected children. (See section Human Immunodeficiency Virus Infection.)

Enterovirus Infections

Enteroviruses are common enteric pathogens in children and give rise to a wide variety of clinical states:

1. Poliovirus
   Paralysis
   Aseptic meningitis
   Nonspecific febrile illness
2. Coxsackie virus, group A
   Herpangina (types 2, 4–6, 8, 10)
   Acute lymphonodular pharyngitis (type 10)
   Vesicular stomatitis with exanthem (hand, foot, and mouth disease) (types 5, 9, 10, 16)
   Nonspecific febrile illness with rash (types 2, 4, 9, 16, 23)
   Aseptic meningitis (most types, usually 7, 9)
   Nonspecific febrile illness, usually during summer months (most types)
3. Coxsackie virus, group B
   Pleurodynia (Bornholm disease) (types 1–6, mostly 3 and 5)
   Aseptic meningitis (types 1–5)
   Myocarditis or encephalomyocarditis, particularly in neonates and infants (types 1–5)
   Nonspecific febrile illness
   Mild paralysis (types 1–6)
   Benign pericarditis (types 1–5)
   Conjunctivitis (types 3 and 5)
4. ECHO viruses
   Aseptic meningitis (many types, usually 4, 6, 9, 30)
   Febrile illness with rash (types 4, 9, 16, and others)
   Nonspecific febrile illness (most types)
   Summer diarrhea of infants and young children (types 4, 9, 11, 17–20, and others)
   Conjunctivitis (types 2, 9, 11, 16, 30)

Characteristically the enteroviruses inhabit the gastrointestinal tract. Infections with enteroviruses are common and perennial in tropical and subtropical regions but tend to have a seasonal peak in the summer and autumn in temperate climates.

Poliovirus Infections; Poliomyelitis

Poliomyelitis is an acute infectious disease that may affect the central nervous system, resulting in the destruction of motor neurons with the production of flaccid paralysis. The poliovirus is an RNA-containing spherical particle, 28 nm in diameter. Three antigenic types are known: 1, 2, and 3.

Extensive poliomyelitis epidemics are usually due to type 1 virus. Smaller outbreaks have been attributed to type 3, and occasional sporadic cases of the disease have been associated with type 2 virus. Human beings are the only natural hosts. In many countries national immunization campaigns have virtually eliminated the disease, but in countries where campaigns have not been mounted, poliomyelitis and its sequelae are still prevalent.

PATHOGENESIS. In human disease the virus enters via the mouth. Primary multiplication occurs in the pharynx and gastrointestinal tract. The virus can be cultured from the throat early in the disease and disappears after about a week. Stool cultures produce virus for several weeks after infection. Antibody to the virus appears in the blood within 7 to 10 days of infection, often before paralysis has occurred. After multiplying in the lymphoid tissue of the intestine, the virus may then invade the central nervous system either by the blood stream or by retrograde spread along axons. Typical lesions are produced in the anterior horn cells, leading to cellular destruction through the phases of chromatolysis and neuronophagia. Perivascular collections of inflammatory cells are usually visible. The virus tends to spread along axons that have been subjected to trauma. If tonsillectomy is performed when virus is present in the pharynx, there is a risk of bulbar poliomyelitis. There is also a high incidence of paralysis in limbs in which intramuscular injections have been given during the incubation period of poliomyelitis.

CLINICAL MANIFESTATIONS. Infection of a susceptible individual with poliovirus may result in one of the following responses: (1) asymptomatic or inapparent infection, (2) abortive poliomyelitis or mild illness, (3) aseptic meningitis (nonparalytic poliomyelitis), or (4) paralytic poliomyelitis.

Asymptomatic or Inapparent Infection. The individual remains well, but the virus may be grown from throat washings or feces. The development of immunity may be shown by a rise in the serum antibody titer. This accounts for 90 to 95% of all infections with the virus.

Abortive Poliomyelitis or Mild Illness. After an incubation period of 3 to 6 days an illness develops that may be characterized by sore throat, low-grade fever, malaise, drowsiness, nausea, vomiting, and headache in various combinations. These symptoms usually last for 24 to 72 hours and are followed by recovery. In such cases clinical diagnosis of poliomyelitis cannot be made unless virological or immunological evidence is obtained. This form of illness accounts for 4 to 8% of poliovirus infections.

Aseptic Meningitis (Nonparalytic Poliomyelitis). In this variety of the disease, in addition to the symptoms and signs just described, the patient acquires meningismus with severe headache, stiffness of the neck and back, a positive tripod sign, and a positive Kernig's sign. The cerebrospinal fluid (CSF) shows a pleocytosis ranging from 10 to 1000 cells/ml; the cells are mainly polymorphonuclear leukocytes early in the course of the disease but change to predominantly lymphocytes within 24 hours. The CSF protein level is usually raised slightly. Nonparalytic poliomyelitis may last as long as 10 days, and most patients recover completely. In some patients, however, paralytic poliomyelitis supervenes.

Paralytic Poliomyelitis. The incubation period is 7 to 14 days but may be as short as 4 days. This form of poliomyelitis is characterized by flaccid paralysis resulting from partial or complete destruction of lower motor neurons in the spinal cord and occasionally in the brain stem. Initially there is pain, stiffness, and spasm in the unaffected antagonist muscles, with incoordination of muscle action in the affected limbs. Deep tendon reflexes may be exaggerated early in the disease, but they soon become lost. The distribution of clinical paralysis is characteristically asymmetrical and haphazard. The disease is frequently classified into spinal, bulbar, bulbospinal, and encephalitic forms. In the spinal form there is weakness of the neck, abdomen, trunk, diaphragm, thorax, or extremities. Bulbar poliomyelitis implies weakness in the motor distribution of one or more of the cranial nerves, and there may be dysfunction of the centers of respiration and circulation. Bulbospinal poliomyelitis combines these two forms. In encephalitic poliomyelitis, drowsiness, disorientation, and irritability occur in conjunction with muscular paralysis. Muscular involvement is usually maximal within a week of onset of paralysis. There is then a slow recovery phase, and for periods up to about 1 year following such an illness some recovery of function may occur; however, various degrees of flaccid paralysis and atrophy of muscle groups are frequently left as a permanent sequel of the irreversible destruction of anterior horn cells. Paralytic poliomyelitis accounts for only 1 to 2% of infections during epidemics.

MANAGEMENT OF POLIOMYELITIS. Paralytic poliomyelitis has been almost eradicated in areas where live oral poliovirus vaccine (Sabin) is given to infants and children routinely. When the disease occurs, treatment is supportive. The rapid progression of the bulbar or spinal forms, particularly with involvement of the respiratory muscles, requires intensive care, the use of respirator, tracheostomy, intravenous fluids, blood chemical determinations, and expert nursing and psychological handling. After the acute phase, rehabilitation measures are employed.

Prevention is best accomplished by administration of the trivalent live oral polio vaccine (OPV). The primary immunization series consists of OPV doses given at 2, 4, and 18 months of age. A booster dose is given before the child enters school. In areas of high endemicity or during epidemics of poliomyelitis, immunization can be initiated as early as 2 weeks of age. The risk of paralytic disease in immunologically normal vaccine recipients has been estimated at one case per 520,000 first doses and one case per 12.3 million subsequent doses of OPV. The trivalent formalin-inactivated poliovirus vaccine (IPV) is used primarily in households with an immunologically deficient individual, unimmunized adults, and individuals infected with the human immunodeficiency virus.

Coxsackie Virus Infections

HERPANGINA. Herpangina is a disease caused by Coxsackie virus, group A, types 1–10, 16, and 22. It occurs most commonly in young children, who usually suffer an abrupt illness with fever, anorexia, and malaise and with a specific complaint of sore throat. The characteristic lesion of herpangina commences as a small papule, which rapidly undergoes vesiculation and rupture within approximately 24 hours, finally appearing as a shallow, ulcerated lesion 3 to 5 mm in diameter. The lesions are confined to the fauces and the soft palate. The ulcers persist for several days and then heal gradually over a period of 2 to 3 weeks. When such faucial lesions are observed, with or without other symptoms (meningismus, upper respiratory tract symptoms, muscular aches and pains, fever, or anorexia), a diagnosis of Coxsackie A infection can be made on clinical grounds.

ACUTE LYMPHONODULAR PHARYNGITIS. This disease, caused by Coxsackie virus, group A, type 10, appears predominantly in young children and manifests as a febrile illness associated with sore throat, headache, general lassitude, and anorexia. The characteristic lesion, occurring on the uvula, the posterior pharynx, and the fauces, is a raised, discrete, whitish, solid area, without vesiculations, surrounded by a zone of erythema. The lesions may be differentiated from those of herpangina by the fact that they do not ulcerate. Also, in acute lymphonodular pharyngitis, rhinorrhea, cough, tracheitis, skin eruptions, otitis media, and cervical adenitis typically do not occur. The disease lasts from 4 to 14 days. The incubation period is considered to be about 5 days. Treatment is symptomatic.

VESICULAR STOMATITIS WITH EXANTHEM (HAND, FOOT, AND MOUTH DISEASE). This disease is caused by Coxsackie virus, group A, types 5, 9, 10, and 16. Children under 10 years are most frequently affected. The illness involves a mild fever and soreness of throat and mouth. These symptoms last for 2 or 3 days and are followed by pharyngeal lesions consisting of red macules, which progress to vesiculation and ulceration. The lesions occur on the pharynx, soft palate, buccal mucosa, tongue, and gingiva. At the same time, a maculopapular rash develops. This progresses to superficial vesicles, 0.5 to 1.0 cm in diameter, containing clear, watery fluid. The limbs, hands, and feet are the usual sites of the skin lesions, which last for 3 or 4 days and regress spontaneously. Buttock lesions are also common. Treatment is symptomatic.

PLEURODYNIA (BORNHOLM DISEASE; EPIDEMIC MYALGIA). This disease is caused by Coxsackie virus, group B, types 1 to 6. Sporadic cases associated with Coxsackie virus, group A, types 1, 2, 4, 6, 9, and 16, as well as several echoviruses may also occur. It is characterized by acute pleuritic pain and a tendency to occur in epidemics. It may be confused with other forms of pleurisy although the presence or absence of epidemics, the clinical and laboratory evidence supporting the presence of other conditions, and the benign nature of pleurodynia are usually sufficient for differentiation.

NEONATAL MYOCARDITIS AND ENCEPHALOMYOCARDITIS. This potentially lethal disease is generally caused by the Coxsackie virus, group B, types 1 to 5. Occasionally cases due to Coxsackie virus, group A, types 1 to 3 and 9, have been identified in children with myocarditis. The disease is most common in neonates and usually commences abruptly within the first 8 days of life. It may be preceded by a brief episode of diarrhea or be associated with a concurrent epidemic of diarrhea in the nursery. Cardiorespiratory embarrassment is manifested by tachycardia, tachypnea, dyspnea, cyanosis, and peripheral circulatory collapse. The heart is dilated, and the electrocardiogram shows changes consistent with myocarditis. Signs of pulmonary and systemic edema may be present. Many affected infants move rapidly to a fatal outcome.

ECHO Virus Infections

ASEPTIC MENINGITIS SYNDROME. Aseptic meningitis is one of the most common manifestations of enterovirus infections and has been associated with all members of the enterovirus group. Sporadic cases can be identified only on the basis of viral studies. During epidemics, however, a specific cause for the syndrome is more easily suspected. Aseptic meningitis may be caused by a variety of other agents.

CLINICAL MANIFESTATIONS. The disease is usually of acute onset, and the presenting manifestations, particularly in older children, are headache and vomiting; in infants, irritability may be the dominant feature. The child is feverish and may display symptoms suggesting a specific viral infection.

Clinical examination usually reveals nuchal rigidity. The disease sometimes progresses to mild muscle weakness, or to severe muscle paralysis when a poliovirus is the infecting agent. The Coxsackie group B viruses may be associated with mild paralysis from which the patient usually recovers quickly and completely.

Examination of the CSF reveals pleocytosis, ranging from 20 cells to several thousand cells. Early in the disease these are predominantly polymorphonuclear leukocytes, but later they are replaced by mononuclear cells. The CSF protein level is normal or slightly raised, and the glucose is normal. Bacteria are not seen or grown. Culture of CSF for virus occasionally reveals the etiological agent, but the stool is a much more dependable source.

Because many diverse organisms may produce similar clinical features, careful history-taking, clinical examination, and CSF studies must be undertaken before any child with fever and stiff neck is diagnosed as suffering from aseptic meningitis. Other viral causes of this syndrome include mumps, arboviruses, herpesviruses, measles, and rubella. Incipient or partially treated bacterial meningitis may closely mimic both the clinical and the cerebrospinal fluid findings of aseptic meningitis; tuberculous meningitis, leptospirosis, syphilis, Lyme disease, systemic histoplasmosis, coccidioidomycosis, candidiasis, toxoplasmosis, trichinosis, and the invasion of meninges by tumors represent nonviral causes of aseptic meningitis that need to be considered. Meningeal irritation from a contiguous lesion such as a cerebral abscess may cause a similar clinical picture.

Treatment. The treatment is symptomatic, with analgesics and the maintenance of fluid balance. The prognosis is entirely favorable provided the syndrome does not herald the onset of poliomyelitis.

FEBRILE ILLNESS WITH RASH. Some enteroviruses give rise to nonspecific febrile illnesses accompanied by exanthems. Generally they occur in early childhood, although occasional cases are seen in older children and adults. In most of these illnesses the incubation period is short, and the rash is nonspecific and may be quite variable, ranging from maculopapules to vesicles or petechiae. Occasionally, during epidemics, there may be accompanying diarrhea suggesting ECHO virus infection, or aseptic meningitis suggesting either ECHO or Coxsackie infection. Occasionally, the lesions are specific enough to allow a distinct infecting virus to be diagnosed — for example, vesicular stomatitis with exanthem caused by Coxsackie group A virus (types 5 and 16). Most enteroviral illness with exanthems are self-limited and require no more than symptomatic treatment.

NONSPECIFIC FEBRILE ILLNESSES. In addition to the syndromes of febrile illness with rash, all members of the enterovirus group may give rise to self-limited febrile illnesses of short duration that are not associated with specific clinical features. In these circumstances a diagnosis of en-terovirus infection is possible in clinical practice only when contacts are known to suffer from one or another of the well-defined syndromes or when specific virus isolations have been made from contacts.

Viral Respiratory Illness

In most parts of the world acute respiratory disease is by far the most common ailment suffered by humans. Different patterns of illness may be caused by the same virus, and conversely, several different viruses may give rise to what appears to be a single clinical syndrome. Some correlations, however, can be made.

Years ago, influenza viruses A and B were the only agents with a proved relationship to acute respiratory illness, but an ever-growing list of agents is now associated with respiratory tract infection. These agents include parainfluenza viruses, enteroviruses, adenoviruses, and respiratory syncytial viruses among others.

Influenza Virus Infections

The influenza viruses belong to the family Orthomyxoviridae (RNA viruses), which comprises three morphologically similar but antigenically distinct groups, influenza A, B, and C. Epidemics are usually caused by influenza A or B.

EPIDEMIOLOGY. Influenza occurs in epidemic or pandemic form. New epidemic strains of influenza A virus appear every 1 to 3 years associated with minor changes in the enveloped glycoproteins of the virus, the hemagglutinin and neuraminidase, by a process of point mutation and selection in a partially immune population — a phenomenon called antigenic drift. Every 10 to 40 years, however, a new pandemic strain of influenza A arises in humans in which one or both of the enveloped glycoproteins are completely different antigenically from those of the preceding strain and with which the population has no prior experience. Such a major change in antigenic profile is described as antigenic shift, and the new virus spreads rapidly around the world as an influenza pandemic.

Influenza B viruses are responsible for small localized outbreaks or epidemics, but less frequently than influenza A viruses. Influenza C viruses cause mild upper respiratory tract infections, more akin to the common cold, and probably as small localized outbreaks. Both influenza B and C viruses exhibit minor antigenic variation or drift, but not antigenic shift.

The spread of virus within the community during pandemic and epidemic influenza is not well understood. Children generally have a higher incidence of infection and may be an important source of spread.

TRANSMISSION. Influenza viruses are transmitted by airborne droplets of the respiratory secretions of infected hosts and by direct contact. Virus can be detected in nasopharyngeal secretions before the onset of symptoms and for at least 5 days after the illness has developed.

CLINICAL FINDINGS. Influenza infections caused by influenza A and B viruses are commonly asymptomatic, may cause only a slight fever, or may result in the typical prostrating illness that is characteristic of major epidemics. After an incubation period of 1 to 2 days, the typical acute disease has an abrupt onset with a rapid rise in body temperature to 38 to 40°C. The early symptoms usually include a dry, unproductive cough, a severe generalized or frontal headache, malaise, and shivering, and these are rapidly followed by aching muscles in the limbs and back, joint pains, anorexia, and nausea. Respiratory symptoms may be entirely lacking, or, if present, most prominent after the systemic symptoms and fever have subsided, usually 3 to 4 days after onset. A rather more productive cough may persist for up to 1 to 2 weeks, and convalescence may be prolonged by lassitude, malaise, and depression. The symptoms in children are generally similar to those found in adults, although there is a lower incidence of myalgia whereas nausea and vomiting are more frequent and maximal temperatures may be higher. A wide range of respiratory and neurological symptoms have been reported among infants and young children admitted to hospitals. Febrile convulsions, vomiting, coughing, diarrhea, and anorexia are the most common presenting features, with gastrointestinal symptoms prominent in young infants.

COMPLICATIONS. The main complications of influenza involve the lower respiratory tract and the cardiovascular and central nervous systems. The major complications arise from secondary bacterial infections of the ear, paranasal sinuses, bronchi, and lungs. Bronchitis, bronchiolitis, laryngotracheobronchitis (croup), and pneumonitis may result from secondary infection with streptococci, staphylococci, pneumococci, or *Haemophilus influenzae*. Secondary bacterial pneumonia may develop, with bubbling rales, consolidation, dyspnea, and radiological opacity either after the acute viral episode, in which case there is usually a biphasic fever pattern, or as a concomitant infection. *Streptococcus pneumoniae* has been the most commonly isolated pathogen, but staphylococcal and progressive influenza pneumonias are the most feared because they tend to run a fulminating and often fatal course. Primary influenza pneumonia may account for up to 20% of all cases of influenza-associated pneumonia, although it is relatively rare in infants and

young children. The pathological features include epithelial necrosis in the mucosa of the respiratory bronchioles, damage to alveolar cells, necrosis of the capillary walls, and thrombosis, with edema and hemorrhage into the alveoli. Clinically there is a relentless course of continued fever, leukocytosis, dyspnea, hypoxia, and cyanosis.

Neurological and cardiac complications are less frequent than and not as well documented as those of the respiratory tract. Although influenza A has been implicated in myocarditis, pericarditis, encephalitis, transverse myelitis, and the Guillain-Barré syndrome, the virus has seldom been isolated from the heart muscle or brain. Acute myositis and rhabdomyolysis with renal failure have been described.

Influenza A and B have both been closely described with Reye's syndrome, a pediatric disease with a high mortality characterized by acute encephalopathy with fatty degeneration of the viscera. Children with influenza should not consume salicylate-containing medications because of the strong association between salicylate use and Reye's syndrome in these patients.

LABORATORY DIAGNOSIS. Laboratory diagnosis is made either by recovery of the virus from throat washings and garglings obtained within 2 to 6 days of the onset of symptoms or by serological procedures (or both). In the latter case, blood is collected at the height of infection and again a fortnight later. A fourfold or greater rise in influenza-specific IgG titers using hemagglutination inhibition, neutralization, complement fixation, or ELISA tests is diagnostic. Rapid diagnosis by detection of influenza antigens in nasopharyngeal secretions by immunofluorescence is possible. Laboratory diagnosis is directed primarily at establishing the presence of the disease in the community.

IMMUNITY TO INFLUENZA. Because influenza A and B viruses undergo antigenic drift (see above), in which the outer antigenic components change with time, immunity tends to be relatively short-lived. Nevertheless, immunity gained from a natural infection may provide protection against reinfection by epidemic strains of the same virus type for several years; however, when new pandemic strains of influenza A arise by antigenic shift (see above), immunity gained by exposure to preceding strains is ineffective and does not provide any protection against the new strain.

The killed influenza vaccines (whole or split) currently available contain different viral subtypes. The composition of the vaccine is periodically modified to include prevalent influenza strains. Only the split (subvirion) vaccine should be used for children 12 years of age or younger. The vaccine has an estimated efficacy of 70 to 80% in normal individuals but is less in immunosuppressed patients. High-risk groups of children such as those with chronic pulmonary

398

disease, cardiac disease, hemoglobinopathies, and immunosuppression should be immunized against influenza. Children with symptomatic human immunodeficiency virus (HIV) infection, chronic metabolic and renal diseases, and those on long-term aspirin therapy (e.g., rheumatoid arthritis, Kawasaki disease) should be considered potentially at risk for complicated influenza disease and may thus benefit from the vaccine. The vaccine should be administered in the fall before the influenza season begins so as to derive maximal benefit.

TREATMENT. Amantadine given orally for 2 to 5 days diminishes the severity of signs and symptoms in influenza A disease only. Acetaminophen should be used for fever reduction. Aspirin use should be avoided because of its association with the subsequent development of Reye's syndrome in patients with influenza. Supportive measures such as supplemental oxygen and mechanical ventilation may be required for hospitalized children suffering from influenza pneumonia. Amantadine given prophylactically may diminish the spread of influenza A among exposed individuals.

Adenovirus Infections

The adenoviruses are common infecting agents in young children, causing a spectrum of mild respiratory illnesses with rhinitis and pharyngitis. Latent infection is also common, and virus can be recovered frequently from adenoidal and tonsillar tissue removed at operation. A more severe respiratory tract illness (pharyngoconjunctival fever) affects children in epidemics during the summer months. Such outbreaks are principally due to adenovirus type 3. Epidemics of adenovirus infection, which also occur in army recruits, assume the form of a catarrhal illness of the upper respiratory tract associated with headache, fever, malaise, and anorexia. Adenoviruses may also cause laryngotracheitis, bronchiolitis, pneumonia with or without pleural effusion, and a pertussis-like illness. Epidemic conjunctivitis and keratoconjunctivitis due to infection with adenovirus type 8 have also been described.

PHARYNGOCONJUNCTIVAL FEVER. Pharyngoconjunctival fever (nonbacterial pharyngitis, nonstreptococcal exudative tonsillitis) presents as a debilitating illness with high fever, sore throat, persistent cough, frequently with purulent sputum, headache, myalgia, rhinitis, and conjunctivitis. The pharynx, fauces, and tonsils are injected, and an exudate that is difficult to distinguish clinically from that due to acute streptococcal tonsillitis may be observed. The temperature may reach 40°C, and the illness lasts 4 or 5 days. In certain cases rhonchi and crepitations are audible in the lung fields; some patients have radiographic evidence of pneumonia. Parts of this syndrome complex may occur in isolation; particularly acute follicular conjunctivitis may occur alone and be due to several adenoviruses, including types 3, 6, 7, 10, 15, 16, or 17. Conjunctivitis, whether occurring alone or in association with pharyngitis, may last from a few days up to 3 weeks. Cervical lymphadenopathy may also be present. Laboratory investigations reveal a normal or slightly elevated leukocyte count; usually there is a slight neutrophilia. Cultures of throat swabs grow normal respiratory tract flora; this is often the only way streptococcal tonsillitis can be excluded. The disease is self-limiting, and recovery is complete without sequelae. Treatment is supportive, and antibiotics have no influence on the course of the illness. Adenoviruses of serotypes 40 and 41 have also been implicated in the development of gastrointestinal illness in infants and young children. Adenovirus particles have been identified in the stool by electron microscopy. The diarrhea caused resolves spontaneously after a somewhat longer course than that associated with rotavirus.

Parainfluenza Virus Infection

The parainfluenza viruses are RNA viruses, belonging to the paramyxovirus group. In some respects their characteristics resemble those of influenza viruses, and in other ways they are similar to the viruses of Newcastle disease and mumps. They are subclassified into four types (1, 2, 3, and 4). Each type can cause acute respiratory tract disease in human beings. The parainfluenza viruses are most important as respiratory tract pathogens during infancy and childhood; they cause a wide spectrum of diseases ranging from inapparent infections to life-threatening involvement of the lower respiratory tract. Infections with parainfluenza virus type 4 are almost always mild and limited to the upper respiratory tract, causing symptoms of coryza and mild sore throat. Parainfluenza virus types 1, 2, and 3 are most frequently associated with croup in infancy, but may also cause bronchiolitis in young infants or viral pneumonia in infants and children.

When the infection is not severe, the usual early symptoms are "brassy" cough and fever of about 38 to 39°C. The predominant physical findings are injected fauces and pharynx, rhinitis, and occasionally cervical lymphadenopathy. The illness lasts for 2 or 3 days and then subsides spontaneously.

Severely affected infants may develop inspiratory stridor due to laryngeal obstruction ("croup" syndrome), as well as the brassy cough, fever, and injection of the fauces. On auscultation of the chest, coarse crepitations are usually heard. The onset of the illness is frequently sudden, particularly at night, and severe respiratory distress may develop rapidly. The initial treatment is oxygen therapy with increased humidity, but emergency surgical relief of laryngeal obstruction by nasotracheal intubation or tracheostomy may be needed (see Chapter 10). Although the syndrome is usually due to infection with a parainfluenza virus, it may be produced by respiratory syncytial virus, and occasionally by other viruses.

Following infection with any of the parainfluenza virus types, incomplete immunity is induced. Reinfection with these viruses occurs throughout life, giving rise to recurrent minor illness, usually with upper respiratory tract symptoms indistinguishable from those of coryza.

Respiratory Syncytial Virus Infections

Respiratory syncytial virus is another member of the paramyxovirus group, giving rise to a wide spectrum of respiratory illnesses. Respiratory syncytial virus infections tend to occur in epidemics but occasionally are sporadic. In adults, the virus is a cause of coryza. In infancy it is the chief cause of serious infection of the lower respiratory tract such as bronchiolitis and pneumonia, with occasional fatalities (see Chapter 10).

Mumps (Epidemic Parotitis)

The mumps virus, a paramyxovirus, causes an acute infectious process characterized by nonsuppurative enlargement of the salivary glands, particularly the parotid, and occasional inflammation of other organ systems.

EPIDEMIOLOGY. Man is the only reservoir of infection. The virus, present in secretions prior to clinical onset of disease, is transmitted by the respiratory route. The incubation period may range from 12 to 25 days, though 16 to 18 days is usual. The period of communicability extends from 4 days before to one week after clinical onset of symptoms. About 33 to 50% of infections are subclinical in nature. The large percentage of subclinical infections together with the presence of infectious secretions prior to the onset of clinical disease accounts for the efficient transmission of this agent. Following inoculation of the respiratory tract, viremia and localization to other organs may occur.

Primarily a disease of children, it enjoys worldwide distribution with peak incidence occurring in late winter and spring. Endemic in most urban populations, the natural epidemiology of this infection has changed due to effective immunization of children in infancy, and it is now uncommon in the United States. Lifelong immunity follows natural infection and durable immunity can also be achieved by immunization with the live attenuated vaccine. Passage of maternal antibody confers passive immunity on the newborn which may last for 6 to 8 months.

CLINICAL MANIFESTATIONS. Prodromal symptoms such

as fever, anorexia, and discomfort in the salivary glands are rare in children. The acute onset of parotid swelling may be the first indication of infection. Pain and trismus are common. Malaise, fever, and anorexia are not infrequently associated. The glandular swelling usually resolves over a period of 5 to 7 days without sequelae. Aseptic meningitis and meningoencephalitis are the most common complications of mumps and may occur in the absence of other clinical manifestations of infection. Orchitis typically occurs in the postpubertal patient. It is usually unilateral and only when bilateral can it rarely be implicated as a cause of subsequent sterility. Deafness, pancreatitis, nephritis, oophoritis, and mastitis are all infrequent complications.

MANAGEMENT. Management is supportive. Attention should be paid to nutrition and fluid intake and analgesia given if necessary. This is usually a mild infection in children.

Measles (Morbilli, Rubeola)

Measles is an acute, highly infectious disease characterized mainly by respiratory symptoms and a typical skin rash. The measles virus, an RNA virus, has been classified as a paramyxovirus.

PATHOGENESIS AND PATHOLOGY. The virus enters via the respiratory tract. It is present in the blood and the nasorespiratory secretions by the time of onset of the prodromal catarrhal phase and persists until about 2 days after the onset of the rash. Tiny grayish-white vesicles (Koplik's spots) occur on the buccal mucosa and may be identified at this time.

Skin lesions are essentially a reaction of the capillary bed to the invading virus. A general inflammatory reaction of the pharyngeal, buccal, respiratory, and conjunctival mucosa occurs, and this extends to involve the lymphoid tissue of the tracheobronchial system. Interstitial pneumonitis due to the virus may develop.

Encephalomyelitis is an uncommon but severe complication whose histological features are scattered petechiae, round-cell infiltrations, and later patchy demyelination of the brain and spinal cord.

EPIDEMIOLOGY. The disease is endemic throughout the world, and in unvaccinated communities occurs in epidemics every 2 or 3 years. During an epidemic a high proportion of the nonimmune child population contracts the disease. When measles is introduced into a family, at least 80% of previously uninfected children in the family experience the infection. Transmission is spread by droplet inhalation, particularly during the prodromal and catarrhal phases of the disease. The reservoir of infection is the acutely ill patient; the "carrier state" does not occur. One attack of the disease usually confers lifelong immunity. Good passive immunity is acquired by the infant of a previously infected mother. This persists until the age of 5 or 6 months. Vaccination has altered the epidemiology of this infection by shifting the age at peak incidence from school-age children to other groups such as unvaccinated preschoolers, adolescents and young adults who had received the less effective killed vaccine, and those immunized before their first birthday, a time when maternal antibodies can inhibit the development of a durable immune response.

CLINICAL MANIFESTATIONS. The disease has an incubation period of 14 days (range, 10–19 days) between exposure to the virus and onset of the rash. A preeruptive phase lasts for up to 10 days and consists of a respiratory tract illness that becomes increasingly more severe as the prodrome progresses. During this stage a mucoid nasal discharge, conjunctivitis, a dry cough, and fever that may reach 39 to 40°C develop. Toward the end of this phase Koplik's spots are seen on the buccal mucosa. They are confined to the inner surfaces of the cheeks and consist of tiny (0.1–0.3 mm) bluish-white vesicular lesions, each surrounded by an erythematous area. Several such lesions are usually seen on each cheek. At this time the pharynx is likely to be injected, and small macules may appear on the conjunctivae. Approximately 48 hours after the appearance of Koplik's spots the exanthem commences, coinciding with the peak of the respiratory symptoms. At the same time the enanthem (Koplik's spots) begins to fade, and it disappears over the following 24 to 48 hours. The exanthematous rash consists of macules that begin as faint reddish spots and rapidly become more florid, usually changing to maculopapules. The rash commences typically behind the ears and progresses to involve the face, neck, trunk, and extremities over the ensuing 24 to 48 hours. In general terms the severity of the rash is a gauge of the severity of the disease. In mild cases of measles the maculopapules are not extensive and begin to fade 3 or 4 days after their appearance, disappearing in the same order that they developed. In more severe cases the lesions become confluent, and for a period the face and trunk may appear to be completely covered with rash, the face usually becoming edematous and swollen. Rarely, hemorrhage may occur into the rash, giving it a purpuric appearance. Such "hemorrhagic measles" is sometimes associated with bleeding from the mouth, nose, and bowel; when this occurs, the term *black measles* is applied.

As the measles rash begins to fade, it is frequently followed by desquamation of epithelium with some brownish discoloration of the skin. There is visible evidence of the fading rash for up to a week in most children. With the appearance and progression of the rash, the upper respiratory tract symptoms and fever reach a climax and then

usually resolve quickly after 2 or 3 days. Direct involvement of the respiratory tract may occasionally be the most prominent feature of the acute illness, becoming manifest as laryngotracheobronchitis (croup), bronchiolitis, or interstitial pneumonia. Lymphadenopathy, particularly of the anterior cervical triangle and the posterior cervical region, is almost universal. The spleen may be enlarged.

Examination of the peripheral blood usually reveals a leukopenia, with a relative lymphocytosis. If secondary bacterial infection supervenes, a polymorphonuclear leukocytosis may develop.

DIFFERENTIAL DIAGNOSIS. Measles must be differentiated from other exanthems. When the regular progression of prodrome, enanthem, and exanthem is taken into account, the diagnosis in most cases is not difficult. Detection of Koplik's spots are often helpful in making the diagnosis.

Rubella is differentiated by the lack of severe respiratory symptoms and the absence of Koplik's spots, the transient nature of the rash, and the presence of enlarged posterior auricular lymph nodes. Similarly, other enterovirus exanthems lack the progressive symptoms of measles, and the rashes are more transient. Exanthema subitum (roseola infantum) is diagnosed by the dramatic subsidence of symptoms with the onset of rash, which again is transient. Infectious mononucleosis may occasionally present with a morbilliform rash but it is differentiated by the lack of Koplik's spots, by the more severe pharyngitis and lymphadenopathy, and by laboratory findings (atypical lymphocytes and positive heterophil agglutination reactions).

COMPLICATIONS. Measles ranks as one of the most severe infectious diseases of unvaccinated children and carries a devastatingly high mortality in underdeveloped countries. Complications include the development of secondary bacterial infections including otitis media, bacterial tracheitis, and pneumonia. Primary measles pneumonia, a severe giant-cell interstitial process, is a cause of bronchiectasis in later life.

Encephalomyelitis is a complication in approximately 1 out of 1000 cases of measles. Symptoms usually develop 2 to 5 days after the appearance of the rash. It is thought, when this time sequence occurs, that the condition is an autoimmune reaction precipitated by measles. Rarely, encephalitic features may commence during the prodrome and then are attributed to the direct action of the virus. Encephalomyelitis manifests as a severe disturbance of cerebral function, usually with convulsions and coma. The mortality is high, being approximately 30%, and in patients who recover there is an equally high incidence of residual motor, intellectual, or emotional impairment. Subacute sclerosing panencephalitis (SSPE) is a devastating degenerative disorder resulting from persistent measles virus infection of the central nervous system and is characterized by deterioration in cognitive functions and seizures leading to death within 6 to 9 months.

Other complications include generalized lymphoid hyperplasia, which may involve the Peyer's patches of the small bowel and cause abdominal colic. Occasionally, catarrhal appendicitis complicates the acute stage of the illness. Myocarditis is an extremely rare complication.

TREATMENT AND PREVENTION. There is no specific treatment for uncomplicated measles; however, when bacterial superinfection is diagnosed, the use of appropriate antibiotics is indicated.

The disease may be modified or prevented following exposure by the administration of immune globulin. This procedure is recommended for susceptible household contacts, especially if less than 1 year of age or immunocompromised. A dose of 0.25 ml of gamma globulin/kg of body weight administered by intramuscular injection within 6 days of exposure usually prevents the disease.

A live attenuated vaccine is available and effective in producing durable immunity. Vaccination is recommended for all children at 15 months of age and for children in epidemic situations at 6 to 15 months to be repeated at 15 months of age. A second dose is given at 4 to 6 years of age on entry to kindergarten or first grade. Side effects of the vaccine include fever and transient rashes occurring 6 to 10 days postinoculation.

Atypical Measles

The atypical measles syndrome was identified in 1965 in subjects who contracted natural measles several years after administration of killed vaccine. Since then there have been further confirmatory series, mostly in young adolescents. Almost all have followed killed vaccine, but a few cases resulting from natural infection following live attenuated vaccine have been reported. Atypical measles has also been described in a series of subjects who were given live attenuated vaccine within 3 months of killed vaccine.

PATHOGENESIS. It is generally accepted that there is an immunological imbalance promoted by the supervention of a "wild" measles virus infection and occasionally by an attenuated measles virus on a previous immune state following killed virus vaccination. Although humoral immunity imparted by killed measles vaccine is short in duration, the cellular immunity induced by the vaccine persists and is enhanced by a natural infection resulting in the manifestation of atypical measles. Measles IgG, antigen, and complement have been detected within skin lesions of atypical measles. An alternative suggestion put forward is that of a generalized Arthus reaction. There is some evidence that an exaggerated lymphocyte reactivity contributes to the adverse clinical response. The syndrome is thought to be due to a persistence of delayed hypersensitivity in subjects whose circulating antibodies have fallen below a protective level.

CLINICAL FEATURES. The clinical features differ from those of natural primary measles infection. The patients are usually older children or teenagers. Early symptoms are malaise, headache, myalgia, cough, and, photophobia. There is usually a high fever up to 40°C. Abdominal pain and vomiting may occur later. The rash is not typically morbilliform. It tends to be polymorphic and to include urticarial, petechial, and vesicular elements. It is usually observed first on the hands and feet and spreads to the limbs and trunk. A frequent accompaniment of atypical measles is pleurisy, causing pleuritic pain and pneumonitis that may persist for weeks. Radiography may demonstrate prominent pulmonary infiltrates in the form of diffuse segmental lesions or nodules, pleural effusion, and hilar gland enlargement. The general symptoms, fever and rash, usually subside within a week, but the pulmonary lesions may persist for months before resolving spontaneously. Before resolution patients may be hypoxemic, as demonstrated by blood gas measurements.

DIAGNOSIS. If the syndrome is not suspected, diagnosis is often difficult. The protean cutaneous manifestations might suggest meningococcemia, varicella, scarlet fever, Rocky Mountain spotted fever, anaphylactoid purpura, infectious mononucleosis, or a drug reaction. Pulmonary features might suggest any number of serious lung disorders, including malignancies, particularly when infiltrates and nodules persist. If the true nature of the illness is not suspected, there is a tendency to overinvestigate the pulmonary component. Once the true nature of the illness is recognized, all that is required is patience until spontaneous resolution occurs.

There is usually a leukopenia with a relative lymphocytosis. There are characteristically high titers of hemagglutination-inhibition and complement fixation antibodies early in the course of the illness. Measles virus is not isolated. Lung biopsies are noncontributory and should not be done.

TREATMENT. Treatment is symptomatic and supportive.

PREVENTION. The syndrome is rare now that the attenuated vaccine is widely used. Persons vaccinated prior to 1967 with either an inactivated or an unknown vaccine should be reimmunized as they are at risk of severe illness if infected with wild virus.

Herpesvirus Infections

There are six distinct herpesviruses that infect humans (see Table 20-3): herpes simplex virus types 1 and 2, Epstein-

Barr virus, varicella-zoster virus, cytomegalovirus, and human herpes virus 6. Herpesviruses are DNA viruses, 100 to 150 nm in diameter.

Herpes Simplex (Herpes Febrilis, Genitalis, Labialis)

Herpes simplex virus is one of the most common agents that infects humans. Between 70 and 90% of adults have antibodies to it. Infection with this virus may produce several well-defined clinical manifestations (gingivostomatitis, keratoconjunctivitis, Kaposi's varicelliform eruption, meningoencephalitis), or it may be subclinical, the virus living with the host as a successful commensal.

PATHOGENESIS AND PATHOLOGY. The main lesions are in the skin and buccal mucous membrane. Proliferation and ballooning degeneration of cells occur with vesicle formation, and intranuclear, acidophilic inclusion bodies are seen. In herpes encephalitis nerve cell destruction, perivascular cuffing, and meningeal reactions occur with intranuclear inclusions in glial cells. Neonatal infections, usually with herpesvirus type 2 from the mother's birth canal, may result in generalized focal areas of necrosis in all organs, particularly the brain, liver, and adrenal glands.

The herpesvirus produces several clinical syndromes, usually classified as primary or recurrent manifestations of the disease. Primary infection occurs in persons without antibody to the virus and may be associated with widespread systemic involvement; however, in most persons the primary infection is not even noticed.

CLINICAL MANIFESTATIONS. Forms in which primary infection may present clinically in children are acute herpetic gingivostomatitis, eczema herpeticum (Kaposi's varicelliform eruptions), herpetic meningoencephalitis, and primary herpesvirus infection in the newborn infant.

Acute Herpetic Gingivostomatitis. This, the most common manifestation, is due to infection with herpesvirus type 1. It occurs in infants and young children 10 months to 3 years of age. The incubation period is short (3–5 days) and is followed by fever, anorexia, and the development of painful vesicular eruptions of the tongue and buccal mucosa. The vesicles erupt and progress to widespread ulceration. The regional lymph nodes are almost always enlarged and tender. The disease is not usually difficult to recognize, but it must be differentiated from herpangina and sometimes from follicular tonsillitis. The stomatitis lasts for 7 to 10 days.

Treatment is mainly supportive, although in severe cases resolution is facilitated by administration of acyclovir at a dosage of 250 mg/m^2 every 8 hours. Careful attention must be paid to fluid intake, as affected babies may refuse to eat or drink and may require intravenous fluids. Acetaminophen may be given for fever and pain. A topical anesthetic solution composed of a mixture of Dyclonine hydrochloride (0.5%) or Benadryl elixir (12.5 mg/5 ml) and Kaopectate in equal parts is helpful in making eating more comfortable. Resolution of the ulcers with complete healing occurs, but a proportion of infected children continue to have manifestations of recurrent herpes.

Eczema Herpeticum (Kaposi's Varicelliform Eruptions). In this condition infection with herpes simplex virus occurs in areas of skin that are the sites of chronic infantile eczema. Vesicles appear abruptly in large numbers over eczematous patches and sometimes spread to surrounding normal skin. They continue to appear for 7 to 9 days. Vesicles may coalesce and give rise to widespread denudations of the epithelium, with a coagulum that may become infected with pyogenic bacteria. Systemic reaction, with fever and debility, usually occurs. Finally the condition subsides, and the affected area is covered with new epithelium. Eczema herpeticum is frequently a manifestation of primary herpes simplex, but repeated milder episodes may have occurred, in which case antibodies to herpes simplex are present in the serum. In severely affected patients, particularly with primary infection, fluid and electrolyte management is of paramount importance as death may occur from loss of fluid, protein, and electrolytes from the denuded skin surface in a manner analogous to that in a patient with a severe burn.

Herpetic Meningoencephalitis. An uncommon form of primary infection with herpes simplex virus is aseptic meningitis or meningoencephalitis. In this form, concomitant evidence of herpes simplex virus infection elsewhere, i.e., stomatitis, keratitis, or liver involvement in newborn infants, may be found. It is frequently acute in onset with a fulminant course leading to death in 70% of untreated patients while survivors typically have severe neurologic sequelae. Acyclovir is the drug of choice and should be given as early as possible after onset of illness.

Neonatal Herpesvirus Infection. Most cases of neonatal herpes are a result of acquisition of herpes simplex virus (HSV) (usually type 2) during passage through an infected birth canal. The risk of transmission from a mother to her newborn is estimated at 40 to 50% for those with primary genital herpes and only about 5% for women with recurrent infections. Neonatal HSV infection may be localized to the central nervous system or to the skin, eyes, and mouth, or it may be generalized in nature involving multiple organs such as the liver, central nervous system, and lungs. The diagnosis is best established by isolation of the virus from one or more body sites. Neonatal HSV infections are associated with high mortality and morbidity rates, especially if left untreated. Acyclovir and vidarabine are both effective, but the former is preferred because it is less toxic and is easier to administer. The mortality rate among treated newborns is about 15 to 20%; however, approximately half of the survivors suffer long-term neurologic sequelae.

Recurrent Herpes Simplex Infection. The usual manifestation of HSV infection is a crop of localized vesicles that appears repeatedly at the same site, often the mucocutaneous junction on the lower lip. The vesicles appear quickly, rupture, and scab. Healing occurs in 7 to 10 days, leaving no scar unless secondary bacterial infection has occurred. In blacks, a transient patch of depigmentation develops at the site. In children, the lesions may become infected with pyogenic bacteria and may be mistaken for impetigo. Commonly called "cold sores," the lesions may be precipitated by a wide variety of stimuli such as upper respiratory tract infections, exposure to sunlight, and trauma. Other sites for recurrent herpes include the genital area and the fingers (herpetic whitlow). Infection of fingers may be due to direct spread when children with facial herpes suck their fingers.

Herpetic Lesions of the Eye

The eye may be the site of a primary or recurrent herpes infection. Conjunctivitis or keratoconjunctivitis occurs. The conjunctiva is injected and swollen, and the preauricular lymph nodes may be enlarged. There is little, if any, purulent exudate. The cornea may be the site of shallow "dendritic" ulcers or a deeper disciform keratitis. Vesicles frequently appear on the lids and are of great value in making the diagnosis. Topical therapy with either trifluridine (1% ophthalmic solution) or vidarabine (3% ophthalmic ointment) is effective. Idoxuridine can be used, but it appears to be less effective and more toxic than the two other preparations. The recurrence rate is not reduced by topical therapy with any of these agents.

Varicella-Zoster Virus

Varicella-zoster virus (VZV) causes both varicella (chickenpox) and herpes zoster (shingles). Morphologically very similar to HSV, the viruses obtained from varicella and zoster lesions are antigenically identical.

VARICELLA (CHICKENPOX). Varicella is characterized by a mild systemic reaction with the appearance on the skin of crops of typical vesicular lesions.

Pathogenesis and Pathology. The virus probably enters via the respiratory tract, circulates in the blood, and finally localizes in the skin. The skin vesicles are similar to herpes simplex lesions and consist of ballooning and degenerating epithelial cells with accumulation of fluid. In the early stages eosinophilic inclusion bodies are found in the nuclei of infected cells. Healing is usually complete, but secondary infection may occur when the lesions are scratched. This sometimes leads to permanent scarring. In the unusual severe cases, hemorrhagic necrosis may occur in the mucous membranes of the mouth, trachea, or intestine. Rarely, encephalomyelitis may occur with perivascular demyelination throughout the central nervous system. Intranuclear inclusion bodies have been found in almost all other organs.

Epidemiology. The disease is highly contagious and is experienced by almost everyone during childhood. Spread is by direct contact or by airborne droplets. The infectious period is from 24 hours before until 6 or 7 days after the appearance of vesicles. The scabs, after the vesicles have dried up, are not infectious. Symptomatic reinfections are rare in otherwise normal individuals.

Clinical Features. The incubation period of chickenpox may range from 10 to 20 days but is usually between 14 and 16 days. Children seldom have prodromal symptoms; fever, rash, and malaise appear together. The typical rash rapidly progresses through the stages of macule, papule, vesicle, and crusting. The vesicles, when present, are thin and fragile and contain clear fluid. They are 2 or 3 mm in diameter with some surrounding erythema. The distribution is predominantly on the trunk, with a few scattered lesions on the limbs. After 24 to 48 hours the crusting gives rise to scab formation that lasts for 5 to 20 days. When scabs finally drop, they leave shallow, pale areas, which disappear in the ensuing few weeks except when secondary infection has occurred. Lesions that progress through this range of changes appear in crops; in the typical attack of chickenpox, three crops appear over 3 or 4 days. Fever, lethargy, anorexia, and headache usually coexist with the rash; they are most prominent in the first 3 or 4 days, when the initial crops are appearing, and resolve when the rash subsides. Pruritus is a common and distressing symptom.

Hemorrhagic varicella is a rare and severe form of chickenpox characterized by high fever and more distressing symptoms than those in the usual attack. Hemorrhage occurs into the vesicles, and many petechiae and ecchymoses appear. This form of chickenpox occurs chiefly in adults but has been seen in children who develop chickenpox while on steroid therapy, or in children with leukemia or the most serious form of immunological deficiency. In a high proportion of children who acquire chickenpox while taking corticosteroids for other diseases, a fulminating hemorrhagic infection develops, usually with encephalomyelitis and a fatal outcome within a few days.

Diagnosis. The diagnosis of chickenpox is usually based on the clinical findings. The presence of VZV can be demonstrated by either culturing the virus from vesicular fluid or by immunofluorescent staining of vesicular scrapings. Serologic diagnosis is based on either detecting VZV-specific IgM or the demonstration of a fourfold or greater rise in VZV-specific IgG titers by complement fixation or ELISA.

Complications. The most common complication is staphylococcal or streptococcal infection of the skin lesions. Central nervous system complications range from aseptic meningitis to fulminant encephalitis. Varicella pneumonia is rare in children. Arthritis, bleeding manifestations, nephritis, and myocarditis are rare complications.

Treatment. Immunosuppressed patients should be treated with acyclovir as early as possible. The use of salicylate-containing medications should be avoided because of the strong association between their use in children with chickenpox and the subsequent development of Reye's syndrome. Antipruritics may be needed to control itching.

Prevention. Individuals at high risk for developing progressive varicella (e.g., immunocompromised patients) should receive varicella-zoster immune globulin (VZIG) prophylaxis within 96 hours of exposure. A live attenuated varicella vaccine has been developed and extensively tested but still awaits licensing in the United States.

Herpes Zoster

Herpes zoster is an uncommon disease in children. When it does occur, the clinical features are very similar to those in adults. The incubation period of 7 to 14 days is followed by malaise, fever, and pain in the skin area along the distribution of a nerve root. A few days later a crop of vesicles appears over the skin supplied by the affected nerve. Occasionally the process spreads to the anterior horn cell of the same segment as the affected dorsal nerve root, resulting in paralysis that is usually temporary. The lesions form vesicles, which become pustular, then dry and scab over a course of 5 to 10 days. Crops of lesions tend to appear for about 7 days and typically start nearest the central nervous system, moving peripherally along the affected dermatome. Except in rare instances the lesions are unilateral. The dermatomes of the second thoracic to the second lumbar nerves are the most common sites to be affected in childhood, although cephalic zoster affecting one of the branches of the fifth cranial nerve may also occur. When the ophthalmic branch is affected (zoster ophthalmicus), lesions appear on the cornea.

COURSE AND PROGNOSIS IN CHILDHOOD. The disease is mild, and postherpetic pain does not occur. Immunocompromised patients with zoster may benefit from acyclovir therapy.

Cytomegalovirus Infection

An estimated 1 to 2% of all newborns in the United States are infected with cytomegalovirus (CMV). About 90% of these neonates are asymptomatic. Symptomatic newborns tend to have serious disease with a mortality rate of 20 to 30%, with most survivors developing serious, long-term neurologic sequelae such as deafness, mental retardation, and visual impairment. In addition, an estimated 5 to 15% of those with asymptomatic, congenital CMV infection develop neurologic abnormalities by 2 years of age. CMV also causes severe, sometimes fatal, infections in immunocompromised hosts involving many organ systems. Like other herpesviruses it tends to become latent — in some cases, for life. Reactivation may occur years after initial infection, particularly following immunosuppressive therapy. Infected hosts may excrete CMV for years.

EPIDEMIOLOGY. The prevalence of CMV in a given population depends on many factors including standard of living, attendance in day-care centers, and sexual activity, among others. In developing countries, most people become infected before they reach puberty. In the United States, seroepidemiologic surveys indicate that about 50 to 60% of women of childbearing age have antibodies to CMV. Higher rates of seropositivity are found among women of lower socioeconomic backgrounds. As many as 70% of 1- to 2-year-old children attending day-care centers excrete the virus.

Transmission of CMV occurs horizontally or vertically. Horizontal transmission occurs when contact with infected saliva or urine occurs. The virus can also be transmitted by sexual intercourse and through blood transfusions. Vertical transmission may occur in utero, during passage through an infected birth canal, or postnatally through ingestion of infected breast milk. Intrauterine transmission may occur after either primary or recurrent maternal CMV infection, but severe congenital disease usually follows primary maternal infection. About half of all newborns exposed to CMV during passage through an infected birth canal acquire the infection but do not shed the virus before 4 to 12 weeks of age.

CONGENITAL MANIFESTATIONS. These are the most serious effects of CMV infections. Fortunately, the proportion of infected infants seriously affected is low. It is estimated that 0.5 to 2.0% of infants may be infected, but less than 10% of these show clinical abnormalities: intrauterine growth retardation, jaundice, hepatosplenomegaly, microcephaly, anemia, and purpura recognized soon after birth. Talipes, cleft lip and palate, congenital heart defects, and inguinal hernias have also been described but are less consistent. The disease is often rapidly progressive, resulting in death within a few days after birth. Surviving infants generally have a poor prognosis. The majority suffer permanent handicaps. The most serious are neurological sequelae of mental and motor retardation, spasticity, epilepsy, impaired vision (but rarely total blindness), and sensorineural hearing loss. Obstructive hydrocephalus has been described. Radiology might reveal intracranial periventricular calcification (especially in infants with microcephaly), pneumonitis, and translucent streaks (celery stalk appearance) in the metaphyses of the long bones similar to those found in infants affected with congenital rubella. Some infants make a surprisingly good recovery but remain stunted in growth. Hepatosplenomegaly may persist for years before subsiding. Occasionally cirrhosis develops. Some infants isolated features, e.g., thrombocytopenia, chorioretinitis, or persistent hepatosplenomegaly detected by routine examination.

DIAGNOSIS. CMV infection cannot be diagnosed with certainty on clinical features alone, as other infective agents (rubella, toxoplasmosis, syphilis) can give similar findings.

Laboratory findings in the first weeks of life may reveal hemolytic anemia, thrombocytopenia, increased levels of direct and indirect serum bilirubin, elevation of liver enzymes, and raised cerebrospinal fluid protein. Specific confirmation of CMV can be made by cytological, histological, virological, and serological techniques. Infected cells have intranuclear inclusions, which can be demonstrated in liver and lung biopsies. Fresh sedimented urine specimens show typical intranuclear inclusions in stained exfoliated cells (owl's eye cells) in 10 to 30% of neonates with confirmed infection.

Virus culture from urine, saliva, throat washings, cerebrospinal fluid, buffy coat cells, and tissue biopsy specimens is the most reliable confirmatory test. Several specimens should be cultured within the first days of life.

Serologic tests for CMV-specific IgG antibodies have to be interpreted cautiously. About 50% of neonates acquire antibodies to CMV transplacentally. CMV infection in an infant can be assumed only if antibodies persist for longer than expected because of natural decay or if the titer is 4 times that of the mother. IgM, if detected, is significant. The best diagnostic test is viral culture in the first 2 week of life because after this time infection could be acquired.

ACQUIRED POSTNATAL INFECTION. Infants infected during passage through the birth canal usually remain well but may excrete virus for weeks. Sometimes they contract pneumonitis. In older infants and children subclinical infections usually develop, but they may have a mild febrile illness with pneumonitis. In older infants and children subclinical infections usually develop, but they may have a mild febrile illness with pneumonitis, hepatosplenomegaly, and transient impaired liver function tests. In adults serious clinical features are uncommon. Fever, malaise, rashes, hepatosplenomegaly, lymphadenopathy, myocarditis, polyneuritis, Guillain-Barré syndrome, thrombocytopenia, hemolytic anemia, and heterophil-negative mononucleosis have been described. Patients on immunosuppressive therapy are more likely to develop these clinical features. Isolation of CMV in the absence of histologic confirmation of viral invasion does not prove that the virus is causing the clinical features.

TREATMENT. There is no effective treatment for congenital infection. Patients with CMV retinitis may benefit from ganciclovir (DHPG), but experience with this drug in children is very limited.

PREVENTION. The ideal prevention is avoidance of contact with infected patients, but this is virtually impossible as most acquired CMV infections are subclinical or have nonspecific features. Attenuated live vaccines are being tried experimentally in adults. Trials of CMV hyperimmune globulin for prophylaxis of seronegative transplant recipients suggest that the preparation may be effective. Maternal antibodies do not necessarily protect the fetus. Infected fetuses in successive pregnancies have been described. Transmission of CMV to preterm infants by blood transfusion can be minimized by using only CMV–antibody-negative donors or blood from which white blood cells have been removed.

Infectious Mononucleosis

This infectious illness, first demonstrated in 1880 as "glandular fever," was shown to be due to the Epstein-Barr virus (EBV), a DNA herpesvirus (see Table 20-3), in 1968. Primary EBV infection in young children differs from the more clinically obvious manifestations of the infection causing "glandular fever" in adolescents and young adults. Like other members of the herpes group of viruses, EBV remains latent in human hosts for indefinite periods of time following primary infection. Saliva is the major reservoir for the spread of EBV. After replication of the virus in the oropharynx, viremia develops and B lymphocytes are infected.

Typical infectious mononucleosis occurs in adolescents and young adults in "advantaged" societies, where young people remain uninfected until teenage years. In this form it is common in college and university students. In "disadvantaged" communities and in developing countries 70 to 90% of children are infected before the age of 6 years, as shown by positive antibodies to EBV. In these communities typical "glandular fever" is rare as a clinical entity, in contrast to protected groups. Subclinical infections are more common than manifest clinical disease.

Peaks of infection in children are less easy to determine. In families, detectable spread is lower than with measles and chickenpox. Young children may develop specific EBV IgM antibodies after minor episodes of upper respiratory infections, tonsillitis, and otitis media. There is probably persistent and intermittent shedding of EBV in all segments of the population. Many clinical manifestations remain unrecognized and may present in forms as diverse as facial palsy, Guillain-Barré syndrome, meningoencephalitis, thrombocytopenic purpura, hemolytic anemia, and hepatitis, and not as typical "glandular fever." EBV does not have the same propensity to cause congenital deformities as CMV.

CLINICAL FEATURES. The prodrome is usually 4 to 6 days, followed by an acute illness with fever lasting 4 days to 3 weeks. Convalescence is usually prolonged and might last several months.

Almost all organ systems are involved, the most common being the hematopoietic system, but usually the liver, spleen, lymph glands, and central nervous system. Typically an adolescent has fever, malaise, sore throat, anorexia, and frequently weakness and prostration. Clinical examination reveals a red throat and enlarged tonsils covered with a grayish-yellow membrane like that of diphtheria. The breath is usually offensive. Simultaneously, or soon afterward, the cervical lymph glands become large and painful and are tender to palpation. Other lymph glands are also enlarged but not to the same extent. Hepatosplenomegaly is common, the spleen being 2 to 4 cm below the left costal margin in 50% of patients. A rash is usually present — sometimes faint maculopapular, occasionally profuse morbilliform and even resembling erythema multiforme. Petechiae are often detected. In severe cases there may be jaundice. The clinical picture might be complicated by features of central nervous system involvement — meningoencephalitis or Guillain-Barré syndrome. A provisional diagnosis of glandular fever is often made but the diagnosis not confirmed by laboratory tests. In these cases other viruses might be the causal agent of the syndrome. When all the features are present in florid form, EBV is usually confirmed as the infecting agent.

COMPLICATIONS. Clinical *hepatitis* is found in about 2% of patients with infectious mononucleosis, but 20 to 40% may show elevated serum transaminase and bilirubin levels.

Thrombocytopenia is a common finding. Hemolytic anemia, glomerulonephritis, and orchitis are uncommon but known complications.

Neurological complications include meningoencephalitis, Guillain-Barré syndrome, transverse myelitis, Bell's palsy.

Cardiac complications include myocarditis, showing lymphocytic infiltration, and sometimes pericarditis. These are reversible and have no sequelae.

Splenic rupture, usually a result of trauma, accounts for a significant number of fatal cases.

Airway obstruction may be due to enormous hyperplasia of lymphoid tissue of Waldeyer's ring. An artificial airway might be required.

DIAGNOSTIC TESTS. Viral isolation is not useful. Nonspecific tests for heterophil antibody (Paul-Bunnell test, slide agglutination reaction) are common and identify about 90% of cases in older children and adults, but they are frequently negative in those younger than 4 years of age. Specific serologic tests detecting antibodies to various components of EBV are also available. Detection of IgM antibodies to the viral capsid antigen (VCA) indicates a recent infection. Antibodies against the early antigen (EA) indicate an acute or recent infection. If antibodies against EBV nuclear antigens are detected, the infection is not acute because these antibodies are not usually found before several weeks to months after onset of illness.

PROGNOSIS. Prognosis is usually good although sometimes the condition can be fatal. Convalescence is often protracted, and the patient may be weak for several months. Attempts to participate in sports may have to be abandoned because of weakness. Body contact sports are not advisable until recovery is complete because of the danger of a traumatic rupture of an enlarged spleen.

TREATMENT. Uncomplicated infectious mononucleosis requires only supportive care. Helpful measures include bed rest, analgesics, antipyretics, and warm saline gargles. Acyclovir reduces the duration of EBV excretion, but its efficacy in improving the clinical illness is uncertain at the present time. Patients with severe airway obstruction may benefit from a short (2–5 days) course of corticosteroids. If the airway obstruction continues to worsen, placement of an endotracheal tube may be needed. Patients with severe and persistent thrombocytopenia may require corticosteroid therapy or even splenectomy, but this situation is rare. Surgery is occasionally required for ruptured spleen. Bacterial superinfections are uncommon but require the administration of effective antibiotics should they occur.

*Other Manifestations of EBV Infections
Including Oncogenic Associations*

Burkitt's lymphoma and nasopharyngeal carcinoma have been associated with EBV infection. The geographical locations of Burkitt's lymphoma and nasopharyngeal carcinoma are significant. Burkitt's lymphoma is almost entirely confined to the tropical rain forest regions of Africa and New Guinea, where malaria is hyperendemic. Nasopharyngeal carcinoma is most prevalent in South China and Southeast Asia. In these endemic areas, infection with EBV occurs in early childhood. Patients with Burkitt's lymphoma and nasopharyngeal carcinoma have EBV antibody titers 10 to 15 times higher than control populations living in the same regions.

Sera from patients with Burkitt's lymphoma and nasopharyngeal carcinoma have antibodies to an early antigen complex. These antibodies occur transiently in the course of the primary EBV infection in childhood. Their continued presence in tumor patients suggests continued ongoing active infection.

Prospective studies of children in Uganda have shown very high levels of EBV antibodies long before tumors of Burkitt's lymphoma develop. The hypothesis has been put forward that perinatal or early infantile infection with EBV may submit these children to the risk of a later development of Burkitt's lymphoma. EBV would thus behave like many tumor viruses whose oncogenic potential is greatly enhanced by neonatal infections. Radiolabeling has provided firm evidence for the presence of EBV-specific DNA in tumor tissue. It is very mysterious that a ubiquitous virus causing so many infections in young people throughout the world should be associated with serious neoplastic disease in Africa, South China, Southeast Asia, and New Guinea. It is controversial whether EBV or a particular strain of it is responsible. Cofactors suggested include hyperendemic malaria, genetic determinants, chromosome 8 translocation with chromosomes 2, 14, or 22, or RNA tumor viruses activating the oncogenic potential of EBV. Cofactors for nasopharyngeal carcinoma might include genetic determinants or environmental associations, e.g., herbs, inhalants, or nitrosamines in salted fish. Interestingly, EBV DNA sequences are found in nasopharyngeal epithelial cells, not in lymphoid cells, in nasopharyngeal carcinoma. Experimental EBV inoculation in primates produces malignant lymphomas of the reticulum and lymphoblastic types in some animals whereas others merely show transient lymphoid hyperplasia.

EBV has also been linked recently to a number of other malignancies such as thymic carcinoma, salivary gland carcinoma, supraglottic laryngeal carcinoma, and tonsillar carcinoma.

Primary EBV infection may cause a severe, and often fatal, illness in males with the X-linked lymphoproliferative syndrome, a disease characterized by a combined variable immunodeficiency and severe susceptibility to this virus. EBV is detected in the saliva, blood, and lymphoid tissues of these patients, but their antibody responses to the viral antigens are poor or absent. The cause of death is usually hepatic failure complicated by bleeding and infection. EBV-associated lymphoproliferative disorders have been described post renal transplantation and, on occasion, post bone marrow or thymus transplants.

A condition described as chronic or recurrent mononucleosis has recently received much attention. It usually occurs in young adults and symptoms include fever, pharyngitis, malaise, headache, lymphadenopathy, and neuropsychological abnormalities. These patients appear to have an enhanced antibody response to the early antigen of EBV, suggesting that they have a reactivated or persistently active EBV infection. Whether EBV is the cause of the syndrome is controversial.

Roseola Infantum (Exanthema Subitum)

Roseola infantum, a benign, acute exanthematous infection of infancy, has a characteristic clinical course that enables it to be identified clinically. The disease is free from complications, and the causative agent is thought to be human herpes virus 6.

EPIDEMIOLOGY. Roseola affects infants and young children between the ages of 6 months and 2 years; it is seen rarely in older children. It appears to attack infants in a sporadic fashion, perhaps because of the presence of immunity among other children in the household. Outbreaks of roseola in nurseries suggest that its attack rate is high among those who have not developed immunity.

CLINICAL MANIFESTATIONS. The incubation period is estimated to be 5 to 15 days. Initially, the clinical manifestations are nonspecific. An infant in the latter half of the first year of life or in the toddler age group may become irritable and anorexic, with features of an upper respiratory tract infection, including a slightly injected throat and nasal catarrh. Usually there is pyrexia of the order of 39 to 40°C. Investigations are often noncontributory, but a blood examination may reveal leukopenia, with a relative lymphocytosis up to 90%. The cervical and occipital lymph glands are generally slightly enlarged. It is rare for a diagnosis of roseola infantum to be made at this stage; usually the child is thought to be suffering from a viral infection of the upper respiratory tract. On the third or fourth day of the illness there is a sudden fall in temperature, the child's general condition improves, and the true nature of the illness is revealed by the appearance of a faint pink macular rash on the trunk, neck, and proximal parts of the limbs. The rash is transient and disappears within 24 hours. This pattern is diagnostic of the disease. The infant makes a rapid recovery without complications. Occasionally febrile convulsions may accompany the preeruptive phase of the illness, but they seldom cause neurological sequelae. Treatment is supportive with antipyretics.

Rubella (German Measles)

When contracted in childhood, rubella is one of the mildest of infectious illnesses. The intense interest centered on the virus stems from the fact that it is a known cause of congenital deformities. The association was first observed in 1941 by Gregg, who recorded a high incidence of congenital cataracts in children whose mothers had contracted rubella in the first trimester of pregnancy. Next it was found that other congenital deformities — notably congenital heart disease, deafness, and eye defects — were common following maternal rubella. Rubella virus is the main virus known to have a consistent relationship with congenital deformities. Because of the teratogenic effects of rubella virus, this fact has great significance, as women in early pregnancy may not realize that they are at risk. Since the widespread use of live attenuated rubella vaccine, the role of rubella virus in causing congenital deformities has become less prominent than that of some other viruses, notably CMV.

Epidemiology

Although sporadic cases of rubella may arise at any time in a community, the disease has a tendency to occur in epidemic form. Because the rash upon which clinical diagnosis is based may be present for no more than a few hours, its recognition is difficult.

Rubella is spread by infected respiratory secretions. The incubation period preceding the appearance of the rash is usually between 13 and 16 days but may be as long as 21 days. Virus can be isolated from the blood and throat of an infected host up to a week before the rash appears, and from the pharynx up to 7 days afterward. The period of infectivity preceding the first recognizable clinical features further adds

to the risk of viral transmission during early pregnancy. Furthermore, infants born with congenital rubella continue to excrete the virus for many months, thus posing a potential hazard for those who come in contact with them.

Clinical Features

Because of the mild nature of rubella and the probable propagation of the virus by those suffering from subclinical infections, the time sequences of clinical features are not definite. Approximately 2 weeks after the infection has been contracted, there may be mild catarrhal symptoms and malaise. At this stage slightly enlarged and tender lymph glands may be noticed in the occipital, postauricular, and posterior cervical regions. The rash of rubella appears simultaneously, but mild symptoms may be present for about 48 hours before the glandular enlargement. The rash is maculopapular, but the macules and papules are smaller and more discrete and have a fainter color than the rash of measles. Sometimes the macules are fine and superficially resemble scarlet fever. The distribution is mainly on the trunk, anteriorly and posteriorly, but the rash may also appear on the face and proximal parts of the limbs. The duration may be quite short and is rarely greater than 48 hours. This rash can often be brought out by the application of heat, as by placing the patient in a warm bath.

Constitutional features are minor. Sometimes there is malaise, anorexia, and the usual vague aches and pains associated with viral infections. Blood examination shows a slight leukopenia with a relative lymphocytosis.

Complications

In all except the fetus, complications are remarkably few. Neurologic complications such as encephalitis, myelitis, and optic neuritis are rare. Thrombocytopenic purpura, myocarditis, and pericarditis have been described on occasion. Polyarthritis is common in adults but rare in children.

FETAL COMPLICATIONS. Congenital heart lesions are most likely to result when infection occurs during the eighth week of pregnancy. These lesions include patent ductus arteriosus, atrial or ventricular septal defects, and pulmonary stenosis.

At the tenth week of pregnancy the eyes are the organs ordinarily affected. The usual complication is cataract; sometimes there is a unilateral retinopathy, microphthalmia, or glaucoma.

Deafness is the chief complication when the infection occurs in the latter part of the first trimester or the early part of the second trimester of pregnancy. Careful assessment of children whose mothers were at risk during pregnancy reveals that partial deafness is more common than was realized on previous observations. This may raise the complication rate from fetal rubella to the order of 30 to 50%. Complications involving the central nervous system, including microcephaly and cerebral agenesis, probably result from rubella in the early part of the first trimester.

Additional complications of fetal rubella with a high fatality rate were reported during the epidemic in the United States in 1964 to 1965. These were congenital thrombocytopenic purpura, jaundice, neutropenia, and hepatosplenomegaly, as well as radiological abnormalities in the long bones.

Delayed manifestations of the congenital rubella syndrome include diabetes mellitus (20% of patients by 35 years of age), thyroid abnormalities (5%), and progressive rubella panencephalitis.

Laboratory Diagnosis

Rubella virus can be grown from throat washings, blood, feces, and urine, but the techniques are cumbersome. Serologic tests are widely available, and the diagnosis can be confirmed by either detection of rubella-specific IgM antibodies or demonstrating a fourfold or greater rise in rubella-specific IgG titers.

Treatment

The treatment of an established case of rubella is entirely symptomatic. The condition is mild, and patients can be managed at home.

The management of a pregnant woman exposed to rubella in the first trimester of pregnancy poses some problems. The risk to the fetus of congenital deformities may be as high as 50%, but for severe deformities it is less than 20%. A decision to undertake therapeutic abortion will be affected by legal, religious, or cultural views.

The live rubella vaccine is now routinely given to children at 15 months of age. Susceptible older children and adults should also be immunized. One dose of vaccine confers long-term immunity.

Smallpox (Variola)

This disease has now been eradicated through effective national vaccination campaigns supported by the World Health Organization.

Yellow Fever

Yellow fever is an acute viral infection characterized by jaundice and hemorrhage from various sites. The disease is found only in the tropical belts of Africa and South America.

Etiology

The virus that causes yellow fever is a flavivirus. The disease is transmitted by a mosquito of the genus *Aedes* after it bites a human host suffering from the active disease. The virus is then incubated in the mosquito for 9 to 12 days and is transferred when another host is bitten. An incubation period of 3 to 6 days occurs before clinical features of the illness develop.

Clinical Manifestations

In areas where the disease is endemic, the attack rate is probably high. It is thought that in most infected hosts a mild subclinical attack develops. When infection becomes clinically manifest, it is probable that the attack is severe, with a high chance of a fatal outcome. The initial features of the illness are nonspecific, consisting of symptoms common to most serious viral infections. The patient suffers from chills, severe headache, backache, pain in the limbs, photophobia, and conjunctival injection. The temperature rises rapidly. Abdominal pain and tenderness, particularly in the epigastrium, and vomiting occur. After 3 days, slowly increasing jaundice develops. Hemorrhages occur in the form of petechiae, bleeding gums, epistaxis, and hematemesis. Cardiac dilatation, hypotension, and oliguria sometimes leading to anuria may develop. On urinalysis, there is heavy albuminuria, and the urinary sediment contains numerous casts. Blood examination reveals anemia and leukopenia. Raised blood urea nitrogen and serum bilirubin levels, with a prolonged prothrombin time, may be demonstrated. Increasing drowsiness leading to coma or convulsions indicates that encephalitis is a complicating feature. The illness lasts about 6 days. If the outcome is not fatal, recovery is rapid and complete.

Immunization

An attack of yellow fever confers a lifelong immunity. It is essential that travelers visiting the yellow fever belts of Africa and South America be immunized against the disease with the 17D vaccine. Immunity lasts for several years. Traditional preventive measures consist of campaigns to control or eradicate the breeding of mosquitoes in endemic areas.

Treatment

There is no specific treatment for yellow fever once the attack has developed. Management is supportive. Patients should be kept completely at rest because of the likely complication of myocarditis and cardiac failure.

Dengue and Dengue Hemorrhagic Fever

Dengue fever is a disease found widely in tropical countries of Southeast Asia and the western Pacific region. It is caused by a group of dengue viruses which are flaviviruses (arbovirus group B) of the family Togaviridae, which includes yellow fever virus (see Table 20-3). There are four distinct antigenic types of dengue virus. Each causes dengue fever in humans through the mosquito vector *Aedes aegypti*. Infection with dengue virus of any specific type confers lifelong immunity to that type. Uncomplicated dengue fever is usually mild or subclinical in children and more severe in adults. The severe form of dengue hemorrhagic fever (DHF) was first recognized in children in Manila in 1953 and subsequently identified in many children in most neighboring tropical countries. It is now a global pediatric infectious disease problem of major dimensions. Viremic humans through rapid travel spread dengue widely throughout the western Pacific region.

Clinical Features

An infant or a young child presents with fever, petechiae, hepatomegaly, thrombocytopenia, hemoconcentration, and shock. The fever usually lasts 2 to 7 days and terminates with a sudden drop in body temperature, clamminess, restlessness, cold extremities, and signs of circulatory failure with fall in blood pressure and imperceptible pulse. The fall in platelet count precedes a hematocrit rise. All degrees of severity occur. Massive bleeding leading to death occurs in about one-third of patients in shock. Mild hemorrhage with petechiae is due to vascular factors and thrombocytopenia, but gross bleeding is due to more complex mechanisms involving not only thrombocytopenia but impaired platelet function, disseminated intravascular clotting (DIC), and coagulation defects from liver dysfunction. This combination of factors leads to multiple organ involvement, irreversibility, and death.

Treatment

The immediate treatment is the same as for shock and circulatory failure. If there are massive hemorrhages, trans-fusion with fresh blood should be given. Salicylates should be avoided, because they can cause bleeding and acidosis.

Rabies

In the United States most cases of rabies result from skunk, raccoon, fox, cattle, cat, dog, or bat bites. Worldwide, the animals involved include wolves, foxes, bats, squirrels, jackals, coyotes, skunks, mongooses, chipmunks, rats, mice, and weasels.

Clinical Manifestations

The usual incubation period is 1 to 3 months, but in rare situations it may be as short as 9 days or as long as a year. The incubation period is related to the site of the animal bite and is considerably shorter when the bite is in one of the proximal areas such as the face.

The initial symptoms are those of a peripheral neuritis involving the nerve used by the virus to travel from the point of entry to the central nervous system. Initial symptoms of pain, tingling, numbness, and weakness progress to diffuse encephalomyelitis and the characteristic pharyngeal and laryngeal spasm known as hydrophobia. Finally, fever, delirium, and convulsions occur, and death ensues. Intensive symptomatic care has led to the report of at least three survivors.

The physician must be aware of the prevalence of rabies virus in his or her own community. This information is usually available from local health departments. Care of exposed individuals includes local care by thoroughly flushing all wounds and cleaning with soap and water, administration of human rabies immune globulin (HRIG) both intramuscularly as well as locally by infiltrating the wound, and actively immunizing patients with the human diploid cell vaccine (HDCV). Five doses of the vaccine are given on days 1, 3, 7, 14, and 28 postexposure.

Children exposed to rabies as a result of animal bites may also need booster doses of tetanus toxoid. Wherever possible, the animal that bit the patient should be turned over to the local health authority in order to determine from clinical observation (and postmortem examination, if it dies) whether or not it was rabid.

Human Immunodeficiency Virus Infection

The family Retroviridae includes viruses whose genetic information is carried in the form of single-stranded RNA contained within an outer glycoprotein envelope. A special enzyme within this envelope, a viral DNA polymerase called reverse transcriptase, allows information to pass in a "retro" direction from RNA to DNA. Through this process of reverse transcription double-stranded DNA is produced and can become integrated into the host chromosome, and remain latent or enter a phase of active viral replication. In 1978 the first of the pathogenic human retroviruses was identified. Human T-cell lymphotropic virus I (HTLV-I) is now recognized as the etiologic agent of adult T-cell leukemia and has been found in association with tropical spastic paraparesis. HTLV-II, identified in 1982, has recently been found to be prevalent among certain groups of intravenous drug users and a relationship with lymphoproliferative disorders has been suggested. The most well known member of this family is the human immunodeficiency virus (HIV-1), previously called human T-cell lymphotropic virus III (HTLV-III), lymphadenopathy-associated virus (LAV), or AIDS-related virus (ARV). This is currently the acknowledged cause of the acquired immunodeficiency syndrome (AIDS). A closely related member of this family, HIV-2 has also been identified in association with a similar immunodeficiency state. Another member of this family, HTLV-V, has been suggested as the etiologic agent of mycoses fungoides, an unusual cutaneous malignancy. Viruses from this family share a common ability to be transmitted by sexual intercourse, by exposure to blood or blood products, by use of contaminated needles, or vertically from mother to offspring. They are associated with the presence of immunodeficiency, malignancies, and progressive neurological disorders.

Epidemiology of Pediatric HIV Infection

HIV infection is now the leading cause of immunodeficiency in infants and children, with 1561 AIDS cases reported as of April 30, 1989. This number is expected to double by 1991. Of children with AIDS, 79% are the product of parents at known risk for infection, 12% received contaminated blood products, 6% are hemophiliacs, and in 3% the route of acquisition is undetermined. These figures will change as the percentage infected perinatally increases and that related to the transfusions decreases. This has serious implications for the delivery of health care to these children as they frequently come from extremely unstable home situations, often the product of young, single, and less educated mothers who are not infrequently coping with the impact of HIV infection on their own health.

Though HIV has been isolated from many body fluids, transmission occurs only by sexual contact, contact with infected blood or blood products, or vertically from mother to infant. As vertical transmission is the main source of HIV infection within the pediatric population, the epidemiology of pediatric AIDS reflects that of the infected mothers and remains concentrated in the larger urban areas where prostitution and intravenous drug use abound. The incidence of HIV infection is 13.6 times higher among black women and 10.2 times higher among Hispanic than among white women, accounting for the disproportionate representation of black and Hispanic children among children with AIDS.

Perinatal transmission rates in the order of 33% have now been reported. Factors influencing the rate and time of transmission remain to be determined. Though a fetal embryopathy suggestive of early infection has been described, its presence has not been accepted by all. Recovery of virus from the early products of conception remains the most convincing evidence of early transmission. Postnatal infection attributed to passage of the virus through breast milk has also been described. In all likelihood transmission will eventually be proved to occur during many stages of pregnancy, delivery, and possibly during the postnatal period if breast feeding is allowed. Of major importance in all studies of transmission is the lack of nonsexual transmission to household contacts, highlighting the fact that in the absence of known risk behaviors, this is not a readily transmissible disease.

Pathogenesis

The virus must enter the host cells by binding to the CD4 receptor present on the surface of T-helper lymphocytes. Attachment is followed by penetration and release of the viral core proteins into the cell. These may then, through the mechanism of reverse transcription, initiate viral replication or become integrated into the host-cell genome and enter a period of latency. The CD4+ cell is one of the main regulator cells influencing other T-cell subsets, B cells, and phagocytic cells. Viral infection depletes these cells with consequent dysregulation of the immune system. Other cells that may also be infected include cells of the monocyte-macrophage line, neural cells, hepatocytes, and possibly also renal cells. The virus thus exerts its effect both by direct cellular invasion and through dysregulation of the immune system.

Clinical Manifestations

The initial manifestations of disease may be subtle and insidious; failure to thrive, lymphadenopathy, slowly progressive organomegaly, an increased incidence of common infections (otitis, sinusitis, pneumonia), or it may present dramatically with the development of an unusual infection such as *Pneumocystis carinii* pneumonia (PCP).

Symptomatic acute infection, with a mononucleosislike syndrome, is rarely if ever recognized in pediatrics. Common clinical features include malaise, fever, lymphadenopathy (which may often regress in the later stages of disease), hepatosplenomegaly, respiratory tract infections, chronic persistent or recurrent diarrhea, failure to thrive with significant delays both in weight gain and in stature, and the presence of persistent mucocutaneous candidiasis.

The development of a lymphoid interstitial pneumonitis occurs in nearly half of all cases of pediatric AIDS but is rarely seen in adults. It may antedate the presence of other features by considerable periods of time and has been regarded as a good prognostic factor. In contrast, neurological involvement as the initial manifestation of disease is a bad prognostic sign. Developmental delay, loss of developmental milestones, motor spasticity, deterioration in cognitive ability, and frank encephalopathy may all occur. When detailed psychometric testing is undertaken, neurological impairment may be detected in over 60% of children with AIDS.

Cardiomyopathy, nephropathy, and myopathy may also occur but are less frequent manifestations of this infection. Hematological manifestations of disease are common. Isolated thrombocytopenia may antedate all other features of disease; similarly, neutropenia and anemia occur but are more often associated with the presence of other features. In contrast to adult patients, malignancies such as Kaposi's sarcoma or lymphoma are rarely encountered.

Children are more likely than adults to develop problems with recurrent bacterial infections. *Streptococcus pneumoniae, Haemophilus influenzae,* and *Salmonella* are frequent pathogens. Mycobacterial infections occur both in adult and pediatric patients. In children, infections with the atypical mycobacteria predominate and may be either localized or disseminated with involvement of virtually every organ system.

Infections with other opportunistic pathogens also occur. Oropharyngeal candidiasis is an almost universal problem faced by these children. Disease progression with involvement of the esophagus, presenting with dysphagia and retrosternal pain, may occur. *Cryptococcus neoformans,* an important cause of meningitis in adult AIDS patients, rarely infects children. Extrameningeal disease including pneumonia, fungemia, and widely disseminated forms of this infection can occur. *P. carinii,* a ubiquitous protozoan, is the most common serious opportunist of pediatric patients. Cough, fever, and tachypnea are its typical symptoms. Hypoxemia, a characteristic feature, may be inapparent initially.

Bilateral diffuse interstitial infiltrates are usually found on chest radiograph. As any number of diverse patterns may be found, however, this diagnosis may neither be definitively made or excluded radiologically. Extrapulmonary disease with *P. carinii* is extremely rare. To confirm the diagnosis of PCP, identification of the organism in the sputum, bronchoalveolar lavage fluid or in a biopsy specimen is required. While recovery of the organism from normally expectorated sputum is unusual, techniques of sputum induction using hypertonic saline have been developed which can avert the need for bronchoscopy. Trimethoprim-sulfamethoxazole (TMP-SMX) is currently the drug of first choice for this infection. Pentamidine, an effective though more toxic drug, can be used when TMP-SMX is contraindicated or where deterioration continues in the face of therapy. The incidence of PCP in high-risk populations may be significantly reduced by the use of prophylactic TMP-SMX or aerosolized pentamidine. Cryptosporidium, a protozoan which causes self-limited diarrheal illness in toddlers, causes intractable diarrhea in patients with AIDS. There is no effective therapy. Spiramycin, an agent of some reported benefit in immunocompetent patients, is disappointing. Use of a period of total gut rest with parenteral nutrition may be beneficial for some. Cytomegalovirus (CMV) can produce serious life-threatening disease such as pneumonia, hepatitis, cholecystitis, enteritis, retinitis, and encephalitis. Ganciclovir (DHPG) has been used to control CMV retinitis and enteritis but has proved disappointing in the treatment of pneumonia. Other members of the herpes family of viruses, HSV 1, 2, and VZV, may all cause serious and recurrent disease in AIDS patients necessitating therapy with systemic agents. The development of varicella in the patient with AIDS should be regarded with the same gravity as its development in other immunocompromised children. Exposure should be avoided where practical. If exposure is documented, the use of varicella-zoster immune globulin (VZIG) is warranted, and if clinical disease develops, therapy with intravenous acyclovir should be instituted.

Laboratory Findings

The complete blood count can be normal. Lymphopenia, a characteristic feature in adults, is less common in children. On lymphocyte subset analysis there is a characteristic depletion of the CD4+ cells with reversal of the CD4/CD8 ratio. Hypergammaglobulinemia or, more rarely, hypogammaglobulinema may occur. Cutaneous anergy is virtually universal. Nonspecific abnormalities of liver function with mild elevations of transaminases are common.

Diagnosis

The initial screening tool is an ELISA, which detects antibody to the virus. If positive, it must be confirmed by repetition and through antibody detection by western blot analysis, a more specific methodology. Viral culture is reserved for investigational use. Assays detecting a structural protein, the P24 antigen, may be useful in establishing the diagnosis both in the rare situation of seronegativity and in young infants, in whom presence of maternal antibody can confound the picture. It may also be used to follow the course of disease or monitor the impact of therapy. The polymerase chain reaction may allow detection of even minute quantities of virus. Once infection is confirmed, a full laboratory assessment of hematological and immunological parameters should be undertaken. As progressive multiorgan involvement is the rule, additional base-line evaluations including chest radiograph, ophthalmological examination, echocardiography, and even computerized tomography of the central nervous system should be considered.

Treatment

The treatment of HIV-infected children has been largely supportive in nature. Nutritional status should be maintained and intercurrent infections promptly treated. Caretakers must be educated regarding initial signs of infection and vigilance for the development of serious infections such as PCP maintained so that early treatment may be initiated. Children at high risk should be considered for PCP prophylaxis. The use of IVIG has been advocated, though not proven, to decrease the incidence of serious bacterial infections. IVIG may be helpful in the management of the thrombocytopenia encountered in this disease. Azidothymidine (AZT) is the only available antiretroviral agents licensed for use in children. A variety of other agents are under investigation. Initial trials of AZT in symptomatic children have proved it to be beneficial. Improvements in clinical parameters such as weight gain, decreases in lymphadenopathy, organomegaly, and neurological deficit have all been detected. Changes in immunological function including increases in CD4 cell count, CD4/CD8 ratio, and decreases in immunoglobulin levels have been reported. These initial results await confirmation in the larger trials that are currently underway. AZT has side effects which are both dose and duration related. While nausea, headache, fever, and malaise have all been encountered, it is the associated bone marrow suppression that is the dose-limiting factor. This together with recent reports of in vitro resistance to AZT make it imperative to develop alternate agents. The most potent member of this family in vitro, ddC, has undergone preliminary study in adults but is associated with serious toxicity, a painful peripheral neuropathy. It may, however, be useful when used in combination with other agents in a way that would limit the total exposure to it. The latest in this group of agents to undergo clinical trial is ddI. It does not appear to be associated with myelotoxicity. As yet it is too early to reach any conclusions regarding its potential role in our armamentarium against HIV infection. Soluble CD4 has now been produced by genetic engineering and is available in a purified form. Administration of CD4 would potentially block all binding sites of the virus and prevent infection. Trials are currently underway in adults and will soon commence within the pediatric population. Ultimately a combination of agents may be necessary for effective control of this disease.

Prevention

HIV infection in pediatrics is a preventable disease. It is not as yet a curable one. Thus, it is clear that major efforts need to be made to prevent the transmission of infection. Children and adolescents must be educated regarding the risks of drug abuse and sexual promiscuity and taught ways of preventing disease transmission. Identification of HIV-seropositive women and counselling them regarding the risk of transmission to their offspring remain difficult issues both ethically and practically. The ultimate goal should be to prevent infection of these future mothers and, thus, eradicate vertical transmission. No vaccines are currently available.

Other Viral Infections

Lymphocytic Choriomeningitis

This condition is a generalized infection of worldwide distribution. It is most common in children, adolescents, and young adults. There have been reports of meningitis in neonates whose mothers were infected. The most prominent clinical features are those of meningitis that is benign and self-limiting. The infecting agent is the lymphocytic choriomeningitis virus (LCMV). It was first isolated in 1934 from a patient with nonbacterial meningitis. Subsequently mice were identified as the host animals. Isolations have also been made from hamsters, guinea pigs, and dogs.

CLINICAL FEATURES. Outbreaks are most common in winter and spring. The incubation period is 6 to 13 days. The illness commences with influenzalike symptoms of fever, headache, malaise, nausea, back pain, sore throat, fatigue, and myalgia. Convulsions may occur in young children. Meningeal irritation does not develop in most patients, and the nature of the infection remains undetermined. When the infection involves the meninges, clinical features are indistinguishable from those of other causes of viral meningitis.

DIAGNOSIS. The origin of the infection and the identity of the virus may be suspected if there is a known contact with mice, guinea pigs, or hamsters. The virus can be isolated from CSF or throat washings. This is the only specific diagnosis. Antibody titers are helpful if a rise in IgG titer can be demonstrated between acute and convalescent sera.

CSF findings resemble those found in meningitis caused by other viruses — enteroviruses, mumps, EBV, arboviruses. Early in the course of meningitis there may be a predominance of polymorphonuclear cells, but in a day or two the pleocytosis is dominated by mononuclear cells, usually 300 to 3000/ml. CSF protein is slightly raised and glucose is low in one-third of patients and normal in the rest. CSF findings return to normal in 2 to 3 weeks.

PROGNOSIS. The course is usually benign and self-limiting in 7 to 10 days, but weakness and fatigue can persist for weeks. A few fatal cases have been recorded. Necropsy has revealed lymphocytic infiltration of meninges and other organ involvement — pneumonia and liver necrosis.

TREATMENT. Treatment is symptomatic and supportive.

PREVENTION. Prevention consists in control of rodents in households.

Coryza (the Common Cold)

Coryza is characterized by nasal catarrh, congested nasal mucosa, and rhinorrhea. Symptoms are uncomfortable rather than distressing, and the condition is self-limiting, lasting from 5 to 10 days. Complications in children usually take the form of bronchitis, which may persist for 1 to 2 weeks. The main concern in childhood is the high infectivity rate and the consequent rapid transmissibility in school children, leading to absenteeism. In infants, nasal obstruction causes feeding difficulties.

The syndrome of common cold is caused by numerous agents, mainly viral. The most important etiological agents in adults are the rhinoviruses, but they are said to be less important in infants and young children, a statement that has not been fully substantiated.

Rhinoviruses are RNA viruses. Over 100 distinct antigenic types have been described. Infection with one type confers long-lasting immunity but does not protect against infection by other types. Transmission is by close person-to-

person contact, aerosol fomites, or by autoinoculation following contamination of the hands.

TREATMENT. There are only supportive measures at the present time.

Molluscum Contagiosum

This condition is caused by a poxvirus. The disease is contracted by direct contact with infected subjects, possibly by fomites, as it is usually found in environments where hygiene is poor. Once established, the lesions spread by autoinoculation.

The lesions are smooth, firm, papular, and shiny, often described as "pearly." Lesions grow slowly and measure 1 to 10 cm in diameter. They tend to have umbilicated centers. They are confined to skin and mucous membranes and are mainly found on the trunk.

DIAGNOSIS. The lesions are typical and should not be confused with warts. The natural history of the illness distinguishes it from chickenpox and skin allergies.

TREATMENT. The lesions resolve spontaneously but may take years to do so, and there is the risk of autoinoculation. They can be easily eradicated by curettage under local anesthesia or by application of corrosive agents, e.g., trichloracetic acid.

Human Parvovirus B19 Infection

Human parvovirus B19 was first discovered in 1975. Infection is commonly asymptomatic. The most commonly recognized clinical illness caused by this virus is erythema infectiosum (fifth disease), a mild childhood illness characterized by a facial rash with a typical "slapped cheek" appearance and a reticulated rash on the trunk and extremities. The virus is also the major cause of transient aplastic crises in patients with sickle-cell anemia and other chronic hemolytic anemias (e.g., beta-thalassemia, hereditary spherocytosis). Other disease associations include polyarthritis, a severe chronic anemia in patients with congenital immunodeficiencies, HIV-related immunodeficiency, or acute lymphocytic leukemia and fetal infections. Pregnant women who develop a parvovirus B19 infection may sometimes suffer fetal death or deliver a newborn with hydrops fetalis, but the majority of fetuses are not adversely affected by the maternal infection. The virus infects erythroid precursors in the bone marrow, and this leads to interruption of normal red blood cell production. Recovery is heralded by the reappearance of reticulocytes in the peripheral smears about 7 to 10 days later. This transient red cell aplasia is clinically inapparent for otherwise normal people but may be sufficient to cause an aplastic crisis in individuals with chronic hemolytic anemias. The diagnosis is usually confirmed serologically by detection of virus-specific IgM or the demonstration of a fourfold or greater rise in virus-specific IgG titers. No specific therapy is available. Intrauterine transfusions may be helpful for fetuses developing hydrops fetalis as detected by ultrasonography.

Verrucae

Warts are caused by human papillomaviruses, DNA viruses 45 to 55 nm in diameter, of the papovavirus family. Transmission is by direct contact, possibly by fomites. Only humans are infected. Recent interest in the transmissibility of human papillomaviruses has centered on their oncogenic potential, particularly that of genital warts, and their relationship to cervical carcinoma and other malignancies.

Hepatitis

Hepatic inflammation may be manifested clinically or biochemically during the course of many infections including CMV, EBV, HIV, and adenoviral infections. This section is concerned with those infections in which hepatitis is the main clinical manifestation of disease, specifically hepatitis A, B, non-A, non-B hepatitis-associated viruses, and the delta agent.

Hepatitis A

The hepatitis A virus (HAV), a small RNA enterovirus, causes a highly contagious but usually self-limited hepatitis.

EPIDEMIOLOGY. Endemic in the community, feco-oral spread is the main route of transmission. Infection is commonly passed amongst household contacts or contacts within closed communities. Transmission within day-care centers is problematic. The congregation of young and, often, untoilet-trained children, who tend to be asymptomatically infected, facilitates rapid spread of infection to older children and adults. Passive immunization by administration of immune globulin may be necessary to avoid a major outbreak. Food, water, and shellfish have all served as vehicles of transmission. Parenteral transmission is rare. After inoculation, the incubation period of 15 to 50 days (average 28–30) is followed by the development of viremia, which precedes the onset of hepatic disease. The period of greatest infectivity is the 2 weeks prior to the onset of symptoms when fecal shedding is maximal. It may persist for up to 12 days after onset of symptoms but rarely persists beyond the time of maximal elevation of liver enzymes. The prevalence of serological evidence of previous HAV infection increases steadily with age, ranging from 5 to 13% seropositivity among children less than 4 years of age to about 50% by the age of 50. The severity of clinical disease is age-related; younger children have mild to asymptomatic disease with increased severity of symptoms with advancing age.

CLINICAL MANIFESTATIONS. The clinical features of hepatitis are not useful in determining the etiologic agent. In most cases of hepatitis A infection is brief and self-limited. Typical features include malaise, fatigue, fever, anorexia, nausea, emesis, icterus, abdominal pain or discomfort, diarrhea, and arthralgias. The urine may be noted to be darker in nature and the stool pale.

DIAGNOSIS. The diagnosis may be evident based on the history of documented exposure and presence of characteristic features. The elevation in liver enzymes is often dramatic in nature with values in excess of 1000 I.U./L not infrequently encountered. Serological confirmation of the diagnosis depends on demonstration of the presence of anti-HAV antibodies. The presence of specific anti-HAV IgM confirms acute infection. It appears early, coincident with the development of symptoms and is short lived. Anti-HAV IgG appears later, often after peak shedding of the virus in the stool, and persists indefinitely. Its presence confirms past but not acute infection.

PREVENTION. Immunoprophylaxis with serum immune globulin (SIG) is effective. Administration to close contacts of infected cases is recommended. Guidelines are available regarding the control of infection in high-risk settings including day-care centers and institutions. They generally involve the implementation of good standards of hygiene together with the administration of SIG to people at risk. School room exposure is not usually regarded as an indication for immunoprophylaxis. Preexposure prophylaxis is recommended for seronegative travellers to areas of high endemicity.

Hepatitis B

Hepatitis B, previously referred to as serum hepatitis, is one of the main causes of chronic hepatitis, cirrhosis, and hepatocellular carcinoma. The etiologic agent, hepatitis B virus (HBV), is a DNA virus whose structure has been well characterized. The viral surface, composed of hepatitis B surface antigen (HBsAg), surrounds a 27 nm core, the hepatitis B core antigen (HBcAg), and a soluble antigen, the hepatitis B e antigen (HBeAg) which also originates in the core. Serological detection of these antigens and of the host's immunologic response to them, the production of hepatitis B surface antibody (HBsAb), hepatitis B core antibody (HBcAb), and clearance of the HBeAg are critical in determining the presence and stage of infection.

EPIDEMIOLOGY. Distribution is worldwide, though the frequency of infection varies considerably from area to area. Highly endemic in Asia, China, and the Far East, it is of low endemicity within the western world. Within the United States, prevalence rates vary from 100% for certain high-risk groups to 5% within the general population. Transmission occurs vertically from mother to infant, sexually, and parenterally. Risk factors for infection include sexual promiscuity, intravenous drug abuse, history of frequent blood transfusions, occupational exposures, and place of origin.

Perinatal transmission is of major importance in pediatrics. Transmission may occur from mothers who acquire their infection near the time of delivery or who are chronic carriers of HBsAg. It takes place primarily at the time of delivery through contact, aspiration, or swallowing of infected maternal blood. Transplacental transmission is rare.

Transmission through the use of infected blood or blood products has decreased since the advent of serological testing of donated blood but is not yet fully eradicated as infective viral particles may occasionally be present at levels below the limits of detection. The incubation period of infection is longer than that associated with HAV, varying from 45 to 160 days (average 60–120). Infectivity may persist indefinitely in carriers. Though infectivity correlates best with HBeAg positivity, individuals who fail to clear their HBsAg remain infective even in the absence of detectable e antigen.

CLINICAL MANIFESTATIONS. The range of clinical symptoms is similar to that observed in those with HAV infections, though the onset of disease may be more insidious, and a subacute course is usual. In most instances, neonates are asymptomatic during the acute phase but are significantly at risk for the development of chronic hepatitis and hepatocellular carcinoma in later life. Hepatitis B may be anicteric in children. Arthralgia and rash may occur early in the course of infection. The Gianotti-Crosti syndrome is a papular acrodermatitis associated with the presence of lymphadenopathy and anicteric hepatitis in young HBV-infected infants.

DIAGNOSIS. The diagnosis is made by detection of hepatitis-associated antigens, and resolution of disease is heralded by their clearance together with the development of an appropriate antibody response. These appear in a predictable sequence such that the stage of infection may be determined. HBsAg and HBeAg are the first serological markers to reach detectable levels appearing coincident or just antedating symptomatic infection. Antibody to core antigen (anti-HBc) is the first evidence of immunological response. When it appears the initial antigens may remain detectable in the serum or have commenced their decline. Occasionally, on serological testing, this is the only detectable marker of infection during the window period between antigen positivity and appearance of the remaining antibodies heralding clearance of infection. At this stage, antigenemia may be present below the limits of detectability, and the patient should be considered potentially infectious. The appearance of anti-HBeAg (HBeAb) first and subsequently anti-HBsAg (HBsAb) indicates successful resolution of infection. Patients who persist as carriers of this infection fail consistently to develop anti-HBsAg (HBsAb).

MANAGEMENT. There is no effective therapy for HBV infectional though a variety of agents including immune modulators are currently under investigation. Prevention is possible and should be our goal. A genetically engineered recombinant vaccine has replaced that obtained from plasma and is devoid of any putative infective risks which limited full acceptance of the original vaccine. It is effective and should be considered for use in all high-risk persons. Hepatitis B immune globulin (HBIG) provides effective temporary prophylaxis when used either pre- or postexposure. Successful prevention of neonatal infection has been achieved by the administration of HBIG in combination with the initiation of an active vaccination schedule within 72 hours of birth.

Delta Hepatitis

The etiologic agent is a defective virus which may only cause infection in the presence of HBV. The delta antigen is detectable in the acute phase of infection, and antibody to it is indicative of past infection.

Non-A, non-B Hepatitis

Hepatitis is also caused by a number of transmissible, but as yet unidentified, agents. In the United States most cases of non-A, non-B hepatitis are transfusion-related while in the Far East the most common cause of non-A, non-B infection is water-borne. Most recently an agent, now designated hepatitis C, has been identified as the etiologic agent of a proportion of transfusion-related cases. The development of screening tests for hepatitis C may eliminate a large percentage of posttransfusion hepatitis.

Bishara J. Freij and Karina M. Butler

Rickettsial, Mycotic, and Protozoan Infections

Rickettsial Infections

Etiology and Epidemiology

Rickettsiae are pleomorphic coccobacilli, but they are also obligate intracellular parasites and cannot generally be grown in cell-free media. For most of them, the natural life cycle involves specific animal reservoirs and multiplication in an arthropod host. Animal-to-human transmission occurs incidentally in association with the ecology of specific arthropod vectors. Knowing the patient's occupational and recreational exposure or his travel history should heighten the index of suspicion for the infection and helps in diagnosis.

Rickettsioses comprise four groups: (1) typhus, (2) spotted fevers, (3) Q fever, and (4) trench fever. Their salient epidemiologic and clinical features are summarized in Table 20-5. In addition, other spotted rickettsial diseases include the North Asian tick-borne disease (caused by *Rickettsia sibirica*), Queensland tick typhus (caused by *R. australis*), and the Fièvre Boutonneuse (caused by *R. conorii*), which occurs throughout Africa, the Middle East, and Mediterranean Europe and India.

Clinical Features

Except for Q fever, common features of rickettsial infections include an acute onset of fever, chills, headache, photophobia, myalgia, prostration, respiratory symptoms, and a generalized rash involving also the hands and soles. The rash is usually erythematous and maculopapular, with rapid progression to petechiae and purpura. In some diseases, a local papular primary lesion with central necrosis (eschar) is found at the site of the arthropod attachment to the human host. Regional adenopathy can be found. The infection can be self-limited, or in severe cases of Rocky Mountain spotted fever or epidemic typhus, multiorgan involvement, encephalitic signs, vascular collapse, and death can occur.

Diagnosis

Rickettsial infections can be confirmed by specific serological tests, either by complement fixation or by indirect immunofluorescent antibodies (IFA). The detection of serum *Proteus* agglutinins (Weil-Felix reaction) is nonspecific and unreliable. Isolation of *Rickettsia* from blood culture may be done with intraperitoneal inoculation of guinea pigs. *R. rickettsii* can be detected by immunofluorescent techniques in infected tissues such as skin lesion biopsy in 50% of the cases.

Clinically, the differential diagnosis includes meningococcemia, viral exanthems, tularemia, leptospirosis, toxic shock syndrome, and Kawasaki's disease.

Treatment

Empiric antibiotic therapy with either tetracycline (for patients older than 8 years of age) or chloramphenicol must be used early to decrease morbidity of the infection, if the suspicion for rickettsial disease is high on the basis of epidemiologic and clinical grounds and without the benefit of serological results, which may take 1 to 3 weeks. Parenteral therapy is advisable in severe cases until the patient is afebrile for at least 2 to 3 days. Total duration of antibiotic therapy is usually 5 to 7 days. Attention should also be given to supportive therapy (e.g., fluids and good nutrition).

Prevention

Control of rickettsial diseases should be aimed at elimination or reduction of ticks and other arthropod vectors and animal reservoirs such as rodents. For Q fever, hygienic practices such as pasteurization of dairy products and adequate desinfection of animal products are important. An effective vaccine exists for epidemic typhus and Q fever for susceptible individuals at risk for contracting the infection by travel or occupational exposure. Infected patients need no specific isolation.

Because of its clinical importance as a cause of morbidity and mortality in the United States, Rocky Mountain spotted fever is discussed here in greater detail.

Rocky Mountain Spotted Fever

There are a few ticks that bite children and may inoculate them with the *Rickettsia rickettsii*. The tick initially acquires this organism from a rodent or from its own tick mother.

Table 20-5. *Epidemiology and Clinical Findings in Common Rickettsial Infections*

Disease	Organism	Animal reservoir	Vector	Geographic distributor	Incubation period (days)	Clinical features (also see text)
Epidemic typhus	R. prowazekii	Humans, body lice, flying squirrels	Body lice	Worldwide	7–10	A recurrent, milder form occurs after a prolonged latent period (Brill-Zinsser disease), not a pediatric problem
Murine (endemic) typhus	R. typhi (mooseri)	Wild rats, mice, other rodents	Rat fleas	Worldwide, sporadic	6–10	A milder disease than epidemic typhus
Scrub typhus	R. tsutsugamushi	Rodent mites	Mites	Asiatic Pacific areas, Japan, India, Australia	6–21	Lymphadenopathy, pneumonitis, myocarditis more common
Rocky Mountain spotted fever ("tick typhus")	R. rickettsii	Dogs, cats, rodents, rabbits, ticks	Wood ticks, dog ticks, Lone Star ticks	Western Hemisphere, especially southeastern US	3–15	Toxicity and neurologic symptoms more common. Rash may be absent initially. Leukopenia and thrombocytopenia common
Rickettsial pox	R. akari	Mice	Mouse mite	Russia, Korea, Africa, some urban areas in US, but very rare	9–14	Mild, self-limiting disease. Primary eschar; generalized papulovesicular rash

Q fever	*R. burnetii*	Sheep, cattle, goats, various arthropods, rodents, birds, cats	Ticks, infected fomites, dairy products	Worldwide	9–28	May be transmitted by contaminated aerosols and fomites. Rash absent; pneumonia and hepatitis common. Can cause endocarditis; Weil-Felix reaction is negative. Rarely, infection can be chronic and relapsing
Trench fever	*R. quintana*	Humans, lice	Body lice	Mexico, N. Africa, Poland, Russia	14–30	Illness may be prolonged, debilitating; relapse common
Ehrlichia	*E. canis*	Dog	*Rhipicephalus sanguineus*, brown dog tick	Recently reported in US, worldwide	13–22	Intraleukocytic parasite. Causes fatal hemorrhagic canine disease. Rash less frequent. Arthralgia, bradycardia, leukopenia, and thrombocytopenia common

Between 2 and 14 days after the bite, the child becomes seriously ill.

Headache, high fever, and chills are prominent for the first 3 days. Then a macular rash, much like the rash of rubeola, appears on the extremities and later extends to other areas. The absence of cough, coryza, and Koplik's spots serves to differentiate Rocky Mountain spotted fever from rubeola. The rash may then become petechial, ecchymotic, confluent, and in a few areas somewhat necrotic. At this point differentiation from meningococcemia is extremely difficult, particularly as headache and drowsiness are prominent in rickettsioses. If the child has meningococcal meningitis along with the meningococcemia, the diagnosis is easy. In the absence of purulent meningitis, one is obligated to obtain appropriate specimens for culture, including staining the petechiae for bacteria, and then institute effective therapy to include the meningococci and the rickettsiae. Ultimately, the results of blood culture and specific complement fixation tests establishes the correct diagnosis.

Because rickettsial infections involve endothelium all over the body, one may now find a wide range of symptoms, e.g., jaundice, convulsions, cardiac failure, pneumonitis, and shock. Prompt institution of antirickettsial therapy with the tetracyclines or chloramphenicol (or both) usually leads to prompt clinical improvement. There may be times when corticosteroid therapy and intravenous fluids including blood and plasma may also be necessary. Digitalization is rarely indicated. Intravascular coagulation with depletion of clotting factors may occur. Judicious use of heparin may be useful.

Because of delay in the development of antibodies, serological tests are of little value in early diagnosis. Biopsied skin samples must be tested using immunofluorescent techniques. If the diagnosis is suspected treatment must be instituted without delay for this life-threatening infection.

Chinh T. Le

Mycotic Infections

Coccidioidomycosis

Coccidioidomycosis has many features suggestive of tuberculosis. It is limited to well-defined areas in California, the southwestern United States, Mexico, and South America.

During the acute phase, headaches, fever, and cough are the predominant symptoms. An erythematous rash, similar to many of the common exanthems, may be seen during this phase. Erythema nodosum may occur later. Rarely, the infection becomes disseminated, with the production of pulmonary cavities, osteomyelitis, lymphadenitis, meningitis, and arthritis.

Diagnostic tests include complement fixation and skin tests as well as isolation of the organism on culture. Elevation of the erythrocyte sedimentation rate and the findings on chest x radiographs may be suggestive of primary tuberculosis.

For patients with mild or moderate disease, no treatment is required. In severe cases, amphotericin B may be needed.

Histoplasmosis

Histoplasmosis is caused by *Histoplasma capsulatum*, a fungus that is widespread in certain geographical locations, especially in the Mississippi and Ohio River valleys. Asymptomatic infections, measured by the presence of a positive skin test or circulating antibodies, are very common in these areas. Progressive disease may occur and seems to be more severe in children less than 4 years of age.

The facultative intracellular parasite grows in the soil, and its spores are inhaled by humans. Pulmonary involvement, including enlarged hilar lymph nodes, and multiple calcifications are the most common lesions seen. The skin, bone marrow, mucous membranes, liver, and spleen may be involved in the acute disseminated form of the disease, resembling reticuloendotheliosis or acute leukemia. Leukopenia and some degree of anemia are often seen in active infections.

The diagnosis is best made by isolating the organism from cultures of the lesions or bone marrow. Complement fixation tests are useful for following the progress of the infection. The histoplasmin skin test should be interpreted with caution. It may be used for epidemiological purposes, but a positive test may indicate current or old infection. There is also a high frequency of false-positive tests, especially in adults, during an active infection. The histoplasmin skin test also affects the interpretation of the serological tests, which are usually more helpful to the physician.

The disease is usually self-limited, and only severe infections should be treated with amphotericin B.

Other Mycotic Infections (Table 20-6)

Actinomycosis produces a chronic low-grade, granulomatous type of inflammatory reaction in the affected tissue or organ.

Blastomycosis is a rare pediatric problem that is very similar to tuberculosis.

Cryptococcosis (torulosis) is primarily a chronic disease

Table 20-6. Mycotic Infections

Disease	Organism	Clinical and laboratory picture	Diagnosis	Therapy
Actinomycosis	*Actinomyces israelii*	Low-grade granulomatous type of inflammatory reaction, usually involving cervical, pulmonary, and abdominal area	Biopsy	Penicillin or tetracycline along with surgery
Blastomycosis	*Blastomyces dermatitidis*	Similar to tuberculosis; primarily respiratory; may produce erythema nodosum	Isolation of organism; skin tests and serum complement fixation tests	Amphotericin B or ketoconazole
Nocardiosis	*Nocardia asteroides*	Pulmonary disease with hematogenous spread; resembles tuberculosis	Isolation of organism	A sulfonamide (? amikacin initially) q TMP/SMX, cycloserine, or erythromycin
Cryptococcosis	*Cryptococcus neoformans*	Primarily CNS in patients with abnormal host defenses; CSF exam resembles that of tuberculous meningitis	Isolation of organism; india ink stain of CSF	Amphotericin B plus flucytosine
Sporotrichosis	*Sporotrichum schenckii*	Deep skin infection spreading to lymph system	Isolation of organism	Potassium iodide, amphotericin B

of the central nervous system characterized by remissions and exacerbations. The disease is becoming more prevalent and is now seen in immunocompromised patients.

Nocardiosis is caused by an acid-fast organism belonging to the Actinomycetaceae family and accounts for many misdiagnosed cases of pulmonary tuberculosis.

Superficial Mycotic Infections

Mycotic organisms may also cause superficial skin infections. Some of these are discussed in Table 20-6. The reader is also referred to Chapter 22.

CANDIDIASIS (MONILIASIS). Infection with *Candida albicans* is a very common pediatric problem. Many normal young infants develop thick white plaques on the gums, mucous membranes of the mouth, and tongue. *Candida albicans* is also a common cause of protracted diaper rash with discrete borders, unresponsive to the usual treatments for ammoniacal dermatitis. It can be confirmed by the examination of skin scrapings. This lesion responds nicely to local nystatin, clotrimazole, or miconazole.

Gastrointestinal moniliasis develops after prolonged antibacterial therapy. Oral and perianal lesions may accompany this form of the infection, which is usually asymptomatic and subsides spontaneously. Serious infections involving the lungs and esophagus may occur but are extremely rare. Persistent moniliasis suggests a defect in resistance, as in

thymic aplasia, or a metabolic abnormality, such as Addison's disease, hypoparathyroidism, or multiple endocrinopathies. The first sign of the last three disorders may be moniliasis of the fingernails. Disseminated or severe infection, may be treated with amphotericin B and flucytosine.

Mohsen Ziai

Protozoal Infections

Amebiasis

Amebiasis is caused by *Entamoeba histolytica*, an intestinal protozoan. Its habitat is the colon, where it lives in the mucosa and submucosa, but it may be transported to other organs, especially the liver. Amebiasis occurs worldwide but is more frequent in the tropics and subtropics. There are two main morphologic stages of the organism — the motile trophozoite and the cyst. Infection occurs after feco-oral transmission of the cyst form.

Intestinal Amebiasis

The disease encompasses a clinical spectrum ranging from only the passage of cysts in an asymptomatic carrier to frank dysentery with colicky abdominal pain and fever accompanied by the passage of trophozoites. The cecum and rectosigmoid colon are most commonly affected. Flask-shaped ulcers with undermined edges are seen, and occasionally the ulcers penetrate through the serosa. In chronic amebiasis intermittent diarrhea and pain or vague discomfort and tenderness in the right or left iliac fossa occur. A granulomatous mass (ameboma) may be palpable in the right iliac fossa.

Hepatic Amebiasis

Hepatic amebiasis follows intestinal amebiasis either during the phase of acute diarrhea or long after the intestinal symptoms have subsided. The trophozoites reach the liver through the radicles of the portal vein, and produce multiple microscopic necrotic foci which may coalesce to form an amebic liver abscess, most frequently in the right lobe. This abscess is filled with a characteristic brownish (anchovy color) pasty material in which trophozoites are scarce.

Symptoms and signs include anorexia, chills, fever, right upper quadrant abdominal pain and tenderness, hepatomegaly, and symptoms of right basilar pneumonia. Jaundice occurs occasionally. Complications include rupture into the pleural space, lung, or peritoneal cavity.

DIAGNOSIS. Trophozoites are identifiable in fresh stools. Specimens obtained by proctoscopy or a fleck of feces obtained from the rectum on a gloved finger may be more useful. It is important to be familiar with the morphological features of E. histolytica and to differentiate this organism from Entamoeba coli. A distinguishing feature is the presence of intracytoplasmic red blood cell debris in the former. Cysts are more easily visualized when the smear is stained with Lugol's iodine solution.

Several serodiagnostic tests are available commercially, but the method of choice is indirect hemagglutination (IHA). IHA titers correlate well with active infection, and the test is most useful in the differentiation of extraintestinal amebiasis from systemic diseases with similar manifestations. Also, stool examinations are usually negative in extraintestinal disease.

TREATMENT. See Table 20-7. The chemotherapeutic agents used are either luminal (nonabsorbable, e.g., diloxanide) or extraluminal (absorbable, e.g., metronidazole), and treatment with the latter alone may not eradicate organisms in the gut lumen.

Toxoplasmosis

Infection with Toxoplasma gondii can be asymptomatic or symptomatic. Symptomatic infection is the disease toxoplasmosis. The majority of infection is asymptomatic; for plasmosis. The majority of infections are asymptomatic; for example, about 50% of the population of the United States is seropositive. The organism is an obligate intracellular parasite that exists in three forms. The tachyzoite or proliferative form is present in acute infection and is responsible for tissue damage. The tissue cyst form is a quiescent infection that can persist lifelong in various organs without causing symptoms. The oocyst is the form shed only in feces of members of the cat family, the definitive host for toxoplasma, and can survive for long periods in water or moist soil. The infection is acquired by ingestion of oocysts that have undergone sporulation or tissue cysts in undercooked meat, especially pork and lamb. Infection may also be acquired transplacentally, resulting in congenital infection. Estimates of the incidence of congenital toxoplasmosis in the United States have varied from 1 in 1000 to 1 in 8000. The incidence is highest when the mother acquires her infection in the third trimester, although severity of disease in the infant is greatest when maternal infection is acquired during the first trimester.

Clinical Features

CONGENITAL TOXOPLASMOSIS. Disease in the newborn varies from clinically inapparent, in most cases, to abortion, stillbirth, or premature or term birth with symptoms. Fever, hydrocephalus or microcephalus, jaundice, hepatosplenomegaly, chorioretinitis, intracerebral calcifications, and cerebrospinal pleocytosis are considered to comprise the classic syndrome of congenital toxoplasmosis. Other common findings include a macular, papular, or petechial rash, pneumonitis, thrombocytopenia, and myocarditis. Many newborns, especially premature infants who look normal at birth, go on to develop sequelae, most commonly chorioretinitis, in the second and third decades of life. Seizures or severe neurologic disability are other late sequelae.

ACUTE ACQUIRED TOXOPLASMOSIS. This occurs in about 10% of postnatally infected individuals, unless the infection is related to an outbreak from spread of oocysts, where more than half the infected people may become symptomatic. The illness is a self-limited one. Nonsuppurative and discrete lymphadenopathy, fever, malaise, sore throat, and hepatocellular damage constitute a picture that can simulate infectious mononucleosis or lymphoma.

DISEASE IN IMMUNODEFICIENT INDIVIDUALS. Infection in immunodeficient patients is acquired either from reactivation of latent infection or by acquiring toxoplasma from a donor organ. Toxoplasma encephalitis or disseminated toxoplasmosis can occur.

Table 20-7. Treatment of Protozoal Infections

Infection	Drug of choice	Alternatives	Comments
Malaria P. vivax, P. ovale	Chloroquine phosphate 10 mg base/kg/day PO (max. 600 mg) stat, then 5 mg base/kg 6, 24, and 48 hr later, followed by primaquine phosphate 0.3 mg base/kg/day for 14 days (max. 15 mg/day)	Hydroxychloroquine sulfate	Primaquine may cause servere hemolysis in G6PD-deficient individuals; check status before treatment
P. malariae	Only chloroquine, as above		
P. falciparum			
Chloroquine susceptible	Only chloroquine, as above		
Chloroquine resistant	Consult CDC for up-to-date guidelines and for parenteral quinine if indicated (see phone numbers in text)		
Toxoplasmosis (congenital)	Pyrimethamine + sulfadiazine or trisulfapyrimidines + folinic acid	Spiramycin	
Pneumocystosis	Trimethoprim (20 mg/kg)-sulfamethoxazole (100 mg/kg) PO or IV divided q6h for 14 days	Pentamidine isethionate, trimetrexate	
Giardiasis	Furazolidone 8 mg/kg/day (max. 400 mg) divided q8h for 10 days	Quinacrine, metronidazole	
Amebiasis			
Asymptomatic	Diloxanide furoate 20 mg/kg/day (max. 1500 mg) PO for 10 days		Diloxanide available CDC only
		Iodoquinol, paromomycin	Iodoquinol has potential for optic neuritis
Intestinal disease and extraintestinal disease	Metronidazole 35–50 mg/kg/day (max. 2250 mg) PO divided q8h for 10 days followed by a luminal agent	Dehydroemetine, chloroquine	

Laboratory Diagnosis

Serodiagnostic methods are the most readily available but are not infallible, and it is important to attempt to isolate the organism or visualize its histology. Several tests are commercially available or available in state reference laboratories. The Sabin-Feldman dye test was the gold standard for detection of IgG antibodies but has now been superceded by indirect immunofluorescent antibody (IFA) tests. The IFA and other types of assays are widely available but not well standardized. Testing for IgM antibody should be relied upon only when done in selected reference laboratories with extensive research experience in the use of the assay. Tests for detection of antigen have also been developed but are performed only in specialized laboratories. Because of the complexity of serodiagnosis and of the difficulty of recovering the organism from tissues, infectious disease consultation should always be obtained to assist in the diagnosis of toxoplasmosis. Prenatal diagnosis of toxoplasma infection in the fetus is now possible, involving identification of maternal acute infection followed by fetal blood and amniotic fluid sampling. This has importance for prognostication as well as for the possibility of treating the infection in utero by administration of antibiotics to the mother.

Treatment

See Table 20-7. The use of spiramycin is considered investigational by the FDA.

Giardiasis

Giardiasis is a diarrheal illness caused by *Giardia lamblia* and is the most common protozoal illness and the most commonly identified intestinal parasitic infection in the United States. *G. lamblia* exists in two morphologic forms. The trophozoite is a pear-shaped, discoid organism with paired nuclei, which give it its characteristic "owl-like" appearance, and a rapid motility produced by its eight flagellae. The cyst is an ovoid structure with two to four nuclei. Transmission occurs by fecal-oral contamination, by oral-anal sexual transmission, and from pets. Giardiasis also occurs in outbreaks traced to drinking water, most commonly mountain streams contaminated fecally by wildlife.

Clinical Features

Giardiasis is a subacute illness in normal children. Mild, persistent, or relapsing diarrhea, often associated with abdominal distension, cramping, or flatulence, is the most common presentation. Older children may complain of upper gastrointestinal symptoms suggestive of acid-dyspepsia. It is also complicated as a cause of the chronic malabsorption syndrome, although its role here is possibly as an exacerbating factor for an underlying illness. Knowledge of the host-parasite relationship in giardiasis is rudimentary, and the factors that determine persistence of disease in a chronic form in certain hosts are unknown. Carriage may occur asymptomatically; therefore, the presence of parasites in the stool should be interpreted in light of other circumstantial evidence. Children attending day-care centers and cystic fibrosis patients are high-risk groups for the disease.

Diagnosis

The most readily available diagnostic method is an examination of a wet-mounted specimen of stool stained with iodine. Trophozoites are visible, however, only on fresh specimens, and cyst excretion is often intermittent and does not correlate with severity of disease. A stool antigen detection method, an ELISA, was recently made commercially available and is being evaluated clinically. The most sensitive methods are invasive techniques that provide a direct examination of the upper small-intestinal habitat of the organism, which should be employed in the differential diagnosis of chronic malabsorption or of chronic diarrhea of unknown cause. A specimen of duodenal juice can be obtained by intubation and aspiration or by the use of the string test. The latter involves swallowing a string-attached capsule which can be recovered a few hours later. Small bowel biopsy may be done endoscopically and used for a touch preparation for trophozoites and for histopathologic examination. Detection of serum antibodies is still investigational.

Treatment

Treatment of asymptomatic carriers is controversial. Drugs for the treatment of the disease are listed in Table 20-7. Relapses are common.

Malaria

Malarial infections are caused by four species of a protozoan of the genus *Plasmodium*. There are two distinct syndromes. *Plasmodium falciparum* malaria is severe and sometimes fatal but is readily amenable to treatment while disease caused by *P. vivax*, *P. malariae*, or *P. ovale*, is mild and can relapse repeatedly. Intrauterine transmission can result in congenital malaria.

Epidemiology

Malaria is distributed widely in Southeast Asia, Africa, and Central and South America. The prevalence of the disease is governed primarily by the density of the mosquito population. The female *Anopheles* mosquito is the vector.

Pathogenesis

The intracellular parasite completes its life cycle in two hosts: human beings (asexual or intermediate phase) and female *Anopheles* mosquitoes (sexual or definitive phase).

PREERYTHROCYTIC STAGE. Sporozoites injected into the human host by the bite of an infected mosquito invade hepatic cells. Small cysts, each with thousands of merozoites, are formed in a few days. The cysts rupture to release merozoites which then infect erythrocytes. In ovale and vivax malaria, some merozoites may enter hepatic cells again and cause future relapses (exoerythrocytic stage).

ERYTHROCYTIC STAGE. The merozoite feeds on the cytoplasm of the erythrocyte and grows into a trophozoite and then into a schizont containing 8 to 30 merozoites. The erythrocyte ruptures, liberating pigment, red cell debris, and merozoites causing fever. Some merozoites enter new erythrocytes and several cycles of merozoite to schizont to merozoite are repeated. Some parasites do not divide but change to male or female forms (gametocytes) within the red cells. This is the only form that infects the mosquito.

MOSQUITO STAGE. In the insect's stomach the parasites undergo fertilization, burrow through the stomach, and form oocysts on its outer wall. These cysts mature to contain a large number of sporozoites. The sporozoites travel to the salivary glands from where they infect human beings.

Clinical Manifestations

The typical attack consists of chills with a rapid rise of fever, accompanied by systemic symptoms including headache, nausea, vomiting, delirium, and myalgia. This is followed by a prolonged diaphoretic phase. The classic single-brood infection causes paroxysms of periodicities of 72 hours (quartan) in *P. malariae* infection and 48 hours (tertian) in all others. Multiple brood infections, however, can cause any fever pattern, including daily (quotidian) fever.

Anemia, jaundice, splenomegaly, herpes labialis, and postural hypotension are also common. Falciparum malaria can be complicated by cerebral malaria and by blackwater fever. In the latter condition there is massive intravascular hemolysis, hemoglobinuria, and acute tubular necrosis leading to renal failure.

Diagnosis

The diagnosis is confirmed by identification of the malarial parasite in the peripheral blood smear. Color plates of morphological details for various stages of each species should be consulted for identification. These are printed in most infectious disease texts and clinical laboratory manuals. Species identification is important because it has implications for treatment.

Treatment

Refer to Table 20-7. The treatment indicated may depend on the geographic origin of the patient. This information is available from the Centers for Disease Control (CDC) (404) 488-4046; nights, weekends, and holidays (404) 639-2888.

Prophylaxis

The CDC now provides constantly updated information on prevention of malaria for travelers, including details pertaining to children and lactating women 24 hours a day by calling (404) 639-1610.

Pneumocystis carinii Pneumonia

Pneumocystis carinii, generally considered a protozoan, although it resembles a fungus in its staining characteristics, is now a major cause of pneumonia in immunocompromised patients. It is most commonly encountered in association with the AIDS. At least three morphological forms are identifiable on light microscopy, cysts, intracystic "sporozoites," and extracystic "trophozoites." The proposed life cycle includes dissolution of the cyst to release up to 8 intracystic bodies (sporozoites) which assume a pleomorphic morphology (trophozoites) when released. The latter develop into the thick-walled cysts. Pneumocystis organisms are occasionally observed in the lungs of normal hosts at autopsy, where their clinical significance and epidemiological importance in the transmission of disease are unknown. Transmission probably occurs by inhalation, and the occurrence of intrauterine transmission is controversial.

Clinical Features

The clinical course varies, but may broadly be placed in two categories. An epidemic, infantile form, which occurs as outbreaks in premature, debilitated, and, especially, marasmic 2- to 6-month old infants, has an insidious onset, usually without fever, with a slow progression of cough, and respiratory distress over 1 to 4 weeks. Pathologic findings include extensive interstitial plasma cell infiltrates. The second is the sporadic form of the disease seen in high-risk immunosuppressed patients. This may also begin insidiously, but more often has an acute onset with fever and rapid progression of respiratory symptoms. Untreated patients have a fatal outcome more often than in the epidemic form. Interestingly, patients with AIDS, although profoundly immunosuppressed, have a more insidious onset and milder respiratory symptoms than other patients with the sporadic form of the disease. A conspicuous physical finding in pneumocystis pneumonia is often the absence of adventitious sounds despite other evidence of severe respiratory involvement.

Diagnosis

RADIOGRAPHIC. No pattern of infiltrates on the chest radiograph is characteristic, and this study is occasionally normal. Bilateral perihilar infiltrates, spreading to become more peripheral and reticulonodular in appearance is the most common pattern seen early in the disease.

INVASIVE TECHNIQUES. At the present time open lung biopsy is the most reliable method of diagnosis. Pathologic examination of the specimen should include staining for the cyst wall, such as the methenamine-silver nitrate method of Gomori. Transbronchial biopsy, endobronchial brush biopsy, and transthoracic percutaneous needle aspiration are methods undergoing evaluation.

SEROLOGY. An initial report about the use of countercurrent immunoelectrophoresis for the detection of *P. carinii* antigenemia has not been replicated. Other serologic methods are not useful for diagnostic purposes.

Treatment

Prophylaxis is considered necessary in immunocompromised patients. A single dose of trimethroprim-sulfamethoxazole given 3 days/week, has been demonstrated to be equally efficacious as a once daily regimen. Recurrence rates are high. See Table 20-7.

Cryptosporidiosis and Isosporiasis

Cryptosporidium sp. and *Isospora belli* are newly recognized causes of diarrhea in children. They constitute major causes of morbidity in immunosuppressed patients and are frequently being implicated in the etiology of diarrhea in normal children attending day-care centers and in water-associated outbreaks. Profuse watery diarrhea occurs, and in compromised hosts, severe abdominal symptoms, weight loss, and dehydration are common. In patients with AIDS, involvement of the biliary tract may occur, with symptoms suggesting cholangitis. Methods of diagnosis include identification of the oocyst in stool smears by a modified acid fast stain, and a recently described fluorescent antibody staining technique. Optimal treatment has not been established for treatment of cryptosporidiosis, but the investigational use of spiramycin should be considered. Isoporiasis can be satisfactorily treated with oral trimethroprim-sulfamethoxazole.

Sunil K. Sood

Spirochetal Infections

Syphilis

Syphilis is caused by *Treponema pallidum,* a thin, motile spirochete. It is acquired by sexual contact, and can be transmitted transplacentally or perinatally, causing a con-

genital infection that can affect all organ systems. After a steady decline, syphilis has been on the increase again in several areas in the United States since the late 1970s.

Clinical Manifestations

ACQUIRED SYPHILIS. Following an incubation period of about 3 weeks (range, 10–90 days), the primary stage of the infection appears as one or more ulcerative lesions (chancre) of the skin and mucous membranes, most commonly in the genital area, although any part of the body may be involved. Infection may also occur without chancre. Secondary syphilis usually appears 6 to 12 weeks after infection, characterized by a diffuse erythematous maculopapular or pustular rash in 80% of the patients, generalized adenopathy (50%), and mild constitutional symptoms. Less frequently, there are signs and symptoms of uveitis, periostitis, glomerulonephritis, arthritis, meningitis, cranial neuritis, anemia, and splenomegaly. These manifestations may disappear spontaneously within months or a year, with subsequent clinical latency. In about a third of untreated cases, tertiary syphilis (usually not a pediatric disease) develops years after the initial infection, characterized by the development of gummatous lesions and cardiovascular and neurological diseases.

CONGENITAL SYPHILIS. Transmission to the fetus or infant is common during the first year following an untreated maternal infection and is less frequent during latent and tertiary syphilis. Transplacental infection usually occurs after 16 to 18 weeks of gestation. It causes abortion or stillbirth in 40% of affected pregnancies and frequently leads to intrauterine growth retardation, prematurity, and infection affecting multiple organ systems. Examination of the umbilical cord may show a necrotizing funisitis.

Disease manifestations are often divided in two groups:

1. *Early congenital syphilis* resembles the secondary stage of the acquired infection in its clinical spectrum with high infectivity and potential curability with antibiotics. Usually it presents at 2 to 5 weeks of age with maculopapular or bullous eruptions, a mucosanguinous nasal discharge, fissures around the mouth (rhagades), anogenital condylomas, nephrosis, hepatosplenomegaly, hemolytic anemia, thrombocytopenia, pneumonitis, and failure to thrive. About 50% of infected infants have CSF abnormalities even in the absence of clinical neurological disease. Osteochondritis and periostitis (usually of the long bones) develop in 100% of cases within the first 3 months of life (Parrot's pseudoparalysis).

2. *Late congenital syphilis* is analogous to late acquired syphilis because it results from destructive stigmata of previously active disease. It appears after 2 years of age, is noninfectious, and poorly antibiotic unresponsive. Sixty percent of untreated infants remain latently infected without overt clinical signs, while about 40% show a variety of tertiary stigmata such as poor growth, keratitis, uveitis and chorioretinitis, neurosensory deafness, Hutchinson's teeth and Moon's mulberry molars, maldevelopment of the nose and mandible resulting in "bulldog" facies, osseous involvement (saber tibia), and bilateral hydrarthrosis (Clutton's joints). Meningovascular neurosyphilis, paresis and tabes, hydrocephalus and mental retardation may also be seen.

Diagnosis and Evaluation

A clinical history and thorough physical examination of the patient and investigations of all personal contacts is essential. Diagnostic tests include dark-field or immunofluorescent demonstration of *T. pallidum* from moist cutaneous or mucosal lesions or from the placenta by an experienced observer. Serological tests for syphilis (STS) include the Venereal Disease Research Laboratory (VDRL) and the rapid plasma reagin (RPR). If positive, specific confirmatory treponemal tests must be done, such as the fluorescent treponemal antiabsorption (FTA-ABS) test, which is most frequently used, the *T. pallidum* microhemagglutination assay (TP-MHA), and the *T. pallidum* immobilization (TPI) test. These treponemal tests are not specific for syphilis, because patients with other spirochetal diseases may also show positivity. The VDRL, however, is uniformly nonreactive in Lyme disease.

Contrary to the specific treponemal tests which remain positive for life even after successful therapy, the VDRL or, the RPR are useful for following response to treatment or reinfection. With adequate treatment, one should see a four--fold decrease in titers and seronegativity within 1 to 2 years after treatment for primary or secondary syphilis. Con-1 versely, titer rise suggests infection or relapse.

In the newborn, testing of the serum from the infant rather than the cord blood is preferred. A positive STS in a newborn may be due to passive transfer of maternal antibodies, usually at a lower titer than in the mother's blood. The STS becomes negative in 4 to 6 months (but up to 1 year or longer for FTA-ABS test). Other evaluations should include CSF examination (with a quantitative VDRL, not RPR test), and radiologic studies of long bones.

Treatment

Treatment recommendations are listed in Table 20-8 for various stages of the disease. Penicillin is the drug of choice, and efforts should be made to skin test and desensitize the penicillin-allergic patient rather than to use a therapeutic regimen of unknown efficacy such as erythromycin, especially in the pregnant woman. It is important to emphasize that therapeutic regimens are being reexamined because of reports of frequent CSF invasion by *T. pallidum* in early syphilis and in asymptomatic patients with normal CSF parameters, and of inadequate penicillin levels in the CSF with benzathine penicillin. Furthermore, the rate of treatment failure may be high among women with secondary syphilis and among women treated in the last trimester of pregnancy. Maternal treatment follow-up is extremely important and should include monthly quantitative VDRL or RPR and retreatment of those who do not show a decrease in titer in a 3-month period. For asymptomatic infants whose mothers were treated adequately with a penicillin regimen during pregnancy, treatment is not necessary. If follow-up cannot be ensured, however, some consultants recommend treatment with benzathine penicillin (50,000 I.U./kg IM in a single dose) or a 10-day regimen of aqueous crystalline or procaine penicillin if neurosyphilis cannot be excluded.

Follow-up of all infants should be done at 1, 2, 4, 6, and 12 months, with STS performed at 3, 6, and 12 months after treatment until the serum VDRL or RPR becomes negative. Retreatment should be given to children with persistent, stable, low titers, to those with a reactive CSF VDRL at 6 months, and to those with persistent or recurrent clinical disease.

Usually the prognosis is favorable if early and adequate treatment is given. A thorough developmental evaluation should be done during early childhood on all patients treated for congenital infection, and prolonged surveillance well into adult life is advisable.

Prevention

Like other sexually transmitted diseases, syphilis can only be controlled by a comprehensive effort in sex education and early detection and treatment of infection, including adequate prenatal care, contact investigation, and treatment of sexual partners. Children and teenagers with syphilis should also be evaluated for sexual abuse. Drainage, skin, and blood precautions are recommended for isolation of patients with primary and secondary syphilis but not for patients with tertiary disease with no skin lesions. Testing for concurrent infections such as HIV is also recommended.

Table 20-8. Treatment Recommendations for Syphilis

Stage	Treatment of choice	Alternative therapy
Early acquired (primary, secondary, and latent of less than 1-year duration)	Benzathine penicillin G, IM, 50,000 IU/kg (max. 2.4 MU) single dose[a]	Tetracycline 500 mg PO qid for 15 days, [b] or erythromycin 500 mg po Qid for 15 days[c]
Latent syphilis[d] (duration indetermined, or > 1 year)	Benzathine penicillin G, IM, 50,000 IU/kg (max. 2.4 MU/dose) weekly for 3 consecutive weeks	Tetracycline 500 mg PO qid for 30 days,[b] or erythromycin 500 mg PO qid for 30 days[c]
Neurosyphilis	Aqueous crystalline penicillin G, IV 50,000 IU/kg/day, q4h (max 2.4. MU/day) for 10 days, followed by benzathine penicillin G, IM, 50,000 IU/kg/dose weekly for 3 weeks.	Procaine penicillin G, 2.4 MU/day, IM, for 10 days, plus probenecid, followed by 3 weekly doses of benzathine penicillin G.
Congenital syphilis	Aqueous crystalline penicillin G, 50,000 IU/kg/day, IV or IM, q12h for 10 days	Aqueous procaine penicillin G, 50,000 IU/kg/day, IM, for 10 days.

[a] See text regarding recent concerns with benzathine penicillin G. IM = intramuscular injections, MU = million units.

[b] Tetracycline not to be used in children ≤ 8 years of age.

[c] Efficacy not proven.

[d] CSF examination is suggested for patients who receive therapy other than penicillin for syphilis of more that 1-year duration to exclude asymptomatic neurosyphilis.

Lyme Disease

Etiology and Epidemiology

First described in Europe early this century, Lyme disease is now known to be caused by *Borrelia burgdorferi,* a spirochete identified in 1982. It is transmitted by arthropod vectors, especially *Ixodes* ticks, Lone Star and other ticks, although insects such as the deer and horse flies and mosquitoes may also be involved. Animal reservoirs include deer, wild mammals, birds and rodents, ticks, and less commonly, cattle, and pet dogs and cats. The disease occurs widely throughout Europe, USSR, and Australia. In the United States, endemic foci exist in the Northeast, upper Midwest, and portions of California, Oregon, Utah, and Texas, corresponding mainly to the distribution and the incidence of *Borrelia* infection in the tick population (1–4% on the West coast, up to 40–100% in the Northeast). Cases occur mainly in the spring and summer. Maternal transmission resulting in intrauterine infection has also been described.

Clinical Manifestations

Classically, Lyme disease has been divided into three stages.

The *first stage* follows an incubation period of 3 to 32 days after a tick bite (which may not be recognized or recalled). It begins with a red macule at the site of the bite, expanding to form a large annular erythematous lesion with partial central clearing (erythema chronicum migrans) in about two-thirds of patients. Secondary annular lesions, conjunctivitis, arthralgia, fever, adenopathy, and "flu-like" and meningoencephalitic symptoms may develop.

The *second stage* comes 2 to 12 weeks after inoculation manifested by neurological symptoms (meningitis, cranial, and peripheral neuritis) in 10 to 15% of the cases and cardiac involvement in less than 10% (myocarditis, arrhythmias).

In about 50% of patients not previously treated, oligoarthritis develops weeks to years after the first stage of disease, especially in patients who did not have erythema chronicum migrans. It usually affects large joints, may be acute or recurrent and if untreated, may be chronic in about 10% of patients. Late central nervous system, cardiac, and hepatic disease can also be seen in this *tertiary phase.*

Intrauterine infection can result in congenital heart disease, cortical blindness, stillbirth, and abortion.

Diagnosis

Culture of *Borrelia* can be done in special Kelly's medium at 30 to 36°C and hypercarbic conditions, but this remains difficult. Animal inoculation and silver and specific immunofluorescent stains may also detect the organism in infected tissues. Serology (IFA or ELISA tests) is the most available diagnostic tool but suffers from lack of sensitivity (especially early in the infection, when only 30–40% of cases are positive after 3 weeks of symptoms), specificity (cross-reactivity with other spirochetal infections), and inter-laboratory variability. Furthermore, antibiotic therapy early in the infection results in abrogation of the serological titers; therefore, Lyme borreliosis remains a clinical diagnosis, especially early in the first stage of the disease.

Treatment and Prevention

Patients with suspected Lyme disease on epidemiologic and clinical grounds should be treated without waiting for results of serologic tests, because treatment given early can avert subsequent complications. The antibiotic recommendations according to the stages of the infection are given in Table 20-9. For cases not responsive to standard regimens, treatment with chloramphenicol, cefotaxime, or ceftriaxone have been reported to be effective in uncontrolled studies. Adjunct antiinflammatory therapy for carditis and arthritis should be given as necessary.

Preventive measures against Lyme disease include awareness of exposure in endemic areas, avoidance of ticks through the use of protective clothing and insect repellents, and rapid tick removal if bitten. Prophylactic antibiotics after a tick bite are not recommended, especially in areas of low endemicity and if the tick attachment is known to be short.

Other Spirochetal Infections

See Table 20-10.

Chinh T. Le

Other Parasitic Infections

Parasites that infect human beings can be divided into three major categories: (1) helminths, (2) ectoparasites, and (3) protozoa.

This discussion deals briefly with some of the more common helminths or parasitic worms that may infect children. For more detailed discussion, the reader is referred to more specific texts.

Because diagnosis, especially serodiagnosis, and treatment are often investigational and constantly updated, and because information on rarely encountered parasites is often not readily accessible, the Centers for Disease Control, Division of Parasitic Diseases, provides information to physicians at 404-639-3356 (404-639-2888 nights and weekends).

Human beings are the *definitive* host when they harbor the adult worms, allowing them to complete their reproductive cycle, and the *intermediate* host when they harbor the larval stages. For some helminths, e.g., *Taenia*, human beings are the exclusive definitive host. Involvement as an intermediate host is sometimes an accidental event, e.g., cysticercosis and echinococcosis.

Platyhelminthes (Flatworms)

Cestodes (Tapeworms)

The cestodes have a common morphology: (1) a scolex or head that attaches them to the mucosa by means of suckers and in some worms hooks, (2) a neck that is an area of metabolic activity and growth, and (3) a ribbon-like body that has no gastrointestinal tract but absorbs nutrients from its surface. The body consists of progressively maturing segments (proglottides) arising from the neck. Terminal proglottides become gravid, detach, and release large numbers of eggs.

Table 20-9. Antibiotic therapy of Lyme borreliosis

Erythema migrans
  Adults: tetracycline. 250 mg qid for 10–20 days
  Children > 8 yr: tetracycline. 40–50 mg/kg/day for 10–20 days
  Children < 8 yr: phenoxymethyl penicillin or amoxicillin. 50 mg/kg/day for 10–20 days (in case of penicillin allergy: erythromycin. 30 mg/kg/day)
Neurologic manifestations
  Meningitis: penicillin G. 200,000–300,000 IU/kg/day (up to 20,000,000 IU) intravenously for 10 days
  Isolated facial nerve palsy or other neuropathy
    As sole manifestation, treat as for erythema migrans
    With spinal fluid abnormality, treat as for meningitis
Arthritis
  Initially:
    Children > 8 yr: tetracycline. 40–50 mg/kg/day for 30 days
    Children < 8 yr: phenoxymethyl penicillin or amoxicillin. 50 mg/kg/day for 30 days
  If no response or in case of recurrence:
    Penicillin G. 200,000–300,000 IU/kg/day (up to 20,000,000 IU) intravenously for 10–14 days
Pregnancy: penicillin G. 200,000–300,000 IU/kg/day (up to 20,000,000 IU) intravenously for 10 days

Table 20-10. *Spirochetal Infections of Medical Importance*

Disease	Organisms	Distribution	Mode of transmission	Clinical features	Diagnosis	Treatment
Endemic treponematodes (endemic syphilis, yaws, pinta)	*Treponema pallidum*; *T. pertenue*, *T. carateum*	Eastern Mediterranea, Asia, and Africa (endemic syphilis); tropical areas (yaws); Central and S. American (pinta)	Nonvenereal, person to person, indirect contamination, *no* congenital transmission	Variety of acute and chronic mucocutaneous lesions, bony involvement with endemic syphilis and yaws	Dark field examination, serologic tests indistinguishable from venereal syphilis	Single IM dose of benzathine penicillin 0.6–1.2 million IU; mortality low
Relapsing fever	*Borrelia sp.*	Louse borne: Africa, Asia, and S. America; tick-borne: worldwide foci	Louse; soft-shelled ticks	Recurrent episodes of paroxysmal fever, flu-like illness for 2–9 days, alternating with asymptomatic intervals of 1–54 days (median, 18 days). Rash, jaundice, anemia, myocarditis may occur with louse-borne disease	Spirochetes can be seen on blood smear during febrile paroxysm; animal inoculation of patient's blood	Erythromycin or tetracycline for 5–10 days. Mortality rate: 0.5% of untreated cases of louse-borne disease

Disease	Organism	Distribution	Source/Transmission	Clinical features	Diagnosis	Treatment
Leptospirosis	*Leptospira*	Worldwide	Farm and pet animals; wildlife reservoirs, especially rodents. Indirect contact or ingestion of food contaminated by animal urine	Asymptomatic or biphasic illness, first "flu-like" with conjunctional suffusion, then with fever and meningeal symptoms. Severe azotemia and liver failure in Weil's disease	Blood, urine, CSF cultures onto Fletcher's medium; guinea pig inoculation with patient's urine; serological tests	Parenteral penicillin or tetracycline. Alternatives: chloramphenicol, streptomycin, erythromycin
Spirillary rat-bite fever (Sodoku)	*Spirillum minus*	Asia and Japan	Bite from infected rat, mouse, squirrel, or weasel; contaminated milk or water	Relapsing fever following a rat bite. Regional lymphadenitis, systemic symptoms, rash	Isolation of organism in special medium or animal inoculation	Procaine penicillin or oral tetracycline for 7 days

TAENIA SOLIUM (PORK TAPEWORM) AND TAENIA SAGI-NATA (BEEF TAPEWORM). The former is the only tapeworm infection likely to be commonly encountered in pediatric practice in the United States, along with its occasional complication, cysticercosis. Tapeworm infections are acquired when insufficiently cooked pork or beef (<56°C) harboring cysticerci is eaten. Cysticerci develop into adult worms that live in the small intestine and reach an average length of 2 to 3 meters for the pork tapeworm and 4 to 10 meters for the beef tapeworm. Gravid proglottides are excreted in the feces, and the eggs are ingested by the intermediate host, the pig and the cow respectively, where they hatch in the intestine and develop into cysticerci in the tissues.

Clinical Manifestations. Symptoms of taeniasis include abdominal discomfort, nausea, loss of weight, and passage of gravid proglottides from rectum. Eosinophilia may occur transiently. *T. saginata* infection is of little clinical significance except for the very rare occurrence of intestinal obstruction. *T. solium* infection is clinically significant because of the occurrence of cysticercosis.

Cysticercosis. The human can become an intermediate host for *T. solium* as a result of autoinfection. This occurs either from ingestion of the eggs by fecal contamination of food or possibly from release of eggs by the adult worm in the intestine. Thus, numerous larvae or cysticerci arise, and they hematogenously spread into various organs. Cerebral cysticercosis may result in seizures, cerebral edema, and death. In children, however, the cerebral lesions tend to be single and self-limiting and neurological symptoms usually resolve within a month.

Diagnosis. Taeniasis is diagnosed by the characteristic morphology of eggs on fecal wet mount examination, preferably enhanced by concentration, and the two species can be distinguished from one another. Definitive identification is by pathological examination of the gravid proglottides. Soft tissue cysticercosis can occasionally be diagnosed on plain radiographs. Computerized tomography is the most sensitive method of identifying the acute inflamed and the healing calcified lesions of cerebral cysticercosis. An ELISA using *T. solium* cysticercus as antigen, available at the Centers for Disease Control, detects antibody in 60 to 90% of serum or CSF specimens from patients with cysticercosis.

Treatment. For treatment of Taeniasis refer to Table 20-11. In view of the self-limiting course of most cases of childhood cysticercosis, treatment may not be necessary. Praziquantel given orally has some demonstrated efficacy in severe cases of cerebral cysticercosis. Because treatment can exacerbate cerebral edema, concomitant corticosteroid therapy has been suggested.

ECHINOCOCCUS GRANULOSUS (HYDATID DISEASE). Human hydatid disease is caused by the larval stage of *Echinococcus granulosus,* a common intestinal tapeworm of the dog in many parts of the world where sheep and cattle are closely associated with dogs. The adult worm measures 3 to 6 mm and the body consists of 2 to 5 segments.

Life Cycle. Eggs passed in dog feces can infect several mammals, including man. The liberated embryo, the oncosphere, burrows through the intestinal wall and reaches various tissues through the lymphatics or blood vessels, most commonly the liver and lungs. The embryo produces the hydatid cyst, which contains a colorless or yellowish fluid surrounded by an active germinative layer, which produces new scolices. Daughter cysts may arise inside the original cyst. Many scolices may be produced by the germinative layer. The cyst can become very large. Rupture of the cyst results in the liberation of the free scolices and daughter cysts, which are capable of initiating secondary cysts wherever they may become implanted. The life cycle is maintained when dogs ingest scolices by feeding on the viscera of infected livestock.

Clinical Manifestations. The symptoms of hydatid cyst resemble those of a slow-growing tumor. Secondary infection of the cyst may occur. Operative or traumatic rupture of the cyst can result in anaphylactic shock.

Diagnosis. The use of imaging techniques may be the most helpful means of diagnosis. Serological tests and the Casoni skin test are not very sensitive or specific. Needle exploration should not be attempted lest the cyst rupture and anaphylaxis result. Excision biopsy provides the definitive diagnosis.

Treatment. Surgery is the treatment of choice. Mebendazole is effective in a limited number of patients with inoperable disease.

OTHER CESTODES OF SIGNIFICANCE.
Diphyllobothrium latum (fish tapeworm)
Hymenolepis nana (dwarf tapeworm)

Trematodes (Flukes)

Most trematodal infestations are not indigenous to the Western Hemisphere but may occasionally be seen in immigrants, especially Southeast Asians, and travelers. The adult forms range from a millimeter to 7.5 cm in length and infect vertebrates. The intestinal flukes, e.g., *Fasciolopsis buski* are not common in the United States. The lung and liver flukes, e.g., *Paragonimus westermani* and *Clonorchis sinensis,* are seen in people from Southeast Asia. The blood flukes (schistosomes) use aquatic snails as their intermediate hosts. *Schisto-*

Table 20-11. Treatment of Helminthic Infections

Organism	Drug of choice	Alternatives	Comments
Taenia saginata and *Taenia solium*	Niclosamide, 11–34 kg: 1g; > 34 kg: 2 g	Praziquantel	Praziquantel not approved by FDA for treatment of adult worms
Cysticercosis	Praziquantel 50 mg/kg/day for 14 days		Not usually necessary in children (see text)
Ascaris lumbricoides	Pyrantel pamoate 11 mg/kg once (max. 1 g) *or* mebendazole 100 mg bid for 3 days (only for age > 2 yr)	Piperazine citrate 75 mg/kg for 2 days (max. 3.5 mg/kg/day)	
Visceral larva migrans	Thiabendazole 25 mg/kg bid (max. 3 g/day) for 5 days	Diethylcarbamazine (investigational)	Not usually necessary
Enterobius vermicularis	Pyrantel pamoate 11 mg/kg once (max. 1 g) *or* mebendazole 100 mg once (only for age > 2 yr)		Repeat treatment in 2 weeks
Trichinella spiralis	For intestinal phase: thiabendazole 25 mg/kg bid for 5 days (max. 3 g/day)	Pyrantel pamoate 11 mg/kg (max. 1 g) for 4 days, mebendazole	Risk of Herxheimer-like reaction, steroids used concomitantly
	For tissue phase: mebendazole	Thiabendazole	Doses not established
Ancylostoma duodenale and *Necator americanus*	Mebendazole 100 mg bid for 3 days (only for age > 2 yr)	Pyrantel pamoate 11 mg/kg (max. 1 g) for 3 days	

soma mansoni is the only species present in the Western Hemisphere, chiefly in South America and the Caribbean. Despite immigration and travel, the absence of susceptible snails has precluded establishment of endemic foci of *S. mansoni* in the United States.

These parasites constitute one of the most important public health problems in many countries of the world. For details the reader is referred to more specific texts.

Nemathelminthes

Nematodes (Roundworms)

Nematodes range from a fraction of a millimeter to a meter or more in length, with cylindrical, elongated bodies tapering at both ends. Their body wall consists of a noncellular, tough hyaline layer, and they possess a pseudocoelom in which the digestive system and the organs of reproduction are located.

ASCARIS LUMBRICOIDES. Ascariasis is acquired by eating fecally contaminated food. Ingested eggs hatch into larvae, which burrow through the intestinal wall. The larvae are carried to the right side of the heart and to the lungs via the lymphatic and blood vessels. In the lungs, they penetrate the alveoli and pass on to the intestine by way of the trachea, esophagus, and stomach. In about 2 to 3 months, the worms become mature in the small intestine. Adult worms measure 15 to 25 cm. Their eggs are excreted in the feces.

Clinical Manifestations. Respiratory symptoms result if numerous larvae migrate simultaneously (ascaris pneumonia). The presence of the adult worms usually causes no significant clinical symptoms, but abdominal pain and malabsorption can occur. Often the first manifestation is passage of the worms from rectum or by regurgitation in vomitus. Heavy ascaris infections may result in obstruction or perforation of the small intestine, peritonitis, or acute appendicitis.

Diagnosis. Specific diagnosis is based on finding characteristic eggs in the feces. Peripheral eosinophilia is common in ascaris pneumonia.

Treatment. See Table 20-11.

VISCERAL LARVA MIGRANS (TOXOCARIASIS). The life cycle of a dog ascarid, *Toxocara canis*, resembles closely that of *Ascaris lumbricoides*. If the embryonated eggs are ingested by an unnatural host such as a human being, the larvae take an aberrant course of migration and become encapsulated in the muscles and organs such as liver, lungs, brain, and kidney. Maturation never occurs and migration continues until the host inflammatory response overcomes the larvae. It is not clear whether other toxocariae such as *Toxocara cati,* a cat ascarid, also cause the visceral larva migrans syndromes.

Clinical Manifestations. Two distinct syndromes, ocular and visceral, occur. Retinal granuloma formation can simulate retinoblastoma and result in unnecessary enucleation. Visceral involvement manifests as a multisystem disorder including fever, hepatosplenomegaly, respiratory symptoms, marked eosinophilia, and hypergammaglobulinemia. Prognosis is usually good.

Diagnosis. Demonstration of larvae on biopsy is the only certain method of diagnosis. Serological tests are investigational and are confounded by cross-reactions with other nematodes.

Treatment. See Table 20-11.

ENTEROBIUS VERMICULARIS (PINWORM). Enterobiasis is the most common human helminthic infestation and is common in children in the United States. The worms are white and are 2 to 12 mm long. The eggs are easily identifiable under the microscope. Infection is acquired by ingestion of eggs. Adult worms inhabit the cecum, where they reproduce sexually. The gravid female migrates toward the rectum, deposits the embryonated ova on the perianal folds, usually at night, and often returns to the large intestine. Perianal itching results, and eggs adhere to the fingers and fingernails, enabling reinfection or contamination of fomites.

Clinical Manifestations. Perianal pruritus, especially nocturnal, and occasionally vulvitis resulting from migration of worms along the perineum, are the symptoms. Appendicitis has occurred. Two alleged but unproved symptoms attributed to enterobiasis are enuresis and teeth-grinding.

Diagnosis. Eggs are easily seen on transparent adhesive tape applied perianally and then affixed to a microscope slide.

Treatment. See Table 20-11. All household members should be presumed to be infected. Hand-washing and trimming of fingernails should be stressed.

TRICHINELLA SPIRALIS. The adult worms inhabit the small intestine of various mammals, while the larvae are found encysted in the voluntary muscles of the same animal that harbors the adult parasite. Sources of infection in the United States are pork, beef contaminated with pork, and bear meat. Pork is not routinely inspected for trichinosis; cooking to 77°C destroys *Trichinella*. The encysted larvae develop into adult worms after ingestion. The viviparous females, 3 to 4 mm long, bore through the intestinal wall and deposit the fully developed larvae in the mucous membrane or intestinal lymph spaces. Hematogenous spread, primarily to skeletal muscle, especially the diaphragm, the tongue, and the eye muscles occurs. In the muscle, the larva lies between and parallel to the long axes of the muscle fibers and assumes the characteristic spiral form. An oval cyst is formed around the larva that eventually may become calcified.

Clinical Manifestations. Initial gastrointestinal symptoms can be severe, and small ulcers can occur in the proximal ileum. Following penetration most infections are asymptomatic. Multiple systemic manifestations characterize symptomatic invasion. A febrile illness with myalgia, periorbital edema, weakness, and eosinophilia is most typical and often diagnostic. Occasionally, pulmonary involvement, myocarditis, and cerebral edema, possibly the result of immunologic reactions, cause serious illness.

Diagnosis. Typical clinical manifestations and marked eosinophilia are the best diagnostic clues. Biopsy of a tender muscle is conclusive. Serological tests are available but not always useful.

Treatment. See Table 20-11.

ANCYLOSTOMA DUODENALE AND NECATOR AMERICANUS (HOOKWORM). Infections caused by *Ancylostoma duodenale* and *Necator americanus* are clinically indistinguishable but geographically distinct — they are the so-called Old World and New World hookworms, respectively. The worms are cylindrical, 8 to 13 mm long, and curved at the anterior extremity. The habitat of the adult worms is the small intestine, where they attach themselves to the mucosa and feed on mucous membrane and red blood cells. Eggs are laid by the female, and pass with the host's feces onto the soil, where first-stage larvae hatch from the eggs and feed on organic matter. They then molt and transform into infective filariform larvae, which are capable of penetrating unbroken human skin. The larvae enter the lymph and blood venules and are carried to the heart and then to the lungs. They penetrate the alveolar capillaries to enter the pulmonary alveoli, migrate to the bronchi and trachea, and are then swallowed. They reach maturity in the small intestine. *A. duodenale* may also establish infection if ingested.

Clinical Manifestations. Itching and a papular eruption may occur at the site of penetration. An initial acute intestinal phase of symptoms is followed by the quiescent infestation than can result in severe anemia.

Diagnosis. Specific diagnosis is based on finding the characteristic eggs in the feces. The species are indistinguishable by examination of the eggs, but a presumptive diagnosis of the species can be made on the basis of geographic origin of the patient.

Treatment. See Table 20-11.

Other Nematodes of Significance

Ancylostoma duodenale and *Uncinaria stenocephala* (hookworms causing cutaneous larva migrans)
Stronglyloides stercoralis (strongloidiasis)
Trichuris trichiura (whipworm)
Wuchereria bancrofti, Brugia malayi, Loa loa, and *Onchocerca volvulus* (the filarial worms)

Sunil K. Sood

References

General References

Beaver, P. C., Jung, R. C., and Cupp, E. W. *Clinical Parasitology* (9th ed.). Philadelphia: Lea & Febiger, 1984.
Drugs for Parasitic Infections. In *The Medical Letter on Drugs and Therapeutics.* New Rochelle, NY: The Medical Letter, Inc. 1988. Vol. 30, P. 15.
Feigin, R. D., and Cherry, J. D. (Eds.) *Textbook of Pediatric Infectious Diseases* (2nd ed.). Philadelphia: Saunders, 1987. Pp. 2001–2079.
Gantz, N. M., Gleckman, R. A., Brown, R. B., and Esposito, A. L. *Manual of Clinical Problems in Infectious Diseases.* Boston: Little, Brown, 1986.
Mandell, G. L., Douglas, R. G., and Bennett, J. E. *Principles and Practices of Infectious Diseases* (2nd ed.). New York: Wiley, 1985.
Moffet, H. L. *Pediatric Infectious Diseases* (3rd ed.), Philadelphia: Lippincott, 1989.
Nelson, J. D. (Ed.). *Current Therapy of Pediatric Infectious Disease* (2nd ed.). St. Louis: Mosby, 1988.
Oski, F. A., D'Angelis, C. D., Feigin, R. D., and Warshaw, J. B. *Principles and Practices of Pediatrics.* Philadelphia: Lippincott, 1990.

Bacterial Infections

ACIP Statement. Use of BCG vaccines in the control of tuberculosis. *M. M. W. R.* 37:663, 669, 1988.
American Academy of Pediatrics, Committee on Infectious Diseases. Tuberculosis, and Diseases due to Nontuberculous Mycobacteria. In *Report of the Committee on Infectious Diseases* (21st ed.). Evanston, IL: American Academy of Pediatrics, 1988. Pp. 429–451.
American Thoracic Society. Treatment of tuberculosis and tuberculosis infection in adults and children. *Am. Rev. Respir. Dis.* 134:355, 1986.
Klein, J. O., Feigin, R. D., and McCracken, G. H. Jr. Report of the task force on diagnosis and treatment of meningitis. *Pediatrics* 78[Suppl. II.]: 959, 1986.

Patel, R. A., et al. Sequence analysis and amplification by polymerase chain reaction of a cloned DNA fragment for identification of *Mycobacterium tuberculosis. J. Clin. Microbiol.* 28:513, 1990.
Sande, M. A., Scheld, M., and McCracken, G. H. Jr. and the Meningitis Study Group. *Pediatr. Infect. Dis.* 6:1, 1987.
Snider, D. E., Bridbord, K., and Hui, F. Research towards global control and prevention of tuberculosis with an emphasis on vaccine development. *Rev. Infect. Dis.* 11 [Suppl. 2]: S335, 1989.
Snider, D. E., Rieder, H. S., Combs, D., et al. Tuberculosis in children. *Pediatr. Infect. Dis.* 7:271, 1988.
Word, B. M., and Klein, J. O. Current therapy of bacterial sepsis and meningitis in infants and children: A poll of directors of programs in pediatric infectious diseases. *Pediatr. Inf. Dis.* 7:267, 1988.

Viral Infections

Bakshi, S. S., and Cooper, L. Z. Rubella. *Clin. Dermatol.* 7:8, 1989.
Balistreri, W. F. Viral hepatitis. *Pediatr. Clin. North Am.* 35:637, 1988.
Blumberg, E. A., and Molavi, A. Herpes zoster. *Clin. Dermatol.* 7:37, 1989.
Centers for Disease Control. Risks associated with human parvovirus B19 infection. *M.M.W.R.* 38:81, 1989.
Centers for Disease Control. Mumps prevention. *M.M.W.R.* 38:388, 1989.
Falloon, J., Eddy, J., Wiener, L., and Pizzo, P. A. Human immunodeficiency virus infection in children. *J. Pediatr.* 114:1, 1989.
Feigin, R. D., and Cherry, J. D. (Eds.). *Textbook of Pediatric Infectious Diseases* (2nd ed.). Philadelphia: Saunders, 1987.
Feldman, S. Varicella zoster infections of the fetus, neonate, and immunocompromised child. *Adv. Pediatr. Infect. Dis.* 1:99, 1986.
Freij, B. J., and Sever, J. L. Herpesvirus infections in pregnancy: Risks to embryo, fetus, and neonate. *Clin. Perinatol.* 15:203, 1988.
Freij, B. J., South, M. A., and Sever, J. L. Maternal rubella and the congenital rubella syndrome. *Clin. Perinatol.* 15:247, 1988.
Gustafson, T. L., et al. Measles outbreak in a fully immunized secondary-school population. *N. Engl. J. Med.* 316:771, 1987.
Kohl, S. Herpes simplex virus encephalitis in children. *Pediatr. Clin. North. Am.* 35:465, 1988.
Markowitz, L. E., et al. Patterns of transmission in measles outbreaks in the United States, 1985–1986. *N. Engl. J. Med.* 320:75, 1989.
Nelson, J. D. (Ed.). *Current Therapy in Pediatric Infectious Disease* (2nd ed.). Toronto, Decker, 1988.
Russo, T., and Chang, T.-W. Eruptions associated with respiratory and enteric viruses. *Clin. Dermatol.* 7:97, 1989.
Spector, S. A., and Dankner, W. M. Rapid viral diagnostic techniques. *Adv. Pediatr. Infect. Dis.* 1:37, 1986.
Suga, S., et al. Human herpesvirus-6 infection (exanthem subitum) without rash. *Pediatrics* 83:1003, 1989.
Sumaya, C. V. Epstein-Barr virus infection: The expanded spectrum. *Adv. Pediatr. Infect. Dis.* 1:75, 1986.

Tabor, E. Etiology, diagnosis and treatment of viral hepatitis in children. *Adv. Pediatr. Infect. Dis.* 3:19, 1988.

Rickettsial, Mycotic, and Protozoal Infections

Burgdorfer, W. The enlarging spectrum of tick-borne spirochetoses: R. R. Parker Memorial address: *Rev. Infect. Dis.* 8:932, 1986.

Dammin, G. J. Erythema migrans: A chronicle. *Rev. Infect. Dis.* 11:142, 1989.

Eichenfield, A. H., and Athreya, B. H. Lyme disease: Of ticks and titers. *J. Pediatr.* 114:329, 1989.

Guidelines for the Prevention and Control of Congenital Syphilis. *M.M.W.R.* 37 Suppl. 1. 1988.

Jacobs, R. F. Tick exposure and related infections: *Pediatr. Infect. Dis.* 3:612, 1988.

Musher, D. M. How much penicillin cures early syphilis? *Ann. Intern. Med.* 109:849, 1988.

Rocky Mountain spotted fever — United States, 1987. *M.M.W.R.* 37:388, 1988.

Parasitic Infections

Beaver, P. C., Jung, R. C., and Cupp, E. W. *Clinical Parasitology* (9th ed.). Philadelphia: Lea & Febiger, 1984.

Drugs for Parasitic Infections. In *The Medical Letter on Drugs and Therapeutics*. New Rochelle, NY: The Medical Letter, Inc. 1988. Vol. 30, p. 15.

Feigin, R. D., and Cherry, J. D. (Eds.). *Textbook of Pediatric Infectious Diseases* (2nd ed.). Philadelphia: Saunders, 1987. Pp. 2087–2134.

Nelson, J.D. (Ed.). *Current Therapy in Pediatric Infectious Disease*. St. Louis: Mosby, 1988.

21

Allergic Conditions

Allergic disorders constitute a large percentage of the problems seen in the general pediatric practice. More than 6 million children are thought to have allergic rhinitis, and approximately 2 million have atopic dermatitis. Of the approximately 10 million people in the United States with asthma, 50% of those are under 16 years of age. It is estimated that 80% of patients with childhood asthma have an allergic component. In sufficiently afflicted patients, allergic manifestations may appear shortly after birth and may continue during childhood and on into adulthood.

An allergic individual reacts in an abnormal fashion to substances that ordinarily do not cause problems for normal persons. The substance that causes the abnormal reaction is called IgE, formerly known as reagin, or skin-sensitizing antibody. Briefly, the basic mechanism is production of IgE on exposure to antigens that are responsible for hypersensitivity in the particular patient. The most important biologic property of IgE is its strong affinity for binding to membrane receptors located on homologous mast cells and basophils. These cells release histamine, SRS-A, neutrophilic and eosinophilic chemotactic factors, and other mediators of the immediate hypersensitivity reaction, after bridging of adjacent surface-bound IgE molecules by an allergen. Dilation of blood vessels, changes in the smooth muscle of the respiratory tract, and secretion by mucous glands follow.

Allergic symptoms can be distressing to the child. The pruritis associated with atopic dermatitis, the nasal obstruction, repetitive sneezing and rhinorrhea of allergic rhinitis, and the dyspnea and cough associated with asthma are difficult to bear in an acute episode. More frustrating for the patient is the tendency for allergic disorders to be chronic and recurrent.

There are two main approaches to the diagnosis and treatment of allergic disease: symptomatic and preventive. Which approach the physician takes depends on the amount of difficulty the patient incurs with the disease. Both approaches will be explored as each specific problem is discussed.

Allergic Respiratory Disease

Allergy respiratory disease may affect both the upper and lower respiratory tract and adjacent tissues, including the conjunctivae, middle ear, and eustachian tube. Rhinitis, sinusitis, conjunctivitis, serous otitis media, eustachian salpingitis, bronchitis, and asthma are common presenting disorders. These problems may exist singly or in various combinations. One may see a 6-year-old who has episodes of nasal obstruction, sneezing, rhinorrhea, and conjunctivitis restricted to one season of the year, who at the age of 9 years suddenly experiences his first episode of expiratory wheezing, cough, and dyspnea during his peak allergic season, and then at age 12 begins to have episodes of wheezing during the rest of the year. Thus, a child with seasonal rhinitis (pollenosis) may become a teenager with chronic asthma.

Infants and children with these clinical patterns all have symptoms that are produced by inflammatory changes within the respiratory epithelium—in the nose, sinuses, pharynx, or bronchial tree. The exposure in an allergic individual of the respiratory epithelium to contact with an allergen or antigen leads to symptoms that do not occur when a nonallergic patient is exposed to the same potential allergen. The tendency of the allergic patient to react to potential allergens may be demonstrated by abnormal reactivity in an organ other than that in which principal symptoms occur. This is the basis of allergy skin testing.

The underlying immunologic or physiologic aberrations responsible for these clinical observations are more obscure. Szentivanyi and Fishel have postulated that the underlying defect is an autonomic imbalance, specifically, beta-adrenergic blockade. Such a defect could have multiple manifestations mediated through abnormalities in intracellular levels of cyclic-AMP (cAMP). According to this theory, it is the beta-adrenergically activated cAMP system that is both the most important restrictive influence regulating the IgE immune response and the dominant regulator of the effector cells (smooth muscle, exocrine gland, and nerve cells) responsible for the observed clinical manifestation.

Vagal hyperactivity has also been postulated to play a role, especially in the etiology of bronchospastic disease.

Allergic Rhinitis

Allergic rhinitis is the most common allergic disorder. Symptoms include nasal obstruction, nasal discharge, sneezing, and periorbital edema. On examination, extreme pallor and bogginess of the nasal mucous membranes are apparent. Allergic rhinitis may be seasonal when it is attributable to sensitivity to a specific pollen or mold, or perennial when it is attributable to dust mite, cockroach, animal, or food sensitivities. Allergic rhinitis during the first few months of life is most often due to food allergy, and cow's milk is the chief offender. Parents may note that the infant has a continual cold and that nasal obstruction is severe enough to interfere with nursing. Inhalant allergy to either dust or mold has been reported in infants as young as 6 months of age and can lead to symptoms of allergic rhinitis. Pollen sensitivity is unusual until after the child has experienced one or more pollen seasons.

Children with allergic rhinitis often demonstrate nasal congestion, with sniffling, itchy nose, postnasal discharge, and mouth breathing. They rub their noses in a characteristic way, by pushing up on the nasal cartilage against the nasal septum with the palms of their hands; this is termed the allergic salute. They may complain of sore throat, the result of mouth breathing, and drying of the oral mucous membranes. They frequently clear their throats; in some children, this continual throat clearing can lead to a behavioral tic. Postnasal discharge may lead to a hacking cough that is slight at first but may become more pronounced, eventually overshadowing the nasal symptoms.

Children with perennial allergic rhinitis often suffer from recurrent otitis secondary to eustachian salpingitis and dysfunction. Acute and chronic sinusitis is being recognized with increasing frequency in children with allergic rhinitis. Unrecognized sinusitis may underlie treatment failure in some patients with chronic rhinitis or asthma.

Increased nasal symptoms are frequently seen in children with allergic rhinitis after exposure to airborne irritants (cigarette smoke, perfume) or with exposure to sudden changes in air temperature. This vasomotor phenomenon is much more frequent in allergic children than in nonallergic children.

Asthma and Cough-Variant Asthma

In asthma and cough-variant asthma, hypersensitivity has spread from the upper respiratory tract to include the lower respiratory tract. These conditions may be preceded by a period of allergic rhinitis. In cough-variant asthma, pulmonary function tests (PFTs) may reveal airway hyperreactivity prior to the onset of clinically apparent asthma. Cough may be provoked by exercise, cold air exposure, and by the inhalation of allergens and airborne irritants. The cough is frequently nocturnal and severe enough to awake the patient from sleep. Often, it is only when the patient begins to experience chest tightness, and expiratory wheezing is noted by the physician, that the diagnosis of asthma is made.

Asthma is the major life-threatening problem with which physicians have to deal in allergic respiratory tract disease. The morbidity and mortality of children's asthma is increasing in some studies, despite advances in diagnosis and treatment. Asthma is the number one cause of school absences, accounting for more than 30% of lost school days. In addition, approximately 40% of chronic disease office visits for children are related to asthma.

In the typical asthma episode, the child initially develops a tight hacking cough, followed by gradually increasing wheezing and associated dyspnea. There is flaring of the alae nasi, the accessory muscles of respirations are brought into play, and anxiety, air hunger, tachypnea, and cyanosis are seen. There may be associated abdominal pain and vomiting.

On examination, the chest is found to be hyperresonant to percussion, and bilateral expiratory wheezing is audible. At times, however, breath sounds are decreased, a warning that ventilation is inadequate. This lack of wheezing may be falsely interpreted as less severe disease. Atelectasis or pneumothorax, or both, may occur, with mediastinal shift to the side of atelectasis or to the side opposite the pneumothorax. If hyperexpansion is severe, the liver and spleen may be felt below the costal margin.

In infancy, asthma is often confused with acute bronchiolitis. When bronchiolitis occurs for the first time in an infant, it is usually secondary to viral infection, most frequently the respiratory syncytial virus. If symptoms are not recurrent, there is little chance that the infant has asthma. If the infant responds to respiratory tract infection repeatedly in this manner, he is probably suffering from asthma.

If a strong family history for allergic disease is not present and if symptoms are not progressive in intensity and are mild and infrequent, there is little need for extensive diagnostic procedures. On the other hand, if there is a strong family history for allergy and if symptoms cause a great deal of difficulty, recur progressively at more frequent intervals, and become more severe in intensity, then complete allergy investigation is suggested.

Initially, a careful history is required. This should include an attempt to relate allergic symptoms to particular foods, time of day, day of week, and season of the year, and to the presence of infection, physical activity, or emotional stress.

The history should include a description of the patient's bedroom, type of bedding, whether or not the patient shares the bedroom with a sibling, type of heating or air conditioning system, and presence of animals or cigarette smokers in the home. A detailed family history for allergy should be obtained. An inquiry as to past treatments, including drugs, is important, as are the results of such treatment.

Careful physical examination, including evaluation of the patient's growth and development, should be performed. Examination of the nose, careful examination of the skin to note areas of eczema, and a complete examination of the chest are required.

Recent refinements in PFTs have provided a means for objective evaluation of airway obstruction in patients with asthma. PFTs before and after inhalation of bronchodilators or bronchial challenge testing with cold air or methacholine may reveal airway abnormalities that are not otherwise apparent. X-ray studies, when indicated, depend on the specific situation but may include examination of the sinuses as well as the chest.

In children who present with recurrent symptoms, a sweat test should be considered to rule out cystic fibrosis. In children with asthma complicated by infection, quantitative immunoglobulin measurements should be done to rule out hypogammaglobulinemia. Patients may even have abnormalities of a specific immunoglobulin subclass, despite normal total immunoglobulin levels.

Allergy Skin Testing

There are many approaches to techniques of skin testing, and the reader is referred to larger texts. Generally speaking, one should test only with allergens likely to be present in the patient's environment. Skin tests are of particular value for detection of allergy to inhalants and are less useful for food sensitivities. In selected instances, however, food tests may be helpful. It may be emphasized that skin tests are not by themselves indicative of clinical sensitivity but should raise the index of suspicion or prompt further investigation.

Following completion of tests and evaluation, a report session is scheduled with the parents, and the positive items are explained to them. Foods that are suspected of causing symptoms can be removed from the diet and carefully reintroduced in order to confirm clinical significance. If the child has dust-mite sensitivity, the preparation of a dust-free room is advised. Dust-proof encasings for pillows, mattresses, and box springs are essential. Quilts and chenille spreads are not allowed. Rugs and all dust-catching items, such as stuffed toys, are removed from the room. If the child reacts to household animals, the animal is removed.

Symptomatic Treatment of Allergic Disease of the Respiratory Tract

Antihistamine drugs, often combined with oral vasoconstrictors, have their greatest use in allergic rhinitis. They often give almost complete relief of symptoms at the onset of the allergic illness, but the patient may develop tolerance to the drugs, requiring larger doses or a change to another drug. Prolonged use of vasoconstrictor nose drops is discouraged, as these may cause severe rebound congestion in the nasal mucosa, far worsening the original rhinitis. The use of nose drops should be restricted to a maximum of 4 days, with a 7-day interval before they are used again. Proper positioning of the patient in the head-down position is also important to derive maximum benefit. Corticosteroids are also effective; however, oral or parenteral administration is generally not advisable because of associated suppression of the hypothalamic-pituitary-adrenal axis. Topical administration of dexamethasone may have similar undesirable effects after prolonged use. The newer nasal steroid preparations, beclomethasone and flunisolide, reportedly topically effective and less likely to cause systemic side effects, are now available. Cromolyn sodium nasal spray is also beneficial.

Epinephrine may be used to control acute symptoms of asthma. Because of the rather short duration of action, repeated injections at 20-minute intervals may be necessary. If the epinephrine successfully relieves the acute episode, however, the use of a 1 : 200 aqueous suspension of epinephrine may give prolonged relief.

Increasingly, selective beta$_2$-adrenergic agents (isoetharine, metaproterenol, terbutaline, and albuterol) are becoming available for both oral and inhalational use; however, intermittent positive pressure (IPPB) administration of the agents affords no advantage over simple nebulization and may increase risk of pneumothorax.

Theophylline may also be used intravenously, via bolus or by continuous infusion for acute management of serious episodes of asthma, or orally for prophylactic or symptomatic control. Serum theophylline measurements are suggested, given the variations in theophylline clearance in the pediatric age group.

Cromolyn for inhalation is a particularly useful therapy in pediatric asthma because of its effect on reducing both the early and late phases of the immediate hypersensitivity reaction. The late phase reaction is a source of the inflammatory changes that occur in the airway.

Corticosteroids have dramatically changed the symptomatic treatment of asthma. They can be used in the acute phase of the attack in relatively large doses intravenously, then continued orally or rapidly tapered, depending on clinical circumstances. Like cromolyn, corticosteroids reduce the late phase response and are of importance in controlling airway inflammation.

Despite the most complete management, a small group of patients with asthma continue to have moderate to severe difficulty. It may be necessary to maintain these patients on long-term steroid therapy to alleviate their symptoms. The smallest dose of corticosteroids consistent with the patient's comfort should be used. An every-other-day schedule has the advantage of reducing the risks of toxic effect, as does the use of inhaled corticosteroid preparations.

Immunotherapy

The child is immunized only with those substances that give him difficulty, to which he has reacted on skin testing, and for which the efficacy of hyposensitization has been demonstrated.

In general, the objective of immunotherapy is to increase the dose of antigen on a weekly basis to the maximum tolerated dose, and then to maintain the patient on that dose as maintenance therapy. The length of therapy depends on response. Patients not responding to immunotherapy within 1 to 2 years should be carefully reevaluated. Ineffective programs of immunotherapy should not be continued. Bacterial vaccines have not proven efficacious. Immunotherapy with mold extracts has not been adequately studied in a controlled manner. Immunotherapy with pollen, cat, and dust-mite allergens, however, has been shown to be clinically effective.

The exact mechanisms by which immunotherapy affects the patient is unknown. An elevation of allergen-specific IgG during immunotherapy has been observed; this may act as a blocking antibody. Suppression of IgE production and alteration of mast cell and basophil responsiveness has also been postulated.

Atopic Dermatitis

Atopic dermatitis is a disorder of the skin seen in infancy and childhood. It is generally held to be allergic in nature. Often associated or confused with it is a type of dermatitis, seborrheic dermatitis, which is seen in early infancy. There does not appear to be a strong allergic component in seborrheic dermatitis.

Atopic dermatitis is usually seen after the introduction of new foods into the infant's diet. It is infrequent in breast-fed babies but may appear after the mother stops breast feeding and places the infant on cow milk–based formula. It may also be seen after commercial milk formula is replaced by whole milk. Egg is another food that may have an etiologic role in the development of atopic dermatitis.

Clinical Manifestations

Atopic dermatitis in infancy usually starts as a rather intense inflammation over the cheeks. Eczematous lesions spread from the cheeks to other areas of the face. It is common to find lesions on the flexoral surfaces of the body as well, particularly the antecubital and popliteal fossae.

Seborrheic dermatitis often begins as a thick scaly eruption over the scalp and forehead but may also be seen on the anterior chest wall, around the umbilicus, and in the diaper area. The chief lesions of seborrheic dermatitis are yellowish scales. In contrast to allergic eczema, the lesions of seborrheic dermatitis do not appear to be pruritic.

Atopic dermatitis may become crusted and weeping, and is often secondarily infected. Bacterial infection of the eczematous areas is most often caused by staphylococci and secondarily by streptococci. This type of infection may be managed by systemic antibiotics. More severe infections of eczematous areas are those caused by viruses; vaccinia, herpes simplex, and varicella viruses are the most serious offenders.

Diseases to be distinguished from either allergic eczema or seborrheic dermatitis include Letterer-Siwe disease, phenylketonuria, Wiskott-Aldrich syndrome (eczema, bloody diarrhea, chronic otitis media, thrombocytopenia, and dysgammaglobulinemia), X-linked agammaglobulinemia, and hyper-IgE syndrome.

Treatment

The treatment of atopic dermatitis focuses on allergic factors, infectious elements, and local and systemic treatment of the rash itself. These three aspects all must be considered.

Local treatment should initially be aimed at dealing with the skin inflammation. Burow's solution is frequently of benefit. If there is a great deal of infection, appropriate antibiotics are administered systemically. Pustules and vesicles are clues to the presence of *Staphylococcus,* whereas cellulitis often indicates a streptococcal infection.

Corticosteroids may be used topically or systemically. The child with generalized atopic dermatitis is probably best managed by using systemic steroids. Prednisone is administered until the inflammation subsides and then is tapered. Steroids are contraindicated in viral infections, such as varicella, vaccinia, or herpes.

As pruritis and subsequent excoriation is a prime factor in persistence of the rash, antihistamines should be used to alleviate itching. Unintentional scratching while the patient is asleep frequently occurs; therefore, it is important to continue antipruritic therapy throughout the night. Trimming the fingernails also helps to reduce excorition. Coarse clothing and bedding (wool) should be avoided.

Allergic management again depends on the extent of the patient's disease. It may be possible to discover an offending food by an elimination diet; however, nearly half the infants and children with atopic dermatitis have negative reactions to scratch testing with common foods. Immunotherapy is not of proven therapy in the management of atopic dermatitis. In fact, exacerbations may occur after immunotherapy.

Nevertheless, skin testing and immunotherapy with inhalant allergens may be justified for concurrent allergic respiratory disease.

In the majority of cases, eczema remits and disappears by the time the child is 3 years old. In more than 30% of affected children, however, other manifestations of allergic disease usually become apparent as the child grows older.

Urticaria and Angioedema

Urticaria and angioedema are common but usually self-limiting problems in pediatrics. These are caused either by substances that act directly by histamine release or by those that are sensitizing and, therefore, truly allergenic. Physical agents, including heat, cold, light, and trauma, can also cause urticaria in certain persons.

In the usual case of urticaria, an irregular blotching red rash, which is raised and pruritic, occurs suddenly. The rash is often first noted after a warm bath, with distribution around pressure points on the body, such as the waist where a tight belt has been worn. Depending on the underlying cause, there may or may not be accompanying fever.

Angioedema is a firm, nonpitting type of edema that appears usually on the face over the lips, eyes, or cheeks, and less commonly over the extremities; it is not as pruritic as urticaria. Angioedema can produce life-threatening symptoms if the airway is involved, in which case there can be respiratory obstruction and death.

A hereditary form of angioedema is due to a deficiency of C_1 esterase inhibitor, which acts to inhibit the esterase produced by activation by the first component of complement. This disease usually begins in childhood. Attacks may be life-threatening. Anabolic steroids, such as Danazol, stimulate production of the deficient protein and control the condition if taken prophylactically.

While specific allergens, such as shellfish or penicillin, can sometimes be demonstrated to cause urticaria, most cases have no demonstrable cause. Chronic idiopathic urticaria can continue for weeks or months and may be difficult to treat. Skin testing and desensitization are not usually helpful in diagnosis or treatment.

Treatment

The treatment of urticaria is basically symptomatic. Use of antihistamines and epinephrine often relieve the symptoms quickly. Corticosteroids may be used in severe or resistant cases but do not exert their influence for several hours after administration.

Anaphylaxis

Anaphylaxis is an acute, often severe generalized allergic reaction involving multiple organ systems. Skin manifestations include urticaria and angioedema. There may be upper and lower respiratory involvement, as well as cardiovascular abnormalities, including pulse variations and hypotension. There is usually a clear-cut temporal relationship of exposure to the offending allergen. Formerly, anaphylactic reactions were most often seen after administration of animal (horse) serum. Today, drug allergies account for many such reactions. Other important causes include insect stings, administration of allergenic extracts for hyposensitization therapy, and reactions to blood transfusion.

Stinging Insect Anaphylaxis

The availability of purified venom extracts from the common stinging insects (bee, yellow jacket, hornet, and wasp) of the order Hymenoptera has vastly improved the diagnostic and therapeutic management of stinging insect hypersensitivity. Positive immediate intracutaneous reactions to dilute concentrations of these venoms correlate well with hypersensitivity in the face of a supporting clinical history. Immunotherapy with these extracts has resulted in protection against anaphylactic reactions to subsequent stings in clinical trials. The use of whole body insect extracts can no longer be justified for the treatment of stinging insect hypersensitivity.

Food Allergy

The wide variety of adverse reactions to foods complicates any discussion of food allergy. In the broadest sense, adverse reactions to foods include all clinically abnormal responses to food ingestion, whereas "food hypersensitivity" (or allergy) should be reserved for those reactions with an immunologic basis.

"Food intolerance" may be used for reactions not proved to be immunologic. Food intolerances may include allergic, pharmacologic, and idiosyncratic food reactions.

True food allergy has been reported as far back as the time of Hippocrates, who described gastric upset and urticaria after cow's milk exposure. Food allergies can provoke dermatologic, respiratory, and gastrointestinal symptoms, and at times can be responsible for acute anaphylactic reactions. The most common offending foods are cow's milk, eggs, peanuts, true nuts, wheat, soy, fish, shellfish, tomato, and corn. Diagnosis requires demonstration of an adverse reaction by history or by challenge testing and detection of allergen-specific antibodies by skin testing or in vitro methods. Positive skin tests or in vitro tests to food allergens without demonstration of a clinical reaction is not diagnostic, as either may occur in nonallergic individuals.

Scott B. Valet

References

Adverse Reactions to Foods. NIH Publication No. 84-2442. An AAAI and NIADD Report. July, 1984.

Middleton, E., et al. (Eds.). *Allergy Principles and Practice* (3rd ed.) St. Louis: Mosby, 1988.

Oski, F. A., D'Angelio, C. D., Feigin, R. D., and Warshow, J. B. *Principle and Practicer of Pediatrics.* Philadelphia: Lippincott, 1990.

Symposium on Pediatric Allergy. *Pedatr. Clin. North Am.* 30:5, 1983.

22

The Skin

Accurate diagnosis of a skin disorder requires acquisition of pertinent historical information, thorough examination of the skin (including mucous membranes, hair, and nails), and evaluation of other organ systems. Histopathologic assessment can be invaluable in some instances. It is usually, however, the recognition of lesional morphology and the configuration and distribution of an eruption that ultimately permits the physician to arrive at the correct diagnosis.

Nevoid Lesions

Café au Lait Spots

These lesions are sometimes present at birth but more often appear during the first few years of life and consist of light tan to dark brown sharply demarcated macules of uniform color and variable size. When numerous, they suggest a diagnosis of neurofibromatosis. They also occur with increased frequency in tuberous sclerosis. McCune-Albright syndrome, Bloom's syndrome, and the multiple lentigines syndrome.

Mongolian Spot

This lesion is probably the most frequently encountered pigmented lesion in the newborn infant, occurring in more than 90% of black, Oriental, and Indian infants and in less than 5% of white infants. The usual site is the lumbosacral area; however, the back, shoulders, and legs may also be involved. The lesions are macular, blue to slate gray, ill-defined patches of variable size and number. They represent collections of melanocytes in the dermis, presumably arrested in migration from neural crest to epidermis. Usually they fade gradually during the first few years of life.

Occasionally these lesions persist into adulthood or appear later in life. A persistent lesion on the face is called nevus of Ota; one on the shoulder, nevus of Ito.

Pigmented Nevi

Melanocytic nevi can be either congenital or acquired. Congenital nevi vary in size from very tiny lesions to large lesions (giant hairy nevi) covering a significant portion of the body surface. The color may be variegated, the surface may be

444

irregular, and there may be a profuse growth of coarse hair from the lesion. Congenital pigmented nevi should be removed early in life because of the increased risk of malignant melanoma arising in these lesions.

Acquired nevi may be junctional, compound, or dermal, terms that relate to the location of the nevus cells within the skin. Junctional nevi are flat, brown to black, sharply demarcated lesions that reflect increased numbers of melanocytic cells at the dermoepidermal junction. Compound and dermal nevi are raised, dome-shaped, dark brown to skin-colored lesions in which the melanocytic cells are found in both epidermis and dermis (compound) or solely within the dermis (dermal). Acquired nevi need be removed only if they constitute a nuisance to the patient, generate undue anxiety, or exhibit changes suggestive of malignant transformation. Any nevi that are removed should be subjected to careful pathological examination.

Vascular Nevi

Nevus Flammeus (Port-Wine Stain)

This flat, smooth, pink-purple lesion is present at birth. It is made up of mature capillaries and, therefore, does not fade with aging. Laser treatments have been successful in selected patients. Cosmetic creams are also available to cover unsightly lesions. These lesions may be found in Sturge-Weber syndrome (see Chap. 13).

Flat, pink vascular stains (salmon patches) are very common in the newborn infant. The facial lesions fade completely during the first few months of life and require no treatment. Those on the nape of the neck may persist into adult life.

Strawberry Hemangiomas

These elevated, sharply demarcated, bright red, soft tumors are composed of immature vascular elements (Fig. 22-1). They may be present at birth but more often appear within the first few weeks of life. Initially they may increase in size, but ultimately they involute. Treatment is unnecessary for small lesions; those that are extensive or impair function may require intervention. A short, intensive course of systemic corticosteroid therapy or intralesional injection of steroid may halt expansion and bring about a more rapid involution of such lesions.

Cavernous Hemangiomas

These tumors, which are raised, poorly circumscribed, and blue to purple in color, are composed of large, dilated

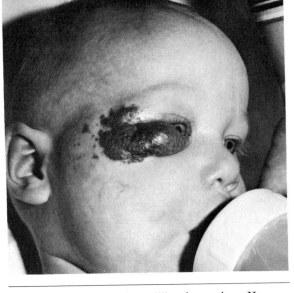

Fig. 22-1. Discrete, elevated, capilliary hemangioma. Nevus flammeus is also frequently found in the periorbital area.

vascular spaces (Fig. 22-2). They are often present at birth and have an initial growth phase. Usually they regress spontaneously. Extensive lesions may be associated with thrombocytopenia secondary to sequestration of platelets and the findings of disseminated intravascular coagulation. Systemic corticosteroid therapy is helpful in some instances.

Hereditary Disorders

Ichthyoses

The ichthyoses are a group of congenital keratinizing disorders. The skin is rough, thickened, and covered with white, gray or brownish scales. The patterns of involvement and the distribution of scales depend on the particular type of ichthyosis. In the most common variety, ichthyosis vulgaris, an autosomal dominant condition, the extensor surfaces of the extremities are the most severely affected. Pruritus may be present and is aggravated by extremes of temperature and dryness.

Treatment consists of a daily bath with a nondrying cleansing agent, followed immediately by application of a lubricating ointment. Urea and lactic acid preparations, vi-

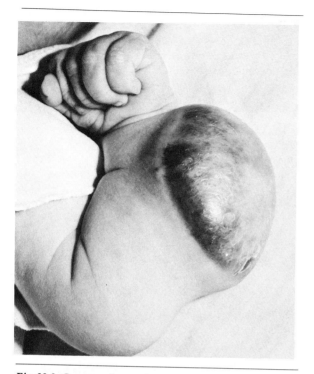

Fig. 22-2. Cavernous hemangioma on the forearm with beginning fibrosis noticeable on the surface. This infant had Kasabach-Merritt syndrome.

tamin A acid, and propylene glycol incorporated in a gel are some effective topical agents.

Ectodermal Dysplasia

Many varieties of this condition are seen in combinations of hypoplastic or absent sweat glands, hypotrichosis, abnormalities of dentition, alteration of the nails, and dry skin. In one form, hypohidrotic ectodermal dysplasia, heat intolerance is a problem because of the inability to sweat. Avoiding exposure to hot environmental temperatures is the only treatment.

Ehlers-Danlos Syndrome and Cutis Laxa

Ehlers-Danlos syndrome, which is now known to include at least 10 different variants, may be manifested by hyperelasticity of the skin, hyperflexibility of the joints, and extreme fragility of skin and systemic vasculature. Wound healing is abnormal, and there is formation of freely movable sub-cutaneous fatty nodules. The patient should be protected against injury.

Cutis laxa is characterized by inelastic, loose skin, which hangs in baggy folds. There may be widespread degeneration of elastic fibers in the skin, lungs, and other organs in the autosomal recessive type. An autosomal dominant type, which has a more benign prognosis, and an X-linked recessive type have also been described.

Adenoma Sebaceum

The lesions are yellowish, elevated, fibroangiomatous papules 1 to 5 mm in diameter, usually distributed symmetrically over the nose, cheeks, and nasolabial folds. These lesions, along with white leaf macules, shagreen patches, periungual and cutaneous fibromas, are markers for tuberous sclerosis, an autosomal dominant multisystem disease.

Incontinentia Pigmenti

This rare hereditary disorder is manifested by whorls and streaks of brownish pigmentation on any body surface and may be quite generalized in distribution. The onset of the disease is during the early months of life, at which time the eruption is vesicular. Hyperkeratotic, verrucous lesions represent the second stage and finally progress to the pigmented stage. They may fade with increasing age. The disorder occurs only in females. Neurological and ocular abnormalities, alopecia, and anomalies of dentition may be associated.

Epidermolysis Bullosa

This group of disorders is manifested by the appearance of bullae over pressure points or at sites of trauma. Lesions may occur anywhere on the body. The more severe forms of the disease may cause extensive scarring, deformity of the fingers and toes, and loss of the nails. All forms of the disease are inherited, and it is important to distinguish scarring from nonscarring types because the prognosis depends on the type and severity of the disease. Heat and warm weather appear to exacerbate the disorder in most patients. Complications include chronic anemia, growth failure, ulcerations and strictures of the mucous membranes, defective dentition, and secondary infection. There is no satisfactory therapy, but protection from trauma and heat, appropriate antibiotics, attention to nutritional needs, early dental care, and plastic procedures, when necessary, all improve the quality of life for the patients.

Diseases of the Newborn Infant

Milia

These superficial epithelial inclusion cysts are often present on the face of the normal term infant or in the oral cavity (in which case they are known as Epstein's pearls). Clinically they appear as 1- to 2-mm white papules, on the forehead, cheeks, and nose, on the central palate and gingivae, or, occasionally, on the penile skin. They exfoliate spontaneously within a few weeks after birth. Milia also may develop in older children as a result of injury to the skin.

Sebaceous Hyperplasia

This physiological skin change is most frequently detectable on the forehead, cheeks, nose, and chin of term infants as a profusion of tiny yellow macules and papules. They are believed to result from maternal androgenic stimulation and involute spontaneously, disappearing within the first month or two of life.

Aplasia Cutis

Also known as congenital absence of skin, these lesions are sharply marginated, solitary or multiple depressed areas of variable size, most often located on the vertex of the scalp just lateral to the midline. Similar lesions are occasionally found elsewhere on the body surface. The depth of the defect varies; when severe, all layers of the skin may be absent. The lesions heal with scar formation and remain hairless throughout life. In some families this congenital defect has been transmitted as a heritable trait.

Erythema Toxicum

This common, transient disorder of the first few days of life is manifested by white papulopustules, 1 to 3 mm in size, on an erythematous base that may occur on any body surface. Systemic symptoms are absent. A peripheral eosinophilia in the range of 7 to 15% is present in approximately half the cases. Demonstration of eosinophils on Gram's stain of the exudate distinguishes this lesion from that of pyoderma. The distribution of the eruption is also a helpful feature because the papules tend to be scattered, while those of pyoderma group themselves in the flexor areas, particularly in the diaper region and axillae. The cause is unknown. Treatment is unnecessary.

Bullous Impetigo

See Chapter 9.

Staphylococcal Scalded Skin Syndrome

The term *toxic epidermal necrolysis* is now limited by dermatologists to a severe form of erythema multiforme, not staphylococcal in origin. See Chapter 9.

Generalized Seborrheic Dermatitis

Seborrheic dermatitis of infancy can be localized or generalized and consists of nonpruritic erythematous plaques with branny or greasy-appearing surface scale. Common sites are the diaper area, axillae, neck folds, and retroauricular areas. Thick scale is usually present in the scalp. The onset is usually sometime after 2 weeks of age and may occur as late as 3 months.

The scalp dermatitis may be treated by daily use of an antiseborrheic shampoo and ointment containing 3% sulfur. A similar preparation may be used for the skin; however, a topical steroid such as 1% hydrocortisone or 0.025% triamcinolone ointment 3 times a day is more effective. The disorder usually responds rapidly to treatment but may recur up until 10 to 14 months of age, when it usually abates spontaneously.

Subcutaneous Fat Necrosis and Sclerema Neonatorum

Subcutaneous fat necrosis usually occurs in the otherwise healthy full-term infant and has been attributed to cold exposure or undue trauma sustained during labor or delivery. The lesions are circumscribed nodular areas of induration, with a woody consistency and a violaceous hue. Necrosis with extrusion of the liquefied material is an occasional complication, as is secondary calcification. The size and number of lesions are extremely variable. The prognosis is excellent, and residual sequelae are rare.

Sclerema neonatorum is more common in premature or debilitated infants and may have a similar etiology. The skin is nonpitting, inflexible, and mottled; it may be involved over the entire body, resulting in generalized boardlike rigidity. Affected infants frequently succumb to the underlying disease. It should not be confused with edema neonatorum, which is a pitting edema of the lower extremities and trunk and does not represent a primary alteration of fatty tissue.

Diseases of Infectious Etiology

Viral Diseases

VERRUCAE. Verrucae on the general body surface are of two types: the flat wart (verruca plana juvenilis), which is a soft, small, often multiple lesion, and the common wart (verruca vulgaris), which is horny, filiform, or conical. Sites of predilection for the latter are the hands and feet; juvenile flat warts are most commonly seen on the face and backs of the hands. When on the plantar and palmar surfaces, warts are flat, round, and exceedingly hyperkeratotic with depressed central cores. Verrucae on the mucous membranes are soft, moist, and polypoid and are called condylomata acuminata. They are all of viral etiology and mildly contagious.

Destruction of verrucae is accomplished by freezing with liquid nitrogen, curettage and desiccation, formalin soaks, and keratolytic agents (Duofilm). Cantharidin, 0.9%, in equal parts of acetone and flexible collodion may also be used. The necrotic debris and blisters produced by these agents should be trimmed off to prevent further dissemination of viral particles and spread of infection. Condylomata acuminata should be treated by freezing with liquid nitrogen or by 20% podophyllin in tincture of benzoin applied every few days until the lesions have disappeared. All of the blistering agents should be confined to the warty tissue to prevent needless destruction of surrounding normal skin. Spontaneous resolution of these lesions is not uncommon.

MOLLUSCUM CONTAGIOSUM. The lesions are sessile, pearly white, often umbilicated papules, which are seen on all body surfaces and vary in size from one to several millimeters (Fig. 22-3). The disorder is contagious, and once it is contracted dissemination by autoinoculation is usual. The

Fig. 22-3. Multiple noninflammatory papules of molluscum on the lateral chest wall and in the axilla.

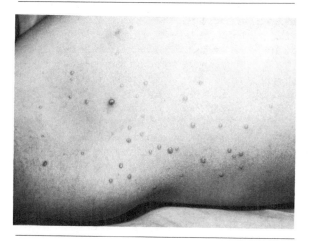

etiological agent is a virus. Treatment is by incision and expression of the contents of the individual lesions or by judicious application of a blistering agent to individual lesions.

Fungal Infections

CANDIDIASIS. *Candida albicans* is a common cause of yeast infections in infants and children. Sites of predilection are the mouth (thrush), diaper area, intertriginous areas, and the paronychial skin. The organism is usually acquired at birth and may colonize the gastrointestinal tract as a relatively harmless saprophyte.

In the oral cavity candidiasis is typified by plaques of white, cheesy material on a friable, erythematous base. In the diaper area and flexures candidal infections consist of brightly erythematous plaques that may be dry and scaly or erosive and weeping. Satellite vesicles, pustules, and small erythematous scaly lesions are a usual feature. In candidal paronychia the typical changes are swelling and erythema of the posterior nail fold and dystrophy of the nail beginning proximally. Candidal infections also occur as persistent mucocutaneous lesions and granulomas in patients with defective immunity.

The diagnosis is made with relative ease by demonstrating the pseudomycelia and budding yeasts on a potassium hydroxide preparation of scrapings, a Gram's stain of pus, or a culture of the intralesional material on blood or Mycosel agar. Treatment with nystatin, amphotericin B, haloprogin, or an imidazole is usually effective. Recurrences are common if predisposing factors such as constant moisture (e.g., thumb sucking) or an underlying dermatitis is present. Patients receiving immunosuppressive agents and those with debilitating diseases are particularly susceptible to candidal infections.

TINEA VERSICOLOR. This superficial fungal infection is characterized by multiple nonpruritic, superficial, scaly macules that may be hypo- or hyperpigmented. The back and the anterior surface of the chest are the primary sites of involvement (Fig. 22-4). Diagnosis is aided by the yellowish fluorescence seen under Wood's lamp and by demonstration of the hyphae and spores of *Pityrosporon orbiculare* on examination of scales in 10% potassium hydroxide. This fungus cannot be cultured on routine media. Removal of the infected upper horny layers is accomplished by the use of various peeling agents or by application of selenium sulfide (Selsun) overnight for 3 consecutive nights. An antifungal agent such as haloprogin, miconazole, or clotrimazole, applied twice daily for 2 or 3 weeks, is also effective. Although temporary cure may be obtained, affected persons are prone

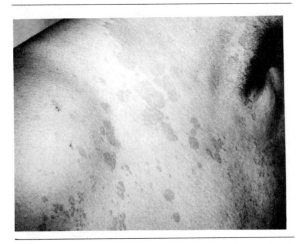

Fig. 22-4. *Sharply demarcated, hyperpigmented, scaly macules of tinea versicolor in a typical distribution.*

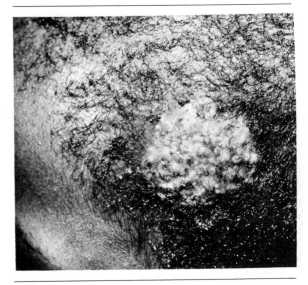

Fig. 22-5. *Circumscribed boggy mass studded with pustules in the scalp. This kerion has been caused by* Trichophyton tonsurans.

to recurrence because the causative organism is a normal saprophyte.

DERMATOPHYTOSIS (RINGWORM). The dermatophyte infections are confined to the epidermis, the hair, and the nails. The three related groups of fungi that are the causative agents are *Microsporum, Epidermophyton,* and *Trichophyton.* These organisms proliferate only in the keratinous structures.

Tinea Capitis. Tinea capitis is caused by either *Microsporum* or *Trichophyton* species. Pathognomonic signs are patchy alopecia, scaling, and broken hairs. The lesions may have papulovesicular erythematous borders or may appear as simple scaling with a few broken hairs. Acute inflammation with edema, pustules, and granulomatous swelling is called kerion (Fig. 22-5). Blue-green fluorescence with a Wood's lamp is diagnostic of *Microsporum* infections. Examination of a plucked infected hair with 10% potassium hydroxide demonstrates clusters of small spores on the outside of the shaft (ectothrix) in *Microsporum* infections and larger spores inside the hair (endothrix) if *Trichophyton* is the causative agent. The species are easily identified by culture. Differential diagnosis includes consideration of seborrhea, psoriasis, and pyoderma. Lack of scaling and inflammation distinguish alopecia areata. The treatment of choice is microcrystalline griseofulvin 15 mg/kg/day. Ingestion with a high-fat meal and the use of a microcrystalline preparation increase intestinal absorption significantly. Additional measures such as shaving the head are unnecessary; however, treatments with an antiseborrheic shampoo decrease spore

shedding. Griseofulvin is usually required for 6 to 12 weeks but should be continued until culture of the infected area is negative. Loss of fluorescence is not a reliable indication of cure.

Tinea Corporis (Tinea Circinata). Tinea corporis is ringworm of the nonhairy skin and may be caused by any of the *Trichophyton, Microsporum,* and *Epidermophyton* species. The lesions are circinate plaques with erythematous, papulovesicular, scaly borders, often with central clearing (Fig. 22-6). Involvement of any body surface may occur, although tinea cruris (ringworm of the groin) is seen most commonly in adolescent males. A potassium hydroxide preparation of scale from the active border of the lesion and positive culture confirm the diagnosis. Localized areas may be treated with topical antifungal agents. Treatment with oral griseofulvin is often more effective (see Tinea Capitis), the usual course of treatment being 2 to 4 weeks.

Tinea Pedis (Athlete's Foot). Tinea pedis is seen infrequently in childhood but more commonly during adolescence. The *Trichophyton* species and *Epidermophyton floccosum* are the etiological agents. Predisposing factors include trauma to the feet and hyperhidrosis, as well as individual susceptibility. The clinical lesions range from vesicopustules, with marked fissuring and inflammation, to mild erythema and scaling. Pruritus and burning may be troublesome. Toenails may be involved and act as a reservoir for

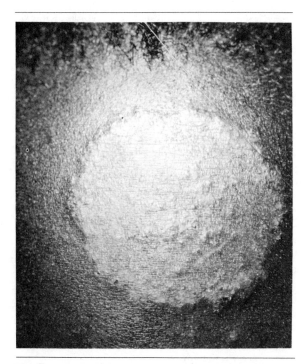

Fig. 22-6. Circinate lesions of tinea corporis with active elevated papular border and scaly center.

reinfection. Diagnosis is made by potassium hydroxide preparation of scales and by culture of the organism. Differential diagnosis includes consideration of contact dermatitis from shoe materials, atopic and dyshidrotic eczema, pyoderma, and hyperkeratosis. Treatment should include meticulous drying of feet and avoidance of occlusive shoes and heavy socks. Acute inflammatory lesions may require frequent tap-water soaks and antibiotics for secondary bacterial infection. Topical antifungal agents or griseofulvin given orally in therapeutic dosages (see Tinea Capitis) may be used. Therapy with griseofulvin is usually required for 4 to 6 weeks but may have to be continued for a longer period, particularly if there is involvement of the nails.

Diseases Due to Parasites

SCABIES. Scabies is produced by the mite *Sarcoptes scabiei* and is characterized by extremely pruritic vesicular and papular lesions. The mite burrows through the stratum corneum, producing linear tracks that are the hallmark of this disease. The ova are deposited within the burrows and hatch

into larvae in 3 or 4 days. The sites of predilection are the interdigital surfaces, the axillary, cubital, and popliteal folds, and the inguinal region, as well as the areolae in the female (Fig. 22-7). Facial lesions are rare, except in infants, who frequently also have lesions on the palms and soles. Excoriation and secondary infection are common because of the intense itching, which is most troublesome at night. The diagnosis is confirmed by mineral oil scrapings from the lesions and microscopical identification of the live mite, eggs, and fecal pellets.

An effective treatment is gamma benzene hexachloride (Kwell), which should be applied to the entire body for 8 hours and repeated in 1 week. If this medication is not available, a 6% sulfur ointment may be used for 3 con-

Fig. 22-7. Erythematous papules, vesicles, and nodules of scabies with accentuation in the axilla, a common distribution in infants and toddlers.

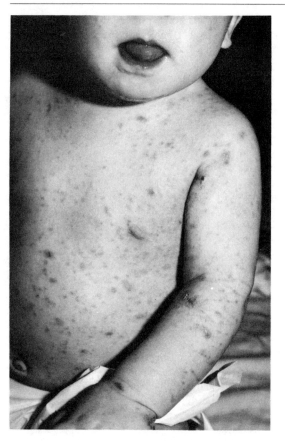

secutive 24-hour periods; however, this may produce an irritant dermatitis in patients with sensitive skin. Infants under 6 months of age should be treated with sulfur ointment because of the hazards of absorption of gamma benzene hexachloride. All contacts should be examined for infection and treated if affected.

PEDICULOSIS. Three varieties of lice may infect humans; the head louse, the body louse, and the pubic louse. Each shows a predilection for its particular area and rarely migrates to other regions of the body. All produce a pruritic, papular dermatitis, which may become severely excoriated. In addition, the louse is a carrier of typhus, relapsing fever, and trench fever.

Pediculosis Capitis. Pediculosis capitis, the most common type of infestation, is manifested by an intensely pruritic dermatitis of the scalp, which may become secondarily infected, resulting in enlarged regional lymph nodes. Diagnosis is made by identification of the ova (nit), a small gray nodule attached to the hair shaft. The most effective treatments are Rid and Kwell, applied once as a shampoo for 5 minutes and rinsed out. Nits may be removed from the hair shafts by a warm 1:1 vinegar-water rinse followed by combing with a fine-toothed comb.

Pediculosis Corporis. Pediculosis corporis is manifested by erythematous macules, wheals, and excoriated papules that are often impetiginized. Sites of predilection are the upper back and pressure areas from tight clothing. Sparing of the hands and feet is important in differentiating this infestation from scabies. The diagnosis is confirmed by identification of the lice and nits in the seams of clothing. The insect is present on the skin only when foraging. Lice on the body can be eradicated by an application of gamma benzene hexachloride lotion or by dusting with 10% DDT powder. The clothing should be boiled and dusted with DDT powder, particularly along the seams.

Infection with the pubic louse is rare in childhood; however, this parasite may also be found in the eyelashes. Infestation of the eyelashes may be treated with physostigmine ointment or petrolatum applied thickly twice daily for a week.

CREEPING ERUPTION (LARVA MIGRANS). This disease is characterized by serpentine, erythematous inflammatory lesions produced by burrowing larvae of a variety of parasites. The principal etiological agents are the cat and dog hookworms. The larvae are acquired from contact with sand or dirt contaminated by infected feces. The lesions are pruritic and may become quite numerous. Local treatment by freezing the larvae with ethyl chloride or solid carbon dioxide is somewhat effective; however, topical application of thiabendazole suspension 4 times daily until the lesions have

cleared is the treatment of choice. Thiabendazole, 25 mg/kg by mouth, twice daily for 2 days, is also a successful therapeutic measure. Common side effects are anorexia, nausea, vomiting, and vertigo.

Pyoderma

Impetigo contagiosa, the most common type of pyoderma, is characterized by discrete vesicles that become pustular and covered with thick, moist, amber-colored crusts. These lesions are often indolent and spread by autoinoculation. The etiological agent is the beta-hemolytic streptococcus. The term *ecthyma* is used for penetrating lesions, which heal with scarring. Scalded skin syndrome is a severe bullous form of staphylococcal etiology that becomes widespread and may cause constitutional symptoms. Bullous impetigo, characterized by superficial blisters that, when ruptured, leave a thin, varnishlike crust, is the localized form of this type of infection. Superficial folliculitis involves the hair follicle primarily and localizes to the scalp or extremities. Furuncles and carbuncles also arise in the hair follicle. Erysipelas is a well-defined superficial, streptococcal dermal cellulitis and lymphangitis producing toxic symptoms and requiring systemic antibiotic therapy.

Treatment consists of hot-water soaks to effect removal of crusts, and incision and drainage of pustular lesions. Scrubbing with soap or germicidal agents may aid debridement. Systemic antibiotics (preferably penicillin or erythromycin) or appropriate antibiotic ointments should be administered until the lesions have cleared.

Hypersensitivity Diseases

Eczema

See Chapter 19.

Urticaria and Angioneurotic Edema

See Chapter 19.

Erythema Multiforme

Erythema multiforme is a hypersensitivity reaction that may be related to antecedent or concurrent infection or to systemically administered drugs or may be of unknown etiology. The polymorphic cutaneous manifestations (erythema multiforme minor) include symmetrically distributed erythematous macules, papules, vesicles, and bullae, and urticarial lesions (Fig. 22-8). The target lesion (rings of

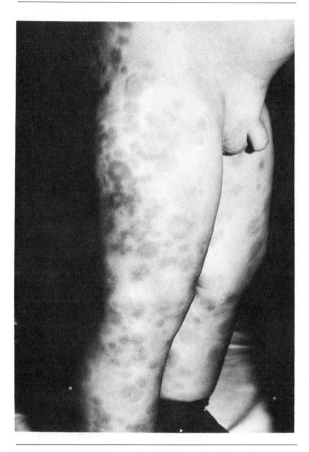

Fig. 22-8. Erythematous urticarial lesions of erythema multiforme scattered over the legs. Note several target lesions.

erythema alternated with a healing clear zone) is pathognomonic when present. Prodromes of malaise, fever, upper respiratory tract symptoms, joint pain, and vomiting may precede the rash.

Mucous membrane involvement (erythema multiforme major, Stevens-Johnson syndrome) may accompany the above lesions or may be the sole manifestation. The intensely painful vesicles result in eroded lesions with crusted or pseudomembranous exudate on the lips, tongue, buccal mucosa, and genitalia and occasionally in nasopharynx, esophagus, and tracheobronchial tree. A purulent conjunctivitis complicated by corneal ulceration may occur, which if not properly managed can lead to blindness. Systemic manifestations may be severe, with prostration, high fever, chills, and occasionally lymphadenopathy and splenomegaly. Laboratory tests are not helpful. The duration of the clinical course is variable and depends on the severity of involvement. Mortality ranges from 1 to 10%; the overall recurrence is approximately 20%. Therapy is supportive; occasionally, systemic steroids may be useful in aborting an attack. Good nursing care of the involved mucous membranes and particularly of lesions involving the eyes is essential. Local antibiotics can be applied to the eye lesions. Systemic antimicrobial therapy is reserved for patients who have secondary bacterial infection. Whenever there is a known provoking agent such as certain sulfonamide drugs, it should be withdrawn. The most severe form of erythema multiforme is called toxic epidermal necrolysis, in which full-thickness necrotic epidermis separates from the underlying dermis over large areas of the body (Fig. 22-9). This

Fig. 22-9. Drug-induced toxic epidermal necrolysis. Sharply marginated erythema, flaccid bullae, and areas of denudation are all visible.

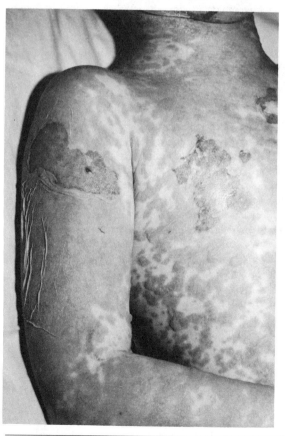

reaction is rare in children and, when it occurs, is almost invariably a drug reaction. The patients suffer all the complications of burn patients, and the death rate is high. Fastidious supportive care and isolation techniques are critical for survival.

Erythema Nodosum

The lesion, as named, is a pale red, discrete nodule, 1 to 3 cm in diameter, that is warm and tender to the touch. Lesions may coalesce to form fluctuant masses. Older lesions show a bruiselike discoloration of the skin with thickening and fine cigarette-paper scale. The anterior aspect of the lower legs is the site of predilection. Prodromes of malaise, fever, chills, migratory joint pain, and pharyngitis may be present. An elevated erythrocyte sedimentation rate is usual while the lesions are active. The cause of this condition is unknown although it is thought to be a hypersensitivity reaction. It is commonly associated with tuberculosis, coccidioidomycosis, streptococcal infections, sarcoidosis, regional enteritis, lymphogranuloma venereum, and therapy with a variety of drugs. Attention should be directed toward diagnosis and treatment of the underlying disease. The skin lesions are self-limited but may be treated with nonsteroidal antiinflammatory agents.

Papular Urticaria (Lichen Urticatus)

This disease occurs principally during the summer months in children between the ages of 2 and 7 years. The lesions are clusters of inflamed wheals that become papular or vesicular and are intensely pruritic (Fig. 22-10). Impetiginization secondary to excoriation is a frequent finding. The eruption occurs predominantly on exposed areas, and duration varies from a few days to 2 or 3 years. Papular urticaria is a persistent, delayed hypersensitivity reaction to insect bites. Effective treatment requires elimination of the incriminated agent from the environment. Cure may be exceedingly difficult. Treatment of patients and all pets with an insecticide spray or dusting powder and spraying of houses and furniture are the most successful therapeutic measures. Antihistamines are relatively ineffective. Itching may be relieved by topical applications of a corticosteroid preparation.

Drug Eruptions

The entire spectrum of cutaneous reactions may be seen in drug sensitivities causing skin eruptions. No single drug produces an invariably typical pattern. The main offenders are the barbiturates, anticonvulsants, and antibiotics.

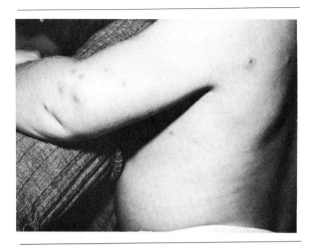

Fig. 22-10. Grouped erythematous wheals surmounted by a tiny vesicle characteristic of flea-bite dermatitis.

Contact dermatitis is an inflammatory reaction to a specific sensitizing agent or to a primary irritant. Poison ivy (*Rhus toxicodendron*) dermatitis is the most prevalent allergic contact dermatitis in childhood. Erythema, edema, and intensely pruritic vesiculobullous lesions are seen several hours to days after contact. The eruption is initially distributed in exposed areas. Other surfaces may later be involved by transference of the sensitizing compound via the hands or clothes. Linear streaks usually consisting of vesicles result from direct contact with the plant or secondary spread of the sensitizing material by scratching. Once the antigen has been removed by cleansing of the skin, the eruption cannot be spread further. Healing occurs in approximately 2 weeks in the absence of secondary infection. Several other members of this plant family cause a typical rhus dermatitis, including poison oak (*R. diversiloba*), mango, Japanese lacquer, and India marking ink.

Many other substances have been implicated in causing contact dermatitis, including the various topical medicaments (particularly the anesthetics, antihistamines, penicillin, and sulfonamides). Among other agents, metals, dyes, paints, rubber, fabric finishers, and plastics are frequent offenders. Patch testing with proper concentrations of these substances affords the best means of establishing an etiology.

Treatment is based on the stage of the eruption. An acute dermatitis requires cool-water soaks and topical corticosteroids. A severe reaction responds promptly to a brief course of systemic steroids. If the lesions are secondarily infected, the use of appropriate antibiotics is mandatory.

Environmental Diseases

Miliaria

Miliaria results from occlusion of the sweat-duct pore, with secondary sweat retention. While individuals of all ages may be affected, in the temperate zones infants and young children are more prone to this disorder. Peak incidence is during the warmer and more humid months.

Retention of sweat in the outermost horny layers resulting in minute, crystal-clear noninflammatory superficial vesicles is called miliaria crystallina. The deeper vesicular and pustular lesions with surrounding erythema are called miliaria rubra. Duration is variable, depending on environmental conditions; exacerbations and recurrences are frequent. Superficial resemblance to papular urticaria, candidiasis, or folliculitis may pose a diagnostic problem. Absence of puncta and whealing excludes papular urticaria; a negative Gram's stain helps to rule out infection.

The underlying principle in treatment of this disease is elimination of the predisposing environmental conditions. Lightweight clothing, limited physical activity, and ventilation help to effect a cure. Topical therapy is generally unsuccessful.

Diaper Dermatitis

Diaper dermatitis is a diffuse, scaly erythema with papular, vesicular, and pustular lesions confined to the lower abdominal, perineal, and gluteal regions (Fig. 22-11). Occasionally, ulcerations or nodular granulomas are seen. An irritant dermatitis may be produced by maceration from wet diapers and fecal contamination.

The differential diagnosis of diaper-area eruptions is usually not difficult. Seborrheic dermatitis may be recognized by flexural involvement, greasy yellow scale, and associated cradle cap. Rarely, a contact dermatitis from detergents, diaper rinses, plastic pants, or medications may occur. Sparing of creases and folds is a helpful differentiating feature. Miliaria is frequently seen during summer months. Candidiasis and bacterial infections are readily diagnosed by their clinical appearance and by the findings on Gram's stain and culture of the exudate obtained from the lesions. Histiocytosis X, syphilis, or acrodermatitis enteropathica may occasionally present in this manner.

Local hygienic measures are important and should include maintenance of dryness by frequent changing of diapers, removal of occlusive plastic pants, and application of protective ointments. Topical corticosteroid creams result in rapid healing; fluorinated agents should be used with great care or not at all in the diaper area.

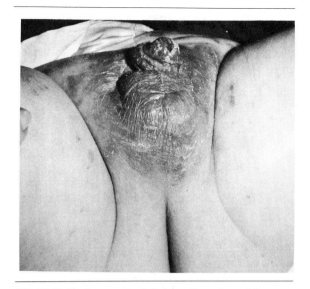

Fig. 22-11. Erythematous scaly irritant diaper dermatitis.

Diseases of Unknown Etiology

Seborrhea

This disorder is most commonly seen in adolescents. The sites of predilection are the scalp, eyebrows and eyelid margins, periauricular skin, and facial, axillary, and intercrural folds. Shampoos 2 or 3 times weekly with an antiseborrheic shampoo containing sulfur and salicylic acid or tar is generally effective for scalp involvement. When inflammation is marked, a topical corticosteroid preparation may also be used.

Pityriasis Rosea

This benign, self-limited disorder is prevalent in late childhood and early adulthood. The herald patch, an erythematous, scaly plaque varying in size from 1 to 10 cm in diameter precedes the generalized eruption by 4 to 6 days. The latter lesions resemble the herald patch in morphology but are smaller, are more ovoid, and run along the skin lines (Fig. 22-12). The rash is usually asymptomatic. The duration is usually 4 to 6 weeks but may be as long as 12 weeks.

Differential diagnosis includes consideration of secondary syphilis, drug eruption, seborrhea, psoriasis, and lichen planus. In most cases, treatment is unnecessary.

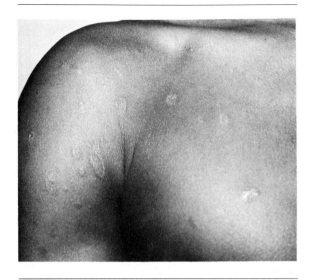

Fig. 22-12. Ovoid scaly lesions of pityriasis rosea. Note the herald patch (larger lesion) on the upper arm.

Keratosis Pilaris

This common condition is characterized by accumulations of keratotic material at the follicular orifices, giving the affected skin a nutmeg-grater-like appearance. The sites of predilection are the extensor surfaces of the thighs and arms. The most practical treatment is the use of a keratolytic agent (e.g., 3–5% salicylic acid ointment or a 10–20% urea cream twice daily).

Lichen Planus

The characteristic lesion of lichen planus is a small, flat-topped, angular, polygonal papule, capped by a fine scale. The lesion has a deep violaceous hue. Lines of papules occurring in the distribution of scratch marks (Koebner's phenomenon) are an identifying feature. Oral involvement is manifested by lacy white streaks on the buccal mucosa or less commonly on the tongue. The eruption is extremely pruritic and may occur on any body surface. Biopsy is diagnostic. Localized disease may be controlled by the application of a topical corticosteroid preparation. In generalized disease, a short course of systemic corticosteroids may be necessary for control. The duration is variable; the recurrence rate is 10 to 20%.

Urticaria Pigmentosa

The eruption of this disease is in the form of small, ovoid, reddish-brown macules, papules, or nodules, 0.5 to 2.0 cm in diameter, which urticate when stroked. Occasionally, bullous lesions are seen in infants. Some patients have only a solitary plaque (mastocytoma); in others, the lesions may be widespread. In the systemic form of this disease the patient may exhibit lymphadenopathy, hepatosplenomegaly, or bony lesions. Episodes of flushing associated with headache, dizziness, nausea, vomiting, and diarrhea are frequently seen.

There is an accumulation of mast cells in the involved tissues. Symptoms are attributed to the massive release of histamine from the cells. Prognosis is dependent in part on age at onset. Periactin in appropriate dosage may be helpful in allaying symptoms; other antihistamines may also be of some benefit.

Psoriasis

Psoriasis is a common skin disorder affecting approximately 2% of the population. Onset can be at any age but occurs more often in late childhood and adolescence. The eruption is characterized by brightly erythematous, circumscribed plaques, which gradually increase in size and are topped by a thick, silvery scale (Fig. 22-13). On removal of the scales, there is an oozing of blood from the capillaries. The sites of predilection are the extensor surfaces of the extremities and the scalp; in childhood, however, a generalized (guttate) eruption may occur. Pitting of the nail plates as well as dystrophic changes and onycholysis are helpful diagnostic signs.

The lesions may be treated locally by application of a corticosteroid ointment (0.1% triamcinolone 3 times daily). The use of topical coal tar preparations with or without ultraviolet light may be beneficial. Scalp lesions respond to frequent use of a tar shampoo as well as a keratolytic agent (salicylic acid in Nivea oil; Baker's phenol and saline solution) and topical steroid in the form of a gel or lotion.

Acne

Acne is essentially a disease of adolescence. Comedones, papules, pustules, nodules, and cysts are all present, depending on the severity of the disorder. Plugging of the pilosebaceous canals with keratotic debris and sebaceous secretion results in the comedo or "blackhead." When obstruction is complete, the follicular epithelium may tear and allow extravasation of material into the dermis. It is thought that the

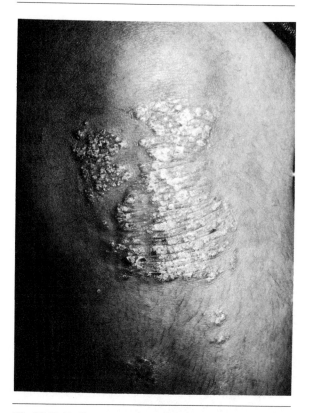

Fig. 22-13. Erythematous scaly psoriatic plaque on the knee.

anaerobic bacillus *Propionibacterium acnes* plays a role in the development of these inflammatory lesions by evoking a neutrophilic response. Hormonal factors are necessary for the development of acne, but the specific etiological role of these substances remains unclear.

While therapy is by no means curative in all cases, effective control can usually be obtained. Thorough cleansing of the involved skin 2 or 3 times a day with mild soaps containing sulfur and salicylic acid is helpful. A variety of commercial preparations (including topical vitamin A acid and benzoyl peroxide) are available for drying and peeling of the involved areas. Their therapeutic effect is presumably due to the unplugging of follicular orifices and to reduction in the numbers of organisms in the follicles and on the cutaneous surface. Clear cosmetic preparations containing these agents are available for use during the day. The use of non-water-based cosmetics should be discouraged. Oral tetracyclines or erythromycin may be helpful in pustular acne. Alternatively, topical antibiotic preparations (particularly Cleocin and erythromycin) in a nonocclusive vehicle are available and effective in treating inflammatory acne. The use of irradiation, stringent diets, oral vitamin A, and thyroid hormone is unwarranted.

Vitiligo

Vitiligo is an acquired disorder of pigmentation. The lesions are depigmented macules that often have a hyperpigmented border. The distribution is frequently symmetrical, and the face, elbows, knees, hands, feet, and genitalia are sites of predilection. If hair-bearing areas are affected, the hair within the patch becomes depigmented.

The cause of vitiligo is unknown although an autoimmune mechanism has been hypothesized, in part because the disorder may coexist with other autoimmune conditions. Repigmentation may occur spontaneously but is usually only partial, and generally the disorder is progressive. The lesions must be differentiated from nevoid pigmentary conditions, postinflammatory hypopigmentation, scleroderma, and other rare cutaneous disorders. Occasionally, a positive family history is obtained. Treatment is difficult and involves the combined use of a photosensitizing drug (psoralen) and exposure to ultraviolet light. Repigmentation cannot be guaranteed, and response is slow. Skin stains and makeup may also be offered for this extremely distressing cosmetic problem.

Alopecia Areata

This nonscarring type of alopecia is one of the most common causes of hair loss in childhood. Typical lesions are round or angular hairless areas devoid of erythema, scaling, or other signs of inflammation. Solitary or multiple plaques may develop on the scalp but occasionally also involve the eyebrows, lashes, and body hair. A minority of affected individuals have extensive hair loss involving the entire scalp and body hair as well. Patients are symptom-free, and the alopecia develops without preceding local changes. A nail dystrophy consisting of pitting, stippling, or ridging of the nails may accompany extensive hair loss.

The cause of alopecia areata is unknown although an autoimmune mechanism has been postulated. The family history is positive in a significant percentage of patients. The disorder must be differentiated from tinea capitis, traction alopecia, trichotillomania, and the scarring alopecias (e.g., lupus erythematosus, morphea). The usual course is one of spontaneous remission although recurrences are common. Topical corticosteroids and anthralin are the only safe modes of therapy for children; however, their efficacy is questionable.

Granuloma Annulare

This benign, asymptomatic skin disorder is most typically represented by solitary or multiple rings of firm, skin-colored, or violaceous papules. The central area of skin may be normal in appearance or slightly atrophic. These lesions develop most frequently on the dorsal hands and feet and over the digits, ankles, and wrists. A subcutaneous variant consists of deep-seated, skin-colored nodules, ordinarily found in the scalp, in the pretibial skin, and around the knuckles.

Differentiation from tinea corporis, rheumatoid nodules, tumor nodules, and panniculitis is most important. Skin biopsy shows degeneration of collagen with a surrounding granulomatous mononuclear infiltrate. Because spontaneous involution within months to years is the rule, treatment is unnecessary. There are no associated systemic complaints.

Juvenile Xanthogranuloma

The xanthomatous lesions of this benign condition are pink, orange, or yellow dome-shaped papules and nodules that may be present at birth or appear during infancy. The lesions may be solitary or numerous and occur with greatest frequency on the scalp, face, upper trunk, and proximal arms. They occasionally occur in the eye and, very rarely, in other organs. Blood lipid levels are always normal. A skin biopsy is diagnostic, demonstrating the lipid-laden histiocytes and a characteristic cell called the Touton giant cell. Because regression within months to years is expected, treatment of the skin lesions is not required.

Morphea

Also known as focal or localized scleroderma, the lesions of morphea consist of solitary or multiple plaques of relatively round or linear configuration. The affected skin has a scarred appearance and feels hidebound on palpation. Early lesions may have an active inflammatory violaceous border.

The cause of morphea is unknown. Occasionally there are associated abnormalities, contractures of the involved extremity, or hemiatrophy of the face with scarring alopecia of the scalp. Sometimes hypergammaglobulinemia, antinuclear antibody, and rheumatoid factor are associated abnormal findings. Progression to systemic scleroderma is rare but has been known to occur. The natural course is one of spontaneous involution after months to years of activity. On resolution the skin may soften and acquire a hypopigmented, translucent appearance. There is no known effective treatment.

Nancy B. Esterly

References

Hurwitz, S. *Clinical Pediatric Dermatology*. Philadelphia: Saunders, 1981.

Hurwitz, S. Pediatric dermatology. *Dermatol. Clin.* 4:1, 1986.

Schaehner, L. A., and Hansen, R. C. *Pediatric Dermatology*. New York: Churchill Livingstone, 1988.

Solomon, L. M., and Esterly, N. B. *Neonatal Dermatology*. Philadelphia: Saunders, 1973.

Solomon, L. M., Esterly, N. B., and Loeffel, E. D. *Adolescent Dermatology*. Philadelphia: Saunders, 1978.

Weinberg, S., Leider, M., and Shapiro, L. *Color Atlas of Pediatric Dermatology*. New York: McGraw-Hill, 1975.

Weston, W. L. *Practical Pediatric Dermatology (2nd ed.)*. Boston: Little, Brown, 1987.

23

Disorders of Behavior and of Emotional and Cognitive Development

The task of preventing, recognizing, and managing behavior problems rests in large part with the physician who cares for children. There are, of course, many others — teachers, social workers, other health and service professionals — who share in this responsibility with the parents or other caretakers of the child. The pediatrician plays a control role, in the effort to identify abnormal behavior in its incipiency. The advantage of knowledge of the family and the child prior to the onset of disturbing behavior is invaluable. The pediatrician's base of experience and appreciation of the wide variability in the behavior of children and their parents makes possible sensitive evaluation of deviations and integration of the physical as well as the emotional aspects of a patient's problem. Above all, most problems can be handled without referral to a child psychiatrist — a happy fact in view of the expense and, in many areas, the limited availability. Indeed, patients usually prefer to have their own physician look after them. Often, if the physician feels the need for referral, this may be accomplished with a variety of nonphysician mental health counselors who are fully possessed of the necessary expertise and who are prepared to work in tandem with the physician.

A knowledge of child development is basic to the understanding of child rearing. The patterns of development are reliable guidelines, and the adaptive socialization processes that enable a child to live competently in society — "training procedures," if you will — are most likely to succeed when carried out in relation to the developmental status. A child responds best to a training procedure when it is introduced at a time in tune with the developmental status, be it for control of bowel or bladder, for undressing, or the like. Premature attempts are generally unsuccessful and may lead to unnecessary strain, particularly if the parent is distressed by the failure of accomplishment. On the other hand, if one waits too long, it may be difficult to alter behavior that has by then become habitual.

The imposition of "training" is but one of many sources of "problems" for the child. The response depends on the nature and intensity of the particular situation, the genetic makeup, the developmental status, and the earlier experiences under similar circumstances, particularly those that were anxiety-provoking. Most childhood problems, like adult problems, seem evanescent and are soon suppressed, but the cumulative effect of those innumerable mini-experiences becomes a major factor in the response to new experience and in the development then of the potential for problem situations.

Problematic behavior may arise as a result of undesirable environmental circumstance — an insufficiency, perhaps, of the four emotional staples of life: affection, acceptance, attention, approval. On the other hand, the primary etiological factor may be innate, as in the case of a child with a specific reading disability. The child's awareness of an inability to compete in school and to live up to expectation may lead to an unhappy situation that may not be readily eased by even the most sensitive approaches of parents and school. Of course, children who have suffered brain damage may have a degree of cerebral disorganization that will seriously modify reaction to the environment.

Management of behavior disorder, however, requires consideration of the personalities and emotional makeup of the parents regardless of primary etiological factors. The family as a unit and the interactions of the individuals within that unit must be understood. If approaches are to be directive, suggestion must be offered in ways acceptable to all. The domineering mother may need curbing, but a direct confrontation is likely to be unsuccessful. She may respond better to the notion that she is "trying too hard," that this is commendable but not always in the best interest of the child, and that children need to learn to make their own decisions than to the charge that she is "bossy" and "overwhelming." At the same time, one may recommend that she find outlets outside the home — for example, in community work — so that her interests and energies are diffused. In any event, this work with the family demands in full the exercise of the art of medicine.

Some broad and general concepts of child rearing should be shared with the parents. Preventive discussion is helpful if it merely succeeds in sealing the bond between pediatrician and family, and it usually goes well beyond that:

1. Children learn more by example than by precept. The parental example provides a major portion of the pattern on which children model their adult attitudes, modes of social behavior, and, most important, character.
2. Children respond to firm and consistent guidance. Parental indecisiveness and vacillation confuse them and, in turn, make them unsure of themselves.
3. Kanner crystallized the basic needs of children in the four A's: affection, acceptance, approval, and attention.
4. Children respond best to quiet management; shouting and hitting reveal a parent's frustration and lack of control of a situation.
5. Parents should recognize that there is no one "right" way

to bring up children. There are many ways. The wisdom about a universal "right" way is not yet upon us.
6. Children are basically the same all over the world although cultural variations modify their behavior to at least some extent.

Certain circumstances are more likely than others to give rise to behavioral disorder. Among these are very young or very old parents, a long period of infertility or frequent miscarriages, severe maternal illness, very low birth weight, parental discord, and distorted parental attitudes such as rejection, overdomination, overprotection, and overindulgence. In addition, certain routine events of life may provoke difficulty if the constellation of factors — inherent drives, growth and developmental status, parental attitudes — has an unfortunate confluence. Certain complaints — fire setting, encopresis — suggest a need for greater concern than do others. The present chapter touches on many of these matters, but the reader is warned that the coverage is extremely limited. In any event, as a thread through it all, the pediatrician is clearly at greatest advantage when there is a sound, continuous, understanding relationship with the family. The exercise of spontaneity in daily living and the need to be free of the constraint of rigid rules of child rearing can be strongly suggested to parents. The value of their individual common sense can be indicated and supported and then, one trusts, appropriate pediatric intervention can help when it becomes necessary.

There is a further and more important need, however. Just as the pediatrician should make the effort to encourage a certain spontaneity and to support the parent's exercise of common sense, so must the pediatrician use that same common sense without too heavy an overlay of personal value judgment. The physician loses power as a counselor when value judgment is translated into conventional wisdom for the parents and the child. There is a need to preserve some humility.

In fact, it is said that one pediatrician, confronted on his very first day in practice with, "Is it all right for our 3-year-old daughter to see my husband and me in the nude?", was able to find in the library papers supporting the positive and negative responses in about equal abundance. It is hoped that, though young in practice, he found the courage to say, "I don't know," and to explore with the parent solutions that might respect the common sense, judgment, and needs of everyone involved.

The essential point to be made is that the child is a seething complex of processes, physical and behavioral, each progressing as its own pace, some more rapidly, some more slowly. The brain develops relatively quickly — packaged in a body that grows at a slower rate in terms of weight and height — and, quite obviously, at a rate much faster than that of the genitalia. That sensitive brain in the immature-looking "package" has a keen awareness of the nuances of behavior of parents, teachers, and, indeed, all else in the environment. It is perhaps the failure to appreciate the highly developed central nervous system and the consequent sensitivity and ability to learn that may entrap parents: "How can a child understand my hesitation in responding to the questions about sex?" Indeed, everything happens in a developmentally ordered sequence, be it the progression of height and weight, the development of the immune response, or the appreciation of the meaning of death.

Much contention between parents and children stems from the best of intentions. Parents want to do a good "job." Those whose lives are reasonably well organized socially and who themselves have received ample shares of attention, approval, affection, and acceptance have, as a rule, the best interests of their children at heart. They may not always have the information that might provide greater understanding of the issues of childhood and point the way to the avoidance of problems. There is also a matter of hubris. It is quite human to want the world's approval for the way our children behave and to want to receive credit for that. Inevitably, it is also quite human to seek some vicarious fulfillment in the accomplishments of our children. These desires are generally innocent enough, but they sometimes lead to trouble.

Feeding

Children usually eat very well during the first year of life. After all, from birth to that first birthday they may gain as much as 15 pounds, tripling their birth weight. In the second year of life, the same children may gain but 2 to 4 pounds. There is a lesser need for food and, in spite of vigorous activity, an *apparent* loss of appetite. It may also be that the consistency and variety of food have not been changed to keep pace with the baby's maturing task and that too much milk is offered and taken. The 640 calories in a quart of milk make up more than half the daily need of a 2-year-old, and, as a consequence, fewer solids might be eaten.

Given these not uncommon circumstances, the highly developed brain to which we have alluded makes the child acutely aware of parental concern and perhaps oversolicitude. The antennae are sensitive. Parents, on the other hand, not well educated about food and caloric requirements and bombarded with propaganda about the importance of diets, begin to coax, cajole, bribe, and even threaten

their children in an effort to get them to eat. The youngsters come to enjoy the attention received in this way and exploit their parents' concern. This contest and the child's emerging desire for independence may lead to daily — indeed, several times a day — conflict and ultimately to undue preoccupation and the genesis of emotional problems. Everyone is unhappy. The role of the pediatrician, then, is obvious, first as an educator and second as a prod to parental planning that, given the facts, can best depend on common sense. It is also possible to offer practical suggestions: Discontinue bland baby foods, use the more interesting "grown-up" foods, limit the intake of milk. Actually, these efforts, too, are simply an extension of the assertion of self on the part of the parents and a support of their refusal to yield to the blandishments of the baby food advertisements.

Sleep

Common attitudes toward sleep are expressed in the tendency, early in the life of an infant, to describe that baby as "good" who sleeps according to a schedule convenient to the parents, the implication being that a baby who sleeps in a less adult-adapted way is "bad." The baby does not know of "good" or "bad," and there is a normal variation in the time it takes to learn the schedule convenient to the parents. The parents' concern in this regard may be sensed by the baby, however, and here, too, is a source of difficulty if the parents define normality in the sleeping situation as a "problem" because it does not suit their adult-oriented need. The effort to force change inevitably causes at least some trouble.

In addition, problems related to sleep may begin when infants are 6 to 9 months old, at just the point when they have identified quite clearly the maternal figure in life and let go of that figure only reluctantly. Children who a few weeks earlier could be tucked in and put to sleep readily now clamber to a standing position in the crib and scream when left alone. They are worried about the separation and cannot think in an abstraction which allows the concept that the maternal figure may be available in the next room. The separation seems like a permanent one as the figure retreats. At this juncture children learn quickly enough the potency of an activity which is, after all, under their own control — crying. It can be used as a weapon, and parents are well advised to be firm and to set limits gently but consistently. During infancy and toddlerhood and even at older ages children begin to express the wish to stay awake, to sleep in their parents' bed, to be fed or entertained during the conventional sleep hours. As a matter of fact, the firmness and the limits are as essential here as they are in most situations that might fall under the rubric of "discipline."

Toilet Training

In toilet training, again, the child has master control. The social need is obvious. The parental sense of achievement and pride when the child is trained is also obvious. Here, too, the child may exploit the too eager, too readily frustrated parent.

The child, of course, should not be toilet trained until there is developmental readiness. This implies the ability to sit firmly on the toilet, awareness that the bowel or bladder is filled, ability to hold the stool or urine, ability to release the sphincters at an appropriate time, and some understanding of the social implications. All of these aspects of development obviously do not mature at the same time; however, it is not inappropriate to begin training some time from 15 to 18 months of age.

Keep in mind the milieu in which this takes place. The early years are, after all, exciting ones. The young child is acquiring a large fund of knowledge about the material world, and if the habit of going to the toilet is not established reasonably early, some children may refuse to leave their interesting explorations and play in order to go to the bathroom. Here again, consistency and gentle firmness are helpful.

The child is placed on the toilet at times when defecation or urination may be expected. The parent can sense this in observing carefully the daily routines of the child. A word — "toilet," perhaps — should be repeated during the move to the bathroom. The child should be kept on the seat for just a few moments. If there is success, there should be encouraging approval. On the other hand, nothing should be defined as failure, and the child should not be given signs of disapproval. If that particular child has habits of voiding and defecation that are unpredictable, it may pay to use the toilet in relation to events of the day — on rising in the morning, after meals, after nap time. At first, the child may be placed on the toilet 4 or 5 times a day; later, the intervals may be lengthened.

The important point is that there should not be a sense of urgency and insistence, or efforts at bribery or signs of disapproval from those persons who, after all, are the most significant in the world to that child. A relatively relaxed approach is rewarding in that the child does not then learn a need to exploit the parents' too eager desire and the parent does not in turn voice disapproval over something that ought not to be shrouded in guilt.

Thumb Sucking

The generation of guilt over the common behaviors of childhood is a pitfall to be avoided. These may be behaviors, however, that parents may define as inappropriate and may, therefore, attempt to suppress, with untoward results. Finger sucking, for example, is a common habit of infancy, ordinarily starting relatively early. The thumb comes in contact with the mouth, and the sensation is found pleasant, is repeated, and may become habitual. Perhaps, too, the discomfort of teething may stimulate the sucking or, if it starts somewhat later in life, the simple imitation of a younger sibling. Certainly the habit is equally common in artificially and naturally fed infants. Regardless, it usually becomes less frequent during the second year of life so long as there is no vigorous adult intervention. Sometimes, however, it persists into the school years.

We cannot adopt a simplistic approach to this habit. There is a preoccupation with the mouth during the first year or more of life, and thumb sucking can be immensely gratifying to the child who needs oral gratification more than most. The understanding of this innate need can help to reinforce the facts that the habit is probably innocuous and that restraints, scolding, shaming, and punishments are not only useless but unjustifiable. They can only serve to injure relationships and generate guilt where none is necessary. There is, after all, nothing to be ashamed of. The worst that can happen is that the thumb may on occasion be excoriated and then become infected. The infection can be treated. It is also feared but not necessarily proved that thumb sucking displaces the permanent teeth, increasing the need for the services of the orthodontist.

If the habit persists, the reasons may be complex, and the pediatrician may be helpful in searching for a greater understanding. The alert physician should be sensitive to the knowledge that the more than ordinary preoccupation with the thumb may be a "flag" warning of more entrenched problems in the family and in its relationships. This, however, is much often the exception than the rule. A low-keyed approach is, therefore, best, one designed to calm the concern of the parents and relieve their possible persistence in trying to force a stop to the habit.

Enuresis

Enuresis occurs in as many as 15% of children, and in a goodly number of these there is persistent day as well as night wetting. As a rule, the incidence of enuresis has been high among close relatives of the patient. Spontaneous remission generally takes place during early adolescence or, on occasion, sooner, although urgency may persist throughout life. Rarely, a few persons continue to wet during adulthood.

There is evidence that the basis for enuresis is genetic. Studies of twins indicate that concordance is significantly greater in monozygotic than in dizygotic twins, and family studies suggest that the closer the relationship to the enuretic patient, the higher the discovered incidence of enuresis.

Basically, the sense of urgency in response to a full bladder is much more intense in the enuretic individual, who can control micturition, but with much greater difficulty than the "normal" person. Deep sleep (hypersomnia) is also a frequent accompaniment of enuresis. Given these perhaps innate conditions, a heavy weight of empirical evidence indicates that emotional factors may influence the enuresis. It is doubtful, however, that they ever *initiate* it; probably, too, they are more likely to play a role when day wetting is present.

Of course, the urine of each of these patients must be examined. The differential diagnosis includes diabetes mellitus, diabetes insipidus, and congenital anomalies of the urinary tract. On occasion, epilepsy with convulsions solely during the night may be confused with enuresis.

The first step in management is an explanation to the parents and patient of the nature of the wetting, emphasizing that the condition is inborn, that it is not based on an emotional disturbance, and that it does not represent willful misbehavior. Parents must be warned against shaming, scolding, threatening, punishing, and the like.

Imipramine hydrochloride is effective in controlling the symptom when given in adequate dosage. A suggested starting dose for an 8-year-old is 25 mg once a day after the evening meal. This may be increased by 25-mg steps weekly, if necessary, up to 75 mg a day. The child is kept on a maintenance dose for about 8 weeks, and then the amount is gradually tapered. If enuresis recurs, a second full course of treatment may be given. The drug should *not* be given with monoamine oxidase inhibitors, and its accidental ingestion in large quantities is hazardous. It must be carefully stored and kept from the roaming hands and eyes of children.

Fears

Parents consult the physician about many of their children's fears, often with an insistent need to resolve the "problem" quickly. Certainly, an intense fear obstructing life's usual course needs deep exploration. Nevertheless, parents must realize that fear is essential to survival. In this regard, an attempt to look at the object of fear through the child's eyes is helpful. After all, what is unreasonable to an adult is quite often reasonable to a child, and the essential thing is to learn

that fear need not be abolished but, rather, disciplined. Thus, the most competent adult uses fear wisely. The child, to learn this lesson, needs the parents' warmth and reassurance. Ridicule of a fear is crushing, and repeated exposure to an object of fear is humiliating and intensely debilitating. It is really not proper to throw a child into the water to teach swimming. Gradual, reassuring introduction without the urgency of a time limit is much more appropriate and usually leads to pleasure in water play. Thus, one wisely takes the moderate approach to the management of fears in the course of growing up.

Death

Children begin to think about death early. Often, the loss of an elderly relative or a pet provokes this preoccupation. Here is an exemplar of the circumstance in which children take their cues from adults. It is obviously difficult to convey an inexplicable concept, an abstraction, to the child. Parents who have firm religious beliefs communicate their ideas best. In any event, it pays to be simple and honest. Children do not necessarily have to have a total explanation, and it is all right to share one's own uncertainties. Children understand and have a "feel" for our uncertainties and our fears. It is vital to think these problems through as best we can, to know where and how we stand, and to be straightforward. Then communication with children on an appropriate level becomes possible.

Sexuality

Parents must first try to understand themselves. They should try to be well informed and comfortable in discussing the subject of sexuality. Then they can begin to communicate with their children. The simple matter of masturbation in the young, for example, may produce much anxiety as the result of a parental response that engenders guilt in the child. Parents who are relatively secure in their own sexual roles function better, and hence masturbation can be kept essentially innocent. It must be realized, however, that excessive masturbation may point to a greater problem. And, of course, the nature and intensity of problems may vary from culture to culture.

Unfortunately, the area of sexual learning is often restricted by parental reluctance to discuss the subject. Parents must be encouraged to provide guidance. This communication, coupled with the child's observation of the parents in the home, can lead to good learning. If the parental relationship is poor, the pediatrician needs to assume that family counseling may be helpful.

Illness

Parents often feel guilty whenever a child of theirs becomes ill—more guilty, of course, when the illness is serious or fatal. The pediatrician must understand and attempt to relieve the guilt. All questions, no matter how impertinent they may seem, should be answered patiently and the effort made to discover what prompted them.

Children, too, view illness and hospitalization as essentially punitive experiences. Hospitalization, therefore, should be avoided whenever possible. Still, if it is necessary, allowing the mother or father or both to stay at the hospital with the child may help (see Chap. 2).

Tics

Tics or habit spasms are abrupt, purposeless, involuntary movements that may or may not simulate a purposeful act. Mild tics, principally eyelid twitchings, are common in young children and are transient. Later on, they may be more persistent and may last for years, finally disappearing. Occasionally they persist throughout life.

A rare type of tic has been described by Gilles de la Tourette. Severe jerking movements, usually involving the face and neck muscles as well as the extremities, are accompanied by grunting sounds, coprolalia, and echolalia. The outlook in this circumstance is difficult but sometimes manageable with drug therapy. Referral to a child psychiatrist or neurologist interested in the problem is suggested.

Tics are, for the most part, responses to stress. The attempt to alleviate those that are most troublesome requires a search for sources of tension in the home, at school, and among peers. Tranquilizing drugs—for example, diphenhydramine and chlorpromazine—may help to allay anxiety but, in the severe circumstance, are merely "crutches," sometimes constructive aids that cannot substitute for an active effort to discover an appropriate therapeutic intervention.

Lying

The young child possesses neither the knowledge nor the experience to distinguish imagery from reality, fiction from fact. Play becomes real, and fairy tales and fables are vivid. There are, then, a variety of circumstances that may provoke misrepresentation. Time and guidance are needed to establish more mature criteria in separating truth from invention.

Older children may exaggerate or fabricate to enhance their status in a group. Any fisherman or golfer can recognize this common practice; it is ordinarily excusable, and not a major defect of character. Still, if a child has frequent resort to this kind of misrepresentation, an effort must be made to identify and to strengthen actual assets that can supplant the false or magnified pretenses.

A child may engage in deliberate, even malicious, falsification to avoid punishment or reprisal. Social custom condemns this expedient, at least in theory. It demands that honesty and courage be developed and that children learn to bear responsibility for their behavior. Children have difficulty in separating "white lies" from the pernicious type, and their parents are their best models in this regard.

Ultimately, the child must learn to understand that lying is undesirable and generally intolerable behavior. First, parents should show consistent disapproval. Second, parents should make sure they do not provide the example, which the child follows. They must be careful to avoid exaggerations and frequent use of the white lies so often used to guard against the pressures of society. They really do need to be truthful in the child's presence, and this conduct helps them to be appropriately truthful in all circumstances. Third, situations should not be created that invite lying. The child who has transgressed should be told so, not quizzed about the behavior. Finally, if the situation is severe, the pediatrician should examine the family structure carefully for evidence of the underlying disharmony that is most certainly there.

Stealing

Stealing is common in childhood. The child will not appreciate that it is inappropriate until that attitude is taught. The moral concept that underlies societal disapproval is not inherent; in fact the common first reason for "taking things" is the inability to distinguish between personal possessions and possessions of others. The 2-year-old, however, can begin to make that distinction. The desire to buy candy and sodas for schoolmates in order to win their favor, an inordinate need to possess, or a compulsion to annoy parents may convert innocence into a disturbing habit. The example of parents who are themselves not strictly honest may, above all, be a moving force.

In any event, it must be made abundantly clear to the child that stealing is wrong, that it is unfair to others, and that it cannot be tolerated. Further, the parents must examine themselves and be certain of the example of their own behavior. Opportunities for stealing should be restricted. Money should not be left casually about the house. Finally, a review of the home and school environment should be made to seek out other reasons that may contribute to this behavior.

Aggression and Timidity

The aggressive drive essential in the natural endownment of each of us is widely variable in its expression. It is possible, even in the very young, to recognize the entire spectrum from the timorous to the bold, and, of course, modifying influences begin to operate early.

The aggressive child who destroys maliciously, assaults peers, and challenges the authority of seniors is always worrisome. Social practice strives to blunt such drives and rechannel the obviously abundant energy. A young child can be provided a suitable play setting with puppets and toys, which may then be objects for the expression of feelings. Parents and teachers must set firm limits and indicate with consistency alternative patterns of behavior.

On the other hand, the shy and withdrawn child is frequently first described as the perfect child, quiet, unobtrusive, and "a pleasure to have in the class." Unable to obtain relief from inner tension by overt behavior, such a child often turns to daydreaming and fantasy. Because society does not, in the long run, value reclusive behavior, it is well to work to give the child, too, the opportunity for an outward expression of feelings.

School Phobia

School phobia, the dread of going to school, is not uncommon. The child awakens on school days in a state of acute anxiety, often presenting somatic complaints—nausea and vomiting, anorexia, pallor, headache, and abdominal pain. The fear of school is often superficially attributed to a strict teacher, a school bully, fear of academic failure, or fear of a poor performance before an admired teacher. These situations are sometimes real; they are more often allegations that mask the reality. The main reason for school phobia is fear of separation from the home, a fear fostered by the mother most often who, for reasons of her own, wants to keep the child with her. In any event, it cannot be easily dismissed and must be carefully studied.

Discussions with the mother attempt to loosen the tie with the child. The situation, however, must be explained in terms that she can accept. The child must return to school quickly. Delay increases the difficulty. Tranquilizers (e.g., chlorpromazine) may be helpful transient aids, but they cannot substitute for clarification of the conditions giving rise to the phobia. The outlook for cure and future development is, fortunately, good in the younger child.

School phobia has a deeper-seated origin in the emotional life of older children or adolescents. It is harder to treat and is less readily amenable to the usual procedures. In the long run, these children, too, usually respond to proper and consistent management. Nevertheless, there must always be an undercurrent of concern that schizophrenia underlies the school phobia of the adolescent, and the persistenece of symptoms should force a consideration of this possibility.

Constipation

Constipation occurs with some frequency, perhaps in as many as 7% of children. It is slightly more frequent in girls than in boys. Fortunately, parents are not always greatly worried by the symptom and do not, therefore, resort to inappropriate use of cathartics or enemas. Some parents, however, may have inordinate concern and sometimes "invade" the child unnecessarily.

Constipation may indeed pose a real problem; the passage of stools may be painful and accompanied by bleeding. General symptoms of abdominal pain, restlessness or apathy, chilly sensations, and headache are sometimes present and may be promptly relieved by evacuation of the stool. At times, the stools are so large as to obstruct the toilet, and fecal soiling may accompany the constipation with fair frequency.

The anal sphincter is often found to be lax on rectal examination. The rectum itself is filled with hard, irregular masses, which are removed with difficulty. These masses may usually be felt in the left lower quadrant of the abdomen.

There is a probable genetic contribution to constipation. Certainly there is significantly greater concordance in monozygotic than in dizygotic twins, and there is a high incidence of constipation in close relatives. Presumably this predisposition expresses itself in increased water absorption from the colon. Nevertheless, it is difficult to separate the "nature/nurture" issues in the causation of this problem. The sensitive child may, in fact, react to the concern of the parent with a more intense disregard of the need to defecate.

One factor influencing the severity of constipation is the promptness with which the predisposed child responds to the weak call to defecate. The eager, active child may delay spending the time necessary to empty the rectum. Failure of response may be exaggerated by a fear of sitting on a strange toilet, by painful fissuring, by a desire to annoy a parent, or by some latent, poorly understood anxiety.

Reliable data on the persistence of childhood constipation into adult life are lacking. The condition probably improves spontaneously because the frequency in adult males is lower than in boys.

The physician must first be certain that there is no significant and correctable physical problem. An assessment of the family's attitude toward the symptom is also necessary. Discussion with the parents and the child (depending on age) may include the explanation of its possible genetic basis, emphasizing that constipation does not necessarily represent willful behavior and reassuring the parents that the physical effects are without the general significance and that the outlook, especially in boys, is good. A daily stool is really not essential!

Cathartic procedures are usually unnecessary and should be avoided if possible. If pain is present for any reason—the passage of hard stools, anal fissuring, hemorrhoids—a stool softener can be effective. The general rule, however, dictates that manipulative procedures—enemas, laxatives—should be undertaken only with conservative care and continued for the shortest time possible. It is easy to create dependency, and it is disturbing to encounter the family in which the enema has become ritual.

Encopresis (Fecal Soiling)

Encopresis is most often associated with constipation. The large, firm, irregularly shaped stool fills the rectum, and bits of stool are from time to time passed into the underclothing.

The soiling that accompanies daytime enuresis has a different character. The stools are soft, and the soiling may occur several times a day.

There is a psychogenic basis in a significant number—although a minority—of cases. In this event, the onset is later than when encopresis is associated with constipation. The stools are of normal consistency, and the rectal examination is normal. The stools are usually passed into the clothes, but they may also be deposited in a special bureau drawer, on a piece of paper, or in other "favored" places. These are obviously disturbing behaviors and demand careful attention.

Psychogenic encopresis has been attributed to the lack of parental affection, the extreme of parental rejection, and, often, to overly demanding parental rules and regulations. It is reported on occasion in children who have been moved to strange new homes, but the symptom is then usually transient.

Treatment of encopresis associated with constipation consists of explanation, education, and a sparing resort to enemas (hypertonic phosphate solutions). An enema is often required to evacuate the rectum. Attention to diet and an understanding of the possible constitutional contribution can then support the patience necessary to the transition to a regular, painless evacuation. The physician should direct the cautious use of enemas and stool softeners and should, during this period, be in contact with the family.

Children with encopresis associated with day wetting usually respond nicely to imipramine. The greatest difficulty in understanding, diagnosis, and management, then, is occasioned by the child with psychogenic soiling. A study of the family is necessary—parents and children—and ultimate treatment must involve the entire group, preferably as a unit. In fact, the point can be made here that the family is truly the patient when the child presents with a behavioral problem, be it major or minor.

Depression

Depression is a more common disorder of children that has been generally recognized. The characteristic mood of sadness and unhappiness is often masked by aggressive, resistant behavior and by somatic complaints. In fact, physicians and parents seldom think of depression as a problem of childhood.

Still, quarrelsome behavior, rudeness, resistence to learning and refusal to go to school are common reactions of the depressed child. Interest in games and hobbies lapses. The child has a soiled self-image. Poor appetite and weight loss, headache, and stomachache are frequent.

Depressive episodes may be a reaction to an unfavorable family environment, a bereavement, a scholastic reverse, or poor athletic performance—just about any of the unmet needs or transitional events associated with growing up; or the depression may be unrelated to life experience (endogenous depression) and may suggest a genetic predisposition. Depression in one or both parents is not infrequent; however, the cycle of manic-depressive psychosis rarely manifests itself during childhood. The important concern is recognition of a largely unacknowledged, common childhood affliction. The pediatrician does well to include the possibility quite consistently in the differential diagnosis of emotional disorder.

The conscientious search for causes must be made, and, along the way, antidepressant drugs (e.g., imipramine and amitriptyline) may be helpful. Medication is given in gradually increasing amounts, continued for a month or more after improvement has taken place, and then gradually decreased. Obviously, the pediatrician needs to consult with the psychiatrist in the exaggerated, unrelieved instance.

Sleepwalking

Sleepwalking or somnambulism may occur in as many as 6% of children. It sometimes begins in early childhood and may continue to and through adolescence. The variation in persistence is considerable. Episodes usually take place during the early hours of sleep. Young children wander about aimlessly; they may go to their parents' room or to the bathroom, usually aware of the environment but apparently indifferent to it. Arousal is difficult, and, following the episode, amnesia for the specific event is common.

The frequency of episodes varies widely. Some children walk but once or twice a year; others, several nights a week. The child is deeply asleep. An electroencephalogram (EEG) may show, at the outset, a paroxysmal burst of high voltage and slow activity. An EEG, however, contributes little if anything to management and is *not* suggested as a routine study.

Sleepwalking is often familial. Studies in twins suggest a genetic basis in that monozygotic twins are concordant for sleepwalking more often than dizygotic twins. In any case, there is no effective therapy. Reassurance coupled with attention to the child's sleep setting and removal of potential accident hazard are most helpful.

Delayed Speech

Children ordinarily start to speak—that is, to use words with meaning—by 12 to 14 months, but delays of up to 2½ years in otherwise normal children are not unusual, and in most individuals further speech development takes place normally. Occasionally, children fail to speak until the third birthday or later. A number of causes are to be considered.

Mental retardation is the most frequent of these and the main concern; however, an otherwise uncomplicated developmental delay is a not uncommon reason for failure to talk by 3 to 3½ years. The children are otherwise normal and understand spoken words and gestures as expected and desired. They may begin to say words at the usual time, but the words are used sparingly, are often mispronounced, and are not put together into sentences. When speech is acquired, it is at first poorly expressed and difficult to comprehend. In fact, the improvement is slow and may not be fully carried out until the child is 8 years old. Successful speech attainment, however, is usually complete, hampered on occasion by a lisp or some persistent cluttering. These delays are about 3 times as frequent in boys as in girls, are often familial, and are not infrequently associated with a later reading difficulty.

Deafness, partial or complete, should be consistently suspected in the child with delayed speech. Early detection is important because among other needs, remedial measures may help greatly in the development of speech. Auditory verbal imperception (failure to understand the spoken word) and high-frequency hearing impairment may also interfere with the development of speech.

Brain injury may lead to delayed speech in a number of ways. For example, children with congenital athetosis are hampered by poor muscle coordination. Or the injury may involve areas that govern language or interfere with speech by a disorganizing effect on cerebral function. Moreover, such injury may retard speech through an associated retardation in general mental development or an associated hearing defect.

Early infantile autism and, certainly, other instances of emotional deprivation or limitation often result in delayed speech, as is frequently evident in the child reared in the impersonal atmosphere of an institution. Transfer to a warm home is followed by improvement. Histidinemia, a rare familial overflow aminoaciduria, is often associated with delayed speech. The list of possibilities, therefore, is broad, and, while the frequency of some is limited, one must be certain that the child with a pattern of delayed speech is carefully examined and understood. Correctable problems must be managed as soon as possible; in the event of an uncorrectable problem, the child and family need sympathetic, consistent support.

Developmental Dyslexia

Developmental dyslexia refers to a condition in children who have difficulty in learning to read despite normal intelligence, age-appropriate motivation, and adequate instruction. It affects possibly 10% of children and is about 4 times as frequent in boys as in girls. Other language disorders—spelling, writing, and speech problems (e.g., delayed speech, cluttering speech)—frequently accompany dyslexia. A history of language disorders in other members of the family is common. An association of developmental dyslexia and alterations in lateral dominance—left-handedness, ambidexterity, crossed dominance—is often mentioned in the literature but has not been proved. In fact, most left-handed and ambidextrous children do not have dyslexia. The child's emotional reaction to a poor scholastic performance is often prominent, fed perhaps by an almost palpable realization of frustrated inherent competence, and is usually the reason for consultation with the physician.

Developmental dyslexia has a genetic basis. Studies of twins demonstrate more than 70% concordance in monozygotic twins and 29% in dizygotic twins. There is also a high incidence of reading difficulty in near relatives. The emotional reaction of the child to this learning difficulty depends in part on the attitude of the parents and the personality of the child. The parents, at least those who are unaware of the genetic imperative, may even regard the child as stupid or unwilling to try to learn. The child may react with aggressive behavior (hitting a younger sibling, staying away from school, rudeness to parents), with bravado, with depression, or with feelings of low self-esteem. The diagnosis is strongly suggested by the demonstration of a wide discrepancy between the low verbal and the higher performance scores on the Wechsler test.

Children who receive no special training improve spontaneously during adolescence, sometimes earlier. Some learn to read like normal individuals; others continue throughout life to be slow readers and poor spellers. A follow-up study of a group of boys of high I.Q. (mean I.Q., 131) who had reading problems in childhood revealed that they followed careers comparable to those of boys who had not had similar difficulty and who, in fact, had had consistent competence in reading.

Nevertheless, remedial tutoring for reading should be sought from teachers familiar with the field. The quality of the child's early years can be supported and much reinforced. The pitfalls of unproved therapeutic regimens—for example, the already discredited eye-training exercises recommended by some optometrists—should be carefully addressed and avoided.

There are other reasons for reading difficulty. An environment in which interest in conversation and in reading is low is chief among these, and television, perhaps helpful in exposing the child to speech, requires no feedback on the part of the child. Reading difficulty has also been suggested as the sole manifestation of some brain injuries and as a more frequent finding in children who had been exposed to two or more complications—prematurity *and* abnormalities—during the prenatal and perinatal periods (e.g., toxemia of pregnancy, bleeding during pregnancy). The studies in this regard are subject to challenge, however, and the contention that a focal brain lesion at or before birth is capable of causing reading problems is at least open to dispute. Finally, a variety of hearing and visual impairments can obviously contribute to reading retardation, and, of course, mental retardation may be the most frequent cause.

Developmental Hyperactivity (Attention Deficit Disorder)

Developmental hyperactivity is frequently at the root of apparent behavioral deviation in children. Much more common in boys than in girls, it presents as greatly increased, tireless activity, sometimes obvious in infancy. The activity is accompanied by distractibility, a short attention span, emotional outbursts, and a low tolerance for frustration. These problems of the hyperactive child are intensified when school begins and the child is expected to sit still. If learning disability is present, a not unusual circumstance, scholastic problems are particularly exaggerated. Fortunately, improvement in hyperactivity often takes place spontaneously during adolescence.

Physical examination reveals little that is helpful. A number of "soft" neurological signs have been described, but their clinical significance is unclear and their frequency is really no greater than in normal children. Developmental hyperactivity, however, can be distinguished from other forms of overactivity by the characteristic constellation of findings: onset early in infancy; ceaseless, tireless activity; and, most important, a favorable and consistent response to methylphenidate hydrochloride (Ritalin). The response to drug therapy allows activity that varies within a wide range but not to the extreme or with the insistency seen in the untreated developmentally hyperactive child; and, since drug therapy allows activity to be directed toward purposeful ends, the hyperactivity is controllable.

Hyperactivity is also seen in emotionally disturbed children, but it is not continuous and is often interspersed with periods of quietness. There are other sources of hyperactivity, and the rubric *minimal cerebral dysfunction* has been used to designate syndromes of developmental origin as well as those due to cerebral damage. The term is useless and confusing. It is certainly distasteful and frightening to parents, and it is so misleading that some schools have included children so labeled in groups with seriously brain-injured children and relegated them unnecessarily and disadvantageously to special classes. Indeed, the diagnosis of minimal cerebral damage can be made only when there is a history of probable injury to the brain and when neurological signs are clearly present.

Developmental hyperactivity does respond promptly to methylphenidate hydrochloride. An initial dose of 5 mg twice daily, after breakfast and after lunch, may be increased to 20 mg if necessary for a favorable response. The absence of a reasonably prompt response mandates that causes of hyperactivity other than developmental be sought.

After several months of improved behavior the status of the child should be reviewed and the dosage of the drug titrated with the schedule and need of the child and the family. The possibility of an associated learning disability must not be forgotten, and attention to this possibility must be the continuous sensitive concern of the physician and the teacher. Obviously, then, the care of the child with developmental hyperactivity is facilitated by the cooperation, the teamwork, of the professionals involved in the life of the child. Each must be prepared to recognize the special contribution of others and to yield the direction of cure in those moments suited to a particular expertise.

Mental Retardation

Mental retardation is usually organically based but always, inevitably, invested with a newly emotional overlay. It involves about 3% of the population in the Western world, about one-sixth of whom are gravely affected. It respects neither sex, race, nor social position. It presents a problem in diagnosis and a more formidable one in management and planning. In addition, it provides an elusive, even abrasive, puzzle in human values. For the retarded, the principle of equality is meaningless if we employ the conventional standards of wealth, power, popularity, influence, or intellectual achievement; all these are beyond their grasp. Deprived, thus, of so many of the objectives of society, the retarded are necessarily dependent on the rest of us for assistance in the preservation of that other human birthright, personal dignity and individual respect.

It is hard to define mental retardation precisely because of its wide spectrum of etiological factors and the variable circumstances that reveal its existence. In an average school setting, the pace of scheduled progress and the level of scholastic demand soon expose the handicap of the retarded and cripple their performance. In an adult situation, many of these people, possessing positive personality attributes, may melt into the anonymity of the unskilled or semiskilled labor group, particularly in a rural setting. The defintion employed in the *American Journal of Mental Deficiency* (January, 1961) has the advantage of succinct clarity: "Mental retardation refers to subaverage general intellectual functioning which originates during the developmental period and is associated with impairment in adaptive behavior." The I.Q. is a convenient measurement to estimate the degree of subnormality. Reasonably accurate when applied to a general population, it becomes increasingly imprecise as one moves to the fringes or applies it to those with brain injury. The irregular test profiles so frequently obtained from persons with mental retardation suggest that the condition is neither global nor uniform and that it often impairs different modalities of performance unequally. Mental retardation is discussed in much greater detail in Chapter 4.

Conclusion

The foregoing are but a few examples of the kinds of behavioral and emotional problems that may affect children and their parents. Obviously, the range of these problems is wide. Some of them are relatively minor; others are tragic in their intensity; all of them soil the quality of life to some extent and all of them can be eased by the positive intervention of the pediatrician, other physicians, and other health professionals. There have been recurring themes in the consideration of the problems, and similar themes run through potential discussions of others that have not been addressed. The exercise of common sense and the absolute mandate for effective teamwork among professionals who serve children are perhaps the most common. Mature judgment can question conventional wisdom and lead to planning that may be more suited to a particular individual. Certainly, no rules are so rigid that they cannot be bent or broken if the circumstance warrants. *Finally, although the reader must be warned that this chapter barely touches on all these problems,* there is in any such problem in childhood the basic requirement for mutual respect between the patient and physician and for a sensitive understanding that does not allow casual disregard of the seemingly trivial. The smallest of points can too readily build up or seem to build up so that the experience of the child and the family is made less happy. There is, of course, no Eden of experience, and achievement of competence as an adult requires some balance of gratification and frustration along the way. The pediatrician can be a help in this regard and, indeed, effective collaboration with psychologists, psychiatrists, teachers, social workers, as well as child and family, can be extraordinarily facilitative. In this way, with effective collaboration, the limits of individual competence are immeasurably extended.

Henry M. Seidel

References

Adams, P. L. *Primer of Child Psychiatry* (2nd ed.). Boston: Little, Brown, 1982.

Adams, P. L., and Fras, I. *Beginning Child Psychiatry*. New York: Brunner/Mazel, 1988.

Allmond, B. W., Jr., Buckman, W., and Gofman, H. F. *The Family Is the Patient, An Approach to Behavorial Pediatrics for the Clinician*. St. Louis: Mosby, 1979.

Balint, M. *The Doctor, His Patient and the Illness*. New York: International Universities Press, 1972.

Friedman, S. B., and Hoekelman, R. A. (Eds.). *Behavioral Pediatrics: Psychosocial Aspects of Child Health Care*. New York: McGraw-Hill, 1980.

Kanner, L. *Child Psychiatry* (4th ed.). Springfield, IL: Thomas, 1972.

Oski, F. A., D'Angelis, C. D., Feigin, R. D., and Warshaw, J. B. *Principles and Practicer of Pediatrics*. Philadelphia: Lippincott, 1990.

Robson, K. S. (Ed.). *The Manual of Clinical Child Psychiatry*. Washington, DC: American Psychiatric Press, 1965.

24

Adolescence: A Perspective

Adolescence is a unique process whereby the child gradually becomes the adult. It is a critical time of development encompassing physical, sociological, and psychological aspects of human life. It begins with the changes of puberty and ends when an autonomous young adult emerges, one who can function at intellectual, sexual, and vocational levels acceptable to society. The health care system has recently focused attention on this age group and on the medical-psychological needs it experiences. Some of these needs are unique to adolescence while others are shared with other age groups of the human life span. It is important that health care providers not ignore the teenager, for the way youth successfully or unsuccessfully complete their unparalleled metamorphosis determines their ultimate adaptation to adult life. Certainly, anything that can be done to aid this process in a positive direction is important for all concerned. It is, thus, natural that persons interested in health care issues of children should extend their concern to these individuals in the second decade of life.

It is important that the person who works with youth recognize the basic fact that teenagers are neither adults nor children. They are human beings at variable physiological

and psychological stages of development, attempting (or they should be attempting) to understand (or "negotiate") many confusing and changing aspects of their lives such as separation from parents ("emancipation"), improved thinking skills, peer values, drug experimentation, and concepts of sexuality (heterosexual and homosexual). Overt physical illness affects this progress in variable ways. Adolescence is made even more difficult because youth are at different maturational stages, and some are at different stages even if at the same chronological ages. Thus, in assessing health care needs, one learns to react to each young person according to his or her individual level of maturation, and not the chronological age per se. Paramount to this approach is recognition of the specific pubertal and psychological changes of adolescence.

Pubertal Changes of Adolescence

Specific central nervous system maturation occurs during and at the end of latency, causing a rise in various hormones (adrenal androgens, testosterone, estrogen) with resultant biological changes termed puberty. It is as yet unclear what causes this critical stimulation of the hypothalamic-pituitary-adrenal-gonadal axis ("pubertal axis"), but it is part of the complex, more generalized biological clock of life that governs many aspects of human change: fetal growth, parturition, onset of puberty, cellular aging, and death of the cell as well as of the organism. The phenomenon of puberty has many facets, including amygdala maturation, reduced hypothalamic sensitivity to gonadal steroids, possible pineal gland dysfunction, adrenal androgen secretion, attainment of a critical weight, midcycle, luteinizing hormone (LH) surge (which induces ovulation), and others. These terms all describe different aspects of puberty but do not explain its origin.

It is interesting to note that the pubertal axis is normally intact in utero and throughout childhood, yet exactly what awakens or energizes the system at the usual time remains to be understood. If the clinical signs of puberty develop prior to age 8 or 8½ in the female, or prior to age 9 or 10 in the male, it is termed *precocious*. If puberty starts after 14 to 15 in the male or female, it is termed *delayed*. Precocious and delayed puberty are discussed elsewhere in this book.

Though the physical changes can *begin* at different ages, a general or sequential pattern is usually involved in the male or female. Thus, once early puberty is established, individuals take 2 to 4 years to gain 25% of their final height as well as 50% of their final weight. Major organs double in size while lymph tissue regresses. Specific changes also occur in the genital system, with growth of breasts, pubic hair, penis, and testicles. A useful scale (sexual maturity rating or Tanner stages I–V) has been developed to categorize the genital changes. Stage I is prepubertal level, stage V is an adult level, and stages II, III, and IV are inbetween maturational stages. These will be reviewed for the female and the male.

Sexual Maturity Ratings in the Female Adolescent

Thelarche or *breast budding* is the first clinical sign of puberty in females and places the individual at a Tanner stage (sexual maturity rating or SMR) of II (2). Though is usually occurs between 11 and 11½ years in this country, it has a wide range of normal: 8.0 to 14.5 (15) years. Stage III (3) describes a small breast (beyond the "bud" stage), while SMR IV (4) has a "double-contoured" appearance in which the areola and nipple form a separate mound on the actual breast tissue. Stage V (5) is a further development, with a larger, single-contour appearance. Some females remain at stage III or go from III to V directly, or note breast change beyond III only with pregnancy.

As the individual progresses beyond SMR II, other aspects of puberty are also noted, and in some cases correlated to the specific stage. For example, she often reaches peak height velocity between breast stages II and III; this has a range of normal between 10 and 14 years. *Menarche,* or the onset of menstruation, often occurs in late SMR III or early IV, with a range of normal between 10 and 17 years. There is usually limited height gain after menarche, and axillary hair often develops in later pubertal stages (III–V). Clinical variations are common.

Finally, *pubarche,* or the onset of pubic hair, usually begins after thelarche and has a normal range of 9 to 14 years. Many clinicians also stage the pubic hair growth: I–none; II–limited immature hair; III–dark, curled type; IV–adult type of hair; and V–adult type and distribution that defines the normal triangular female escutcheon. Correlating pubertal events with pubic hair stages has not proved to be as useful as correlating them with breast stages.

Sexual Maturity Ratings in the Male Adolescent

Stage II in the male refers to growth of the testes (beyond 2.5 cm in diameter) often in association with a stippled, coarser appearance to the scrotal sac. SMR II usually occurs between 11.0 and 11.6 years of age, but there is a normal range of 10 to 14.8 years. Further growth of testes along with penile growth (usually in length) defines the male SMR III, while stage IV describes even further growth of both (especially increased penile width). "Adult-sized" genitalia define stage V, which has a normal range between 13 and 18 years. Also, stages have been developed for pubic hair development similar to those reviewed for the female. Stage V (pubic hair) notes the diamond-shaped appearance to the hair distribution, with extension along the linea alba to the umbilicus.

Once SMR II (testicular growth) is noted in the male, other pubertal changes eventually follow in the normal individual. The male peak height-growth velocity is usually between stages III to IV and IV to V, with a normal age range of 11 to 16.6 years. It should be noted that the growth spurt occurs later in the pubertal sequencing in males than females. Other changes also occur in the mid to late stages: nocturnal emissions, axillary hair, facial hair, and muscular development.

Because various situations and even disease states occur more often in certain Tanner stages, such ratings are a useful guide for clinicians when evaluating teenage patients. For example, a 13-year old male with SMR II may have a good potential for growth while a male with SMR IV has only a limited growth potential, even though he is the same age. A 14-year old female who has just developed stage II would not be expected to menstruate, because menarche usually occurs 1 to 3½ years after thelarche in stage III or IV. Also, certain orthopedic disorders often occur during rapid growth stages in SMR II and III: Osgood-Schlatter disease, slipped capital femoral epiphysis, or scoliosis. Laboratory tests may also correlate: Alkaline phosphatase levels peak in SMR II females and SMR III males, while hematocrit and uric acid levels rise in males during stages II to V. Thus these stages have clinical usefulness and are important to keep in mind. Division of adolescence into three psychological stages is also important.

Psychological Stages of Adolescence

The main psychological changes are summarized by division of adolescence into three stages: early, middle, and late. Though not all youth fit easily into one of these three groups, they do provide a useful guide for clinicians seeking to characterize their teenage patients. Some youth seem to act like early adolescents in some respects and middle adolescents in others. Cultural and economic factors can affect these groups as well. Thus, it is advisable for clinicians to apply such stages to the patients they see, taking into account as many of these additional factors as possible.

Early adolescence usually occurs between 10 and 14 years of age, when the individual is undergoing the main changes of puberty. Early adolescents are often concerned with bodily function of changes, are just beginning the process of emancipation (separation from parents), and are learning to get along with peers of the same gender. They also have "concrete" operational thinking skills, with which they can deal with simple "here and now" issues, but are not capable of applying abstract or future-oriented skills. A medical history session, for example, usually consists of many questions by the clinician and an equal number of short (often monosyllabic) answers by the "concrete" young adolescent. It is often advantageous and time-saving to have this individual fill out a medical questionnaire (with "yes" or "no" responses) and then discuss the positive answers in detail. This procedure can also be of considerable educational benefit to young adolescents, who are often very interested in the functioning of their bodies.

Middle adolescence is frequently noted between ages 14 and 18, though it can occur at earlier or later chronological times. It is a period when most biological changes are complete (or being finalized), and youth become more concerned with issues of adolescence: further autonomy, more dependence on peer group influences, and exploration of various heterosexual issues. It is a time when parents often feel that they have lost some control of their youth and that

peer group standards are too predominant. It is the time most adults associate with "adolescence," in which there is challenge to adult moral codes and authority, as well as experimentation with drugs and sexuality issues. Sexually transmitted diseases (STDs) and adolescent pregnancy are major health care issues. Transient depression (mood swings) and lowered school performance are also noted in many individuals.

Middle adolescents are also in a further maturation stage in their thinking process—the Piagetian "formal" operational level. That is, they can think and reason like most adults. They can think about the future, use reverse logic, and even reflect about thinking itself. The main limiting factor now is lack of experience. Many begin to fantasize about various aspects of their lives, and some spend a considerable part of their time in such activity. Thus, improved cognitive ability coupled with limited experience and a desire to test values to discover which can be accepted combine to create a potentially difficult adolescent phase.

It is impossible to estimate all the problems youth have during this psychological stage. Certainly not all teenagers have great perplexity. Though a few seem to have no overt problems, most experience some worries and others go through considerable turmoil. It is a time when many youth do not receive health care, or if they do, it is only limited care. They may, for example, seek only a brief sports physical to play on a team, or go to a venereal disease clinic only with an acute complaint. Every opportunity should be utilized to get these individuals into some health care system and to provide comprehensive care. Successful adaptation to adult life necessitates successful neogtiation of middle adolescence. The health care profession as medical advisers and even as general counselors may be of substantial help to youth at this time.

Fortunately, most teenagers progress beyond middle adolescence into the final youth stage, *late adolescence*. This usually occurs between 18 and 21 years of age but can be much earlier or later depending on many factors such as pubertal maturation, results of childhood experiences, overall health, presence of chronic illness, overprotective or rejecting parents, cultural influences, social and economic background, intelligence level, and vocational (educational) preparation. It implies that the individual has become comfortable with most aspects of middle adolescence. It is a time to prepare for adult vocational and sexual roles, as well as to finalize the emancipation process. Thinking ability does not usually advance, per se, but does become tempered by more experience with life in general. Many variations are noted. For example, many persons who are 17 to 20 years of age are just entering formal operation thinking, while some remain at a concrete level during adulthood. Thus the clinician must individualize his or her approach to the teenage patient, whatever the chronological age.

Legal Rights of Adolescents

Anyone involved with youth (including parents, teachers and health care professionals) must realize that American laws are now recognizing the fact that minors (youth) do have some legal rights. Understanding these rights, especially when specific issues arise, is often difficult because the laws are frequently general, vague, and nonspecific. Different states disagree on certain details, and thus one needs to be familiar with current local laws. Definition of "the law" tends to be a compilation of various statutes, Supreme Court rulings, or decisions (state and federal) as well as interpretation of law philosophy, which covers areas not always specifically covered by an identified law at the local, state or federal level.

Only recently has official law identified rights of minors (those under age 21). The first 100 years of United States' history was marked by a legal philosophy that parents had essentially complete autonomy over their children. In this "era of parental autonomy," children were expected to obey parents and were punished by parents or other individuals (as the police) if disobedience occurred. Toward the end of the 19th century a shift in legal philosophy developed which ushered in the "era of child welfare." The laws then reflected the concept that children were different from parents and needed to be protected from parents. If the legal guardian abused these privileges, punishment of the adult was then possible. Thus juvenile courts developed and child labor was forbidden to some extent. Minors, however, were still not allowed to make contracts of their own. Common law tradition has often held that to treat a minor without appropriate parental consent means that one is committing an "unauthorized touching," which legally could be called "assault and battery."

Much of this legal philosophy continues today, but it has become a very complex issue in the light of recent legal cases. In 1967 the "era of rights of minors" began with a well-known legal case—*In re: Gault*. This involved a 15-year-old male who was sentenced by a court to several years of institutionalization after being convicted of placing obscene phone calls to a teacher. The boy's parents brought forth a successful countersuit, claiming the original trial was not legal because it violated the minor's rights on various grounds (as no official legal representative, no cross-examination, and others). The Danforth Case (1976) placed the minor's rights against the parent's rights. In this

case of a late adolescent seeking an abortion from a qualified physician, the state court ruled:

The State may not impose a blanket provision requiring the consent of a parent or person in loco parentis as a condition for abortion of an unmarried minor during the first twelve weeks of her pregnancy . . . The State does not have the Constitutional authority to give a third party an absolute, and possibly arbitrary, veto over the decision of the physician and his patient to terminate the patient's pregnancy. Minors, as well as adults, are protected by the Constitution and possess Constitutional rights . . . Any independent interest the parent may have in the termination of the minor daughter's pregnancy is not more weighty than the right of the competent minor mature enough to become pregnant.

Such issues are quite complex and far from being resolved, especially the abortion issue. It seems clear, however, that youth can give consent for medical treatment in some situations and do not necessarily have to involve parents in the cases. In general it is best to involve parents in such matters, but such is not always possible or feasible. A nonofficial legal concept has emerged over the past generation—the *mature minor doctrine*. This implies "emancipated" minors may seek and receive some medical treatment; however, the interpretation of "emancipation" can be vague and vary according to different criteria that have been used in various states (Table 24-1). Being familiar with one's own state rules and philosophy is strongly recommended for those who deal with such teenagers.

Parent(s) and youth under 18 can make a verbal or written contract declaring emancipation. Its legality would depend on the circumstances. In general individuals over age 18 are allowed to initiate such contracts while those under 18 are not. If an individual 16 or 17 years of age seeks medical treatment, understands the physician's recommendations, and explains why parents are not to be involved, the physician can then document this, declare the patient to be an emancipated minor in need of treatment, and proceed

Table 24-1. Various Criteria for Emancipation

1. Age (often over 18, but varies from 14–19)
2. Marriage
3. Parenthood
4. Runaway status (financially independent)
5. Individuals away from the home with parent's permission
6. Individuals at home who are "essentially independent"
7. Education (as high-school graduates)
8. Member of armed forces
9. Certified by physician and others

with appropriate medical treatment. Some consultants recommend having a second physician sign this document also, but one needs remember it is not an official, legal statement. The individual who is between 13 and 15 years of age represents a very complex legal situation, even if he or she appears to be fully "emancipated." Minors in need of emergency care, as determined by a physician, can always be treated. Youth who present with possible sexually transmitted disease, pregnancy, or drug abuse can also be evaluated and treated without parent's consent or knowledge if necessary. There never has been a successful lawsuit against a physician treating a minor over 15 years of age for any purpose if the minor consented to the treatment. Also there has not been a successful lawsuit against a physician treating a minor of any age for contraceptive-relative services. When treating minors without parent's approval, the youth should be reminded of their obligation to follow through with medical recommendations and to consider the cost of such health care.

Thus there are some legal rights which the youth has, though the situation currently remains complex and in a state of constant legal flux. Problems of sterilization (especially with mentally subnormal youth), abortion, sexual assault, mental health, health record privacy, payment issues, and others remain critical concepts for individuals involved in the health care issues of adolescents.

Health Care Issues of Adolescence: Overview

Health care issues arise during adolescence, and many of them are reviewed in this chapter or elsewhere in this book. As previously noted, learning to *relate* to the youth is often critical in order to discover the actual medical-psychological problems that may be present. Some of these are missed if the physician and youth do not cooperate in a situation of mutual respect. The young (early) adolescent may want to have the parent(s) directly involved in all decisions, while middle and late adolescents often wish more autonomy. Sometimes a delicate balance must be reached by the clinician who deals with both youth and parents. Working effectively with both groups may be very difficult in some situations; however, even the "rebellious" middle adolescent is likely to relate to a nonjudgmental adult figure (the clinician) who offers confidential, honest, and professional advice.

The clinician does have an advantage, knowing that the patient is often concerned over middle adolescent issues. Many youth are relieved to "find" adults (apart from parents) who are willing to discuss these matters. Part of the goal of the health care professional should be to help youth,

if possible, continue their journey through adolescence and not become fixed at one or another age (or substage). Various factors can contribute to this delay: chronic illness, overprotective or rejecting parents, harsh peer criticism, limited sexual functioning, physical handicaps, delayed puberty, intellectual subnormality, reduced socioeconomic background, unresolved childhood conflicts, and many others. Clearly, a specific clinician does not have the time or expertise to deal with *all* problems. But the individual who likes this age group and attempts to discover underlying problems in these patients can still be of considerable help. Referral to appropriate community resources may be the most significant step one can take in certain situations.

How often should an adolescent be seen for evaluation of health care issues? This author recommends that the "healthy" teenager be seen at least 3 times during adolescence for a "well-adolescent" health care visit. Thus, a meticulous health screening (with psychomedical questionnaire and physical examination) can be done once during each of the adolescent stages (early, middle, and late). The goals can be a bit different depending on the clinician and the individual patient. The finding of a specific problem or recommendation of a therapeutic regimen may necessitate more frequent evaluations.

Such examinations can be a learning experience for youth, as previously noted. The hearing-vision screening is usually important, while documented immunizations should be sought, indicating that the individual is protected against diphtheria, tetanus, polio, rubella (especially in the female), mumps (especially in the male), and measles. Select teenagers may need additional immunizations against influenza, pneumococcal disorders and others. Health screening should be done especially in young adolescents between Tanner stages II and IV, who are at the greatest risk for scoliosis and significant curvature changes. Individuals in middle adolescence (regardless of age) should be carefully screened with regard to issues such as parent-teen conflicts, school difficulty, depression, sexuality issues, sex-related problems (such as STDs or pregnancy), and drug use or abuse (including cigarettes, marijuana, and alcohol). Late adolescents may need guidance about vocational concerns, especially if there is a chronic illness or other condition limiting their potential. Screening often identifies a problem, and the health care professional can then arrange referral to the most appropriate community resource.

Many other questions arise in this area. For example, what about breast examination? Clinicians should examine the breast when the patient is in Tanner II or beyond. Youth in general should become more aware of their bodies and thus be taught breast self-examination in females and testicular self-examination in males from early adolescence on. When is a pelvic examination necessary for a teenager? It should be done in an individual of any age who presents with a possible STD or pregnancy, as well as abdominal pain of uncertain etiology. The person should be screened for sexual activity, especially if he or she appears to be in conflict over various midadolescent issues. Teenagers identified as being sexually active need pelvic examinations with STD screening (such as cervical culture for *Neisseria gonorrhoeae* and *Chlamydia trachomatis*) every 6 to 12 months. They also need an initial and periodic Papanicolaou smear, but the frequency of this procedure in healthy individuals is debatable. The asymptomatic, nonsexually active individual need not have a routine pelvic examination until 15 to 18 years of age, depending on the views of the physician and the patient. The patient whose mother received diethylstilbestrol (DES) during pregnancy needs a pelvic screening by a gynecologist at menarche or sooner if symptoms (such as pain or bleeding) develop. The issue of acquired immunodeficiency syndrome (AIDS) testing remains controversial.

Finally, whatever screening is done, one should always be prepared to listen to the specific concerns being presented. Usually the teenager should be seen alone. The youth may present with a "smoke-screen" defense. They come with one complaint when they are really concerned over something else. For example, a young woman may arrive with a vague story about abdominal pain, but she is really worried about being pregnant. The art of listening to all cues of the history–physical examination process is always at the heart of the patient-physician relationship.

Interviewing the Adolescent

It is important to seek a good rapport with the teenager so you can identify her current concerns and so she will return in the future for routine health screenings and for specific problems. Youth need a health care professional to trust and many physicians do want youth to trust them. Unfortunately many patients leave childhood and their early doctors at the same time; this is regrettable, because both groups need each other! Many of our youth have no identified physician; though they often do not appreciate their parents, most adolescents do want a trusted adult to rely on when inevitable questions arise. Growing up is not easy—financial pressure, parental divorce, unemployment, latch-key kids, and other current realities of life all add up to the tragic conclusion that our youth are placed under considerable and potentially harmful stress. Having a trusted health care professional to rely on can be very important—whether one gives specific advice/treatment or helps the

youth find the most appropriate physician or counselor or both.

A major difference between the traditional interview with a child and a teenager is that the physician sees the patient alone at some point during the interview. The first time this is done, both patient and parents may be very surprised and even resistant; however, a clear explanation of your motives usually clears the way. Some professionals prefer to start meeting alone when the patient is in earlier childhood—as early as 6 or 7 years of age, even if only for a few minutes. Getting the patient and parents accustomed to this interview technique can be helpful as a preparation for later.

The length of this interview (average of 30 minutes) can vary, depending on the patient's age, reasons for the visit, concerns of the parent versus the child and others. The 10-year-old may not be very vocal; however, variations do occur between the garrulous 10-year-old versus the silent 12-year-old or the angry 14-year-old. Allowing the youth to have their own time is the main technique to use. When evaluating a young teenager with a parent, you can see them together at first, but save some time for the teenager alone. Encourage the youth to answer his or her own questions while with the parent, but interviewing alone may be the only way to identify concerns. When placed with the parent, the teenager may be silent while the mother or father dominates the conversation. It may take a few attempts at private interviewing for him or her to open up, after becoming accustomed to this technique. Thus, the earlier you introduce this concept, the sooner you may be rewarded with positive patient responses! As the child or teenager gains in trust for you and also gains in cognitive abilities, he or she will be more likely to answer your questions. A private interview with the parent may be helpful as well. A summary session with both together can be useful to present your initial conclusions and recommendations.

Further Interview Techniques

When interviewing the teenager, try to be honest and natural. It is important that you like the patient — if you do not like children and adolescents, the patient will pick up your negative "vibrations" and interfere with your attempts to establish a rapport. Children and youth generally respond best to the honest professional who acts in a natural manner. Questions should be aimed at their cognitive level, whether concrete or formal operational. Having the patient complete a medical/psychosocial questionnaire that is aimed at their age and cognitive level can save the professional much time in identifying positive response, while showing the patient (and parents) what questions you feel are important. Encourage the patient to ask questions and TAKE THE TIME TO ANSWER THEM, whether about body changes, medical issues, human sexuality, or others. It is important that the professional understand normal events of puberty and adolescence — especially the wide variety of normality; this gives the physician confidence in his or her attempts to help youth.

When talking to the patient, NEVER ASSUME what the patient is thinking or feeling — try to find out! Start with "neutral" questions about topics such as sports, music, or art before pursuing sensitive or potentially embarrassing topics such as dating, coital activity, or pregnancy. After some general discussion, medical topics can be reviewed (headaches, visual problems, etc.); this can be followed by inquiries about friends, family, and school. The health questionnaire can be very helpful in this process. Eventually, early adolescents should be asked about girlfriend or boyfriend issues, menstruation, dating, etc. Depending on the responses received, further questions can be presented. In the very least, the physician should clearly grant the patient permission to deal with these and even more sensitive issues alone and in confidence. Some physicians like to use a "third-party" approach: "Amy, it is common for some not to like school. Do any of your friends feel this way? What about you?"

Keep alert to nonverbal cues, such as those observed between the patient and parent, the parent and you, or the patient and you. Observe the body language given off by the patient, the parent, and even you! Both positive and negative body language can be noted. Point it out when observed. For example, you may ask: "Amy, I noticed you seemed angry when your mother said you misssed 10 days of school. What were you angry about? Do you get along with your mother? Many argue with their parents. What about you?" Educating the patient about possible issues may open up a very meaningful dialogue, if you have clearly given your patient permission to talk.

Allowing such an open dialogue is the main thrust of this interview. It is worthwhile to have a room filled with "adolescent ambiance" such as teen-oriented posters and brochures. It is advisable, if possible, to see teenagers during office hours not filled with babies and small children (e.g., late afternoon or early evening); however, the QUALITY of the interview is more important! Those who see youth must deal with the teenager as an individual who should be respected on his/her own merits and as a separate entity from the parents. If the teenager trusts you, she or he will put up with the lack of a "perfect" adolescent environment.

Barriers to Successful Interviews

Of course, your efforts to develop a "meaningful" dialogue can be frustrated by many factors. The patient may not be ready to talk, she may talk constantly but without meaning, she may be very upset and only cry, and she may see you in a very angry-resistant mood. The interviewer, as always, must remain patient. Remember, the teenager does not have the experience of the adult; however, they still need your help even if they offer resistance. Many techniques have been suggested for these difficulties, but none are foolproof! Always allow your concern for the patient to show through, and allow your clinical judgment to be the best guide. Do not become angry with the patient and do not be judgmental. Keep your personal difficulties out of the interview. It is not your obligation to "convert" the patient to your way of thinking. It is your obligation to grant "neutral" advice and to allow her to find her own way.

If she does not wish to talk, respect that and suggest a later discussion. If she talks constantly without direction, structure the interview. If she is angry, point that out and see if you can diffuse some of it. Give her a chance to agree or disagree with the "facts" which her parent(s) presented. If she states "I don't know" to a question, ask for clarification — whether she means she lacks sufficient knowledge to answer or does not want to discuss that topic or any topic. If she is crying, be prepared with a box of tissues and offer silent support. Again, a warm, honest approach usually wins over your patient sooner or later! Understanding the family dynamics may give you invaluable clues, explaining the way she or the parent is acting. If you have the privilege of having followed this family for several years, you are in a better position than others to understand what is going on. If you set up counseling sessions, work out the ground rules. Many counselors have found it useful for the patient to keep a daily, written log of feelings for you to review at a later date; this is especially helpful for the patient having difficulty expressing feelings during the initial interview.

The issue of confidentiality is vital to the interview process, especially as the patient arrives on adolescent shores. One should never promise total or absolute confidentiality. You should never say to the patient or family that anything the child or teenager says to you will be held in the strictest secrecy. The patient may alert you to suicidal thoughts or homicidal tendencies which must be shared with parents. Some patients will test you and you may fail! As previously noted, do not guess what your patient is thinking or feeling.

You can, however, alert the patient and parents to the fact

that you want to honor the teenager's confidentiality, and will, under most situations. If you feel, however, you must disclose information from a private conversation, the patient must be notified and the reason(s) given. Openly reserve the right to disclose information if you feel it is necessary. Give the patient and family concrete examples demonstrating various points which you wish to make.

Adolescent Sexuality

Any discussion of adolescent health care issues should include adolescent sexuality. Youth go through various stages in acquiring an "adult" sexual identity. It is important to note that human beings are sexual individuals from birth to death, and teenagers must follow the same pattern. Thus, issues of sexuality occur early in life, with erections noted in males even in utero, with masturbation being commonplace in the 2 to 4 age group, and with a common curiosity noted in most children about physical differences between the sexes. Children can be taught about their bodies according to their own maturational levels. The clinician can encourage parents to come to grips with their own sexuality concepts and pass them on to their offspring. Children should be taught proper names for genital parts, and health screening of children should include evaluation of both male and female external genitalia at any age. Children and parents can be prepared, to some degree, for the eventual inevitable changes of adolescence. Thus the preparation of teenagers to learn about their own sexuality starts in childhood.

The hormonal events of early puberty create new sexual feelings in young teenagers, while middle to late adolescents go through various sexuality experimentation. Societal attitudes can have considerable influence in this regard. Masturbation, homosexuality, dating, and even coital activity become reality for many. It is usually not until late adolescence that actual acceptance of sexual roles (heterosexual or homosexual) takes place, with establishment of permanent sexual relationships occurring in late adolescence or early adulthood.

How the individual clinician reacts to this phenomenon is highly variable. All clinicians, however, note that, though many teenagers are not sexually active, there are millions of youth in the United States who are coitally experienced and in need of specific contraceptive information and methods. Though abstinence can always be offered to youth, many choose to be and remain coitally active, with an annual result of over 1 million pregnancies and millions of STD cases among the American teenage population. Thus, well-adolescent health care should include questions about the

patients' sexual development and, as appropriate to the situation, a thorough and honest discussion about sexuality and even contraception, if they state they want to become or are to continue to be sexually active.

Certainly, *contraception* during adolescence is often a complex and emotionally charged issue. The contraceptive *choice* of the young person depends on many factors: cognitive development, a specific choice of using or not using contraceptive methods, knowledge of specific methods, results of medical screening (determining which method seems safe for the individual), the specific sexual pattern, the patient's moral or religious views, and even the clinician's professional and moral views about adolescent sexuality and contraception. Methods to consider include abstinence, barrier types (diaphragm, cervical cap, condom, vaginal contraceptives), oral contraceptives, postcoital contraception, injectable contraceptive (such as depomedroxyprogesterone acetate), and rhythm methods.

The health care provider should consider many aspects of this issue. For example, does prescription of contraceptives to youth mean that one condones or accepts teenage sexual activity? Do physicians have to give contraceptives to sexually active youth? Should one refer such individuals to other sources if the physician is unable or unwilling to provide contraceptive information or methods? Indeed, the subject can become very complex. Sometimes the clinician has three entities to contend with: the teenager, the parent, and the clinician's own adolescence.

Adolescent Pregnancy

There has been considerable discussion recently concerning the phenomenon of the pregnant teenager. Many underlying factors emerge: the recent increase in sexual activity among youth, earlier maturation, societal attitudes toward sexuality (including the influence of the media), motivations for pregnancy, and the limited knowledge of the youth regarding sexuality and contraceptions.

Early adolescents are often developmentally unable to relate coital activity with pregnancy and delivery of a baby 9 months later; the ability to think beyond the present, as previously noted, is limited in many individuals. They often cannot use contraceptive methods effectively. Some become pregnant out of Oedipal conflicts with parents or because of domination by older youth or even through incest. Middle adolescents may become pregnant as part of their attempts to manipulate the environment, either by getting even with someone (a parent or boyfriend) or simply to improve what is perceived as a limited life situation. Though often intellectually capable of assuming effective contraceptive roles, they often refuse, because the pregnancy may represent an acting-out phenomenon or power struggle issue. Others become caught up with the magic thinking process; they believe they are magically immune from the consequences of a specific action (as pregnancy from coitus). The motivations of late adolescents may be similar to those of middle adolescents or resemble those of young adult women — purposeful failure to use effective contraceptives, desire to solidify a sexual relationship, or others.

Clearly, even if prevention is not always possible, identification of a pregnant teenager is important. Early referral for adequate prenatal care significantly reduces maternal and perinatal complications for youth of all ages. Thus, when obtaining a history from teenagers, note the presence or absence of coital activity and review the menstrual history. Always ask about the last normal menstrual period in postmenarchal youth. Ask about pregnancy symptomatology: morning sickness, urinary frequency, breast swelling or tenderness, and other symptoms. The pelvic examination and laboratory studies (such as urine and serum pregnancy tests) are helpful in confirming the diagnosis.

Medical as well as psychosocial assessment and support are necessary for the pregnant teenager. Support personnel include obstetrician-gynecologist, nurse midwife, pediatrician, or family physician, social worker, nurse, community health individual, nutritionist, and psychologist. There are also many support facilities that may help prenatally or postnatally: vocational-educational training programs, counseling groups (addressing parenting skills or marriage skills), drug abuse programs, child care facilities, contraceptive services, and so on.

Without adequate prenatal and postnatal attention, medical and psychosocial complications associated with teenage pregnancy are considerable. Some of the risk factors in this regard include short interpregnancy period (with repeat teenage pregnancies), low financial status, food faddism, drug abuse (e.g., cigarette smoking, alcohol abuse, heroin addiction), weight loss during pregnancy, severe psychosocial difficulties, presence of an STD, and abuse of the pregnant youth by family or boyfriend.

Problems that may occur or be increased in the pregnant teenager who is not receiving good care include bleeding complications, severe anemia, toxemia, cephalopelvic disproportion with difficult labor, urinary tract infection, increased social difficulty (with more drug abuse and suicide), family disruption, low self-esteem with early repeat pregnancy, and limited educational-vocational attainment.

Finally, there may be increased morbidity in the baby: prematurity, congenital defects, handicaps (mental and physical), increased illness in the first few years, poor parenting with resulting undersocialization, possible child abuse (neglect), and limited educational-vocational achievement of the child. Early pregnancy diagnosis and care (prenatal and postnatal care) by interested and knowledgeable health care professionals can reduce some of these potential complications.

Sexual Abuse and Assault

Sexual abuse and assault of teenagers is a serious and growing problem of many societies, with thousands (or perhaps hundreds of thousands) of annual victims. *Rape* is a legal term referring to carnal knowledge (or any penile penetration during coitus) of a female without her consent, and with the use of force, fear, or fraud. *Statutory rape* refers to coitus with a female below the age of consent (16 to 21 years). *Sexual assault* defines sexual contact (manual, genital, or oral) with the victim's genitalia, without consent and with the use of force, fear, or fraud. *Incest* means there is coital contact between a young victim (child or young teenager) and a blood relative.

Factors that contribute to the sexual abuse or assault of teenagers include being alone late at night, frequent hitchhiking, drug abuse, and running away. General and local genital injuries are common, especially with young individuals. Pregnancy and STDs may also occur. Severe emotional reactions can develop, including acute reactions (such as shock, dismay, or denial) and chronic reactions (such as depression, phobias, and sexual dysfunction). Failure to receive psychological help may result in a severely disruptive life-style, with developmental arrest and chronic emotional difficulties. Males also may be victims of sexual abuse and assault, comprising 5 to 10% of most large assault series.

Adolescents who are seen within 48 to 72 hours of a sexual assault (or rape) need a careful physical and emotional assessment by a trained health care professional. Many areas have rape crisis centers with individuals specialized in this sphere. The use of a specific protocol designed by local experts is invaluable for dealing with the situation. The examiner obtains a history and then performs a thorough physical examination, including a pelvic examination. The examiner also collects material to observe personally for spermatozoa identification (and motility) and acid phosphatase, as evidence for the presence of semen and, thus, coital activity. Other materials collected from the victim, including aspirates, blood, and clothes, are sent to a local forensic laboratory. Medicolegal pictures are taken, and signed consent is obtained.

General treatment is given for the injuries. The individual is often treated as a gonorrhea and chlamydia contact (and screened for syphilis). The victim is also evaluated for other STDs. Tetanus toxoid is given if necessary. Measures for genital injury include an antiseptic douche, warm sitz baths, hydrocortisone cream, and oral analgesics. Surgical repair of injury or antibiotic therapy may also be necessary. Pregnancy prevention measures should not be forgotten. Finally, arrangements must be made for follow-up emotional support for the victim and, often, for the family. Because of the increasing numbers of victims, a general sexual history should inquire about the possibility of previous sexual assault or abuse. Individuals with a history of this, even if not in the immediate past, also need a careful psychosocial assessment and counseling.

Incest

Incest is a special type of sexual abuse that is underreported and not clearly understood. These are more than 5000 reported cases per million population each year in the United States, but the correct figure may be much higher. Many types are noted and numerous etiological theories proposed. Information, however, remains limited. Concern with incest is from religious, ethical, medical, and societal points of view. Society and religion have always condemned incest on moral grounds, and there is concern over resultant psychological problems of the involved parties, as well as over the increased morbidity (and mortality) noted among the offspring.

The classic situation is *father-daughter incest,* in which there is a domineering father figure, a weak mother figure, and the involved female child or adolescent who submits to the abuse. Here the parents have marked sexual difficulty, and the mother condones (often passively) the incest. Usually this begins at age 10 and a chronic pattern then ensues. Subsequent daughters may become involved as the original abused child leaves the home. Most authorities stress that this phenomenon should be viewed as part of generalized family disruption and turmoil. The daughter may display evidence of genital symptomatology or acting-out behavior; however, in some instances there is no overt evidence of difficulty. A high degree of suspicion is required to make the diagnosis, and once it is made, the situation must be reported as child abuse. Therapy should be available for all three involved individuals — father, daughter, and mother. The impact of this situation on the rest of the family must also be considered. The goal in most cases is to repair the family disruption, if possible, and prevent further occurrences.

Recent evidence indicates that sibling incest is more common than was previously estimated. Again, only limited information is currently available. Current thinking is that mother-son incest is quite rare. A high index of suspicion is necessary for all these cases and rests on a careful psychomedical assessment of all youth by health care professionals. Referral to qualified local resources is then important. Clearly, further studies in this area are needed.

Drug Abuse

The abuse of drugs among youth represents a serious problem for society. It cannot be eliminated but must be controlled. It may represent simple adolescent experimentation or overt use that markedly interferes with the young person's negotiation of adolescence itself, and thus significantly interferes with potential as an adult. It may be an expression of adolescent conflict and contribute to parent-youth altercations, transient situational disorders, juvenile delinquency, personality trait disorders, sexual acting out, and depression. Because of the high drug use among youth, health care professionals who deal with teenagers must become knowledgeable in this area. Numerous drugs are used: marijuana, tobacco, alcohol, hallucinogens (such as lysergic acid diethylamide, phencyclidine), stimulants (such as amphetamines, cocaine), barbiturates, narcotics (such as morphine, heroin), inhalant substances (such as aerosol sprays, gasoline, glue), and many others.

Currently there is frequent use of marijuana, alcohol, tobacco, and cocaine with enormous negative effects on youth and society. It is imperative that teenagers, health care professionals, and society itself be aware of these consequences. Careful assessment of the drug use pattern of each user seen is important. Our youth must receive accurate information about drug use, and particular attention must be given to the individual who "abuses" drugs. Abusers may be defined as persons who use a substance to such an extent that it affects them medically or interferes with their functioning in society.

Prevention and treatment of drug abuse are complicated tasks, because the causes of abuse are numerous and complex. Attention to psychological factors is important, and alternatives to the drug abuse must be offered. Underlying psychological problems (depression, for example) must be identified and treated. The abuse may be a reflection of many of society's problems, thus complicating the clinician's task even more. Evaluation and therapy of adolescent drug abuse represents challenging aspects of the field of adolescent medicine itself. The discipline of *adolescent medicine* states that medicopsychosocial elements of disease must be considered when caring for adolescents. Therapy of the drug abuse phenomenon represents a classic example of this important concept.

Donald E. Greydanus

References

Committee on Adolescence. Adolescent pregnancy. *Pediatrics* 83: 132, 1989.

Greydanus, D. E. Depression in adolescence: A perspective. *J. Adol. Health Care* 7:109S, 1986.

Greydanus, D. E. Disorders of the Adolescent. In M. Ziai (Ed.). *Pediatrics* (3rd ed). Boston: Little, Brown 1984.

Greydanus, D. E. Risk-taking behaviors in adolescence. *J.A.M.A.* 258: 112, 1987.

Greydanus, D. E., and Shearin, R. B. *Adolescent Sexuality and Gynecology*. Philadelphia: Lea & Febiger, 1990.

Hofmann, A. D., and Greydanus, D. E. (Eds.). *Adolescent Medicine* (2nd ed.). Norwalk, CT: Appleton-Lange, 1989.

Johnson, J. Sexually transmitted diseases in adolescents. *Prim. Care* 14: 101, 1987.

MacKenzie, R. G. and Jacobs, E.A. Recognizing the adolescent drug abuser. *Prim. Care* 14:225, 1987.

Schonberg, S. K. (Ed.). *Substance Abuse: A Guide for Health Professionals*. Elk Grove Village, IL: American Academy of Pediatrics, 1988.

Strasburger, V. C., and Greydanus, D. E. (Eds.). *Adolescents at Risk: Problems and Solutions. State of the Art Reviews: Adolescent Medicine*. Philadelphia: Hanley & Belfus, 1990.

Tanner, J. M. *Growth at Adolescence* (2nd ed.). Oxford: Blackwell, 1962.

Appendix A

Differential Diagnosis

1. States of Unconsciousness

Unconsciousness lasting 20 minutes or longer constitutes a true medical emergency. Immediate supportive therapy to prevent hypoxia and prompt etiological diagnosis to ensure proper specific therapy are mandatory. In known epileptic patients postictal unconsciousness lasting longer than 1 hour strongly suggests the presence of some intercurrent acute disease state and, hence, calls for immediate and complete diagnostic evaluation.

Clinically, several levels of impaired consciousness may occur. The somnolent patient can be aroused by gentle shaking or by a raised tone of voice; when aroused, such a patient responds to commands or questions rationally, but briefly, before again falling asleep. The stuporous patient requires stronger stimuli for arousal and, when aroused, does not respond rationally. In semicoma and deep coma the patient cannot be aroused by any stimulus. In semicoma, corneal reflexes, pupillary response to light, and cochleoorbicularis and retinoorbicularis as well as motor response to pinprick on face or limbs are still present. In deep coma even these reflex reactions disappear, leaving the patient in the deepest level of unconsciousness compatible with life. The GLASGOW scale is an excellent measure for the evaluation of patients with altered states of consciousness.

The conscious state is maintained by the central reticular formation, which extends from the medulla oblongata through the pons, midbrain, and dorsal hypothalamus to the reticular nuclei of the thalamus. These interconnected nuclei act as an alerting system that keeps the cerebral cortex in a state of wakefulness when incoming stimuli are received. Lesions affecting the infratentorial portion of the central reticular formation (in pons and medulla) cause deep, unwavering coma, which is usually accompanied by disturbances of circulation and respiration. Upper brainstem and thalamic injuries (supratentorial) are more likely to cause lighter levels of unconsciousness that fluctuate and are often associated with seizure activity. Mention should also be made of a stuporous state termed akinetic mutism in which the patient lies with eyes open and muscles relaxed but without voluntary activity; although obviously out of contact, such a patient responds briefly to painful stimuli. Akinetic mutism is associated with lesions of the third ventricle.

Both focal lesions of the brain and systemic disorders (toxic, infectious, or metabolic) that affect the brain diffusely may cause coma. Whatever the cause of the patient's disease, it is the effect of a disease upon the central reticular formation that leads to impairment of consciousness. Because events may move rapidly—for better or for worse—the unconscious patient must be repeatedly examined at frequent intervals. Particular attention should be paid at each examination to changes in the level of unconsciousness, to cardiovascular and respiratory function, and to the development of focal neurological signs.

Examination of the Unconscious Patient

The physician's very first duty is to make certain that the unconscious child has an unobstructed airway and that cardiopulmonary function is adequate. Then the other resuscitative steps listed below are carried out.

1. Establish a clear airway. Begin mouth-to-mouth resuscitation if patient is not breathing spontaneously or respiratory air exchange is grossly inadequate.
2. Check carotid pulse; if it is absent, carry out external cardiac massage.
3. Evacuate stomach and begin continuous gastric suction.
4. Cannulate vein for administration of parenteral fluids, blood, plasma, and drugs as indicated.
5. Control seizures (protect patient from self-injury until seizures are controlled).
6. In cases of multiple trauma or severe infection, type and crossmatch blood, begin treatment for shock, control external bleeding, splint fractured limbs, give tetanus prophylaxis.
7. Do meticulous physical examination and emergency laboratory tests to ascertain need for specific emergency therapeutic procedures.
8. Remember that lack of oxygen and glucose for brain metabolism can lead to permanent damage; use these whenever in doubt. If blood for determination of sugar has already been obtained, intravenous administration of glucose can do no harm while the diagnosis of possible hypoglycemia is being established.

The physician then quickly proceeds to a more thorough examination of the patient.

The aim of this examination is to determine whether one is dealing with disease localized to the central nervous system or with some systemic disorder. Often the history available in the emergency situation is inadequate or inaccurate so that prime reliance must be placed upon a complete physical examination. First, the level of unconsciousness is determined (see above). Unconscious patients must be moved and turned en bloc until the presence or absence of injury to the spine can be determined. Children with spinal injuries must never be flexed.

Turning now to detailed examination, one first makes a general inspection of the patient, paying particular attention to the following points:

1. Is there evidence of external injury anywhere? Falls and automobile accidents often produce multiple injuries; in such cases there may be minimal external evidence of injury in the presence of life-threatening internal injury (hemothorax, pneumothorax, ruptured abdominal solid or hollow viscus). These internal injuries take precedence over most other problems.
2. Is there external evidence of both old and fresh injuries? If so, the battered child syndrome must be considered. Old scars and fresh bleeding of the tongue suggest previous

Table A1-1. *Guide to Etiological Diagnosis of States of Unconsciousness (Including Coma) in Infancy and Childhood*

Etiology	Clinical findings and useful procedures	Etiology	Clinical findings and useful procedures
Primary Intracranial Disorders *Acute head trauma* Cerebral concussion, cerebral edema, contusion, laceration, hemorrhage, epidural hemorrhage, subdural hemorrhage or hematoma, subarachnoid hemorrhage	Clinical observations, possible imaging studies	**Primary Intracranial Disorders** *Convulsive disorders* Idiopathic epilepsy	Postictal unconsciousness rarely lasts more than 1 hr before improvement occurs; focal signs do not persist; previous history of seizures usually obtained; CSF normal; EEG usually helpful
Space-occupying lesions Subdural hygroma; brain abscess, cyst, or tumors	Enlarging head, bulging fontanel, lateralizing signs, vomiting, headache, preceding history of ataxia, slow but progressive diminution of consciousness, cranial nerve palsies, papilledema; sudden coma may follow hemorrhage in tumor	Febrile seizures	Occurs in younger children during acute febrile episode as fever is rising
Vascular lesions Congenital vascular malformations (aneurysms, Sturge-Weber syndrome)	Sudden onset of headache, seizures, and neurological signs in previously well child; imaging procedures need to be considered, cautious lumbar puncture	**Systemic Disorders Affecting Central Nervous System Infections** Acute bacterial meningitis	Infant signs vague and atypical; in older infants and children signs related to increased intracranial pressure, meningeal irritation, and systemic infection; shock and purpura may be present
Thrombosis of dural sinuses	Sudden onset of convulsions, unconsciousness, and rigidity followed shortly by vomiting, bulging fontanel, distention of scalp veins in a chronically malnourished infant with acute dehydration (diarrheal disease) In septic thrombosis associated with otitis media, infections of scalp, skull, sinuses, face; signs superimposed on those of sepsis; possible early exophthalmos, ocular nerve palsies, edema of orbit, engorgement of retinal veins	Tuberculous meningitis	Onset insidious over 1–3 wk; malaise, anorexia, apathy followed by signs of increasing intracranial pressure (vomiting) and decreasing consciousness; convulsions late and intractable
		Viral and post infectious encephalitis	Nonspecific prodromata of respiratory, gastrointestinal, and skin manifestations followed by seizures and unconsciousness History of preceding infection or exposure; onset of hyperpyrexia and convulsions followed by unconsciousness; cerebellar signs common in varicella
		Toxic encephalopathy and acute brain swelling due to severe systemic illnesses and infections	Evidence of primary infection

Table A1-1. (Continued)

Etiology	Clinical findings and useful procedures	Etiology	Clinical findings and useful procedures
Systemic Disorders Affecting Central Nervous System Infections		**Metabolic and Endocrine Disorders**	
Acute cerebral malaria	Delirium followed by unconsciousness; temperature may reach 43°C; prior history of malaria, transfusion, or travel helpful Repeated blood smears may be necessary to demonstrate parasites Blood smear for parasites	Hypernatremia (diarrheal disease, excessive salt intake, diabetes insipidus)	Progressive loss of consciousness together with hyperirritability, leading ultimately to coma and convulsions Serum electrolytes necessary for diagnosis
Metabolic and Endocrine Disorders		Hyponatremia ("water intoxication"); occurs most commonly after inappropriate water and electrolyte administration or syndrome of inappropriate ADH; hyponatremia, hyperkalemia, and shock characteristic of salt-loosing congenital adrenal hyperplasia	Weakness, hypotension, nausea, vomiting, hypotonia, restlessness progressing rapidly to coma and convulsions Serum electrolytes: sodium less than 120 mEq/L, but symptoms may occur at higher concentration of sodium if rate of fall is rapid
Diabetes mellitus (diabetic coma)	Kussmaul respirations, pallor, dehydration, vomiting, abdominal signs, cherry-red lips, acetone odor on breath; look for needle-puncture wounds High blood sugar; acetone, diacetic acid, and sugar in urine; history very important	Children with cystic fibrosis may lose electrolytes by sweating CO_2 narcosis Carbon monoxide intoxication	Cherry-red color of lips, face; loss of consciousness without convulsions (acute poisoning); antecedent history of headache, easy fatigability, hyperirritability in chronic exposure; history of inhalation of automobile exhaust fumes, smoke, or exposure to heating system with defective ventilation; spectroscopic examination of blood diagnostic
Hypoglycemia (insulin reaction, adrenal failure, etc.)	Unconsciousness often associated with convulsion, preceded by sense of fatigue, sweating, tachycardia, headache, pallor, speech and visual aberrations, tremulousness, weakness; pattern repetitive in individual patient; signs vague in infants. Blood sugar low (do not wait for results; give IV glucose—results may be dramatic and life-saving) Hypocalcemia and hypomagnesemia are very rare	Hypoxia; obstruction of airway; severe pulmonary disease; CNS disease involving respiration regulation in medulla	Restlessness, mental confusion, disorientation, coma, convulsions, decerebrate rigidity; serious hypoxia may be present in absence of visible cyanosis

Metabolic and Endocrine Disorders

Severe metabolic acidosis; diarrhea, vomiting; renal tubular disorders; salicylism and other poisonings	Serum electrolytes and various urine tests
Endocrine disorders (Addison disease, salt-loosing congenital adrenal hyperplasia, etc.)	Systemic manifestations of primary disease may usually not be obvious by time unconsciousness occurs; Blood sugar, serum electrolytes (Na, K, Cl, HCO_3), urea
Hepatic coma (severe hepatitis—toxic infections, parasitic infestation of liver, or biliary obstruction with cirrhosis, Reye syndrome)	Coma seen only in severe liver failure; characteristic "flapping tremor," jaundice may be absent; abnormal liver-function tests, raised blood ammonia must be looked for

Blood dyscrasias

Intracranial hemorrhage due to deficiency of various coagulation factors, thrombocytopenia, and severe infections	Platelet and coagulation studies; possible bone marrow study
Sickle-cell disease (hemoglobin SS)	Sudden onset of localizing signs and unconsciousness due to occlusion of cerebral vessels by thrombi; hemoglobin typing, sickle-cell preparation diagnostic

Cardiovascular disorders

Cardiac arrhythmias	Careful monitoring of the heart rate and rhythm clinically and by ECG
Anaphylactic shock; shock due to blood loss; endotoxin shock	Careful history
Embolic phenomena — fat, septic, air	Careful history; examination of blood and urine for fat; blood culture; cardiac evaluation

Renal diseases

Acute glomerulonephritis	Careful history; urinalysis, blood pressure; Foul smell of breath
Uremia, chronic nephritis, toxic nephropathy	Urinalysis, serum electrolytes, and blood urea nitrogen

Physical agents

Heat stroke	Prolonged (hours) exposure to great heat; abrupt onset of cessation of sweating, hyperpyrexia ($> 41°C$), muscular rigidity, convulsions followed by coma; must be differentiated from heat exhaustion (temperature normal) due to excessive loss of electrolytes in sweat; accurate history, body temperature, serum electrolytes
Toxic agents (including drug overdose)	Careful history and toxicology studies

convulsions. Needle-puncture scars suggest the use of insulin or narcotics.

In hot climates hyperpyrexia and hot, dry, red skin should suggest the possibility of heat stroke. The hyponatremic infant may show the classic loss of skin turgor, hypotonia, and evidences of peripheral vascular collapse. Look at the conjunctivae, the oropharynx, and the skin for early petechial and purpuric rashes; lesions differing in size strongly suggest meningococcemia. Erythematous eruptions may be associated with both viral and severe bacterial infections.

Smell the breath for alcohol, acetone, cyanide, ammonia, and urea. Is there flaring of the alae nasi as in pneumonia? Characterize the respiratory pattern—Cheyne-Stokes (coma due to effect on medullary respiratory center), Biot (increased intracranial pressure), or Kussmaul (acidosis). An enlarged spleen may mean cerebral malaria or a cerebral accident due to sickle-cell disease. Rapidly enlarging liver, kidney, or spleen signifies trauma to the organ. Boardlike rigidity of the abdomen suggests generalized peritonitis with septicemia. By the time most systemic disorders have progressed to the point of causing unconsciousness, there is evidence outside the nervous system that indicates the generalized nature of the patient's disease.

In examining the nervous system in the unconscious patient, one should pay special attention to the head, the eye grounds, and localizing neurological signs. Inspect the head for evidences of trauma, enlargement, or depressed fracture. Note whether blood or spinal fluid is oozing from nose or ears. Increased intracranial pressure may be suggested by a bulging fontanel or engorged scalp veins. Examine the eyes carefully. Do the eye grounds show engorgement of vessels, papilledema, hemorrhages, old chorioretinitis, or changes suggestive of leukemia or bacterial endocarditis? In the semicomatose patient, weakness or paralysis is best detected by the patient's withdrawal response to pinprick. In deep coma one can detect differences in muscle tone by raising and dropping each extremity; the paralyzed extremity drops like a dead weight. Pathological reflexes, hyperreflexia, and spasticity are more likely to be associated with primary intracranial disease, while hyporeflexia, absence of focal neurological signs, hypotonia, and deep sleep are usually associated with systemic disease. Nuchal rigidity suggests meningeal irritation due to infection or bleeding or the meningismus of severe infections.

Medical History

In cases of suspected head trauma obtain as accurate a description of the accident as possible. Recent failure to take anticonvulsant medication usually leads to seizures and postictal unconsciousness. Ingestion of certain household products and drugs in toxic amounts or drug abuse may cause coma. The onset of unconsciousness may be delayed a few hours, or it may follow several months of toxic ingestion (lead encephalopathy, chronic mercury poisoning).

Determine whether or not the onset of unconsciousness has been sudden. If it has been gradual, have there been suggestive cerebellar signs, motor abnormalities, or behavior disturbances in the recent past that might point to tuberculous meningitis, or an intracranial space-occupying lesion? Environmental exposure to carbon monoxide, certain insecticides, and lead should also be determined. Careful history of substance abuse is essential. The family history may reveal the presence of seizure disorders or diabetes mellitus in other members of the family.

Emergency Laboratory Tests

Urinalysis (including metabolic and toxicology studies).

Blood tests, including a smear (for malaria, sickle-cell disease, etc.), toxic substances analysis, chemical studies, and cultures, when indicated, are the most helpful laboratory procedures.

Save *vomitus* for specific analysis if there is suspicion of poisoning.

Imaging studies. Computed axial tomography (CAT) scanning and magnetic resonance imaging (MRI) have revolutionized the diagnosis of many intracranial disorders. Skull and chest x-ray films are also indicated in coma of uncertain cause.

Cerebrospinal fluid examination is most helpful when indicated. If papilledema is present, consult with a neurologist or neurosurgeon. Even when no papilledema is found, lumbar puncture should be carried out with the greatest of care.

Mohsen Ziai and J. Julian Chisolm, Jr.

---

2. Increased Intracranial Pressure

Palpation of the fontanels and use of the tape measure for frequent and regular measurements of head circumference are among the well-established habits of the good pediatrician. The large head associated with increased intracranial pressure is observed only under the age of 3 years. After this time, the cranial vault does not increase in size with intracranial hypertension, although the sutures may be forced open, causing the so-called cracked-pot sound. Significant papilledema is not expected in small infants with increased intracranial pressure because the sutures are open and compensate for the increasing pressure, but the bulging fontanel, "setting sun" sign of the eyes, and rapidly enlarging head reveal its presence. The underlying process, however, is often associated with certain other fundoscopic abnormalities such as chorioretinitis and hemorrhages, making this examination mandatory. Craniosynostosis may cause increased intracranial pressure, with irritability, vomiting, and a peculiar head shape, due to failure of the skull to enlarge properly with growth of the brain. Prompt x-ray diagnosis and neurosurgical treatment are required.

Slowly Progressive Intracranial Pressure

Enlarged head must be differentiated from megalencephaly and normal variations in head size. Whenever true enlargement of the head is detected, every effort must be made without delay to discover its underlying cause in order to prevent, whenever possible, further brain damage.

The first diagnostic consideration is to establish whether the problem is due to a space-occupying lesion (i.e., tumor, abscess, cyst, hematoma) or to an abnormality related to cerebrospinal fluid (CSF) circulation. There obviously may be a combination of these, e.g., a tumor obstructing CSF flow.

A simple procedure, often overlooked, is transillumination of the head. Much information can be obtained by this clinical maneuver in the diagnosis of hydrocephalus, subdural hematoma, cysts, and other localized lesions. More elaborate imaging techniques are presently available.

Brain abscess in childhood is usually a complication of cyanotic congenital heart disease or secondary to middle ear infection. The presenting signs are often those of a space-occupying lesion rather than an infectious process unless the abscess ruptures and causes meningitis. Subdural hematoma or effusion is common in infancy following head trauma or pyogenic meningitis. Signs and symptoms may be vague and include failure to thrive, vomiting, irritability, and fever. Specific neurological deficits are seldom present. Laterally bulging parietal areas and retinal hemorrhages, when present, are highly suggestive of this condition. Only by subdural tap can one be certain of the diagnosis. Other evidences of trauma, such as skin bruises and fractured bones, suggest that the cranial difficulties may also be traumatic. Child abuse should be suspected by the alert pediatrician. Most brain tumors in childhod are located in the posterior fossa and usually present with unsteady gait, other

cerebellar signs, and cranial nerve palsies as well as intracranial hypertension of early onset. Most of the remainder are in the suprasellar region, causing visual defects and signs related to pituitary involvement. In areas where hydatid disease is common, chest x-ray examination and skin tests should be carried out in an older child with unexplained increased intracranial pressure.

Intracranial hemorrhage is rare in childhood after the neonatal period. When seen in infancy, child abuse should be considered. When it is present, a bleeding disorder or a vascular malformation should be suspected. Listening to the skull with the stethoscope is sometimes very rewarding. Hums and bruits may be elicited, pointing to the presence of vascular malformations or arteriovenous fistulas.

Cutaneous lesions such as café au lait spots or neurofibromas may suggest the probable nature of an intracranial lesion. Increased intracranial pressure may be a complication of tetracycline therapy in early infancy, overdosage of vitamin A, steroids, and certain other drugs. Following otitis media one may see brain abscess, dural sinus thrombosis, acute bacterial meningitis, cerebritis, or pseudotumor cerebri. It is essential, therefore, to inquire about and look for any evidence of middle ear infection.

Ancillary investigations to establish the nature of intracranial lesion include echoencephalography, subdural puncture, skull x-ray films, imaging studies, electroencephalography, and tracer brain scan techniques. Lumbar puncture must be carried out with discretion and utmost care to avoid the serious complication of brain herniation.

Whenever meningitis or encephalitis is suspected, the examination of CSF becomes mandatory immediately.

Solomon J. Cohen

3. Convulsions

Alterations in cortical electrical activity result in convulsive seizures. The underlying causes for this phenomenon are many and may be related to intracranial lesions or systemic affections leading to changes in neuronal metabolism. Those cases in which the cause is unknown are called idiopathic. The causes of convulsions are summarized below.

1. Central nervous system (CNS) disorders
   a. Prenatal disorders (e.g., vascular malformations, porencephaly)
   b. Infections (e.g., meningitis, encephalitis, tetanus)

c. Intracranial space-occupying lesions (e.g., hematoma, tumor, cyst, abscess)

d. Intracranial hemorrhage (e.g., subarachnoid or intra-cerebral hemorrhage)

e. Cerebrovascular accidents (e.g., embolism, thrombosis)

f. Cerebral trauma

g. Acute cerebral edema (e.g., acute glomerulonephritis, allergic cerebral edema)

h. Degenerative (e.g., cerebromacular degeneration, leukodystrophies)

i. Brain damage due to other causes (e.g., anoxia, hypoglycemia, phenylketonuria)

2. Toxic (e.g., lead encephalopathy, Metrazol)

3. Metabolic
   a. Hypoxia
   b. Hypoglycemia
   c. Hypocalcemia
   d. Uremia
   e. Inborn metabolic errors (e.g., maple syrup urine disease)

4. Fever

5. Idiopathic

6. Conditions simulating convulsive seizures
   a. Breath-holding spells
   b. Fainting
   c. Narcolepsy and cataplexy
   d. Hysterical attacks

It is apparent that there are numerous possible causes for convulsive seizures. A systematic approach is, therefore, needed for the analysis of each case. Many affections that cause convulsions are also considered in the differential diagnosis of coma (see App. A, Sec. 1). In assessing the problem of a child with convulsions, it is helpful to consider the following points: age, type of seizure, history, physical examination, and laboratory findings. More details on specific convulsive disorders are found in Chapter 14.

Age

In general, there are sharp differences in the underlying causes of convulsions at different ages. In the neonatal period the most frequent cause is perinatal injury to the brain due to hypoxia or traumatic hemorrhage. Second in frequency is irritation of the brain caused by certain chemical abnormalities such as an elevated serum bilirubin level or a decreased blood sugar or ionized calcium value. Congenital anomalies of the brain can also cause neonatal seizures and be confused with birth injury. Meningitis, neonatal tetanus,

pyridoxine dependency, and narcotic withdrawal (in infants of addicted mothers) constitute some of the other causes.

From 1 month to 3 years of age the most frequent cause of convulsions is fever. In most cases this is a simple febrile seizure; however, seizures from any cause can be precipitated by fever. Previous brain injury often results in seizures beginning at this age. Acute illnesses associated with convulsions include meningitis, diarrhea with electrolyte disturbances, ingestion of toxic chemicals, subdural hematomas, and hypoglycemia. Seizures due to brain diseases affecting function such as phenylketonuria, tuberous sclerosis, and Sturge-Weber syndrome usually begin at this time. Finally, many patients with idiopathic epilepsy have their first seizures before 3 years of age.

After the third year, increasing numbers of "idiopathic" cases appear, but residual brain damage may also be manifested for the first time by a convulsion. Hypoglycemia, renal disease with uremia or hypertension, other metabolic or degenerative diseases, brain tumors, and meningitis should be considered at this age too.

Type of Seizure

Grand mal and focal motor seizures occur at all ages, but some convulsive problems are age-specific. These are listed below.

In the newborn period a seizure may consist only of apnea, rigidity, sucking, or unresponsiveness. Most such episodes are not seizures, however, and a correct interpretation usually requires a concurrent electroencephalographic (EEG) tracing.

From 1 month to 3 years one may see minor motor seizures (massive myoclonic jerks, head drops, sudden eye rolling, or akinetic spells). They are often associated with the EEG picture of hypsarrhythmia and may be due to any cause (e.g., metabolic, birth injury, idiopathic). These seizures usually imply a grave prognosis.

Simple febrile seizures are generally limited to this age. The prognosis is excellent if the fever is high, the seizure is brief (less than 5 minutes) and generalized, and the neurological examination and EEG are normal.

Breath-holding spells (see p. 279) are not considered convulsions but occur at this age and have to be considered in the diagnosis.

After the third year one may see petit mal seizures involving simple staring spells. These require a 3-second, spike-dome EEG pattern for diagnosis. Temporal lobe (or psychomotor) seizures usually start after this age. Focal sensory seizures cannot be recognized before this time because younger children cannot describe the sensation.

History

Proper description and chronology of the spells and the surrounding events (see p. 278) are very helpful in establishing the daignosis. Because the seizures are seldom witnessed by the physician, it is essential to obtain this history from a reliable observer. A full medical, obstetrical, neonatal, and developmental history is likewise essential in disclosing the nature of possible underlying conditions such as trauma, infection, and hypoglycemia. The family history is also important in the evaluation.

The most important function of the history is to differentiate the true convulsion from conditions that resemble it. Breath-holding spells are always preceded by anger, fright, or pain and are accompanied by apnea (usually in expiration). Vasovagal attacks (ordinary fainting) may be caused by fatigue, by long standing, by poorly aerated, warm rooms, and by anxiety. Hysterical attacks may be difficult to establish, but fortunately they often occur in the presence of the examiner, providing an opportunity to observe a few suggestive features. These may include bilateral motor seizures with preservation of consciousness and speech, or total physical and speech paralysis with presumed awareness of all events.

Physical Examination

Examination of a convulsing child should be swift and confined to essentials; further evaluation is then carried out when the patient's condition permits. Many patients are lethargic, confused, or agitated for a short time after the seizure, but these postictal changes, while important to note, may be only temporary. Muscle atrophy or persistent neurological signs suggest preexistent brain injury or malformation. The skin may show signs of trauma or infection (rash, petechiae), or disclose the nature of underlying neurological disease (tuberous sclerosis or Sturge-Weber syndrome). Cyanotic heart disease or evidence of infection in sinuses or mastoids suggests brain abscess. A bulging fontanel or stiff neck accompanies meningitis. Papilledema or retinal hemorrhage may suggest a brain tumor or subdural hematoma, while chorioretinitis is found in toxoplasmosis or cytomegalic inclusion disease. Jaundice in the newborn infant may lead to kernicterus with apathy, hypotonia, and then opisthotonos; Chvostek's sign is present in tetany.

Laboratory Findings

Laboratory investigations may give valuable information about a patient with convulsions, but they should be ordered with discretion.

Blood counts and urinalysis may indicate the presence of an underlying systemic illness. Lead poisoning, for example, is usually accompanied by anemia, stippled cells on smear, with stippled normoblasts in the bone marrow, and excretion of sugar and coproporphyrin in the urine. Special tests for phenylpyruvic acid or other amino acids in urine may also be indicated.

An emergency blood sugar determination at the time of a seizure or a fasting blood sugar at a later occasion is necessary to document hypoglycemia. One or two normal values do not rule out this disease, however. Serum calcium and blood urea nitrogen measurements are indicated when parathyroid or renal disease is suspected. All these studies, as well as measurement of the serum bilirubin value, are usually indicated in the newborn infant with convulsions.

Lumbar puncture is one of the most important tests, primarily performed for the early detection of infections of the CNS. Lead poisoning may give an increased CSF pressure and protein but a normal cell count. The procedure should be carried out very cautiously, if at all, when there is evidence of increased intracranial pressure because of possible danger of brain herniation.

X-ray studies of the skull may show separation of the sutures, erosion of bone, and abnormal calcifications.

Electroencephalography is helpful in the diagnosis of epilepsy and diseases that affect cortical functions. Specific EEG patterns are usually observed in such conditions as petit mal, temporal-lobe epilepsy, and sometimes minor motor seizures.

When a structural lesion of the CNS is suspected, MRI or CCT (computerized cranial tomography) should be done if available.

William T. McLean, Jr. and Spyros A. Daxiadis

---

4. Failure to Thrive and Dwarfism

Satisfactory growth in accord with presumed genetic potential is the most sensitive index of a child's good health. Failure to achieve this growth potential is called dwarfism. Shortness of stature, combined with an even greater deficit in weight, usually indicates long-standing undernutrition or disease and is called failure to thrive. Measurements of height and weight should, therefore, be made periodically, recorded on standard charts (see Chap. 3), and compared with the child's previous measurements. The size of siblings, parents, and other blood relatives, as well as marked individual variations in the pattern of growth, must be taken into account. Infants who have gained weight excessively in the first year of life often do not gain much, if anything, during the second or third year. A significant number of children grow slowly for several years but eventually achieve their expected genetic potential. Although they usually lag behind their peers, their heights and sexual maturation ages correspond well to their radiological bone ages. They can, therefore, be considered constitutionally late maturing (delayed adolescence with retarded growth spurt). The duration of growth in such cases is prolonged as if to compensate for its slow rate.

If the patient's height is satisfactory, the finding of unexpectedly low weight usually reflects one of two things: a particular somatic type or a recent period of illness or anorexia.

If height and weight are both significantly but proportionately reduced, the child has a deceptively healthy appearance. The etiological factor may be genetic, a prenatal uterine disturbance, or a long period of previous ill health or undernutrition. If the body proportions are abnormal for age, and particularly if the extremities are short, the cause can usually be found in some disorder that affects the development of bone. Abnormalities of the skeletal system, both clinically and radiologically, would be expected in such cases.

In the following outline the most common causes of failure to thrive and dwarfism are given.

1. Intrauterine disturbances
   a. Placental dysfunction
   b. Fetal infection
   c. Severe maternal undernutrition
2. Primordial or genetic factors
   a. Racial or familial
   b. Sporadic without congenital anomalies
   c. Progeria
   d. With craniofacial anomalies
   e. With severe brain defects
3. Chromosomal abnormalities
   a. Trisomy syndromes (e.g., Down syndrome)
   b. Gonadal dysgenesis
4. Insufficient intake or utilization of food
   a. Poverty, neglect, or ignorance
   b. Feeding problems (e.g., psychological, insufficient lactation, physical defects interfering with sucking or swallowing)
   c. CNS diseases (e.g., brain damage, mental retardation, subdural hematoma)
   d. Inborn errors of metabolism (e.g., galactosemia, glycogen storage disease, maple syrup urine disease, cystinosis, urea cycle defects, multiple carboxylase deficiencies)
   e. Infections (e.g., urinary tract infections, tuberculosis, malaria)
   f. Specific nutritional deficiencies (e.g., vitamins, iron, zinc)
   g. Renal acidosis of any origin
   h. Hepatic insufficiency
   i. Loss of nutrients through the stools (e.g., cystic fibrosis of the pancreas, celiac disease, protein-losing enteropathy, steatorrhea following diarrheal episodes or giardiasis)
   j. Diabetes mellitus, diabetes insipidus
   k. Malignancies
5. Endocrine disorders
   a. Hypothyroidism
   b. Hypopituitarism
   c. Sexual precocity with early epiphyseal fusion
   d. Addison's disease
   e. Cushing's syndrome
6. Disorders of oxygenation leading to anomexia
   a. Congenital malformations of the heart
   b. Chronic pulmonary disturbances
   c. Blood dyscrasias (e.g., Cooley's anemia)
7. Inflammatory bowel disease
8. Constitutional delay in adolescence
9. Disturbances of bone
   a. Chondrodystrophies
   b. Osteogenesis imperfecta
   c. Rickets due to any cause
   d. Renal osteodystrophy
   e. Diseases of the spine (e.g., tuberculosis, congenital malformations)

The pediatrician's first responsibility is to determine whether growth is indeed poor, and if so whether it has been poor from the time of intrauterine existence, since birth, or from some later date. A detailed history and complete physical examination are of great importance. Data on birth weight and length, as well as subsequent measurements if available, should be diligently obtained and organized, as should measurements of siblings, parents, and close blood relatives. The dietary history should be detailed, with an attempt to get accurate figures on volume of intake and composition of food (particularly of milk feedings) and conversion of these figures to total calories and grams of protein. Accurate estimates of losses due to regurgitation and vomiting are important, as are descriptions of stool frequency, character, and volume. Estimates of water intake and urine output are often vital. Thirst needs to be differentiated from hunger. It is important to know whether the

Table A4-1. Expected Findings in Some of the Causes of Dwarfism

Finding	Hypothyroidism	Constitutional delay	Hypopituitarism	Primordial dwarfism	Gonadal dysgenesis
Family history	Occasionally	Often	None	Occasionally	None
Birth weight	Normal	Normal	Normal	Often low	Often low
Hypoglycemia	None	None	Often	None	None
Dental eruption	Delayed	Minimally delayed	Delayed	Normal	Normal
Facial features	Cretinoid	Slightly immature	Juvenile	Normal, progeroid, or pinched	Normal or peculiar
Dwarfing	Minimal to marked	Minimal to marked	Minimal to marked	Minimal to marked	Marked
Sexual development	Infantile	Delayed	Infantile	Normal	Infantile except sexual hair
Body structure	Chubby	Normal	Normal	Subcutaneous tissue decreased	Normal or peculiar
Skeletal proportions (U/L ratio)	Immature	Slightly immature	Normal	Normal	Normal
Bone age	Delayed (1+ to 4+)	Delayed (1+ to 2+)	Delayed (2+ to 4+)	Normal or delayed (1+)	Normal or delayed (1+)
Water tolerance	Usually normal	Normal	Often delayed	Normal	Normal
Insulin sensitivity	Normal	Normal	Often positive	Normal	Normal
Buccal smear	Normal	Normal	Normal	Normal	Usually abnormal
Serum thyroxine	Usually low	Normal	Often low normal	Normal	Normal
Growth hormone	Normal	Normal	Often abnormal	Normal	Normal

Source: Modified from R. M. Blizzard, The differential diagnosis and treatment of short stature at adolescence. *J. Iowa Med. Soc.* 54:219, 1964.

appetite is decreased, normal, or excessive. An exploration of the emotional climate at home is often indicated.

During the examination, the child must be adequately exposed. Attention must be given to the various measurements and their proportions, posture, attitude, fat distribution, and pigmentation. The physical examination must be thorough and include examination of the ocular fundi, the blood pressure, and rectal examination. Certain other telltale signs such as the shape and position of the external ears, abnormalities of the external genitalia, and breast development in young females must also be noted.

Throughout the world by far the most common cause of poor growth is inadequate food intake due to unavailability of food (or the means to acquire it) or ignorance about feeding infants and children. The diagnostic value of the response to an adequate diet under controlled conditions must not be overlooked. It often makes a series of difficult and expensive examinations unnecessary. When the mother is healthy and well nourished, exclusive breast feeding supports normal infant growth for at least 6 months, often longer. Among the ill-nourished poor of many parts of the world the growth of breast-fed infants commonly begins to falter between 2 and 4 months of age, often sooner. When exclusive breast feeding is prolonged beyond 6 months, a slowing of growth is very common but good health is generally maintained. If supplementation of inadequate breast milk is attempted with bulky, protein-poor foods, overt malnutrition develops, with a significant mortality. Success in catch-up growth among the survivors depends on the diet and environment during later childhood but can be complete.

Regardless of what has caused "failure to thrive," the earlier its onset and the longer its duration, the greater is the risk of significant stunting. Intrauterine infection or undernutrition (see Chap. 9) results in a small size at birth and a poor prognosis for growth.

Most congenital physical and metabolic defects become apparent in early infancy. Acquired disease can be dated to the time of a detectable fall in the slope of the growth curve or by the evaluation of the height and bone age already achieved. Weight is a much less reliable index in this type of evaluation, as it can be rapidly regained during a period of relative well-being.

Laboratory Tests

Tuberculin test, urinalysis, and blood counts often rule out some of the relatively common disorders. Anemia and a high erythrocyte sedimentation rate may be the first clues to the diagnosis of inflammatory bowel disease. The blood urea nitrogen, serum electrolytes, and blood pH may assist in the diagnosis of renal disorders. Determination of the total serum protein is helpful when malnutrition is suspected. Serum calcium and inorganic phosphate determinations are needed in the diagnosis of rickets, parathyroid disease, hypercalcemia, and vitamin D intoxication. The glucose tolerance test and other tests of hormonal homeostasis are important in the diagnosis of pituitary disorders, diabetes mellitus, and glycogen storage diseases. Celiac syndrome and other malabsorptions are ruled out by the appropriate tests of the stools and intestinal function. On the basis of the history and physical examination and these preliminary tests, more specific laboratory examination may be indicated.

Estimation of the radiological bone age is important, particularly in assessing the prognosis for "makeup" growth. A bone age in agreement with or in advance of the chronological age (e.g., in sexual precocity with early epiphyseal fusion as in primordial dwarfism) carries a poor prognosis, while a markedly retarded bone age (e.g., in constitutionally delayed adolescence or in juvenile hypothyroidism) implies better potential for growth. Studies of the urinary tract are essential to the diagnosis of renal conditions that may not have produced any biochemical abnormality, as in many cases of hydronephrosis. X-ray examination of the chest is needed in the diagnosis of pulmonary tuberculosis, cystic fibrosis of the pancreas, and many cardiovascular conditions, particularly congenital heart diseases. When cardiac malformations are suspected, electrocardiograms and ultrasound studies may also prove useful. Imaging studies of the head may be valuable, particularly in the neonatal period when the presence of intracranial calcification suggests the possibility of toxoplasmosis and cytomegalic inclusion disease.

More elaborate procedures, such as chromosomal testing, examination of the urine for aminoaciduria, and tests of endocrine function, are among the later steps in the diagnostic approach. Among the endocrine causes of dwarfism, hypothyroidism is the most common. In this condition, the prognosis for mental development may depend on early diagnosis and therapy. Table A4-1 summarizes the expected findings in some of the more obscure causes of dwarfism.

Mohsen Ziai and George G. Graham

5. Dyspnea

Respiration is the most elemental human need; it is made possible by adequate ventilation. Any observed or perceived alteration in ventilation manifested by labored, difficult, or ineffective breathing is called dyspnea. Dyspnea can result from alterations in the lung parenchyma, the airways, or the chest wall.

Specific terms describe the various breathing patterns. Bradypnea: slow respiration; hypopnea: shallow breathing; hyperpnea: deep breathing; orthopnea: preference of a sitting position with continued increased respiratory effort as in congestive heart failure; tachypnea: rapid, shallow breathing; trepopnea: preference for a lateral recurrent position as with pleural effusions or pneumothorax.

Upper airway obstruction is manifested by alterations in the inspiratory cycle. Tracheal tugging and suprasternal, intercostal, sternal, and subcostal retractions can be present. Agitation and apprehension commonly accompany moderate to severe upper airway obstruction. Inspiratory stridor is the cardinal sign. Chronic upper airway obstruction can be recognized by pectus excavation.

Expiratory dyspnea is normally associated with intrathoracic airway lesions, specifically, airway obstruction or loss of airway or lung elastic recoil. The former's hallmark is wheezing.

Chest wall abnormalities can be seen with neuromuscular disease, congenital abnormalities, and orthopedic problems. The infant is prone to respiratory fatigue because of the relative instability of the thin, flexible chest wall. Both diaphragmatic and intercostal muscle fatigue can lead to respiratory failure. A practical classification for the causes of dyspnea is as follows:

1. Mechanical factors
   a. Airway obstruction (e.g., foreign body, congenital malformation, infections, inflammation or iatrogenically created lesions, bronchospasm, extrinsic airway compression)
   b. Diaphragmatic dysfunction/elevation by phrenic nerve injury, fatigue, or ascites
   c. Respiratory muscle fatigue or weakness (e.g., prematurity, poliomyelitis, myasthenia gravis, Guillan-Barré, muscular dystrophy)
   d. Bony defects of the thoracic cage (e.g., kyphoscoliosis, meningomyelocele)
   e. Limitation of movement such as pneumothorax, hemothorax, pyothorax, pleural effusions
   f. Splinting of the chest secondary to fractures, trauma, or surgery
2. Parenchymal factors
   a. Restrictive lesions (e.g., decreased lung surface area as in hyaline membrane disease, bronchopulmonary dysplasia, hypoplastic lungs, fibrosing alveolitis)

b. Interstitial disease with alveolar-capillary block (e.g., viral infections, lymphoid interstitial pneumonitis, pneumocystis pneumonia, collagen vascular disease, autoimmune disease, interstitial fibrosis)
   c. Decreased elasticity and destruction of normal architecture as in emphysema
   d. Loss of function tissue (e.g., atelectasis, tumor, pneumonia, cystic fibrosis)
   e. Alteration in pulmonary blood flow (e.g., intrapulmonary shunting, pulmonary hypertension, pulmonary embolism, congenital heart disease with shunting, congestive heart failure)
   f. Shock lung (ARDS)
3. Central or metabolic causes
   a. Acidosis
   b. Drugs (e.g., salicylates, bromides)
   c. Head trauma

In an attempt to elicit the cause of dyspnea, the physician must remember that there may be a combination of causes. It is sometimes difficult to determine the most important of these factors without adequate observation of the patient's course and of the effect of therapy. A careful history and physical examination are always needed, and selected laboratory examinations such as chest roentgenogram and electrocardiogram offer additional aid. Sudden dyspnea usually suggests a mechanical cause involving the respiratory organs, such as obstruction of airways, pneumothorax, atelectasis, or embolism. Chronic pulmonary or cardiac insufficiency can be recognized and its nature detected by the presence or absence of clubbing of the fingers, signs of congestive cardiac failure, cough, hemoptysis, emphysema, and other specific clinical findings. The differential diagnoses of cyanosis and of congestive cardiac failure are discussed elsewhere (App. A, Secs. 6, 7).

James E. Clayton and Mohsen Ziai

---

6. Cyanosis

Cyanosis is a bluish discoloration of the skin or mucous membranes or both. It may be central or peripheral. The central type is characterized by cyanosis of the skin, the mucous membranes of the mouth, and the conjunctivae. The oxygen saturation of the systemic arterial blood is diminished, but cyanosis is usually not recognized until the oxygen saturation is below 85%. Because cyanosis is recognizable when 5 g/100 ml of unsaturated hemoglobin is present in the systemic arterial blood, it may not be detected in individuals with severe anemia. In contrast, it is more easily observed in the presence of polycythemia. Besides the level of desaturated hemoglobin, other factors play a role in determining the presence and degree of cyanosis: skin color, skin thickness, and blood flow. Peripheral cyanosis results from blood stasis, as in newborn infants and in subjects exposed to cold environments. It is usually not seen in the oral and conjunctival mucous membranes, and the systemic oxygen saturation is normal. Cyanosis may be caused by methemoglobinemia. In the neonatal period it is particularly important to rule out sepsis and hypoglycemia.

Recognition of Cyanosis

A minor degree of cyanosis is not readily recognized if conditions are not optimal. A good light, preferably daylight, is essential. Comparison of the patient with normal controls is especially useful in a nursery. The hemoglobin and hematocrit values are typically elevated. Transcutaneous measurement of PO_2 is a painless indirect test of blood oxygen. Direct intraarterial blood gases are more precise, but care should be taken that the infant is quiet and relaxed. Blood gases are useful, especially in infants, but the arterial specimen should be drawn after the baby has ceased crying and is relaxed in order to obtain reliable data.

Having decided that the patient has central cyanosis, the physician must determine whether the patient has primary cardiac or respiratory disease. Cyanotic congenital heart disease usually becomes apparent in infancy and often in the neonatal period. The distinction between cardiac and respiratory causes of cyanosis may be difficult. A useful test is the inhalation of 100% oxygen while the arterial PO_2 is being measured. An intracardiac right-to-left shunt is rarely associated with a rise in arterial PO_2 above 150 to 200 mm Hg. By contrast, a greater rise in arterial PO_2 indicates a pulmonary cause of the cyanosis.

Cyanosis Resulting from Respiratory Disease

UPPER AIRWAY OBSTRUCTION AND MECHANICAL INTERFERENCE WITH VENTILATION. A low alveolar PO_2 may result from aspiration of a foreign body or inhalation of amniotic fluid or mucus during delivery or congenital anomalies of the lower respiratory tract. Congenital anomalies of the larynx and trachea or vascular ring may result in inspiratory stridor and retractions, which are apparent in the suprasternal area as well as the chest.

DIFFUSION DEFECT. In the immediate postnatal period one has to consider the acute respiratory distress syndrome and persistent fetal circulation. Pneumonia also may occur at any age including the first few days of life, with signs of a diffusion defect (see Chap. 9, The Newborn Infant). Blood gases and response to oxygen inhalation tend to be similar to the findings in acute respiratory distress syndrome. The chest roentgenogram may show signs of pneumonia, and blood cultures may be positive. Another condition in the small infant associated with diffusion defects is bronchopulmonary dysplasia, but in this case there has been preceding respiratory distress.

CHRONIC PULMONARY PROBLEMS. These are discussed in Appendix A, Section 8.

Cyanosis Resulting from Heart Disease

There are three circumstances that allow for cyanosis in the child with heart disease: (1) when there is a septal defect and the right-sided pressures exceed the left (e.g., tetralogy of Fallot); (2) when there is common mixing of pulmonary venous and systemic venous blood (e.g., single ventricle); (3) when there is transposition of the great arteries and the right ventricle is connected directly to the aorta. In addition, left-sided heart failure resulting in pulmonary edema may cause cyanosis, but this is more akin to pulmonary parenchymal disease; i.e., the response to oxygen inhalation is greater than in the presence of right-to-left shunting (Tables A6-1 to A6-3).

Table A6-1. Timetable of Typical Onset of Signs and Symptoms in Cyanotic Congenital Heart Disease

Age	Sign or symptom
1st week	Transposition of great arteries with patent foramen ovale and patent ductus arteriosus
	Mitral and/or aortic atresia
	Pulmonary atresia with intact ventricular septum
	Pulmonary valvular stenosis with small right ventricle
	Tricuspid atresia
1st month	Total anomalous pulmonary venous return
	Asplenia with multiple anomalies
	Pulmonary atresia with ventricular septal defect (VSD) (pseudotruncus arteriosus)
	True truncus arteriosus
2nd to 6th months	Tetralogy of Fallot

Table A6-2. Increased Pulmonary Markings

Congenital heart disorder	Cardiac silhouette and size	Other radiological features	Typical ECG features
Transposition of great arteries	Heart size initially normal Right ventricular enlargement by end of first week Usually prominent right atrium develops; left atrial enlargement with VSD or VSD + pulmonary stenosis	Pulmonary vascular markings initially normal, increasing with increasing heart size because of predominant right-to-left mixing	Initially normal Right ventricular hypertrophy before end of first week
Mitral and/or aortic atresia	Moderate to marked right ventricular and right atrial enlargement	Increased pulmonary arterial and venous markings	Right axis deviation; right ventricular hypertrophy often with Q and V_3R and V_1; right atrial enlargement
Total anomalous pulmonary venous return	Moderate to marked cardiac enlargement involving mainly right ventricle and right atrium; in supracardiac type, "snowman" appearance not seen in early infancy; in cardiac type there may be anterior indentation of esophagus by dilated coronary sinus; in infradiaphragmatic type, small heart and large liver	Increased pulmonary arterial and sometimes venous markings	Right axis deviation; right ventricular hypertrophy and right atrial enlargement
Persistent truncus arteriosus	Mild to marked enlargement; absent main pulmonary artery segment; right aortic arch in 25–50% of cases; in some instances anterior shelf formed by right ventricle making angle with aorta in RAO view	Pulmonary arterial markings increased High takeoff of left pulmonary artery	Normal or right QRS axis and left or biventricular hypertrophy; left atrial enlargement

Differential Diagnosis of Cyanosis

While two-dimensional echocardiography provides a reliable anatomical diagnosis, the clinician requires that all measures of the patient fit together with the proposed diagnosis. The historical data, the auscultatory findings, the chest x-ray film, and the electrocardiogram must be reconciled with the anatomical observations obtained from echocardiography.

History

In the neonate, early signs of congenital heart disease may be minimal. It is necessary to have a high index of suspicion in

the prompt diagnosis of congenital heart disease in the neonate, as many neonates deteriorate rapidly after the first symptoms. In the cyanotic neonate prompt examination using two-dimensional echocardiography is mandatory and in general clarifies the diagnosis. Cardiac catheterization may be urgently required to enable appropriate surgery to be performed without delay. An initial indication of heart disease may be a dusky appearance not readily recognized. Tachypnea is often an early sign of distress in the neonate. Other signs, such as failure to feed well and change in activity, may be subtle features. Intermittent cyanosis appearing when the infant cries suggests temporary reversal of a left-to-right shunt. Cyanotic spells are virtually pathognomonic of tetralogy of Fallot.

Table A6-3. Reduced Pulmonary Vascular Markings

Congenital heart disorder	Cardiac silhouette and size	Other radiological features	Typical ECG features
Tetralogy of Fallot	Size normal; concave main pulmonary artery segment; rounded, sometimes elevated apex	Right aortic arch in ±25%; lung fields may show bronchial artery pattern	Right axis deviation; right ventricular hypertrophy
Severe valvular pulmonary stenosis			
a. With intact ventricular septum, normal-sized or enlarged right ventricle	Normal cardiac silhouette; size normal or slightly enlarged	Left aortic arch	Right axis deviation; right ventricular hypertrophy; may be right atrial enlargement
b. With small right ventricle	Size small or normal	Small tricuspid valve on angiocardiogram	Mild to moderate left axis deviation; left ventricular hypertrophy; right atrial enlargement
Tricuspid atresia	Normal size, or slightly enlarged; concave main pulmonary artery segment; rounded apex	Right aortic arch in less than 10%; may be prominent superior vena cava	Left axis deviation, rarely normal; left ventricular hypertrophy; P tricuspidale, right and left atrial enlargement
Pulmonary atresia with intact ventricular septum			
a. With small right ventricle	Normal size; rounded apex; concave main pulmonary artery segment		Normal or slightly left axis deviation; left ventricular hypertrophy; right atrial enlargement
b. With large right ventricle	Mild to gross enlargement; concave main pulmonary artery segment		Normal or right axis; may be right ventricular hypertrophy
Asplenia syndrome (usually left-sided superior vena cava, single atrium, single ventricle, TGA, pulmonary atresia or stenosis)	Size variable; main pulmonary artery segment may be small because of pulmonary stenosis or atresia	Midline transverse liver; pulmonary isomerism; left-sided superior vena cava; symmetrical bronchus pattern and bilateral "right" lungs	Right ventricular hypertrophy

Physical Examination

The cyanotic neonate with congenital heart disease does not necessarily have a heart murmur. When no murmur is heard in an infant with suspected congenital cyanotic heart disease, one should look for other signs of cardiac disease. A prominent cardiac impulse and the presence of a gallop rhythm suggest heart disease. Evidence of congestive heart failure such as distended neck veins, hepatomegaly, peripheral edema, tachypnea, dyspnea, and pulmonary rales is noted.

X-ray Study and Electrocardiography

In the newborn period a chest x-ray film is often not especially helpful. Interpretation of the amount of pulmonary vasculature is difficult, and estimations of the heart size are as much a reflection of what happened in utero for 9 months as they are of what happened in the hours or days since birth. The electrocardiogram provides one more measure of the patient that adds to the profile of information even though it is rarely diagnostic by itself.

Echocardiography and Cardiac Catheterization

Modern echocardiography provides an anatomical diagnosis that is highly reliable in cyanotic patients. In general, cardiac catheterization is done to confirm the diagnosis and to document details pertinent to surgical success.

Mohsen Ziai

7. Congestive Heart Failure

Congestive heart failure is a symptom complex, conveniently divided into right- and left-sided congestive failure.

Left-Sided Congestive Failure

Left-sided congestive heart failure is characterized by respiratory phenomena, tachypnea, dyspnea, and pulmonary rales. These signs and symptoms may result from pulmonary disease or from pulmonary edema caused by cardiac failure. It is often not possible to be certain whether the symptoms result from a cardiac or a pulmonary problem, and on these occasions the physician must treat the child for both possibilities. In infants, pneumonitis complicating left-sided myocardial failure is common, particularly in babies with ventricular septal defects. Chest x-ray films demonstrating an asymmetrical area compatible with pneumonitis point toward primary lung disease while evidence of bilateral symmetrical haziness compatible with pulmonary edema suggests congestive heart failure. Left ventricular myocardial failure is the major cardiac cause of left-sided congestion, but obstructions in the left atrium or at the mitral valve, though less common, produce the same symptom complex.

Elevated pulmonary venous pressure is characteristic of left-sided congestive failure and may be inferred from the plain chest x-ray picture because of linear basilar densities (Kerley's B lines) resulting from lymphedema. Otherwise, clinical suspicion of increased pulmonary venous pressure is based on an increased respiratory rate, fine pulmonary rales, or outright dyspnea, possibly worse in the upright position and clearly aggravated by exercise or excitement. In the first month of life in infants of normal birth weight, tachypnea at rates of 60/min or higher should be interpreted as resulting from left-sided congestive failure until other causes such as pulmonary parenchymal disease can be documented. Alternatively, tachypnea in the newborn can result from severe arterial hypoxemia, as in infants with a transposition of the great arteries.

An important concomitant of left-sided heart failure in an infant is dilatation of the patent foramen ovale. If the left-sided failure is severe, the left atrial pressure is high, the flap of the foramen ovale may become incompetent, and a considerable left-to-right shunt may appear. This additional cardiac work load aggravates an already bad situation and may result in a rapidly downhill course. Deterioration may occur in a very few hours, especially early in infancy and commonly in babies with coarctation of the aorta or those

with critical aortic stenosis. With vigorous anticongestive treatment the downhill spiral may sometimes be broken and an equally dramatic recovery observed.

Right-Sided Congestive Failure

Pulmonary venous hypertension (left-sided failure) is the main cause of right-sided heart failure via the mechanism of reflex pulmonary arterial hypertension. Pulmonary arterial hypertension results from vasoconstriction and obstruction of small peripheral pulmonary arteries causing the right side of the heart to supply a normal cardiac output at ever-increasing pressure.

Right-sided congestive failure is clinically suggested by distended neck veins, hepatomegaly, splenomegaly, and rarely ascites or peripheral edema. While the symptom complex usually results from intrinsic heart disease, the symptoms are nonspecific, and myocardial and valvar function may be normal. An infant with pericardial effusion may simply be unable to get enough blood into the right side of the heart to supply the demand. Combined superior and inferior vena caval obstruction, as is sometimes seen following Mustard's operation, may produce right-sided congestion despite normal intracardiac pressures.

When there is right-sided heart failure without left-sided disease, the higher right atrial pressure may force open the foramen ovale, with resulting right-to-left shunting. The patient suffers from hypoxemia but is unlikely to experience right-sided congestion, because only part of the cardiac output must pass through the right side of the heart and the lungs. Cardiac output is maintained and right ventricular work is decreased, though at the cost of hypoxemia. Thus, any tendency for the right ventricle to fail is compensated by increased right-to-left shunting. For this reason pure right-sided cardiac failure is rarely seen in infants.

Intrauterine Congestive Failure

Intrauterine congestive failure results in hepatosplenomegaly, peripheral edema, and anasarca. Because the ventricles function in parallel in fetal life, the number of causes of congestive failure are limited. Primary myocardial disease, valvar regurgitation, anemia, and arrhythmias are likely possibilities to account for the discovery of hydrops at birth.

Congestive Failure in the First Month

In the newborn period, the sudden change from a circulation with ventricles in parallel to a circulation with ventricles in series uncovers cardiac anomalies that did not cause trouble in fetal life. Prior to birth, the right ventricle carries as much as double the blood carried by the left ventricle. Postnatally the two ventricles carry equal amounts of blood. Hence, the load on the left ventricle is increased at birth. Moreover, the abrupt exposure to extrauterine life is associated with a requirement for higher systemic pressure and an increased demand for output, approximately double that required in fetal life. Thus, in the normal situation, the output from the left ventricle may be increased threefold at birth. Consequently, any significant cardiac abnormality is tolerated poorly. Over the course of the first weeks the adjustments to produce the needed cardiac output have been made and the probability of developing congestive heart failure because of a congenital anomaly becomes more remote. In this age group congestive failure may be very deceptive and in early stages present with food intolerance, tachypnea, cough, or increased perspiration. Generalized or pitting edema is rare and the best manifestation of fluid retention is unexplained weight gain in the face of inadequate intake.

Congestive Heart Failure After Newborn Period

Congestive failure appearing after the first weeks of life is usually the result of acquired diseases such as tachypnea, arrhythmias, myocardial disease, or progressively self-aggravating lesions such as atrioventricular valve regurgitation. Congestive failure following surgical procedures is perhaps the most common cause of congestive failure after the newborn period.

Mohsen Ziai

8. Chronic Pulmonary Problems

A careful and complete history is the first step in the investigation of a chronic or prolonged subacute pulmonary problem. The symptoms may be continuous but are more likely to be intermittent or evanescent. Subtle symptoms frequently appear shortly after birth or in early infancy but are often mistaken for or obscured by the frequent upper and lower respiratory infections seen in the young child. Chronic pulmonary problems are often secondary to dysfunction of other systems, i.e., neurologic defects, cardiac defects, gastrointestinal problems, or more global immunological defects.

Cough

Cough is the single most common acute and chronic respiratory symptom. It can be caused by irritation anywhere in the respiratory system as well as from esophageal irritation. The most frequent source for persistent nocturnal cough is sinusitis or adenoitis with postnasal discharge. Cough that is extinguished by sleep is usually psychogenically induced.

Although most cough in children sounds productive, this is misleading. Because of the proximity of the larynx to the oropharynx and nasopharynx, poorly cleared secretions, formula, or regurgitated gastric contents may simulate purely bronchial produced secretions. Any degree of persistent mucopurulent discharge suggests an infectious etiology, either alone or in conjunction with an underlying functional or anatomic obstruction, such as bronchiectasis or an alteration in host defenses. Cough as a "wheeze equivalent" should strongly be considered in the otherwise well child in whom a detailed evaluation has revealed no other overt cause.

Wheezing

Wheezing is almost as frequent a chronic complaint as cough. The sound is produced by partially obstructed airways, usually in the third through sixth division of airways. Polyphonic wheezing with many different pitches of sound is created by diffuse airway disease such as fluid aspiration, bronchiolitis, viral pneumonia, congestive heart failure with pulmonary edema, asthma, cystic fibrosis, or bronchiectasis. Monophonic wheezing is synonymous with stridor.

Stridor

Stridor is classically produced by a partially obstructed central airway. If the source is extrathoracic, the sound is more prominent during inspiration, and if the sound is heard enhanced during expiration, the source is usually intrathoracic, i.e., distal to the thoracic inlet. In either case an intraluminal mass, mural abnormality, or extramural compression can cause the symptom. Laryngeal and tracheal lesions such as laryngomalacia, vocal cord pareses, subglottic stenosis, tracheal stenosis, hemangiomas, granulomas, papillomas, and adenomas may cause inspiratory stridor. Expiratory stridor and wheezing may be generated by vascular rings, tracheoesophageal fistulae, tracheomalacia, anomalous vessels, adenopathy, or mediastinal masses extrinsically compressing the central airways. Foreign bodies, bronchial stenosis, and congenital cartilaginous defects are additional intrinsic sources.

Table A8-1. *Differential Diagnosis of Chronic Pulmonary Problems*

Etiological factors	Cause	Clinical features	Diagnostic procedures
Recurrent viral infections	Respiratory syncytial virus (RSV) and adenovirus chiefly; basic susceptibility due to lack of previous exposure	Affects infants and children in early school years, bronchiolitis or interstitial pneumonia; may cause apnea in children less than 3 months of age; respiratory syncytial virus prevalent in winter months	Chest x ray (signs may be minimal — characteristically, patchy clouding, or hilar streaking); nasal smear or washings for EIA or IFA for RSV; absence of leukocytosis unless secondary infection present
Recurrent bacterial infections	Chronic upper airway obstruction		
	1. Adenoid and tonsillar hypertrophy	See Chapter 10	
	2. Allergic rhinitis with secondary infection	See Chapter 21	
	Tracheal or bronchial obstruction		
	1. Postrepair of tracheoesophageal fistula, or with H-type fistula	Previous history of repaired tracheoesophageal fistula	Bronchoscopy; barium swallow
	2. Vascular ring	Affects young infants: recurrent "croup," wheezing, stridor, occasionally dysphagia; costal retraction; extension of head	Barium swallow (indentation of esophagus); bronchoscopy helpful in revealing external tracheal pulsations; cardiac catheterization with arch study is definitive
	3. Bronchostenosis from endobronchial tuberculosis	Recurrent pneumonia in same lobe; previous history of tuberculosis or contact	Positive tuberculin skin test; bronchography; bronchoscopy
	4. Foreign body in bronchus or aspiration of food	High degree of suspicion, history can be unsteady; wheeze, especially if unilaterally present; persistent pneumonia or unilateral hyperlucency	Fluoroscopy or inspiratory, expiratory and decubitus films may show air trapping; bronchoscopy, diagnostic and therapeutic
	5. Aspiration of oil or other irritating substances, e.g., zinc stearate powder	Chronic lung symptoms, tachypnea	Chest x ray; careful history
	Esophageal abnormalities		
	1. Achalasia	Dysphagia may be inconspicuous; nocturnal regurgitation with gurgling may precede sudden onset of pneumonia; postprandial cough and discomfort	Esophagography (shows dilated esophagus with failure to empty) and esophagoscopy
	2. Hiatal hernia leading to esophageal stricture	Vomiting from early months of life; possibly hematemesis	Barium swallow
	3. Chalasia; gastroesophageal reflux	Reflux of formula; recurrent pneumonia; failure to thrive; nocturnal cough; recurrent wheezing	Esophagography; pH probe studies; esophageal manometry; pulmonary milk aspiration scans

Etiological factors	Cause	Clinical features	Diagnostic procedures
	Altered host response to infection		
	1. Chronic anemia		
	2. Immunodeficiency disorders	Recurrent pneumonia, especially pneumococcal; other severe bacterial infections may be familial; persistent interstitial pneumonia with tachypnea; relative hypoxemia	Measurements of the serum immunoglobulins and IgG subclasses; tetanus and diphtheria titers; skin tests for delayed hypersensitivity; HIV studies; white cell studies
	Left-to-right shunts with congenital heart disease	Occur most often with left-to-right shunt with pulmonary hypertension; clinical signs essential in diagnosis	Chest x ray and electrocardiography; further cardiac studies if indicated
Viscid mucus and bacteria	Cystic fibrosis	Failure to thrive; pulmonary symptoms of cough, recurrent pneumonia, and wheezing; onset during first few months to first few years of life; usually but not always associated with typical frequent stools; may be familial history	Elevated sweat chlorides, stool trypsin (absent or low); chest x ray, serum isoamylase, genetic studies
Specific infections	Complicated primary tuberculosis	See Chapter 20	Chest x ray; tuberculin and BCG skin test; gastric washings for acid-fast bacillus culture
	Mycotic (see Chap. 20)	Occur in endemic areas; skin and other ectodermal involvement in some	Skin tests; identification of the fungus by direct examination or culture
	Aspergillosis (allergic bronchopulmonary aspergillosis [ABPA])	Underlying chronic pulmonary disease (asthma, cystic fibrosis); shifting infiltrates on x ray, eosinophilia, central bronchiectasis, brownish fleck or plugs in expectorant	*Aspergillus* hyphae in secretions; skin reactivity to *Aspergillus* antigen; IgE determinations and IgG precipitating antibodies against *Aspergillus;* positive sputum culture
	Protozoal and parasitic		
	1. *Pneumocystis carinii* (see Immunodeficiency States, Chap. 19)	Occurs in premature infants and debilitated patients or those with immunodeficiency conditions; presence of emphysema	Identification of the organism by staining the tracheal aspirates or bronchial washings; needle or open lung biopsy less commonly necessary
	2. *Taxocara cati, T. canis* (visceral larva migrans)	Multiple pulmonary infiltrations; hepatosplenomegaly; sometimes skin and ocular manifestations	Severe eosinophilia and hyperglobulinemia are present; larvae may be demonstrated in biopsy specimen
	3. Hydatid disease (echinococcosis)	Rupture of the cyst causes discharge of watery fluid by coughing; grapelike particles may be coughed up; hydatid thrill may be present	Chest x ray (may show cystic mass); eosinophilia may occur; skin test and serological tests helpful

Etiological factors	Cause	Clinical features	Diagnostic procedures
	4. Amebiasis (amebic abscess)	Not necessarily associated with intestinal symptoms, may have pleural effusion	The abscess fluid is "anchovy sauce" in color
	5. Chlamydial pneumonia	Usually in infants; conjunctivitis may precede symptoms by 2–3 weeks; infant has cough, tachypnea, increased secretions, usually no fever; may last for weeks or months	Chest x ray; diffuse interstitial infiltrates and areas of atelectasis; specific cultures
Noninfectious, mechanical, or tissue necrosis	Pulmonary fibrosis 1. Parenchymal	May follow atelectasis, bronchiectasis, or pulmonary necrosis of any cause; may lead to pulmonary insufficiency and cor pulmonale	X ray of chest, electrocardiography
	2. Immotile cilia syndrome (50% associated with situs inversus)	Recurrent productive cough with bronchiectasis; sinusitis; otitis media	Phase microscopy of cilia, electron microscopy of cilia biopsy
	3. Bronchopulmonary dysplasia (BPD)	Development of chronic lung disease in infants who were premature and treated with high ventilatory pressures and high partial pressure of oxygen; these infants require prolonged oxygen therapy and are subject to poor weight gain and cor pulmonale	Chest films reveal areas of hyperaeration with areas of atelectasis and coarse reticular patterns; ECG may show right heart strain (as a late finding)
	4. Idiopathic pulmonary hemosiderosis	Recurrent episodes of cyanosis, dyspnea, cough, and perhaps hemoptysis, anemia, or pallor, not accompanied by systemic hemosiderosis; may also present with fever and mimic recurrent bacterial pneumonias; rusty sputum	Chest x ray (may show picture resembling miliary tuberculosis or pulmonary shadows that change during the acute episodes); hemosiderosis-laden macrophages; low serum iron
	5. Congenital cystic disease of the lungs	May cause mechanical problems, often of acute nature, or become infected; frequently forms incidentally	Suspected by x-ray examination of the chest
	Sarcoidosis	Lymphadenopathy, ocular and skin manifestations as well as multiple pulmonary symptoms; tachypnea; wheezing; clubbing	X rays of the chest and of hands and feet; blood studies for the detection of hypercalcemia, hyperproteinemia, hyperglobulinemia, eosinophilia, and leukopenia; negative tuberculin; elevated angiotensin-converting enzyme
Allergic or nonspecific	Chronic bronchial asthma	See Chapter 21	

Tachypnea

Persistent tachypnea is usually a sign of respiratory insufficiency but may have cardiac etiology as well. Resting tachypnea with minimal increase in work of respiration usually suggests a diffuse small airway process, interstitial process or alveolar involvement. Tachypnea with associated increased work of respiration as manifested by use of accessory muscles of respiration suggests obstructive airway disease.

Weight Loss

Weight loss is common in the older child with prolonged pulmonary disease particularly if it is of infectious etiology. Younger children and infants have growth deceleration as a primary manifestation. This is usually caused by increased caloric utilization from increased work of respiration as well as the energy costs of host defense mechanisms. Cystic fibrosis is the best example of this. Impaired appetite is a frequent presenting symptom of both acute and chronic disease processes in children.

Hemoptysis

True hemoptysis is rare but is still seen with bronchiectasis, particularly in cystic fibrosis. Primary tuberculosis, hemangiomas, bronchial adenomas, papillomas, and lung abscesses are other common causes. Hemoptysis is seen with idiopathic pulmonary hemosiderosis and Eisenmenger's complex.

Signs

Physical examination should be carried out with a differential diagnosis (Table A8-1) formulated by the diagnostician in order to seek specific confirmatory signs.

Upper airway obstruction and infection are important associated findings in many cases of chronic pulmonary disease. Nasal polyps and tender sinuses suggest cystic fibrosis. Hyperactivity, tonsillar and adenoidal hypertrophy associated with sleep disturbances and snoring suggest chronic nocturnal hypoxemia and cor pulmonale. Persistent coarse stridor suggests glottic level obstruction. Persistent resting tachypnea suggests interstitial lung disease; in the chronically ill or malnourished child, immunodeficiency states should strongly be considered. Persistent lobar pneumonias can be caused either by mechanical obstruction of clearance, i.e., foreign bodies, bronchiectasis, sequestration, or infected lung cyst, or by immunodeficiency states,

particularly granulocyte disorders. Chronic pharyngitis, hoarseness, and nocturnal cough with multilobar or perihilar infiltrates are consistent with gastroesophageal reflux with microaspiration. Multilobar pneumonias in neurologically impaired children is frequently a result of direct aspiration. Increased anteroposterior (AP) diameter of the chest is a sign of obstructive airway disease. Pectus excavatum is often associated with upper airway obstruction.

Examination of the cardiovascular system is important but usually only reveals the relatively late finding of cor pulmonale. An accentuated single second heart sound heard best at the pulmonic post is indicative of pulmonary hypertension. A fourth-heart-sound gallop may also be present. High-flow left to right shunts have an increased incidence of associated lower respiratory infection. Cyanosis, polycythemia, and clubbing are usually late findings.

In evaluating chronic pulmonary disease after physical examination, the next most valuable tool is the chest radiograph. Serial chest films with AP and lateral projections are essential to provide documentation of progression or resolution of the disease process. High kV airway films can also be quite useful. Arterial blood gas evaluation remains the gold standard for evaluation of respiratory function, but digital oximetry is much easier and generally quicker for screening purposes. Pulmonary function studies are of significant value in the child older than 7 or 8 years. Newer measurement techniques have limited practical application for general use. Bronchography has largely been replaced by computerized axial tomography and flexible fiberoptic bronchoscopy. Bronchoalveolar lavage, cytology, and direct culture techniques have allowed earlier diagnosis of chronic interstitial processes. Skin testing for tuberculosis with a control is still an essential part of all evaluations. Specific skin testing is usually dictated by geographic locale.

James E. Clayton and Mohsen Ziai

9. Fever

It seems appropriate to begin a discussion of fever in infants and children by quoting DuBois' aphorism: "Fever is only a symptom and we are not sure it is an enemy. It may be a friend." Proper management of the febrile child depends on the recognition of underlying cause; therefore, a logical approach in differential diagnosis is based on careful clinical appraisal of the patient.

Low-Grade Fever

It is easy to confirm the presence of high fever, but the evaluation of persistent low-grade temperature elevations may pose difficult problems. The body temperature in such cases is preferably measured in the morning, afternoon, and evening after a period of rest for several successive days. Before taking the temperature one should be sure that the child is exposed to room temperature in light clothes for at least 15 minutes. These observations lead to one of the following conclusions: (1) that there is no abnormality of body temperature (one may then proceed to reassure the family) or (2) that the temperature elevation, even though low-grade, is real (an underlying pathological condition should then be suspected and a thorough search made). When there is any doubt about the patient or the family producing false temperature readings, the temperature of a freshly voided specimen of urine may provide additional information.

Physical Examination

The degree of care with which the physical examination is conducted, including the child's full exposure under a good light and the use of properly functioning instruments, often determines the physician's success or failure in interpretation. Examination must be thorough and always include the visualization of the eardrums. Such subtle signs as a postnasal discharge, mild icterus, a fading skin rash, or a faint cardiac murmur or friction rub may constitute the only clues to correct diagnosis.

Interpretation of Fever

Acute febrile illnesses are most often due to infections, and by far the most common are infections involving the respiratory tract. A thorough examination of the ears, sinuses, mouth, pharynx, adenoids, tonsils, larynx, and lungs is essential in every febrile child. Of the bacterial infections outside the respiratory tract, infections of the urinary and gastrointestinal systems are the most important to look for, particularly because the signs and symptoms produced by these do not necessarily point to the area of involvement. Persistent low-grade fever suggests chronic infections, regional enteritis, collagen diseases, blood dyscrasias, and tumors. Brain-damaged children characteristically have poor temperature control, which at times may cause confusion.

The daily temperature chart may suggest certain diagnostic possibilities. When there are large daily variations of

fever, such conditions as septicemia, miliary tuberculosis, rheumatoid arthritis, pyelonephritis, malaria, lymphoma, and leukemia should be considered. Kala-azar often gives two daily peaks of temperature elevation. Unlike the stepladder curve in adults, typhoid fever in children may have a more acute onset with temperature spikes. In Kawasaki's disease, the fever is quite characteristic, with temperatures of 39 to 40°C lasting more than 5 days and is poorly responsive to antipyretics. Table A9-1 summarizes some of the causes of temperature elevation in infancy and childhood.

Perplexing diagnostic problems may be encountered during the prodromal stages of the so-called childhood infections such as measles and chickenpox. Specific inquiry about exposure to these and other infections as well as certain specific signs (e.g., Koplik's spots in measles) may save the patient and family discomfort and the physician embarrassment.

Roseola infantum usually produces high fever in infancy. The physical examination is unrevealing except for occipital lymphadenopathy, and the diagnosis can be suspected only on the basis of a leukopenia and the relatively healthy appearance of the infant in spite of high fever. Confirmation comes when the erythematous rash on the trunk briefly appears, 3 to 4 days after the onset of the fever and concomitantly with the disappearance of the fever.

Miliary tuberculosis can be a very deceiving infection because the typical x-ray findings may be absent during the early stages. A positive tuberculin test and even a slight hepatosplenomegaly should alert the physician to this possibility. A thorough search for tubercles in the retina as well as certain laboratory investigations can usually confirm the diagnosis.

It is best to begin with a tuberculin test, urinalysis, and white blood count and differential. The absence of pyuria does not rule out the possibility of pyelonephritis, and a urine culture and bacterial colony count are needed to exclude this diagnosis. If these are negative, erythrocyte sedimentation rate and an x-ray film of the chest should be obtained. In early infancy, when signs of meningitis are nonspecific, the examination of CSF is mandatory when the cause of fever is uncertain. Blood cultures are essential in the diagnosis of septicemia, but usually several are needed over a 24-hour period. The phase of bacterial multiplication is usually reflected by a concomitant rise in fever.

In fevers of obscure origin, it is always helpful to save some of the patient's serum in cold storage, as a number of laboratory findings may be more logically interpreted in the light of changes that may occur (e.g., rise or fall in antibody

Table A9-1. Differential Diagnosis of Fever

Cause of temperature variation	Most important findings	Cause of temperature variation	Most important findings
Physiological (following markedly increased activity, heavy eating, excitement, etc.)	Flushed facies, increased blood pressure and pulse rate	Collagen diseases (lupus erythematosus, rheumatoid arthritis, rheumatic fever, dermatomyositis, periarteritis nodosa, Kawasaki's disease, etc.)	Multiple organ involvement; familial tendency in some cases; splenomegaly; serological tests and on occasion biopsy can be helpful
Infections			
1. Bacterium	Chills, splenomegaly, sometimes petechiae; white cell count, ESR; blood culture	Tissue necrosis (e.g., infarctions, gangrenes, presence of blood in body cavities)	Depends on location
2. Localized abscess (hepatic, cerebral, lung, osteomyelitis, empyema, perinephric, subdiaphragmatic, appendiceal, renal, peridental, etc.)	Localized signs of inflammation and abscess formation. Abscess may be concealed in some cases of toxic shock; depends on site of abscess; aspiration, culture, nuclear scan, and other imaging procedures such as sonogram and CAT scan can be very helpful in localization	Dehydration from any cause	Loss of skin turgor; sunken eyes, cracked lips, dry tongue; decreased urinary output. In cases where the urinary output remains good check specific gravity; check chemistry of body fluids
		Heat stroke	History; flushed face, nausea and vomiting, restlessness, headache; possible convulsions and coma; hyperpyrexia
3. Localized infections (meningitis, encephalitis, endocarditis, hepatitis, pneumonia, enteritis, pyelonephritis, etc.)	Localized signs of inflammation; in toxic shock the typical rash, postural hypotension, and use of tampon may provide the clue; depending on site of infection, cultures; cardiac and renal ultrasound in suspected cases are helpful	Central nervous system disorders (e.g., cerebral hemorrhage, brain tumors, congenital maldevelopment of brain, dysautonomia)	Specific neurological symptoms depending on location of lesion; may follow brain surgery

4. Specific infections
  a. Acute (typhoid, diphtheria, tularemia, rickettsial, tetanus, common exanthems, infectious mononucleosis, etc.)
  b. Subacute and chronic tuberculosis, brucellosis, syphilis, histoplasmosis, malaria, kala-azar, etc.
	Depends on specific infection

Neoplastic diseases (leukemia, lymphoma, etc.)	Pressure symptoms; enlargement of lymph nodes, liver, and spleen; bone marrow aspiration; imaging detection of possible areas of involvement and mestastasis; biopsy
Unknown Kawasaki's disease	Fever lasting several days; mucocutaneous lesions, conjunctival injection, rash, lymphadenopathy, irritability, thrombocytosis, elevated ESR, sterile pyuria hydrops of the gallbladder, possible cardiac involvement
Inability to sweat (usually due to ectodermal dysplasia)	Absence of teeth, hair, sweat, mammary and sebaceous glands; atrophic rhinitis, cataracts; a sex-linked hereditary trait
Hemolysis (e.g., transfusion reactions, congenital hemolytic anemias, hemolytic uremic syndrome)	Signs of extramedullary hematopoiesis, icterus, hemoglobinuria, appearance of peripheral blood smear. Repeat crossmatching in case of transfusion reactions; reticulocyte count, hemoglobin electrophoresis, and Coombs' test
Allergenic and toxic agents (poisonings)	History of drug ingestion and exposure to toxic and allergenic substances; specific toxic signs (e.g. dilatation of pupils in atropine poisoning); blood and urine studies for suspected drug

titers). The necessity of specific tests for brucella, malaria, kala-azar, typhoid fever, fungal diseases, etc., depends on the prevalence of such illnesses in the community as well as the patient's associated clinical findings. In the absence of positive etiology of illness, examination of bone marrow may be carried out, including culture and cell morphology. Several serological examinations can also be helpful in obscure fevers. Rheumatoid arthritis in young children may be heralded by a septic temperature curve and marked leukocytosis for weeks or months before the joint problems make their appearance. Similarly, in the early stages of Hodgkin's disease, fever may be the only manifestation.

Ali Akbar Velayati, Mohsen Ziai, and
Spyros A. Doxiadis

10. Pain in the Extremities

Pain in the extremities is a common pediatric problem that is often explained after careful history and physical examination. The first step is an attempt to determine the origin of the pain — bones, joints, ligaments, tendons, or soft tissue. The examination should be performed only after careful observation. Be slow and gentle, beginning with the normal extremity. The child's ability to move the affected limb spontaneously is assessed, with careful observation of facial expression.

Trauma constitutes one of the most common reasons for pain. Child abuse should be considered in a child with frequent or multiple fractures. Another frequent cause is muscular fatigue, which usually appears at bedtime and disappears during the day. The pain that follows known trauma, obvious evidence of cellulitis, draining osteomyelitis, or swelling of the joints in a boy known to have hemophilia pose few problems in diagnosis. Often, however, the underlying condition is not so obvious and needs careful consideration of different factors.

Infectious Diseases

Pyogenic infections involving the bones, joints, and soft tissues constitute serious and urgent problems in pediatrics. A septic process in the joint may be caused by any of the pyogenic bacteria that infect the skin or upper respiratory tract. Salmonellosis, which may cause osteomyelitis and arthritis, must be particularly considered in a black child suspected of having sickle-cell disease. Chronic meningococ-

cemia, brucellosis, Lyme disease and rat-bite fever caused by *Streptobacillus moniliformis* may be confused with rheumatoid arthritis. Tuberculosis is an especially important disease to consider in patients who have involvement of only one joint without the acute manifestations of a systemic infection. The origin of infection may at times be outside the affected extremity, as in psoas abscess. A septic process in the hip joint is a true emergency. Careful clinical evaluation of joint mobility and x-ray findings may suggest the need for prompt aspiration of the joint fluid, institution of surgical drainage, and medical therapy in order to prevent ischemic necrosis of the femoral head. The prompt diagnosis of osteomyelitis may prevent irreversible damage to the child's potential growth and mobility. This diagnosis must be considered in every child who presents with fever, pain, leukocytosis, and swelling in an extremity even though the characteristic x-ray findings may be inapparent. Radioisotope scans are positive before radiographic changes occur. Among other infections that can cause muscle and joint pain are typhus, Rocky Mountain spotted fever, syphilis, leptospirosis, dengue, and Lyme disease.

Rheumatic Fever and Collagen Diseases

Rheumatic fever is difficult to diagnose when the usual signs and symptoms are not present. The disease is now preventable, and after having made the diagnosis, one is committed to administering penicillin prophylaxis for life. Conditions simulating rheumatic fever include systemic lupus erythematosus, periarteritis nodosa, and rheumatoid arthritis. In rheumatoid arthritis, usually small joints, characteristically more than one, are affected, and the response to salicylate therapy is less impressive than in rheumatic fever. A skin eruption (known as rheumatoid rash), splenomegaly, lymphadenopathy, and chorea are among the helpful findings. Subcutaneous nodules are not characteristic of any of the collagen diseases but are more commonly seen in severe forms of rheumatic fever and in chronic rheumatoid arthritis. Although laboratory examinations are not specific in collagen diseases, the LE cell preparation, C-reactive protein, antistreptolysin-O titer, erythrocyte sedimentation rate, electrocardiograms, antinuclear antibody (ANA), Coombs' test, and latex fixation test are among the preliminary steps in laboratory diagnosis.

Blood Dyscrasias

Chronic hemolytic anemias such as Cooley's anemia may be associated with bone pain. The vascular crises of sickle-cell disease are commonly manifested by pain in the extremities. Leukemia is frequently associated with pain in the bones or articulations. Any disease that causes bleeding tendency, such as thrombocytopenia, hemophilia, and other coagulation defects, may cause pain in the extremities.

Neoplastic Diseases

Neuroblastoma commonly metastasizes to the bone. Osteoid osteoma may make itself known by awakening the child at night. Any suspicion that a bone tumor may be present should lead to immediate radiographic investigation in an attempt to reduce the high mortality associated with this condition. Ewing's type of bone sarcoma may mimic osteomyelitis.

Aseptic Necrosis

Various names are assigned to diseases included under aseptic necrosis according to the location of the lesion (see Chap. 15). X-ray films of the affected extremity are usually diagnostic.

Neurological Disturbances

Pain in an extremity may precede the muscle weakness and the reflex changes of poliomyelitis. Pain in the legs with ascending weakness, hypoactive deep tendon reflexes, and sensory changes suggest the syndrome of polyneuritis. Consider also reflex sympathetic dystrophy.

Occlusive Vascular Diseases

Thromboses, occlusions, Raynaud's syndrome, and embolic phenomena may produce pain in the affected area.

Disturbances of Vitamin Metabolism

Excessive administration of vitamins such as vitamin A, or a deficiency of vitamins such as is seen in scurvy or complicated rickets, may produce pain in the extremities.

Allergic Conditions

Serum sickness, drug reactions, or urticaria may produce joint symptoms. Anaphylactoid purpura is characterized by purpura, arthralgia, and crampy abdominal pain. Post–rubella vaccine arthralgia in adolescents may be an allergic phenomenon.

Miscellaneous Diseases

Pathological fractures may be seen in conditions such as osteogenesis imperfecta, osteoporosis due to prolonged steroid therapy, and osteochondrosis. Acrodynia is a rare disease characterized by swollen red hands and feet and accompanied by apathy, irritability, photophobia, excessive perspiration, and hypertension. It is caused by mercury intoxication. Periarticular conditions, such as tumors, synovitis, and bursitis, may produce joint manifestations. Gout (hyperuricemia) almost never occurs before puberty except under unusual circumstances, as in treated leukemia, the Lesch-Nyhan syndrome, or glycogen storage disease. Slipped femoral epiphysis must be considered when there is history of rapid growth or obesity. Pulmonary osteoarthropathy rarely is manifested by pain in the extremities. Benign postviral myositis with elevated CPK enzymes is now being recognized more frequently.

Solomon J. Cohen and Mohsen Ziai

11. Vomiting

Vomiting is one of the most common symptoms in children and may be the first symptom of any one of a number of common infections, such as pharyngitis, otitis media, pneumonia, or urinary tract infection, when it is usually associated with fever, or it may indicate one of many other diverse conditions. Vomiting is a key symptom in the early phases of Reye syndrome and presumably reflects increasing intracranial pressure. Vomiting is important clinically because its persistence may lead to severe metabolic derangements.

In very young and debilitated infants, vomiting presents the added hazard of aspiration because of their poor neuromuscular coordination. To prevent this, the infant must be positioned properly, either on one side or in the prone position, but not supine. The patient's age is of importance. For example, in the neonatal period, "spitting up" or regurgitation of small amounts of vomitus is usual and of little pathological significance; however, several congenital malformations that cause gastrointestinal obstruction become evident at this age. These conditions may be fatal unless treated early.

The character of vomiting may be informative. Projectile vomiting is usually associated with gastrointestinal obstruc-

506

tion or with increased intracranial pressure. The vomitus that contains unchanged food with no gastric juice is esophageal. Vomitus containing curds of milk, but no brown or green color, comes from the stomach. The newborn infant who vomits greenish material probably has intestinal obstruction below the ampulla of Vater. Bloody vomitus may be red or coffee-ground in character. In the immediate neonatal period it is often due to ingestion of maternal blood during delivery, which can be differentiated by the alkali denaturation test (Apt test). In older children bloody vomiting is usually caused by rupture of esophageal varices and by peptic ulcer — rarely, by diaphragmatic hernia. Fecal vomiting suggests peritonitis or intestinal obstruction. It is not possible to give a complete differential diagnosis of this extremely common problem. What follows summarizes some of the important considerations. The reader must consult larger references for more detailed discussions.

Etiologic Diagnosis of Vomiting

Neonatal Period and Infancy

Some spitting up is not unusual in this age group. The main problem is to distinguish the common regurgitation from the faulty feeding by an unexperienced mother, tensions and environmental factors, and certain serious causes. In the latter situation various warning signs may serve to alert the physician to perform certain investigations and institute appropriate therapy. These consist of irritability, drowsiness, fever or hypothermia, bilious vomiting, abdominal mass, peristaltic waves moving from right to left, failure to pass meconium, dehydration, abdominal distention, presence of neurological signs such as seizure activity, signs of increased intracranial pressure, abnormal bleeding, jaundice, failure to gain weight, or detectable abnormal odor. Some of these signs are suggestive of life-threatening situations, e.g., mechanical obstruction requiring surgical intervention; sepsis requiring specific investigations and antimicrobial therapy; intracranial bleeding or other forms of CNS pathology; metabolic inborn errors such as galactosemia, salt-loosing adrenal hyperplasia in an otherwise normal male, organic acidemia, urea cycle defects, and allergy or intolerance to certain foods; urinary tract anomalies with obstruction; and renal failure. Vomiting and food intolerance may also be a sign of cardiorespiratory problems such as cardiac failure. All environmental factors, toxic substances, and drugs to which the infant or the mother may have been exposed must be investigated.

Early Childhood and Adolescence

As the child becomes older, psychologic and emotional factors assume increasing importance along with infections, particularly those related to the gastrointestinal tract (e.g., appendicitis, infectious diarrhea, and hepatitis). Migraine can present with vomiting as do several other CNS problems (e.g., meningitis, encephalitis, and pyelonephritis), which must always be looked for in a febrile child. Severe pain as in torsion of the testis or ovary or renal colic may present with vomiting. With increasing incidence of intoxication and substance abuse, this possibility must always be kept in mind. Finally, it must be emphasized that missing the diagnosis of intestinal obstruction, appendicitis, or pelvic inflammatory disease in the sexually active adolescent female can have catastrophic consequences.

Ali Akbar Velayati and Mohsen Ziai

12. Abdominal Mass

Solid neoplastic lesions of the abdomen are relatively common in childhood, and their timely detection can be lifesaving. In the early stages, when there is still a reasonable chance for cure, subjective complaints are often lacking. Palpation of the abdomen must, therefore, be carried out on every occasion that a child is brought to the physician.

Once a solid abdominal mass has been discovered, it becomes the physician's responsibility to expedite definitive therapy (usually surgery). Injudicious palpation is potentially dangerous, as it may cause dissemination of tumor cells by the trauma of examination. In teaching hospitals it is especially important to keep this in mind. Several diagnostic procedures can be considered according to the patient's age and other clinical findings. These should include urinalysis, hemogram, skeletal survey, chest film, and intravenous pyelography. An ultrasound and x-ray investigations of the small and large intestines and examination of bone marrow may be desirable in some cases. These tests should be completed within 24 hours of admission, holidays not withstanding, and early surgical exploration carried out.

A solid mass that is not readily identifiable as an organ or part of an organ is likely to be either of renal origin or neuroblastoma.

The differential diagnosis of abdominal mass in the pediatric age group is summarized in Table A12-1.

Solomon J. Cohen

Table A12-1. Differential Diagnosis of Abdominal Mass

Etiological factors	Clinical findings	Investigations
Splenomegaly (discussed on p. 529)		
Hepatomegaly (discussed on p. 518)		
Renal malformations (multicystic and polycystic kidney disease)	Possible signs of renal disease; fever, pain, pyuria if kidney is infected	Urinalysis, urine culture, ultrasound
Hydronephrosis	Recurrent urinary tract infections, hypertension, and a smooth, movable mass in the flank	Urinalysis and urine culture; ultrasound, VCUG
Neoplastic tumors		
Neuroblastoma (sympathicoblastoma)	Occasional pain, fever, and anorexia; metastasis to orbit, skull, liver, or chest; can pass midline; calcification may occur within tumor; hematuria infrequent	Bone scan, bone marrow examination; urinary excretion of vanillylmandelic acid may be increased; IVP (caliceal outline not distorted; calcification frequent); bone metastasis common; surgical exploration
Wilms' tumor (embryonal adenosarcoma, nephroblastoma)	Possible hematuria and hypertension; hemihypertrophy and congenital malformations; does not pass midline	IVP (shows distortion of pelvis and calices; kidney is enlarged; calcifications are rare); lung metastases common; bone scan
Leukemia	Most often of the acute variety, with bleeding, pallor, lymphadenopathy, and splenomegaly	Examination of bone marrow and of peripheral blood
Lymphomas including Hodgkin's and lymphosarcoma	Unexplained fever; pressure symptoms or interference with normal physiology (e.g., causing malabsorption)	Examination of bone marrow; biopsy of the lesion; lymphangiography
Primary hepatomas	May be associated with hepatic cirrhosis, thalassemia, hepatitis B	Liver scan, biopsy, alpha-fetoprotein
Ovarian neoplasms	Functioning tumors produce signs of sexual precocity	Calcification and teeth in x-ray of the abdomen in teratomas; test for gonadotropins in the urine
Miscellaneous (tumors of adrenal glands, retroperitoneal sarcoma and teratoma, etc.)	Depends on type of tumor	Biopsy
Inflammatory		
Pyogenic abscess (appendiceal abscess most common)	Right lower quadrant mass; history of fever, vomiting, irritability, diarrhea, anorexia for 2 wk; mass is tender and palpable on rectal examination	WBC (leukocytosis); barium enema; exploratory laparotomy; gallium scan
Tuberculosis	Cold abscesses; ascites; multiple solid masses	Tuberculin test; bacteriological procedures
Amebic cyst	Usually in the liver; may rupture through the diaphragm, giving empyema	Demonstration of the organism; aspiration of characteristic "anchovy sauce" cyst fluid
Hydatid disease	Usually in the liver unless rupture of original cyst has occurred	Skin and serological tests
Cysts (dermoid, urachal, mesenteric, pancreatic, enteric, choledochal, vitelline duct cyst, etc.)	Depends on location	X-ray examination helpful in some cases and ultrasound

13. Abdominal Pain

Abdominal pain is a frequent ailment in childhood. In infants and preverbal children the complaint of abdominal pain must be deduced from the patient's appearance and behavior, and the physician should not necessarily accept the parent's interpretation.

Pain may arise from the abdominal wall or the structures within the abdominal cavity or be referred to the abdomen from adjacent parts of the body. A subjective element enters into any complaint of pain, and an appreciation of the emotional state of both patient and informant is always helpful. The primary classification of abdominal pain into (1) organic and (2) functional, or (a) medical and (b) surgical, is practical. Pain due to organic disease can usually be explained, whereas the cause of functional pain is often mysterious; the distinction between medical and surgical types of pain promptly leads to different courses of action.

Detailed analysis of the symptom of abdominal pain and examination of the abdomen alone rarely yield conclusive diagnostic evidence; it is important to inquire about associated symptoms and to perform a general physical examination. In the case of recurrent, intermittent, or periodic pain it is essential to obtain adequate information about the frequency of episodes, their duration, the site and character of the pain, and the presence of associated symptoms such as vomiting, headache, constipation, and anorexia, as well as factors that precipitate, exacerbate, or alleviate the pain.

Acute abdominal pain demands a detailed description of clinical events leading up to its onset, with careful recording of associated symptoms such as fever, headache, vomiting, constipation or diarrhea, or complaints referable to the respiratory or genitourinary tracts. Certain investigations may be needed to elucidate the cause of abdominal pain. These should include a urinalysis and white blood cell and differential count.

The important features of some of the more common causes of abdominal pain in childhood are listed below.

I. Acute abdominal pain
   A. Arising from the gastrointestinal tract
      1. Inflammatory lesions. These are usually accompanied by fever, vomiting, anorexia, and alteration in bowel habit. Pain is poorly localized and colicky in nature, but peritoneal involvement or abscess formation produces localized pain and tenderness.
         a. Acute appendicitis. This occurs at any age, but ordinarily at school age; onset is acute with fever, periumbilical colic, and vomiting. Pain later becomes constant and localized to the right lower quadrant. Local tenderness and guarding are found in this area.
            Diagnosis in very young children or in children with a retrocecal appendix is particularly difficult. Though rare in infancy, appendicitis should be considered whenever there is moderate fever, abdominal pain, distention, and localized abdominal tenderness. In the case of a retrocecal appendix, diarrhea or crampy pain may be the only abdominal symptom, and tenderness may be elicited only in the right flank, by deep pressure over the cecum, or by rectal examination. In many cases of appendicitis tachycardia and polymorphonuclear leukocytosis are present. The diagnosis of appendicitis is primarily clinical, but urinalysis and white cell count should always be done.
         b. Acute enteritis. May occur at any age, more commonly in infancy. Onset is acute, with fever, vomiting, diarrhea, and colicky pain. Stools are loose, watery, perhaps blood-stained, and smelly. Dehydration occurs rapidly. The abdomen may be distended, with diffuse tenderness and increased bowel sounds.
         c. Inflammatory bowel disease (Crohn's type). Rare in infancy and preschool age, and uncommon at school age. It may sometimes present with features similar to those of acute appendicitis but most often produces fever, weight loss, and intermittent crampy abdominal pain.
      2. Obstructive lesions of the intestine. The pain is colicky, except in newborn infants, in whom pain is usually not apparent, and is associated with abdominal distention and absolute constipation. Vomiting is prominent and is often bilious, occasionally fecal, depending on the site of obstruction. Bowel sounds may be initially increased but become diminished or absent when ileus supervenes. Plain x-ray films of the abdomen, showing dilated, gas-filled loops of bowel with fluid levels, are the most useful investigation.
         a. Newborn period. Obstruction may be

caused by a variety of lesions such as atresia or duplication of the bowel, annular pancreas, meconium ileus, necrotizing enterocolitis (NEC), or Hirschsprung's disease.
  b. Infancy
    (1) Intussusception. Common during the first year, intussusception is coincidental with the introduction of solids in diet. Colicky, spasmodic abdominal pain, vomiting, constipation, and passage of blood-stained mucus ("currant-jelly stool") are characteristic. Abdominal mass is palpable in many cases; rectal examination may reveal the tip of the intussusception. Contrast enema is most useful in diagnosis and may cure the condition in its early phases.
    (2) Incarcerated or strangulated hernia. Symptoms and signs of intestinal obstruction are present. Palpable inguinal hernia is present in the majority of cases.
    (3) Volvulus with malrotation of gut. Signs of intestinal obstruction with abdominal distention are prominent. Plain abdominal x-ray film identifies distended loop or gut and may confirm malrotation.
    (4) Foreign bodies, undigested food, and masses of ascarides are occasional causes.
  c. Childhood. Intussusception is usually secondary to primary lesions (e.g., polyp, lymphadenitis, hemorrhagic lesion of anaphylactoid purpura). Obstruction due to hernia also occurs. Obstruction is occasionally due to adhesions from previous abdominal operations and may be the presenting manifestation of inflammatory bowel disease or neoplasms of the gastrointestinal tract. At all ages intestinal obstruction (paralytic ileus) may complicate peritonitis, perforation of the gut, gangrene of the gut, severe dehydration with hypokalemia, and intoxication with ganglion-blocking drugs.
B. Arising from the liver and biliary system
  1. Inflammatory lesions
    a. Acute hepatitis. Fever, vomiting, and anorexia with tenderness over the liver are usually evident. Pain may precede jaundice, bili-

rubinuria, and pale stools. During the preicteric phase of the disease, leukopenia is the rule.
    b. Acute cholecystitis. Rare in childhood; affects school-age children; sometimes preceded by history of vague abdominal pains, anorexia, and vomiting.
  2. Obstructive lesions. Biliary stone is uncommon except in children with chronic hemolytic anemia. Choledochal cyst is a rare cause of biliary colic.
C. Arising from the urinary tract
  1. Inflammatory lesions
    a. Acute pyelonephritis. Sometimes presents with fever, flank pain, or diffuse abdominal pain. Urinalysis shows pyuria, bacilluria, and occasionally hematuria.
    b. Acute cystourethritis. Pain is suprapubic, associated with frequency of micturition and dysuria. Urinalysis shows pyuria, bacilluria, and sometimes hematuria.
  2. Obstructive uropathy
    a. Ureteric calculus. Typical ureteric colic is present; renal stones may be silent or produce vague flank pain, while vesical calculi give rise to vague suprapubic pain or dysuria.
    b. Hydronephrosis, hydroureter. Acute dilatation of the pelvis of the kidney may cause acute abdominal pain without infection, but usually pain is due to infection of the urinary tract complicating a preexisting anomaly. Urinalysis and radiographic examination of the urinary tract are valuable investigations.
D. Arising from the genital tract
  1. In females. Pelvic inflammatory disease may occur in adolescent girls, usually due to gonococcal infection. Also gonococcal perihepatitis (Fitz-Hugh Curtis syndrome) can present as acute abdominal pain. Ovarian pain due to torsion or neoplasm may be acute.
  2. In males. Torsion of the testis gives acute pain, which may be referred to the abdomen in the case of scrotal or inguinal testes; the pain is truly intraabdominal if the testes are undescended.
E. Arising from the pancreas
  Acute pancreatitis is rare; pain is often referred to the back. Estimation of serum amylase is a useful diagnostic test.
F. Arising from vascular lesions

1. Allergic vascultis (anaphylactoid purpura)
2. Mesenteric thrombosis
3. "Sickle-cell" crisis

G. Acute abdominal pain for which the mechanism is uncertain

1. Mesenteric adenitis. May mimic acute appendicitis, but there is usually evidence of pharyngitis or tonsillitis. Laparotomy reveals questionably enlarged and inflamed mesenteric glands.
2. Measles. Acute abdominal pain is common during the prodromal and exanthematous stage of measles. Occasionally true acute appendicitis occurs with typical signs during measles.
3. Diabetes mellitus. In diabetic precoma acute abdominal pain is sometimes a major manifestation; considerable leukocytosis accompanies the syndrome. Urinalysis reveals glycosuria and acetonuria; blood glucose concentration is elevated.
4. Acute rheumatic fever. Acute abdominal pain is occasionally prominent at onset of this disease. Other manifestations of the disease are usually present together with history of preceding streptococcal infection.
5. Acute porphyria. This is not usually manifest in childhood.

H. Extraabdominal causes of acute abdominal pain

1. Arising from the thorax
   a. Acute pneumonia. Lobar pneumonia, especially of the lower lobes, may be complicated by abdominal pain.
   b. Epidemic myalgia (coxsackievirus infection; pleurodynia).
   c. Diaphragmatic pleurisy.
2. Arising from the spine and spinal cord. Pain referred along the spinal nerves may be referred to the abdomen from irritative lesions of spinal nerve roots in herpes zoster, osteomyelitis of the spine, intraspinal and extraspinal neoplasm, epidural abscess, and myelitis.
3. Arising from muscles, tendons, and joints adjacent to the abdomen.

II. Subacute abdominal pain

Pain may be of considerable severity but is usually insufficient in degree to merit designation as an instance of "acute abdomen."

A. Arising from the gastrointestinal tract

Intestinal colic is caused presumably by spasm of the intestinal musculature:

1. Infantile colic (see Chap. 12).
2. Lead intoxication. In this condition colicky pain may be associated with constipation, anorexia, and irritability. There is a history of pica. Investigations show anemia, basophilic stippling of erythrocytes, coproporphyrinuria, radiological evidence of lines of increased density at the ends of the long bones, and radiopaque material in gut (if recent ingestion), with increased concentrations of lead in blood and urine.
3. Peptic ulceration. Acute ulcers in infancy are usually painless. Chronic duodenal ulcer is found most often in boys of school age. Family history of peptic ulcer is common. Upper abdominal pain is the main complaint, and epigastric tenderness is expected. X-ray examination of the upper gastronintestinal tract and endoscopy are the most useful diagnostic procedures. Infection with *Campylobacter pylori* may be associated.
4. Intestinal parasites. Vaguely localized intestinal colic may be symptomatic of infestation with roundworms, hookworms, and tapeworms. Fresh stools should be examined for evidence of parasites.
5. Food intolerance. Abdominal pain perhaps due to disorders of gut motility is generally ascribed to food intolerance; and acute abdominal pain is a side effect of many medications.
6. Incomplete intestinal obstruction. Pain is prominent and episodic; vomiting often occurs; constipation is not absolute, and abdominal distention is variable. The causes are numerous:
   a. Congenital malformations of the gastrointestinal tract.
   b. Postoperative adhesions.
   c. Inflammatory processes, such as regional enteritis.
   d. Neoplasms of gastrointestinal tract are rare in children, but sarcoma or lymphoma may be seen.
7. Pain of presumed psychogenic origin. It is usually periumbilical but may also be in the lower quadrants. It is common at school age and may be a manifestation of school phobia. The colon may be palpable and tender. Constipation, vomiting, and headache may be associated.

History of "stress" between patient and environment (home or school) can usually be elicited. Family history of emotional disorders and characteristic personality patterns are discernible.

B. Arising from the liver and biliary system

The lesions mentioned under acute pain (p. 508) may often present with pain of moderate severity and should be investigated in the same way.

C. Arising from the urinary tract

In addition to the conditions previously mentioned under acute pain, there are

1. Acute glomerulonephritis. Hematuria, edema, and hypertension are found; flank pain is not uncommon; urine shows hematuria, proteinuria, and casts. Urine output is diminished, and some azotemia is present.

2. Acute pyelonephritis. Pain is usually in the flanks. Pyuria and bacilluria are found.

D. Peritoneal inflammation

1. Primary peritonitis. Rarely, this may complicate septicemia or states of reduced resistance (e.g., nephrotic syndrome).

2. Secondary peritonitis. This is a sequel of inflammatory lesions of the gastrointestinal tract such as appendicitis or perforation of alimentary tract due to infection, ulceration, or trauma.

Patient rapidly becomes "toxic," and abdominal distention, paralytic ileus, and dimished bowel sounds develop. If patient is receiving corticosteroids, pain may be less prominent.

III. Recurrent or intermittent abdominal pain

This common cause of referral to the pediatrician often challenges clinical judgment and diagnostic acumen. In the majority of cases no organic disease is found. Certain well-defined clinical entities exist, and if these are recognized, the patient may be saved expensive and uncomfortable investigations or surgical procedures.

A. "Periodic syndrome"

Recurrent abdominal pain may occur in attacks in combination with vomiting, headache, pallor, and anorexia. The attacks have a definite periodicity and may be accompanied by fever. If they are severe, the patient may be pale, look as if he were in a toxic condition, and be dehydrated. Ketonuria is present if the vomiting is intractable. The attacks last for a day or two and then pass away. Affected children are often nervous, and the attacks appear to be precipitated by emotional stress, but allergy may well be implicated as an alternative explanation. If headache is prominent, migraine may be diagnosed. In people from the Middle East, particularly in Ashkenazi Jews but also in other ethnic groups, familial Mediterranean fever often manifests itself as periodic fever and abdominal pain.

B. "Attention-seeking" pain of preschool children

The complaint of pain is unaccompanied by objective signs of abdominal distress, fever, diarrhea, or vomiting. Characteristically the pain is localized by the child to the periumbilical region or umbilicus, is of brief duration, and often occurs at mealtimes. A history of food refusal rather than true anorexia is common, and the parents may admit to having forced food. Abnormal physical signs are absent, and the child is usually healthy in appearance and development.

C. Recurrent abdominal pain of school children

In this age group a great variety of abdominal pains are encountered. Generally, if the pain is of short duration, poorly localized, or localized to the center of the abdomen and is not associated with disturbance of general health, bowel function, or appetite, a functional cause is reasonably suspected. If careful and complete physical examination yields no abnormal physical signs, and urinalysis is repeatedly normal, the question of psychogenic pain due to emotional problems at home or school should be explored. Other investigations such as complete blood count, plain abdominal roentgenogram, and erythrocyte sedimentation rate are warranted, but more extensive investigations should not be done without proper indications. Abdominal pain associated with bowel dysfunction, generalized abdominal tenderness, and a palpable colon may be attributed to "irritable bowel syndrome."

D. Recurrent abdominal pain in adolescent girls

In adolescence, ovarian pain and dysmenorrhea are commonly related to emotional problems and tension. A comprehensive history, with evaluation of the patient's total physical, emotional, and environmental status, is usually more valuable than laboratory investigations or surgical procedures. Gynecological cause may sometimes be suspected because of unequivocal physical abnormalities.

When ovulation is established, "mittelschmerz" with pain and tenderness in the lower quadrants due to rupture of the ovarian follicle with hemorrhage may also be seen in older adolescent girls midway between menstrual periods.

Thomas E. Oppé

---

14. Jaundice

Normally, the concentration of bilirubin in the vascular and extravascular tissues of the body (except for the gallbladder) is not sufficient to be recognized visibly. Yet there is a brisk daily turnover of endogenously formed bilirubin, 6 to 8 mg/kg during neonatal life and 3 to 4 mg/kg thereafter. About 80% of the daily formation of bilirubin is derived from catabolism of the hemoglobin in senescent erythrocytes by the reticuloendothelial system. This fraction of daily bilirubin production is derived from the porphyrin ring of hemoglobin and is cleared from the circulation by the liver. Serum bilirubin concentrations normally remain below 1.2 mg/100 ml; however, a number of conditions in infancy and childhood interfere with the normal balance in bilirubin metabolism between formation and hepatic clearance and lead to its accumulation in the circulating plasma. When the binding capacity of plasma albumin for bilirubin approaches saturation, significant amounts of bilirubin diffuse into and accumulate within extravascular tissue spaces, including subcutaneous tissue, resulting in visible jaundice.

Clinically, one recognizes jaundice or icterus by the yellow hue of the skin and sclerae. This visual correlation becomes increasingly evident as the serum bilirubin rises and roughly correlates with the serum concentration of bilirubin. Other organic anions (such as fatty acids and some drugs), which also bind to albumin, can compete with bilirubin for its albumin-binding sites. This competition results in more protein-free bilirubin in the plasma water. The free bilirubin diffuses into extravascular tissue and, in some neonates, causes damage to the central nervous system. This condition is known in its acute form as kernicterus and in more subtle forms as bilirubin encephalopathy. Thus, the amount of bilirubin in the extravascular space is multifactorial in its determinants, only one of which is the serum concentration of bilirubin.

The differential diagnosis of clinical jaundice is most sensibly approached by consideration of its two fundamental causes, overproduction and undersecretion.

Overproduction of bilirubin is primarily a consequence of excessive hemoglobin catabolism:

$$\text{Protoheme} \xrightarrow[\text{microsomal heme oxygenase}]{\text{NADPH}} \text{Biliverdin IX}\alpha + \text{Fe} + \text{CO}$$

$$\text{Biliverdin IX}\alpha \xrightarrow[\text{biliverdin reductase}]{\text{NADPH}} \text{Bilirubin IX}\alpha$$

The tetrapyrrole moiety from 1 g of hemoglobin is normally catabolized by miscrosomal heme oxygenase to yield 36 mg of bilirubin. When hemolysis is present, the formation of bilirubin from hemoglobin can exceed the excretory capacity of the liver, resulting in "retention" jaundice, which is manifest by the accumulation of nonconjugated bilirubin in the circulating plasma.

Undersecretion of bilirubin can occur from either a failure of uptake of bilirubin from the sinusoidal circulation or impairment of enzymatic conjugation of bilirubin to its more polar derivative, primarily bilirubin diglucuronide, and impaired secretion of conjugated bilirubin into the biliary tree, thus permitting regurgitation of conjugated bilirubin into the plasma. The regurgitation of bilirubin from the liver after its conjugation is reflected by an elevation of the concentration of the "direct"-reacting fraction of the total bilirubin in the serum.

In many clinical situations associated with jaundice, the hyperbilirubinemia is a consequence of both overproduction and impairment of hepatic secretion of bilirubin.

The total concentration of serum bilirubin consists of the conjugated ("direct"-reacting, as measured by van de Bergh's test) and unconjugated ("indirect") fractions. Either fraction may predominate when the total serum bilirubin is elevated. These measurements are helpful in determining the underlying cause of the jaundice in individual patients. For example, the jaundice associated with hemolytic disease is associated with "indirect" hyperbilirubinemia of the plasma, while in hepatitis the direct-reacting fraction of the serum bilirubin is significantly elevated. Conjugated bilirubin, which is more water-soluble, can be filtered across the glomerulus and is, therefore, associated with bilirubinuria.

The jaundice of early infancy creates one of the greatest problems in differential diagnosis, because all infants have some degree of hyperbilirubinemia during the first week of life, and it is of sufficient magnitude to produce visible jaundice in one-third of neonates. In full-term infants, a serum bilirubin in excess of 7 mg/100 ml is associated with visible jaundice. In premature infants, the paucity of subcutaneous fat allows greater visibility of the red hue of the underlying capillary bed and obscures the yellow coloration of the skin due to jaundice. Blanching of the skin by light pressure allows visibility and recognition of jaundice in such infants.

The many causes of hyperbilirubinemia due to underlying pathological disorders during neonatal life are itemized in

Table A14-1. The presence of neonatal jaundice is a potentially valuable clinical sign of a number of illnesses and should not be casually dismissed as physiological. Jaundice should be considered abnormal in the neonatal period until proved otherwise if (1) it appears before 36 hours of life, (2) it persists beyond 10 days of age, or (3) the serum bilirubin concentration exceeds 12 mg/100 ml.

Overproduction of Bilirubin

Fetal-Maternal Blood Group Incompatibilities

This is the most common cause of early intense jaundice and results when, during pregnancy, there is leakage of erythrocytes from fetal to maternal circulation. If the fetal erythrocytes are of a different antigenic type, particularly with reference to Rh and ABO blood group antigens, the maternal reticuloendothelial system forms antibodies (IgG immunoglobulins) against them (maternal sensitization). These antibodies can cross the placental barrier into the fetal circulation, where they are bound to fetal erythrocytes. Such Rh antibody–coated erythrocytes undergo sequestration and rapid destruction within the fetal reticuloendothelial system. Infants affected by Rh antibody sensitization develop pallor from anemia, a rapidly appearing jaundice, and hepatosplenomegaly. If the anemia is severe, generalized edema (fetal

Table A14-1. Causes of Neonatal Hyperbilirubinemia

A. Overproduction of bilirubin
1. Fetal-maternal blood group incompatibilities resulting in isoimmunization
2. Extravasation of blood into body tissue spaces
3. Polycythemia
4. Hemoglobinopathies, erythrocyte membrane and enzyme defects
5. Induction of labor
6. Increased enterohepatic circulation of bilirubin
B. Undersecretion of bilirubin
1. Inborn errors of metabolism
2. Hormones and drugs
3. Prematurity
4. Hepatic hypoperfusion
5. Obstruction of the biliary tree
6. Cholestatic syndromes
C. Combinations of overproduction and undersecretion
1. Bacterial sepsis
2. Intrauterine infections
3. Congenital cirrhosis

hydrops) may be evident at birth. Laboratory findings include normoblastemia and reticulocytosis in the peripheral blood smear, hemoglobin concentrations at birth as low as 2 g/100 ml, rapidly rising serum bilirubin concentration, and, characteristically, a positive direct Coombs' test of the circulating erythrocytes. ABO incompatibility is usually milder in presentation. Hydrops is rare, and anemia is less frequent. The hemolysis is intravascular and complement-mediated. More often, such infants become clinically manifest as babies whose serum bilirubin exceeds 12 mg/100 ml on day 3 of life, and hepatomegaly is frequent. Their cord blood samples may exhibit a positive direct Coombs' test and microspherocytosis of their erythrocytes. A reticulocytosis greater than 10% may be present at 48 hours. In more severe instances, hemoglobinuria may be present. In ABO incompatibility, fetal disease may occur in the first pregnancy, in contrast to Rh disease, which usually spares the first-born.

Extravasation of Blood

Erythrocytes outside the capillary bed (e.g., cephalohematomas or ecchymoses) undergo accelerated destruction with conversion of the hemoglobin to bilirubin by tissue macrophages. Jaundice associated with formation of bilirubin from such sources can be significant but does not occur within the first 2 days of life. Diagnosis is usually made on physical examination, though occult bleeding (e.g., intracranial, intestinal, or pulmonary hemorrhage) has similar effects. Swallowed blood can also be responsible for hyperbilirubinemia, because the microsomal heme oxygenase in intestinal epithelium can metabolize hemoglobin to bilirubin, which is transferred to the portal circulation rather than excreted directly into the intestinal lumen.

Polycythemia

The hyperbilirubinemia often associated with polycythemia becomes manifest after 48 hours of life and is characterized by abnormally elevated hematocrits (above 65% by venipuncture). Presumably, the normal rate of destruction of red cells results in increased bilirubin production because of the absolute increase in the red cell mass. Polycythemia may result during placental separation when bleeding occurs from the maternal circulation into the fetus (maternal-fetal transfusion). In the case of twin births, polycythemia may result from fetal-fetal transfusion. The polycythemic twin is plethoric, while the other twin is pale and anemic. Often they are discordant in size.

Hemoglobinopathies, Erythrocyte Membrane and Enzyme Defects

Hereditary spherocytosis usually goes unrecognized during the neonatal period, but hemolytic crises do occur and are associated with elevations in the serum bilirubin level and a decreasing hematocrit. In these cases the peripheral blood smear reveals the characteristic abnormal red cell morphology. A family history of spherocytosis or gallstone disease in early life (under 40 years of age) in related individuals may be the only means of distinguishing familial spherocytosis from ABO hemolytic disease if the infant and mother happen to have different ABO blood types and the cord blood is not available for a Coombs' test for the presence of antibody-coated cells.

Nonspherocytic hemolytic anemias include drug-induced hemolysis, erythrocyte enzyme deficiencies (glucose 6-phosphate dehydrogenase [G-6-PD] deficiency, pyruvate kinase deficiency, and others), alphathalassemias, and vitamin K and bacterially induced hemolysis. The clinical manifestations of anemia and hyperbilirubinemia can range in severity from intrauterine death with hydrops fetalis (alpha-thalassemia) to mildly exaggerated neonatal hyperbilirubinemia (some variants of G-6-PD deficiency) to insignificant hyperbilirubinemia and no anemia. It is important to remember that drugs or other substances responsible for hemolysis may be transferred to the fetus or infant transplacentally or via breast milk.

Induction of Labor

Induction of labor by means of oxytocin in term pregnancies is often associated with pathological hyperbilirubinemia. Infusion of 5% glucose to the mother is rapidly metabolized and may represent a hypotonic infusion of fluid to the mother and her fetus that results in hypotonicity of the fetal and neonatal circulation. The erythrocytes swell in response to the osmotic gradient, resulting in increased osmotic fragility. Accelerated sequestration of these spherocytic erythrocytes by the reticuloendothelial system increases bilirubin production.

Increased Enterohepatic Circulation of Bilirubin

During fetal life and at birth, the intestinal tract is sterile. Bile pigment is, therefore, excreted in the stool as bilirubin rather than urobilin, the product normally formed by bacterial reduction of bilirubin. Furthermore, the fetus and neonate do have demonstrable beta-glucuronidase within the intestinal lumen; this may hydrolyze bilirubin glucuronides, which are secreted by the liver into the intestine. The nonconjugated bilirubin resulting from the glucuronidase activity can be absorbed from the gut. Several clinical diseases or conditions that are characterized by delayed evacuation of meconium or stool are associated with hyperbilirubinemia during neonatal life. The delay allows for greater absorption of bilirubin from the gut. In contrast to upper bowel obstructions (e.g., duodenal atresia, tracheoesophageal fistulas, and annular pancreas) that can be anticipated at birth because of polyhydramnios and copious and bile-stained gastric aspirates or vomitus in the first 24 hours of life, obstruction of the distal small bowel or colon (e.g., Hirschsprung's disease, meconium ileus, meconium plug syndrome) is often heralded by abdominal distention, failure to pass meconium in the first 24 hours of life, and hyperbilirubinemia. The increased incidence of hyperbilirubinemia associated with fasting involves more than just delayed passage of meconium stools. Decreased bile flow, substrate depletion for conjugation of bilirubin, and increased enterohepatic circulation all contribute to this hyperbilirubinemia.

Undersecretion of Bilirubin

In a number of conditions, bilirubin is presented to the liver normally; however, a subsequent step in its metabolism prevents normal secretion, resulting in pathological jaundice.

Inborn Errors of Metabolism

Following its uptake by the hepatocyte, bilirubin is enzymatically converted to bilirubin diglucuronide according to the following reactions:

(1) Uridine diphosphate glucose + NAD →
    Uridine diphosphate glucuronic acid + NADH + H^+
(2) Uridine diphosphate glucuronic acid + bilirubin →
    Bilirubin monoglucuronide + uridine diphosphate
(3) Uridine diphosphate glucuronic acid
    + bilirubin monoglucuronide →
        Bilirubin diglucuronide + uridine diphosphate

The soluble enzyme uridine diphosphate glucose dehydrogenase, which catalyzes step 1 above, has reduced activity in neonatal liver and has been implicated in physiological jaundice. No other clincial disturbance has been reported associated with this enzyme. Steps 2 and 3 are catalyzed by uridine diphosphate glucuronosyl transferase (UDPGT). Complete absence of UDPGT activity for bilirubin is seen in the rare genetic disturbance known as the Crigler-Najjar syndrome, type I. Affected infants develop intense persistent jaundice in the first few days of life. Their lifelong jaundice has been treated with phototherapy and experimental blockage of the enterohepatic circulation. A less severe deficiency of the glucuronyl transferase sometimes referred to as type II can be treated by phenobarbital, which causes enhanced excretion of conjugated bilirubin in the bile and serves to distinguish these two types of hereditary jaundice. The inheritance of the two types also differs. Type I is autosomal recessive, while type II is autosomal dominant. Gilbert's syndrome, another autosomal dominant disorder involving impaired conjugation of bilirubin, has been estimated to occur in 2 to 6% of the population. The role this disorder may play in neonatal jaundice has not been established. Dubin-Johnson syndrome and Rotor's syndrome are rarely recognized during neonatal life. Both disorders are characterized by elevations of conjugated bilirubin and are of autosomal recessive inheritance. Dubin-Johnson syndrome is characterized by a deficiency in canalicular secretion of conjugated bilirubin and other anions. Rotor's syndrome is associated with a defect in hepatic storage of anions. Both defects result in the regurgitation of conjugated bilirubin into the circulation.

Patients with galactosemia, an autosomal recessive disorder, usually will exhibit exaggerated jaundice on day 3 and thereafter, once lactose is included in the diet. Lack of galactose 1-phosphate uridyl transferase in these patients leads to accumulations of galactose 1-phosphate. This substance is believed to be hepatotoxic and in the first week of life is associated with nonconjugated hyperbilirubinemia. Affected infants show a reducing substance (galactose) in their urine, other than glucose, if their diet contains lactose. Definitive diagnosis rests on the demonstration of the enzyme deficiency in erythrocytes. Infants with galactosemia often develop bacterial sepsis during neonatal life.

Tyrosinosis and hypermethioninemia are two disorders of amino acid metabolism that, like galactosemia, are better known for the associated hepatic injury that occurs after neonatal life, when the liver disease is manifest by jaundice characterized by the presence of both unconjugated and conjugated hyperbilirubinemia. In neonatal life, jaundice is predominantly nonconjugated. These disorders are diagnosed by appropriate urine and serum amino acid analyses. Some of the tyrosinemias are relieved by appropriate dietary restriction. The large urinary excretion of methionine in hypermethioninemia is associated with the odor of cabbage and prompts the eponym "New England boiled dinner."

Alpha$_1$-antitrypsin (A$_1$AT) is a glycoprotein, synthesized only in the liver, that inhibits elastase and numerous other enzymes. Genetic deficiency of A$_1$AT rarely is recognized during the first week of life. More usual is a presentation

with conjugated hyperbilirubinemia at 6 weeks of age, although most patients do not show signs of this deficiency until they develop cirrhosis or pulmonary emphysema in early adulthood. Various phenotypes are recognized by the serum protein electrophoretic pattern. Protease inhibitor (Pi) MM is the most common phenotype, occurring in 80 to 95% of the population, and is associated with normal serum levels of A$_1$AT. Pi ZZ patients have the lowest A$_1$AT levels (15% of normal) and the highest incidence of liver disease in infancy. MZ, SZ, and MS have intermediate levels of A$_1$AT, and rare case reports of liver disease in infancy exist. Diagnosis is made by demonstrating a low A$_1$AT level in serum, compatible phenotype, and characteristic liver histology showing PAS-positive diastase-resistant globules within the hepatocytes.

Hormones and Drugs

The unconjugated hyperbilirubinemia of hypothyroidism may exceed 17 mg/100 ml and is persistent. Jaundice may precede the other manifestations of hypothyroidism. The basis for the jaundice is not entirely understood, but animal studies have shown the need for thyroxine for hepatic clearance of bilirubin. The definitive diagnosis can be made by demonstrating low T$_4$ and elevated thyroid-stimulating hormone (TSH) levels in the affected infant's serum. Hypopituitarism and anencephaly also manifest pathological jaundice because of low circulating levels of thyroxine; however, here TSH levels are low and inadequately stimulate the thyroid gland to synthesize thyroxine.

The jaundice associated with infants of diabetic mothers is probably multifactorial in origin. Prematurity may be a factor. If hypoglycemia is present, substrate deficiency for glucuronidation may result. Poor hepatic perfusion may be caused by circulatory insufficiency (due to respiratory distress syndrome, persistent fetal circulation, or cardiomyopathy). Polycythemia and increased enterohepatic circulation of bilirubin (secondary to delayed evacuation of meconium) may also be contributory factors.

Reports exist of one or more siblings from the same parents who experienced profound neonatal hyperbilirubinemia associated with the in vitro inhibition of UDPGT by both maternal and infant serum. The substrate used for this in vitro assay, in what has come to be known as the Lucey-Driscoll syndrome, was o-aminophenol. It is assumed that similar inhibition of bilirubin glucuronidation took place and was related to gestational hormones.

Some drugs depend on the same uptake and conjugation sites as bilirubin for hepatic clearance. Novobiocin usage has been associated with greater incidence and severity of neonatal hyperbilirubinemia and is believed to interfere with hepatic clearance of bilirubin. It would seem prudent to avoid all such drugs both in neonatal life and at the time of delivery in mothers.

There is an increased incidence of neonatal jaundice in breast-fed, as compared with formula-fed, infants. Characteristically, a nonconjugated hyperbilirubinemia begins once the milk "comes in" after the third day and persists beyond discharge from the hospital. Recent data shows infants that are breast-fed have higher levels of bilirubin during neonatal life and it is of greater duration. In some breast-fed infants the neonatal jaundice occurs in the first 3 days of life. This occurs when there is delay in the production of breast milk and no nutritional supplementation is given the infant. The jaundice becomes severe during the neonatal hospital stay and is accompanied by an 8 to 10% weight loss. Hyperbilirubinemia in the infant promptly resolves with adequate caloric and fluid intake. The more profound and protracted neonatal hyperbilirubinemia associated with breast feeding is associated with high concentrations of β-glucuronidase in the maternal milk. The ingested enzyme enhances the enterohepatic circulation of bilirubin in the infant. Currently, the diagnosis of breast-feeding jaundice involves either reduction or substitution of breast feeding by formula and a subsequent decline of serum bilirubin within 48 hours. In some centers, the breast milk can be assayed for its inhibitory activity. Reinstitution of breast feeding is unlikely to cause a rise in serum bilirubin, although mild hyperbilirubinemia may last for weeks. Acute kernicterus has not been described in this variety of prolonged hyperbilirubinemia, but whether more subtle forms of bilirubin encephalopathy occur is unknown.

Prematurity

Hyperbilirubinemia is seen frequently in premature infants and usually occurs after the third day of life when serum concentrations exceed 12 mg/100 ml. Bromsulphalein (BSP) clearance data indicate deficiencies for both uptake and secretion of bilirubin. Conjugation is also probably impaired both because of inadequate glycogen stores to supply UDPGA as substrate and because of reduced UDPGT. Bilirubin clearance improves rapidly with extra-uterine life and is independent of gestational age or birth weight.

Hepatic Hypoperfusion

Inadequate perfusion of the hepatic sinusoids can often produce serum bilirubin levels greater than 12 mg/100 ml on or after the third day of life. This may result from portal vein thrombosis, congestive heart failure, or patency of the ductus venosus as seen in respiratory distress syndrome. Blood in the portal circulation can bypass the hepatic sinusoids via a patent ductus venosus. Surprisingly, cyanotic heart disease is rarely associated with serum bilirubins greater than 12 mg/100 ml, indicating that hypoxia per se seems to have little role in the pathogenesis of neonatal hyperbilirubinemia.

Obstructive Jaundice

The diseases that produce obstruction within the liver or biliary tree generally do not become manifest until 4 to 6 weeks of age. During intrauterine life, bile pigment must reach the fetal intestines in some manner because there are no reports of infants whose meconium was not normally bile-pigmented. Obstructive jaundice usually presents with a history of progressively pale stools and darkening of the urine from bilirubinuria. The serum bilirubin consists of both unconjugated and conjugated bilirubin. The latter reflects the regurgitation of bilirubin that has been metabolized in the liver but not excreted. During neonatal life, any infant who develops conjugated bilirubinemia in excess of 1.5 mg/100 ml should be considered to have liver or biliary tract disease.

The usual posthepatic extrahepatic biliary atresia and the syndromatic intrahepatic atresias of Alagille are not encountered during the first week of life unless the pulmonary stenosis in the latter produces cardiopulmonary symptoms. Patients with the trisomy 18 syndrome have severe hypoplasia of the extrahepatic tree; conjugated hyperbilirubinemia may develop in them if they survive.

The cause of biliary atresia is unknown. Pathological examination suggests that many cases result from sclerosing inflammation of the ductular tissues, which may begin in fetal or neonatal life. It has been proposed that biliary atresia and idiopathic neonatal hepatitis have the same cause. Extensive hepatocellular injury can so reduce bile flow that bile ducts may be narrowed and considered atretic. A recently developed mouse model for biliary atresia has been produced by rheo-3 virus infection of sucklings and has been helpful in working out the relationship between biliary atresia and neonatal hepatitis.

Choledochal cyst may present in the late neonatal period with the classic triad of jaundice, pain, and abdominal mass. The mass may be difficult to distinguish form the liver, although transillumination of this cystic dilatation of the common bile duct may be demonstrable. Ultrasound, computed tomography, and percutaneous transhepatic cholangiography can be useful in establishing the diagnosis. Laparotomy with excision and revision of the ducts can successfully remove the obstruction. Choledochal cyst can be considered one of the diseases of connective tissue whose predominant pathology involves the hepatobiliary system. The other diseases in this spectrum include congenital hepatic fibrosis and Caroli's disease (cystic dilatation of the intrahepatic biliary tree). These diseases usually do not present in the neonatal period.

Although it is unusual, obstructive jaundice can develop in patients with cystic fibrosis as early as the second week of life. They may have a history of delayed passage of meconium. They have thick, tenacious bile, which is felt to cause obstruction. Needle biopsy shows characteristic eosinophilic plugs in the portal bile ducts. Fibrosis and cirrhosis are generally not encountered this early in life. Elevation of the sweat chloride concentration is diagnostic unless the infant is edematous, in which case the chloride concentration can be normal.

Extrahepatic compression of the biliary tract by any intra-abdominal mass or fibrous band from fetal peritonitis can lead to conjugated hyperbilirubinemia. Diagnostic workup is similar to that for a choledochal cyst, though laparotomy may be necessary to confirm this diagnosis ultimately.

Cholestatic Syndromes

Most of the familial cholestatic syndromes do not present during the first week of life as abnormal conjugated hyperbilirubinemias, but they may do so shortly thereafter. Byler's disease is progressive, and elevated serum bile acids are seen. In one familial disorder of bile acid metabolism, coprostanic acid, a C_{27} rather than C_{24} bile acid, is secreted. This bile acid is normally found only in alligators. Both of these disorders exhibit progressive hepatic insufficiency and lead to early death.

One well-documented example of cholestasis is that associated with phototherapy, the bronze baby syndrome. Patients receiving phototherapy develop bronze-colored skin and associated elevations of serum bile acids and conjugated bilirubin. The disorder clears when phototherapy is

Table A14-2. Simple Diagnostic Procedures in the Preliminary Identification of the Cause of Neonatal Jaundice

Type of jaundice	Test	Information provided
Jaundice before 36 hr	Hematocrit	Anemia or polycythemia
	Blood typing and Coombs' testing of infant and maternal blood	Isoimmunization
	Peripheral blood smear and reticulocyte count	Hemolysis, abnormally shaped red cells, thrombocytopenia, leukopenia
Jaundice associated with serum bilirubin > 12 mg/100 ml	Hematocrit, blood typing, Coombs' testing, peripheral blood smear, and reticulocyte count	Hemolytic disease
	Urine for bacterial culture, abnormal cells, and reducing substance	Sepsis CMV Galactosemia
	Measurement of conjugated bilirubin	Hepatic disease
	Review of medications to mother and infant	Hemolysis, delayed hepatic clearance
	Review of dietary intake, weight gain, and stooling pattern	Fasting or starvation, intestinal obstruction, increased enterohepatic circulation
	Family history of jaundice	Gilbert's syndrome
Persistent jaundice beyond 10 days	Urine analysis for bacterial culture, reducing substance, amino acids, bile pigments	Late sepsis Galactosemia Tyrosinemia Hepatic disease

stopped. No known permanent sequelae have been reported, although one infant expired with the disorder.

Cholestasis associated with parenteral alimentation is also well recognized in neonatal life. It usually requires 2 or more weeks of parenteral alimentation before the concentrations of conjugated bilirubin and bile acids become elevated in serum. The amino acids in the parenteral fluids may be what is responsible for the cholestasis. It generally resolves when hyperalimentation is stopped.

Combinations of Overproduction and Undersecretion

A number of diseases that occur during neonatal life are associated with jaundice due to both accelerated formation of bilirubin and impairment of its hepatic clearance. The conjugated bilirubin exceeds 1.5 mg/100 ml in these situations.

Bacterial sepsis causes hemolysis on account of the hemolysins released by bacteria. The endotoxins released during gram-negative bacteremia acutely reduce canalicular bile formation in experimental studies. Hence, both overproduction and undersecretion of bilirubin occur in bacterial sepsis, resulting in elevated concentrations of conjugated and nonconjugated bilirubin. Jaundice is rarely a cardinal sign of sepsis, and when it occurs, it is often later in its course.

A number of *intrauterine infections* result in hepatitis and hyperbilirubinemia: toxoplasmosis, rubella, cytomegalovirus (CMV), herpes simplex, syphilis, *Listeria* hepatitis, and other as yet unidentified agents. In hepatitis, the obstruction to bile flow can be as complete as in biliary atresia. Hepatomegaly is often found, with prominent extramedullary hematopoiesis in the liver. Thrombocytopenia is common. The affected infants are often full-term, but small for gestational age, indicating the intrauterine onset of the disease and its interference with organogenesis. Malformations involving the eye, central nervous system, and heart are common. Specific IgM measurements and other serological tests can be helpful in establishing the diagnosis. The characteristic giant cells seen on biopsy in neonatal hepatitis can also be seen in noninfectious liver disease.

A poorly understood group of patients are born with a well-established hepatic fibrosis and *cirrhosis* at the time of birth. Standard serological evaluations generally do not provide a diagnosis. Prognosis is likely to be poor, with patients succumbing to hepatic failure at an early age.

Table A14-2 summarizes some of the useful procedures

that can readily be performed and are helpful in orienting the physician to the pathogenesis of the infant's jaundice.

Glenn R. Gourley and Gerard B. Odell

References

Gourley, G. R., and Arend, R. A. β-glucuronidase and hyperbilirubinaemia in breast-fed and formula-fed babies. *Lancet I:* 644-1986.

Gourley, G. R., and Odell, G. B. Bilirubin Metabolism in the Fetus and Neonate. In E. Lebanthal (Ed.). *Human Gastrointestinal Development.* New York: Raven, 1989. Pp. 581–621.

Odell, G. B., and Gourley, G. R. Hereditary Hyperbilirubinemia. In E. Lebenthal (Ed.). *The Textbook of Gastroenterology and Nutrition in Infancy* (2nd ed.), New York: Raven, 1989. Pp. 949–967.

Poley, J. R. The Liver. In C. M. Anderson, V. Burke, and M. Gracey (Eds.). *Paediatric Gastroenterology* (2nd ed.). Melbourne: Blackwell, 1987. Pp. 529–658.

Poland, R. L., and Odell, G. B. Physiologic jaundice: The enterohepatic circulation of bilirubin. *N. Engl. J. Med.* 284:1, 1971.

15. *Hepatomegaly*
Normal Palpability of the Liver

The liver is normally palpable in many infants and sometimes even in older children. Because of the irregular shape of the organ and its variation in position with the level of the diaphragm, it is difficult to arrive at a norm for clinical purposes. In general, the liver edge is usually felt less than 2 cm below the costal margin in the right midclavicular line of the newborn infant and about 1 cm below the costal margin throughout childhood. In assessing the size of the liver, it is helpful to note the upper limit of dullness to percussion in the right midclavicular line. The normal-sized liver may become palpable if it is pushed down by conditions in the thorax, such as emphysema, or if there is visceroptosis, as in rickets. Also, Riedel's lobe (advanced tongue-like projection of right lobe of liver), which is a simple anatomical variation, may be mistaken for hepatomegaly or even for a kidney tumor. Similarly, enlargement of the left lobe may be mistaken for the spleen or an enlarged left kidney.

In many well-fed normal babies the thick abdominal wall and the softness of the liver make palpation difficult on routine examination. If the liver is easily felt in a well-nourished older child, it should be investigated. In developing countries, however, where children commonly suffer from malnutrition, infections, and infestations, ascertaining whether or not a palpable liver represents an important physical sign is often difficult.

Common Causes of Hepatomegaly

The exact nature of hepatomegaly can be elicited only by total evaluation of the patient, and sometimes after follow-up with appropriate treatment. Palpation should be used to estimate not only the size of the liver but also the degree of firmness and irregularity of the liver edge.

In general, increases in the size of the liver result from the trapping of blood, as in congestive cardiac failure, from hepatic edema, obstruction to the outflow of bile, swelling of the liver cells, abnormal deposition of substances, granulomatous reactions, reticuloendothelial hyperplasia, increase in fibrous tissue, or space-occupying lesions. The following outline may be helpful in the differential diagnosis of hepatomegaly.

I. Newborn infants
   A. Most of the conditions causing neonatal jaundice
   B. Neonatal infections (e.g., syphilis, septicemia)
   C. Congestive heart failure
   D. Infant of diabetic mother
   E. Inborn errors of metabolism (e.g., glycogen storage disease, galactosemia)
   F. Tumors (e.g., hemangioendothelioma)
II. Infants and children
   A. Nutritional causes (e.g., kwashiorkor, deficiency of iron, vitamin B_{12}, folic acid, and thiamine — beriberi; also hypervitaminosis A, dirt eating)
   B. Blood disorders (e.g., hemolytic anemias, nutritional anemias, and leukemias)
   C. Infections and infestations
      1. Bacterial (e.g., tuberculosis, brucellosis, liver abscess)
      2. Protozoal (e.g., kala-azar, malaria, amebiasis, toxoplasmosis)
      3. Helminthic (e.g., hydatid disease, visceral larva migrans, schistosomiasis, liver flukes)
      4. Mycotic (e.g., actinomycosis, histoplasmosis, cryptococcosis)
      5. Spirochetal (e.g., syphilis, leptospirosis, relapsing fever)
      6. Viral (e.g., infectious and serum hepatitis, yellow fever, ?infectious mononucleosis)
   D. Cirrhosis, including postnecrotic scarring, biliary cirrhosis due to chronic obstruction, hemosiderosis, and cystic fibrosis of the pancreas
   E. Inborn errors of metabolism (e.g., glycogen storage disease; galactosemia; gargoylism; Tangier disease — absence of beta-lipoproteins; Wilson disease)
   F. Lipoidosis (e.g., Gaucher disease, Niemann-Pick disease)
   G. Congestion (e.g., portal hypertension, congestive cardiac failure, tricuspid atresia, constrictive pericarditis)
   H. Connective tissue disease (e.g., systemic lupus erythematosus, rheumatoid arthritis, periarteritis nodosa)
   I. Neoplastic disease
      1. Liver tumors (e.g., sarcoma, carcinoma)
      2. Generalized tumors (e.g., lymphoma, neuroblastoma, Wilms tumor, retroperitoneal sarcoma)
   J. Cysts and benign tumors (e.g., adenoma, congenital polycystic disease of liver, focal nodular hyperplasia)
   K. Toxic factors (e.g., cytotoxic drugs, carbon tetrachloride, Reye syndrome)
   L. Miscellaneous factors (e.g., amyloidosis, sarcoidosis, reticuloendotheliosis, nephrosis)

Mohsen Ziai and V. Balagopal Raju

---

16. Melena

The passage of blood from the rectum necessitates a medical investigation. Profuse bleeding can rapidly cause anemia and shock, in which case prompt transfusion of blood and other supportive measures may have to precede definitive diagnosis and specific treatment. In the neonatal period melena may be caused by the passage of swallowed maternal blood (see Table A16-1).

Isolated lesions within the gastrointestinal tract are distinguished by the absence of bleeding or other abnormal signs elsewhere. If the bleeding site is small or the gut is not involved in any other pathological process, no symptoms or signs other than hemorrhage are elicited. Bleeding of this nature may be profuse, as from a Meckel's diverticulum or from single or multiple polyps. It is often recurrent. When blood is visible in the stool, the site of bleeding is usually the lower bowel, but if there is only occult blood, a lesion in the upper gastrointestinal tract should be suspected.

Table A16-1. Causes of Rectal Bleeding

Cause	Main clinical findings	Valuable diagnostic tests
Swallowed blood		
Neonatal	No evidence of disease; possibility of swallowed maternal blood	Estimation of fetal hemoglobin in the stool (Apt test)
Infants and children	No history or signs of gastrointestinal disease; preceding epistaxis, upper respiratory tract infection, operation; identification of bleeding site	
Damage to intestinal mucosa		
Mucosa previously abnormal		
Hiatus hernia	Under 2 yr: vomiting, hematemesis, anemia	Contrast studies of upper gastrointestinal tract, ultrasonography
Meckel's diverticulum	Any age: recurrent, severe bleeding	Ultrasonography
Duplication of gut	Any age, usually under 2 yr	X-ray of chest; laparotomy
Chronic peptic ulcer	Age 9 yr and above: family history of ulcer; history of abdominal pain	Contrast studies of stomach and duodenum; endoscopy
Mucosa previously normal		
Acute bacterial dysentery	Fever, diarrhea, dehydration; stools contain mucus and pus	Microscopical examination of stool, culture of rectal swab; blood culture
Amebic dysentery	Diarrhea; abdominal pain	Microscopical examination of stool
Hookworm infestation	Abdominal distention, anemia, edema	Microscopical examination of stool
Medications with aspirin, cortico-steroids; poisoning with iron	History of ingestion or administration of the drug; hematemesis	Identification of agent in blood or urine
Poisoning with domestic or horticultural substances	History of exposure, hematemesis, and vomiting	Inspection of the home environment
Traumatic lesions		
Swallowed foreign body, after intestinal biopsy, proctoscopy, or sigmoidoscopy; foreign body inserted in rectum	History of preceding event	X-ray studies for opaque foreign body; endoscopy
Anal fissure	Usually under 2 yr; history of constipation; crying on defecation	Inspection of anal orifice
Endogenous disease present		
Carbohydrate intolerance (disac-charidase deficiency)	Infancy; cow's milk feeding; profuse diarrhea, vomiting, failure to thrive	Examination of stool for pH, sugars; intestinal biopsy, with histochemical estimation of enzymes
"Milk allergy"	Vomiting, diarrhea, failure to thrive	Exclusion of cow's milk; eosinophilia; milk antibodies
Ulcerative colitis	Usually over 5 yr; history of diarrhea, foul, mucus-containing stools	Microscopical examination of stool, endoscopy of lower gastrointestinal tract
Regional enteritis	Usually over 5 yr; history of pain; sometimes palpable mass	Contrast studies of GI tract; endoscopy
Cushing-Rokitansky ulcer	Signs of acute disease of midbrain or brain stem, after neurosurgical operation	
Neoplasm of gut		
Polyps		
Single	Usually under 2 yr; bleeding only	Rectal examination; endoscopy
Multiple	Usually over 2 yr; family history	X-ray studies of gastrointestinal tract; laparotomy
Lymphosarcoma	Pain, bleeding, mass sometimes	X-ray; laparotomy

Table A16-1. (Continued)

Cause	Main clinical findings	Valuable diagnostic tests
Vascular abnormalities		
Esophageal varices	History of exchange transfusion or liver disease; hematemesis; signs of extrahepatic portal hypertension or chronic liver disease	Endoscopy; contrast studies of esophagus
Strangulation of gut		
Intussusception	1st yr of life: pain prominent; palpable mass; child previously well	Contrast enema; laparotomy
Malnutrition with volvulus	Signs of intestinal obstruction	Plain film of abdomen; laparotomy
Strangulated hernia	Signs of intestinal obstruction, palpable hernia	Operation
Allergic vasculitis	Usually over 5 yr; pain prominent; manifestations of purpura elsewhere	X-ray studies of gastrointestinal tract if intussusception suspected
Familial telangiectasia	Small telangiectases, if present, on skin	
Bleeding disorders		
Newborn period		
"Hemorrhagic disease"	Third to fifth day of life; multiple hemorrhages	Prothrombin time
Thrombocytopenia	History of thrombocytopenia in mother; history of maternal rubella; presence of severe hemolytic disease	Platelet count; elucidation of cause of thrombocytopenia
Later period		
Thrombocytopenia		
Primary	Acute or chronic idiopathic thrombocytopenic purpura	Platelet count; bone marrow examination
Secondary	Signs of leukemia, aplastic anemia; history of drug ingestion	Platelet count; bone marrow examination
Coagulation disorders	Usually males; previous history or evidence of bleeding disease	Bleeding and clotting time; specific tests of coagulation

Peptic ulceration is a rare cause of *melena* and is often combined with hematemesis. Apart from acute ulceration in the neonate, peptic ulcers occur most frequently in school-age boys from families with a history of the condition. Bleeding is usually preceded by symptoms of abdominal pain, which is often not typical of peptic ulceration in the adult, being less related to hunger and less clearly relieved by food and alkali.

Inflammatory processes involving the mucous membrane of extensive areas of the gastrointestinal tract are usually accompanied by diarrhea, and the blood is mixed with loose, often offensive stool. Perhaps the main cause of bloody diarrhea is acute dysenteric infection with *Salmonella* and *Shigella* organisms. The onset is acute, and diarrhea is accompanied by colicky abdominal pain and fever.

Hemorrhage is a complication of typhoid ulceration of the ileum and may occur without diarrhea; it is rare in childhood. Severe hookworm infestation can produce anemia and hypoproteinemia as well as blood loss in the stool.

Inflammatory bowel disease is a condition of uncertain origin involving the small and large bowel. It usually affects adolescents and young adults but may occur at any age. Typically, there is a history of intermittent diarrhea before the characteristic foul-smelling, blood-stained stools appear. Colicky abdominal pain is common, and affected children soon lose weight and become chronically ill. Ulcerative colitis (large bowel disease) is associated with bleeding more commonly than Crohn's disease (mainly affecting small bowel).

Vascular lesions of the gut occur in primary form with allergic vasculitis (anaphylactoid purpura); rarely the alimentary features of the disease, colicky pain and melena, exist without cutaneous manifestations. Venous bleeding is either due to esophageal varices occurring as a result of portal hypertension or secondary to impairment of venous drainage or strangulation of the gut.

Intussusception, occurring mainly in infants during the first year of life, is a common entity. The onset is usually acute, with colicky abdominal pain, vomiting, and constipation. Mucus and blood, forming a "currant-jelly stool," are passed by rectum, and a mass can often be palpated either abdominally or upon rectal examination. Congestion with bleeding and ultimately gangrene of the bowel are found in the late stages of strangulated hernia, volvulus with malrotation, and thrombosis of the mesenteric vessels.

Melena may be the only manifestation of a bleeding disorder and may be a feature of any condition characterized by spontaneous hemorrhage. Exclusion of this possibility must, therefore, form part of the investigation of any patient with melena. If there is bleeding from multiple sites or if simple hematological tests suggest a generalized bleeding disorder, further investigation should be made to elucidate the specific nature of the disorder.

Trivial bleeding manifested by small amounts of visible blood on the stool or spotting of the diaper or pot is rarely of major significance. If it is associated with constipation and pain at defecation, inspection of the anal orifice will probably reveal an abrasion at the mucocutaneous junction. When no fissure is apparent, a mild proctitis due to irritation from hard stools may be assumed. The readiness with which bleeding can be induced from the delicate mucous membrane is demonstrated by the bleeding that frequently occurs even with gentle digital examination. Perianal fissures and scarring that are not readily explained should arouse suspicion of child abuse in children of both sexes.

Diagnosis of the cause of melena is rarely a problem when rectal bleeding is combined with other revealing symptoms or signs, but it can be exceedingly difficult when melena is the only manifestation of disease. Judgment is required when considering the study of a patient presenting intermittent mild or moderate bleeding. Contrast x-ray study and endoscopy of the gastrointestinal tract are the most revealing investigations. Less invasive procedures such as abdominal ultrasound examination, radioisotope scanning, and CT scan may provide diagnostic information. A single severe hemorrhage or recurrent small hemorrhages will demand such investigations, and if they are negative, a diagnostic

laparotomy must be considered. Table A16-1 summarizes the important causes of rectal bleeding in infants and children.

Thomas E. Oppé

17. Edema

Differential Diagnosis of Edema

Localized Edema

Regional edema is found in all diseases involving the lymphatic system: infections (acute or chronic); thrombophlebitis; parasitic infestation (filariasis, causing elephantiasis); neoplasms, either primarily involving the lymph nodes or metastatic; and irradiation or surgical removal of the lymph nodes. Palpebral and periorbital edema may be one of the presenting signs of infectious mononucleosis.

TRANSITORY EDEMA. A transitory edema in the newborn infant is often seen in the head, around the eyes, and on the backs of the hands and feet. Premature infants may have localized edema even when they are dehydrated in other parts of the body.

EDEMA OF THE NEWBORN AND SCLEREDEMA. Often found in weak or premature infants, scleredema may either develop as a "pitting" edema beginning on the distal parts of the extremities or appear as a pale, cool, wax-hard swelling starting on the lateral surfaces of the thighs and buttocks and around the shoulders, gradually spreading to the rest of the body including the face. This latter condition is similar to sclerema neonatorum, but it is characterized more by edema than by hardening of the subcutaneous tissue.

GONADAL DYSGENESIS. Newborn infants with gonadal dysgenesis (Turner's syndrome) often have pitting edema of distal parts of the extremities and the backs of the hands and feet.

BILATERAL RENAL AGENESIS. This rare disorder may be diagnosed by early dyspnea (congenital hypoplasia of the lungs) and "Potter's face" with edema, wideset eyes and epicanthus, and low-set ears. The baby does not void at all and dies within the first few hours of life, often from pulmonary hypoplasia.

IDIOPATHIC HEREDITARY LYMPHEDEMA. Idiopathic hereditary lymphedema (Nonne-Milroy disease) is a congenital defect of the lymph channels. Edema of one or both of the lower extremities is often present at birth; more rarely, the arms are involved. Later the edema may increase to become generalized. When the abdominal lymphatics are malformed, ascites and a severe hypoproteinemic edema occur.

Localized lymphangioma should not be confused with lymphedema. Lymphangiomas are soft and give the impression of a vague tumor. They usually appear in the neck and on the extremities.

ANGIONEUROTIC EDEMA. Angioneurotic edema or giant urticaria is either an allergic manifestation or a hereditary disease with rapidly developing edema, most often around the head, hands, or feet. If the oropharyngeal region or larynx is involved, it may be fatal. Closely related to this condition is the edema found in serum sickness, and in allergic purpura (Henoch-Schönlein syndrome). In cases of angioneurotic edema it is important to carry out both qualitative and quantitative assays for Cl esterase inhibitor deficiency as this is now a potentially treatable condition.

Generalized Edema

HYDROPS FETALIS. Hydrops fetalis is a disorder with extreme degrees of edema, ascites, and hydrothorax, often leading to fetal or neonatal death. It is seen in connection with severe erythroblastosis fetalis associated with anemia, rapidly increasing jaundice, bleeding tendency, and serological evidence of Rh sensitization. Hydrops is presumably caused by cardiac insufficiency due to anemia, but hydrops fetalis has also been described in a variety of other conditions such as intrauterine infections, congenital heart or lung diseases, congenital nephrosis, fetal neuroblastoma, placental hemangioendothelioma, alpha-thalassemia, maternal diabetes mellitus, and toxemia and in patients with Down syndrome.

NEPHROSIS. Nephrosis is characterized by a gradual onset of edema, first noticed in the face. Later the edema appears generalized. Marked ascites, massive albuminuria, hypoproteinemia, elevated serum cholesterol, and other laboratory abnormalities are present.

GLOMERULONEPHRITIS. In the acute phase edema may be seen as puffiness around the eyes and swelling of the ankles, except in severe cases with anuria, in which more generalized edema is found. Other typical findings are hematuria, fever, malaise, headache, oliguria or anuria, and hypertension with encephalopathy and cardiac decompensation. The edema is caused by a decreased filtration and excretion of water and sodium. In the subacute or nephrotic phase, with low plasma protein and sodium retention, massive edema and ascites may be found with hypertension and azotemia.

CARDIAC DISEASE. In children, cardiac disease takes the form mainly of congenital heart diseases and rheumatic heart disease; here edema is often a minor finding and mostly seen in severe decompensation. The edema is first noted on the backs of the hands and feet. Other and more important signs are dyspnea, rales, cyanosis, cardiac murmurs, and an enlarged liver. It is essential to remember that small infants and newborns in cardiac failure may not manifest overt signs of edema and the only sign of fluid retention may be inappropriate weight gain.

CUSHING DISEASE. In Cushing disease, either primary or induced during steroid treatment, the patients have general edema due to salt and water retention. Typical findings are moon face, striae, and elevated urinary excretion of 17-hydroxycorticosteroids.

HYPOTHYROIDISM. In hypothyroidism, myxedema of the skin may be seen, primarily in the face.

MALNUTRITION. Edema is seen in severe malnutrition, such as protein-energy deficiency (kwashiorkor), in vitamin B_1 deficiency (beriberi), with cardiac failure, and in patients with liver cirrhosis. Liver disease due to any cause with resultant hypoalbuminemia is an important cause of generalized edema.

Mohsen Ziai and Bent Friis-Hansen

---

18. Ascites

Clinical Manifestations

The most important clinical sign of ascites is the increased size of the abdomen. Symptoms of respiratory distress may also be observed. The fluid may accumulate slowly. The first sign is increase in the distance between the xiphoid process and the umbilicus. With marked distortion there is bulging of the abdomen to both sides when the patient lies in the supine position. A wavelike impulse can be noted when one side of the abdominal wall is tapped sharply while the other hand is placed on the opposite side. On percussion it is possible to determine the shifting level of intraabdominal fluid. Clinically it is difficult to determine the presence of small quantities of ascitic fluid. In adults the limit is 1000 ml. Plain abdominal roentgenograms can be of great diagnostic help. Small quantities of ascites (as little as 100 ml) can be detected by abdominal ultrasonography. This technique can also show the presence of ascites prenatally.

The most common causes of prenatal and neonatal ascites are erythroblastosis fetalis, obstructive urinary tract malformations, peritonitis due to intestinal rupture, and hepatic and cardiac failures.

Table A18-1. Guide to the Etiological Diagnosis of Ascites in Infancy and Childhood

Disease	Clinical manifestations	Investigations	Ascitic fluid
Chronic cardiac failure; myocarditis; congenital heart malformation	Other signs of cardiac decompensation; history of preceding streptococcal or other infections	Chest x-ray, electrocardiogram (ECG), antistreptolysin-O (ASO) titer, erythrocyte sedimentation rate (ESR)	Transparent; protein content low; cells: few epithelial or absent
Constrictive pericarditis	Dyspnea, tachypnea visible; increased venous pressure; small pulse pressure; enlarged spleen and liver	Chest x-ray, ECG	Transparent; protein content low; cells: few epithelial or absent
Obstruction of portal veins (glands, tumors, thrombosis—prehepatic, intrahepatic, or posthepatic)	Hepatosplenomegaly; evidence of collateral circulation and esophageal varices	Liver function tests; splenoportography; liver biopsy; laparotomy; determination of leukocytes and thrombocytes	Transparent—color sometimes unusually yellow; protein content low; cells: few epithelial or absent
Hepatic cirrhosis	Universal edema; signs of hepatic damage in addition to depletion of protein synthesis; signs of portal hypertension as above	Liver biopsy and function tests	Transparent or slightly cloudy; protein content moderate; cells: few or absent
Nutritional protein deficiency	Generalized edema; signs of vitamin deficiencies	Serum and urinary protein; cholesterol	Transparent or slightly cloudy; protein very low; cells: few or absent
Nephrotic syndrome	Universal edema	Serum and urinary protein; cholesterol	Transparent or slightly cloudy; protein content extremely low; cells: few or absent
Acute peritonitis (primary or secondary)	Acute onset, often with high fever, vomiting, and diarrhea; abdomen distended, painful; later ileus, icterus	WBC (leukocytosis); abdominal x-ray; blood, throat, and stool cultures	Turbid to purulent, sometimes reddish (streptococci); protein content high; cells: numerous, polymorphonuclear; bacteria may be present
Tuberculous peritonitis	Main symptoms of a chronic illness; slowly developing distention of abdomen; rarely, pains	Tuberculin skin tests; lung x-ray; culture of bacilli; laparotomy	Turbid; protein content high; cells: increased, mainly lymphocytes
Intraperitoneal tumors or metastases (compression; see "Obstruction of portal veins" above)	Involvement of general health; tumor detected elsewhere	Blood count; ESR; abdominal x-ray before and after insufflation of O_2 retroperitoneally	Clear to turbid; protein content increased; cells slightly increased (malignant cells may be present)
Chylous ascites	Distention of abdomen; dyspnea increasing in infancy or after trauma	Plasma protein (may be low)	Milky white, fat-containing protein content elevated
Peritoneal bleeding	Trauma; acute distention of abdomen; pains; signs of hypovolemic shock	Hemoglobin	Bloodlike appearance
Pancreatic duct rupture	Trauma or infection, tenderness, slightly distended abdomen	Amylase determination in blood and urine	Turbid; amylase test positive

Pathogenesis

The interchange of fluid between the blood and the tissue space is controlled by the balance between the capillary blood pressure and the osmotic pressure of the plasma proteins retaining fluid in the vascular compartments. Accordingly, the two factors that mainly cause an increase in intraperitoneal fluid (transudate) are hypoproteinemia (below 2.5 g of albumin/100 ml) and increased portal capillary pressure. The latter serves to localize the fluid retained in the peritoneal cavity rather than in the periphery. Also, the retention of water and electrolytes due to renal failure or to excess secretion of antidiuretic hormone and aldosterone can cause an accumulation of ascitic fluid.

Intraperitoneal infections, tumors, and metastases may produce exudate in the peritoneal cavity. Rupture of the corresponding lymphatic vessels may fill the peritoneal cavity with chylous fluid. Leakage of fluid into the peritoneal cavity may result from lesions of the pancreatic duct. Bleeding of ruptured parenchymatous organs causes hemoperitoneum.

Diagnostic Examinations

The following examinations of ascitic fluid are important: turbidity (inflammation or chylus), color (bloody, bile-stained), protein (high in inflammation), specific gravity (inflammation, > 1.020), cytological studies (bacteria, cells) after centrifugation of the fluid, and culture.

Differential Diagnosis

Other conditions causing distention of the abdomen must be excluded. These include gaseous distention of the intestine encountered in children with paralytic ileus, megacolon, acute gastric dilatation, different types of tumors, especially cysts, and extreme distention of the urinary bladder (Table A18-1).

Paracentesis of the peritoneal cavity is often necessary; the quality of fluid obtained from an ovarian cyst cannot exclude the diagnostic mistake. Paracentesis is performed with a trocar or needle under aseptic conditions and local anesthesia. A good site for paracentesis is at a point one-third of the distance between the anterior iliac spine and the umbilicus; another possibility is the vertical or almost vertical position near the midline below the umbilicus.

Niilo Hallman and Erkki Savilahti

References

Riazi, J., and Dale, J. T. Ascites. In M. Ziai (Ed.), *Bedside Pediatrics*. Boston: Little, Brown, 1983.

Wyllie, R., Chasu, T. S., and Fitzgerald, J. F. Ascites: Pathophysiology and management. *J. Pediat.* 97:167, 1980.

19. Hypertension

The measurement of blood pressure (BP) must be included in every routine and complete physical examination. Recently, the NIH Task Force on Blood Pressure Control issued revised guidelines concerning the prevalence, diagnosis, and management of hypertension in infants and children. The importance of primary (essential) hypertension in children is now fully recognized, although secondary etiologies with well-described pathophysiologies are always carefully considered, particularly in infants and younger children. There is a need for early identification of primary hypertension so that adequate surveillance, specific measures of hygiene and pharmacologic management of fixed hypertension may be instituted in a timely fashion. Certain conditions should call the clinician's attention to the possibility of hypertension in a child: abdominal bruit or masses, active or historical renal disease or lesions (trauma, pyelonephritis, nephritis, proteinuria, hematuria), neurofibromatosis, familial dysautonomia, failure to thrive, heart failure, Turner syndrome, premature birth and umbilical artery catheterization, endocrine disorders (thyroid, adrenal), ambivalent genitalia, orbital tumors, and prolonged orthopedic injuries with casting.

Measuring and interpreting BPs in infants and children is rendered difficult by the following problems: patient anxiety/restlessness, variable arm sizes requiring the use of appropriately sized cuffs, artificially generating Korotkoff sounds by heavy pressure on the stethoscope, and developmental changes in BP for children. Many automated devices which use Doppler or oscillometric techniques provide accurate systolic BP measurements in infants and children for whom auscultatory BP measurements may be difficult to obtain; however, only the Dynamap oscillometric unit has been shown to be reliable for diastolic BPs. All BP measuring devices require frequent calibration to guarantee their accuracy (standard remains the mercury manometer). Errors in cuff selection can be minimized by selecting the largest cuff that fits the child's arm. The cuff bladder should be long enough to completely encircle the circumference (with or without overlap) and wide enough to cover 75% of

Table A19-1. Guide to the Etiological Diagnosis of Hypertension in Infancy and Childhood

Disease	Clinical findings	Investigations
Renal disease		
Acute glomerulonephritis	History of preceding streptococcal infections; mild edema, headache, discoloration of urine, oliguria; cardiac failure, hypertensive encephalopathy, uremia, coma; ophthalmoscopical findings	Urinalysis; creatinine; blood urea nitrogen (BUN) high; antistrep serologies, erythrocyte sedimentation rate (ESR); serum complement (C_3, C_4)
Chronic nephritis	Not common in pediatric age group; history of acute glomerulonephritis or allergic purpura may not be present; anemia, poor growth, and signs of chronic renal failure	CBC urinalysis, proteinemia, total CO_2, creatinine vitamin D ($1,2,5$-OH_2), BUN, serum phosphorus; renal functions, renal ultrasound, and renal biopsy
Nephritis associated with collagen disease	Multiple organ involvement and fever	FANA and DANA; white blood cell (WBC), and hemoglobin (Hgb)in lupus (leukocytosis in periarteritis); serum complement; urinalysis; electrophoretic pattern of serum proteins; renal biopsy; specific antibody titer (ANCA, etc.)
Pyelonephritis	In acute cases fever, urinary symptoms, abdominal or back pain; chronic cases usually asymptomatic	Urinalysis; bacterial colony count more diagnostic; ultrasound, VCUG, DMSA renal scan
Polycystic kidney; ectopic kidney; hypoplastic kidney; horseshoe kidney; hydronephrotic kidney	Except for the possible presence of palpable mass, asymptomatic during early stages	Urological studies beginning with ultrasound, DTPA renal scan
Renal vascular anomalies and thromboses	Clinical manifestations variable according to degree of involvement	Urinalysis, renin (PRA), split-function tests, DTPA renal scan, Doppler ultrasound
Primary arteriolar disease of the kidney	Progressive renal failure; retinal changes	Renal biopsy
Wilms' tumor	Palpable mass, occasional hematuria	Ultrasound, CT, MRI or exploration
Other	Clinical evidence of cystinosis, amyloidosis, diabetes; history of irradiation or familial or hereditary nephritis; porphyria	Specific tests for the diseases; renal biopsy
Cardiovascular disease		
Coarctation of the aorta (very important)	In early stages asymptomatic, but may produce cardiac failure; sometimes associated with gonadal dysgenesis; blood pressure higher in upper extremities; femoral pulsations weak	Chest x ray for evidence of collateral circulation; MRI, echocardiography, aortography
Cardiac runoffs; anemia; thyrotoxicosis; aortic regurgitation; patent ductus	These are fairly easily differentiated clinically; systolic pressure is high, but diastolic is not	Echocardiography, thyroid function tests
Neurological diseases		
Space-occupying lesions: abscess, cysts, hematoma, tumors	Signs of increased intracranial pressure; specific neurological signs	Skull x ray, computed axial tomogram (CAT scan) with contrast enhancement, MRI
Edema of brain	Intracranial hypertension plus history of trauma, infection, or intoxication (lead)	CAT scan and toxicological studies, MRI
Poliomyelitis Poliomyelitis	Paralysis, bulbar signs, stiff neck	Lumbar puncture; search for virus in CSF or elevated antibody titer in serum or elevated antibody titer in serum

Table A19-1. (Continued)

Disease	Clinical findings	Investigations
Encephalitis	Impairment of sensorium and specific neurological signs, stiff neck	As above
Riley-Day syndrome (familial dysautonomia)	Intermittent hypertension; absence of tears; skin rashes; excessive perspiration; postural hypotension	None
Poisoning		
Lead	Encephalitic signs, coma, convulsions; pallor; history of pica or exposure to lead	Examination of urine for glucose and coproporphyrin; x-ray (for evidence of lead lines in long bones and opaque material in abdomen); urine and blood lead content; blood studies for anemia; stippled erythrocytes; examination of CSF for protein cells, pressure elevation
Acrodynia	Nervous symptoms; irritability; erythema of hands and feet; vasomotor phenomena	Urinary mercury excretion
Vitamin D	History of excessive ingestion; anorexia, vomiting, constipation, thirst, polyuria	Bone x-rays; serum calcium and phosphorus; 25-OH vitamin D
Endocrine and metabolic diseases		
Inborn errors of urea cycle	Mental retardation	Blood ammonia
Pheochromocytoma	Intermittent or persistent hypertension, anxiety, palpitation, headaches, rapid pulse and dilated pupils, precipitation of attack by abdominal pressure	Urinary catecholamines; Regitine test; sonogram; CT scan, laparotomy; ^{131}I-MBIG scan
Cushing's syndrome	"Moon facies," "buffalo" type of obesity; striation of skin, back pain; weakness; hirsutism	Bone x-rays (detection of osteoporosis); glycosuria, hyperglycemia, corticosteroid excretion in urine; [131]I-19-iodo-cholesterol scan
Corticosteroid therapy	History of steroid therapy plus above	
Adrenogenital syndrome	Excessive growth, pseudohermaphroditism in female; large penis, small testicles in male; salt-losing syndrome; response to cortisone	Bone age; urinary steroid studies; serum 17-hydroxyprogesterone
Other low-renin hypertensions	Dexamethasone-suppressible hyperaldosteronism; apparent mineralocorticoid excess	Detection of 11-ketoreductase deficiency
Hyperthyroidism	See "Cardiac runoffs" above	
Aldosteronism	Periodic paralysis; large urinary output; hypertension only in secondary form, not in primary congenital aldosteronism	Pitressin (vasopressin) administration; examination of urine for specific gravity; serum sodium and potassium
Hypercalcemia — idiopathic; immobilization	Peculiar facies, mental retardation; supravalvular aortic stenosis; "elfin facies"; immobilization with high milk intake; anorexia, headache, and vomiting	Elevated serum calcium; increased excretion of calcium in urine
Essential hypertension (rare)	The only signs may be related to the elevation of blood pressure; family history often positive	Elimination of all other causes; cold pressor test; renin profile with urinary sodium excretion

the upper arm length. Smaller cuffs may result in an artificially elevated BP, whereas cuffs slightly wider than necessary should not mask hypertensive levels of BP. A comfortably seated child (infants may be supine), and proper inflation/deflation technique are equally important. When possible both the fourth and fifth Korotkoff phases should be recorded with the phase I sound (systolic).

Blood pressure standards have been recently modified based on several reasonably well-conducted studies with compatible data; however, no normative BP data obtained from a probability sampling of United States children are available at present. The probable etiology of hypertension in children varies with age. In newborns, renal artery thrombosis, renal artery stenosis, congenital renal malformations, coarctation of the aorta, and bronchopulmonary dysplasia are common. Infants to 6-year-olds often present with renal parenchymal diseases, coarctation of the aorta, and renal artery stenosis, whereas preadolescent children usually have renal artery stenosis, renal parenchymal diseases, and primary hypertension in that order. Finally, adolescents usually present with primary hypertension or renal parenchymal diseases. Table A19-1 reviews the clinical findings and suggested investigations in some detail.

Mohsen Ziai and Robert Fildes

References

Dillon, M. J. Investigation and management of hypertension in children. *Pediat. Nephrol.* 1:59, 1987.

Report on the Second Task Force on Blood Pressure Control in Children — 1987. *Pediatrics* 79:1, 1987.

---

20. Lymphadenopathy

The lymphatic tissue forms a larger percentage of total body weight during infancy and childhood than in adult life. The frequency of infections in childhood and the child's intensive lymphatic response to infections contribute to easy palpability of lymph nodes during early life. Not realizing these facts, many parents are alarmed by the incidental discovery of enlarged lymph nodes in their children.

It is important for the physician to distinguish this normal lymphatic hypertrophy from pathological conditions and to reassure the family, who usually are worried about the possibility of a malignant disorder or serious infection such as tuberculosis. It is equally important to consider the possibil-

ity of an underlying disease process whenever true lymphadenopathy — that is, more than small shotty nodes — is present.

Lymphadenopathy is considered localized when the nodes in only one region are affected, and generalized when at least the cervical, axillary, and inguinal nodes are enlarged. In palpating the lymph nodes one must pay attention to their size and consistency and whether or not they are matted together. The presence of heat, tenderness, or fluctuation in the affected area and mobility of the overlying skin are additional signs of clinical importance. When the deep lymph nodes are increased in size, they may encroach on other organs or tissues, causing pressure symptoms — for example, cough in the case of mediastinal involvement. In such cases the x-ray findings usually disclose the presence of lymphadenopathy. The causes of lymph node enlargement are summarized here.

I. Localized
  A. Infections
    1. Pyogenic (e.g., staphylococci, streptococci)
    2. Tuberculosis and atypical mycobacteria
    3. Postvaccination (e.g., BCG)
    4. Tularemia, plague, brucellosis, cat-scratch disease
    5. Spirochetal (e.g., syphilis, rat-bite fever)
    6. Viral (e.g., granuloma inguinale, lymphopathia venereum, rubella, AIDS)
    7. Protozoal (e.g., toxoplasmosis, trypanosomiasis)
    8. Fungal (e.g., dermatophytosis, histoplasmosis)
  B. Malignant neoplasms
    1. Primary (e.g., Hodgkin's disease)
    2. Metastatic (e.g., carcinoma of thyroid, neuroblastoma)
  C. Others (e.g., Kawasaki disease, sarcoid, benign giant lymph node hyperplasia, sinus histiocytosis)
II. Generalized
  A. Infections
    1. Acute (e.g., generalized skin infections, septicemia, common contagious diseases, infectious mononucleosis, kala-azar)
    2. Chronic (e.g., tuberculosis syphilis)
  B. Connective tissue diseases (e.g., systemic lupus erythematosus, rheumatoid arthritis)
  C. Hypersensitivity states (e.g., serum sickness, drug reactions)
  D. Neoplastic and storage diseases
    1. Malignant neoplasms (e.g., reticulum cell sarcoma, leukemia)

2. Reticuloendothelioses (e.g., Letterer-Siwe disease)
3. Storage diseases (e.g., cystinosis, Niemann-Pick disease)
E. Granulomatous diseases (e.g., sarcoidosis)
F. Other (e.g., mucocutaneous lymph node syndrome — Kawasaki disease)

It is apparent that there are many causes for generalized lymphadenopathy, whereas localized lymph node enlargement is seen only in neoplastic and infectious diseases. Localized pyogenic infections of lymph nodes, such as retropharyngeal abscess, are among examples of interesting aspects of infections in early life. The finding of localized posterior cervical nodes is of special diagnostic significance in some diseases such as rubella or trypanosomiasis, while occipital lymphadenopathy occurs particularly in roseola infantum. Sometimes during the early stages of a systemic malignant disease one can find glandular enlargement confined to only one region (e.g., in Hodgkin's disease).

In a child with enlarged cervical lymph nodes it is particularly important to consider the possibility of a bacterial upper respiratory tract infection, commonly with beta-hemolytic streptococci, with late secondary involvement of the glands, and tuberculosis or infection with atypical mycobacteria. Usually the presence or absence of tenderness, heat, and redness over the affected area favors one of these diagnostic possibilities. It is wise to remember that these two types of infections may coexist and to direct the treatment toward both possibilities when any uncertainty exists. In countries where unpasteurized milk is used, cervical tuberculosis is common. Skin infections over the face and scalp may lead to enlargement of regional lymph nodes, such as periauricular and posterior auricular glands. Adenovirus conjunctivitis often causes a characteristic enlargement of the preauricular lymph node known as the oculoglandular syndrome.

Involvement of the inguinal nodes is commonly seen because of the frequent traumatic lesions in the lower extremities. One should not overlook the possibility of bone and joint tuberculosis in such cases. Axillary lymphadenopathy may be secondary to a portal of entry through the skin of the hands or arms, complications of BCG vaccination, and cat-scratch disease.

A thorough history and meticulous physical examination often lead to recognition of these and other possible portals, such as contact with rodents in rat-bite fever and tularemia. Skin testing for tuberculosis is mandatory in all cases. Other skin tests depend on the specific infections that are suspected.

Many laboratory examinations can be performed to elucidate the nature of underlying illness, particularly in generalized lymphadenopathy. One can begin with a hemogram, erythrocyte sedimentation rate, and an x-ray film of the chest. If a neoplastic disease is suspected, bone marrow examination and biopsy of the gland generally constitute the initial steps; they must be performed without delay.

In the presence of acute localized lymphadenopathy and a negative tuberculin test, one should use antibiotics, particularly penicillin or a synthetic penicillinase-resistant derivative. The response to this treatment, with decrease in signs of inflammation and size of the gland, may be diagnostic of a pyogenic infection.

Ali Akbar Velayati and Mohsen Ziai

---

21. Splenomegaly

The tip of the spleen is usually palpable in premature infants and in about 30% of full-term infants. It may be felt in children up to 3 or 4 years of age. Thereafter the spleen is palpable only when enlarged to about two or three times its average size. Palpability due to an ectopic location or a depressed diaphragm is rare.

Technique of Palpation of the Spleen

Palpation is easiest with the patient supine and turned slightly to the right. The patient places his left hand under his left flank. The examiner's hand is superficially pressed to the left and above the level of the umbilicus, toward the left costal margin, or it is kept stationary at this position, relying on the movement of the diaphragm to push the organ against the fingers. Palpation must be carried out gently; otherwise an enlarged soft spleen, as in typhoid, will be missed. If palpation is too vigorous, occasionally rupture of the spleen and hemorrhagic shock may follow — particularly in infectious mononucleosis. Helpful pointers in identifying the spleen are a notch on the anteromedial margin like that on a big coffee bean, its location over the intestines, and its movement with the diaphragm during respiration.

Causes of Splenomegaly

The significance of splenomegaly depends on the underlying disease. In general, diseases that cause hyperplasia of the lymphoid and the reticuloendothelial system involve the spleen and result in splenomegaly. As the bulk of the spleen is reticuloendothelial, it participates in blood formation when extramedullary hematopoiesis is needed; splenic enlargement, therefore, results. Because of the vascular arrangements of the spleen, splenomegaly due to enlargement and distention of the sinusoids occurs whenever there is increased pressure in the portal or splenic veins. The various causes of splenomegaly are as follows.

A. Primary disorders of the spleen
  1. Cysts
  2. Tumors — hemangioma, lymphangioma, hamartoma, other benign tumors
  3. Hemorrhage in spleen
     a. Trauma
     b. Subcapsular hemorrhage, as in infectious mononucleosis
B. Infectious splenomegaly (see below)
C. Congestive splenomegaly
  1. Cirrhosis of the liver due to any cause (infections, inborn errors of metabolism, cholestasis, cystic fibrosis, malnutrition, toxins, etc.)
  2. Splenic or portal vein thrombosis
D. Blood dyscrasias
  1. Hemolytic anemia
  2. Leukemia
  3. Extramedullary hematopoiesis — osteopetrosis
  4. Thalassemia
  5. Sickle-cell disease (sequestration crisis)
E. Granulomatous splenomegaly
  1. Sarcoidosis
  2. Chronic granulomatous disease with susceptibility to infections
F. Infiltrative splenomegaly
  1. Metastatic neoplasms — lymphomas, Hodgkin disease
  2. Histiocytosis — Letterer-Siwe disease, reticuloendotheliosis
  3. Storage diseases
     a. Amyloidosis
     b. Niemann-Pick disease
     c. Gaucher disease
     d. Mucopolysaccharidoses
G. Hypersensitivity states
  1. Serum sickness
  2. Collagen vascular diseases — lupus erythematosus, rheumatoid arthritis, etc.

Primary Disorders of the Spleen

Primary conditions involving the spleen such as cysts, hemangiomas, lymphangiomas, and other tumors are rare.

Diagnosis is made by the process of elimination. Radioactive turnover rates measured by scintillation counters over the spleen have proved valuable for diagnosis. Abdominal ultrasound can be very helpful in cases of splenic cysts, and abdominal CAT scan can assign density values and improved resolution in cases of infiltrative splenomegaly and injuries to the spleen. Traumatic rupture of the spleen or spontaneous rupture following subcapsular hemorrhage produces the symptoms of shock and local tenderness, but splenomegaly follows trauma without rupture.

Infectious Splenomegaly (Acute Splenic Tumor; Acute Splenitis)

Splenomegaly occurs with infections in which the infectious agent is blood-borne or there is intensive antigenic stimulation with hyperplasia of the reticuloendothelial and lymphoid systems. Splenomegaly may occur with acute, subacute, and chronic infections due to bacteria, viruses, fungi, rickettsiae, and protozoa. Some of the infections that may cause splenomegaly are as follows.

A. Acute
  1. Bacterial — septicemia, enteric fever, typhoid, tularemia, and plague
  2. Rickettsial — typhus fever
  3. Viral — infectious mononucleosis, cytomegalic inclusion disease, etc.
B. Chronic
  1. Bacterial — bacterial endocarditis, brucellosis, syphilis, and miliary tuberculosis
  2. Generalized mycotic — histoplasmosis, coccidioidomycosis
  3. Protozoal — toxoplasmosis, kala-azar, malaria, schistosomiasis, and visceral larva migrans

Common bacterial causes are septicemia, subacute bacterial endocarditis, typhoid fever, brucellosis, congenital syphilis, and miliary tuberculosis. The most frequently encountered viral infection is infectious mononucleosis.

Chronic infections include generalized mycotic infections such as histoplasmosis. Protozoal infections giving rise to marked splenomegaly, such as kala-azar and malaria, usually occur in endemic areas.

Congestive Splenomegaly

Obstruction of the venous system of the spleen may have many causes, hepatic cirrhosis being the most common.

Portal thrombosis of the extrahepatic vein has been traced

to omphalitis in the newborn infant or to other distant or regional infections. In a few cases it has followed abdominal injury. Important, clinical manifestations are those of "hypersplenism" — anemia, leukopenia, and thrombocytopenia with marked, firm splenomegaly and tendency to severe hematemesis from rupture of esophageal varices.

Some helpful pointers in the diagnosis of intrahepatic obstruction are the presence of a history suggesting liver disease and the finding of hepatomegaly, ascites, and abnormal liver function tests. A confirmatory diagnostic procedure is liver biopsy.

Splenomegaly in Blood Dyscrasias

Splenomegaly is common in hemolytic anemias, particularly when the disorder is congenital, as in erythroblastosis, hereditary spherocytosis, and Cooley's anemia, because of both extramedullary hematopoiesis and increased blood destruction. In sickle-cell disease one finds splenomegaly in the early stages; as the disease progresses there is a virtual disappearance of the spleen (autosplenectomy) on account of infarctions.

Infiltrative Splenomegaly

Infiltrative splenomegaly may be caused by a variety of diseases, among them the "storage" diseases, such as Gaucher disease, which may cause massive splenomegaly. Usually these diseases involve many organs and systems, including the viscera, skeletal system, and nervous tissue. Radiographic examination of the chest and skeleton, bone marrow aspiration, or biopsy usually reveals various foam cells or other underlying disorders.

Ali Akbar Velayati, Mohsen Ziai, and Fe del Mundo

References

Dale, J. T. Splenomegaly. In M. Ziai (Ed.), *Bedside Pediatrics.* Boston: Little, Brown, 1983.

---

22. Pallor and Anemia

Pallor is commonly but not necessarily associated with anemia; it occurs when there is vasoconstriction and edema. Patients who are in shock appear pale, and chronic diseases

such as rheumatic fever, ulcerative colitis, and celiac syndrome are associated with pallor. Sallow complexion may be familial or ethnic. The diagnosis of anemia therefore depends on laboratory confirmation.

Ninety-five percent of all childhood anemias are diagnosable by means of a complete history, a thorough physical examination, and a relatively minor amount of laboratory work. Accurate techniques in the preparation and examination of the patient's blood smear by an informed individual, a reticulocyte count, and mean corpuscular volume (MCV) are essentials to correct diagnosis.

Basic Causes of Anemia

There are four basic processes causing anemia in childhood: blood loss, blood destruction, failure of blood production, and bone marrow replacement.

Blood Loss

Blood loss is the cause most likely to be revealed by the history. Usually patients and their families are not only aware of but also alarmed by evidence of acute blood loss. Evidence to support the presence of chronic blood loss can be elicited by specific questions as to color of stools, bruising, nosebleeds, and so forth. It is also essential to examine the stools for evidence of occult bleeding in patients.

Blood Destruction

Patients with hemolytic states may or may not be visibly jaundiced, but they invariably have a history of sallow complexion and perhaps "muddy" sclerae. For a patient with a palpable spleen, a family history of other members with chronic anemia or gallstones or both increases the possibility of chronic hemolysis. Confirmation of this diagnosis is accomplished by laboratory tests showing bizarre red cell morphology (spherocytes, sickle cells, target cells, inclusion fragments) and elevation of the reticulocyte count, indirect-reacting serum bilirubin, and urine urobilinogen; specific identification of the type of hemolytic anemia can then be made utilizing the definitive tests.

Failure of Blood Production

The third major cause of anemia — failure of production — especially requires an accurate history. Cells may not be produced because the necessary building blocks (iron, folic acid, protein) are unavailable; because the patient is unable to absorb those building blocks ingested (because of diarrhea, pernicious anemia, celiac disease); or because, having ingested and absorbed the necessary building blocks, he is unable to incorporate them into normal red cells on account of a metabolic disorder (hypothyroidism, uremia, rheumatoid arthritis). Investigations for this wide variety of conditions are diverse, but the history and physical examination can eliminate many of the possibilities. It is significant that close to 90% of the anemias in children due to production failure result from nutritional iron deficiency.

Bone Marrow Replacement

Not all diseases of bone marrow replacement are malignant; in aplastic anemia the marrow is replaced with fat, but the condition is nevertheless life-threatening. Diagnosis must be confirmed by bone marrow aspiration. Osteopetrosis is presently one of the conditions that are being treated with bone marrow transplantations.

Causes of Anemia in Relation to Age

The age of the patient at onset of the disease is an important consideration. The diagnostic approach to anemia is simplified if one classifies the pediatric age group into five major divisions: 0 to 7 days; 1 week to 3 months; 3 months to 2 years; 2 years to 6 years; over 6 years. If one plots the five age groups on the horizontal against the aforementioned classifications on the vertical, the significance of age in the etiology of anemia becomes apparent (Table A22-1).

Birth to 7 Days

In the newborn infant blood loss represents a leading cause of anemia, second only to erythroblastosis fetalis. Blood loss may occur before the baby is born, as in prenatal bleeding, fato-fetal, or fetal-maternal transfusion. If mother and infant are of different blood groups, this accident can be confirmed by demonstrating the baby's blood cells in the maternal circulation. In monozygotic twins one twin may contribute the majority of his blood volume to the other; one infant is then born with a polycythemic hematocrit level, and the other is at the same time near shock from blood loss. The more obvious bleeding from premature separation of the placenta, placenta previa, and even occasionally from the cord itself should alert the physician to anemia. The possibility of internal hemorrhage, particularly after a breech delivery, should be carefully considered. Time is precious if lifesaving therapy is to be effective. From the second through the fifth day of life the infant may suffer from hemorrhagic disease of the newborn caused by the absence of vitamin K. Serious neonatal infections may also be heralded by a bleeding tendency. Unexplained bleeding likewise demands immediate investigation for other bleeding disorders, most of which are hereditary.

Erythroblastosis fetalis due to Rh sensitization of the mother by her fetus was previously the major cause of hemolysis in the newborn. ABO incompatibility is another frequent offender. Because of skin pigmentation, anemia or jaundice suggesting a hemolytic process may be easily overlooked. Hemolysis secondary to sepsis may be an insidious complication of the newborn period. The neonate often fails to give the classic warning signs of infection, such as elevation of temperature or pulse. Subnormal temperatures are not uncommon but are hard to evaluate; the pulse, already rapid, may not increase perceptibly. Respirations are normally somewhat irregular, particularly in premature infants. Loss of appetite in the older infant is of no value at such an early age. If hemolysis and anemia are present and erythroblastosis fetalis can be ruled out, the infant should be considered to have an infection until proved otherwise. This possibility demands careful investigation into the maternal, delivery, and postpartum history; careful examination and bacteriological cultures taken from the blood stream or other suspicious areas as well as prompt institution of appropriate antimicrobial therapy are also mandatory. A third occasional source of anemia at this age is a hereditary red cell defect such as spherocytosis, and glucose 6-phosphate dehydrogenase deficiency (see Chap. 16).

Table A22-1. *Differential Diagnosis of Pediatric Anemias and Pallor According to Their Frequency*

Cause	0–7 days	1 wk–3 mo	3 mo–2 yr	2–6 yr	Over 6 yr
Blood loss	+ + +	+	(±)	(±)	(±)
Blood destruction	+ + + +	+ + + +	+ +	+	+
Production failure	—	+	+ + + +	+	+ + +
Bone marrow replacement	—	—	+	+ + + +	+ + +

Failure of red cell production does not occur in the first weeks of life, and anemia secondary to bone marrow replacement, such as that seen in congenital leukemia or reticuloendotheliosis, is exceedingly rare at this age.

The First 3 Months

Hemolysis is the major cause of anemia. In infants with maternal-fetal blood incompatibility, the incompatibility may be recognized early; however, if the infant is not exchange-transfused, so that the original problem of unremoved circulating antibodies remains, or if the infant is exchange-transfused with adult donor blood having a lower hematocrit value than that of the infant, these factors may lead to moderately severe anemia. Crises due to hereditary hemolytic processes may occur even this early in life. Of more significance is the large number of young infants who suffer hemolysis associated with infections, usually of the lungs or genitourinary tract. Particularly in the latter case the infectious process may be missed until the child becomes extremely pallid from the anemia. For practical purposes, in this age group it is possible to ignore the anemias secondary to failure of blood production or bone marrow replacement. Except under the most unusual circumstances of depleted maternal iron stores, multiple pregnancies, and prematurity, the infant under 3 months of age does not show anemia due to iron deficiency. Tumors and leukemia are also very rare at this early age.

From 3 Months to 2 Years

Blood loss in subjects between the ages of 3 and 24 months is uncommon except from a Meckel's diverticulum. Nevertheless, the stools must always be examined for gross or occult blood in anemic patients. The congenital hemolytic anemias are present at birth and can be recognized if one searches for them; crises are usually associated with infections, making the hemolytic process more overt. In this age group acute acquired hemolytic anemia secondary to infection is not uncommon. Hemolytic-uremic syndrome may be one of the consequences of infection.

The most significant cause of anemia in this age range continues to be pure iron deficiency. The amount of iron in the body ready for incorporation into newly made red cells may be greatly reduced if the infant was premature or born of a mother with depleted iron stores caused by multiple pregnancies, bleeding, or poor diet. When the infant with a poor iron reserve fails to eat foods rich in iron, iron-deficiency anemia results. Even in the presence of adequate

iron storage, the infant who is not given a diet containing iron may become deficient. Premature infants are most prone to this difficulty, as they are born before the end of the third trimester, during which they normally secure the bulk of their iron stores. In addition, the growth of the premature infant is exceptionally brisk during the first year of life, and because the blood volume must parallel this growth spurt, there has to be adequate iron to fill the rapidly increasing red cell mass. Milk contains little bioavailable iron; supplemental food and, possibly, iron may be needed. Rarely do children suffer from such severe protein deficiency that they are unable to make adequate red cell precursors. Deficiency of vitamins, such as vitamin B_{12}, folic acid, and vitamin C, must be considered a possible cause of anemia in certain areas of the world. The incidence of malignancy in children up to 2 years of age remains moderately low.

From 2 to 6 Years

As seen in Table A22-1, a marked shift in the cause of anemia occurs in this age group. Whereas in the first 2 years of life stress is placed on loss or destruction of blood, and later on the lack of proper nutrients for normal, healthy blood production, in children over 2 years of age these factors become less important. The hereditary hemolytic processes should already have been recognized in infancy; the acquired hemolytic states are uncommon, but the ingestion of drugs, sprays, poisons, chemicals, and so forth must nevertheless be considered as a possible cause of sudden hemolysis. Unless mentally deficient or unable to obtain the proper nutrients for socioeconomic reasons, children over 2 years do not usually acquire dietary iron deficiency. If an iron-deficient picture appears, one must search very carefully for slow, chronic, unsuspected blood loss. Simple investigation for intestinal parasites is often rewarding.

The bone-marrow-replacement diseases cause many of the anemias seen in the preschool child. Of these the prime offender is acute leukemia. Lymphosarcoma, lymphoma, metastatic neuroblastoma, and metastatic Wilms' tumor constitute some of the other important causes.

The School Child

In the child of school age, the peak incidence of acute leukemia has been passed and the incidence of most malignancies is on the downgrade. Blood loss is indeed to be considered as a cause of anemia in menstruating adolescent girls, and iron replacement is to be considered even in the absence of overt anemia when iron deficiency is suspected on clinical (e.g., poor school performance) or laboratory tests. The hemolytic anemias (particularly of the congenital variety) should long since have been diagnosed. Acquired hemolytic anemias are rare, but occasionally an acquired autoimmune hemolytic process is seen in a child. Hemolysis may occur secondary to lupus erythematosus, rheumatoid arthritis, or leukemia but seldom does so. One expects adequate production of red cells at this age, and an ample dietary intake. Statistically, however, one finds the chief cause of anemia in the school child to be inadequate red cell production secondary to metabolic disorders or diseases of other organs. Therefore, a careful search must be made for underlying disease such as chronic infection, collagen disease, uremia, endocrine disturbances, or inflammatory bowel disease.

In this age range a complete failure of production of red cells as well as other blood elements may be seen. A small percentage of these children may have Fanconi's type of aplastic anemia, in which there are associated congenital defects and a late-appearing aplasia of the bone marrow. The larger number of cases of aplastic anemia are idiopathic in etiology, although they may be due to drugs, toxins, or poisons, which must be diligently sought for and eliminated. Diagnosis in the anemic school-age child demands scrutiny for underlying disease.

Mohsen Ziai and Ali Akbar Velayati

References

Miller, D. R., Pearson, H. A., Bahner, R. L., and McMillan, C. W. (Eds.). *Smith's Blood Diseases of Infancy and Childhood* (5th ed.). St. Louis: Mosby, 1989.

Nathan, D. G., and Oski, F. A. (Eds.). *Hematology of Infancy and Childhood* (3rd ed.). Philadelphia: Saunders, 1987.

---

23. Bleeding and Purpura

The preliminary investigation of a suspected bleeding disorder is neither difficult nor expensive. Because it does require both a venipuncture and bleeding time in order to be comprehensive, however, it should be reserved for appropriate circumstances.

Questions about recurrent epistaxis are probably the most common ones asked of pediatricians concerning bleeding. In the absence of other features such as a positive family history, a past history of some other bleeding manifestation, or the physical presence of extensive bruises or petechiae, the likelihood of a bleeding disorder is extremely remote. Similarly, a history of easy bruisability without any significant family or past history, and without petechiae or deep hematomas, does not usually warrant a bleeding investigation except in the infant.

A strong family history of bleeding or bruising does merit a screening evaluation, especially in males. A past history of hemarthrosis, bleeding following tonsillectomy and adenoidectomy, post-dental-extraction bleeding, unexplained hematuria, or umbilical stump bleeding warrants evaluation. Questioning should try to establish any relationship between aspirin ingestion and bleeding events.

Preoperative screening should be strongly considered when one is planning potentially hazardous major surgery such as cardiac or CNS surgery, or operations known to be bloody such as tonsillectomy and adenoidectomy or scoliosis repair. Patients should be advised against taking aspirin for 10 days before surgery and, if possible, all the other drugs listed under Disorders of Platelets and Blood Vessels, page 315.

Petechiae should always be investigated immediately, as should a spontaneous deep hematoma or a sudden cluster of unexplained fresh bruises. Child abuse is probably a more common cause of these than all the congenital and acquired coagulopathies combined.

Screening Tests

1. Platelet count is normal if 200,000 to 400,000/mm^3 and abnormal if below 175,000/mm^3.
2. Bleeding time should be determined by the Ivy or template method on the forearm. Ear-lobe bleeding time is inaccurate and potentially dangerous. Normal is up to 9½ minutes. The bleeding time should not be measured if the platelet count is below 100,000/mm^3, as it is always prolonged. It is prolonged if there has been any aspirin ingestion within 8 to 10 days. Patients should be warned to avoid aspirin prior to having a bleeding time or specific platelet function test.
3. Prothrombin time (PT) is normal at approximately 12 seconds; laboratories run daily controls. A prolongation up to 2 seconds beyond control is acceptable.
4. Partial thromboplastin time (PTT) is normal at approximately 37 seconds; laboratories may vary. Any prolongation beyond the upper limit should be investigated further.
5. Factor XIII assay (clot stability test) should be undertaken on children with umbilical stump bleeding or bleeding in association with poor wound healing.

Specific Tests

1. Platelet function tests have variable laboratory normals. They should be done if the bleeding time is prolonged without exposure to antiplatelet drugs (see Disorders of Platelets and Blood Vessels, page 315). Decreased aggregation to epinephrine, ADP, or collagen suggests an unknown drug effect or a congenital platelet dysfunction.

2. Fibrinogen assay is normally greater than 0.200 g/100 ml. It should be done if the PT or PTT is prolonged, or disseminated intravascular coagulation (DIC) is suspected.

3. Fibrin split products should be determined if there is any suspicion of DIC. Several different assays are available, with normal being 0 to 1 : 4. Titers 1 : 8 or higher suggest DIC or some other (rare) cause of increased fibrinolysis.

4. Factor VIII coagulant activity test should be done if PTT is prolonged; normal is 60 to 150%. If DIC is suspected, a decreased factor VIII is confirmatory. The test is diagnostic of hemophilia A or von Willebrand disease. It may be placed in a ratio with factor VIII antigen to determine carrier status of hemophilia (VIII:C/VIII:Ag is approximately 0.5) or to differentiate hemophilia (VIII:C/VIII:Ag is very low) from von Willebrand disease (VIII:C/VIII:Ag is approximately 1.0).

5. Factor IX, XI, and XII assays are done if PTT is prolonged and PT is normal. A subcategory of factor XII, Fletcher factor, may be assayed if the above are normal.

6. Factor VII assay is called for if PT is prolonged and PTT is normal.

7. Factor X, Factor V, prothrombin, and fibrinogen are assayed if PTT and PT are prolonged and a deficiency in the common pathway is suspected.

8. Inhibitors to factors VIII, IX, and XI may be assayed if a patient with any of the hemophilia syndromes fails to respond to an adequate infusion.

9. Lupus anticoagulant can be assayed in a patient with nonspecific systemic disease, a prolonged PT or PTT, but no bleeding.

10. Thrombin time measurement is a less common and indirect method of determining the availability of fibrinogen or the presence of heparin. The heparin effect may be nullified by measuring the reptilase time.

11. Clot lysis test is used when a high titer of fibrinolysin is suspected. The euglobulin lysis test is more sensitive.

12. Antithrombin III, protein C, and protein S assays are done if hypercoagulability is suspected.

The abnormalities of the screening tests seen in the clinical context should give a good indication as to which specific tests provide a definitive conclusion. When a hereditary disorder is suspected, testing of other family members sometimes provides a clearer answer than tests on the propositus.

John T. Truman

---

24. Obesity

Obesity is the most frequent nutritional disturbance in children of the advanced countries and causes much disability. Many obese children feel embarrassed about their appearance and become emotionally disturbed. They may develop flatfeet and knock-knees. Gross obesity may interfere with normal cardiorespiratory mechanisms and lead to the pickwickian syndrome (alveolar hypoventilation, arterial hypoxia, polycythemia, right-sided heart failure, and somnolence). The obese infant carries a greater risk of becoming an obese child than does the infant of normal weight, and the obese child is more likely to become an obese adult. Coronary disease, hypertension, diabetes, and cholecystitis are more frequent in the obese adult, and gross obesity is associated with shortened life expectancy.

Pathogenesis of "Simple" Obesity

Though obesity results when caloric intake persistently exceeds requirements, the cause of the condition is rarely simple. Genetic factors are important, but it is usually not possible to distinguish their effects from those of the environment. For instance, an increased familial incidence of obesity may result from genetic factors, but equally may reflect the family's eating habits.

Psychological Factors

Psychological factors are important. The hypothalamus, which plays a central part in appetite regulation, is under the influence of the cerebrum. Psychological factors influence food intake as well as physical activity. Several psychological mechanisms play a role. Parents may regard a good weight gain in their children as evidence of health and fail to recognize when it is becoming excessive. Some mothers compensate for guilt feelings by overfeeding and overprotecting their children. The giving of food then becomes synonymous with the giving of love. Other mothers, feeling the need to keep their children closely attached to themselves, attempt to maintain this close relationship by bribing the child with delicacies and sometimes even prevent them from taking part in sports. They may keep them away from school for inadequate reasons. In the child who feels unloved, overeating may result from a need for oral gratification or from the wish to gain parents' approval and regain their love.

Physical Inactivity

Low calorie expenditure is as important as high caloric intake in causing the energy imbalance. The hypothalamic appetite-regulating mechanism functions best over a limited range of physical activity. When this is reduced below a certain minimum, the caloric intake is likely to increase rather than decrease. In wealthy countries, children nowadays tend to be physically less active, and in many overweight children inactivity is remarkable. Physical inactivity may result from cerebral palsy, primary muscle disease, meningomyelocele, or severe mental retardation. Long periods of confinement to bed predispose to obesity. Once children have become overweight, the accumulation of fat further limits their activity, and they may feel too shy to take part in games.

Diet

Though overweight children eat more than they require, they do not necessarily eat more than other children of their age, sex, and height who are not overweight. The concept of nutritional individuality must be kept in mind; it implies that the same amount of food may not be enough for one child and too much for another of the same age. Real gluttony—that is, eating excessively by any standard—is probably an infrequent cause of childhood obesity.

The possibility that primary metabolic factors play a role in the etiology of obesity continues to be investigated.

Effects of Overnutrition

Overnutrition not only causes excessive deposition of depot fat but also accelerates growth in height, skeletal maturation, and the onset of puberty. The misconception that obesity in boys is frequently associated with delayed or incomplete pubertal development arises because the base of the penis is

Table A24-1. Differential Diagnosis of Obesity

Cause	Mechanism responsible for obesity	Clinical findings	Investigations
"Simple" obesity	Usually multifactorial: diet, environmental, psychogenic, physical inactivity (habit or enforced), genetic	Height usually above average; early onset of puberty; striae, particularly in adolescent	None usually required
Cushing's syndrome and prolonged administration of corticotropin, hydrocortisone, or analogues	High levels of glucocorticoids, gluconeogenesis	Height usually below average; "moon" facies, "buffalo hump," hirsutism, plethoric skin, acne, striae; hypertension	Bone x-ray (osteoporosis); glucose tolerance (impaired); levels of corticosteroids in blood and urine (high); tests of adrenal-pituitary axis
Hypothalamic lesions	Gross disturbance of appetite-regulating centers	History of meningitis, encephalitis; symptoms of increasing intracranial pressure; hydrocephalus; papilledema; visual-field defects; sexual infantilism	Skull x-ray (suprasellar calcification in craniopharyngioma); brain scan, studies of other hypothalamic functions
Prader-Willi syndrome	Probably hypothalamic disturbance	Short stature, mental retardation, typical facies, small scrotum, undescended testes	Chromosome analysis
Glycogenoses (during first 2 yr of life obesity is a frequent finding)	Hypoglycemia leading to voracious appetite, gluconeogenesis	Height usually below average; hypoglycemic attacks; hepatomegaly	Fasting hypoglycemia; lactic acidosis; confirmation by enzyme studies

surrounded by rolls of fat and the organ, therefore, appears small. Overnutrition stimulates adrenocortical activity; therefore, striae and a mild degree of hypertension are frequent findings, especially in the adolescent.

Differential Diagnosis

The diagnosis of "simple" obesity is easy and can usually be made on clinical grounds (Table A24-1). A child whose weight is more than 20% above the average for normal children of the same age, sex, and height is likely to be obese as long as edema and unusual muscular development, such as occurs in athletes, can be excluded. Measurement of skinfold thickness with calipers is useful in confirming the presence of excess fat. If the child is above average height for age and neurological signs, papilledema, and marked hypertension are absent, a confident diagnosis of "simple" obesity can be made.

When the child is below average height, primary endocrine and metabolic disturbances such as hypothyroidism, Cushing syndrome, pseudohypoparathyroidism, and the glycogenoses need to be considered. Obesity is not invariable in any of these conditions. In Cushing syndrome the typical "moon face" and "buffalo hump" over the shoulders may suggest the diagnosis.

Gross lesions of the hypothalamus, such as craniopharyngioma, are rare causes of obesity and should be considered when there are symptoms of increased intracranial pressure and lcoalizing signs such as visual-field defects and papilledema. Excessive thirst, somnolence, and failure of pubertal development may also occur.

In the Prader-Willi syndrome, hypotonia, feeding difficulties, and slow weight gain in early infancy are followed by the onset of obesity. Other features of the syndrome are mental retardation, short stature, and an abnormally small scrotum with failure of testicular descent. The condition occurs in both sexes, but the diagnosis is more difficult in girls. Kyphoscoliosis and diabetes mellitus may develop, and the obesity may become gross and shorten life. The condition may be associated with an abnormality of chromosome 15.

Otto H. Wolff

References

Keller, S. R. Obesity. In M. Ziai (Ed.), *Bedside Pediatrics*. Boston: Little, Brown, 1983.

Lloyd, J. K., and Wolff, O. H. Obesity. In D. Hull (Ed.), *Recent Advances in Paediatrics,* No. 5. London: Churchill Livingstone, 1976. P. 305.

25. *Abnormal Sexual Development*

Normal Sexual Development

Normal embryological sexual differentiation into one of the two typical sexes (male and female) is dependent on the following.

1. Normal sex chromosomal components from the time of fertilization — that is, XX (female) or XY (male). Two X chromosomes are required to sustain differentiation of the ovary. Testicular differentiation is dependent on the H-Y antigen, present on the surface of all male cells, and the product of testis-inducing genes. These genes probably reside within a small section of the Y chromosome, although certain inconsistencies imply that the genes may be on the X or on autosomes and that the genes in the Y may be regulatory.
2. Normal development of the gonadal anlage occur during the first weeks of embryogenesis and further differentiation of this bipotential gonad, which contains both medulla (testicular) and cortex (ovarian). This occurs about the eighth week of fetal life.
3. Normal development of the internal duct system into male structures (wolffian structures) requires the presence of normal fetal testicular tissue with special secretions to produce male differentiation. The fetal testis secretes a polypeptide hormone called the müllerian inhibiting factor (MIF). This substance obliterates the müllerian structures. Development of the wolffian structures depends on the testosterone secretion by the fetal testis around 10 to 11 weeks. In the presence of ovarian fetal gonads or the absence of gonads, the female internal system (müllerian) necessarily predominates, with formation of fallopian tubes, uterus, and upper vagina, and generally the female phenotype.
4. Normal development of the external genitalia is from the urogenital sinus and surrounding structures. Fusion occurs, with enlargement of the genital tubercle and formation of the penis and penile urethra, under the influence of fetal testicular secretion in the normal male (or other anomalous virilizing hormones). In response to testosterone and DHT, the genital tubercle enlarges to form the penis and penile urethra. The masculine differentiation of the external genitalia is dependent on cytosol receptors

for testosterone within the cells and on dihydrotestosterone (DHT), which is produced within the cells of this region by the action of a specific 5-alpha-reductase on testosterone. In the absence of testosterone and DHT the urogenital sinus remains open, with slight evagination, to form the normal female external organs.

Abnormal Sexual Development

Disturbances in the above order of events leads to abnormal sexual development, with the presence of ambiguous genitalia at birth. The ambiguity is of variable degree and conformity to one sex or the other may be very close. Indeed, in some forms of "intersex" the sexual structures may be virtually identical to the normal male or female structure but at variance with the basic chromosomal and gonadal sex (i.e., the phenotypic sex may not be particularly ambiguous). The levels of disturbance are as follows.

Abnormalities of Sex Chromosomes

If the chromosomes are other than XX or XY, normal gonadal differentiation may not occur; there may be variable malformations of the genital ducts. Numerous abnormal combinations of sex chromosomes may occur, varying from XO (absence of one sex chromosome) to XXX and XXXXY or combinations wherein one of the sex chromosomes is abnormal in structure (as by partial deletion, or because of isochromosomes of the long or short arms). In the presence of a single Y, regardless of other chromosomal abnormalities, gonadal differentiation is likely to be testicular and the sex structures male, although the testes may not be entirely normal in structure or function at the time of puberty. In various combinations of X, as in XO without a Y chromosome, sexual differentiation is female except that normal gonadal tissue is almost entirely absent.

Abnormalities of Gonadal Differentiation

In true hermaphroditism, all other factors, including sex chromosomes, are often normal, but — for unknown reasons — the gonads do not develop in one direction. Both ovarian and testicular elements are present; the genital structures are likely to be ambiguous, although at times they may strongly resemble the structure of one sex or the other. In some male fetuses the testes, which otherwise are apparently entirely normal in appearance, do not secrete the fetal androgen.

Abnormalities of Hormones

When other factors are normal, unusual and contradictory hormones may conflict with the basic sex — especially in the female human fetus exposed to androgenic hormones. The possible sources may be exogenous androgens or some progestins administered to the mother; maternal tumors that secrete androgen during pregnancy; and congenital adrenal hyperplasia in the female, in which fetal adrenal cortex secretes abnormal androgens that affect development of the external genitals. The reverse situation is most rare in male fetuses with this condition; the gonads and chromosomes are in agreement with the basic sex, and the internal genital organs are not affected.

Intersex

The most common forms of intersex are classified as follows.

Chromosomal Intersex

The principal form is known as gonadal dysgenesis (Turner syndrome) and is accompanied by an XO sex chromosome component. The phenotypic sex is almost always clearly female, with normal external genitalia and a uterus. The expected clinical features are short stature, edema, hypertension, webbed neck, "doll" facies, high-arched palate, and failure of secondary sexual development. The diagnosis is confirmed by chromosomal karyotyping. At the time of puberty, estrogen levels remain low; gonadotropin levels are elevated. In so-called mixed gonadal dysgenesis there may be remnants of testicular tissue. In this form of the disease the essential cytogenetic lesion is mosaicism, including an XO stem and another stem with a Y. While the internal structures are predominantly female, in a few instances there is a mixture with the male. The external genitalia are variable, sometimes resembling those in females with clitoromegaly and at other times very much male. There is likely to be virilization at the time of puberty in such cases, and the incidence of malignancy in the gonadal remnant is high.

In the phenotypic male, the usual form is XXY (Klinefelter syndrome). The external genitals are normal. Gynecomastia may occur at puberty, testicular biopsy reveals seminal tubule fibrosis, and sterility is the rule. Different degrees of mental retardation may be present. Variants of this syndrome include XXXY and other more complicated abnormal combinations of sex chromosomes. The buccal smear is usually positive, denoting a double X as well as a Y chromosome; it may be doubly positive, as in XXXY.

True Hermaphroditism

True hermaphroditism is rare and can be diagnosed only by gonadal biopsy. The sex chromosomes are usually normal and most often XX. There are no recognizable hormonal abnormalities until later life, when either androgens or estrogens may predominate, depending on the major gonadal elements present (if they function). The external as well as the internal genital structures are likely to be ambisexual. Examination of the gonads in true hermaphroditism has shown that the testicular elements contain the male-determining H-Y antigen whereas the ovarian components do not.

Hormonal Intersex

If all elements are normal for clear sex differentiation, the female fetus may have been inundated by inappropriate masculinizing hormones. The most common cause is congenital adrenal hyperplasia, which can be diagnosed by markedly elevated levels of serum 17-OH progesterone in the usual form of the disease. Only in this form of human intersexuality are these hormonal disturbances to be found. The female with this condition shows a normal XX karyotype. The male is usually normal at birth with respect to the genital organs, and there is no ambiguity, except in some rare forms of congenital adrenal hyperplasia due to 3-hydroxysteroid dehydrogenase deficiency and 17-hydroxylase deficiency. In these forms the male may not have achieved completely masculine differentiation of the external organs. In either sex there may be a salt-losing tendency with vomiting, leading to severe dehydration during the first weeks of life. This disorder can be properly recognized only by hormonal studies. Another helpful differential feature is that progressive virilization occurs only in this disorder; it continues after birth, and there is early appearance of sexual hair, rapid growth, and advanced bone age.

The female fetus may develop ambiguous external genitalia if the mother has taken drugs such as testosterone or progesterone during pregnancy. The history is essential in making the diagnosis. Serum hormonal studies on the infant are always normal, and the karyotype is normal XX. This condition is never progressive after birth.

Failure of the fetal testis to secrete the MIF would lead to the persistence of female internal structures (e.g., uterus) in an otherwise male individual. Failure of the fetal testis to secrete testosterone as a result of a number of specific enzymatic defects leads to incomplete male differentiation.

Another example of incomplete male differentiation of the external genitalia is the result of defective 5-alpha-reductase. At birth the subject has a bifid scrotum and a blind vaginal pouch, but the wolffian structures are well developed and there is no uterus. Strangely, in this condition at the time of puberty definite virilization occurs, and contrary to the usual effect of rearing as girls there is often a change to male gender identity.

Testicular Feminizing Syndrome

This is a condition in which the subject has a normal male chromosome XY complement and morphologically normal testes, but the external genitalia are female. The fetal testes have functioned properly but have not induced the usual male differentiation of the genital tract due to testosterone "resistance" of the fetal cells. This "resistance" is due to absence of cytosol receptors for testosterone within the fetal cells or to a cytosol-testosterone complex that fails to translocate to the appropriate chromatin sites within the nucleus. This condition is seldom recognized at birth. Frequently the testes are palpable as inguinal masses; therefore, this condition needs to be considered in any newborn female with palpable inguinal masses. At puberty the individual has normal female breast development due to conversion of testosterone to estradiol. Sexual hair does not develop due to the testosterone and androgen resistance. There is a blind vaginal pouch. The uterus is absent because the fetal testes normally secrete müllerian inhibitary factor (MIF), which suppresses the müllerian elements. There are partial forms of this syndrome.

Assignment of Sex

The most serious mistakes in human medicine concern incorrect sex assignment in the presence of ambiguous external genitalia. In some of the conditions cited above, such as gonadal dysgenesis or Klinefelter syndrome, there is no ambiguity. The most grievous mistake is to assign the male sex to a female whose external genitalia may resemble male structures. This attribution can occur in female adrenal hyperplasia; it may also happen when the abnormal appearance of the genitalia is due to maternal exposure to exogenous virilizing hormones during pregnancy. It is essential in such a female to recognize the correct sex by chromosomal karyotyping if possible, x-ray examination of the internal genital structures by injection of dye into the external orifice, and urinary hormonal studies. Female children with this condition have the full potential for female life, including reproduction, after simple corrective surgery. Medical treatment with cortisone is also indicated in congenital adrenal hyperplasia and may be lifesaving for the affected neonate. This possibility must always be kept in mind. The most common and most drastic errors originate from hasty decisions made on the basis of appearance of the external genitalia alone. The above studies should be carried out by experts in this complex field.

In cases of true hermaphroditism, it is wise to raise the child within the sex that the external genitalia most closely resemble. In difficult cases of this latter type, the decision to raise the child as a female is more practical.

Kathleen M. Link

References

Brook, C. G. D. *Clinical Pediatric Endocrinology.* Boston: Blackwell, 1989.

Kaplan, S. A. *Textbook of Pediatric Endocrinology.* 1989.

William, R. H., Wilson, J. P., and Foster, D. W. (Eds.). *Textbook of Endocrinology.* Philadelphia: Saunders, 1985.

26. Sexual Delay and Precocity

Problems of idiopathic delayed adolescence and of early secondary sexual development are frequently referred for endocrine consultation. Although usually benign, they are distressing to the patient and parent because of the psychological disturbance engendered by the patient's age-mates, who ridicule and tease the child who is physically "different."

The mechanisms responsible for normal adolescence are largely unexplained although they are under intense investigation and the timing of the hormonal events has been described in detail. *Adrenarche* (or pubarche) refers to the adrenal component of adolescence, the mechanism of which is also not explained. The adrenal is the principal source of androgens in the female.

In girls secondary sexual development normally begins between 8 and 13 years. The usual sequence is breast development followed by growth of sexual hair and then menarche. In about 10% of girls the appearance of hair may be first. Menarche usually occurs between 12 and 13 years (range, 10 to 16 years) and is best correlated with osseous maturation ("bone age"). Growth in height is usually only 5 to 10 cm in the majority (75%) of normal girls after menarche.

In males the first sign of puberty is testicular enlargement ($\geq$ 2.5 cm). Normally the appearance of secondary sexual characteristics takes place between 9 and 14 years. Linear growth commonly continues until 19 to 21 years. Over the centuries there has been a tendency toward taller stature and earlier adolescence in both boys and girls. Since 1840, menarche has averaged about 4 months earlier each decade.

Delayed Adolescence (see Table A26-1)

Males and females:

1. Hypopituitarism — may be idiopathic or caused by intracranial lesions (i.e., craniopharyngioma)
2. Hypothyroidism

Table A26-1. Investigation of Delayed Adolescence

Procedure	Comment
Height measurement	Short stature with normal growth rate ($\geq$ 2 in/yr) in normal patient with simple delayed adolescence; short stature with decelerating growth rate in hypopituitarism, hypothyroidism, and chronic malnutrition; short stature with normal or subnormal growth rate in Noonan's, Prader-Willi, and Turner's syndromes, etc.
Bone age	Delayed in simple delayed adolescence; more marked delay relative to height age in hypopituitary and hypothyroid conditions; bone age variable in above syndromes
Buccal smear	Abnormal in Klinefelter's, Turner's syndromes
Karyotyping	Necessary to detect Turner's mosaic
Circulating gonadotropins by radioimmunoassay	Elevated with gonadal insufficiency
Skull x-ray	May reveal craniopharyngioma

3. Chronic malnutrition (i.e., celiac disease, anorexia nervosa) (Crohn's disease)
4. Noonan syndrome — superficially similar to Turner syndrome, but normal buccal smear and normal karyotype for sex likely; features common to Noonan syndrome as opposed to Turner's: right-sided cardiac lesions, ptosis, proptosis, pectus carinatum, cryptorchidism, and mental retardation.
5. Kallman syndrome — anosmia associated with hypogonadotropic hypogonadism; most reported cases in males.
6. Familial delayed adolescence — usually a family history for delayed adolescence in the father or mother or both.

Males:

1. Testicular atrophy in utero or testicular hemorrhage or torsion at or after delivery — may result in prepubertal castration
2. Klinefelter syndrome — occurs in about 1 in 500 live-born phenotypic males; gynecomastia at adolescence a feature
3. Reifenstein's syndrome — hypospadias associated with the absence of virilization and presence of gynecomastia at adolescence
4. Prader-Labhart-Willi syndrome — obesity associated with short stature (patients with exogenous obesity usually tall, with slightly advanced bone age and sexual development); hypotonia in infancy and mental retardation associated with hypogenitalism and development of diabetes
5. Laurence-Moon-Biedl syndrome — also associated with obesity and mental retardation: retinitis pigmentosa and polydactyly or syndactyly also seen in this heredofamilial condition
6. Fertile eunuchs — have active spermatogenesis despite inadequate Leydig cell function

Females:

1. Turner syndrome — occurs in 1 out of 2000 live-born phenotypic females; clinical recognition of typical XO patients easy; mosaic forms offer less or even no chance of clinical recognition; karyotype in order for all otherwise unexplained short girls and in delayed adolescence, particularly when sexual hair appears and persists without evidence of secondary sexual estrogen effect
2. Ovarian atrophy — may be associated with the polyglandular syndrome (hypoparathyroidism, Addison and Hashimoto diseases, and moniliasis)
3. Ovarian atrophy or removal — may also be secondary to torsion surgical removal

In males the great majority of patients have normal but delayed adolescence. Some patients tolerate this psychologically; others become disturbed. The latter can be helped by receiving a temporary acceleration. Testosterone enanthate, 100 mg, can be given for 4 to 6 months without diminishing ultimate height potential.

Early Adolescence

Premature thelarche is fairly common in prepubertal girls. Clinically, unilateral or bilateral breast development occurs. This benign condition is not associated with rapid growth or bone age advancement. In about one-third of patients the condition disappears, in one-third it is stationary, and it may progress in the remainder. It is important to follow the patients to separate the condition from the earliest manifestations of sexual precocity. The LRF stimulation test discriminates between premature thelarche and precocious puberty in the majority of patients.

Premature adrenarche (pubarche) consists in early appearance of pubic hair without other evidence of virilization, and with mild elevation of serum dehydroepiandrosterone sulfate and mild advance in height age and bone age. It must be separated from late onset congenital adrenal hyperplasia and virilizing tumors.

Sexual Precocity (Appropriate Secondary Sexual Development for Sex) (see Table A26-2)

In either sex the ingestion of sex hormones or medications contaminated with sex hormones must be ruled out. Often there is a family history in idiopathic cases. Previous encephalitis or meningitis can advance or delay adolescence. Hamartoma of the tuber cinereum and other CNS space-occupying lesions (neurofibroma in the area of the optic chiasm) may be asymptomatic and discovered only at autopsy. In general, lesions of the posterior hypothalamic area are associated with sexual precocity, while those of the anterior portion cause sexual infantilism. Pinealoma causes sexual precocity in boys more often than in girls. The lesion may destroy the capability of the pineal to produce a substance that would ordinarily inhibit gonadotropin release. Inexplicably, hypopituitarism has been reported with sexual precocity.

In males the production of chorionic gonadotropin by hepatomas has been reported. Testicular Leydig cell tumors and virilizing adrenal adenomas and carcinomas have been

Table A26-2. Investigation of Sexual Precocity

Procedure	Comment
Height measurement and bone age x-ray	Normal in premature thelarche; slight advance with premature adrenarche; marked advance with sexual precocity
Pelvic sonogram	Usually reveals presence of feminizing ovarian tumors or benign ovarian cysts
Neurological; retinoscopic; visual-field examination	May reveal CNS lesion (paralysis of upward gaze with pinealoma; visual field cut with optic neurofibromatosis)
Circulating gonadotropins by radioimmunoassay	Elevated or normal with idiopathic variety; elevated chorionic gonadotropin with chorionepithelioma or hepatoma in males
Circulating or urinary sex hormones	Elevated for age; very high levels of estrogen with granulosa cell tumor
LRF test	Injection of LRF (2.5 mcg/kg; max. = 100 mcg). Measure LH and FSH at 0 min, 30 min, 60 min. Pubertal vs. prepubertal response.

responsible. The enzymatic deficiency form of congenital virilizing adrenal hyperplasia (21-hydroxylase; non-salt-losing type) is a frequent cause. A familial precocious puberty in males also occurs, which is thought to be due to "autonomous" functioning of the testes.

In females granulosa cell tumors have accounted for many cases. Although usually palpable, in several reported cases the tumor was small and was not initially detected. Serum radioimmunoassayable estrogens are generally very high and circulating gonadotropins low. Theca cell tumors and choriocarcinoma are less frequent. Feminizing adrenal tumors are rare. Interestingly, primary hypothyroidism has been found in association with sexual precocity and galactorrhea, all of which were reversible with thyroid treatment. In the McCune-Albright syndrome precocious puberty appears to be caused by cyclic autonomous functioning of the ovaries.

Despite the many pathological lesions associated with sexual precocity, it is estimated that 90% of cases in females and 50% in males are idiopathic, "centrally mediated" (i.e., gonadotropin-dependent) precocious puberty. The luteinizing hormone releasing hormone (LHRH) analogs (LHRHa) have been effective in arresting the progression of secondary sexual characteristics in patients with gonadotropin dependent precocious puberty. Early investigations also indicate that LHRHa treatment may improve the adult stature of children with precocious puberty. Currently, use of LHRHa for treatment of precocious puberty is approved for investigational use only.

Treatments for gonadotropin independent forms of precocious puberty, i.e., puberty associated with McCune-Albright syndrome and familial male precocious puberty, are also under investigation. Testolactone and spironolactone have been effective in short-term studies.

Mohsen Ziai and Kathleen M. Link

References

Brook, C. G. D. (Ed). *Clinical Pediatric Endocrinology*. Boston: Blackwell, 1989.

Pescovitz, O. H. and Cutler G. B. Premature thelarche and central precocious puberty: The relationship between clinical presentation and the gonadotropin response to LHRH. *J. Clin. Endocrinol. Metab.* 67:474, 1988.

Wilkins, L. *The Diagnosis and Treatment of Endocrine Disease in Childhood and Adolescence* (3rd ed.) Springfield, Ill.: Thomas, 1965.

William, R. H., Wilson, J. D., and Foster, D. W. (Eds.) *Textbook of Endocrinology*. Philadelphia: Saunders, 1985.

27. Skin Eruptions

One of the most common pediatric problems is the differential diagnosis of a skin rash. At times it is difficult even for an experienced clinician to choose one of the many etiological possibilities with certainty, and surely it is impossible for us to include all of them in this brief presentation.

An important consideration in any child with a skin eruption is that of a drug reaction, as well as allergic or contact dermatitis. The reader is urged to keep these possibilities constantly in mind. Although we have not included them in Table A27-1, certain comments on drug eruptions are in order.

Table A27-1. *Differential Diagnosis of Common Infectious Exanthems*

Disease	Early symptoms	Eruption			Diagnostic procedures
		Character	Site	Duration of eruption	
Chickenpox	Mild; fever and malaise for less than a day	Crops of macules evolving to papules, vesicles, and crusts	Hairline, face, trunk, proximal extremities, and mucous membranes	1–2 wk	All stages of lesions are present simultaneously in any anatomical area
Erythema infectiosum (fifth disease, Boston exanthem)	None; children appear to be healthy	Intense erythema on face with circumoral pallor; symmetrical maculopapular reticulated rash on extremities	First on face, next day on extensor surfaces of extremities, and 3 days later on flexor surfaces, distal extremities, trunk, and buttocks	3–10 days	Flushed face in an asymptomatic 2- to 12-yr-old; rash may recur at variable intervals
Infectious mononucleosis	Fever, exudative pharyngitis, lymphadenopathy	Rashes occur in approximately 20% of cases, usually but not always maculopapular; rash may be brought about by administration of ampicillin	Mainly trunk; extremities rarely involved	Variable	Atypical lymphocytes, splenomegaly, high titer of heterophil antibodies; liver function tests, possible CSF changes
Enterovirus infections (may present as hand-foot-and-mouth disease) Coxsackie Types 5, 16	Vesicular stomatitis	Maculopapular progressing to vesicular	Buttocks, hands, and feet	3–4 days	Viral studies
Types 2, 4, 9, 16, 23	Nonspecific febrile illness	Variable, usually maculopapular	Variable	3–4 days	Viral studies
ECHO viruses	Fever, upper respiratory and gastrointestinal symptoms; possible aseptic meningitis with type 9	Maculopapules either discrete or confluent; rarely petechial; nonpruritic	Face and neck; then spreading to shoulders, trunk, and extremities	2–8 days	Isolation of virus or rising antibody titers

Table A27-1. (Continued)

Disease	Early symptoms	Eruption Character	Eruption Site	Duration of eruption	Diagnostic procedures
Exanthem subitum (roseola infantum)	3 or 4 days of high, spiking fever, which returns to normal by crisis; occipital lymphadenopathy	Discrete macules appearing as temperature returns to normal	Usually found on chest and trunk, but may spread to extremities and face	Several hours to 2 days	White cell count low
German measles (rubella)	Mild; fever for less than a day; lymphadenopathy in posterior auricular and occipital regions	Discrete measles-like rash on first day; scarlet-fever-like rash on second day, fading on third day	Begins on scalp, face, and neck; rapidly spreads to trunk and extremities	3 days	Rising antibody titers; in the neonate stigmata of the congenital rubella syndrome; viral studies if necessary
Lyme disease	After an incubation of 3–32 days from the tick bite, the typical progression of erythema chronicum migrans as well as fever, CNS, arthritic, and cardiac problems at later stages	Red macule at the site of tick bite expanding as an erythematous, marginated lesion with a clear center (erythema chronicum migrans)	At the site of the tick bite, expanding later	Variable	Culture of *Borrelia* and serologic studies
Measles (rubeola)	3 to 5 days of fever, cough, conjunctivitis, and coryza; Koplik's spots	Discrete maculopapules become confluent in areas of extensive and early involvement	Begins on hairline, face, and neck, spreading to trunk and extremities; disappears in the order of appearance	5–6 days	Rising antibody titers
Meningococcemia	Fever of sudden onset, chills, generalized pain, possible meningeal signs, vomiting	Purpuric or petechial lesions; may begin as maculopapules	Generalized	Variable	Gram stain and culture of skin lesions and body fluids
Rickettsialpox	A papular primary lesion progresses to a vesicle and then an eschar; followed within a week by fever and other symptoms	Tiny vesicles upon firm papules; lesions eventually crust	Generalized, but usually spares soles and palms	5–10 days	Rising titer of complement-fixating antibodies

Staphylococcal scalded skin syndrome (SSSS)	Erythematous scarlatiniform rash in infants and young children followed by exfoliation particularly around the mouth; intense tenderness of the skin	Generalized erythema which resembles scalding with the peeling of the skin (and Nikolsky's sign particularly around the mouth and in flexures)	Periorbital edema and later on cracking of the skin in this area characteristic	Variable	Tissue histology of separated epidermis differentiates it from toxic epidermal necrolysis; culture of *S. aureus* from portal of entry
Rocky Mountain spotted fever	3 or 4 days of usually sudden fever, chills, headache, and muscle pain	Erythematous maculopapules; become hemorrhagic in 1 or 2 days	Appears first on distal parts of extremities, spreading centrally; palms and soles may become involved	2–4 wk	History of tick bite, rising titer of complement-fixing antibody; Weil-Felix reaction
Scarlet fever	Fever, chills, pharyngitis, and vomiting; several hours' to 2 days' duration	Diffuse, erythematous, punctate, blanchable eruption over the body; face is flushed with circumoral pallor; Pastia's sign	Appears first on flexural surfaces, becomes generalized within 48 hr; lesions are most prominent on skin folds, creases, and pressure areas	7–10 days	Clinical evidence of an acute streptococcal or staphylococcal infection; strawberry tongue and exudative pharyngitis
Toxic shock syndrome	Malaise, fever, vomiting, dizziness, "sunburn rash," postural hypotension	Scarlatiniform rash followed by desquamation	Diffuse	Variable	Demonstration of toxin producing staphylococci
Toxoplasmosis	Weakness and malaise for about 1 wk followed by fever, pneumonia, rash (lymphadenopathy, chorioretinitis, encephalitis, etc.)	Maculopapular	Generalized, sparing palms and soles	Variable	Dye test for measurement of neutralizing antibodies or presence of complement-fixing antibodies
Typhoid and paratyphoid fever	Fever, chills, headache, gastrointestinal complaints	Discrete, rose-colored spots; blanching with pressure	Trunk, especially abdomen	3–5 days for each crop	Isolation of organism from stool or blood culture; relative bradycardia is suggestive
Typhus fever	4 to 6 days of high fever, chills, headaches, and generalized pains	Blanchable, maculopapular lesions become petechial	First appears on trunk, then spreads to extremities, sparing face, palms, and soles	2–3 wk	Endemic area; complement-fixing antibodies; Weil-Felix reaction

1. They are caused primarily by anticonvulsants, sulfonamides, and antibiotics, although many other substances, including the antipyretics, antimetabolites, and even antihistamines, may occasionally cause drug eruptions.
2. Although the most common type of drug eruption is maculopapular, resembling measles or scarlet fever, all types of lesions can occur including vesicles, urticarial wheals, and acneiform lesions. Mucous membranes may also be involved (Stevens-Johnson syndrome) (see p. 451).
3. A meticulous and thorough history almost always leads to the discovery of the responsible agent. When in doubt, one must withdraw all medications or possible allergens to elucidate the cause
4. There is no typical finding in drug eruption; even the same drug may produce various clinical manifestations.

Several dermatoses and systemic illnesses such as Kawasaki disease may also resemble the infectious exanthems (Table A27-1). Again, a thorough history and follow-up study of the patient usually clarifies the problem. The reader is referred to the chapter on skin disorders as well as larger texts for further study. Further specific infections are discussed in greater detail elsewhere in the text.

Ali Akbar Velayati, Mohsen Ziai, and Nancy B. Esterly

References

Aicardi, J. *Epilepsy in Children — International Review of Child Neurology.* New York: Raven, 1986.

Dreifuss, F. E. *Pediatric Epileptology.* Boston: John Wright–PSG, 1983.

Swaiman, K. F. *Pediatric Neurology — Principles and Practice.* St. Louis: Mosby, 1989.

Volpe, J. J. *Neurology of the Newborn — Major Problems in Clinical Pediatrics* (2nd ed.). Philadelphia: Saunders, 1987. Vol. 22.

Appendix B

Emergencies, Trauma, and Poisoning

Proper management of emergencies in pediatric practice requires immediate access to certain materials and equipment (Table B-1). Such equipment includes suction apparatus, a laryngoscope, endotracheal tubes, and oropharyngeal airways in infant and child sizes. Also needed are cutdown trays, scalp vein needles, syringes and needles of various sizes, assorted types of parenteral fluid solutions, plasma, whole blood, corticosteroids, epinephrine, atropine, and parenteral antibiotics. A dose chart of the drugs commonly needed for pediatric emergencies should also be readily available (Table B-2).

The physician must formulate an organized approach in order to deal effectively with emergencies. The following procedures must be carried out in virtually all pediatric emergencies. Conduct the physical examination swiftly while the salient features of history are being obtained from the informant. Record the vital signs, including blood pressure. Pay careful attention to proper airway and positioning of the patient to avoid suffocation and aspiration of vomitus. Evacuation of the stomach by nasogastric tube suction helps and can prevent aspiration of gastric contents in unconscious patients with impaired airway protective reflexes.

(Acute gastric distension in traumatized children [secondary to aerophagia] can compromise diaphragmatic function and air exchange.) Assess the adequacy of ventilation by observing chest wall expansion and by auscultation of breath sounds. Assess the adequacy of circulation by verifying the presence of palpable pulses and the quality of peripheral perfusion with capillary refill time less than 2 seconds. In febrile patients, search for the presence of petechiae (especially on hands, feet, and conjunctivae). Check the anterior fontanel in infants. A sunken anterior fontanel is a good indication of dehydration, while a bulging firm fontanel indicates intracranial hypertension secondary to meningitis, subdural or other hematomas, hydrocephalus, or cerebral edema. Look for bleeding in nose, ears, or mouth. Assess the patient's level of consciousness and note the presence or absence of meningeal signs. The heart, lungs, and abdomen must always be examined. The patient must be weighed nude whenever possible. A weight estimation chart (see Table B-2) is useful for initial management in acute life-threatening emergencies. Drug and fluid dosages are guided by body weight, and response to therapy may be later assessed by change in body weight. Draw enough blood for

Table B-1. Equipment Guidelines According to Age and Weight

Equipment	Premie (1–2.5 kg)	Neonate (2.5–4.0 kg)	6 Months (7.0 kg)	1–2 Years (10–12 kg)	5 Years (16–18 kg)	8–10 Years (24–30 kg)
			Age (50th percentile weight)			
Airway—oral	Infant (00)	Infant/small (0)	Small (1)	Small (2)	Medium (3)	Medium/large (4/5)
Breathing						
Self-inflating bag	Infant	Infant	Child	Child	Child	Child/adult
O₂ ventilation mask	Premature	Newborn	Infant/child	Child	Child	Small adult
Endotracheal tube	2.5–3.0 (Uncuffed)	3.0–3.5 (Uncuffed)	3.5–4.0 (Uncuffed)	4.0–4.5 (Uncuffed)	5.0–5.5 (Uncuffed)	5.5–6.5 (Cuffed)
Laryngoscope blade	0 (Straight)	1 (Straight)	1 (Straight)	1–2 (Straight)	2 (Straight or curved)	2–3 (Straight or curved)
Suction/stylet (F)	6–8/6	8/6	8–10/6	10/6	14/14	14/14
Circulation						
BP cuff	Newborn	Newborn	Infant	Child	Child	Child/adult
Venous access						
Angiocath	22–24	22–24	22–24	20–22	18–20	16–20
Butterfly needle	25	23–25	23–25	23	20–23	18–21
Intracath	—	—	19	19	16	14
Arm board	6"	6"	6"–8"	8"	8"–15"	15"
Orogastric tube (F)	5	5–8	8	10	10–12	14–18
Chest tube (F)	10–14	12–18	14–20	14–24	20–32	28–38

Source: L. Chameides (Ed.). Textbook of Pediatric Advanced Life Support. Dallas: American Heart Association, 1988. P. 105. By permission of the American Heart Association, Inc.

Table B-2. Resuscitation Medications, by Weight and Age, for Infants and Children 0 to 10 Years

Age	50th Percentile weight (kg)	Epinephrine		Atropine		Bicarbonate*	
		mg	ml	mg	ml	mEq	ml
Newborn	3.0	0.03	0.3	0.1	1.0	3.0	6.0
1 Month	4.0	0.04	0.4	0.1	1.0	4.0	8.0
3 Months	5.5	0.055	0.55	0.11	1.1	5.5	11.0
6 Months	7.0	0.07	0.7	0.14	1.4	7.0	7.0
1 Year	10.0	0.10	1.0	0.20	2.0	10.0	10.0
2 Years	12.0	0.12	1.2	0.24	2.4	12.0	12.0
3 Years	14.0	0.14	1.4	0.28	2.8	14.0	14.0
4 Years	16.0	0.16	1.6	0.32	3.2	16.0	16.0
5 Years	18.0	0.18	1.8	0.36	3.6	18.0	18.0
6 Years	20.0	0.20	2.0	0.40	4.0	20.0	20.0
7 Years	22.0	0.22	2.2	0.44	4.4	22.0	22.0
8 Years	25.0	0.25	2.5	0.50	5.0	25.0	25.0
9 Years	28.0	0.28	2.8	0.56	5.6	28.0	28.0
10 Years	34.0	0.34	3.4	0.68	6.8	34.0	34.0

Volume (ml) is based on the following concentrations:
  Epinephrine—1 : 10,000 (0.1 mg/ml)
  Atropine—0.1 mg/ml
  Bicarbonate—≤ 3 months = 4.2% solution (0.5 mEq/ml)
          > 3 months = 8.4% solution (1 mEq/ml)
* The use of bicarbonate in cardiac arrest is controversial. Good ventilation must be established before bicarbonate is used.
Source: L. Chameides (Ed.). *Textbook of Pediatric Advanced Life Support*. Dallas: American Heart Association, 1988. P. 103. By permission of the American Heart Association, Inc.

typing and crossmatching at the same time that the initial blood specimen is obtained for such key measurements as hematocrit, pH, electrolytes, blood sugar, and serum calcium levels. Empiric treatment with glucose and naloxone is appropriate in convulsive patients. Unless a properly secured intravenous needle is easily placed, it is often necessary to perform a saphenous vein cutdown. In cases of trauma, control any external bleeding, splint fractures, and administer tetanus prophylaxis. Repeated evaluation of the patient's condition constitutes the most important principle in the management of trauma.

It is essential to develop proficiency in pediatric techniques. Learn how to begin intravenous infusions and how to obtain blood from small infants. Become proficient in intubating with a laryngoscope and endotracheal tube. Know how to perform mouth-to-mouth resuscitation and how to administer closed cardiac massage. These are truly lifesaving techniques and must be mastered by anyone dealing with children. In learning them, develop an attitude of calmness, assurance, and technical proficiency while working under pressure.

Causes and Prevention

In most areas of the world, accidents and poisonings are the leading causes of death in children over the age of 1 year. In the United States approximately 23,000 deaths a year in children under 14 are caused by accidents, and there are 100 to 150 times as many serious injuries from the same causes.

Physicians must concern themselves not only with providing the best possible treatment in these accidents but also with taking the lead in preventing them.

Motor Vehicle Accidents

Efforts are being made by many groups to curb the increasing carnage from motor vehicle accidents. Early education of children in the dangers of driveways and streets must be reinforced by firm discipline continuously applied by parents throughout childhood. Adequate driver education in high schools, disciplined behavior of young passengers, and insistence on the use of safety belts can reduce injuries to motor vehicle occupants. For infants, the use of approved car seats is strongly urged from birth onward and is legally mandated in many states. The conduct of a teenage driver is a corollary of his past home training and sense of responsibility. For these reasons, family guidance by the physician over the years can play a vital role in accident prevention.

Fires, Explosions, and Burns

Many agencies are working toward methods of fireproofing children's clothing, Christmas trees, and other flammable materials. Two-thirds of young children fatally burned sustain the injury at a time when there is no adult in the home. Many burns result from careless play in proximity to open flames. These facts emphasize the need for constant supervision of young children by a responsible adult.

Falls and Drownings

Another frequent source of danger — falls — can be eliminated by removal of hazards (toys and so forth, carelessly left about) in the home and by the use of gates at the tops of stairways. Infants and toddlers most often drown in unguarded outdoor pools and water-filled washtubs or basins indoors during unsupervised moments. Drowning and other water accidents can be reduced in older children and adolescents by early instruction in swimming, lifesaving, and resuscitation and by insistence on responsible behavior in swimming areas. Legislation to require fences with self-closing gates surrounding all private residential swimming pools, preventing access from within or without the house, is a political priority with pediatricians concerned about water safety.

Acute Traumatic Injury

The following is a brief consideration of acute traumatic injury with particular reference to intrathoracic and intraabdominal injuries. Acute head injuries (see Chap. 14) and fractures (see Chap. 15) are discussed elsewhere. The following general principles apply to the early management of serious visceral trauma.

Injuries are often multiple, especially following motor vehicle accidents and falls from a height. Serious internal injuries may be associated with minimal external evidence of trauma to the overlying skin and muscles. The presence of shock in a child with obvious acute head injury almost always indicates severe trauma elsewhere. In the absence of external bleeding, signs of occult injury within the chest or abdomen must be rigorously sought. Tension pneumotho-

rax and hemothorax often accompany visceral trauma and can mask serious upper abdominal trauma. The stomach is more likely to be ruptured if the child has eaten recently. Sharply circumscribed blows (e.g., impact with post, ball bats, stair rails, steering wheels) are most likely to cause injury directly beneath the site of impact, while crushing injuries (child run over by moving vehicle or pinned under a falling object) are more likely to injure fixed intraabdominal structures at a distance from the site of impact. Initial blood loss cannot be accurately estimated, and internal hemorrhage may continue undetected; therefore, clinical evidence of circulatory sufficiency is the most important guide to the adequacy of transfusion and fluid resuscitation. Easily palpable pulses, rapid capillary refill in the distal extremities, and resolution of tachycardia indicate adequate cardiac output. Adequate urinary output (0.5–1.0ml/kg/hour) is the most reliable clinical index of adequate circulation and should be measured hourly. The usual error is undertransfusion. Excessive transfusion results in increased venous pressure, which is most easily detected by engorgement of the neck veins or enlargement of the liver. When in doubt about the need for further fluid resuscitation, place a catheter for measurement of central venous pressure. Unless the value is elevated (i.e., > 10 mm Hg), further fluid administration is indicated in the presence of clinical signs of low cardiac output.

When the severely injured child is first seen, the following order of procedure is recommended: (1) Establish a patent airway, followed by cardiopulmonary assistance as needed; (2) type and crossmatch blood; (3) start intravenous fluids and transfusion of blood to combat shock; (4) empty stomach and begin continuous nasogastric suction; (5) control external hemorrhage; (6) splint fractured limbs; (7) administer tetanus prophylaxis for penetrating wounds; (8) begin serial recording of vital signs; and (9) examine for evidence of tension pneumothorax and hemothorax — these injuries are frequent in trauma to the trunk and require immediate relief by closed drainage through a thoracotomy. Whenever doubt exists, diagnosis can be confirmed be needle aspiration through the chest wall. Upon completion of these emergency procedures, it is vital for the physician to obtain a detailed history of the accident and to make frequent complete physical examinations of the patient, looking particularly for localizing signs. An accurate history provides important clues to the types and sites of injuries sustained.

The immediate course of the patient following laceration of liver or spleen depends on whether the laceration carries through the capsule of the organ at the time of injury. The splenic capsule is more easily lacerated than the hepatic capsule. Once the capsule is lacerated, there is rapid exsanguination into the peritoneal cavity, and immediate laparotomy is required as well as simultaneous transfusions through multiple sites until the bleeding is controlled on the operating table. Subcapsular lacerations of liver and spleen progress more slowly and may give rise to progressive anemia and organ enlargement. Nonoperative management, with intensive monitoring of vital signs and organ size, may be acceptable in the absence of progression and in the presence of a good response to initial resuscitative measures.

Immediate operative repair is indicated for rupture of a hollow viscus (stomach, intestine, bladder, ureter). Persistent, severe abdominal tenderness and pain rather than pneumoperitoneum are the early signs of rupture of the intestinal tract. Rupture of the bladder may be suspected by the presence of urine in the peritoneal cavity and persistent hematuria. It is seen particularly in association with pelvic fractures.

Retroperitoneal bleeding, laceration of the pancreas, and mesenteric avulsion are usually the result of crushing injuries. They cause profuse and prolonged bleeding and diffuse signs of peritoneal irritation. They should be suspected particularly when there is difficulty in restoring and maintaining the circulation.

In cases of intraabdominal and thoracic trauma, the patient's best interests are served by prompt operative intervention. Each of the following is a valid indication for immediate exploratory laparotomy in suspected trauma: (1) continued blood loss without obvious source, as indicated by difficulty in restoring and maintaining circulation and basal urine output; (2) four quadrant peritoneal taps positive for blood, urine, or air; (3) evidence of peritoneal irritation; (4) abdominal mass or organ enlargement; and (5) persistent abdominal tenderness and pain. Negativity of these signs does not preclude serious intraabdominal injury. For example, four quadrant abdominal taps may be negative in subcapsular laceration of a solid viscus, retroperitoneal hemorrhage, or simple failure to recover the fluid with a needle. The patient's general condition may make it impossible to demonstrate peritoneal irritation or abdominal pain and tenderness. The decision for early operation must therefore be based on a comprehensive evaluation of both the accident and the patient's course immediately thereafter. Undue emphasis must not be given to the presence or absence of any particular physical signs or laboratory findings.

The management of acute renal trauma is considered separately because early operation is indicated only in the presence of massive bleeding, and renal function is best conserved by nonoperative intervention. Massive bleeding is usually indicated by a rapidly enlarging flank mass and rapid deterioration due to shock. If nephrectomy is contemplated, intravenous pyelography is essential prior to operation to make certain that a functioning kidney is present on the contralateral side. Even after a period of conservative management, subtotal or total nephrectomy may still be necessary; however, in a number of cases recovery takes place without removal of kidney substance.

Child Abuse and Neglect

Intentional physical abuse by adults is a significant cause of injury, disability, and death in young children. The "battered child syndrome" encompasses a variety of physical injuries suffered by children at the hands of their caregivers, often in a setting of social instability resulting from mental strife, financial distress, drug and alcohol abuse, or mental illness. Children with congenital malformations, prematurity, or hyperactivity are at increased risk.

Children presenting with traumatic injury secondary to abuse can be identified by characteristic clinical findings (Table B-3) or by suspicious parental behavior, such as a delay in obtaining medical care, harsh or punitive manner, or failure to maintain adequate preventive care through regular well-child checkups and immunizations. The history given by the caregiver is often incompatible with the nature of the injuries.

Child neglect may present with malnutrition, chronic recurring or inadequately treated illnesses, or a high frequency of accidental injuries because of poor supervision.

The clinician must maintain a high level of surveillance and suspicion for child abuse and neglect and is legally mandated to report it to child protection authorities when it

Table B-3. Clinical Manifestations of Child Abuse

Behavioral	Fearful behavior in the presence of the perpetrator, withdrawn, sad affect, decreased activity
Physical Finding	Retinal hemorrhages with chronic subdural hematoma (shaken baby syndrome)
	Unkept appearance of child
	Circular (cigarette) burns
	Scalding injury of buttocks and perineum
Radiographic	Multiple fractures of varying ages
	Bucket handle fractures
	Chronic subdural hematomas

552

is suspected. Hospitalization with involvement of a comprehensive health care team including social workers, physicians, nurses, child life workers, nutritionists, psychologists, and occupational and physical therapists is often indicated in suspected child abuse or neglect. Because many such cases require court-directed remedies, including removal from the custody of the parents, the physician must be prepared to serve as a legal witness. Only through such comprehensive intervention will the suffering of the hundreds of thousands of abused and neglected children in America be reduced.

Thermal Injuries

Burns may be caused by heat, electricity, or caustic substances. The resultant injury may vary from simple erythema to a third-degree burn, which includes damage to both superficial and basal layers of the dermis. In deep dermal injuries there is considerable loss of plasma constituents at the burn site. Some of this fluid escapes from the body, but a much larger portion is sequestered at the site of injury.

Certain practical points in relation to thermal injuries in children require emphasis:

1. It is common to underestimate the severity of burns in children. Infants, in particular, should be admitted to the hospital with all but the most trifling burns.
2. When the area of burn exceeds 5% of the body surface, the risk of shock is significant, and hospitalization is mandatory.
3. All burns of the face, hands, feet, and genitalia require hospitalization.

FIRST-AID MANAGEMENT. A burned child is wrapped in clean cloth and transported to the hospital. A burned limb may be wrapped with plastic sheeting. Speed is of utmost importance to prevent shock. On arrival at the hospital the need for endotracheal intubation is assessed. The upper airway is most liable to injury in smoke inhalation, blasts, and burns of face, neck, and upper thorax. An indwelling catheter in the bladder is often needed to monitor urinary output. At this time fluid requirements for the first 48 hours are estimated.

FLUID THERAPY. The fluid losses that occur in burns are (1) obligatory burn edema, (2) insensible losses, and (3) extrarenl losses (e.g., vomiting). Obligatory burn edema accumulates rapidly in the injured tissue during the first 12 hours. Subsequently, accumulation of fluid is slower, and the point of maximal sequestration is reached 48 to 96 hours after the injury. Thereafter the sequestered fluid is resorbed, and, in the presence of good renal function, it is completely

delivered by the end of the first week. During the period of edema resorption, parenteral fluid administration must be limited to maintenance requirements. As much as one-half of the patient's extracellular fluid volume can be sequestered in severe burns. By the seventh day of treatment a 5 to 10% weight loss but no more may be tolerated. Ideally, early hyperalimentation should induce a modest weight gain by the end of the first week. Pulmonary burns or tracheostomy increase insensible water losses. Flame burns tend to produce less burn edema than scalds.

The amount of edema fluid sequestered is closely related to that body-surface area (square meters) sustaining second-degree and third-degree burns. The area burned (square meters) is equivalent to the child's total surface area (square meters) multiplied by the percentage burned (%). The child body-surface area is determined from nomograms on the basis of weight and height, and the percentage of area sustaining second-degree and third-degree burns is estimated according to charts such as the one shown in Figure B-1. In calculating fluid and transfusion requirements, one must never estimate a burned area as more than 50% of total body surface. During the first 24 hours, calculate replacement at a rate of 4 ml/kg/% burn given as Ringer's lactate. Give one-half of this during the first 8 hours and the other half during the remaining 16 hours after the burn. Calculate from the actual time of burning, not the time of arrival in hospital.

NUTRITION. Early hyperalimentation substantially improves prognosis and in a number of cases may obviate the need for later grafting.

MANAGEMENT OF BURN AND CONTROL OF INFECTION. The initial therapy of a burned patient must include adequate sedation by morphine or meperidine. Tranquilizers should never be used as they may complicate the management of shock. Adequate tetanus prophylaxis should be provided. The prophylactic use of antibiotics remains controversial; however, bacteriological studies on admission and periodic surveillance cultures of burn wounds and the nasopharynx are not controversial. Parenteral administration of prophylactic antibiotics initially for short duration may be undertaken at the physician's discretion.

Caustic Substances

Caustic substances are fixed to tissue upon contact and may cause chronic scarring and strictures. The principal injuries are to the eye and esophagus. Ingestion also results in burns of the oropharynx and stomach. The severity of the injury is more dependent on the concentration of the substance than on the amount ingested. Because they cause penetrating

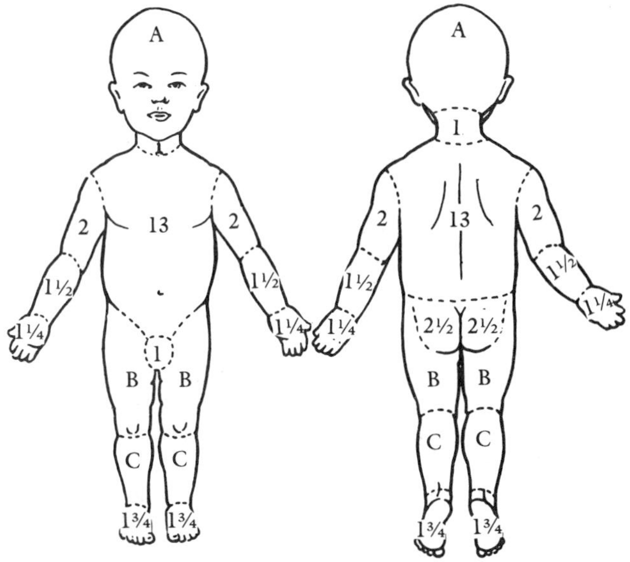

Area	Age 0	1	5
A = ½ of head	9½	8½	6½
B = ½ of one thigh	2¾	3¼	4
C = ½ of one leg	2½	2½	2¾

Fig. B-1. *Relative percentages of areas affected by growth. (From C. C. Lund and N. C. Browder, The estimation of areas of burns.* **Surg. Gynecol. Obstet.** *79:356, 1944. By permission of* **Surgery, Gynecology & Obstetrics.)**

injuries that usually include the muscular layer, alkaline salts cause the more serious disability. Any chemical compound with a pH greater than 8 can cause caustic burns. Severe corrosive injury of the esophagus usually causes severe pain in throat and chest, fever, leukocytosis, and excessive salivation within a few hours, so that diagnosis is not difficult. Death, when it occurs, is usually the result of mediastinitis and empyema. The treatment of severe esophageal burns is prolonged, difficult, and beyond the scope of this text. Less severe caustic burns can also lead to esophageal stricture and thus give the greatest difficulty in diagnosis. The mouth and pharynx may initially be free of burns. Chronic stricture in such cases can be prevented by prompt diagnosis and early institution of therapy. Careful esophagoscopy very soon after the ingestion offers the best means of detecting the presence of burns early. When this is not available, esophageal bougienage should be started within 48 hours and

continued for 10 to 14 days. By the tenth to fourteenth day, early narrowing of the esophagus can be detected by x-ray with barium swallow. Corticosteroid administration in small doses (2.5 mg hydrocortisone/kg/day or equivalent) can prevent lesser burns from producing strictures, if begun within a few hours of the injury. In such cases antibiotics should be given.

Stephen R. Keller and Thomas E. Cone, Jr.

Poisonings

Several hundred poison information centers are now located throughout the United States, Canada, and several European countries. These centers have ready access to current reference data on the toxicology of drugs and numerous household products. United States law requires that labels on containers of hazardous substances include the generic name, first-aid instructions, and other information that can facilitate speedy identification of the contents and institution of proper treatment in case of accident.

Most accidental poisonings occur in preschool children. Items ingested by children are frequently neither in their original containers nor in their customary storage places. All medicines and those household products that are quite toxic if ingested (i.e., corrosives, bleaches, polishes, and rodenticides) should be locked in special cabinets or stored in areas out of children's reach. Old medicines and household products should be discarded by flushing them down the toilet. The newer "palm and turn" safety closures (and strip packaging) for drugs are effective in limiting entry by small children and should be specified on prescriptions. The physician's role is to persuade the family to take the necessary precautions. Physicians should limit prescriptions to the amounts of medication required for immediate use only. The generic name of the drugs should appear clearly on all prescription labels to facilitate identification in case of accident.

The goals in the treatment of acute poisoning are fivefold: (1) identification of the material ingested; (2) removal of the noxious material from skin or intestinal tract; (3) inactivation of what cannot be removed from the gut (i.e., precipitation of ferrous iron with sodium bicarbonate instilled into the stomach following gastric lavage or induced emesis); (4) acceleration of the excretion of the portion absorbed; and (5) use of appropriate general supportive measures to counteract the toxic effects of the material until it is sequestered or excreted. Unfortunately, few specific antidotes are available. Prompt removal of the noxious material can greatly reduce morbidity and, in some cases, be lifesaving. To be effective some first-aid steps must be performed in the home before the child is transported to the hospital emergency room; for example, ingested caustic substances (lye, oven cleaner) are fixed to tissue virtually on contact so that effective inactivation can be accomplished only if milk or egg is given immediately to bind the material. Do not give acids. If caustic materials or substances that are absorbed through the skin (certain insecticides, phenolic derivatives, methyl salicylate) are spilled on skin, clothing, or eyes, the contaminated clothing should be promptly removed and the child should be copiously rinsed all over under running water, redressed in fresh clothing, and then brought to the emergency room.

Syrup of ipecac (30-ml bottles) is available in pharmacies in the United States without prescription. This drug may be used for prompt induction of emesis in the home, but only after consultation with a physician, poison center, or hospital. Attempting to induce emesis by placing a spoon handle or finger in the child's throat is almost uniformly ineffective.

Syrup of ipecac* is safe and usually effective, but the more concentrated fluid extract of ipecac must never be given. Induction of emesis by any method is contraindicated in unconscious or convulsing patients and following the ingestion of caustic substances or hydrocarbons. The effectiveness of syrup of ipecac is enhanced if its administration is immediately followed by administration of 100 to 200 ml of water.

The following are valid indications for gastric lavage: (1) removal of substances for which induced emesis is contraindicated (except caustics); (2) unconscious or convulsing patients; (3) failure of syrup of ipecac to empty the stomach; (4) removal of substances of unknown chemical composition; (5) instillation of binding or precipitating agents when indicated after lavage. Careful lavage with tap water is suitable in most instances; 50 to 100 ml of tap water should be introduced and withdrawn repeatedly until 1 liter is used. Gastric lavage is contraindicated after ingestion of caustics because it is ineffective and carries the risk of perforation of the esophagus. When hydrocarbons are removed from the stomach by lavage, a cuffed endotracheal tube should be placed to prevent aspiration.

Parents should be instructed to bring the material ingested by the child and its container to the hospital. Initial vomitus, urine, and blood should be saved until the need for chemical analysis is determined. The use of chelating agents, buffers, alkalinizing salts, and specific antidotes to hasten inactivation and excretion of toxic substances is highly selective and must be considered in relation to specific poisonings. Activated charcoal is particularly useful for binding alkaloids until removal by lavage. Charcoal binds ipecac and should not be administered until after emesis occurs. Cathartics are not generally necessary, and their use in young children may be negated by paralytic ileus or may complicate fluid and electrolyte therapy in the seriously ill. Therapeutic techniques must be judiciously employed since most drugs and procedures have inherent risks and so should be used only to the extent justified by the need in each case. For example, peritoneal dialysis and exchange transfusion are rarely indicated except in severe renal failure, so that a concerted effort should be made to restore renal excretory capacity before their use is contemplated.

A few of the more serious and common types of accidental poisoning in children are described briefly below. For detailed treatment protocols and further information on these and other intoxications the references at the end of

---

*The usual dose in a child 1 to 5 years of age is 15 to 20 ml repeated once if the child has not vomited in 15 minutes.

Appendix B should be consulted. In particular, physicians should acquaint themselves with the specific problems indigenous to their locale.

Aliphatic Hydrocarbons, Aromatic Hydrocarbons, Terpenes

Aliphatic hydrocarbons, as exemplified by kerosene, gasoline, and Stoddard solvent, are used as fuel for light, heat, and machinery, as components of paint thinners, dry-cleaning agents, and furniture and floor polishes, and as vehicles for pesticides. Benzene, xylene, and toluene typify the aromatic hydrocarbons; these compounds are found in paint removers, degreasing cleansers, lacquers, pesticides, airplane glue, and other plastic-binding products. Terpenes are the important toxic ingredients of turpentine and pine oil products and are most likely to be found in the home in paint thinners, paint and wax removers, and spot removers. Hydrocarbons of different classes may be found in the same products. The main toxic effects of all hydrocarbons are exerted on the lungs and central nervous system (CNS). Induction of emesis is contraindicated in all types of hydrocarbon ingestion, but cautious gastric lavage is indicated in terpene and aromatic hydrocarbon ingestion. Milk, oils, alcohols, and digestible fats must never be given as they may promote intestinal absorption of hydrocarbons.

Because aliphatic hydrocarbons are poorly absorbed from the gastrointestinal tract, ingestion and retention of several ounces are required to produce systemic toxicity. On the other hand, they are irritating to pharynx, esophagus, and stomach, and aspiration of a few milliliters into the lung can produce a fatal chemical pneumonitis, which is the principal toxic effect of this class of substances. Furniture polishes containing "mineral seal oil" deserve special comment for they produce a severe prolonged pneumonitis not unlike chronic lipoid pneumonia.

Aromatic hydrocarbons are readily absorbed by all routes including skin, lung, and gastrointestinal tract. The lethal dose of benzene by ingestion in adults is estimated at 15 ml. Because this class of substances is readily absorbed from the stomach, gastric lavage with tap water is indicated and may be followed by the instillation of mineral oil after the lavage returns are clear. The main acute toxic effects of aromatic hydrocarbons are upon the CNS, the heart, and, to a lesser extent, the pulmonary system. Aliphatic hydrocarbons cause CNS depression, but aromatic hydrocarbons cause CNS excitation followed by depression. Aromatic hydrocarbons can sensitize the myocardium to the effects of epinephrine with resultant ventricular fibrillation. Epinephrine and related compounds are, therefore, contraindicated. Toluene is usually the substance responsible for the toxic nervous system manifestations seen in adolescent "glue sniffers."

Terpenes are well absorbed via skin, gastrointestinal tract, and respiratory tract. The lethal adult dose by ingestion is estimated as 15 ml. Milk or other digestible fat must never be given in such cases, as it promotes absorption. Emesis is contraindicated, but gastric lavage with tap water should be carried out promptly in all cases, and mineral oil may be instilled via the tube following lavage. These compounds cause gastroenteritis and pulmonary and renal irritation, but their main toxic effect is depression of the central nervous system.

Iron Salts

Acute iron intoxication nearly always requires immediate hospitalization for proper therapy. The estimated lethal dose of ferrous or ferric iron is 0.3 g/kg of body weight, which is the amount of iron contained in three ordinary medicinal 5-grain ferrous sulfate tablets. Iron salts are absorbed throughout the gastrointestinal tract. Severe vomiting and diarrhea occur early and are often bloody. The vomitus often contains partially digested tablets. Teeth may be stained black. Considerable blood loss may result from widespread gastrointestinal hemorrhage. The onset of systemic manifestations (shock, hepatic injury, anuria) may be delayed for as long as 6 to 12 hours. Sometimes, after a brief period of apparent improvement, collapse recurs 24 to 48 hours after acute ingestion in severe cases. Emesis should be promptly induced, and this should be followed by lavage with sodium bicarbonate solution. Because ferrous and ferric carbonate are insoluble, a small amount of sodium bicarbonate should be instilled into the stomach following lavage. Administration of plasma, whole blood, and parenteral fluids is necessary for the prevention of shock and the correction of the systemic acidosis usually present. Deferoxamine, a chelating agent for iron, is highly useful both diagnostically and therapeutically.

Salicylate Poisoning

Salicylate is available in flavored pediatric tablets (75 mg), in standard adult tablets (0.3 g), and in solution as methyl salicylate (4.4 g/teaspoonful). Oil of wintergreen (91% methyl salicylate) constitutes the greatest hazard, because even 1 teaspoonful contains a potentially lethal dose. In a previously healthy child, acute ingestion of 200 mg/kg or more is likely to produce poisoning serious enough to require hospitalization. In a child with an intercurrent illness, a lesser dose can have the same effect.

In clinical practice, reliable estimates of dosage can rarely be obtained, so that serial serum salicylate levels are the most reliable predictors of severity, particularly after a single excessive ingestion. Done's nomogram, found in many therapeutic manuals, is useful in such cases. Serum salicylate is plotted against time after ingestion in this nomogram. Thus, a serum salicylate level of 80 mg/100 ml 4 hours after ingestion and a level of 60 mg/100 ml 12 hours after ingestion both portend severe and potentially fatal poisoning and indicate the need for prompt hospitalization. Because of the state of health of the child at the time of ingestion has an important bearing on the severity of intoxication produced by a given dose, these values should be scaled down when intercurrent illness is present. Even antipyretic doses can produce acute poisoning after a few days if given continuously to a sick child. In chronic poisoning, there may be little correlation between serum salicylate and severity. In such cases, clinical evaluation, the severity of acidosis, and particularly the presence of CNS manifestations (hyperirritability, hyperexcitability, coma, or convulsions) take precedence and call for prompt treatment. At the other end of the spectrum, falling or stable levels of serum salicylate of less than 30 mg/100 ml during the first 8 hours after ingestion in an otherwise healthy child usually mean little difficulty.

The metabolic effects of salicylate are complex. It stimulates the CNS and in particular the respiratory center, with resultant hyperventilation and reduction of plasma carbon dioxide tension (PCO_2). This effect is of less clinical import in children under 4 years of age because metabolic acidosis very quickly supervenes. A profound water loss can result from hyperventilation, diaphoresis, and vomiting. Both hypoglycemia and hypokalemia may occur. Not infrequently these symptoms are mistaken for pneumonia, bronchiolitis, or asthmatic bronchitis; the administration of more aspirin can lead to a fatal outcome in such cases. Unrecognized, salicylism proceeds eventually to coma and convulsions. Antipyretic doses of aspirin is a significant cofactor in Reye's syndrome. The drug is easily detected in urine and gastric aspirate with the ferric chloride test.

Lavage or induced emesis should be performed even many hours after ingestion, because absorption, although usually rapid, may be slow, particularly in the case of methyl salicylate. Following this, therapy is directed at correcting the metabolic aberrations, replacing the water deficit, and accelerating the excretion of the drug in the urine. In mild cases promotion of a water diuresis may be all that is required. At the other end of the spectrum, when renal failure supervenes or parenteral fluid therapy fails to reduce serum salicylate rapidly enough, peritoneal dialysis with 5% salt-poor albumin or hemodialysis may offer the only hope of survival. Most cases fall between these two extremes and respond to careful parenteral fluid therapy.

Barbiturates and Tranquilizers

Mortality from barbiturate intoxication results mainly from pulmonary complications (atelectasis and infection), cardiovascular collapse, and renal failure. It is not generally appreciated that barbiturate overdosage causes dilatation of the peripheral vascular bed, which is not responsive to epinephrine, and that the onset of shock may be delayed. Proper management must be aimed principally at the prevention of brain damage due to hypoxia. Oxygen is necessary. An open airway must be maintained, by tracheostomy if necessary. The circulation must be supported with fluids, plasma, and in severe cases levarterenol. Analeptics are usually useless and may be harmful in barbiturate intoxication. Osmotic diuresis with mannitol can hasten urinary excretion and reduce the period of coma. Mannitol is especially useful in barbital and phenobarbital intoxication because these drugs are eliminated almost entirely by the kidney. Alkalinization of the urine with sodium bicarbonate also increases urinary excretion of these drugs. Such steps are not so effective in the elimination of barbiturates that are handled mainly by the liver.

The same general principles apply in the treatment of poisoning due to numerous tranquilizers. This group of drugs can also cause hypotension so that levarterenol may be required to maintain the circulation. Similarly, the onset of hypotension may be delayed, postural in nature, and sudden in onset.

Lead Poisoning

There have been substantial reductions in exposures of the general population to environmental lead during the past decade. Concurrently, clinical and experimental research has revealed adverse health effects, particularly on neurodevelopment in the fetus and young child at blood lead concentrations (PbB) previously considered "safe." Exposures to the fetus associated with umbilical cord PbB levels greater than 10 μg/100 ml of whole blood, even in the absence of significant postnatal overexposure to lead, are significantly associated with impairment in mental development persisting to at least 2 years of age. Increase in integrated PbB levels during the first 3 years of life from 10 to 31 μg Pb/100 ml are significantly related to an average reduction in IQ at 4 years of age of seven points throughout the IQ range. From the public health viewpoint, the implication is as follows: for overexposed populations, there is a general downward shift in IQ with substantial reduction in the numbers of individuals with superior intelligence as well as a substantial increase in the number of individuals classified as mentally retarded. The main effect of lead on neurodevelopment is an increased incidence of short attention span, reading disability and impairment in auditory processing. Likewise, epidemiological studies show subclinical impairments of balance and growth rate. With the substantial reductions of lead in air, food, and water, average PbB in the United States population has decreased from 16 μg Pb/100 ml to an estimated 6 μg/100 ml during the past decade. It now appears that the most pervasive sources of overexposure to lead in the U.S. are exposure to particulate lead in surface soil, household dust, and lead paint in poor condition on older housing. An estimated 2.4 million preschool-aged children how have PbB greater than 15 μg/100 ml, including an estimated 200,000 with PbB in excess of 25 μg Pb/100 ml. An estimated 52% of currently occupied United States housing has lead paints on exposed interior and exterior surfaces. Where the paint is intact, this represents a potential hazard. Where the paint is defective and scaling, it represents an immediate hazard. The principal route of entry of lead from soil, dust, and paint is the hand-to-mouth route, which makes the preschool child the population group most sensitive to these sources because of the normally high level of hand-to-mouth activity during this age period.

The physician is likely to encounter children suspected of lead toxicity in two ways: (1) asymptomatic children identified in screening programs, and (2) symptomatic children in whom lead poisoning must be considered in the differential diagnosis. For asymptomatic children with moderately increased blood lead concentration (i.e., 15–50 or 60 μg Pb/100 ml), lead in soil, dust, and defective old paint in their home and play areas are the most likely sources of lead. Symptomatic lead poisoning is generally associated with some concentrated source of lead, such as excessive ingestion of lead paint or consumption of acidic foods and beverages from improperly lead-glazed ceramicware. The most important aspect of treatment is identification of the environmental source of lead for a particular child and separation of the child from that source. Children must be kept away from lead-contaminated soils. Wet housecleaning methods only should be used in order to suppress dust, because many lead-containing particulates are too small (less than 100 microns) to be trapped efficiently by standard vacuums. This is difficult in old deteriorated housing. When extensive renovations in old housing are undertaken, young children and pregnant women must live elsewhere. The diet should be reviewed. An appropriate diet is an adequate mineral, low-fat diet. Excessive milk intake should be avoided. Dietary deficiencies in iron, calcium, copper, and zinc, as well as excessive milk and fat intake, may enhance the absorption of lead from the intestinal tract. Occupational histories of all adults in the house should be obtained, as lead workers who wear their workclothes home may contaminate the dwelling with lead-bearing dusts. Cases of lead toxicity in young children have been traced to this source. In all cases, long-term follow-up throughout the preschool years is indicated, according to Centers for Disease Control (CDC) guidelines. Psychometric evaluation prior to entry to school is indicated to identify any learning handicaps that may require special educational attention. Blood lead and erythrocyte protoporphyrin measurements should be drawn with lead-free equipment and the samples analyzed in laboratories regularly carrying out these tests and performing successfully in blind interlaboratory proficiency testing programs, such as those sponsored by the CDC and laboratories approved by the Occupational Safety and Health Administration (OSHA).

Lead-pigment paints have already been mentioned as a "high dose" or concentrated source of lead. Such paints may contain 1 to 70% lead, so that tiny flakes hold a highly toxic dose. For example, a paint flake weighing 10 mg and containing 10% lead would provide an oral dose of 1000 μg Pb or at least 20 times the amount of lead normally consumed each day from food, uncontaminated water and usual ambient air. Balance studies show that a young child is in positive lead balance if the dietary intake of lead exceeds 5 μg Pb/kg/day. Other high-dose sources of lead that account for sporadic cases of symptomatic lead poisoning include ingestion of lead fishing weights, lead curtain weights, lead shot (which, if retained in the stomach, slowly dissolve), jewelry painted with lead to simulate pearl, inhalation (sniffing of leaded gasoline), use of oriental cosmetics and medicines (al kohl, surma), chewing of lead painted toys and cribs, use of lead nipple shields, ingestion of ashes from painted wood or storage battery cases, inhalation of fumes from burning battery casings in the home, use of improperly lead-glazed dishware, drinking of soft well water conveyed in lead pipes, and taking of certain folk medicines. When an index case traceable to one of these sources is found, cluster testing should be carried out to evaluate all others similarly exposed. Several of these high-dose sources have been associated with clinical illness ranging from colic to gross aggressive antisocial personality disorders to acute lead encepholopathy with coma or intractable convulsions. Untreated, acute lead encepholopathy has a mortality of 66%, while early recognition and modern chelation therapy can reduce the mortality to less than 2%. The risk of irreversible mental deficiency, chronic convulsive disorder and severe behavior disorder is great in survivors of lead encephalopathy. Permanent CNS sequellae may also follow recurrent colic. Because chelation therapy begun after the onset of symptoms probably does not reduce the occurrence of permanent sequellae, it is most effective if initiated on the basis of metabolic abnormalities in the preclinical stage.

Lead is a potent inhibitor of sulfhydryl enzymes. It produces important pathological changes as well as functional alterations in the brain, kidneys, bone, and hematopoietic system. It inhibits the formation of heme. Raised levels of heme precursors in blood (zinc protoprophyrin) and urine (coproporphyrin, delta aminolevulinic acid) provide metabolic evidence of toxicity in both the clinical and preclinical stages. Measurement of these metabolites facilitates preclinical diagnosis and intervention.

Lead poisoning usually has an insidious onset over a period of 3 to 6 weeks with anorexia, anemia, hyperirritability, incoordination, and the subtle loss of recently acquired skills. These symptoms often suggest a behavior disorder. They may also be erroneously attributed to iron deficiency anemia, which is commonly seen in young children with plumbism. In this regard, iron deficiency is associated with microcytic erythrocytes, whereas lead toxicity is not. As the disorder progresses, these symptoms intensify, gross ataxia may occur and the onset of acute encepholopathy is indicated by the appearance of signs of increased intracranial pressure (forceful and intractable vomiting, lethargy, stupor, coma, and convulsions). Infrequently, convulsions and coma occur without warning. Differential diagnosis must consider meningitis, encephalitis, and other causes of increased intracranial pressure (brain tumor, brain abscess). The peripheral neuropathy seen in adults is uncommon in children. One-half of the reported cases of peripheral neuropathy in children have been reported in those with sickle-cell disease. The so-called "lead line" sometimes found in the gums of affected adults is rare in children. Early recognition requires a high index of suspicion, as there are no pathognomonic abnormalities on either physical examination or the usual tests of blood and urine. Positive diagnosis requires specific laboratory tests, of which the most important is a blood lead concentration determined on venous blood and drawn with special lead-free needles and syringes and determined in a qualified laboratory. Recent experimental studies indicate that the calcium disodium EDTA mobilization test for lead is not without hazard, because a single injection of this drug in chronically poisoned rats results in an increase in brain lead. Detailed use of chelating agents is beyond the scope of this text, but may be found in the references listed at the end of Appendix B.

Summary

It is obvious from the foregoing discussion that there must be continuous effort in the area of prevention if the incidence of accidents and poisonings is to be reduced. Specifically, physicians can contribute a great deal by following these suggestions.

1. Make accident prevention a routine part of their regular health care.
2. Observe hazards in and around the house when on home calls and suggest corrective measures.
3. Give careful instructions when talking to the family and prescribing medications so as to reduce the risk of accidents, exposure to injurious agents, overdosage, and careless handling, or ready accessibility of harmful drugs to children.
4. Study the causes of medical emergencies and accidents, particularly where the involved individuals appear to be "accident prone"; the use of this knowledge with the family and others can help to prevent similar conditions in the future.
5. Emphasize ways to prevent accidents as well as to treat them in accident-case presentations before hospitals, medical societies, and medical students.
6. Assist health departments and other agencies in developing educational programs and community projects, such as poison information centers and distribution of health-education material illustrating the dangers of various types of accidents.

J. Julian Chisolm, Jr.

Management of Common Complaints Presenting as Emergencies

Although emergency room experience lends credence to the contention that parents are usually more frightened than their children are hurt, there are still a large number and variety of illnesses and injuries in infants and children that require immediate and urgent treatment. These guidelines are a compilation of recommendations intended to outline a systematic approach to the pediatric emergency room patient. They are *not* intended as dogma.

Acute Abdominal Pain in the Child and Adolescent

The evaluation of abdominal pain in the emergency department is challenging, in part because of the extremely large differential diagnosis, and because the history may be limited by the patient's ability to communicate.

DIAGNOSIS. Diagnostic evaluation begins with careful history-taking to characterize the nature, acuity, localization, and severity of the complaint, as well as any risk factors present for specific etiologies (e.g., sexually active adolescent female with abdominal pain may have ectopic pregnancy or pelvic inflammatory disease, commonly caused by *Chlamydia*).

Cautious but complete physical examination, beginning with the part of the abdomen of least concern to the child, is the cornerstone of differentiation between a surgical abdomen and a problem requiring medical management only.

Differential diagnosis is carefully reviewed in Appendix A (pages 479–546). Commonly required diagnostic studies in emergency department evaluation are:

1. Complete blood count (CBC), differential count, erythrocyte sedimentation rate
2. Urinalysis
3. Stool guaiac

Additional studies that may be indicated are:

1. Abdominal flat and upright radiographs
2. Chest x ray
3. Pelvic exam with endocervical cultures for *N. gonorrhea* and *Chlamydia trachomatis* and *Chlamydia* antigen detection
4. Pregnancy test (beta-HCG)
5. Barium enema and upper gastrointestinal series
6. Abdominal ultrasound

Anaphylaxis

Anaphylaxis is the most dangerous and serious manifestation of IgE-mediated allergy. The anaphylactic reaction most commonly occurs following allergenic extract injection in allergic children on desensitization programs. It may occur following a variety of exposures to drugs, food, stings, or inhalants. The symptoms of anaphylaxis are usually conjunctival and oral mucosal swelling, hypotension, laryngeal edema with stridor, and bronchospasm characterized by wheezing. Arrhythmias and cardiac arrest may occur especially in the hypoxic patient.

Treatment is as follows:

1. Oxygen is given by mask.
2. Epinephrine 1 : 1000, in a dose of 0.01 ml/kg (maximum 0.3 ml) should be given subcutaneously. The effect may be transient, and the dose can be repeated at 20-minute intervals. For severe reactions and shock, 0.1 ml/kg of 1 : 10,000 epinephrine should be administered IV.
3. The area of the offending injection or sting site may also be infiltrated with epinephrine to decrease absorption, and a tourniquet should be applied proximately.
4. Bronchospasm unresponsive to epinephrine should be treated with aminophylline, 5 mg/kg IV over 20 to 30 minutes. Nebulized aerosol beta-adrenergic bronchodilators may also be administered to treat refractory bronchospasm (e.g., albuterol, 0.02 ml/kg (up to 0.5 ml) diluted in respiratory saline 3.5 ml.
5. IV fluids are given as normal saline or plasma expanders to maintain blood pressure and perfusion.
6. Antihistamine in the form of diphenhydramine, 2 mg/kg IV or 5 mg/kg/day divided q6h by mouth, is administered for therapy of urticaria.
7. Steroids (prednisone 2 mg/kg PO or methylprednisolone 2 mg/kg IV) may be of help in later management of bronchospasm and should begin on admission to the hospital. Outpatient steroid therapy may also be useful.
8. Cardiac and respiratory monitoring should continue until the patient is out of danger.

Bronchial Asthma

In an asthmatic attack bronchospasm, mucosal edema, and mucous secretions result in bronchiolar narrowing, atelectasis, and impaired gas exchange. Usually the patients are hypoxic and may begin to retain CO_2 as well (the hallmark of respiratory failure). Anxiety and agitation often compound the physiological process, hypoxia occurs, leading to more agitation, and a vicious cycle is set up.

The evaluation should include a careful history of duration of the attack, concomitant illnesses, course and severity of previous attacks, and dosages of all current and past medication.

The physical examination should include vital signs, level of awareness, cyanosis, breath sounds, air movement (a patient with asthma and respiratory distress without wheezing should be considered in impending respiratory failure), pulsus paradoxus, use of accessory respiratory muscles, and hydration status. The laboratory evaluation should include at least CBC, urine analysis (UA), venous pH, and PCO_2. The chest x-ray film may be misleading if the patient is not well hydrated.

TREATMENT
A. Outpatients with mild to moderate attacks
    1. Quiet nonstressed approach and surroundings

2. O_2 by ventimask; oral fluids
3. Albuterol 0.5 ml in 3.5 ml respiratory saline by hand-held oxygen-driven nebulizer device. May be repeated every 20 minutes.
4. For patients with insufficient air movement to allow absorption of nebulized bronchodilators, epinephrine 1 : 1000, 0.01 ml/kg/dose (max. 0.3 ml) subcutaneously every 20 minutes up to 3 doses or until clear.
5. Sus-Phrine 0.005 ml/kg SQ × 1 (maximum 0.15 ml) when clear (optional)
6. Theophylline 5 mg/kg/dose q6h (until current illness is resolved if this is the first attack)
7. Augment previously utilized medication regimen for chronic asthmatics. This frequently requires initiation of a short course of oral prednisone (1 mg/kg/day for 5–7 days) if the child is already receiving beta-adrenergic and/or theophylline therapy.

B. Outpatients with mild to moderately severe attacks who fail to clear (consider admission at this point)
1. IV fluids — maintenance plus deficit; usually 1¼ maintenance fluids until urine is isotonic
2. O_2, 40% by ventimask or more if indicated by low-pulse oximeter values
3. IV aminophylline 5 mg/kg slow bolus over 20 to 30 minutes
4. Albuterol 0.5 ml in 3.5 ml of sterile H_2O

If at this point there is still wheezing, it does no service to the patient to continue emergency department therapy and the patient should be admitted.

C. Severely ill patients who are still symptomatic
1. Hospitalization, O_2, monitoring of ECG, pulse oximetry
2. Arterial blood gases
3. Hold postural drainage until air entry improves
4. IV fluids; albuterol q1–4h
5. Aminophylline continuous drip (1.1 mg/kg/hr); follow with blood levels to assure therapeutic levels of 10 to 15 mg/100 ml and to avoid toxicity (level > 20)
6. Methylprednisolone 1 to 2 mg/kg/dose q6h IV.

Extraordinary measures include pediatric intensive care unit (PICU) management with arterial line, continuous beta-adrenergic aerosol, isoproterenol drip, or positive pressure ventilation.

Bronchiolitis

Bronchiolitis is commonly seen in infants under 2 years of age. The etiology is usually respiratory syncytial virus with a peak seasonal incidence from December through February. Parainfluenza, influenza, and adenovirus are other significant etiologic agents. The pathophysiology is one of small airway obstruction with hyperinflation and hypoxemia. On examination these infants are found to be tachypneic with retractions and often with cough, coarse rales, and wheezing. There is usually a preceding illness characterized by coryza, cough, and possibly fever. In infants less than 8 weeks of age, apnea may be the presenting sign of RSV bronchiolitis.

Treatment includes the following:

1. Hospitalization is indicated for respiratory distress, hypoxemia, patient or parental fatigue, and dehydration.
2. Humidified O_2 is given, as are IV fluids if respiratory rate is greater than 70 — otherwise by mouth.
3. Rapid detection of RSV antigen in nasal secretions by EIA or direct immunofluorescence facilitates treatment with ribavirin (an antiviral agent administered by nebulization) in high-risk patients (Table B-4).
4. In infants with apnea, severe respiratory failure, or fatigue ($PCO_2 \uparrow$, $PO_2 \downarrow$, pH $\downarrow$), assisted ventilation is indicated.
5. Antibiotics are indicated if the infant has an associated otitis, pneumonia, or other bacterial infection, which is commonly seen.
6. Corticosteroids have not been shown to be beneficial, though in patients with previously existing reactive airway disease they may be of benefit.
7. A trial of aerosolized bronchodilator is often helpful.
8. Isolation is required, including gown, glove and mask precautions.
9. Cough suppressants and decongestants are contraindicated.
10. Patients with recurrent bronchiolitis should have further allergy and pulmonary evaluation.

Cardiac Arrest

The underlying factors in cardiac arrest may be unknown as the patient is rushed to the hospital in the unconscious state,

Table B-4. Infants at High Risk for Respiratory Failure with RSV Infection

1) Infants less than 6 weeks old (or prematures less than 46 week postconception)
2) Infants with underlying cardiopulmonary disease (e.g., bronchopulmonary dysplasia, cyanotic heart disease)
3) Immunocompromised host

blue and limp. The following is a general scheme for managing an apparent cardiac arrest (i.e., inaudible heart sounds, nonpalpable cardiac impulse and peripheral pulses). In such highly anxiety-producing situations it is always helpful to organize thoughts via the ABCD mnemonic.

A. *Assess:* State of ventilation, circulation, pupils. *Airway:* Clear secretions, foreign bodies, oral airway, or endotracheal tube. *Acquire* help: The secretary or nurse should place an urgent page for respiratory therapy, anesthesiologist, and other experienced staff. Avoid overcrowding with personnel.
B. *Breathing:* Facilitate ventilation
   1. Administer 100% oxygen with an Ambu bag through either a well-fitting face mask or an endotracheal tube with positive pressure ventilation.
   2. If relatively inexperienced or unskilled, do not waste time intubating a patient in the initial moments of the resuscitation.
   3. Initially give two slow full breaths, then ventilate the patient at a rate of 12 to 30 times/minute depending on the age of the patient.
   4. For certain causes (e.g., epiglottitis) an emergency tracheotomy or endotracheal intubation may be indicated.
   5. Insert a nasogastric tube as soon as circulation is established with external cardiac massage.
C. *Circulation*
   1. Administer external cardiac massage.
      a. In infants, provide support by surrounding chest with hands and using thumbs to compress the midsternum. *Warning:* Compression of ribs may cause fracture.
      b. In older children, always use a cardiac arrest board. The heel of the hand should compress the sternum.
      c. The depth of sternal compression should reach about 0.5 to 1 inch in infants and 1 to 1.5 inches in children.
      d. In young infants the rate of compressions should be 100/minute. In older children it should be 80 to 100/minute.
      e. There should be roughly one breath for every five compressions of the thorax.
   2. Continue to reassess the state of ventilation, circulation, and pupils to determine efficacy of the resuscitation.
D. *Drugs*
   1. Establish a reliable intravenous or intraosseous route and ECG monitor early in the resuscitation.

   a. One may use intravenous or intraosseous epinephrine in a dose of 0.1 ml/kg 1:10,000 dilution. Endotracheal administration with 3 ml normal saline flush followed by bag ventilation may also be effective.
   b. Sodium bicarbonate 1 to 2 mEq/kg may be given empirically in an unwitnessed or prolonged arrest. Repeat doses should be guided by pH measurement via arterial blood gases, and given only for persistent metabolic acidosis (pH < 7.25).
   c. Atropine 0.01 mg/kg (minimum 0.1 mg) for bradycardia.
   d. Narcan (0.4 mg/1-ml ampule) 0.01 mg/kg IM or IV (maximum 2 mg); repeat every 2 to 3 minutes prn × 3.
   e. Calcium chloride (10%) 0.1 ml/kg for known hypocalcemia of hyperkalemia.
   f. Dextrose to correct hypoglycemia (50% dextrose in water), 1 ml/kg.
E. *Etiology*
   1. The underlying cause of apparent cardiac arrest may suggest other emergency measures, such as control of bleeding, colloid and electrolyte replacement, use of pressor agents, and D.C. countershock.
   2. An assistant should be dispatched to speak with the parents and survey the patient's past medical record. The latter should be obtained at once from the physician of the institution in which the patient has a medical record.
   3. Obtain arterial blood gas, serum electrolytes, glucose, BUN, calcium, Hgb, hematocrit, WBC, differential count, and platelet count.
   4. Obtain a chest x ray for endotracheal tube placement and cardiopulmonary evaluation.
   5. Notify responsible service, physician, and parents; consider support for family (i.e., clergy, baptism).
   6. Keep infant warm.
   7. Crossmatch blood.
   8. Record data and drug intervals during arrest.

Croup

The patient with the typical barking cough, inspiratory stridor, and supraclavicular retractions of laryngotracheitis (croup) can become a real pediatric emergency. The challenge is to distinguish mild croup from severe croup and epiglottitis from other forms of croup.

A. History. A sudden onset with rapid progression is typical of epiglottitis. Croup is usually of slower onset, often at night, with a low-grade fever and a seal-bark cough.

B. Physical examination. A thorough but fast, gentle, and atraumatic examination should be performed.
   1. Assess degree of respiratory deprivation. Look for cyanosis, extreme retraction, poor air exchange, altered mental status (all are indications for immediate treatment and admission).
   2. Visualization of the epiglottis is hazardous, and vigorous attempts may precipitate sudden death from laryngospasm in children with epiglottitis. If a child has a history compatible with epiglottitis, assume its presence until proved otherwise, and initiate institutional protocols for anesthesia and otolaryngology consultation.
C. Laboratory studies.
   Anteroposterior and lateral neck films are useful to rule out foreign body and epiglottitis. The trachea in croup reveals subglottic edema with narrowing of the extrathoracic trachea. A clinical diagnosis of epiglottitis obviates the need for x-rays, since visualization of the larynx under anesthesia is mandatory (see below).
D. Treatment and follow-up.
   1. Mild cases with no other source of infection are treated as follows:
      a. Cold steam vaporizer, preferably with a makeshift tent over bed or crib, is used.
      b. Sometimes steaming up a bathroom and sitting in it with patient is helpful. Outdoor air can also be therapeutic.
      c. Antibiotics and corticosteroids generally are not indicated in the treatment of uncomplicated mild croup. Sedatives should be used with great caution, if at all.
   2. Moderate and severe cases (inspiratory stridor at rest following mist treatment) should be admitted.
      a. Blood gases should be obtained to determine whether respiratory failure or fatigue is present.
      b. The child should be placed in a cool mist tent with O_2.
      c. IV fluids are needed in severe croup because of the hazards of aspiration.
      d. Steroids may be of some benefit in severe croup, in a dose of 0.6 mg/kg dexamethasone IV q6h for a total of four doses.
      e. Otolaryngology or anesthesiology consultation should be obtained in children with severe croup, hopefully before the child needs airway assistance.
      f. Racemic epinephrine by nebulization may give dramatic relief; however, beware of the recurrence of airway narrowing which occurs ½ to 3 hours following the first dose of 0.5 ml diluted to 3 ml with sterile water or saline.

Epiglottitis

Epiglottitis is an acute bacterial infection of the epiglottis and glottic soft tissues caused by *Hemophilus influenzae* type b in 95% of the cases. It occurs most commonly in children from 2 to 7 years of age and presents with fever, inspiratory stridor, severe sore throat with drooling, and pronounced use of accessory muscles of respiration. Two particularly notable aspects of this disease are its rapid progression (6–8 hours) and characteristic appearance. Children with epiglottitis usually look frightened, sit upright, and may cling to their parents; in contrast, the child with croup is irritable and climbs from crib to mother's arms with astounding speed.

Epiglottitis is a medical emergency. Treatment is aimed at defusing this potential bomb quickly and with quiet efficiency. As soon as the diagnosis is suspected, the ear, nose, and throat (E.N.T.) and anesthesiology services should be notified and operating room personnel mobilized.

1. Initial evaluation should note respiratory rate, pulse, temperature, color, stridor, and retractions. Duskiness and cyanosis indicate advanced ventilation obstruction.
2. A portable lateral neck roentgenogram (physician with patient) is obtained. The epiglottis appears as a "fat thumb" if involved.
3. If there is a questionable x-ray picture *and* if the patient is not cyanotic and in minimal to mild respiratory distress, direct peroral examination of the epiglottis may be performed with caution.
4. Intubation is the treatment of choice, carried out in the operating room by an experienced anesthesiologist with the child under light anesthesia. Blood cultures followed by ceftriaxone 50 mg/kg/dose q12h IV are performed. The child should be transferred to an intensive care unit for further treatment and observation should the tube happen to become displaced.

Distended Abdomen in Infancy

A. This complaint can be regarded as the equivalent of the more familiar abdominal pain in older children.
   1. In the respective age group, each is the single most important complaint involving both pediatrician and pediatric surgeon.
   2. Each may be due to a large number and variety of conditions.

3. In each, the important decision usually is whether surgery is indicated, to be deferred, or to be avoided altogether.
4. Careful observation and repeated examination are often required.
5. In each, x-ray examination frequently plays an important role.

B. Normal distention is mild in degree, diffuse, symmetrical, soft (seen typically in premature infant after feeding). It is regarded as the "ileus of prematurity" by some pediatric surgeons.

C. Abnormal distention is moderate to marked in degree, sometimes local and asymmetrical, tense.

D. Distending substance.
   1. Gas — may be inside and outside intestine.
   2. Liquid — inside and outside intestine.
   3. Solid — organ, neoplasm.
   4. "Cyst" — hydronephrosis, hydrometrocolpos, ovarian tumor.

E. Diagnostic signs.
   1. Vomiting (regurgitation). Bile in vomitus usually indicates organic obstruction.
   2. Absence of stools.
   3. Presence of imperforate anus; tense, tender inguinal swelling.
   4. Periumbilical redness; suggestive of staphylococcal sepsis or intraabdominal necrosis and cellulitis.
   5. Heme-positive stools; seen in necrotizing enterocolitis (NEC), anal fissures, and rectal trauma from thermometers.
   6. "Residuals" — significant amounts (one-third to one-half) of prior feeding remaining in stomach.
   7. Tenderness on palpation; suggestive of NEC or peritonitis.
   8. X-ray examination.
      a. Flat, upright, lateral, upside-down views.
      b. Various positions after ingestion or retrograde injection of opaque media, intravenous urography.
      c. *Note:* Repeat films at 2- to 4-hour intervals (same gas configuration means obstruction).
      d. Air-fluid levels.
      e. Granular appearance of meconium suggests meconium ileus.
      f. Adventitious calcium suggests meconium peritonitis.
      g. Isolated distended loops, intestinal wall edema, peritoneal free air can be seen in NEC. Pneumatosis intestinalis is diagnostic of NEC.

F. Differential diagnosis.

1. NEC.
2. Meconium (plug) constipation.
3. Megacolon (aganglionic).
4. Meconium ileus.
5. Meconium peritonitis.
6. Imperforate anus.
7. Ileal atresia.
8. Volvulus.
9. Spontaneous rupture of stomach.
10. Hydrometrocolpos.
11. Strangulated hernia.
12. Hydronephrosis.
13. Neoplasm.
14. Splenic cyst.
15. Enteritis.
16. Sepsis with ileus.
17. Mesenteric cyst.
18. Neonatal ascites.
19. Megacysts.
    a. Primary.
    b. Secondary to posterior urethral valves.

Diabetic Ketoacidosis

Diabetes is a relatively common pediatric problem and is seen occasionally by most practitioners. The children have a deficiency of insulin, as a result of which hyperglycemia, ketonemia, and acidosis develop. In fact, they may not be diagnosed until they present to the emergency department with coma, Kussmaul respirations, and dehydration. There are very few other entities that cause glucosuria and ketonuria, but aspirin intoxication and hypernatremic dehydration should always be considered. The acute management of diabetic ketoacidosis is discussed in Chapter 7.

Eye Emergencies

The great majority of complaints involving the eye result from foreign bodies in the eye and other trauma.

A. Foreign bodies.
   1. Patient can usually recall when the foreign object entered the eye and complains of a scratchy sensation when the eye is moved — whether the object is on the inner aspect of the upper lid or attached to the cornea. There may be a secondary conjunctivitis, but often there is none. Some degree of lacrimation is usual.
   2. Satisfactory examination requires adequate light, a magnifying glass, and cooperation on the part of the patient. The upper lid should be everted. The exam-

iner should be prepared to remove the foreign body at this point. An ophthalmologist should be called in consultation when the foreign body cannot be wiped off the cornea with a wet cotton wisp. One or two drops of ophthaine* in the eye provides the necessary anesthesia.

B. Abrasions and lacerations.
1. Superficial abrasions and lacerations of the cornea are painful lesions that may be difficult to visualize without the use of fluorescein. The tip of a specially prepared strip of paper is placed inside the lower lid of the anesthetized eye for 5 to 10 seconds. Blinking spreads the dye over the cornea and leaves a green stain where the corneal epithelial cells have been damaged or lost.
2. Simple abrasions may be treated with antibiotic ointment four times a day and patching of the eye. Follow-up examination to verify healing should be performed daily.

C. Contusions.
1. Contusions of the eye that result in subconjunctival hemorrhage alarm parents but are not serious in themselves and require no treatment. Visual acuity should be checked for evidence of intraocular injury. When the blow has been a severe one with resulting periorbital swelling, bony deformity, or extensive subconjunctival hemorrhage, intraocular injury should be suspected and consultation with an ophthalmologist should be obtained. Vision may be normal even in the presence of serious eye injury.

D. Signs of serious ocular injury.
1. Blood in anterior chamber.
2. Distortion, dilation, or paralysis of pupil.
3. Shallow anterior chamber in comparison with other eye.
4. Black fundus reflex.
5. Gray shadows in the fundus.
6. Limitation of movement or diplopia.
7. Ciliary flash type of conjunctivitis with most intense erythema surrounding the cornea and fading toward the periphery.
8. Proptosis.

Foreign Bodies

Children have been accused by their parents of introducing foreign bodies into all of the natural body orifices. Sometimes the accusation proves to be well founded, sometimes false. The physician is obliged to look.

*Proparacaine hydrochloride, ophthalmic solution 0.5%.

A. Esophagus.
1. Esophagoscopy under general anesthesia and direct-vision removal of the foreign body may be necessary.
2. Papain-containing meat tenderizer may be used for esophageal obstruction from meat if the ingestion took place less than 6 hours prior to emergency department visit.

B. Trachea and bronchi.
1. If obstruction is complete, in infants, four sharp interscapular back blows should be administered until the foreign body is dislodged. Chest thrusts may be tried if back blows are unsuccessful. Abdominal thrusts (Heimlich maneuver) to the subxyphoid area in rapid sequence are used in children over 1 year of age.
2. Partial obstructions cause inspiratory stridor, mimicking croup, and cause choking if located in the relatively narrow glottic (vocal cord) region.
3. Lateral neck films and inspiratory, expiratory films with fluoroscopy or manual abdominal compression to ensure expiration are helpful in revealing air trapping in the obstructed segmental lobe caused by an endobronchial foreign body.
4. Attempts to remove foreign bodies with bronchodilators or postural cupping are hazardous as the obstructing object can be dislodged into the trachea, causing a complete airway obstruction.
5. Rigid bronchoscopy is the ideal method for removal of a tracheobronchial foreign body.

C. Intracutaneous and subcutaneous foreign objects.
1. The great majority of these are either wood splinters, fragments of glass, or needlelike metal objects.
2. Wood splinters are usually identified and removed with little difficulty. More than one may be present and easily overlooked.
3. Glass fragments are often multiple, small, and difficult to find. Some glass is sufficiently opaque to make x-ray examination worthwhile in all cases.
4. Metallic foreign objects are usually in the subcutaneous tissue and are the most difficult to find. Success in localizing and removing them may require that the procedure be carried out under the fluoroscope. A Berman locator, if one is available, is a big time-saver and usually obviates the necessity of moving patient and sterile equipment to the x-ray department.
5. Under certain circumstances, search for a foreign body is likely to do more harm than good: the object is tiny, it is causing no discomfort, it fails to

show on x-ray examination, the point of entrance is no longer visible. With adoption of a watch and wait attitude, it is necessary *infrequently* to drain pus that has collected around the foreign body. The location of the latter is thus identified, and it is removed along with the pus that surrounds it.

D. Nose.

The presence of a nasal foreign body is a likely possibility in a child with unilateral mucopurulent discharge. Often the parents will have noticed a foul smell to the child's breath.

1. Soft material and small hard objects that lie anteriorly in the nostril can usually be removed with forceps.
2. Topical application of Neosynephrine ⅛% to the nasal mucosa may reduce edema sufficiently to allow removal of the foreign body more easily.
3. Consultation with an otolaryngologist should be obtained if simple extraction is unsuccessful.

Hematuria

See also Chapter 13, The Genitourinary System.

A. Diagnostic workup.
   1. On all patients.
      a. Careful history. Especially seek past history of hematuria, recent infection, trauma, and family history of renal disease.
      b. Physical examination — blood pressure, weight, presence of edema (mother may be best judge), flank tenderness, evidence of trauma to flank or urethra, observation of urinary stream (in males), abdominal mass.
      c. Young females (2–6 years) with hematuria may in fact have a vaginal or urethral foreign body.
      d. Urinalysis with determined hunt for casts.
      e. Blood counts, sedimentation rate.
      f. Urine culture.
   2. Patients with gross hematuria or clear history of trauma to flank should have a consultation with a pediatric surgeon or urologist.
   3. Patients with hematuria unexplained by obvious trauma or infection should be referred for further evaluation by an appropriate pediatric specialist outside the emergency department setting.
B. Management.
   1. Patients with genitourinary trauma should be referred immediately to the pediatric urology service.
   2. Patients who are very ill with acute glomerulone-

phritis as well as any patient with hypertension or oliguria should be admitted to the hospital. Patients with a recurrence of glomerulonephritis should also be admitted as they may well require kidney biopsy.
   3. Patients who require a very extensive diagnostic evaluation should probably be admitted to the hospital.

Acute Renal Failure

Acute renal failure has a number of causes that can be divided into prerenal (perfusion defect such as volume depletion), postrenal (as in obstruction from urethral valves), and renal injury secondary to toxins or renal necrosis. One of the major causes of acute renal failure is the hemolytic-uremic syndrome (HUS). This syndrome occurs most often in young children following an upper respiratory infection or diarrheal illness and presents with edema, pallor, and often bloody diarrhea. Laboratory studies reveal the classic triad of microangiopathic hemolytic anemia, azotemia, and thrombocytopenia. Oliguria or anuria, with accompanying azotemia, acidosis, and electrolyte disturbances, are characteristic. Additional complications are seizures and hypertension. See Chapter 13 for additional discussion on acute renal failure.

Hemorrhage and Anoxia

A. Immediate lifesaving measures are required for two basic conditions:
   1. Hemorrhage (continuing blood loss).
   2. Oxygen deprivation.
B. Hemorrhage. Life-threatening hemorrhage in children is caused far less often by sharp instruments than by blunt trauma with consequent laceration of an organ and by spontaneous bleeding (bleeding peptic ulcer, bleeding Meckel's diverticulum).
C. Steps to be taken immediately for external bleeding:
   1. Direct pressure on bleeding point.
   2. Application of hemostat.
   3. Hematocrit (may be normal in early hemorrhage on account of vasoconstriction and volume contraction).
   4. Blood typing and crossmatching.
   5. Elevation and wrapping of limbs.
   6. Administration of type O blood, plasma, or albumin until type-specific blood is available.
D. Occult blood loss. Increasing pallor and pulse rate and falling hematocrit mean blood loss, the location of which may not be obvious.

1. There may be gastrointestinal bleeding from peptic ulceration (duodenum, Meckel's diverticulum).

2. Hemoperitoneum in the newborn period may be diagnosed by aspiration of blood from the abdominal cavity.

3. Trauma resulting in fracture of pelvic bones may result in considerable blood loss into the pelvis extraperitoneally. Blood typing and crossmatching is always done in anticipation of this.

4. Blunt trauma to the abdomen may cause lacerations of spleen or liver — rarely both — with consequent hemorrhage into the peritoneal cavity. The liver laceration is by far the more urgent, requiring rapid preparation for a laparotomy.

5. Patients with infectious mononucleosis are at risk for traumatic or even spontaneous splenic rupture and should refrain from contact sport and vigorous activities.

E. Oxygen deprivation. Patients with oxygen deprivation usually have a mechanical cause for the deprivation.

1. Airway obstruction is ordinarily due to narrowing of the airway at the level of the larynx either by a foreign body or by inflammation (infection, burn). In either case, bypassing the involved area by a tracheostomy tube may be necessary and requires a special skill and a supply of tracheostomy tubes of various sizes.

2. Encroachment on the lung volume and ability to expand may be due to air (pneumothorax), fluid (hydrothorax), viscus (elements of the gastrointestinal tract through a diaphragmatic hernia), or elevation of the diaphragm as in ascites of the newborn. When the lung is compressed and exchange volume limited, oxygen requirements may be met in full or in part by supplying high-concentration oxygen as a temporary measure pending a definitive procedure. Both air and fluid should be aspirated with needle and syringe when there is likelihood of localization. X-ray examination indicates the site for thoracentesis. In newborns, transillumination often "lights up" the side of the pneumothorax.

Lacerations

A. Skin. Treatment of skin lacerations varies greatly, depending on the type, extent, and location of the laceration and on the presence of other injuries such as a fracture or severed tendon. It is directed toward the restoration of normal anatomy and involves:

1. Careful cleansing of the surrounding skin and application of sterile drapes. It is almost impossible to avoid contamination of suture material without covering the area immediately surrounding the wound with sterile drapes. A convenient way to do this is to use a paper towel in which a hole of appropriate size and shape has been cut before it is placed over the wound. Useful also, especially on the face, is the application of Mastisol around the wound to hold the drape in place should the head be turned.

2. Administration of a local anesthetic. Local skin anesthesia is obtained most rapidly and with least pain if one uses a 2% rather than 1% solution of anesthetic (Xylocaine is rapid in action and nontoxic in the amount required for most lacerations) and a 26-gauge needle. Start the injection in the subcutaneous tissue immediately under the skin margin and inject slowly.

3. Inspection, exploration, and cleansing of the wound. Exploration of every laceration that extends through the skin is very important and can be done adequately only after the administration of a local anesthetic. The actual depth of the wound is determined. Involvement of bone and tendon is sometimes a surprise finding. Foreign material and devitalized subcutaneous tissue are identified and removed.

4. Debridement of devitalized tissue including (if primary healing and good cosmetic result are desired, as with facial lacerations) excision of contused skin margins. Many lacerations of children are caused by blunt rather than sharp objects. Thus contusion of skin margins and healing with a broad scar result if the involved skin is not excised. Gauze pads well soaked with antiseptic solution are used routinely to cleanse the depth of the wound immediately prior to closure. Irrigation is used rarely. Excision of grossly dirty wounds is more effective.

5. Control of bleeding. Where oozing persists and where a large area of subcutaneous tissue is exposed, insert rubber tissue drain for 24 to 48 hours.

6. Closure. In general, use the finest material that does the required job. Nylon is usually best for most minor lacerations.

7. Application of a dressing. This, too, should be no bulkier than necessary to do the required job. Dressings applied to fingers and hands should be held in place by gauze extending to and tied at the wrist. Adhesive sticks best if the skin to which it is to be applied is treated with some adhesive base that is

allowed to dry. When the laceration lies over a joint, a splint should be incorporated in the dressing to prevent motion.

8. Administration of tetanus toxoid. Patient should be given tetanus toxoid (0.5 ml) if none has been administered within the last 8 years.

9. Parents should receive instructions:
   a. To keep the dressing clean and dry.
   b. To arrange for change of dressing if it becomes wet.
   c. To report immediately any evidence of infection (pain, swelling, red streaks radiating from wound, fever). Arrangements should be made for future removal of sutures.

B. Special sites.

1. Tongue. Do not suture when wounds are small and edges remain in good approximation — the usual situation. Sutures, when necessary, should consist of fine catgut placed below the level of the mucosa.

2. Lips. Through-and-through lacerations should be sutured at skin end of wound only, unless there is a flap of mucosa that must be fastened down — loosely. Vermilion borders must be sutured exactly for good cosmetic results if the laceration extends to facial skin.

3. Scalp. All scalp lacerations that require suturing should be explored carefully for evidence of injury to the skull.

4. Fingers. Tendon and nerve involvement should always be suspected and their integrity demonstrated — if possible, prior to treatment of the laceration, but always before closure of the skin defect.

5. Face. A good cosmetic result is important. Hence, the most experienced person available should perform or supervise the treatment. Eyebrows should not be shaved as their subsequent regrowth may well be distorted.

6. Tendons. Of prime importance is the fact that a severed tendon is often overlooked. Evidence of a severed tendon, even when such an injury is strongly suggested by the location and depth of a laceration, may be difficult to elicit in a small child. With the exception of partially severed expanded portions of extensor tendons on the back of the hand, all tendon lacerations should be sutured in the main operating room. A laceration involving the flexor tendons of the fingers should be cleansed and sutured and repair of the tendons deferred.

C. Puncture wounds. These differ from linear lacerations in that they cannot be cleansed except superficially.

Hence chance alone (the nature of the instrument, the site and depth of penetration, the bacteria and foreign material introduced) determines whether the wound heals without significant infection. Surprisingly, it usually does. The superficial cleansing mentioned above may involve a cruciate incision of the skin margins and excision of the corners thus developed. This should be done under local anesthesia. A probe should be inserted into all puncture wounds to determine their depth. Occasionally, the presence of a foreign object is revealed.

D. Dog bites. The typical dog bite consists of several puncture wounds, some of them large, some small, and all prone to infection. They should not be sutured, even though, as when on the face, the temptation to suture is great. Suturing of the occasional linear laceration following careful cleansing and mechanical debridement may be attempted with good chance of primary healing. The wounds in all cases should be examined no less frequently than every 2 days. Antibiotics should be given. *Pasteurella multocida* is a commonly found cause of dog bite infections.

E. Miscellaneous.

1. Schedule for removal of sutures:
   a. Face and scalp — 5 days.
   b. Upper extremities, anterior chest, abdomen — 7 days.
   c. Back, lower extremities — 10 to 14 days.

2. Elbow, knee, and hand lacerations usually require application of a posterior splint.

3. History of unconsciousness requires skull x-ray examination and admission to hospital.

Meningitis

The clinician should always have a high index of suspicion for meningitis especially in children less than 1 year of age, in whom the meningeal signs may be absent. "When in doubt — tap." See also Chapter 20.

A. Definite indications for a lumbar puncture are the following:

1. Meningeal signs, e.g., nuchal rigidity, Kernig's, Brudzinski's.

2. Full fontanel (usually a late sign).

3. Paradoxical irritability, e.g., infant who is irritable when picked up, quiet, when left still on table.

4. Unexplained fever or lethargy in an infant less than 6 months old.

B. Analysis of spinal fluid.

1. Cell count and differential defines any existing pleiocytosis; the presence of neutrophils suggests a bacterial infection, while mononuclear cells are suggestive of viral infection or other inflammatory processes.
2. Decreased CSF glucose (< 50% of blood glucose) suggests bacterial infection.
3. Increased CSF protein is significant for any inflammatory process.
4. Culture and sensitivity provides definitive diagnosis in bacterial meningitis.
5. Adjunctive testing for bacterial antigens by latex agglutination is often helpful in early differentiation among the common pathogens (*S. pneumonia, H. influenzae* type b, meningococcus, or group B streptococcus).
6. In experienced hands, Gram's stain of CSF may be diagnostic if organisms are present in significant numbers.
7. Acid-fast culture, viral cultures, Wright's stains can be done on the fluid when appropriate, but not routinely.
C. Further workup if spinal fluid is consistent with meningitis and if patient cannot be admitted immediately:
1. Obtain blood cultures, complete blood count, nose and throat cultures, electrolytes, BUN, blood sugar, and chest x-ray film (if patient is not too sick).
2. Consider obtaining blood for type and crossmatch, skull x-ray films, prothrombin time, sedimentation rate.
D. Preparation for admission.
1. After cultures are obtained, first dose of antibiotics can be given in the emergency department.
a. Ceftriaxone, 50 mg/kg body weight, by intravenous infusion over ½ hour, to be continued q12h pending culture and sensitivity results.
b. In infants less than 8 weeks of age, ampicillin 50 mg/kg IV, repeated q6h and cefotaxime 25 mg/kg IV, to be continued.
c. Recent evidence suggests that administration of dexamethasone 0.15 mg/kg IV, beginning with the first dose of antibiotics and continuing q6h for 4 days, reduces the incidence of profound hearing loss in children with *H. influenza* type b meningitis.
2. Physician should accompany any sick meningitic patient to the ward.
3. The ward staff and head nurse should be notified of any meningitis very early so that prompt admission can be expedited.
4. Fluids may need to be restricted to two-thirds maintenance if evidence for SIADH (↓ serum Na$^+$, ↑ urine osmolarity) appears. Of primary concern is establishment of adequate intravascular volume via isotonic crystalloid or isotonic colloid bolus infusion during the emergency phase of treatment. These should be given until adequate circulation is produced (easily palpable pulses, warm distal extremities, capillary refill time < 2 seconds) in order to prevent cerebral infarction secondary to sludging and cerebral vaso-occlusive disease. Inotropic support (e.g., dopamine) may also be required. Keep serum glucose concentration above 75 mg/dl.
5. Watch for complications: cerebral edema (early), subdural effusions (later), pericarditis, septic arthritis.
6. Watch for seizures and early signs of increased pressure (sixth and third nerve palsies).

Orthopedic Problems

A. Fractures.
1. The type and severity of the injury usually suggest the likelihood of injury to bone. Even though the history and physical examination may suggest only a sprain or soft tissue contusion, the physician attending the patient should not hesitate to request an x-ray examination — especially if the injury was incurred in an auto accident.
2. When a fracture of an extremity is obvious clinically, the physician checks the circulation and sensation distal to the fracture, applies a temporary splint, and elevates the injured extremity.
3. Following the x-ray examination the physician should examine the films personally.
4. With few exceptions, definitive care of fractures is the responsibility of the orthopedic surgeon.
5. When fracture of the pelvis seems likely, blood should be drawn for hematocrit and immediate typing and crossmatching. Frequent determination of blood pressure and pulse rate are required due to the risk of occult retroperitoneal bleeding.
6. Portable x-ray evaluation in the emergency department is preferred in all patients with significant trauma.
7. Occasionally, as with elbow injuries in small children, bilateral x-ray films should be ordered to facilitate comparison to the unaffected side.
8. Care of depressed skull fractures is the responsibility of the neurosurgeon. Care of facial fractures is the responsibility of the plastic surgeon.
9. In the case of a simple fracture of the clavicle in a small child, treat the injury by applying a figure-of-eight splint.

10. Whenever a plaster splint is applied, the patient should be instructed to report to the physician on the following day for a "cast check."

B. Sprains.

1. In all instances in which a severe sprain is the clinical diagnosis, x-ray examination of the involved part should be obtained. Always consider the possibility of fractures.

2. If the patient is seen within a few minutes of the time of injury, an ice pack should be applied for 30 minutes in an effort to minimize swelling from hemorrhage and edema.

3. With fracture ruled out, the emergency department physician will treat the injury with splint (elastic bandage, "webroll" with elastic bandage support or plaster), crutches, and medication to relieve pain, depending on the circumstances.

C. "Nursemaids' elbow" or dislocation of the radial head. This common entity is difficult to recognize if the physician is not aware of it. X-ray examination is negative when the parts are not ossified. (The dislocation is usually reduced with 90-degree flexion of the elbow and supination of the forearm.) The reduction may happen during the initial examination, making confirmation of the diagnosis and aftercare difficult.

D. Slipped capitular femoral epiphysis. This should be the primary diagnosis in all patients whose chief complaint is painful hip. They should be sent to the x-ray department non-weight-bearing, regardless of their previous activity.

E. Other causes of hip pain.

1. Toxic synovitis of the hip. It is important to rule out more serious lesions such as monarticular arthritis, tuberculosis, and coxa plana. Treatment is bedrest until synovial reaction subsides.

2. Osteochondrosis of the hip (Legg-Calvé-Perthes disease). Early diagnosis and treatment are important to prevent permanent deformity.

F. Osgood-Schlatter disease. Pain localized to the region of the tibial tubercle, aggravated by squatting and running, in the early teenage years is a common complaint. The physician should arrange for x-ray examination (both knees) and refer the patient to an orthopedic surgeon.

G. Septic arthritis. When this diagnosis is suggested by fever, toxicity, exquisite pain and tenderness of the joint, effusion, and near immobility, the investigations should include blood counts, sedimentation rate, x-ray examinations, blood culture, and synovial fluid examination (note that this may constitute a true medical emergency).

H. Hemophilia with joint bleeding. The involved joint should be elevated, splinted, and ice-packed. Both the orthopedic surgeon and the hematologist become involved in the continuing care. Clotting factor infusion may be indicated.

Pharyngitis

See Chapter 20.

Pneumonia

A. Diagnosis in infancy.

1. Infants usually present with abruptly rising fever, restlessness, vomiting, diarrhea, and respiratory distress; often there is no history of coughing.

2. On physical examination the infant may have rapid shallow respirations, grunting, cyanosis, flaring of alae nasi, abdominal distention, splinting, retractions, diminished breath sounds, and a palpable liver. Rales and fever need not be present in children with pneumonia. Clinical signs of pneumonia may well precede radiographic findings.

3. Respiratory syncytial virus bronchiolitis may progress to pneumonia and in young infants contributes to significant morbidity and mortality. Apnea is commonly associated with RSV infection in infants less than 2 months old. (Nasal secretions may be rapidly tested for RSV antigen by EIA or direct immunofluorescence.)

4. Chlamydial pneumonia is seen in infants 1 to 3 months of age and presents with staccato cough, rales, and often a history of a preceding conjunctivitis. Eosinophils may be present on the peripheral blood smear.

B. Diagnosis in older children.

1. Many present with headache, fever, malaise, hacking cough, chest pain, abdominal pain.

2. Physical examination may reveal tachypnea, retractions, flaring of the nostrils, diminished breath sounds. Rales are usually heard. Pneumonia may simulate an acute abdomen.

3. The patient may present with fever and toxicity and without detectable respiratory signs and symptoms.

C. Workup.

1. A chest x-ray examination often confirms the clinical diagnosis and may yield additional information (e.g., pleural effusion, pneumatoceles, cardiac enlargement) of great importance in diagnosis and management.

2. Blood counts may be helpful (e.g., eosinophilia in chlamydia, lymphocytosis in pertussis, monocytosis

in tuberculosis, neutrophilia with immature forms in bacterial infection).

3. Cultures. Whenever possible, sputum should be cultured and gram-stained. A child in toxic condition should also have a blood culture. Pleural effusions should be tapped and cultured.

4. Tuberculin test. It is an inviolable law that every patient with pneumonia have this test performed and read by a doctor 48 hours later. Nasal secretions may be rapidly tested for RSV antigen by EIA or direct immunofluorescence. Nasal secretions may also be tested for *Chlamydia* antigen. Rapid diagnostic tests are now available for many of the pathogens which cause pneumonia in children.

Latex agglutination testing of the urine may detect antigens of *S. pneumonia, H. influenzae* type b, Group B streptococcus, and meningococcus. Serologic testing for IgM (early phase) antibodies specific for *Mycoplasma pneumoniae,* Epstein-Barr virus, and cytomegalovirus are also available.

5. Cold agglutinins may be useful in suspected mycoplasmal pneumonia. Bedside cold agglutinins can be noted quickly by putting an equal amount of whole blood into a sodium citrate vacutainer and placing the tube in ice. After 5 minutes, the presence of cold agglutinins may be detected by small clumping of adherent groups of erythrocytes, easily seen when the vacutainer is held up to the light and the tube is rotated.

D. Therapy.
1. Antimicrobials.
   a. Penicillin is the usual starting drug for pneumococcal or meningococcal pneumonia. It can be given parenterally (intramuscularly) until definite clinical improvement occurs (ordinarily 1–3 days), then orally for 7 to 10 days. Erythromycin is becoming popular as initial therapy because of its activity against gram-positive bacteria, chlamydiae, and mycoplasmas.
   b. Specific diagnosis allows treatment as follows:
      (i) Erythromycin for *Mycoplasma* or *Chlamydia.*
      (ii) Cefuroxime or ceftriaxone for *H. influenza* type b.
      (iii) Inpatient therapy with aerosolized ribavirin in high-risk patients with RSV disease (age < 6 weeks, underlying heart or lung disease in older infants).
2. Physical therapy. The physician can teach parents how to perform postural drainage with cupping. If it

seems appropriate, patients can be referred to a physical therapy clinic, or a visiting nurse can help in the home. Physical therapy is particularly important in pneumonia with atelectasis.

3. Bronchodilators. Oral or aerosolized bronchodilators are sometimes useful adjuncts in the treatment of pneumonia, especially where there is hyperinflation (or other evidence of bronchospasm) and in pneumonia with atelectasis.

F. Follow-up.
1. Parents should be in close contact with the physician during the first few days of illness. Infants should be seen daily at first.
2. Arrangements should be made for a purified protein derivative (PPD) reading in 2 days and a follow-up chest x-ray examination in 2 to 3 weeks.
3. Patients with recurrent pneumonia or persistent atelectasis should be further investigated.

G. Criteria for admission of patients with pneumonia.
1. Significant respiratory distress or toxicity.
2. Cyanosis.
3. Age less than 6 months.
4. Staphylococcal pneumonia, e.g., pneumatoceles on x-ray film.
5. Pleural effusion.
6. Inadequate care at home.

Psychiatric Emergencies

A. The common psychiatric complaints include acute anxiety state, suicide attempt, school phobia, fire setting, conflict with parents, and running away.

B. It is useful and important for the physician to take a complete history, although this procedure is not always feasible in a busy emergency room. He should spend some of his time alone with the child.

C. A complete physical examination should be performed tactfully. This should include a thorough neurological examination.

D. One should appreciate the desperate, often humiliating, nature of the visit and provide ample support, consolation, and reassurance to parents and child.

E. The physician should patiently help the parents and the child talk about what has been happening.

F. A psychiatrist should be called both to evaluate and treat the acute situation and to arrange follow-up care. In general, the psychiatrist should be sought after the physician has seen the patient.

G. Use of medications should be avoided unless clearly indicated for the control of extreme anxiety or psychomotor excitement. Below are some suggested drugs and their stat doses.

1. Chlorpromazine (Thorazine), 0.5 mg/kg of body weight intramuscularly. Contraindicated in phencyclidine intoxication.
2. Valium, children 2 to 5 mg/dose; adolescents 5 to 10 mg/dose.

H. Children showing bizarre behavior should be carefully evaluated from the point of view of drug ingestion. The most commonly seen ingestion causing bizarre behavioral disturbances is phencyclidine (PCP, angel dust, Kay Jay). These patients have distorted sensory input and often need pharmacological assistance as well as a quiet, nonthreatening environment. Haloperidol (Haldol) has been useful in these situations, 0.5 to 2.0 mg, or Valium.

I. Adolescents and children may present with what appears to be acute psychotic reaction with marked dystonic posturing. In this situation one should consider an acute extrapyramidal reaction from phenothiazine ingestion. The treatment of choice is diphenhydramine (Benadryl) 2 mg/kg IV. This is both a diagnostic and a therapeutic attempt; if the signs are due to phenothiazine, a complete but temporary response is noted. The patient should then be given a 2- to 3-day course of oral Benadryl to prevent recurrence.

Seizures

A. Acute management of status epilepticus in older infants and children.
1. Supportive measures. Lay patient on side; suction as needed. Give oxygen if patient appears hypoxic. Use soft mouth gag or plastic airway.
2. Observe seizure carefully. If patient is not hypoxic, most seizures need not be stopped instantly, and much can be learned by observing the nature of the convulsion.
3. Laboratory evaluation — Dextrostix, serum glucose, electrolytes, BUN, CA^{2+}, anticonvulsant levels if on therapy, toxic screen, Pb (if history is suggestive), cultures (if febrile). Push dextrose if Dextrostix is less than 30 mg/100 ml, 1 ml/kg of 50% D/W or 2 ml/kg of 25% D/W.
4. Medications.
   a. For a prolonged and *continued* seizure it is best to start with slowly administered diazepam, 0.1 to 0.3 mg/kg IV. By drawing up 0.3 mg/kg in a syringe and giving this dose in three successive increments, one can individualize the dose. *One*

must observe very carefully for evidence of respiratory or circulatory depression (particularly in patients with prior sedation, e.g., phenobarbital).
   b. *Phenytoin,* 5 to 10 mg/kg *IV* slowly. Monitor for cardiac arrhythmias. This may be repeated every 15 minutes to a maximum of 20 g/kg. *DO NOT USE PHENYTOIN INTRAMUSCULARLY.*
   c. *Phenobarbital,* 5 to 10 mg/kg IV over several minutes. Monitor for respiratory depression.
   d. *Paraldehyde,* 0.15 to 0.30 ml/kg by rectum. Dilute 1:2 to 1:10 with mineral oil. Instill as a retention enema using glass syringe and Foley catheter with balloon inflated.
5. For refractory status epilepticus, the anesthesiologist and neurologist should be consulted and the possibility of administering pentobarbital general anesthesia considered.

B. Diagnostic evaluation.
1. CSF examination should be considered in all patients having a seizure for the first time (febrile or not).
2. Patients with known seizure disorders should have the following questions answered in their charts.
   a. Has there been an intercurrent illness?
   b. Was there a lapse or inadequate dose of anticonvulsant medication?
   c. Is there a change in the neurological examination?
   d. Was there a change in the nature of the seizure compared to previous ones?

C. Disposition.
1. First, nonfebrile seizures in children under 12 months and over 6 years should lead to admission for evaluation.
2. One should obtain a neurology consultation for any child who has a prolonged or unusual seizure.
3. Known seizure patients with a marked change in the type or frequency of their seizures should be given an early appointment for further evaluation.
4. Patients with more than two episodes of febrile seizures should be considered for initiation of a daily prophylactic dose of anticonvulsant and should have an electroencephalogram. The choice and dose of drug should be discussed with a neurologic consultant.

Shock

Shock is not a primary disease but, except for control of hemorrhage, demands primary consideration in treatment. The patient who is prostate, pale, cold, sweaty, and hypotensive and whose mental state varies from intense anxiety to deep coma is in a critical clinical status, whatever the basic cause (infection, hemorrhage, trauma). Treatment is directed toward:

1. Ensuring adequate pulmonary oxygen and carbon dioxide exchange.
   a. Check airway to ensure freedom from obstruction.
   b. Increase oxygen in inspired gas.
   c. Provide judicious positive pressure ventilatory resistance if the patient is apneic.
   d. Assess gas exchange by arterial blood gas determination.
2. Restoring adequate cardiac output (normalize capillary refill, blood pressure, heart rate).
   a. Intravascular volume expansion with isotonic crystalloid, colloid, or, in hemorrhagic shock, colloid and packed RBCs. Administer in 20 ml/kg increments until clinical response occurs or signs of fluid overload develop (e.g., distended jugular veins, increased liver size, pulmonary rales, increased central venous pressure).
   b. In cardiac failure (failure to respond to adequate restoration of intravascular volume), initiate inotropic support with dopamine, 5 to 20 μg/kg/minute.
   c. Insert central venous catheter or pulmonary artery catheter to monitor cardiac filling pressures.
3. Evaluating cardiac status.
   a. Check heart rate and rhythm with electrocardiogram.
   b. Check heart size with chest x ray.
   c. Assess function with echocardiogram.

Strangulated Inguinal Hernia

A. Symptoms.
   1. Painful, tender swelling in groin, sudden in onset, and not reduced by gentle taxis.
   2. Scrotal swelling.
   3. Vomiting, abdominal distention (from intestinal obstruction).
B. Differential diagnosis.
   1. Hydrocele of cord is often firm in consistency, but it is not tender and may be moved horizontally.
   2. Acute lymphadenitis causes pain, swelling, and tenderness as strangulated hernia, but onset is not sudden, there is no evidence of intestinal obstruction, and there is no scrotal swelling. *Note:* Parent may insist swelling was sudden in onset.
C. Treatment.
   1. Sedation (after surgical evaluation)

2. Place cold pack on groin and put child in Trendelenburg position for 30 to 60 minutes. Then attempt reduction by taxis. If this is unsuccessful, admit the patient immediately for emergency surgery. If taxis is successful, admit immediately, but for elective surgery.

Subungual Hematoma

Crushing injuries of fingertips are fairly common. One very painful consequence is hemorrhage under the nail. Evacuation of the blood through a small hole in the nail relieves the pressure and the pain. This can be done easily with the red-hot point of a paper clip pressed firmly on the nail over the hematoma. A No. 11 blade may also be used to drill a small hole into the nail after the nail has been prepared with iodine. The nail will be lost, but the loss should usually be allowed to take place spontaneously. X-ray examination for fracture of the distal phalanx should be obtained. If a fracture is present, antibiotics should always be used as this is technically an open fracture.

Tetanus Prophylaxis

Up-to-date recommendations for tetanus prophylaxis are available in the "Red Book" Report of the Committee on Infectious Diseases published by the American Academy of Pediatrics. General guidelines are as follows:

1. A booster dose of tetanus toxoid should be given to all patients with burns (partial thickness and deeper), puncture wounds, human and animal bites, severely contused and contaminated lacerations, deep abrasions, and compound fractures. The booster dose is given unless there is absolute documentation of a minimum of three booster doses in the past and the most recent one being within 5 years of the injury.
2. Patients with clean simple lacerations of face and scalp do not need tetanus prophylaxis.
3. When the injury occurs at approximately the time when the patient should be receiving a booster dose of toxoid, the injury offers a good opportunity to carry out the procedure.
4. Rarely a patient may be seen who has had no prior tetanus prophylaxis and whose injury requires tetanus immunoglobulin 250 to 500 units IM. Tetanus toxoid should be given at the same time in the opposite extremity to start active immunization.

Torsion of Appendix Testis

A. Basis for diagnosis.
1. Sudden, moderately severe pain in one side of scrotum, aggravated by walking.
2. Small hydrocele.
3. Small, very tender mass at upper pole of testis with faint redness of overlying skin.
B. Differential diagnosis.
1. Torsion of spermatic cord. It is sometimes impossible to rule this out. Radionucleotide testicular scan may be helpful in showing diminished uptake in testicular torsion.
2. Epididymitis. This is a rare disease, but such a diagnosis is often made in error.
C. Treatment.
1. Admit for urological consult, as torsion of appendix testis may well be a surgical emergency.

Upper Respiratory Infections

See Chapter 10.
TREATMENT

1. Fever control.
2. Antibiotics. These are indicated only when there are suppurative complications, such as sinusitis, purulent rhinitis, or acute otitis media with effusion.
3. Careful examination of the tympanic membranes, including pneumocitic otoscopy to evaluate mobility, is indicated in all patients with upper respiratory infection, in order to diagnose acute otitis media with effusion.

Fever Control

When significant pathology has been ruled out or appropriately treated, control of fever may be desirable for patient comfort.

1. Antipyretic therapy with acetaminophen 10 to 15 mg/kg orally or rectally may be repeated every 4 to 6 hours.
2. Tepid water sponging to encourage radiant and evaporative heat loss without producing shivering or peripheral vasoconstriction is another option if fever control is urgent (e.g., following a febrile convulsion).

Discharge Instructions for Parents of Children with Minor Head Injuries

Even though your child has been thoroughly examined for evidence of head injury, there are certain signs of trouble that may appear in the next 48 hours. It has been considered safe to allow the child to return home by the examining physician; however, observe your child carefully during the next 48 hours, and let the physician know should any of the following signs of trouble develop. Before leaving the emergency department, be sure that you have had all the signs of trouble listed below explained to you by the examining physician and that all of your questions have been answered.

Signs of Trouble

1. Excessive drowsiness. The child may well be exhausted by the ordeal surrounding the injury but should be easily aroused by methods that you would ordinarily employ to awaken him from a deep sleep. If you cannot arouse him easily, notify the hospital.
2. Persistent vomiting. Children will, in most cases, vomit one or more times following a severe head injury. Should the vomiting recur more than once or twice, or should the vomiting begin again hours after it has ceased, notify the hospital.
3. If one pupil appears to be larger than the other, notify the hospital.
4. If the child does not use either arm or leg as well as previously, or is unsteady in walking, notify the hospital.
5. Should speech become slurred or the child be apparently unable to talk, notify the hospital.
6. If severe headache occurs, particularly if it increases in severity and is not relieved by aspirin, notify the hospital.
7. Should a child complain of "seeing double" or should you detect any failure of the eyes to move together appropriately, notify the hospital.
8. Should a convulsion occur, place the child on one side and where he cannot fall. Be sure there is ample room for him to breathe. Place a firm object between the molar teeth to keep this mouth open. Stay with the child until the convulsion begins to subside, and notify the hospital as soon as possible.

On the night following the head injury, or during any nap, it is advisable to awaken your child (every 3 hours) and look for any of these danger signs.

Stephen R. Keller and Thomas E. Cone, Jr.

References

Bellinger, D., et al. Longitudinal analyses of prenatal and postnatal lead exposure and early cognitive development. *N. Engl. J. Med.* 316:1037, 1987.

Chameides, L. (Ed.). *Textbook of Pediatric Advanced Life Support*. Dallas: American Heart Association, 1988.

Clinical Handbook of Economic Poisoning. Publication No. 476. US Department of Health and Human Services. Government Printing Office, 1963.

Committee on Infectious Diseases, American Academy of Pediatrics. *Report of the Committee on Infectious Diseases*. Evanston, IL: American Academy of Pediatrics, 1988.

Committee on Accident and Poison Prevention, American Academy of Pediatrics. Statement on childhood lead poisoning, committee on environmental hazards. *Pediatrics* 79:457, 1987.

Davis, J. M., and Svendsgaard, D. J. Low-level lead exposure and child development. *Nature* 329:297, 1987.

Fleisher, G., Ludwig, S., et al. (Eds.). *Textbook of Pediatric Emergency Medicine* (2nd ed.). Baltimore: Williams & Wilkins, 1988.

Gosselin, R. E., Smith, R. P., and Hodge, H. C. (Eds.). *Clinical Toxicology of Commercial Products* (5th ed.). Baltimore: Williams & Wilkins, 1985.

Kanakriyeh, M., et al. Initial fluid therapy for children with meningitis with consideration of the syndrome of inappropriate antidiuretic hormone. *Clin. Pediatr.* 26:126, 1987.

Lebel, M. H., et al. Dexamethasone therapy for bacterial meningitis; Results of two double-blind placebo-controlled trials. *N. Engl. J. Med.* 319:964, 1988.

Lovejoy, F. H. Jr., and Chaffee-Bahamon, C. Poisoning in Children and Adolescents. In M. Green, and R. J. Haggerty (Eds.). *Ambulatory Pediatrics*, Vol. III. Philadelphia: Saunders, 1984. P. 165.

McMichael, A. J., et al. Port Pirie cohort study: Environmental exposure to lead and children's abilities at the age of four years. *N. Engl. J. Med.* 319:468, 1988.

Orlowski, J. P., et al. Comparison study of intraosseous, central intravenous, and peripheral intravenous infusions of emergency drugs. *A.J.D.C.* 144:112, 1990.

Piomelli, S., et al. Management of childhood lead poisoning. *J. Pediatr.* 105:523, 1984.

Rumack, B. H., et al. Accidents and Emergencies. In S. S. Gellis, and B. M. Kagan (Eds.). *Current Pediatric Therapy* (12th ed.). Philadelphia: Saunders, 1986. Pp. 652–785.

Index